SYSTEMIC PATHOLOGY / THIRD EDITION

Volume 4   Nervous System, Muscle and Eyes

SYSTEMIC PATHOLOGY / THIRD EDITION

General Editor W. St C. Symmers

Volume Editors

M. C. Anderson **Gynaecological and Obstetrical Pathology**

T. J. Anderson and D. L. Page **Breasts**

B. Corrin **Lungs**

I. Friedmann **Nose, Throat and Ears**

K. Henry and W. St C. Symmers **Thymus, Lymph Nodes, Spleen and Lymphatics**

P. D. Lewis **Endocrine System**

B. C. Morson **Alimentary Tract**

K. A. Porter **Urinary System**

R. C. B. Pugh **Male Reproductive System**

W. B. Robertson **Cardiovascular System**

H. A. Sissons **Bone, Joints and Soft Tissues**

D. Weedon **Skin**

R. O. Weller **Nervous System, Muscle and Eyes**

S. N. Wickramasinghe **Blood and Bone Marrow**

D. G. D. Wight **Liver, Biliary Tract and Pancreas**

SYSTEMIC PATHOLOGY / THIRD EDITION

General Editor   W. St C. Symmers

Volume 4

Nervous System, Muscle and Eyes

EDITED BY

R. O. Weller
BSc PhD MD FRCPath

Professor of Neuropathology, University of Southampton, UK;
Consultant Neuropathologist to the Wessex Region

CHURCHILL LIVINGSTONE
EDINBURGH LONDON MELBOURNE AND NEW YORK 1990

CHURCHILL LIVINGSTONE
Medical Division of Longman Group UK Limited

Distributed in the United States of America by Churchill
Livingstone Inc., 1560 Broadway, New York, NY 10036, and
by associated companies, branches and representatives
throughout the world.

First published 1990

ISBN 0-443-03312-9

British Library Cataloguing in Publication Data

Systemic pathology.—3rd ed.
  Vol. 4: Nervous system, muscle and eyes
  1. Medicine. Pathology
  I. Weller, R. O.   II. Symmers, William St Clair
  616′.07

Library of Congress Cataloging in Publication Data

Nervous system, muscle, and eyes.
  (Systemic pathology; v. 4)
  Includes index.
  1. Nervous system—Diseases.   2. Muscles—Diseases.
3. Eyes—Diseases and defects.   I. Weller, Roy O.
II. Series. [DNLM: 1. Eye Diseases.   2. Muscular
Diseases.   3. Nervous System Diseases.
QZ 4 S995 1986 v. 4]
RB111.S97   1987 vol. 4   [RC347]   616.07 s   89–9854

Printed in Great Britain by BAS Printers Limited, Over Wallop, Hampshire

Preface

Since the last edition of *Systemic Pathology*, advances in clinical investigation of the nervous system and the rapid progress in neuroscience and molecular biology have influenced greatly diagnostic and research pathology of the nervous system, muscle and eyes. The last decade has seen the widespread use and sophistication of computerised axial tomography and magnetic resonance imaging; similar advances have occurred in cerebral angiography and electrophysiological investigation of the nervous system. Biochemistry, pharmacology and molecular biology have all played significant roles in the advancement of our knowledge of the nervous system and of the wide range of diseases affecting the brain, spinal cord, peripheral nerves, muscle and eyes. Pathologists find themselves interposed between basic neuroscience and molecular biology on the one hand and clinical medicine on the other; from this special position, we have shared in the exciting advances in a wide range of related fields of science and technology.

As with the study of other organ systems, improved electron microscopic techniques and more significantly the growth of immunocytochemistry have led to a greater understanding of the normal nervous system and its histopathology. This volume of the third edition of *Systemic Pathology* is written with the aim of creating a working text for pathologists with a more general experience in histopathology and for clinicians and basic scientists who wish to delve into the pathology of the nervous system.

The first four chapters of the book set the general scene for the study and investigation of pathology of the central nervous system. Many of the cellular aspects of the brain cannot be fully appreciated except by electron microscopy; the first chapter, therefore, concentrates upon the cytology and ultrastructural aspects of the normal central nervous system in addition to its pharmacological and physiological features. This is followed by a review of general pathological reactions of the nervous system depicting those features which can be used to analyse the pathology of biopsy and autopsy specimens in order to diagnose specific disease entities. A further chapter on the general pathology of the central nervous system concentrates upon the particular problems which arise in an organ, like the brain, which is not only very sensitive to ischaemia, but is also enclosed within rigid compartments.

A guide to the pathological examination of the central nervous system precedes chapters on specific disease entities. Sections on cerebral vascular disease, and later in the book, on ageing and dementia, cover important areas in the pathology of the nervous system which are widely encountered in general pathological practice and will become even more important with an increasingly ageing population. The chapter on trauma of the nervous system is relevant not only to clinicians treating head and spinal injuries but also to the pathologist confronted by medicolegal problems. Despite advances in diagnostic techniques and in treatment, bacterial, fungal, parasitic and viral infections of the nervous system still present many problems for clinicians and pathologists. Infections are covered in three separate chapters. The effects of the acquired immune deficiency syndrome (AIDS) on the nervous system have become increasingly apparent not only through direct involvement by human immunodeficiency virus (HIV) but also from the fungal, bacterial and viral infections which are associated with the immunosuppression.

The chapter on demyelinating diseases mainly concentrates upon multiple sclerosis, which still presents a major problem with regard to aetiology, pathogenesis and treatment. A review of toxic and deficiency disorders in Chapter 11 illustrates how individuals are affected worldwide and how many advances have occurred in recent years in our knowledge of the basic pathology and biochemistry of toxic disorders of the nervous system.

The consideration of developmental, neonatal and paediatric neuropathology (Chapter 12) takes into account how advances in imaging techniques, biochemistry and molecular biology have increased the scope of diagnosis of neurological damage in utero, in infancy and in childhood. As a result of these advances, there is increasing pressure upon pathologists for detailed clinicopathological correlations in genetic and metabolic disorders. Two important categories of neurological disease, which are often difficult to investigate pathologically, are covered in the next two chapters. Epilepsy is a disabling disorder with many different causes and its study requires careful pathological examination of biopsy or autopsy material. System disorders present the problem of classification which will remain until the causes of these disorders are known. In this volume, an attempt is made to formulate a logical approach to them.

Few texts on the pathology of the central nervous system contain a section on tumours. However, neoplasia is a very important facet of the pathology of the nervous system and advances in imaging techniques have increased the need for accurate clinicopathological correlation. Although the World Health Organization classification of tumours of the central nervous system is closely

followed, problems arise due to the advances that have taken place in the 10 years since it was published. In the light of immunocytochemical investigations of nervous system tumours, a slightly modified version of the WHO classification is used. The pathology is correlated with the clinical aspects in this chapter and in the subsequent chapter on the pineal.

The sections on the peripheral nervous system and on muscle both contain chapters on the normal features, general pathology and special pathology of these tissues on the same basis as the larger section on central nervous system diseases. Muscle and nerve biopsies are increasingly used in the assessment of muscle and nerve disease and close clinicopathological correlation is required for successful diagnosis. This is well illustrated by the large number of neurologists who have a firm interest in the pathology of peripheral nerves and muscle. In this volume, the chapters on peripheral nerve and muscle are written mainly from the pathologist's point of view but with a firm eye on the clinicopathological correlation.

The last section, on the pathology of the eye, is included in this volume as the eye is partly derived from the central nervous system and is functionally very closely allied to the central nervous system. An enormous number of diseases involve the eye; some of these overlap with diseases of the skin. In this section of the book there is a comprehensive guide to the pathology of the eye and a detailed glossary of terms which may be unfamiliar to histopathologists.

Written with trainee and established histopathologists, clinical neurologists, neurosurgeons, ophthalmologists and basic neuroscientists in mind, we hope this volume will prove not only a useful guide and source of information on the pathology of the nervous system, muscle and eyes but also that it will act as a stimulus to research in these exciting fields.

R. O. Weller 1990

Acknowledgements

It would not have been possible to produce this volume without the generous help of many of our clinical and technical colleagues. We would like to thank them and those who have kindly supplied photographs for publication in this book and who are acknowledged in the captions of the appropriate illustrations.

Our special thanks are due to those who were intimately involved in the preparation of material for the manuscripts. Technical help was kindly provided by A. Brady and A. J. Davey (Institute of Psychiatry, London), P. R. Bogue, D. A. Robinson, S. C. Toms, Mrs E. A. Wakefield and P. Walsh (Leeds), T. Gradidge and Miss N. Sullivan (Bristol), P. Langham (Cardiff), P. Bond, R. Hickton and I. J. Bradley (Birmingham), R. H. Hunt, Barbara Davis, P. V. Steart, Jean Buontempo, Sue Cox and Sue Harris (Southampton).

We are grateful for specific advice on manuscripts from Dr R. W. Cox (Institute of Ophthalmology, London), Miss E. E. Kritzinger (Birmingham), Dr Janice Anderson (Cambridge), Dr B. Harding (Institute of Child Health, London), Dr Marie Ogilvie (Edinburgh), Professor J. Hume Adams (Glasgow), Dr I. Janota (Institute of Psychiatry, London), Dr Isabella Moore, Dr A. Lowes and Professor J. Pickard (Southampton).

We especially thank Mrs Susan Milford (London), Mrs S. A. V. Gooch (London), Mrs A. Minto (Birmingham) and Mrs J. Rubython (Glasgow) for their untiring secretarial assistance and Margaret Harris who bore the burden as the Editor's secretary in Southampton.

Lastly, the Editor would like to thank Dr Bill Symmers, senior, for his tremendous enthusiasm and advice in the preparation of the volume and in the editing of the manuscripts and for the many *mots justes*. Our further thanks are due to the staff of Churchill Livingstone, Edinburgh, for all their help and advice.

R. O. Weller 1990

Contributors

J. B. Cavanagh
MD FRCP FRCPath

Emeritus Professor in Applied Neurobiology, University of London; Honorary Consultant in Neuropathology, MRC Toxicology Unit, Carshalton, Surrey, UK

D. I. Graham
MB BCh PhD FRCPath FRCP(Glas) FRS(E)

Professor of Neuropathology, Institute of Neurological Sciences, Southern General Hospital, Glasgow, UK

D. G. F. Harriman
MD FRCP FRCPath

Formerly Reader in Neuropathology, University of Leeds, and Honorary Consultant Neuropathologist, Leeds Regional Health Authority, UK

John Harry
BSc MB BCh MRCPath FCOphth

Consultant Ocular Histopathologist, Birmingham and Midland Eye Hospital; Honorary Senior Clinical Lecturer in Pathology, University of Birmingham Medical School, UK

P. L. Lantos
MD PhD FRCPath

Professor of Neuropathology, Institute of Psychiatry; Honorary Consultant in Neuropathology, Bethlem Royal Hospital, Maudsley Hospital and King's College School of Medicine and Dentistry, London, UK

Paul D. Lewis
DSc MD MRCP FRCPath

Reader in Histopathology, Royal Postgraduate Medical School; Honorary Consultant Neurologist, Hammersmith Hospital; Honorary Lecturer in Neuropathology, Royal Free Hospital School of Medicine, London, UK

R. O. Weller
BSc PhD MD FRCPath

Professor of Neuropathology, University of Southampton; Consultant Neuropathologist to the Wessex Region, Southampton, UK

Contents

PART 3   Muscle

PART 4   Eyes

PART 1

Central Nervous System

Cytology of the normal central nervous system

INTRODUCTION

The central nervous system (CNS) is composed of various types of cell including neurons, glial cells (astrocytes, oligodendrocytes, ependyma and choroid plexus epithelium), blood vessel elements and microglia. Leptomeninges (pia mater and arachnoid mater) surround the CNS, and the pachymeninges (dura mater) form an outer coating which separates the brain from the skull and the spinal cord from the spine.

There are illustrations throughout subsequent chapters which depict many of the histological and macroscopic features of the nervous system. This chapter, however, is more concerned with the basic structure and function of the different cell types in the brain and spinal cord, an understanding of which is a prerequisite for an appreciation of the pathology of the nervous system.

NEURONS

Nerve cells vary enormously in size and configuration. The cerebellum presents the best example of morphological extremes: the Purkinje cells and their impressive dendritic trees dwarf the neighbouring granule cells and their short dendrites (Figs 1.1 and 1.2).

The shape of the nerve cell body, the perikaryon, also varies throughout the central nervous system: pyramidal, polygonal, round, oval and fusiform forms can be distinguished. Neuronal cell processes fall into two categories: dendrites and axons. Whilst a neuron usually has

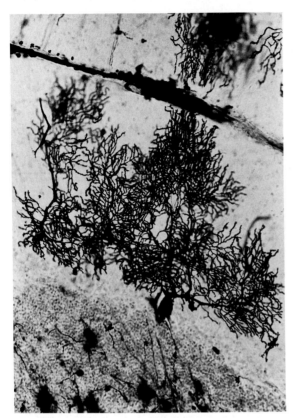

Fig. 1.1 The cerebellar cortex: the dendritic tree of a single Purkinje cell spans the entire thickness of the molecular layer between the pial surface and the granule cell layer (bottom). Golgi-Cox × 160

nuclear profile is occasionally indented. The nucleo- or karyoplasm is separated from the cytoplasm by the nuclear membrane which is composed of two laminae enclosing the perinuclear cisterna: the inner lamina is smooth, whilst the outer one, studded with ribosomes, is frequently continuous with the rough endoplasmic reticulum. Finely granular chromatin is evenly dispersed with some clumping at the nuclear membrane (Fig. 1.3).

The nucleolus is prominent and this helps to distinguish neurons from astrocytes which contain only a small inconspicuous nucleolus. Electron microscopy reveals the nucleolus to be composed of granular and fibrillar constituents. Attached to the nucleolus is the nucleolar satellite or sex chromatin: a dense, coarsely fibrillated body which occurs only in females.

Nuclear inclusions of various types, filamentous, granulofibrillar, tubular and vesicular,[1] often occur in normal neurons and can be occasionally discerned in the light microscope. Variations in nuclear morphology exist according to neuronal type, topography and functional activity. The large vesicular nuclei of the Purkinje cells or the pyramidal cells of the cerebral cortex are in sharp contrast to the small, dense nuclei of the cerebellar granule cells (Fig. 1.2).

only a single axon, the number of dendrites ranges from one to nearly one hundred. The length and arborisation of processes also display considerable individual variations.

Silver impregnation techniques of classical neurohistology, electron microscopy, enzyme histochemistry and more recently immunocytochemistry have all contributed to the understanding of neuronal morphology and function. The previous morphological classifications of nerve cells are now gradually being replaced by classifications based on functions: neurons can be distinguished according to the neurotransmitters they use.

The nucleus

Nerve cell nuclei are round or oval, although the

Cytoplasmic organelles

Nissl substance

This cytoplasmic component is intensely basophilic when stained with cresyl violet or methylene blue. Electron microscopy shows that Nissl substance is composed of stacks of the rough-surfaced endoplasmic reticulum (RER) (Fig. 1.4). The cisternae are usually arranged in parallel arrays and their outer surface is covered by ribosomes. The amount of RER varies from neuron to neuron and appears to be related to the length of the axon: it is particularly abundant in the anterior horn cells of the spinal cord and the pyramidal neurons of the cerebral cortex. It is present not only in the perikaryon but also in the dendrites, but it is absent from the axon hillock and from the axon itself. Since the RER is the site of protein synthesis, its amount is related to the metabolic

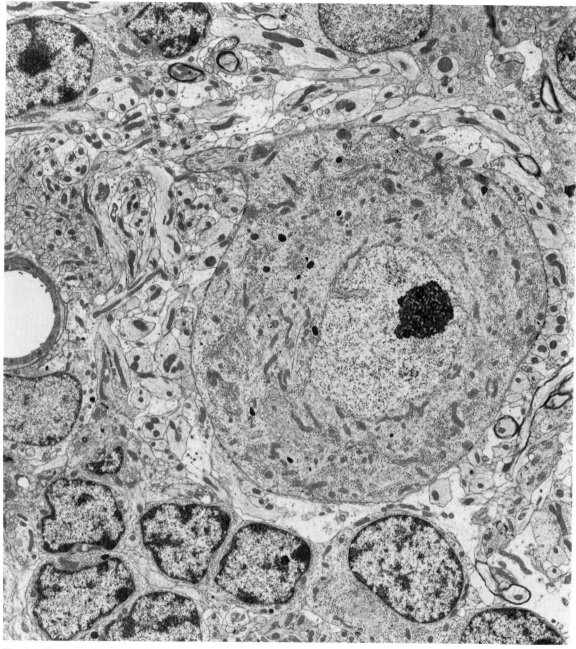

Fig. 1.2 Electron micrograph of the cerebellar cortex showing a large Purkinje cell and several smaller granule cells. × 7000

activity of the cell. The Nissl substance forms an integral component of the neuronal membrane system which is associated with the transfer of membrane molecules amongst organelles, the packaging and transport of exportable protein and energy metabolism.[2] In addition to the membrane-bound particles of the RER, ribosomes are scattered throughout the cytoplasm either singly or in groups as polyribosomes or ribosomal rosettes.

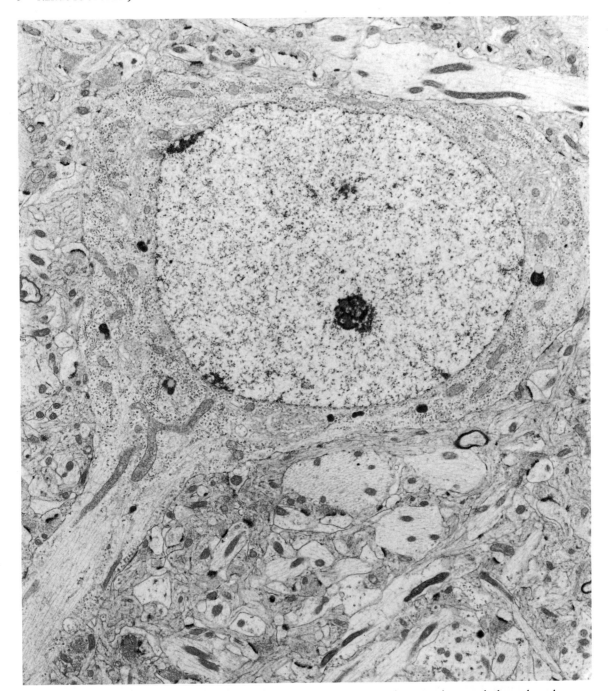

Fig. 1.3 Electron micrograph of a single neuron. The regular, round nucleus contains a prominent nucleolus and evenly distributed chromatin. Astrocyte processes dendrites and synapses are in the neuropil surrounding the neuron. × 10 500

Agranular endoplasmic reticulum and the Golgi apparatus

Cisternae of various lengths which are not covered by ribosomes permeate the cytoplasm. This smooth or agranular reticulum is particularly prominent at the bases of cell processes, where the Nissl substance is sparse, and usually extends into

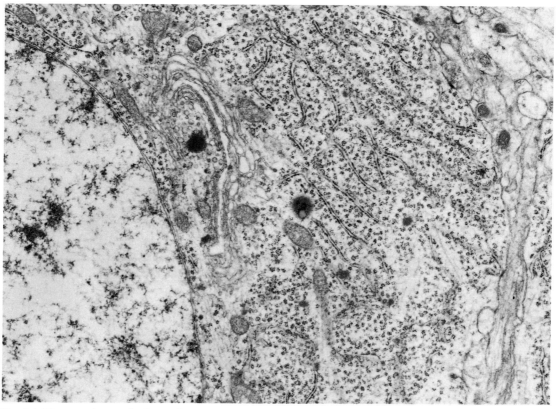

Fig. 1.4 Electron micrograph of part of a neuron: the cytoplasm contains cisternae of rough endoplasmic reticulum (the Nissl substance), masses of polyribosomes, a well developed Golgi complex and several mitochondria. × 16 000

the axon and dendrites. Although the precise function of the agranular reticulum is not known, its widespread distribution within the cytoplasm and its close spatial relationship to the cell membrane suggest a role in intracellular transport.

The internal reticular apparatus of Golgi appears as tortuous anastomosing strands in the light microscope. Located between the nucleus and the cell membrane or at the base of a dendrite, the Golgi apparatus is composed of arrays of closely packed, smooth-surfaced cisternae and numerous associated vacuoles and vesicles (Fig. 1.4). Its curved configuration allows a convex, external forming face and a concave, internal mature face to be distinguished. The internal face of the Golgi apparatus forms an integral part of the GERL system (Golgi apparatus, smooth endoplasmic reticulum and lysosomes): a spatially closely related group of organelles which is devoted to the synthesising and condensing

activity of the Golgi apparatus.[3] This polarisation of the Golgi apparatus, although not evident in all neurons, is thought to serve the efficient transport of materials. The demonstration of concanavalin A binding sites on Golgi membranes strongly suggests that this organelle is concerned with glycoprotein metabolism.[1] The formation of new plasma membranes during mitosis and the maintenance of normal membrane structure in resting cells are important functions of the Golgi apparatus.[4]

The Golgi apparatus itself promotes the movement of membranes: vacuoles fuse to form a cisterna at the forming face, while vesicles are budding off at the mature face. The diameter of these vesicles ranges from 20–60 µm and they are usually smooth-surfaced, round or elliptical. Coated or alveolate vesicles of 50–60 µm diameter are distinguished by their regularly spaced arms or striae. These vesicles are concerned with the transport of hydrolytic enzymes to the lysosomal system. Larger alveolate vesicles, 100 nm in diameter, derived from the cell surface by invagination or pinocytosis, ingest proteins which then are transferred to the lysosomes to be digested. In addition, many neurons, particularly those of the supraoptic and paraventricular nuclei, contain dense-cored, neurosecretory granules up to 150 nm in diameter.

Multivesicular bodies are spherical structures of 0·5 μm in diameter which contain vesicles and an assortment of inclusions. Although frequently associated with the Golgi apparatus, they are not part of these organelles and occur throughout the perikaryon and cell processes. Multivesicular bodies sequester material transported to them by coated vesicles, and hydrolytic enzymes acquired from smaller coated vesicles convert them into lysosomes.

Lysosomes

Primary lysosomes are round or oval, uniformly dense bodies up to 1 μm in diameter, bound by a unit membrane. They contain various hydrolytic enzymes, including acid phosphatase which serves as a marker enzyme for their identification.[3] Secondary lysosomes are larger, more irregular and usually contain various ingested materials.

Lipofuscin granules

Although visible by light microscopy, lipofuscin can be better appreciated in the electron microscope: a single membrane encloses a dense granule and one or two peripheral vacuoles (Fig. 1.3). Lipofuscin or lipochrome is frequently referred to as 'wear-and-tear' pigment, since the number of granules within the neurons increases with age. These granules are end products of intracellular peroxidation and polymerisation of unsaturated fatty acids. Their origin is controversial, but according to the most widely accepted concept they are derived from lysosomes. The precise function of lipofuscin is unknown. Degenerated cytoplasmic constituents contribute to its formation, which requires intracellular oxidants and antioxidants. Lipofuscin is thus the by-product of metabolic activity; it is stored in lyso-

somes and is only disposed of by expulsion during mitosis or by cell death.[5] Since mature nerve cells do not divide, lipofuscin granules accumulate during life. Appearing as light brown granules in haematoxylin and eosin stained sections, lipofuscin can be demonstrated by a variety of fat stains including Sudan black B, Sudan III and Nile blue sulphate. It is acid fast and PAS positive and reduces ferric ferricyanide to Prussian blue (Schmorl's reaction).

Melanin

This pigment is present in the leptomeningeal cells and in the pigmented nuclei of the brainstem. Melanin-containing cells in the leptomeninges are most plentiful over the ventral aspect of the brainstem; this is the area in which the rare primary malignant melanomas most often develop. Two major accumulations of pigmented neurons occur in the brainstem: in the substantia nigra of the midbrain and in the much smaller locus ceruleus of the pontine tegmentum. The cells of the substantia nigra and locus ceruleus are dopaminergic and noradrenergic respectively. Other brainstem nuclei, including the motor nucleus of the vagus, also contain melanin in small amounts.

Mitochondria

These organelles vary considerably in shape and size, depending upon their location within the neurons. They are apparently distributed at random in the perikaryon and also occur in dendrites and axons, including the presynaptic terminals. Mitochondria have a smooth outer membrane and an irregular inner membrane. The inner membrane forms complex folds (cristae); the inner compartment of the mitochondrion is filled with a moderately dense matrix (Fig. 1.3). The inner surfaces of the cristae are rendered uneven by many minute projections, each ending in a knob. The inner and outer membranes differ in composition, structure and function; the electron transport mechanism and many hydrogenases are located in the inner membrane, whereas the monoamine oxidase system is found in the outer membrane.[1]

The cytoskeleton

The neuronal cytoskeleton is composed of three elements: neurofilaments, microtubules and microfilaments.

Neurofilaments. These filaments are 10 nm in diameter and of indeterminate length. They belong to the class of intermediate filaments, their diameter being in between that of the microfilaments (4–6 nm) and that of microtubules (24 nm). Of the five types of intermediate filaments found in animal cells, two occur in the central nervous system: neurofilaments in nerve cells and glial filaments in astrocytes. Although the various types of intermediate filaments appear to be similar morphologically, they are composed of different proteins.

In cross-section, neurofilaments display a central hollow core, surrounded by a wall of 3 nm in thickness. The basic unit of the wall is composed of four globular subunits, each 3·5 nm in diameter, which are linked together by connecting arms of 2·5 nm in thickness. These units are stacked one upon another and rotated in the transverse plane by 45° to each other.[6] In longitudinal section, neurofilaments appear as two dense, parallel lines which enclose the central hollow core. They are dispersed throughout the perikaryon, but tend to accumulate at the base of large processes, into which they extend, forming parallel arrays.

Neurofilaments isolated from the nervous system are formed by three polypeptides with the approximate molecular weights of 70, 150 and 200 kilodaltons.[7] Recent investigation has revealed that immunohistochemical differences may exist between neurofilaments in the perikarya, dendrites and axons.[8]

Although the morphology and biochemistry of neurofilaments have been established,[9] very little is known about their functions. They are intimately related to microtubules, the other component of the neuronal cytoskeleton, and with them they could play a role not only in stabilising nerve cells, but also in axonal transport.[10] Neurofilaments are also major intrinsic determinants of axonal diameter in large myelinated nerve fibres: the expression of a single set of neuron-specific genes encoding neurofilaments directly determines axonal calibre.[11]

Microtubules. Microtubules are of indeterminate length and 24 nm in diameter. Their walls are 6 nm thick and composed of 13 globular subunits, each representing a constituent protofilament.[10] Microtubules are intermingled with neurofilaments both in the perikaryon and in cell processes: the ratio of neurofilaments to microtubules decreases as the axon becomes smaller, and in thin unmyelinated axons usually only microtubules are present. Tubulin, the major protein component of microtubules, is composed of an α and β dimer, each with a molecular weight of 60 000.[12] In an adult brain this protein comprises 10–30% of the soluble protein[10] and more recently a group of microtubule-associated proteins has also been recognised.[13] Many functions have been attributed to microtubules: skeletal support, maintenance of axonal flow, transport of various substances and of cytoplasmic vesicles, cellular contraction and a rôle in mitosis.[1] Microtubules also play a rôle in the maintenance and function of the Golgi apparatus.[14]

Microfilaments. These are not obvious in nerve cells: they have a diameter of 4–6 nm and are composed of actin, a globular protein with a molecular weight of 42 000.[13] Microfilaments, in addition to their stabilising function, also play a rôle in axonal transport.[10]

Synapses

Synapses are specialised interneuronal contacts which can be electrical or chemical. Electrical synapses function by the propagation of electrical impulses and do not require elaborate structural organisation of the plasma membrane and cytoplasmic organelles. These synapses, which are rare in mammals but common in lower vertebrates, are formed by the close apposition of the cell membranes at a gap junction. Chemical synapses, in contrast, utilise various substances—neurotransmitters and neuropeptides—for intercellular communication: this chemical transmission requires a sophisticated subcellular mechanism well demonstrated by electron microscopy. By light microscopy, using silver impregnation techniques, only the profile of the end-bulb or bouton terminal of the axon abutting onto the surface of the perikaryon or dendrite can be seen. A synapse is composed of three constituents: the presynaptic element, the synaptic cleft and the postsynaptic component (Fig. 1.5). Both the pre- and the postsynaptic membranes display densities along the specialised stretch of cell membrane and these, together with the intervening cleft, are referred to as the synaptic junction.

Originally two types of synapse were distinguished on ultrastructural examination of the pyramidal cells of the cerebral cortex. The type I junction is usually extensive, the postsynaptic density prominent, rendering the synapse asymmetrical, and the wide synaptic cleft contains a dense plaque. In the type II synapse, in contrast, the postsynaptic density is less readily identifiable and the narrower cleft does not contain a dense plaque; the overall configuration is symmetrical.[15] The presynaptic element in most cases is an axon,

either at its end (bouton terminal) or along its course (bouton en passant): the axonal terminal can form a synapse with any part of another neuron and thus axo-dendritic, axo-somatic and axo-axonal synapses are distinguished. The presynaptic element, however, does not need to be an axonal terminal and synapses can be formed between any part of two neurons, providing a wide variety of synapses.

The presynaptic element contains the synaptic vesicles which, in turn, are filled with neurotransmitters (Fig. 1.5). The size, shape and content of the vesicles vary, depending upon the type of synapse. The most frequently occurring vesicles are apparently clear, spherical and 40–50 nm in diameter. Elongated or flattened vesicles with clear centres are 20 nm wide and 50 nm long. There have been many attempts to correlate vesicular shape with functional activity:

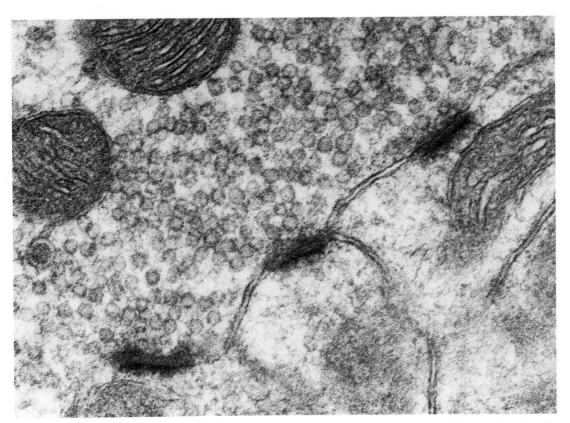

Fig. 1.5 Electron micrograph shows a single presynaptic terminal containing synaptic vesicles and forming three densely-stained synapses.
× 80 000

spherical vesicles occur in excitatory, type I synapses, whilst flattened vesicles are associated with inhibitory, type II synapses. Larger vesicles of up to 60 nm in diameter with a dense core are encountered in areas of catecholamine activity and contain noradrenaline, dopamine or 5-hydroxy-tryptamine. Another, larger dense-cored vesicle, up to 150 nm with a spherical dense core of 50–70 nm in diameter, is most frequently seen in the presynaptic terminals of autonomic ganglia, but also occurs in various parts of the central nervous system intermingled with clear vesicles. The presynaptic element, particularly the axonal terminal, also contains other organelles, including mitochondria, neurofilaments, microtubules, smooth endoplasmic reticulum and glycogen.

The synaptic cleft, separating the pre- and postsynaptic membranes, is 20–30 nm wide and usually contains a dense plaque of intercellular material. In addition, filaments appear to traverse the cleft and contribute to the formation of the plaque.

The postsynaptic membrane is rendered conspicuous by an accumulation of dense material on its cytoplasmic surface (Fig. 1.5). This post-synaptic density, composed of granular material and an occasional filamentous structure, is more pronounced in asymmetrical, type I, synapses. The existence of postsynaptic density is dependent upon the presence of the presynaptic element: if the presynaptic structures degenerate, the postsynaptic density will eventually disappear. The postsynaptic element also contains cisternae of the smooth endoplasmic reticulum and the spine apparatus, which is composed of 2–3 flattened cisternae, separated by plaques of dense material.

The morphological appearances of synapses reflect the functional dynamics of neuro-transmission. Accordingly, in chemical synapses the vesicles contain quanta of the neurotransmitter which is discharged into the synaptic cleft after the vesicle has fused with the presynaptic membrane. Thus, the uptake of calcium into the nerve terminal triggers off a chain of events leading to exocytosis: vesicular apposition, membrane fusion and fission.[16] Although this vesicular or exocytotic hypothesis of neurotransmission[17] provides a plausible explanation for the quantal nature of transmitter release, an increasing body of evidence now suggests that this may not be the only mechanism by which chemical signals in the central nervous system are propagated. Chemical substances may be released from non-synaptic axon terminals and even from regions of nerve cells other than presynaptic axon terminals.[18]

A parasynaptic system is envisaged in which so-called neuroactive or informational substances reach specific target cell receptors by diffusion from release points through the extracellular fluids.[19] The mechanism of exocytosis itself remains poorly understood not only morphologically, but also neurochemically, and various alternative biochemical mechanisms have been considered to explain the release of neuro-transmitters.[20]

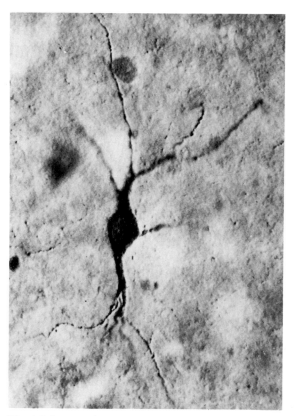

Fig. 1.6 A neuron in the caudate nucleus contains neuropeptide Y.
Immunoperoxidase (peroxidase-antiperoxidase). Interference contrast microscopy × 700
Immunocytochemical preparation lent for reproduction by Dr Yvonne S. Allen, Department of Neuropathology, Institute of Psychiatry, London, UK

There have been attempts to correlate synaptic morphology and function, based on the type of neurotransmitter used.[21] Thus, synapses in the central nervous system can be classified by the combination of electron microscopy and immunocytochemistry into synapses which use acetylcholine, compounds with amine groups (noradrenaline, dopamine, 5-hydroxytryptamine), amino acids (glutamate, γ-aminobutyric acid and glycine) and various neuropeptides (Fig. 1.6).

Neuronal processes

Axons

The transitional zone between the neuronal perikaryon and the axon is the cone-shaped axon hillock. In larger, multipolar neurons the axon hillock lacks Nissl substance, and it is in this region that cytoskeletal elements, the microtubules and neurofilaments, converge to become parallel as they enter the axon. The microtubules then form a fascicle in the initial segment of the axon, a feature which enables axons to be distinguished from dendrites, in which microtubules are more evenly distributed. The more distal portion of the axon may contain various organelles, but granular endoplasmic reticulum and polyribosomes are usually absent. The internal structure of the axon has recently been visualised as a three-dimensional lattice: the longitudinally orientated neurofilaments and microtubules are extensively cross-linked to each other and to the plasma membrane by thin filaments. Similar bridges also connect membrane-bound organelles with the components of the cytoskeleton and with each other.[22]

There is axonal transport of material from the perikaryon towards the periphery (anterograde transport) and to a lesser extent in the opposite direction (retrograde transport).[23] Since the axon terminal, the most active site of neurotransmission, can be far removed from the perikaryon in which proteins are synthesised, this axonal transport is vital for the proper functioning of the nerve cell. Axonal flow has a slow and a fast component, 0·2–8·0 mm and 50–500 mm per day respectively. Fast axoplasmic flow carries organelles, including vesicles and mitochondria, and membrane-bound substances like proteins and neurotransmitters—materials which are essential for synaptic activity. The fast axonal flow is effected by microtubules, but the possibility that some membrane-bound proteins are transported by the smooth endoplasmic reticulum[24] or another tubulo-vesicular system[25] cannot be excluded. Slow flow, in contrast, transports high molecular weight and soluble materials which are involved in the growth and maintenance of the axon. The structural basis of slow transport is controversial, but the movement of the cytoplasmic matrix itself may represent the prime force.[23] Mechanisms of anterograde and retrograde transport are similar: both need metabolic energy, have similar ionic requirements and are sensitive to the same drugs.[23] Both anterograde and retrograde transport can be blocked by low temperatures and suspended by colchicine and vinblastine, agents which disrupt microtubules. The factors which determine the direction of axonal transport remain conjectural: alternatives envisage either two, oppositely polarised transport systems or a single mechanism in which the direction of movement is determined by the nature of the material or organelle to be transported. Investigation of the molecular mechanisms of axonal transport should contribute to our further understanding of this vital neuronal function.[26]

Dendrites

There is wide variation in the number and organisation of these cell processes in the central nervous system. The character of the dendritic tree reflects the afferent neuronal connections and consequently indicates the functional activity of the cell. The complex configuration of dendrites is best appreciated in Golgi preparations; these have allowed the classification of neurons into three groups based on their dendritic arborisations (Fig. 1.1). Isodendritic neurons issue straight dendrites which run in all directions, whilst allodendritic cells are distinguished by shorter, branched dendrites which are restricted in their wavy course. Idiodendritic neurons have a unique dendritic tree characteristic of and determined by their location.[27] A further, more detailed classification of neurons has been achieved by the dendritic branching pattern.[28]

Although clear differences exist, it may not be always easy to distinguish a dendrite from an axon. Dendrites have irregular contours, taper gradually, branch at relatively acute angles, are unmyelinated and contain Nissl substance. Axons, in contrast, display a smoother contour, have a relatively even diameter along their course, branch at obtuse or at right angles, can be myelinated or unmyelinated and lack Nissl substance. The smaller axons and dendrites become, the more difficult is their positive identification; the presence of clustered ribosomes, particularly in association with cisternae of rough-surfaced endoplasmic reticulum, remains the most reliable identifying feature of small dendritic processes.

The dendritic tree represents the most substantial receptive area of the nerve cells. Synapses are formed either on the dendritic trunks themselves or on the dendritic spines, the specialised structures projecting from them. The spines are composed of a stalk or neck which connects the dendrite with the ovoid bulb or head. There is a considerable variation in their configuration, but their overall length appears to be relatively constant at $2\,\mu m$. Spines can also be present on the perikaryon and they are responsible for 43% of the total surface area of the dendrites and the cell body: there are 4000 spines on a single pyramidal neuron.[1] The function of the dendritic spines is still largely unknown. Although they synapse with axon terminals, their role is not restricted to increasing receptive surfaces; they may regulate the excitatory input to a neuron.[1]

The neuropil and the extracellular space

The neuropil is composed of the complex and intricate feltwork of neuronal cell processes. This intermingling and interconnection of myelinated and unmyelinated axons and dendrites may appear random, but these processes form the neuronal circuitry of a particular area. Cell processes of astrocytes, oligodendrocytes and microglial cells further add to the variety of structures in the neuropil (Fig. 1.3).

Cell processes and perikarya, bounded by typical unit membranes, are separated by an extracellular space with an average width of 15–20 nm. Electron-dense markers, electrical impedance and the distribution of radiotracers have conclusively demonstrated the existence of this extracellular space, which constitutes 18–25% of the total grey and white matter.[29]

Myelin

Myelin in the central nervous system is produced by oligodendrocytes (see p. 22–24). The myelin sheath is formed by the spiral wrapping of the cytoplasmic processes of the myelinating cells around axons, and the subsequent extrusion of the cytoplasm leads to a compact, tightly spiralled, multi-layered envelope. Electron microscopy reveals the characteristic structure of the myelin sheath: major dense lines alternate with thinner intraperiod lines to form the repeating units. The major dense line results from the fusion of the thicker, inner leaflet of the oligodendrocytic plasma membrane, whereas the intraperiod line is formed by the apposition of the thinner, outer leaflet of this membrane. Unlike Schwann cells (the myelinating cells of the peripheral nervous system which are concerned with the myelination of a single axon), each oligodendrocyte may provide myelin for many axons. From this it follows that the motion by which the sheath is produced by the myelinating cell may be different in the central and peripheral nervous systems. Whilst Schwann cells can, in principle, lay down myelin by rotating around a single axon, the oligodendrocyte, being in connection with many axons, cannot perform a revolving motion. Consequently, ensheathment takes place by the progressive lengthening of the oligodendrocytic process which encircles the axon completely and an internal mesaxon is formed by apposition of the free edges of the myelinating process. The outermost lamella of the sheath encloses the outer tongue and this, together with the internal mesaxon, represents the tenuous connections which remain between the fully formed myelin and the myelinating cell.

Nodes of Ranvier occur regularly along the course of central myelinated fibres; the segment between two nodes is referred to as internodal myelin, and the region where the lamellae terminate is the paranode. The thickness of the myelin sheath is related to axonal diameter: larger axons are surrounded by thicker myelin sheaths. Evidence from experimental animals has convincingly shown that the formation of myelin is preceded by the proliferation of glial precursors which develop into young oligodendrocytes. The processes of these active oligodendrocytes are frequently wrapped around axons, but this direct connection is difficult to demonstrate in later life.[1] Biologically, the formation of myelin is a two-step process: first, the oligodendrocyte relates to the axon in response to an axonal myelinogenic stimulus and, second, it produces myelin, the volume of which is determined by the internodal axonal surface area.[30]

Myelination in man progresses slowly and generally proceeds centripetally: it commences peripherally and whilst many axons, particularly in the spinal cord, are myelinated at birth, the more central fibres in the frontal and parietal lobes remain unmyelinated well into postnatal life. Completion of myelin formation is achieved largely during the first two years after birth.[31] Immunohistochemistry for myelin basic protein confirms earlier findings of the chronological sequence of myelination: phylogenetically older regions acquire myelin first.[32] The sequential nature of myelination reflects physiological demand: the time and rapidity of myelination are related to the relative significance of a fibre system at various periods of cerebral development.[33]

Biochemically, myelin is composed of alternating layers of proteins and lipids. Of the myelin proteins, a proteolipid protein constitutes approximately 50%, basic protein (the antigenic agent capable of inducing experimental allergic encephalomyelitis) 30%, and an acidic proteolipid protein 20%.[34] Myelin-associated glycoprotein is an acidic, concanavalin A binding minor component which is also present in the cytoplasm of oligodendrocytes before and during myelination.[35] The various lipids to be found in the myelin include cholesterol, phosphatidylethanolamine, phosphatidylserine and phosphatidylcholine, sphingomyelin and glycolipids. Galactocerebroside is the main glycolipid component and the cell membrane of the myelinating cell contains a high percentage of this compound. This suggests that galactocerebroside may play an important role in the successive layering of cell membranes, a process unique to myelination. The demonstration of myelin and its breakdown products will be described in Chapter 2 (see p. 47–48).

Neurotransmitters and neuropeptides

The number of putative neurotransmitters has been dramatically increased during the last decade. In addition to the classical monoamine neurotransmitters (acetylcholine and catecholamines) and a few amino acids, at least 30 neuropeptides have been discovered: all these compounds can act as chemical messengers in the mammalian nervous system.[36] Immunohistochemistry has allowed the precise localisation of these neurotransmitters and neuropeptides and thus contributed to the understanding of how certain regions of the brain work.[37] This expanding knowledge of the relationship between structure and function has been accompanied by the realisation that certain neurological and psychiatric disorders are caused by an imbalance (overproduction or deficit) of these substances. It is for this reason that the distribution of neurotransmitters and neuropeptides is of considerable importance not only to neurobiologists, but also to histopathologists. Neurochemical analyses of post-mortem brains are affected by various factors including sampling, precision of dissection, age, sex, medication, the agonal state of the patient and post-mortem delay.[38]

Of the monoamines, acetylcholine is found in the motor nuclei of the cranial nerves and in the motor neurons of the spinal cord; in these locations it serves as the chemical messenger for neuromuscular transmission. Acetylcholine is also present in the intrinsic pathways within the central nervous system, and cholinergic neurons project in a diffuse ascending system from the medial septal nuclei to the hippocampus and from the nucleus basalis of Meynert to the cerebral cortex.[39] The basal ganglia are rich in this monoamine and the enzymes related to its metabolism: choline acetyltransferase and acetylcholinesterase, the synthesising and catabolising enzyme respectively. Large cholinergic neurons have been recently demonstrated by histochemistry in the human striatum,[40] but only the isolation, purification and immunohistochemical localisation of choline acetyltransferase have made a more comprehensive mapping of cholinergic pathways possible.[41]

There are three catecholamines in the central nervous system: noradrenaline, adrenaline (epinephrine) and dopamine. The noradrenergic system is localised in the brainstem nuclei, the largest of which is the locus ceruleus, the pigmented column of cells in the rostral part of the pontine tegmentum: axons originating from these cells establish extensive connections with the cerebral cortex and hippocampus. The hypothalamus is also rich in noradrenergic fibres.

The adrenergic system, in contrast, is more restricted: cells in the pons and medulla project to other brainstem structures or to the hypothalamus.

The major dopaminergic pathway originates in the pars compacta of the substantia nigra and ascends to the striatum: devastation of this system is the underlying cause of Parkinson's disease.[42] In addition to this nigrostriatal pathway, there is also a mesocortical and mesolimbic dopaminergic system: cells in the ventral tegmentum of the midbrain project to the cerebral cortex and to the limbic areas respectively.

The raphe nuclei form a long, ill-defined chain in the midline of the brainstem; their nerve cells give rise to the serotoninergic system which contains 5-hydroxytryptamine (serotonin) and projects to various sites in the forebrain including the hypothalamus, basal ganglia and medial forebrain bundle, and descends to the anterior and posterior horns of the spinal cord.

γ-aminobutyric acid (GABA), glutamate and glycine are amino acid neurotransmitters. GABA is the principal inhibitory neurotransmitter in the vertebrate nervous system and one-third of all nerve terminals in the rat brain appears to be GABAergic.[36] Moreover, neurophysiology, autoradiography and immunohistochemistry have all demonstrated that inhibitory synapses of the cerebellum utilise GABA and that the major efferent pathways of the Purkinje cells are also GABAergic.[36] GABA is also found in the spinal cord, although glycine is the major inhibitory neurotransmitter at this site. Glycine occurs in the small inhibitory interneurons of the grey matter and acts upon the large motor neurons of the anterior horn.[39] An increasing body of evidence suggests that glutamate is the universal putative excitatory neurotransmitter in the central nervous system. The possibility that some excitatory synapses use aspartate instead of glutamate cannot be excluded: the properties of these amino acids are too similar to allow a clear-cut separation. In the hippocampus, the major afferent pathways and the local interneurons use glutamate, as do the granule cells, the principal excitatory interneurons in the cerebellum.[36]

The last decade has witnessed the discovery of a variety of neuropeptides which may act as neurotransmitters or neuromodulators (Fig. 1.6). The increasing list of these small peptides includes circulating hormones, pituitary peptides, opioid peptides, intestinal hormones, hypothalamic releasing factors and a group of miscellaneous peptides.[36] Some of these compounds have been known to be the products of the endocrine or the neuroendocrine system, whilst other peptides, like the endorphins and enkephalins, have been more recently discovered. The neuropeptides may represent a different mode of intercellular communication from the fast and point-to-point action of amino acids such as GABA and glutamate: they have a slower time course, less precise spatial connections and a wider range of chemical messengers.[36,43] There are now more than 30 regulatory peptides and it is likely that more will be discovered.[44] Recent developments in neurotransmitter research have confirmed the view that neurons of the central nervous system are secretory cells and that the products of this activity represent the chemical signals of interneuronal communication.

It has been recognised that some of the neurotransmitters and neuropeptides are abnormally distributed in a variety of neurological and psychiatric disorders,[45,46] including extrapyramidal abnormalities,[42] Alzheimer's disease,[47] epilepsy,[48] schizophrenia[49] and anxiety.[50]

Histological demonstration of neurons

Nerve cells can be identified in most cases in sections stained with haematoxylin and eosin, but various 'special' methods are used in order to demonstrate particular organelles, cell processes

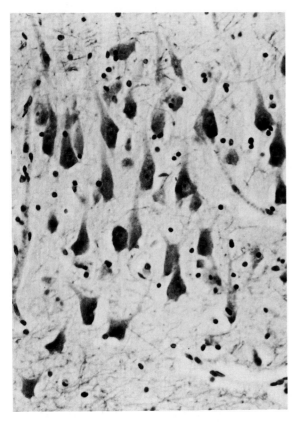

or myelin sheaths (Fig. 1.7). Cresyl violet (Nissl's stain) displays the coarse granular Nissl substance composed of rough endoplasmic reticulum and consequently is ideal for detecting chromatolysis in which Nissl substance is lost (see p. 38–39). This technique, combined with Luxol fast blue for the staining of myelin, is one of the most valuable methods for revealing topographical details in sections of brain and spinal cord.

Since neurofilaments are argyrophilic, there are various silver impregnation techniques for the demonstration of nerve fibres (e.g. Glees and Marsland, Palmgren or Bielschowsky). The Golgi method has, however, remained superior in revealing neuronal configuration in its entirety with all the cell processes (Fig. 1.1).

Immunohistochemistry is extensively used in neurocytology, and the various antigens to be found in neurons and other cells can now be demonstrated by both immunofluorescence and immunoperoxidase techniques[51] (see Table 1.1).

Fig. 1.7 The pyramidal layer of the hippocampus showing neurons, glial cells and capillaries.
Luxol fast blue–cresyl violet × 315

Table 1.1 Immunocytochemical markers in the central nervous system

Cell types	Markers	References	Comments
Neuron	Neuron-specific enolase ($\gamma\gamma$)	58	
	Neurofilament proteins	13, 56, 57	
	Tetanus toxin	54	in vitro only
	Cholera toxin	54	in vitro only
Astrocyte	Glial fibrillary acidic protein	67, 68, 69	
	Glutamine synthetase	95, 100	
Oligodendrocyte	Carbonic anhydrase II (c)	108	
	Galactocerebroside	109	in vitro only
	Myelin basic protein	32, 52	
	Myelin-associated glycoprotein	53	
Ependyma	No immunocytochemical markers at present	—	
Choroid plexus	Carbonic anhydrase II (c)	149	
Microglia	α_1-antitrypsin	128, 129	
	α_1-antichymotrypsin	129, 130	
	Fc receptor	54	in vitro only
	Lysozyme	129, 131	
Endothelium	Factor VIII-related antigen	138	
	Angiotensin-converting enzyme	139	frozen section
Leptomeningeal cells	Fibronectin	54, 55	
	Vimentin (also present in astrocytes and endothelium)	156	
	Desmoplakins	156	

Monoclonal and polyclonal antibodies against these antigens have proved to be valuable in diagnostic work. Monoclonal antibodies against the protein components of neurofilaments are also valuable in the study of abnormalities affecting these organelles[9,56] and in the diagnosis of neuronal neoplasms.[57] Of the three forms of enolase to be found in the central nervous system ($\alpha\alpha$, $\alpha\gamma$ and $\gamma\gamma$), the $\gamma\gamma$ isozyme occurs in nerve cells (neuron-specific enolase) and thus provides an immunological marker for neurons.[58] However, γ-enolase is widely distributed in extraneural tissues and is not a neuron-specific antigen.

NEUROGLIA

The term glia was introduced by Virchow[59] to describe a second cell type whose function was to bind the nerve cells together in the brain. Later Cajal[60] classified the glial cells into three categories: the first and second corresponded to the two varieties of astrocytes (protoplasmic and fibrous), whilst the third 'element' referred to a group of cells which was subsequently shown by del Río Hortega[61] to comprise both oligo-dendrocytes and microglial cells. Del Río Hortega introduced the silver carbonate method, which not only distinguished and separated oligo-dendrocytes from microglia, but also indicated that they were of different derivation. Thus oligo-dendrocytes have a similar neuroepithelial origin to astrocytes, whereas microglial cells originate from mesenchyme. Thus, the term neuroglia should not be applied to microglial cells. Neuro-glia includes only astrocytes, oligodendrocytes, ependymal cells, and the choroid plexus epithelium derived from ependyma.

ASTROCYTES

Of the neuroglial cells, astrocytes are the most varied morphologically and the most versatile functionally. It is traditional and convenient to distinguish protoplasmic and fibrous astrocytes. The difference between these two types is based upon the configuration and the number of processes rather than on the filament content of the

cell body: the processes of fibrous astrocytes are fewer and longer and branch less frequently and at a more acute angle than those of protoplasmic astrocytes.

Protoplasmic astrocytes are found mainly in the grey matter (Fig. 1.8) whilst fibrous astrocytes occur mainly in the white matter of the brain and spinal cord (Fig. 1.9). Fibrous astrocytes, however, are also found in the outer cortical layer, around penetrating arterioles and, together with protoplasmic astrocytes, in the deep grey matter: the inferior olive contains a particularly large proportion of fibrous astrocytes.[62] A variety of fibrous astrocytes, the so-called marginal glia, sends short, robust processes towards the pial surface, and contributes to the formation of the external glial limiting membrane (glia limitans) (Fig. 1.8).

Subdivision of protoplasmic astrocytes in the

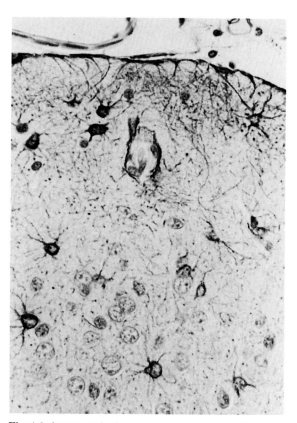

Fig. 1.8 Astrocytes in the cortex demonstrated by glial fibrillary acidic protein. Astrocytic processes project towards the glia limitans and surround a small blood vessel. Biotin-streptavidin immunoperoxidase × 640

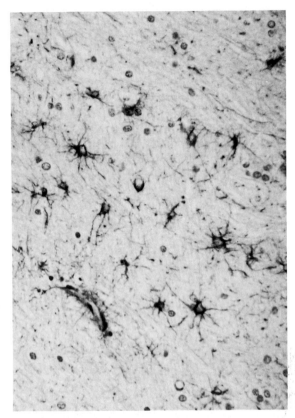

Fig. 1.9 Fibrous astrocytes in the white matter demonstrated by glial fibrillary acidic protein. Biotin-streptavidin immunoperoxidase × 300

grey matter, according to their localisation, into neuronal satellites, interneuronal astrocytes and vascular satellites serves little useful purpose. However, astrocytes of the cerebellar cortex, which are principally of the protoplasmic type, merit separate consideration on the basis of morphological variation and functional difference. The smooth astrocyte is found throughout the cerebellar cortex, the velate or lamellar type chiefly in the granular layer, and the Golgi epithelial cell in the Purkinje and molecular layer.[63] Golgi epithelial cells are in fact the Bergmann glia, whose processes cover large areas of the cell body and dendrites of Purkinje cells. A further type in the cerebellar cortex is the feathered glia of Fañanás: these cells are more superficial than Bergmann cells and their short stout processes do not reach the pial surface. One form of astrocyte which has features of both the protoplasmic and fibrous astrocytes, but is identical with neither, occurs in

the corpus callosum, basis pontis and spinal cord. This intermediate or mixed astrocyte has long fibril-containing processes identical to those of the fibrous type, whilst their shorter processes are more protoplasmic in structure.[64] Astrocytic density varies greatly in various parts of the brain. The ratio of glial cells to neurons, for example, is 4:1 in the striatum and 100:1 in the globus pallidus, accounting for 20% and 40% of the brain volume in these areas respectively.[65] These variations in astrocytic morphology in different parts of the central nervous system are well established, but information has only recently emerged from immunocytochemical and tissue culture work regarding the possible differences in astrocyte physiology and development in various topographical sites in the brain.[66]

Although astrocytes can be identified in haematoxylin and eosin stained sections (see p. 81), the intricate pattern of cytoplasmic processes which render these cells star-shaped can be better demonstrated by the use of special stains (see p. 82). The oval or round vesicular nucleus usually lacks a prominent nucleolus and this feature proves particularly convenient in identifying cells in the cortex: neurons are distinguished by their conspicuous nucleoli. Astrocytic processes cover the external surfaces of the central nervous system, surround blood vessels and abut upon nerve cells. The external glia limitans is formed by stout astrocytic processes which, in turn, are covered by a basal lamina beneath the pia (Fig. 1.8). Similarly, end-feet, the expansions of astrocytic processes, envelop blood vessels and form a limiting membrane around the adventitia of larger vessels. These astrocytic end-feet or foot processes also invest the capillaries, and this intimate relationship has provided the structural basis for the astroglial involvement in the blood-brain barrier. Astrocyte cell bodies can be in close apposition to neurons, and astrocytic processes are frequently seen covering the extensive surfaces of neuronal perikarya and dendrites.

Electron microscopy has revealed that the vesicular astrocyte nucleus contains evenly dispersed, fine chromatin which is occasionally clumped at the nuclear membrane. The nuclear profiles can be somewhat irregular with inden-

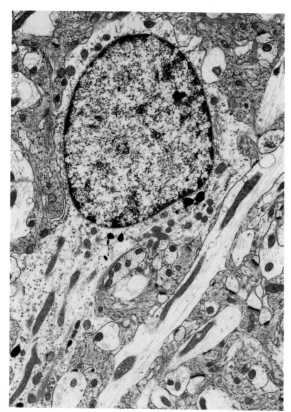

Fig. 1.10 Electron micrograph of a protoplasmic astrocyte. The light cytoplasm contains the usual assortment of organelles but few fibrils.
× 7500

cytes, in which they occur throughout the cell body and extend into the larger processes (Fig. 1.11).

Microtubules, although present, are not plentiful in mature astrocytes. Astrocytes often form specialised cell contacts of the gap junction type (so-called nexus) in which the outer leaflets of the apposed plasma membranes are separated by an interval of 2–3 nm. Adjacent astrocytes are also joined by puncta adhaerentia, where the plasma membranes run parallel, separated by a gap of 25–30 nm.[1]

Astrocytic filaments and glial fibrillary acidic protein (GFAP)

Astrocytic filaments are 10 nm in diameter and indeterminate in length. They are composed of four globular protein subunits, each measuring

tations, and the nucleolus, when present, is small. The cytoplasm is of low electron-density and contains the usual assortment of organelles. The cisternae of the rough endoplasmic reticulum are short, ribosomes few and Golgi complexes not well developed. Mitochondria are present both in the perikaryon and the cell processes, and the larger, more unusual forms are likely to correspond to the gliosomes detected by light microscopy. Glycogen granules are numerous in well-fixed tissues and appear to be concentrated in areas of high synaptic density and near neuronal perikarya. Lysosomes are also seen as electron-dense bodies limited by a single unit membrane. Astrocytic filaments, 10 nm in diameter, belong to the class of intermediate filaments of the cytoskeleton and are conspicuous in the perikaryon and in cell processes. The filaments are present in protoplasmic astrocytes, usually in the form of cytoplasmic bundles (Fig. 1.10), but they are more abundant in fibrous astro-

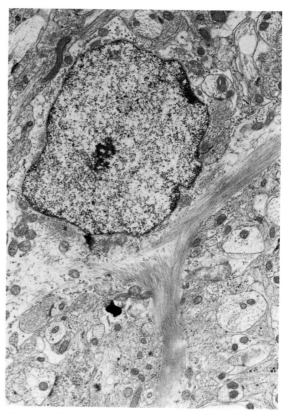

Fig. 1.11 Electron micrograph of a fibrillary astrocyte. Thick bundles of filaments extend into processes.
× 7200

2·5 nm, and linked by a cross-arm 1·5 nm in thickness. These units are stacked upon each other to produce the characteristic configuration: in transverse section a hollow central core is surrounded by a dense wall of 2·5 nm, whilst in longitudinal section two parallel dense lines enclose the lumen.[1,6]

The filaments are composed of glial fibrillary acidic protein (GFAP) which was first isolated in a water-soluble form from glial scar tissue of burnt-out plaques of multiple sclerosis and from hydrocephalic brains.[67] GFAP has a molecular weight in the range of 50 000 daltons and is well characterised chemically.[68] Immunocytochemistry indicates that GFAP may exist in two structural states, diffuse in the cytoplasm or localised to filaments, and these in turn may correspond to the water-soluble and water-insoluble forms, respectively.[69] Metabolic studies of cytoskeletal proteins in cultured astrocytes have revealed that GFAP is amongst the most actively synthesised proteins with a relatively fast turnover,[70] and both the level of synthesis and accumulation of GFAP can be experimentally manipulated.[71] It is present in normal, reactive and neoplastic astrocytes and has become the most reliable immunocytochemical marker by which the identity of astrocytes can be positively established both in diagnostic work and for research.[69] In addition to astrocytes, GFAP can be demonstrated by immunocytochemistry in other cells which contain glial filaments: in reactive ependymal cells, tanycytes, reactive Müller cells of the retina, in the pituicytes of the neurohypophysis[68] and in the glial cells of the enteric nervous system.[72] It is also present transiently during development in the myelin-forming oligodendrocytes of the human fetal spinal cord,[73] and in ependymal cells of human fetuses between the 15th and 40th week of gestation.[74] The function of GFAP has yet to be determined, but experimental evidence suggests an important role in fibrillogenesis which, in turn, is associated with astrocytic differentiation.[75]

Functions of astrocytes

The concept of astrocytic function has changed profoundly during the last 20 years: cells which once were thought to be mere physical supporting elements have been shown to have a wide range of activity in the developing, normal and diseased central nervous system.

Structural support. Virchow's original view of neuroglia[59] as cells which somehow held the neurons together has been supported by successive observations of astrocytic morphology. First, astrocytic processes cover the outside surfaces of the central nervous system, forming the glia limitans, and envelop intraparenchymatous blood vessels, constituting a sleeve of end-feet (Fig. 1.8). Second, astrocytic filaments provide mature astrocytes with a cytoskeleton which stabilises the cell configuration and endows processes with considerable strength (Fig. 1.11). These processes may form bundles which interweave with nerve fibres, particularly in the white matter. Finally, astrocytic processes are often joined together by specialised cell contacts which increase their strength and cohesion. Although microtubules play a role in process formation in differentiating astrocytes, filaments are the organelles which maintain and influence the overall morphology of mature cells.[76]

Repair. The ability of astrocytes to produce abundant filaments is seen in various pathological conditions (see p. 50). Although the formation of glial scar tissue is important in repair of the central nervous system following injury, fibrillary gliosis may occur physiologically in certain areas including the olivary nuclei, the floor of the fourth ventricle, and around both the cerebral aqueduct and the central canal of the spinal cord.

The blood-brain barrier. The structural proximity of astrocytic foot processes to capillaries has provided a morphological basis for the view that astrocytes contribute to the maintenance of the blood-brain barrier (see p. 30).

Isolation of neuronal surfaces. Astrocytes establish intimate spatial relationships with nerve cells. They are occasionally satellites to neurons, but more importantly their processes regularly cover receptive surfaces of the nerve cells, including the perikarya and dendrites. Moreover, astrocytic processes often abound in areas of intense synaptic activity; the most striking example of this phenomenon is to be found in the thalamus, where the synaptic glomeruli are wrapped in astrocytic sheets which form capsules several layers thick. Astrocytic processes are thus not disposed at random, but they conform to a pattern which ensures that receptive neuronal surfaces are protected from non-specific afferent influences.[77] Astrocytes also play a rôle in synaptic remodelling in the mature, normal brain by removing degenerating synapses.[78]

Neuronal development. Evidence for astrocyte involvement in neuronal development originates from both in vivo and in vitro observations. Radial astroglial fibres appear to guide immature, migrating neurons and to form a template for the growth of nerve cells.[79] Neurons of the central nervous system are difficult to grow in primary cultures, unless an astrocyte monolayer is provided or the medium is conditioned by growing astrocyte cultures.[80,81] In vitro studies have also shown that glial cells can influence the projection and branching patterns of nerve cells and may be instrumental in determining the neuronal polarity observed in vivo.[82]

Electrophysiology and ion transport. Recent investigations have revealed that astrocytes are not inactive cells: they respond to K^+ accumulation or release, with changes in intracellular K^+ concentration. Astrocytes can act both as spatial buffers, merely redistributing extracellularly accumulated K^+, and as active accumulators of K^+. These mechanisms complement each other and may enable astrocytes to monitor the extracellular ionic milieu and consequently to control neuronal function.[83] Furthermore, release of potassium ions (K^+) from astrocyte end-feet may play an important rôle in regulating regional cerebral blood flow in response to changes in neuronal activity.[84] It has been demonstrated in primary astrocyte cultures, which are presently the best experimental system for ion transport studies, that not only K^+, but also Na^+ and Cl^- can enter and leave these cells, suggesting that astrocytes contain significant ion transport pathways.[80,85] Under controlled conditions in culture, astrocytes show

both spontaneous action potentials and action potentials induced by current. These responses indicate the presence of voltage-dependent Ca^{2+} channels which may be important in the regulation of excitability within the central nervous system.[86] Furthermore, both glutamic and aspartic acid directly depolarise rat brain astrocytes in primary cultures, suggesting that the electrophysiological effects of excitatory amino acids in situ may not be exclusively a neuronal property.[87]

Creatine kinase (isoenzyme BB) has been shown by immunocytochemistry to be present in human astrocytes. The function of this enzyme in the brain may be related to the increase in respiration and the fall in both ATP and creatine phosphate levels which result from exposure to high potassium concentrations or from electrical stimulation.[88]

Neurotransmitter metabolism. Astrocytes in culture possess receptors for neurotransmitters, and exposure to noradrenaline results in increased levels of intracellular cyclic adenosine monophosphate (cAMP). Adrenergic α- and β-receptors have also been identified on astrocytes, and dopamine, for example, enhances cAMP by activation of β-receptors.[80] Astrocytic processes surrounding synapses could control the levels of transmitters by taking up these compounds, but it remains to be determined whether this uptake is involved in the further metabolism or inactivation of the neurotransmitter.[89] Primary cultures of astrocytes indeed take up dopamine, noradrenaline, serotonin, GABA (γ-aminobutyric acid) and glutamate and have some of the enzyme systems required for their metabolism.[90,91] Astrocytes in culture also respond to histamine and its agonists, but the functional role of histamine receptors remains to be elucidated.[92] However, the wide range of receptors on astrocytes allows these cells to play an important and varied rôle in the central nervous system.[93]

The rôle of astrocytes in the metabolism of glutamate, a putative excitatory neurotransmitter, is well documented. Glutamate is released by neurons at synapses and is taken up by astrocytes in which glutamine synthetase catalyses the reversible formation of glutamine from glutamate and ammonia. Glutamine is freely diffusible and reaches nerve cells in which glutaminase will produce glutamate and thus complete this metabolic pathway. The small glutamate pool in the brain is, therefore, compartmentalised in astrocytes.[94] Immunohistochemical studies have demonstrated that glutamine synthetase is confined to astrocytes, and the amount present in various brain areas correlates well with sites of presumed glutaminergic activity.[95]

Detoxification of ammonia. From the above description it follows that as astrocytes possess glutamine synthetase activity, they are also important in the detoxification of ammonia.[94] (see p. 54).

Phagocytosis. There is now little doubt that astrocytes have pinocytotic and phagocytic functions and by removing various substances, including plasma, particulate material and cell debris from the extracellular space, they contribute to the maintenance of a controlled internal environment (see p. 30).

Immune response. Recent experimental evidence suggests that astrocytes may have a physiological function essential for the generation of immune responses within the brain: they respond to lymphocyte-derived growth factors and secrete immunoregulatory molecules in culture.[96] They can be activated to release prostaglandin E and interleukins. Rat astrocytes appear to be able to present antigen to T lymphocytes in a specific manner which is restricted by the major histocompatibility complex.[97] Astrocytes are stimulated in the presence of γ-interferon, produced by T lymphocytes, to express Ia antigens. Astrocytes and their precursors also respond, in culture, to glial maturation factor and produce interleukin 1; this, in turn, stimulates the proliferation of astrocytes.[98]

Histological demonstration of astrocytes
(see also Ch. 4, p. 82)

The configuration of astrocytes, complete with their cytoplasmic processes, can be demonstrated by a range of specialised histological stains. The older techniques include Mallory's phosphotungstic acid haematoxylin (PTAH), Holzer's crystal violet, Cajal's gold chloride sublimate and del Río Hortega's silver carbonate impregnation.[99] The most widely used method is Mallory's PTAH but, unfortunately, this technique also stains myelin sheaths, smooth muscle fibres and extracellular proteins. The intimate relationship between astrocytes and capillaries is best visualised by Cajal's method: the close apposition of foot processes to the capillary wall is most convincingly shown.

Immunohistochemical techniques, developed more recently, offer superior specificity and sensitivity over conventional staining methods, and are increasingly used in diagnostic and research work. Astrocytic antigens can be demonstrated by both immunoperoxidase and immunofluorescence techniques; and whilst the former is preferred for paraffin sections, the latter is the method of choice for tissue culture preparations. GFAP is now most widely used to identify astrocytes[68] (Figs 1.8 and 1.9), whilst glutamine synthetase, confined to astrocytes in the central nervous system,[95] offers an alternative marker[100] (Table 1.1).

OLIGODENDROCYTES

Oligodendrocytes can be subdivided according to their location: satellite cells are adjacent to neurons in the grey matter (Fig. 1.12) and interfascicular oligodendrocytes occur between nerve fibres in the white matter (Fig. 1.13). In the grey matter (Fig. 1.14), oligodendrocytes are also associated with nerve fibres or are adjacent to blood vessels. Perineuronal oligodendrocytes are functionally similar to those in the white matter. Immunocytochemistry for myelin basic protein and myelin-associated glycoprotein reveals a similar staining pattern for all oligodendrocytes in the normal brain, during remyelination and following trauma.[101] Based on ultrastructural features, particularly on cytoplasmic density, three subtypes can be distinguished: light, intermediate and dark.[102] This separation is arbitrary and these forms represent developmental stages through which oligodendrocytes evolve during postnatal life. Light oligodendrocytes appear to be mitotically the most active and they become smaller and darker as they mature.

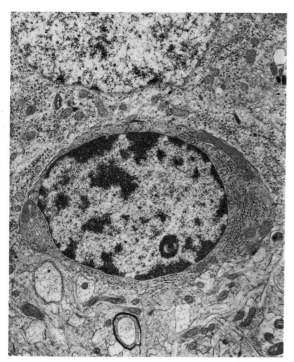

Fig. 1.12 Electron micrograph of a satellite oligodendrocyte. Both the nucleus and cytoplasm are darker than in the adjacent nerve cell (top). The nucleus is round and the cytoplasm contains abundant rough endoplasmic reticulum. × 8000

In sections stained with haematoxylin and eosin (see p. 81), oligodendrocytes can be recognised by their round or oval nuclei which are surrounded by a rim of cytoplasm. Silver impregnation reveals only a few processes, which are usually long and delicate and radiate from the polygonal or spherical perikaryon. By electron microscopy, oligodendrocytes are, in general, darker cells than astrocytes, with an intrinsic density of the cytoplasmic matrix created by tiny granules which occupy all the space between organelles (Figs 1.12 and 1.13). The chromatin in the round, oval or, occasionally, irregular nucleus often forms clumps, which is another difference from the evenly dispersed chromatin of astrocytes. Oligodendrocyte cytoplasm contains abundant rough endoplasmic reticulum, many free ribosomes and a well-developed Golgi apparatus. Mitochondria, lysosomes and heterogeneous inclusion bodies are present. Unlike in astrocytes, however, glycogen granules are not seen in

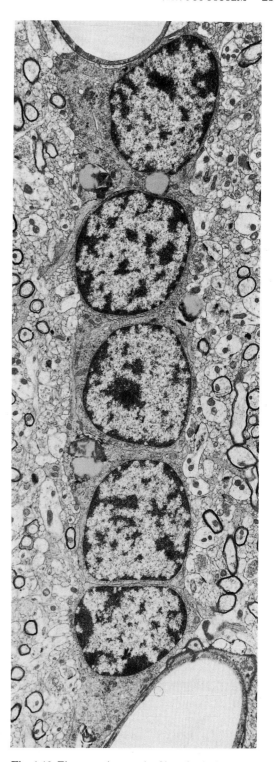

Fig. 1.13 Electron micrograph of interfascicular oligodendrocytes in the white matter. × 4725

oligodendrocytes. There is a striking difference between the cytoskeletons of oligodendrocytes and astrocytes in that the ratio of filaments to microtubules is reversed: oligodendrocytes have many microtubules and only an occasional filament. The microtubules are dispersed at random in the cell body, whilst in processes they are arranged in parallel bundles. The following features distinguish the oligodendrocyte from the astrocyte: greater nuclear and cytoplasmic density, the lack of filaments and glycogen granules, and the abundance of microtubules.

Functions of oligodendrocytes

Two major functions are usually attributed to oligodendrocytes: the formation and maintenance of myelin (see p. 13–14), and the nutrition of neurons. There is now little doubt that the myelin-forming cell in the central nervous system is the oligodendrocyte, which first appears immediately before myelination begins. In the developing brain direct connection can be seen between oligodendrocytes and the myelin sheath as it forms.[103] Biochemical studies have shown that oligodendrocytes, particularly neuronal satellites, can contribute to the nutrition of nerve cells. The metabolic activities of neurons and oligodendrocytes can complement each other in a symbiotic fashion, and these two cell types form a functional unit.[104] Furthermore, mature oligodendrocytes, in vitro, proliferate only in the presence of neurons, indicating that axons are mitogenic for these cells.[105] Tissue culture studies have also shed new light on the functions of oligodendrocytes. Isolated cells synthesise both galactocerebrosides and sulphatides[106] and contain various enzymes including 2':3'-cyclic-nucleotide 3'-phosphodiesterase, carbonic anhydrase, glycerol phosphate dehydrogenase and glucose-6-phosphate dehydrogenase, indicating a high rate of metabolic activity.[107] Oligodendrocytes respond to a variety of lymphokines and other growth factors and thus may be involved in immunological reactions.[98]

Histological demonstration of oligodendrocytes

Oligodendrocytes are usually recognised without

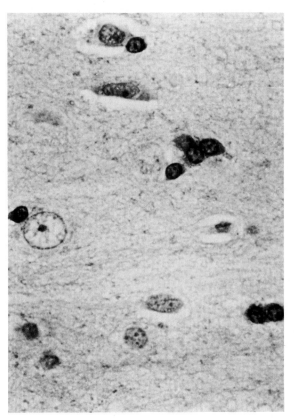

Fig. 1.14 Oligodendrocytes stained for carbonic anhydrase isoenzyme II.
Indirect immunoperoxidase × 960

difficulty in sections stained with haematoxylin and eosin (see p. 81), but silver impregnation techniques to demonstrate cell processes are capricious even in the most experienced hands.[99] Of the immunocytochemical markers, carbonic anhydrase (isoenzyme II or C) appears to be the most promising[108] (Fig. 1.14), whilst the surface marker, galactocerebroside, can be demonstrated in cultured cells[109] and myelin basic protein is present in immature oligodendrocytes during myelination[110] (Table 1.1).

EPENDYMAL CELLS

The ependyma lines the ventricular system, the cerebral aqueduct and the central canal of the spinal cord. These epithelium-like cells are cuboidal or columnar and show characteristic

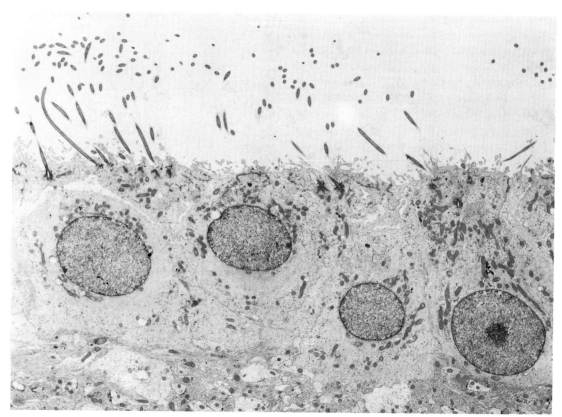

Fig. 1.15 Electron micrograph of the ependymal lining of the lateral ventricle. The round nuclei with evenly distributed chromatin tend to be basal, whilst most organelles are in the apical portion of cells. Cilia and microvilli increase the apical surface area.
× 3000

polarity of cellular organisation (Fig. 1.15). A round or oval nucleus is located in the basal part of the cell, whilst most organelles occupy the apical portion. The cell membrane is specialised according to surface. Thus the lateral membranes of adjacent cells run parallel and are joined together by specialised junctions; the cell membrane at the base of the cell has an irregular contour and rests upon glial fibres; the apical surface is studded with cilia. Ependyma lining the ventricular system varies in its morphology. In general, cells covering the white matter are more flattened and have fewer cilia than those covering grey matter.

Electron microscopy shows that the nucleus contains evenly distributed, fine chromatin and a small eccentric nucleolus (Fig. 1.15). The well developed Golgi apparatus is supranuclear, and mitochondria tend to crowd the apical portion of the cell. The rough endoplasmic reticulum consists of only a few, short cisternae, but free ribosomes are numerous. Multivesicular bodies, lysosomes and vesicles of various sizes are also present. The cytoskeleton is composed of 10 nm intermediate filaments, 4–6 nm microfilaments and occasional 24 nm microtubules. Intermediate filaments are similar to those found in astrocytes, but they do not appear to contain GFAP in normal, mature ependyma. However, ependymal cells in human fetuses contain GFAP transiently between the 15th and 40th week of gestation.[74] The nature of filaments in mature ependymal cells remains an enigma: they may be antigenically different from astrocytic filaments or the binding of GFAP within the filament may have resulted in loss of affinity for the specific antiserum.[68]

Cilia spring from the basal bodies in the apical cytoplasm which can occasionally be seen as blepharoplasts with the light microscope in good PTAH preparations. Each cilium is composed of 9 pairs of microtubules surrounding a central pair. Between the cilia, microvilli and simple cytoplasmic protrusions increase the apical surface area of the cell. The lateral plasma membranes of adjacent ependymal cells often interdigitate, forming gap junctions (nexus), extensive zonulae adhaerentes and occasional tight junctions (zonulae occludentes) toward the apices.

Tanycytes

Tanycytes are modified ependymal cells distinguished by their long, radially orientated and unbranching basal processes which usually reach subependymal capillaries. These cells, which owe their name to their elongated shape, have a somatic portion, which lies in the ependyma and contains the nucleus, a neck portion, which is located in the periventricular neuropil, and a tapering tail. The apical surfaces of tanycytes have more thin cytoplasmic projections and fewer cilia than other ependymal cells and, by electron microscopy, their cytoplasm is somewhat darker and contains fewer filaments and more microtubules.[111]

Functions of ependymal cells

The cilia of ependymal cells beat rapidly during life and this movement may contribute to the circulation of the cerebrospinal fluid (CSF) (Fig. 1.16). The structural organisation of ependyma, with its interdigitations and specialised junctions at the lateral cell surfaces, is suggestive of a supportive function, similar to that performed by astrocytes. As ependyma forms a barrier between the ventricular CSF and the parenchyma of the central nervous system, it is ideally situated to influence the transport of substances. When electron-dense markers, such as horseradish peroxidase and ferritin, are injected into the ventricles they penetrate into the brain between ependymal cells. In addition, these materials are taken up by the ependyma and transported in vesicles and multivesicular bodies, suggesting that other substances in the CSF may follow a similar pathway. As tanycytes connect the ventricular surface and capillaries, it is thought that they

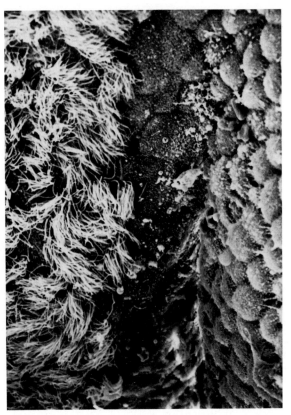

Fig. 1.16 Scanning electron micrograph of the lateral ventricle showing the ependymal surface, studded with cilia (left), and the choroid plexus (right). × 1000

transport material from the CSF to the brain and into the vascular circulation, but their major function is structural.[112] Ependymal cells may perform sensory and secretory functions in various animal species,[1] but evidence for these activities in man is still not available.

MICROGLIAL CELLS

The profusion of names which exist for microglial cells is a good indicator of the controversy surrounding the origin and morphological heterogeneity of microglia. Hortega or Robertson–Hortega cell, cerebral histiocyte, phagocyte, rod cell and mesoglia are synonyms for the microglial cell. It has been established that microglial cells are present in the normal brain;[113] the reactive changes of microglial cells in damaged brain will be considered on pages 57–59.

Microglial cells are ubiquitous in the central nervous system, although they are somewhat more numerous in the cortex than in the white matter. Most appear to be distributed at random, but some are preferentially located near neurons and blood vessels. The nucleus is triangular or elongated and the chromatin pattern is less vesicular than in astrocytes, although not as dense as in oligodendrocytes. Very little cytoplasm is visible in haematoxylin and eosin stained sections, but immunocytochemical techniques and silver impregnation (Table 1.1) demonstrate the cell processes, which are occasionally very long, but less numerous than astrocytic processes (Fig. 1.17). Electron microscopy reveals the usual complement of organelles in microglial cytoplasm. Thus, a few, long cisternae of the rough endoplasmic reticulum, some ribosomes, an active

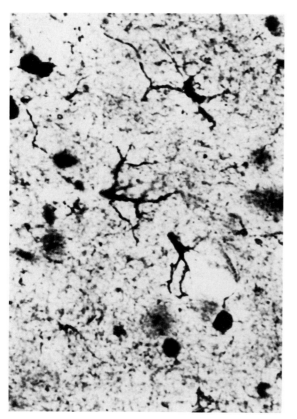

Fig. 1.17 Microglial cells in the cerebral cortex. Scott's silver impregnation × 800

Golgi apparatus, mitochondria, microtubules and a few filaments are seen (Fig. 1.18). The most prominent feature of the cytoplasm is the presence of dense inclusion bodies, mainly lysosomes. The nucleus contains coarsely clumped chromatin, and is often located at one end of the cell, surrounded by a thin rim of cytoplasm, whilst the organelles occupy the opposite pole.

Origin of microglia

The origin of microglial cells has been the subject of long controversy and the problem has yet to be convincingly settled. Various hypotheses have been proposed and include origins from pial, neuroepithelial, pericytic and monocytic cells.[114] A mesodermal or pial origin of microglia suggests that primitive mesodermal cells accumulate beneath the pia and penetrate the brain parenchyma as diverse forms of amoeboid microglia which, during differentiation, retract their pseudopodia and develop branching processes to become mature microglial cells.[61,113] The opposing neuroepithelial theory maintains that microglial cells originate from the primitive cells of the subependymal plate either directly or indirectly through amoeboid microglial cells.[115] Microglioblasts or amoeboid microglia are, in fact, glioblasts derived from the matrix cells and thus, according to this theory, microglial cells would share a common progenitor with astrocytes and oligodendrocytes.[116]

Pericytes are cells closely apposed to the capillary endothelium and enclosed by the basement membrane. Morphological similarities and the phagocytic capacity of pericytes[114] have led to the view that they could be a source of microglia; these cells could migrate into the brain through disruptions in the basement membrane.[117] However, pericytes have been shown to remain anchored to the vascular wall in pathological conditions and do not become transformed into actively phagocytosing microglial cells.[118]

The theory that microglial cells originate from monocytes has attracted many supporters,[113] who maintain that monocytes from the blood enter the brain, in which, conforming to a different environment, they acquire the features of resting microglial cells. That blood monocytes can permeate the

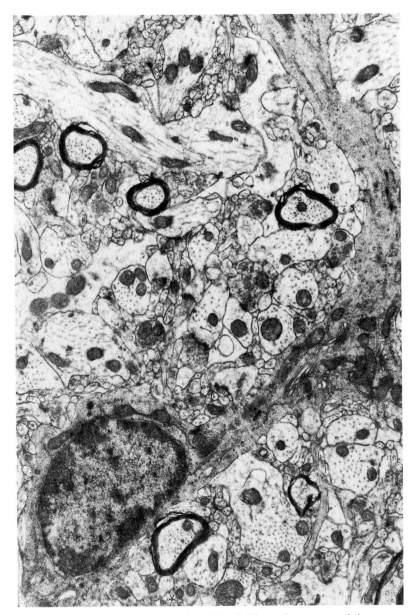

Fig. 1.18 Electron micrograph of a microglial cell. The perikaryon extends into a
long, thick process.
× 5600

brain has been shown using carbon-labelled cells;
thus, the sequential appearance of carbon particles
in monocytes, amoeboid microglia and microglia
strongly suggests that monocytes become microglial cells.[114] However, the infiltration of blood
monocytes into the brains of experimental animals
is age dependent, and the blood-brain barrier may
also play a rôle in preventing monocytes from

entering the brain in large numbers in mature
animals.[119] Moreover, immunological studies have
produced evidence against the monocytic origin of
microglia; microglial cells do not possess monocytic membrane antigens and mononuclear
phagocytic markers.[120,121] However, monocytes
may lose their membrane markers on entering the
brain and then adapt to an entirely different

environment. Monoclonal antibody specific for a macrophage membrane antigen reacts with resting microglia in the brain, indicating functional similarities.[122]

In conclusion, the original concept of a pial origin for microglial cells has not been refuted; on the contrary it has gained new support.[123] However, the possibility of a dual origin, both pial and monocytic, cannot be excluded. It is likely that occasional monocytes can enter the normal brain, and this has been demonstrated in experimental animals and in the adult normal human brain;[124] the relationship of these cells to resting microglial cells has yet to be determined.

Functions of microglia

The function of resting microglia in the normal brain is far from clear. These cells are thought to maintain a close, functional relationship with neurons, axons and myelin sheaths, to regulate the ion and fluid balance of the extracellular space and to transport substances.[115] The presence of Fc and complement receptors and of HLA class II complex on microglial cells suggests that they could play a rôle in the immunological defence of the nervous system.[125,126] Microglial cells have the ability to engulf and ingest various substances, including particulate material, parts of other cells or even whole cells. They are rich in lysosomal hydrolytic enzymes, which enable them to perform phagocytic activity.[127] This potential becomes manifest in pathological conditions (see p. 57–59).

Histological demonstration of microglial cells

Although silver impregnation demonstrates cell processes and gives the most comprehensive picture of microglial cells, the technique only works in expert hands. Enzyme histochemistry for acid phosphatase and non-specific esterase stains lysosomes and thus indicates phagocytic activity. Of the immunocytochemical markers, α_1-antitrypsin,[128,129] α_1-antichymotrypsin,[129,130] and lysozyme[131] are in general use, and an increasing number of monoclonal antibodies is now available[132] (Table 1.1).

BLOOD VESSELS AND THE BLOOD-BRAIN BARRIER

Cerebral capillaries are fundamentally similar to those of other tissues, but there are important differences. There is a paucity of cytoplasmic vesicles in the endothelial cells, and the tight junctions between the endothelial cells differ from those of other tissue capillaries. In addition, astrocytic foot processes surround each capillary. The lumen is lined by endothelial cells which display oval or elongated nuclei located in the thickened part of the capillary wall (Fig. 1.19). The cytoplasm contains the usual set of organelles, of which mitochondria are the most abundant; they constitute 8–11% of cytoplasmic volume as

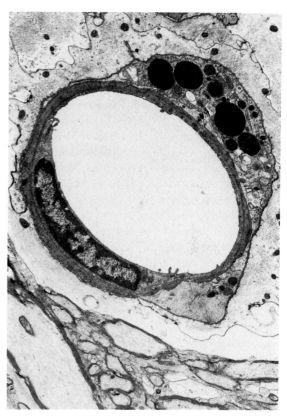

Fig. 1.19 Electron micrograph of a capillary surrounded by astrocytic foot processes. Basement membrane applied to the endothelial cell also encircles the pericyte which contains large, dense cytoplasmic inclusion bodies.
× 8000

compared to 2–5% in the capillary endothelium of other organs.[133] Complex membrane-bound structures, the Weibel–Palade bodies,[134] are difficult to find. Cytoplasmic vesicles are scarce and fewer than in most other capillaries. The structure of the interendothelial connections is variable, but in general the adjacent cell membranes are parallel, and, towards the luminal end, the outer leaflets fuse to form tight junctions (zonulae occludentes).

The endothelial cytoplasm is richly endowed with enzymes, including adenosine tri-phosphatase, nicotinamide adenine dinucleotide, monoamine oxidase, acid and alkaline phosphatases, various dehydrogenases, DOPA decarboxylase and γ-glutamyl transpeptidase.[135] The wealth of these enzyme systems reflects the unique rôle played by the cerebral endothelium in the blood-brain barrier. Moreover, differences in the intensity of various hydrolytic enzymes at the luminal and abluminal cell membrane strongly indicate the polarity of endothelial function in the control of the blood-brain interface. Outside the endothelium lies a continuous basal lamina or basement membrane approximately 40–50 nm thick and composed of an admixture of substances, including type IV collagen, heparan sulphate proteoglycan, laminin and entactin.[136] Astrocytic foot processes abut onto capillaries, forming a complete envelope in most cases (Fig. 1.19): occasionally other cells may have direct contact with the basal lamina. Pericytes are completely surrounded by a duplication of the basement membrane,[137] and are frequently seen extending their processes around the capillary; their cytoplasm contains many lysosome-like bodies. The origin and function of pericytes remain to be established, although the view that they could give rise to microglial cells has gained some support (see above).[117]

Arterioles and small arteries differ from capillaries not only in their larger size, but also by the presence of smooth muscle cells in their walls. Outside the endothelium, one or two layers of smooth muscle cells are transversely orientated and sandwiched between thick basal laminae. Venules resemble large capillaries and the transition between the two types of vessel is difficult to identify.

Histological demonstration of blood vessels

Van Gieson's technique alone or combined with an elastin stain gives good results in demonstrating connective tissue components of vessel walls. The overall pattern of vascularisation is well demonstrated by reticulin stains. Of the enzymes, the alkaline phosphatase reaction reliably identifies endothelial cells both by light and electron microscopy. The immunocytochemical demonstration of factor VIII-related antigen is now routinely used to define endothelial cells.[138] Monoclonal antibodies against endothelial angiotensin-converting enzyme[139] are also available (Table 1.1).

The blood-brain barrier

The concept of a blood-brain barrier was first based upon the observation that intravenously injected vital dyes, like Evans (azovan) blue and trypan blue, entered and stained various organs, but not the brain.[140] Later, ultrastructural studies with electron-dense tracers, such as horseradish peroxidase or lanthanum, demonstrated that tracers do not penetrate the interendothelial cell junctions in the brain, neither are they carried across the endothelial cell by vesicular transport.[141] The morphological basis for the blood-brain barrier appears to reside in two features of endothelial cells: the presence of tight junctions and the paucity of cytoplasmic vesicles. The oversimplified single-membrane model, however, is no longer accepted; intercellular tight junctions, intracellular enzyme systems and the two endothelial cell membranes all contribute to the barrier effect.[29] It has been demonstrated in vitro that astrocytic foot processes, unique to cerebral capillaries, could contribute to the barrier. Astrocytes are essential for the expression of the endothelial enzymes which play a rôle in transport mechanisms[142] and for the induction of barrier properties in vitro.[143]

The blood-brain barrier does not pertain in all parts of the mammalian brain: a few, relatively small and usually periventricular structures are freely permeable to vital dyes and electron-dense tracers. These structures include the area postrema, median eminence, subcommissural organ, pineal gland, subfornical organ, supraoptic crest and neurohypophysis. The blood vessels in these areas have ultrastructural, enzymatic and permeability features which are different from those in other areas of the brain.[144]

It has been realised that the blood-brain barrier is more a regulatory interface between the blood flow and the cerebral parenchyma than a simple rigid physical barrier.[145-147] The passage of a particular substance across the blood-brain barrier may depend upon various factors, including its lipid solubility, electrical charge, molecular size, dissociation constant, affinity for a carrier molecule and the nature of the substance in relation to the capacity of the blood-brain barrier for active transport.[144]

The function of the blood-brain barrier is threefold. First, it prevents or hinders the entry of most water-soluble substances into the brain; the permeation rates are usually determined by lipid solubility. Secondly, the blood-brain barrier promotes the transport of certain materials, including some hexoses and several amino acids, by stereo-specific carrier transport systems which are present in the cerebral endothelium. The transport of various materials across the blood-brain barrier has been recently reviewed.[146-148] Thirdly, the blood-brain barrier plays an important rôle in the volume regulation of the central nervous system. This is achieved by two mechanisms which limit the bulk flow of water across the blood-brain barrier: these are the low hydraulic conductivity of capillaries and the high osmotic activity of the major solutes.[29]

THE CHOROID PLEXUS

The choroid plexus is composed of a vascular fold of the pia mater and an epithelial layer derived from the ependymal lining. There are four choroid plexuses, one in the medial wall of each lateral ventricle and one each in the roofs of the third and fourth ventricles. They have clearly defined attachments to the ventricular wall and their free edges are invaginated into the ventricles. The surface area of the choroid plexus is greatly increased by the many fronds, which in turn consist of tiny villous processes. The arteries

supplying the choroid plexus branch out into capillaries, one for each villus, which then join to form a vein.

The epithelium consists of a single layer of cuboidal cells mounted on a basement membrane; in a few areas, however, pseudostratification or even true stratification may occur. Choroid plexus epithelium can be identified immunocytochemically by the presence of carbonic anhydrase II(c) in the cytoplasm[149] (Table 1.1); this enzyme probably plays a rôle in the production of cerebrospinal fluid (CSF). The round or oval nucleus of the cell is usually centrally located in the cytoplasm, which has the usual complement of organelles. Mitochondria are particularly numerous and are mainly in the apical portion of the cell: they provide the energy necessary for the active transport carried out during production of the CSF. Smooth and coated vesicles of various sizes are seen throughout the cytoplasm and these take part in the transport of materials. The apical surface of the epithelial cell is greatly increased in area by masses of microvilli and occasional cilia which tend to be grouped together. The lateral plasma membranes are bound together by complex connections: by tight junctions (zonulae occludentes) at the apical end, by zonulae adhaerentes, and by intricate infoldings at the basal end. Occasional phagocytes, the epiplexus or Kolmer cells, are seen on the surface of the choroid plexus epithelium; they may play a rôle in keeping this surface free of debris.[1]

The fibrovascular core of the choroid plexus supporting the epithelium contains arachnoid cells; whorls of collagen fibres in the fibrous stroma become calcified with advancing age.[150] Blood vessels of various sizes include small arteries, arterioles, capillaries and venous sinuses. Capillaries in the villi are fenestrated and their endothelial lining is very thin.

Functions of the choroid plexus

The main function of the choroid plexus is the production of the CSF, although a proportion of the CSF, estimated to be 10-20%, is derived from extrachoroidal sources.[151] In man, approximately 500-700 ml is produced every day; of this only 140 ml can be accommodated at any one time:

25–30 ml in the ventricles and the rest in the sub-arachnoid space.[152] Although it has been disputed whether the CSF is the result of passive dialysis or active secretion, evidence now favours the latter mechanism. Factors which are involved in the formation of CSF include pressure, serum osmolality, temperature, age, innervation of the plexus and prostaglandins.[152] The enzyme systems of the choroid plexus and various theories of CSF production have been recently reviewed.[153]

The choroid plexus may also take part in the absorption of materials as demonstrated in experimental animals,[154] but this function has not been unequivocally confirmed. An estimated 10% of the CSF may be absorbed by the choroid plexus.[152]

THE MENINGES

The meninges covering the central nervous system are composed of three layers: the dura mater, the arachnoid mater and the pia mater. The arachnoid and pia jointly form the leptomeninges.

The dura mater (pachymeninx) is a tough, dense membrane which surrounds the brain. It has two extensions: the falx, between the two cerebral hemispheres, and the tentorium cerebelli, separating the contents of the posterior fossa from the rest of the brain. The cranial dura is closely attached to the skull; its two layers, the periosteal and meningeal dura, are fused and separate only to form the venous sinuses. In the spinal canal, however, the dura is separated from the vertebral periosteum by the epidural space, which contains fibro-fatty tissue and an epidural venous plexus.

The dura is formed by dense, interlacing bundles of collagen in which flattened fibroblasts are embedded. The central part contains more cells and occasional blood vessels. Its outer surface is covered by thin, overlapping cell processes and its inner border also has a covering of flattened cells. The subdural space is artefactual, since the dura and arachnoid are closely apposed in life with no appreciable gap between them.[155]

The arachnoid mater has a variable thickness, in places being formed by several cell layers. Its outer, dural aspect is smoother than the inner, pial aspect from which trabeculae emerge to bridge the subarachnoid space. The arachnoid cells are joined together by specialised contacts, including tight junctions, which ensure an effective physiological barrier impermeable to CSF.

The cells of the pia mater are similar to those of the arachnoid, but the pia itself is thinner than the arachnoid. Pial cells form a complete layer joined by desmosomes and gap junctions.[156] The subpial space separates the pia from the glia limitans of the underlying neural tissue and the pia mater separates the subarachnoid space from the perivascular (Virchow–Robin) spaces of the brain[156,157] (see p. 156).

Arachnoid villi are diverticula of the arachnoid mater and the subarachnoid space which extend into veins and venous sinuses of the dura. Arachnoid granulations are larger than villi and are visible to the naked eye, whereas villi are microscopical structures. Each villus or granulation is coated on its venous aspect by endothelial cells and is bathed by venous blood. As the villus or granulation penetrates the dura, it forms a narrow neck which then expands to form a central core composed of channels and collagenous trabeculae. Towards the apex of the granulations there is a cap of arachnoid cells with wide channels running through to the coating endothelium.[158] These structures are a major pathway for the drainage of cerebrospinal fluid, which percolates through the cores of the villi or granulations and is transported across the endothelium into the blood.

THE SUBEPENDYMAL PLATE

The subependymal plate has long been recognised as a layer of primitive cells beneath the ependymal lining of the lateral ventricles in the adult human brain.[159] It is the remnant of the embryonal matrix (the subventricular zone).[160] Studies of the subependymal plate in various animal species have revealed that in the fetus it gives rise to both neurons and glia, whilst after birth it is a source of glial cells only.[161,162] The cells of the subependymal plate display ultrastructural features common to primitive cells: high nuclear–cytoplasmic ratio, dominance of free ribosomes over membrane-bound ribosomes and a general scarcity of organelles.[163] Mitotic activity persists into later adult life in various species, including primates.[164,165] Unfortunately, information on the human subependymal plate is limited, and an extrapolation from experimental animals to man may be misleading.

In addition to the subependymal plate there are other secondary germinal sites in the mammalian central nervous system, including the dentate gyrus of the hippocampus, the olfactory bulb and the external granular layer of the cerebellum. This latter zone, which has been more comprehensively studied than the other two, is formed in fetal life and postnatally continues to produce the neurons of the internal granular layer.[166] The proliferative activity of these secondary germinal zones and the hormonal, nutritional and pharmacological factors which influence cellular turnover have been reviewed.[167]

The presence of the subependymal plate with potential mitotic activity in the adult human brain raises the question of the replacement of glial cells and of their proliferative activity in the normal brain. The view that cells of the adult central nervous system do not divide cannot be maintained any longer[168] as there is convincing evidence that astrocytes and cells of the subependymal plate maintain mitotic activity throughout adult life. Although oligodendrocytes undergo mitosis in pathological conditions,[169] their ability to divide in the normal brain has not been unequivocally demonstrated. Similarly, microglial cells do not appear to be mitotically active in the normal, adult central nervous system. Neurons, ependymal cells, choroid plexus epithelium and pericytes do not divide after they have become differentiated, whilst endothelial cells continue to undergo mitosis during adult life.[168] The low turnover of cells in the adult central nervous system, coupled with the difficulty of positively identifying dividing cells and the occasional cell which is not fully differentiated, makes precise assessment of the mitotic activity of a particular cell type difficult. Moreover, recent tissue culture studies of the developing rat optic nerve have revealed that glial precursors, depending on the composition of the culture medium, can differentiate into either astrocyte or oligodendrocyte even without the influence of other brain cells.[170] If these cells persist into adult life they may retain their differentiation potential and mitotic activity.

REFERENCES

Neurons

1. Peters A, Palay SL, Webster HdeF. The fine structure of the nervous system: the neurons and supporting cells. 2nd ed. Philadelphia: Saunders, 1976.
2. Broadwell RD, Catalda AM. J Histochem Cytochem 1983; 31: 1077.
3. Novikoff AB. In: Hydén H, ed. The neuron. Amsterdam: Elsevier, 1967: 255.
4. Whaley WG, Dauwalder M. Int Rev Cytol 1979; 58: 199.
5. Dolman CL, Macleod PM. In: Fedoroff S, Hertz L, eds. Advances in cellular neurobiology. New York: Academic Press, 1981; 2: 205.
6. Wuerker RB. Tissue Cell 1970; 2: 1.
7. Shelanski ML, Liem RKH. J Neurochem 1979; 33: 5.
8. Dahl D. Exp Cell Res 1983; 149: 397.
9. Schlaepfer WW. J Neuropathol Exp Neurol 1987; 46: 117.
10. Pachter JS, Liem RKH, Shelanski ML. In: Fedoroff S, ed. Advances in cellular neurobiology. Orlando: Academic Press, 1984; 5: 113.
11. Hoffman PN, Cleveland DW, Griffin JW, Landes PW, Cowan NJ, Price DL. Proc Natl Acad Sci USA 1987; 84: 3472.
12. Kalnins VI, Connolly JA. In: Fedoroff S, Hertz L, eds. Advances in cellular neurobiology. New York: Academic Press, 1981; 2: 393.
13. Anderton BH. In: Smith WT, Cavanagh JB, eds. Recent advances in neuropathology. Edinburgh: Churchill Livingstone, 1982; 2: 29.
14. Thyberg J, Moskalewski S. Exp Cell Res 1985; 159: 1.
15. Gray EG. J Anat 1959; 93: 420.
16. Palade G. Science 1975; 189: 347.
17. Katz B. Proc R Soc Lond (Biol) 1962; 155: 45.
18. Vizi ES. Neurochem Int 1984; 6: 435.
19. Schmitt FO. Neuroscience 1984; 13: 991.
20. Cooper JR, Meyer EM. Neurochem Int 1984; 6: 419.
21. Gray EG. In: Clegg NJ, ed. Neurotransmitter systems and their disorders. London: Academic Press, 1978: 1.
22. Hirokawa N, Glicksman MA, Willard MB. J Cell Biol 1984; 98: 1523.
23. Bisby MA. In: Fedoroff S, Hertz L, eds. Advances in cellular neurobiology. New York: Academic Press, 1980; 1: 69.
24. Droz B, Koenig HL, Di Giamberardino L. Brain Res 1973; 60: 93.
25. Holtzman E. Neuroscience 1977; 2: 327.
26. Amos LA, Amos WB, J Cell Sci 1987; 87: 1.
27. Ramon-Moliner E. In: Bourne GH, ed. The structure and function of the nervous tissue. New York: Academic Press, 1968; 1: 205.
28. Abdel-Maguid TE, Bowsher D. J Anat 1984; 138: 689.
29. Fenstermacher JD. In: Staub NC, Taylor AE, eds. Edema. New York: Raven Press, 1984: 383.
30. Blakemore WF. In: Smith WT, Cavanagh JB, eds. Recent advances in neuropathology. Edinburgh: Churchill Livingstone, 1982; 2: 53.
31. Brody BA, Kinney HC, Kloman AS, Gilles FH. J Neuropathol Exp Neurol 1987; 46: 283.

32. Borit A, McIntosh GC. Neuropathol Appl Neurobiol 1981; 7: 279.
33. Richardson EP. In: Haymaker W, Adams RD, eds. Histology and histopathology of the nervous system. Springfield: Thomas, 1982: 146.
34. Seil FJ. In: Fedoroff S, Hertz L, eds. Advances in cellular neurobiology. New York: Academic Press, 1982; 3: 235.
35. Marton LS, Stefansson K. J Cell Biol 1984; 99: 1642.
36. Iversen LL. Proc R Soc Lond (Biol) 1984; 221: 245.
37. McGeer EG, McGeer PL. In: Fedoroff S, Hertz L, eds. Advances in cellular neurobiology. New York: Academic Press, 1980; 1: 347.
38. Perry EK, Perry RH. Life Sci 1983; 33: 1733.
39. Iversen LL. Lancet 1982; 2: 914.
40. Parent A, Csonka C, Etienne P. Brain Res 1984; 291: 154.
41. McGeer PL, McGeer EG, Peng JH. Life Sci 1984; 34: 2319.
42. Marsden CD. Lancet 1982; 2: 1141.
43. Iversen LL. Ann Rev Pharmacol 1983; 23: 1.
44. Polak JM, Bloom SR. Br Med J 1983; 286: 1461.
45. Constantinidis J, Bouras C, Richard J. Clin Neuropathol 1983; 2: 47.
46. Beal MF, Martin JB. Ann Neurol 1986; 20: 547.
47. Rossor MN. Lancet 1982; 2: 1200.
48. Spero L. Lancet 1982; 2: 1319.
49. Snyder SH. Lancet 1982; 2: 970.
50. Braestrup C, Nielsen M. Lancet 1982; 2: 1030.
51. Kennedy PGE. J Neuroimmunol 1982; 2: 35.
52. Itoyama Y, Sternberger NH, Kies MW, Cohen SR, Richardson EP Jr, Webster HdeF. Ann Neurol 1980; 7: 157.
53. Itoyama Y, Sternberger NH, Webster HdeF, Quarles RH, Cohen SR, Richardson EP Jr. Ann Neurol 1980; 7: 167.
54. Raff MC, Fields KL, Hakomori S-I, Mirsky R, Pruss RM, Winter J. Brain Res 1979; 174: 283.
55. Vaheri A, Ruoslahti E, Westermark B, Pontén J. J Exp Med 1976; 143: 64.
56. Anderton BH, Breinburg D, Downes MJ et al. Nature 1982; 298: 84.
57. Trojanowsky JQ, Lee VM, Schlaepfer WW. Hum Pathol 1984; 15: 248.
58. Schmechel D, Marangos PJ, Zis AP, Brightman M, Goodwin FK. Science 1978; 199: 313.

Neuroglia

59. Virchow R. Virchows Arch Pathol Anat 1854; 6: 135.
60. Cajal S Ramón y. Histologie du système nerveux de l'homme et des vertébrés. Madrid: Consejo Superior de Investigaciones Cientificas. Instituto Ramón y Cajal, 1972.
61. Del Río Hortega P. In: Penfield W, ed. Cytology and cellular pathology of the nervous system. New York: Hoeber, 1932; 2: 481.
62. Scheibel ME, Scheibel AB. J Comp Neurol 1955; 102: 77.
63. Chan-Palay V, Palay SL. Z Anat Entwicklungsgesch 1972; 138: 1.
64. Polak M, Haymaker W, Johnson JE Jr, D'Amelio F. In: Haymaker W, Adams RD, eds. Histology and histopathology of the nervous system. Springfield: Thomas, 1982: 363.
65. Treff WM. In: Weibel ER, Elias H, eds. Quantitative Methoden in der Morphologie. Berlin: Springer, 1967: 79.
66. Patel AJ, Hunt A, Tahourdin CSM. Dev Brain Res 1983; 8: 31.
67. Eng LF, Vanderhaeghen JJ, Bignami A, Gerstl B. Brain Res 1971; 28: 351.
68. Eng LF, DeArmond SJ. In: Zimmerman HM, ed. Progress in neuropathology. New York: Raven Press, 1983; 5: 19.
69. Eng LF, DeArmond SJ. In: Fedoroff S, Hertz L, eds. Advances in cellular neurobiology. New York: Academic Press, 1982; 3: 145.
70. Chiu F-C, Goldman JE. J Neurochem 1984; 42: 166.
71. Goldman JE, Chiu F-C. J Neurochem 1984; 42: 175.
72. Jessen K, Mirsky R. Nature 1980; 286: 736.
73. Choi BH, Kim RC. Science 1984; 223: 407.
74. Roessmann U, Velasco ME, Sindely SD, Gambetti P. Brain Res 1980; 200: 13.
75. Bignami A, Dahl D, Rueger DC. In: Fedoroff S, Hertz L, eds. Advances in cellular neurobiology. New York: Academic Press, 1980; 1: 285.
76. Trimmer PA, Reier PJ, Oh TH, Eng LF. J Neuroimmunol 1982; 2: 235.
77. Meshul CK, Seil FJ, Herndon RM. Brain Res 1987; 402: 139.
78. Adams I, Jones DG. Neurobiol Aging 1982; 3: 179.
79. Levitt P, Rakic P. J Comp Neurol 1980; 193: 815.
80. Kimelberg HK. Cell Mol Neurobiol 1983; 3: 1.
81. Assouline JG, Bosch P, Lim R, Kim IS, Jensen R, Pantazis NJ. Dev Brain Res 1987; 31: 103.
82. Denis-Donini S, Glowinski J, Prochiantz A. Nature 1984; 307: 641.
83. Walz W, Wuttke W, Hertz L. Brain Res 1984; 292: 367.
84. Paulson OB, Newman EA. Science 1987; 237: 896.
85. Walz W, Hertz L. J Neurosci Res 1984; 11: 231.
86. MacVicar BA. Science 1984; 226: 1345.
87. Bowman CL, Kimelberg HK. Nature 1984; 311: 656.
88. Thompson RJ, Kynoch PAM, Sarjant J. Brain Res 1980; 201: 423.
89. Schousboe A. In: Smythies JR, Bradley RJ, eds. International review of neurobiology. New York: Academic Press, 1981; 22: 1.
90. Hertz L. In: Lajtha A, ed. Handbook of neurochemistry. New York: Plenum Press, 1982: 319.
91. Kimelberg HK, Katz DM. Science 1985; 228: 889.
92. Hösli L, Hösli E, Schneider U, Wiget W. Neurosci Lett 1984; 48: 287.
93. Murphy S, Pearce B. Neuroscience 1987; 22: 381.
94. Norenberg MD. In: Fedoroff S, Hertz L, eds. Advances in cellular neurobiology. New York: Academic Press, 1981; 2: 303.
95. Norenberg MD. J Histochem Cytochem 1979; 27: 756.
96. Fontana A. J Neurosci Res 1982; 8: 443.
97. Fontana A, Fierz W, Wekerle H. Nature 1984; 307: 273.
98. Merrill JE. Immunol today 1987; 5: 146.
99. Cox G. In: Bancroft JD, Stevens A, eds. Theory and practice of histological techniques. Edinburgh: Churchill Livingstone, 1977.
100. Pilkington GJ, Lantos PL, Neuropathol Appl Neurobiol 1982; 8: 227.
101. Ludwin SK. Neuropathol Appl Neurobiol 1984; 10: 143.
102. Mori S, Leblond CP. J Comp Neurol 1970; 139: 1.
103. Bunge RP. Physiol Rev 1968; 48: 197.
104. Hydén H. In: Hydén H, ed. The neuron. Amsterdam: Elsevier, 1967: 179.
105. Wood PM, Bunge RP. Nature 1986; 320: 756.

106. Szuchet S, Stefansson K. In: Fedoroff S, Hertz L, eds. Advances in cellular neurobiology. New York: Academic Press, 1980; 1: 313.
107. Norton WT. In: Fedoroff S, Hertz L, eds. Advances in cellular neurobiology. New York: Academic Press, 1983; 4: 3.
108. Langley OK, Ghandour MS, Vincendon G, Gombos G. Histochem J 1980; 12: 473.
109. Raff MC, Mirsky R, Fields KL et al. Nature 1978; 274: 813.
110. Sternberger NH, Itoyama Y, Kies MW, Webster HdeF. J Neurocytol 1978; 7: 251.
111. Millhouse OE. Z Zellforsch Mikrosk Anat 1972; 127: 149.
112. Gould SJ, Howard S. Neuropathol Appl Neurobiol 1987; 13: 421.
113. Cammermeyer J. In: Ehrenpreis S, Solnitzky OC, eds. Neurosciences research. New York: Academic Press, 1970; 3: 44.
114. Ling EA. In: Fedoroff S, Hertz L, eds. Advances in cellular neurobiology. New York: Academic Press, 1981; 2: 34.
115. Oehmichen M. In: Smith WT, Cavanagh JB, eds. Recent advances in neuropathology. Edinburgh: Churchill Livingstone, 1982; 2: 83.
116. Kitamura T, Miyake T, Fujita S. J Comp Neurol 1984; 226: 421.
117. Mori S, Leblond CP. J Comp Neurol 1969; 135: 57.
118. Barron KD, Means ED, Feng T, Harris H. Exp Mol Pathol 1974; 20: 344.
119. Ling EA, Penney D. Anat Rec 1979; 193: 604.
120. Oehmichen M, Wiethölter H, Greaves MF. J Neuropathol Exp Neurol 1979; 38: 99.
121. Wood GW, Gollahon KA, Tilzer SA, Vats T, Morantz RS. J Neuropathol Exp Neurol 1979; 38: 369.
122. Mathew RC, Gupta SK, Katayama I, Curtis J, Turk JL. J Pathol 1983; 141: 435.
123. Merchant RE, Low FN. Am J Anat 1979; 156: 183.
124. Oehmichen M. In: Zimmerman HM, ed. Progress in neuropathology. New York: Raven Press, 1983; 5: 277.
125. Perry VH, Hume DA, Gordon S. Neuroscience 1985; 15: 313.
126. Hayes GM, Woodroofe MN, Cuzner ML. J Neurol Sci. 1987; 80: 25.
127. Lantos PL. Acta Neuropathol (Berl) 1974; 29: 45.
128. Isaacson P, Jones DB, Millward-Sadler GH, Judd MA, Payne S. J Clin Pathol 1981; 34: 982.
129. Esiri M, Booss J. J Clin Pathol 1984; 37: 150.
130. Motoi M, Stein H, Lennert K. Virchows Arch (Cell Pathol) 1980; 35: 73.
131. Mason DY, Taylor CR. J Clin Pathol 1975; 28: 124.
132. Rossi ML, Hughes JT, Esiri MM, Coakham HB, Brownell DB. Acta Neuropathol (Berl) 1987; 74: 269.

Blood vessels and the blood-brain barrier

133. Pollay M, Roberts PA. Neurosurgery 1980; 6: 675.
134. Weibel ER, Palade GE. J Cell Biol 1964; 23: 101.
135. Inomata K, Yoshioka T, Nasu F, Mayahara H. Acta Anat 1984; 118: 243.
136. Martinez-Hernandez A, Amenta PS. Lab Invest 1983; 48: 656.
137. Bär T, Budi Santoso AW. Cell Tissue Res 1984; 236: 491.
138. McComb RD, Jones TR, Pizzo SV, Bigner DD. J Histochem Cytochem 1982; 30: 371.

139. Auerbach R, Alby L, Grieves J et al. Proc Natl Acad Sci USA 1982; 79: 7891.
140. Ehrlich P. Das Sauerstoff-Bedürfniss des Organismus. Eine farbenanalytische Studie. Berlin: Hirschwald, 1885.
141. Reese TS, Karnovsky MJ. J Cell Biol 1967; 34: 207.
142. DeBault L. Brain Res 1981; 220: 432.
143. Janzer RC, Raff MC, Nature 1987; 325: 253.
144. Lee JC. In: Haymaker W, Adams RD, eds. Histology and histopathology of the nervous system. Springfield: Thomas, 1982: 798.
145. Rapoport SI. Blood-brain barrier in physiology and medicine. New York: Raven Press, 1976.
146. Bradbury MWB. The concept of the blood-brain barrier. Chichester: Wiley, 1979.
147. Fenstermacher JD, Rapoport SI. In: Renkin EM, Michel CC, eds. Handbook of physiology: the microcirculation. Bethesda: American Physiological Society, 1983; 4: 969.
148. Bradbury MWB. Circ Res 1985; 57: 213.

Choroid plexus

149. Weller RO, Steart PV, Moore IE. In: Walker MD, Thomas DGT, eds. Biology of brain tumour. Boston: Nijhoff, 1986: 115.
150. Alcolado JC, Moore IE, Weller RO. Neuropathol Appl Neurobiol 1986; 12: 235.
151. McComb JG. J Neurosurg 1983; 59: 369.
152. Bargmann W, Oksche A, Fix JD, Haymaker W. In: Haymaker W, Adams RD, eds. Histology and histopathology of the nervous system. Springfield: Thomas, 1982: 560.
153. Masuzawa T, Sato F. Brain 1983; 106: 55.
154. Cserr HF. Physiol Rev 1971; 51: 273.

Meninges

155. Schachenmayr W, Friede RL. Am J Pathol 1978; 92: 53.
156. Alcolado R, Weller RO, Parrish EP, Garrod D. Neuropathol Appl Neurobiol 1988; 14: 1.
157. Hutchings M, Weller RO. J Neurosurg 1986; 65: 316.
158. Upton ML, Weller RO. J Neurosurg 1985; 63: 867.

Subependymal plate

159. Globus JH, Kuhlenbeck H. J Neuropathol Exp Neurol 1944; 3: 1.
160. Angevine JB Jr, Bodian D, Coulombre AJ et al (The Boulder Committee). Anat Rec 1970; 166: 257.
161. Smart IHM. J Anat 1973; 116: 67.
162. Privat A. Int Rev Cytol 1975; 40: 281.
163. Blakemore WF. J Anat 1969; 104: 423.
164. Lewis PD. Nature 1968; 217: 974.
165. McDermott KWG, Koppel H, Lantos PL. Neuropathol Appl Neurobiol 1987; 13: 234.
166. Koppel H, Lewis PD. Neuropathol Appl Neurobiol 1983; 9: 207.
167. Lewis PD. In: Smith WT, Cavanagh JB, eds. Recent advances in neuropathology. Edinburgh: Churchill Livingstone, 1979; 1: 41.
168. Sturrock RR. In: Fedoroff S, Hertz L, eds. Advances in cellular neurobiology. New York: Academic Press, 1982; 3: 3.
169. Ludwin SK. Nature 1984; 308: 274.
170. Temple S, Raff MC. Nature 1985; 313: 223.

Histological and cytological reactions

INTRODUCTION

The pathology of the central nervous system can be considered disease by disease. However, as the nervous system exhibits a limited number of pathological reactions, diagnoses are achieved by the recognition and analysis of these reactions, together with considerations of the anatomy, the clinical history and the age of the patient.

In this chapter, the general pathological reactions of the central nervous system and its constituent cells are described. Subsequent chapters make use of this information to describe particular disease entities.

PATHOLOGY OF NEURONS

SELECTIVE VULNERABILITY

The response of nerve cells to pathological stimuli varies according to site and cell type. The same insult may severely affect particular neurons and certain areas of the nervous system, whilst other cells within the same topographical area or in other regions show little evidence of damage. This *selective neuronal vulnerability* has been most extensively studied in experimental hypoxia. Layers 3, 5 and 6 in the cerebral cortex, CA1 area (Sommer sector) and the end-plate in the hippocampus, Purkinje cells and basket cells in the cerebellum (Fig. 2.1) and the central and basolateral portions of the amygdala are preferentially damaged by hypoxia. Changes also occur in the basal ganglia, but the spinal cord appears to be the region of the CNS most resistant to hypoxia.[1,2]

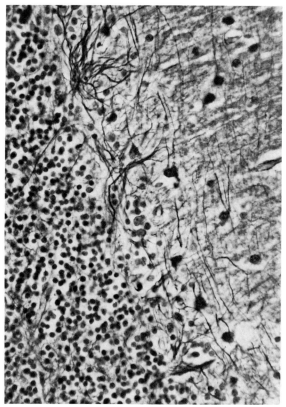

Fig. 2.1 Selective loss of Purkinje cells from the cerebellar cortex is demonstrated by the preserved axons of basket cells ('empty baskets').
Palmgren × 350

Although the assessment of hypoxic damage is more difficult in man than in experimental animals, a similar pattern of neuronal vulnerability has been established in the human CNS.[3,4] Cardiorespiratory arrest, for example, provides a very clear picture of selective neuronal vulnerability in man. The neocortex of the parietal and occipital lobes is more affected than that of the frontal and temporal poles, and the damage is more severe in the depths and at the sides of sulci than on the crests of gyri.[3]

Other examples of selective neuronal vulnerability are the *boundary or watershed infarcts* which develop in the cerebral and cerebellar hemispheres at the boundary zones of adjacent arterial territories. If the cerebral blood flow is reduced, the oxygen supply becomes insufficient in those parts of the arterial territory which are furthest from the origin of the blood vessels: infarction consequently develops at the boundary zone in which small vessels from the two arterial fields anastomose.

The reasons for selective neuronal vulnerability are not known, but it is likely that more than one factor plays a role. Structurally, selective neuronal vulnerability is related to the neuroanatomical connections and cytological features of a given site in the CNS. Neurons of a particular type within the same area of brain, and possessing the same characteristic Nissl substance and protein synthesising capacity, form an anatomical and metabolic unit; neurons within this unit are endowed with similar selective vulnerability to various insults.[5] In order to explain selective neuronal vulnerability, two hypotheses have been formulated.[3] The vascular concept envisages anatomical and physiological features of individual blood vessels as the determining factors, whereas the theory of pathoclisis puts the emphasis on local physicochemical factors. Different neurons have different rates of metabolic activity, and those which are particularly active will suffer first if the demand for oxygen and nutrients outstrips supply. Consequently, the local blood supply, neuronal activity, and the ability of nerve cells to utilise all the essential materials are paramount factors in determining neuronal vulnerability.

NEURONAL LOSS

There is now evidence for a continuous and gradual decrease in the number of nerve cells with increasing age.[6] However, the statement that approximately 100 000 neurons are lost each day of our adult life[7] has not been universally accepted. Precipitate and extensive neuronal loss may also occur in a variety of degenerative diseases, but the assessment of this reduction in neurons presents considerable practical problems. Neuronal degeneration and loss can be readily assessed if small, well-circumscribed nuclei, like the substantia nigra and locus ceruleus, are involved as in Parkinson's disease. The task, however, becomes more difficult in the basal ganglia; as, for example, with the evaluation of neuronal loss from the caudate nucleus and the putamen in Huntington's disease. The widespread decrease of cortical nerve cells which occurs in Alzheimer's disease can be accurately assessed only by means of quantitative morphometry.[8] Special techniques now enable precise and reliable evaluation of neuronal loss and have provided a solid scientific basis for the previously subjective assessment of neuronal populations. In practice, when neuronal loss is not obvious, the astrocytic and microglial response is often a good indicator of preceding neuronal damage (see p. 52).

GENERAL PATHOLOGY OF NEURONS

Chromatolysis

Chromatolysis is the disruption, dispersal and gradual disappearance of the Nissl substance in the neuronal cytoplasm (Fig. 2.2). In sections stained with haematoxylin and eosin, chromatolytic

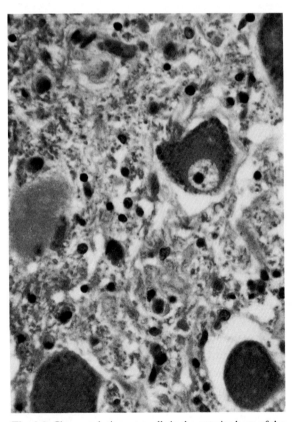

Fig. 2.2 Chromatolytic nerve cells in the anterior horn of the spinal cord.
Haematoxylin-eosin × 500

neurons can be easily recognised: with the loss of basophilic Nissl granules, the cytoplasm becomes uniformly eosinophilic. The process usually starts in the cytoplasm adjacent to the nucleus, whilst a narrow rim of Nissl substance remains at the periphery. This pattern of depletion is *central chromatolysis* which can occur both in physiological conditions, as a result of excessive electrical stimulation, and in a variety of pathological processes. When chromatolysis is caused by raised physiological activity, the Nissl substance can completely recover after an interval of rest; this structural reconstitution usually starts at the periphery of the cytoplasm.

Severance of the axon induces chromatolysis in the parent neuron as an *axonal response*. The Nissl substance disintegrates and disappears, the nucleus is displaced to an eccentric position in the cell and the nucleolus enlarges. The entire cell loses its normal configuration and becomes rounded. These neuronal changes are accompanied by astrocyte hypertrophy and hyperplasia and by local microglial activation.

Electron microscopy of chromatolytic neurons reveals the disorganisation of rough endoplasmic reticulum: the well-ordered arrays of cisternae disintegrate and vesiculate, and ribosomes become detached from the membrane. Cisternae of the smooth endoplasmic reticulum and Golgi complexes are abundant and there is an increase of neurofilaments, microtubules and lysosomes.[9] The nuclear membrane develops deep indentations and the chromatin may become coarsely clumped. Afferent synapses are also affected and the boutons terminaux undergo dark or light degeneration: in the former, more frequent form, the dense matrix contains clumped synaptic vesicles and shrunken organelles; in the latter, there is an excess of filaments in the swollen terminal. These profound ultrastructural changes are accompanied by alterations of enzyme activity and of the physiological state of the cells.[10]

The sequence of perikaryal events following axotomy has been studied in experimental animals and it was found that the severity of changes depended upon the age, species, area affected, type of neurons and nature of the injury. The site of axonal injury is an important factor: the more proximal the damage, the more severe is the degeneration of the perikaryon. Central chromatolysis can, however, develop occasionally without apparent axonal damage; for example in pellagra, despite the obvious changes in the perikaryon, no axonal injury has been demonstrated.[10]

The type of injury determines the outcome of neuronal damage: crush injury of the facial nerve in mice causes chromatolysis which is followed by full recovery in the facial nucleus, whereas complete sectioning of the nerve results in extensive neuronal disintegration.[11]

The mechanism which triggers off chromatolysis after axonal damage has not been established, but it is likely that retrograde axonal transport carries the signals for chromatolysis. These signals could include extracellular proteins taken up at the site of injury, lack of a trophic factor normally derived from the target tissue and endogenous substances usually destined for the terminal but delivered instead to the cell body by the reversed axoplasmic flow.[12]

The amount of the Nissl substance varies according to neuronal type, and many nerve cells, particularly those in the brainstem, have sparse rough endoplasmic reticulum limited to the periphery of the cell body. These normal cells therefore should not be confused with those which have undergone central chromatolysis.

Hypoxic damage and ischaemic cell change

Neurons, perhaps more than any other cells in the body, are dependent upon an adequate oxygen supply. If this requirement is not met, hypoxic neuronal damage develops. The underlying physiological conditions of cerebral hypoxia vary:[2] arrest or reduction of blood flow in the brain, decrease of arterial oxygen tension, reduction of haemoglobin available to bind oxygen, and toxic substances can all cause hypoxic damage. Similarly, since glucose is the principal metabolic substrate of neurons, hypoglycaemia can also lead to morphological changes superficially similar to those of hypoxia, although the distribution and structural details of damage are somewhat different.[13] The causes and mechanisms of hypoxic neuronal damage are discussed in Chapter 5 (see p. 115).

The existing knowledge of hypoxic neuronal damage has been obtained mainly from animal experiments which allow well-controlled sequential studies. The earliest change, observed by electron microscopy, in rodents, monkeys and man is microvacuolation of neuronal cytoplasm.[1] The small vacuoles correspond chiefly to swollen mitochondria; these organelles contain the enzyme systems of respiration and oxidative phosphorylation and appear to be most sensitive to hypoxia. Some vacuoles may also result from the dilatation of the cisternae of the rough endoplasmic reticulum. This stage of vacuolation is followed by gradual and progressive condensation of the cytoplasm and nucleoplasm, leading to the characteristic picture of *ischaemic cell change* in which the cell body is shrunken and can be easily recognised with the light microscope by the intensely and homogeneously eosinophilic cytoplasm. The densely staining nucleus is often triangular in shape and the damaged neurons are frequently surrounded by swollen astrocytic processes. The next stage is heralded by the appearance of *incrustations*, which are heavily stained, small irregular bodies close to the surface of the perikaryon and sometimes on the surfaces of the dendrites. They correspond, at the ultrastructural level, to extremely dense cytoplasmic areas in the peripheral part of the perikaryon and cell processes. The cytoplasm of the neuron at this stage contains an assortment of damaged organelles, including disrupted endoplasmic reticulum and dense mitochondria; many lysosomes and autophagic vacuoles are also seen in the cytoplasm. At a more advanced stage of hypoxic damage, the incrustations progressively disappear and the cytoplasm loses all its normal features: this appearance represents the stage of *homogeneous cell change*. In the final phase, the neuron is seen only as a shrunken, pyknotic nucleus surrounded by a rim of structureless cytoplasm.

The time course of these stages varies in different species. In rats microvacuolation develops after only 5–15 minutes and ischaemic cell change is observed as early as 30 minutes, whereas in rhesus monkeys these stages may take longer to occur, 30 and 90 minutes, respectively.[1] Although hypoxic brain damage represents a progressive chain of events which begins with mild degeneration of organelles and ends in neuronal death, this process is reversible if the hypoxia is mild or is not sustained for long periods. Recent ultrastructural investigations suggest that abnormalities in the Golgi apparatus and cell membrane may represent the point of no return: the failure of the Golgi apparatus to repair or maintain the neuronal cell membrane could be the underlying cause of irreversible neuronal damage.[14,15]

Hypoxic cell damage does not affect all areas of the central nervous system to the same degree; similarly, certain neuronal types are more severely affected than others. In the cerebral cortex, the pyramidal cells in laminae 3, 5 and 6 are affected, in the hippocampus the pyramidal cells, particularly in CA1 area, are vulnerable, and in the cerebellum the Purkinje cells are most susceptible to hypoxic damage. In the striatum, hypoxia is known to affect preferentially the small and medium-sized neurons. In general, hypoxic changes develop more rapidly in small neurons than in larger ones.[1,3]

These morphological investigations have now been complemented by pathophysiological and biochemical studies of hypoxic-ischaemic injury of the brain. Severe and persistent hypoxia leads to energy failure and cellular depolarisation which, when prolonged, is not compatible with cell survival.[16]

Simple atrophy

Simple atrophy is a severe form of neuronal damage which can occur in a variety of degenerative disorders. Neuronal atrophy or shinkage occurs in system disorders such as motor neuron disease, multiple system degenerations, Huntington's disease (p. 382) and Friedreich's ataxia (p. 417). The affected neurons may display changes of varying severity ranging from central chromatolysis to advanced pyknosis. Damage to the neuronal perikarya extends to the cell processes, and axonal degeneration will, in turn, lead to breakdown of myelin sheaths with a consequent astrocytic and microglial response.

Vacuolation

Vacuoles of various sizes may occur in a number of pathological conditions, but they may also rep-resent post-mortem or fixation artefacts in human material. For this reason, their presence in autopsy specimens or poorly fixed biopsies should be interpreted with utmost caution. Moreover, neuronal vacuoles are sometimes difficult to distinguish from swollen astrocytic processes. Intra-cytoplasmic vacuoles usually result from dilatation of the lumina of existing organelles (e.g. endoplasmic reticulum or Golgi complexes) or from mitochondrial damage. Vacuolation of nerve cells occurs in Creutzfeldt–Jakob disease and kuru (see pages 221, 384–388), two spongiform encephalopathies which affect man. These vacuoles of various sizes impart the characteristic appearance to the grey matter and are one of the histological hallmarks of the spongiform encephalopathies.[17]

Satellitosis and neuronophagia

The terms satellitosis and neuronophagia describe

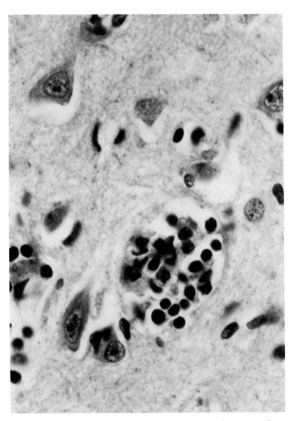

Fig. 2.3 Neuronophagy in the cerebral cortex in a case of herpes simplex encephalitis. Haematoxylin-eosin × 800

two different processes. *Satellitosis* refers to an increase of satellite cells which are normally present adjacent to neuronal perikarya. These cells are chiefly oligodendrocytes, which are particularly prominent around the large nerve cells in the frontal cortex and basal ganglia. Occasional astrocytes and microglial cells may also be found in satellite positions in the normal brain. *Neuronophagia* is the active process by which severely degenerate or dead neurons are surrounded, destroyed and ingested by phagocytic cells (Fig. 2.3).

In some virus infections such as poliomyelitis (see p. 205), polymorphonuclear leucocytes appear first and are later replaced by macrophages. However, neuronophagia in most virus infections and following hypoxic cell damage is characterised by the accumulation of microglial cells around the dead neurons (Fig. 2.3). Neuronophagia is most commonly seen in grey matter areas of the brain and spinal cord, but may very occasionally be seen involving ectopic neurons in the cerebral white matter. Nerve cell death is not always followed by neuronophagy; neurons may die and disappear without much evidence of microglia or macrophages surrounding them.

Lipofuscin accumulation

Increase in neuronal lipofuscin content occurs during ageing and in pathological conditions. It is common to find a large number of lipofuscin particles in the nerve cells of the brains of elderly people, hence the term 'wear-and-tear' pigment (Fig. 2.4). However, ultrastructural demonstration of acid phosphatase within lipofuscin granules in the aged human brain indicates autophagic activity and an active role in cellular metabolism.[18] It has been recognised that lipofuscin is related to lysosomes, and the inhibition of lysosomal enzymes causes a massive and rapid increase of these particles in the brains of young rats.[19] Neurons vary in their ability to acquire and accumulate lipofuscin; it is always present in the neurons of the hippocampus and thalamus, whereas Purkinje cells are almost free of this pigment.[20] In ageing marmosets, lipofuscin is present in neurons, glia, perivascular macrophages and pericytes.[21]

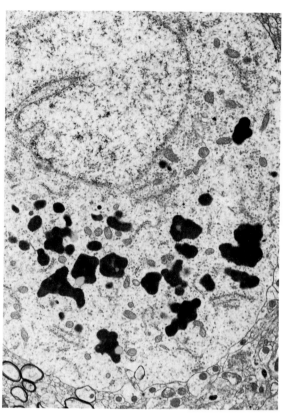

Fig. 2.4 Electron micrograph of a neuron showing accumulation of lipofuscin in the cytoplasm. × 5200

The accumulation of lipofuscin usually begins in the region between nucleus and axon hillock and, as the process progresses, both the nucleus and Nissl substance are displaced towards the periphery. Lipofuscin accumulates not only during ageing, but also in Parkinson's disease, Alzheimer's disease and in lysosomal enzyme deficiencies, including Batten's disease and type IV mucolipidosis (see Ch. 12). Lipofuscin has also been induced in experimental animals: large amounts of this pigment accumulate in the nerve cells of vitamin E deficient rats, or in rabbits following the intrathecal administration of vincristine or colchicine. The pigment in these conditions is thought to be ceroid rather than lipofuscin and although both are lipo-pigments, they differ in autofluorescence, ultrastructure and chemical composition.[22] It is noteworthy that, although cells may accumulate large amounts of lipofuscin, this does not apparently interfere with their viability.

Ferrugination and calcification

Normal neurons in several areas of the brain, including the red nucleus, substantia nigra and subthalamic nucleus, contain iron. Neurons in the vicinity of haemorrhages and contusions and in areas of birth injury display brown or brown–black granules which usually give a positive (Prussian blue) reaction with Perls' reagents. This siderophilia and the intensity of the colour reaction distinguish iron deposits from formalin pigment. In the electron microscope, the iron deposits appear as small electron-dense particles, similar to the subunits of ferritin; they are either membrane-bound in siderosomes or dispersed freely in the cytoplasm.[23] Electron probe investigation of these ferruginated nerve cells has revealed that the deposits are composed of calcium, phosphorus, iron, sulphur and traces of copper and zinc.[24] Intense blue staining of the entire neuronal perikarya with haematoxylin suggests that the deposition of pseudocalcium (an organic protein matrix) and calcium may occur near old infarctions and contusions, but the tinctorial properties of this material in histological sections are inconstant. Although phosphates (and thus, by implication, calcium) are demonstrated by von Kóssa's method, the reaction for iron is strong in most cases. The deep basophilic appearance of these neurons may be due to an organic matrix composed of a mucopolysaccharide complex which precedes the deposition of calcium and ferruginous material. According to the presence or absence of previous tissue damage, it is convenient to distinguish between primary (spontaneous) and secondary accumulation of calcium. The effects of these deposits on the activity of neurons are not known, but cells encrusted with minerals apparently remain viable for years. In experimental animals, axons undergoing Wallerian degeneration display granular deposits of calcium both in the axoplasm and in organelles.[25]

Excessive accumulation of iron occurs in Hallervorden–Spatz disease, in which siderophilic incrustation of nerve cells, astrocytes and micro-glia imparts a rust-brown colour to the globus pallidus and the reticular zone of the substantia nigra. Fahr's disease is a progressive form of excessive deposition of pseudocalcium–calcium throughout the brain and is seen particularly in patients with hypoparathyroidism. In encephalo-facial angiomatosis (Sturge–Weber syndrome), the meningeal vascular abnormality is associated with calcification of the underlying atrophied cortex and, to a lesser degree, of the white matter.

Abnormal neurons

Neurons are postmitotic cells, so they do not divide after reaching maturity, but occasional binucleate (Fig. 2.5) and multinucleate forms do occur. These are seen in developmental malformations and occasionally at the edges of old focal lesions, possibly representing a response to tissue injury. Binucleate neurons are common in

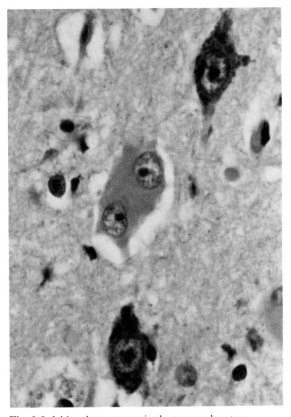

Fig. 2.5 A binucleate neuron in the temporal cortex. Haematoxylin-eosin × 800

hamartomas. Abnormal, primitive neurons, which fail to assume the pyramidal cell shape and to develop the typical dendritic arborisations, are present in tuberous sclerosis[26] (see p. 354), a condition in which giant and binucleate neurons also occur.

DISEASE-SPECIFIC PATHOLOGY OF NEURONS

Alzheimer's neurofibrillary change

This neuronal change, although discernible in sections stained with haematoxylin and eosin, can be best demonstrated by various silver impregnation techniques and by Congo red; the latter renders the tangles of neurofilaments birefringent in polarised light. Alzheimer's neurofibrillary tangles consist of cytoplasmic accumulations of filamentous material which tend to displace the nucleus towards the periphery of the cell. The configuration of neurofibrillary degeneration varies according to the site and type of neuron involved. In pyramidal neurons, neurofibrillary tangles appear triangular or flame-shaped, whilst in the nerve cells of the brainstem, globose forms occur. The finer details of neurofibrillary tangles are revealed in the electron microscope: they are composed of paired helical filaments[27] which in turn are formed by two filaments wound around each other. Each filament has a diameter of 8–12 nm with crossover points every 80 nm, resulting in the characteristic periodicity of a double helix.[28] Negative staining techniques and electron microscopy reveal that each filament is composed of four protofilaments with a diameter of 3–5 nm.[29]

Neurofibrillary tangles most frequently occur in Alzheimer's disease but also develop in normal, ageing brains, in patients with Down's syndrome who survive into adulthood, in postencephalitic Parkinsonism, in the amyotrophic lateral sclerosis (ALS)-Parkinsonism-dementia complex of Guam (see p. 275 & 415) and in dementia pugilistica. There are two diseases in which neurofibrillary changes differ ultrastructurally from those in ageing and in the dementia of Alzheimer type: these are progressive supranuclear palsy and sporadic motor neuron disease. The detailed pathology and

immunochemistry of neurofibrillary degeneration are discussed in Chapter 13.

Granulovacuolar degeneration

This neuronal change is more limited in distribution than Alzheimer's neuronal degeneration: it is virtually restricted to the pyramidal neurons of the hippocampus in the ageing brain and in Alzheimer's disease. It is a cytoplasmic alteration composed of one or more vacuoles of 3–5 μm in diameter. Each vacuole contains a single granule which, in the electron microscope, appears to be a granular core embedded in a translucent matrix. Granulovacuoles can be easily seen in haematoxylin and eosin stains; silver impregnations or Lendrum's phloxine tartrazine stain provide very little additional information. Granulovacuolar degeneration also develops in a variety of diseases, including Down's syndrome, supranuclear palsy, amyotrophic lateral sclerosis-Parkinsonism-dementia complex of Guam, and tuberous sclerosis.[30]

Hirano bodies

These structures are most commonly seen in and amongst the pyramidal cells of the hippocampus. They are present at all ages, but their frequency increases with advancing age. Patients suffering from Alzheimer's disease have significantly more Hirano bodies than normal people of the same age, but the presence of these structures is by no means restricted to this dementing disorder: they have been reported in various neurological diseases, including Pick's disease, motor neuron disease and kuru, and also in animals infected with kuru and scrapie.[31]

Hirano bodies stand out as bright pink homogeneous structures in tissue stained with haematoxylin and eosin. They are circular in cross-section, with a diameter up to 15 μm, and rectangular or spindle-shaped, up to 30 μm in length, in longitudinal sections. Electron microscopy has shown that Hirano bodies are composed of parallel filaments which alternate with longer sheets.[30] They are localised most often in the neuronal perikarya, and rarely in cell processes; and they may give the illusion that they are extracellular.

Pick bodies and Pick cells

These neuronal changes are histological hallmarks of Pick's disease, a progressive dementing disorder (see p. 379). Neurons in cortical layers 2, 3 and 5 become swollen, rounded and pear-shaped. The Nissl substance disintegrates, leaving a homogeneous central area in the cytoplasm, while the nucleus moves to the periphery of the cell. With Mallory's phosphotungstic acid haematoxylin, these cells appear pale, in sharp contrast with the darkly-stained background. Nissl's method confirms the disappearance of the rough endoplasmic recticulum. The swollen cytoplasm contains an argyrophilic inclusion, the Pick body, in silver impregnated sections (e.g. Marsland–Glees or Palmgren technique). Ultrastructural examination of Pick bodies has revealed a heterogeneous structure composed of three types of filaments.[32]

Lewy bodies

Lewy bodies are cytoplasmic inclusions which occur in Parkinson's disease in the pigmented and non-pigmented neurons of the brainstem. They are seen most frequently in the substantia nigra and locus ceruleus and in the dorsal motor nucleus of the vagus, but they are also found in the nucleus basalis of Meynert, the hypothalamus and the intermediolateral column of the spinal cord. Recent investigations have drawn attention to their occurrence in neurons of the cortex and basal ganglia, a finding which has warranted the term diffuse Lewy body disease.[33] Although they are a histological hallmark of Parkinson's disease, Lewy bodies are also seen in other degenerative disorders.[34] The pathognomonic significance of these structures will be discussed in Chapter 15. Affected neurons contain one or more of these intensely and uniformly eosinophilic hyaline bodies. The central cores are often surrounded by a clear peripheral rim, or halo. However, their configuration varies according to the site and type of neuron involved. Although Lewy bodies react with various acidic and neutral dyes, including phloxine tartrazine, Giemsa and Masson stains, they are easily recognisable in haematoxylin and eosin preparations. In the electron microscope, the central core of a typical Lewy body in the sub-stantia nigra is composed of filamentous and granular material surrounded by radially orientated filaments in the peripheral zone.[35] Immunocytochemistry using anti-neurofilament antibodies has demonstrated equivocal staining, but Lewy bodies appear to contain ubiquitin.[36] This small protein plays a rôle in an ATP-dependent proteolytic system responsible for the degradation of short-lived or abnormal proteins in the cells. The filamentous structures of Lewy bodies could be composed of abnormal proteins which, once ubiquitinated, may become targets for rapid degradation.

Lafora, Marinesco and Bunina bodies

Lafora bodies were originally observed in cases of myoclonic epilepsy,[37] and they most frequently occur in the cytoplasm of large nerve cells of the dentate nucleus, substantia nigra and thalamus, and occasionally of the cerebral cortex. Their size varies between 1 and 20 μm, and one or more may be located in the perikaryon or, less frequently, in the cell processes of the neuron. They are round, with a central basophilic dense core and a light peripheral rim. In the electron microscope, the core appears to contain an admixture of filaments 6–8 nm thick, and dense granules resembling glycogen, whilst at the periphery radially orientated filaments are interspersed with degenerate organelles.[38] Lafora bodies show metachromasia with toluidine blue and cresyl violet; they are strongly periodic acid-Schiff (PAS) positive and argyrophilic; they do not stain with Congo red.

Marinesco bodies[39] are acidophilic, intranuclear, fibrillary inclusions which occur most commonly in the pigmented nuclei of the brainstem. Their number increases with advancing age, but their significance in neurological disorders is not known.[40]

Bunina bodies are single or multiple, eosinophilic cytoplasmic inclusions whose configuration varies from a simple round shape to ribbon-like complex forms.[41] They occur in the neurons of the spinal cord, in the motor nuclei of the brainstem and in the Betz cells of the motor cortex in motor neuron disease. Their pathological significance remains controversial.[42]

Viral inclusions

The identification of viral inclusions by light and electron microscopy may be of diagnostic importance. They are often numerous in some types of encephalitis (see p. 196) and can then be easily seen in tissue sections or even in smear preparations, yet in many cases the application of special stains (e.g. phloxine tartrazine) and a thorough ultrastructural search are required. Inclusions which are discernible with the light microscope are formed from many individual viral particles. Viral inclusions are either cytoplasmic or intranuclear. A characteristic cytoplasmic inclusion is the Negri body, an eosinophilic, Giemsa-positive complex structure which is diagnostic of rabies. In poliomyelitis, herpes encephalitis, subacute sclerosing panencephalitis and progressive multifocal leucoencephalopathy the viral inclusions are intranuclear and are found in both neurons and glial cells (see p. 219). Care must be taken to distinguish viral inclusions from a variety of nuclear and cytoplasmic inclusions which are either normal cellular constituents or harmless products of altered metabolism.[43] Virus-like particles have been described in various neurological disorders of non-viral aetiology,[44] and even in patients without evidence of cerebral disease.[45]

Inclusions in lysosomal enzyme deficiency disorders

Neuronal inclusions are common in various lysosomal enzyme deficiency diseases: the morphology and biochemistry of these structures are usually characteristic of a particular disorder (see Ch. 12).

AXONAL DEGENERATION

Axonal or *Wallerian degeneration* was originally described in peripheral nerves,[46] but the mechanism is similar in both the central and the peripheral nervous system (see p. 533).

As a general rule, the more central the lesion, the longer is the segment of the axon which degenerates; damage to the perikaryon itself results in degeneration of the entire axon. The pathological lesions causing anterograde degeneration are commonly infarction, haemorrhage, trauma and tumours affecting the white matter. At the molecular level, an increase of free calcium within the axons stimulates calcium-activated neutral proteases and a massive proteolysis of the cytoskeleton may then follow.[47]

Although the principal axonal changes are similar in all cases, their time course and severity are influenced by various factors including species, age and the fibre systems involved. Axonal degeneration progresses more rapidly in mammals than in cold-blooded animals, and is faster in young animals than in adults; in general, large fibres are affected before smaller fibres. Although various silver impregnation techniques have been developed for the study of axonal degeneration[48] (Fig. 2.6), it is only by electron microscopy in experimental animals that the sequence of events occurring during anterograde axonal degeneration

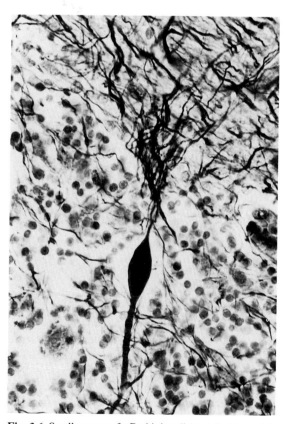

Fig. 2.6 Swollen axon of a Purkinje cell (so-called torpedo) in the cerebellum.
Glees–Marsland × 510

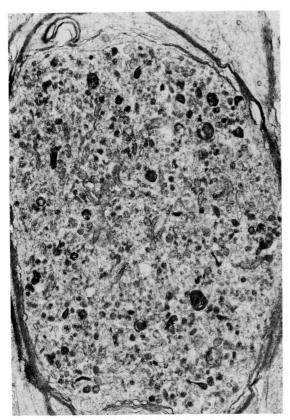

Fig. 2.7 Electron micrograph of a swollen, degenerating axon filled with a mass of abnormal organelles.
× 10 800

has been revealed (Fig. 2.7). As early as two days after axon transection, the axoplasm may become electron-dense and the organelles, particularly the mitochondria, undergo degenerative changes. Other axons may become swollen and appear to contain an increased amount of filamentous material; but even these axons later become shrunken.

Nerve terminals undergo similar degenerative changes and in the electron microscope 'dark' and 'light' or filamentous degeneration can be distinguished. In the first, the boutons become electron-dense and the shrunken mitochondria and synaptic vesicles are clumped together in an ill-defined mass. Other nerve endings may initially become swollen and contain an excess of neurofilaments, but later assume the more typical dark appearance.[48] The degenerating boutons usually remain for a while attached to the post-synaptic membrane, but later they are phago-cytosed by microglial cells and astrocytes. Axonal degeneration is followed by myelin damage: the sheaths become disorganised and fragmented; these changes will be considered later in this chapter (see p. 47).

Retrograde axonal degeneration occurs in the axon and subsequently in the neuronal perikaryon, central to the site of axonal damage. Acute retrograde changes in the perikaryon are seen as severe *central chromatolysis*, with displacement of the nucleus to the periphery and frequently, but not always, swelling of the neuron. Cells thus affected may recover or may disintegrate. The late retrograde changes represent a progressive degeneration, resulting in dark, pyknotic cells which then disappear.

The proximal stump of a transected axon also undergoes degeneration and the nature of this process may vary according to species, age group and fibre system involved. Severed axons become reduced in diameter proximal to the site of injury and may show progressive fragmentation. Changes occurring in the dendrites of cells whose axon has been cut are similar to those developing in the perikaryon itself.

Changes in the axonal transport systems may cause, or contribute to, neurological disease. For example, altered slow transport of neurofilaments can change the axonal calibre, causing either swelling or atrophy. Impaired fast transport occurs in experimental models of distal axonal degeneration (dying-back phenomenon; see p. 540).[49]

TRANSNEURONAL DEGENERATION

Transneuronal or trans-synaptic degeneration occurs in nerve cells deprived of their afferent connections. The fibre systems most often studied are the visual, auditory and olfactory pathways. The de-afferented cells show shrinkage of the nucleus and nucleolus and reduction of dendrites, and this slow but progressive degeneration finally leads to the disappearance of some of the affected cells. Occasionally transneuronal degeneration affects a second neuron in the chain: transneuronal pontine atrophy in man is often followed by shrinkage of the contralateral cerebellar hemisphere which receives a large proportion of ponto-cerebellar fibres.[48] The cause of transneuronal degeneration is the loss or reduction of afferent impulses; the cells survive only if sufficient afferent fibres are preserved to maintain a minimal degree of neuronal activity. Experimentally produced transneuronal degeneration is more dramatic and fulminant in younger animals, and is accompanied by a striking microglial reaction.[50]

Transneuronal or trans-synaptic retrograde degeneration may affect cells whose efferent processes make contacts with neurons which have suffered axonal damage and have consequently undergone retrograde cellular changes. The precise mechanism of retrograde transneuronal degeneration is not known.

MYELIN LOSS

Myelin sheaths are damaged and undergo degeneration in a variety of pathological conditions which interfere with the oligodendrocyte-myelin-axon complex. It is important to distinguish between primary demyelination and secondary loss of myelin. Primary demyelination is a process caused by diseases (e.g. multiple sclerosis—see Ch. 10) which selectively destroy myelin or myelin-forming cells, whilst axons remain relatively well preserved. Secondary demyelination, in contrast, is a consequence of neuronal or axonal damage; the myelin breaks down only after axonal degeneration.[51] In addition, diffuse loss of myelin staining may be seen histologically, associated with destructive lesions of the white matter such as infarcts, tumours and haemorrhages; this loss of staining may be a combination of axonal and myelin degeneration together with oedema of the white matter.

Primary demyelination may result from a variety of factors including mechanical compression, nutritional deficiency (e.g. of vitamin B_{12}), myelinotoxic agents (e.g. diphtheria toxin, lysolecithin, triethyltin), destruction of myelin-forming cells (e.g. cuprizone toxicity), virus infections (e.g. progressive multifocal leuco-encephalopathy) and immunological abnormalities mediated either by sensitised T lymphocytes or by antibodies directed against myelin.[52] Myelin

damage, ranging from small vacuoles to larger areas of demyelination, has been consistently observed in the acquired immune deficiency syndrome (AIDS; see p. 214). The mechanism of this myelin loss is controversial but the human immune deficiency virus (HIV) may be directly involved. In these demyelinating conditions, the myelin is apparently normal prior to the onset of the disorder which eventually leads to its destruction, whereas in *leucodystrophies* abnormal myelin is formed as a consequence of inherited enzyme defects (see Ch. 12). Primary demyelination can involve either a whole internode along a nerve fibre or part of an internode (Fig. 2.8). In the former, the entire length of the internode myelin undergoes vesiculation and fragmentation following the death of the supporting oligodendrocyte, and this event is characterised by an increase of both macrophages, which are seen

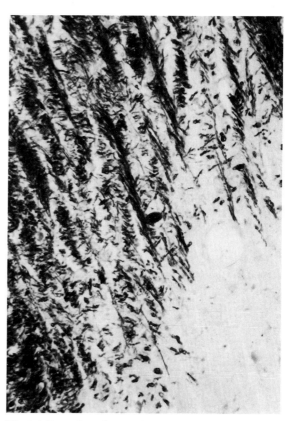

Fig. 2.8 Loss of myelin: myelin sheaths terminate at the edge of a plaque in multiple sclerosis.
Luxol fast blue–cresyl violet × 320

stripping off myelin, and astrocytes which are also engaged in phagocytosis of myelin debris. Partial demyelination, in contrast, is the subtotal loss of internodal myelin. Thinning of myelin may be restricted to the paranodal region or may involve the whole internode, but this change is not associated with oligodendrocyte death or an inflammatory reaction.[51] Demyelinating diseases are discussed in Chapter 10.

Secondary demyelination is a consequence of neuronal damage; the best example of this type of myelin degradation is seen in Wallerian (axonal) degeneration. Severance of the axon is followed by a sequence of myelin disintegration. The myelin sheath first appears to be evenly swollen, but soon becomes fragmented: ballooned, spindle-shaped segments develop which, although initially connected, later become separate fragments and form rows of ovoids. These ovoids gradually disintegrate into smaller globules which mark the original course of the axon. The breakdown of myelin stimulates a strong microglial and astrocytic response and both these cell types are seen to engulf and degrade myelin remnants. Electron microscopy confirms these changes and shows that the first alterations develop at the intraperiod lines, which split with consequent loosening (Fig. 2.9), unwinding, vesiculation and fragmentation of the lamellae.

The time course of myelin degeneration can be followed both in experimental animals and in man. Although the rate of myelin breakdown is slower in the central nervous system than in peripheral nerves, degenerating fibres in the corticospinal tracts can be demonstrated as early as three days after axonal damage in rats[53] and in man.[54]

Various stages of myelin disintegration can be demonstrated by histological stains and impregnation techniques. Myelin sheaths undergoing early degeneration acquire a 'bubbly' appearance in Klüver–Barrera (Luxol fast blue–Nissl) or Weigert (acid haematoxylin) preparations. At later stages various lipid stains—Sudan IV, Sudan black or Scharlach R—demonstrate myelin breakdown products in frozen sections: their optimal use is from 1 to 3 months after central nervous system injury. One very useful technique is Marchi's method, which stains degenerating myelin black. The optimal period is from 20 to 80

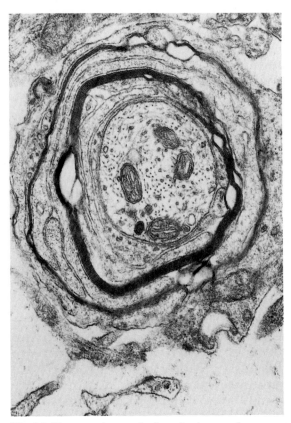

Fig. 2.9 Electron micrograph of myelin damage: the compact myelin lamellae are separated from each other, while the axon appears to be normal in the centre of the field.
× 12 000

days after axonal damage,[55] although a positive reaction may be seen much earlier (3 days) and considerably later (1 year). The method involves the use of potassium bichromate, which prevents osmium from staining normal myelin; subsequent treatment with osmic acid results in black discoloration of degenerating myelin, whilst normal sheaths remain unstained.

REMYELINATION

Remyelination in the central nervous system does not appear to be as efficient as remyelination in the peripheral nervous system. In multiple sclerosis (see Ch. 10) there is minimal remyelination in demyelinated plaques and this may be a result of destruction and loss of oligodendrocytes. Remyelination, however, has been observed following experimental demyelination, provided that the demyelinating stimulus is removed and the oligodendrocytes survive. The prime event in remyelination is probably an axonal signal to which oligodendrocytes respond by multiplication and migration. The replacement of oligodendrocytes and the production of myelin are, however, separate events and the presence of astrocytes may also be necessary for remyelination to occur.[51]

AXONAL REGENERATION IN THE CENTRAL NERVOUS SYSTEM

The concept of regeneration of axons in the central nervous system remains controversial. Although there are examples of successful regeneration in neurosecretory, noradrenergic and unmyelinated cholinergic fibres, central axons usually fail to regenerate despite their capacity for considerable collateral sprouting.[56] In fetal and neonatal mammalian brains, functional recovery occurs after injury, but the evidence for anatomical restitution across a damaged area of brain or cord remains equivocal. It is likely that functional recovery in these brains results from the inherent plasticity by which immature nerve cells establish new connections, or from the continuing growth of axons in developing animals. Moreover, the response to injury differs in the immature and adult brains: in the former, less glial scar tissue is formed, and there is little connective tissue present. These tissue elements are thought to form a mechanical barrier in the path of potential axonal regeneration in the adult brain. However, in the light of experimental evidence,[57] this barrier theory is no longer tenable as an explanation of the failure of central axons to regenerate. Some axons, as stated earlier, do regenerate and, according to the growth factor hypothesis, all would do so if their specific growth promoting agents were present.[58] Such agents could be proteins, polypeptides or enkephalin-type pentapeptides which may activate protein synthesis through cyclic AMP as a secondary messenger. While these growth factors may be operational in the developing brain, they may disappear during ontogenesis, or auto-antibodies may neutralise them. Moreover, central axon regeneration may be inhibited by substances which enter the parenchyma of the CNS from the blood or by metabolites which are produced during degenerative processes.[56] Adult brains, however, may adapt by forming new synapses rather than new neurons, and this reactive synaptogenesis may be an important factor in recovery.[59]

The recently developed methodology of transplantation has opened an entirely new approach to the old problem of regeneration. Fragments of fetal brain or cell suspensions prepared from them are implanted into the brains of animals with the same genetic background.[60] Such intracerebral grafts will establish synapses with the surrounding tissue of the recipient brain.[61] For example, occipital cortical neurons from fetal rats, when implanted into the rostral cortex of newborn animals, extend axons into the corticospinal tracts and maintain them there.[62] Preliminary successful results indicate that selected neuronal systems may be transplanted in order to replace damaged, deficient or lost nerve cells.[63,64] Substantial and persistent memory loss caused by chronic alcohol administration in rats and associated with impaired cholinergic function was reversed by transplants of cholinergic regions of fetal brain.[65]

NEUROTRANSMITTER ABNORMALITIES

Changes in neuronal morphology have provided essential information for the study of diseases of the central nervous system. Recently, it has become possible, by the use of histochemical and immunohistochemical techniques, to achieve a biochemical classification of neurons and to trace pathways between various nuclei in the brain.[66] Neurotransmitters and neuropeptides are localised in particular neuronal groups or brain areas which, in turn, could be preferentially affected in a variety of neurological and neuropsychiatric disorders. Dopaminergic deficit associated with neuronal loss in the substantia nigra in Parkinson's disease, or cholinergic, noradrenergic and serotoninergic deficits related to neuronal decrease in the nucleus basalis of Meynert, locus ceruleus and raphe nuclei, especially in Alzheimer's disease, illustrate this point. Changes in neuronal morphology may be accompanied or even preceded by alterations in neurotransmitter activity, such that an understanding of the pathogenesis of certain diseases of the central nervous system requires knowledge of the biochemistry and chemical pathology of the brain (see Ch. 1).

PATHOLOGY OF ASTROCYTES

REACTIONS TO BRAIN DAMAGE

Astrocytes respond to a wide variety of stimuli, and the cellular changes which subsequently develop are reliable indicators of underlying brain pathology. Despite their physiological versatility and morphological plasticity, the astrocyte

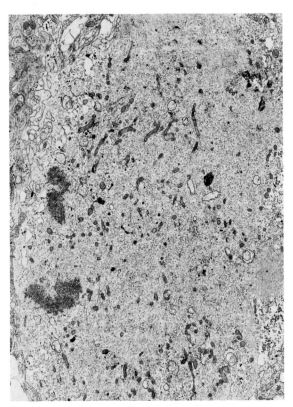

Fig. 2.11 Electron micrograph of a reactive astrocyte in mitosis: the chromatin is not bound by a nuclear membrane and the cytoplasm is crowded with organelles. × 5500

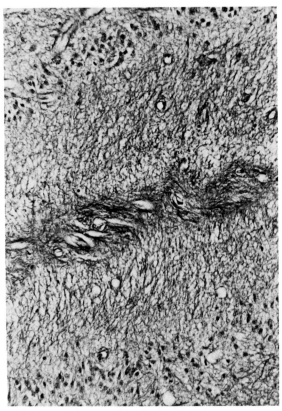

Fig. 2.10 Extensive fibrillary gliosis of the cerebellar cortex; the glial scar extends into and obliterates the space between two folia.
Phosphotungstic acid haematoxylin × 180

response is relatively limited in scope and takes the form of hyperplasia and hypertrophy or degeneration and death. The astrocytic changes depend upon the nature, severity and duration of the underlying pathological process and the site and type of astrocyte. The term *astrocytosis* denotes an increase of both astrocytes and their intracellular fibrils, whilst in *fibrillary gliosis* there is an excess of fibrils and relatively few nuclei, as in old glial scars. In *isomorphous gliosis* the astrocyte fibrils are produced in regular parallel arrangements: this pattern is usually observed in degenerating nerve tracts where the astrocyte processes are orientated by preserved tissue elements. An irregular, disorderly mass of fibrils, *anisomorphous gliosis*, develops around destructive lesions such as infarcts. A glial or astrocytic scar is a mesh of fibrils with very few nuclei and is seen as the end result of tissue damage (Fig. 2.10). It is misleading to compare the repair processes in the CNS to scar formation in the skin and other organs as is so often done: whilst collagen fibres are extracellular products secreted by fibroblasts, astrocyte filaments are intracellular, and remain bounded by the cell membranes of astrocytes and their processes.

Proliferation and *hypertrophy* of astrocytes commonly occur following tissue damage and mark the beginning of the repair process (Fig. 2.11). The former view of astrocytes proliferating by amitotic division has been shown by autoradiography in properly fixed brains to be incorrect: even normal astrocytes in the corpus callosum of rats show their proliferative capacity as they are labelled following the injection of tritiated thymidine.[67] Following injuries, the increase in mitotic activity of astrocytes is both dramatic and fast, reaching a peak 48–72 hours after a stab wound in the rodent brain.[68] The signal which triggers the astrocyte response has not been estab-

lished, but experimental evidence suggests that various factors are involved, including neuronal damage, myelin breakdown, extravasation of proteins, change in the volume of the extracellular space and disturbance of ion transport. It has also been suggested, from observations in experimental stab wounds, that astrocytes react to the disruption of tissue architecture; the response may therefore restore the structural integrity of damaged tissue.[69]

Astrocyte hypertrophy involves both the perikaryon and the cell processes. The cell becomes larger and the nucleus often assumes an eccentric position as the cytoplasm becomes abundant, homogeneous and strongly eosinophilic (Fig. 2.12). The electron microscope reveals a general increase of organelles, amongst which 10 nm intermediate filaments of glial fibrillary acidic protein (GFAP) predominate: the filaments form thick bundles at the periphery of the cell and extend into the processes (Fig. 2.13). This hypertrophy with the concomitant increase in filaments often results in the formation of large cells whose cytoplasm is filled with filaments: these are the *hypertrophic, reactive* (or *gemistocytic*) *astrocytes* (Fig. 2.12). Both glial fibrillary acidic protein (GFAP)[70] and glutamine synthetase[71] are abundant in reactive astrocytes. There is an increase of oxidative enzymes, particularly those involved with glycolysis and the hexosemonophosphate shunt, rather than those of the citric acid cycle.[72,73]

Hyperplasia and hypertrophy of astrocytes are particularly striking in destructive lesions: for example, at the edges of cerebral infarcts and contusions the number and size of astrocytes increase as early as 48 hours (Fig. 2.14). As time progresses, astrocyte fibres become the predominant elements in the cell as a glial scar is gradually formed. Cerebral oedema also elicits a rapid astrocyte response: hypertrophic, reactive astrocytes often stand out histologically in the lace-like pattern of swollen white matter. The progressive changes of astrocytosis and gliosis are seen in a number of diseases which affect the white matter, including multiple sclerosis and leucodystrophies. *Fibrillary gliosis* is the end-stage in the evolution of a multiple sclerosis plaque, and it is the hard sclerotic consistency of these old plaques from which the name of the disease is derived. It

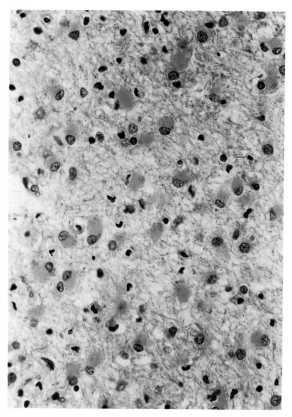

Fig. 2.12 Reactive astrocytes in the subcortical white matter. Haematoxylin-eosin × 350

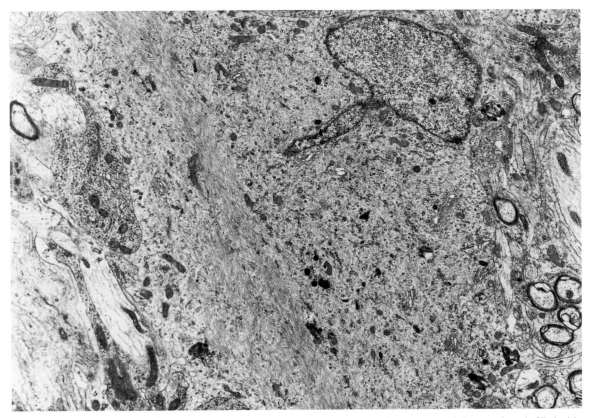

Fig. 2.13 Electron micrograph of a reactive astrocyte. The irregular nuclear profile is eccentric and the cytoplasm is filled with organelles amongst which filaments predominate.
× 7000
Reproduced by permission of Springer Verlag, Heidelberg, from: Lantos PL. Acta Neuropathol (Berl), 1974; 30: 175 (Fig. 1a)

has been convincingly shown in experimental demyelination that astrocytes can not only multiply but are also capable of phagocytosis.[74] Reactive astrocytes around chemically-induced brain tumours engulf breakdown products of myelin and extravasated erythrocytes;[75] they also phagocytose degenerating fragments of myelin following Wallerian degeneration.[76] Astrocytes also contain tissue type plasminogen activator, a serine protease which converts plasminogen to plasmin; this proteolytic enzyme may play a rôle in myelin degradation in demyelinating diseases and in Wallerian degeneration.[77]

Inflammation, particularly in viral diseases, is frequently associated with astrocyte changes (see Ch. 9). Infection of astrocytes by papovavirus in progressive multifocal leucoencephalopathy results in the bizarre cells and hyperchromatic

nuclei which are pathognomonic of this disease (see p. 219) (Fig. 2.15). In *subacute sclerosing panencephalitis* (see p. 212), astrocyte proliferation is vigorous, and astrocyte nuclei are often found in pairs or in small groups. It is of interest that a neurotropic murine hepatitis virus induces expression of Ia antigen on astrocytes in tissue culture, rendering these cells competent to participate directly in the immune response to a viral infection.[78] Astrocytes also play an integral part in the '*gliomesodermal*' reaction seen in cerebral abscesses (see p. 169), in which a fibrous capsule forms around the abscess, but astrocytes are included, particularly at the periphery.

The number of GFAP-containing astrocytes increases in the normal ageing brain[79] and in Alzheimer's disease (see p. 375–376).[80] In Huntington's disease (see p. 382–384), astrocytosis

descending fibre tracts.[84] In experimental cord transection astrocytes also secrete laminin, a major component of the basal lamina, and this may play a rôle in the restoration of cord anatomy.[85]

Astrocytes are less vulnerable than neurons, but may still undergo degenerative changes. In *anoxia* and *ischaemia*, progressive astrocyte changes develop: the cell body becomes rounded and fragmentation of processes (clasmatodendrosis) takes place; finally the cell body becomes swollen and the nucleus pyknotic. Swollen astrocyte processes have been consistently observed around damaged neurons in hypoxia.[86] The swelling of astrocytes is, however, not necessarily irreversible. An ultrastructural study of thermal lesions of the rat cortex has shown that, although astrocytes undergo severe changes, they may revert to normal morphology between 4 and 12 days after cold injury.[87] Swelling of astrocytes may also occur as a

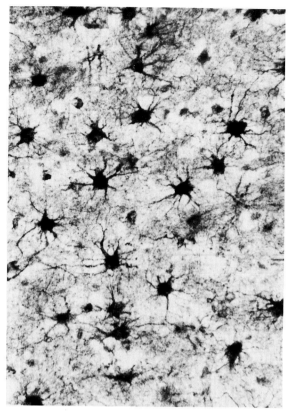

Fig. 2.14 Astrocytosis in the white matter. Cajal's gold chloride sublimate technique × 300

of the basal ganglia is an accepted feature; astrocyte abnormalities may play an important rôle in its pathogenesis and could be responsible for the failure of glial-neuronal interaction.[81] Astrocytes are affected by X-ray or alpha particle irradiation; in the acute stages there is an accumulation of intracellular glycogen which increases up to 48 hours and then gradually disappears.[82] Striking reactive astrocytosis develops in the brains of patients who have undergone radiotherapy for malignant cerebral tumours.

Astrocytes also react when axons are damaged. For example, following transection of the hypoglossal nerve in rats, astrocytes in the medulla show a two-phase response: an increase of thin, lamellar astrocytic processes is followed by a transient hypertrophy and astrogliosis.[83] Gliosis occurs after experimental transection of the spinal cord, as it does in man following injury, and results from the degeneration of the long ascending and

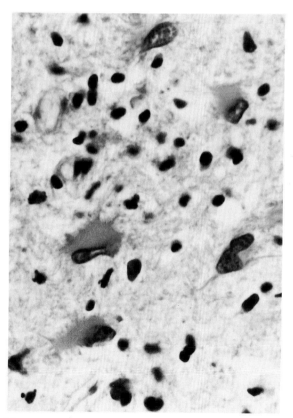

Fig. 2.15 Bizarre astrocytes in a case of progressive multifocal leucoencephalopathy. Haematoxylin-eosin × 800

fixation artefact and care must be taken in the interpretation of such changes in biopsy material.

Alzheimer type I and type II astrocytes

Abnormally large astrocytes with irregular nuclei are associated with liver disease. They are called Alzheimer astrocytes but they have no connection with Alzheimer's disease. The Alzheimer type I astrocyte possesses a giant lobulated nucleus embedded in vacuolated cytoplasm. These cells are rare but are most often seen in Wilson's disease in the corpus striatum (caudate nucleus and putamen). The Alzheimer type II astrocyte occurs more frequently than type I and its distribution is more widespread: the cortex, thalamus, corpus striatum, globus pallidus, substantia nigra, red nucleus and pontine nuclei may all contain these cells. The large, irregular nucleus, displaying a light chromatin pattern and one or two prominent nucleoli, is surrounded by a narrow, inconspicuous rim of cytoplasm. Electron microscopy, revealing degenerative cytoplasmic changes, indicates that the obvious hypertrophy may later be followed by cellular degeneration. A recent review of astrocytes in liver disease has indeed suggested that the astrocyte changes are morphological manifestations of ammonia metabolism: astrocytes initially undergo hypertrophy in order to detoxify ammonia, and the degenerative changes subsequently develop as a consequence of increased metabolic activity. Thus hepatic encephalopathy is the result of the functional failure of astrocytes.[88] Portocaval anastomosis in rats[89] and primates[90] reproduces the same astrocyte changes observed in man. In chimpanzees the cellular abnormalities correlate with ammonia levels and with the severity of clinical signs.

The Opalski cell

The Opalski cell has an abnormally enlarged, ballooned perikaryon in which the dense, relatively small nucleus is peripheral. The nature of this cell remains controversial: astrocytes, neurons and histiocytes have all been considered as its origin,[91] but the evidence in favour of an astrocytic origin is the most convincing. Opalski cells were first described in Wilson's disease[92] and they occur in the cortex, thalamus, globus pallidus, substantia nigra, red nucleus, subthalamic nucleus and, occasionally, in the corpus striatum.

Rosenthal fibres

Rosenthal fibres are carrot-shaped or cylindrical tapering structures which are round or oval in cross-section (Fig. 2.16). They vary in size and can be up to 45–50 µm in length and 10 µm in diameter. Intensely and uniformly eosinophilic in haematoxylin and eosin preparations, Rosenthal fibres stain positively with Mallory's phosphotungstic acid haematoxylin and with Holzer's stain. Electron microscopy shows that they are altered astrocytic processes in which bundles of intermediate filaments mingle with amorphous, granular material.[93]

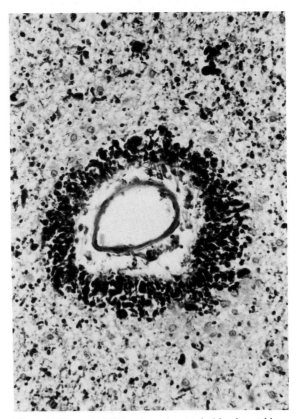

Fig. 2.16 Rosenthal fibres abound around a blood vessel in the white matter of the brain in Alexander's disease. Phosphotungstic acid haematoxylin × 140

Staining of Rosenthal fibres for GFAP varies; small fibres are positive, but larger fibres usually only stain at the periphery and not in the centre.[94]

Rosenthal fibres are common in areas of long-standing fibrillary gliosis and also in slow growing astrocytic and ependymal tumours, particularly in cerebellar astrocytomas (see p. 435). They are a histological hallmark of Alexander's disease (see p. 351) in which Rosenthal fibres occur in abundance throughout the brain, particularly in the subpial, subependymal and perivascular regions.

Corpora amylacea

Corpora amylacea are present in the normal brain and spinal cord: large numbers of these round or oval basophilic structures, with a diameter between 10 and 50 μm, can be seen beneath the pia, under the ependymal lining and around blood vessels (Fig. 2.17). They are PAS-positive, stain with iodine and methyl violet and show metachromasia with toluidine blue. Glycogen can be demonstrated by Best's method and biochemically they contain glycogen-like material with sulphate and phosphate groups.[95] Corpora amylacea are to be found within distended astrocytic processes: electron microscopy has revealed spherical masses of linear and curved profiles.[96] The significance of these structures is unknown. They have not been implicated in any disease entity, but their frequency increases with advancing age and they are often seen in longstanding tract degeneration, particularly in the spinal cord. Corpora amylacea should not be confused with fungi such as cryptococci.

PATHOLOGY OF OLIGODENDROCYTES

The range of oligodendrocyte response to injury is more limited than that of astrocytes, and the significance of some of the changes is not well established. Acute swelling of oligodendrocytes, during which the cytoplasm becomes a clear perinuclear halo, has been observed in hypoxia, ischaemia and trauma, but it also occurs in undamaged brain tissue fixed by immersion. Acute swelling, therefore, could represent artefactual damage or post-mortem change; it can be avoided in experimental material by perfusion fixation. In oligodendrogliomas the cytoplasm can be intensely stained with mucicarmine: the pathological significance of this mucoid change is not known.

Clustering of oligodendrocytes is seen around the large neurons of the deeper layers of the normal cortex and in the basal ganglia; this is *satellitosis* and it should be distinguished from neuronophagy (see p. 40) as it is not usually a consequence of a degenerative process.

The ability of oligodendrocytes to become phagocytic has not been universally accepted, although they become activated and ingest degenerating and foreign material following experimental injury to the brain.[97] A variety of chemical compounds, including cuprizone, isoniazid, 6-aminonicotinamide, triethyltin and hexachlorophane, are known to cause changes in

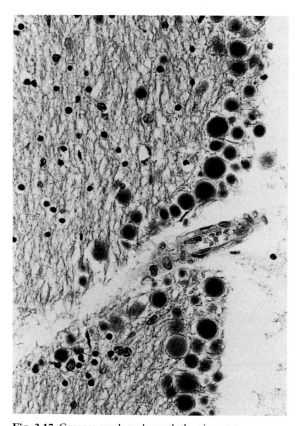

Fig. 2.17 Corpora amylacea beneath the pia mater. Haematoxylin-eosin × 800

oligodendrocytes and their associated myelin sheaths, following systemic administration or direct injection into myelinated fibre tracts (see Ch. 11). The effects depend upon the dose and length of exposure; whether a compound will cause vacuolation of myelin sheaths or cell death with consequent demyelination is influenced by the amount of the compound administered. This suggests that the vacuolation of myelin results from oligodendrocyte intoxication, rather than from a specific myelinopathy.[98] Oligodendrocytes may express major histocompatibility complex class I antigens as a result of impairment of the blood-brain barrier or in the presence of activated T-cells—a phenomenon which has been demonstrated in active multiple sclerosis. This immunological activation means that oligodendrocytes are possible target cells for cytotoxic T-cells.[99] Oligodendrocytes also show abnormalities in rats subjected to portocaval anastomosis: accumulation of filamentous and tubular structures in these cells could reflect disturbance of the metabolism of cytoskeletal proteins brought about by high plasma ammonium levels.[100]

Oligodendrocytes are particularly sensitive to irradiation: acute degenerative changes[101] and total loss of these cells[102] may occur, largely as a delayed effect. Oligodendrocytes are lost from demyelinated plaques in multiple sclerosis (see p. 235), whereas they may increase in some experimental demyelinating lesions.[91] This raises the controversial issue of oligodendrocyte proliferation, since mature oligodendrocytes in the adult mammalian nervous system appear to be postmitotic and thus incapable of division. Experimental evidence, however, shows that mature oligodendrocytes in the mouse brain incorporate tritiated thymidine following trauma and can therefore be presumed to undergo mitotic activity.[103] Tissue culture studies have also confirmed the proliferative potential of oligodendrocytes.[104] Experimental evidence indicates that inflammatory reactions, caused, for example, by trauma or viral infections rather than demyelination, can stimulate the proliferation and differentiation of oligodendrocytes; these cellular processes are influenced by glial growth factors.[105]

Oligodendrocytes may contain viral inclusions, particularly in subacute sclerosing panencephalitis and progressive multifocal leucoencephalopathy (see Ch. 9). Abnormal material can also accumulate in these cells in various lysosomal enzyme deficiencies.

PATHOLOGY OF EPENDYMA

Ependymal cells are relatively inert and show little evidence of proliferation and regenerative activity in pathological conditions. Focal ependymal loss in the lateral walls of the lateral ventricles, ventral surface of the corpus callosum and lateral aspects of the septum pellucidum observed in the human fetal brain is related to normal growth and development, and only more extensive loss should be considered pathological.[106] During development groups of ependymal cells may become detached and form small nests in periventricular brain tissue at the tips and angles of the lateral ventricles and around the cerebral aqueduct and central canal of the spinal cord. In hydrocephalus the ependyma becomes disrupted: the spaces between cells in the periventricular white matter widen and cerebrospinal fluid accumulates beneath the ependymal lining, spreading between myelinated fibres and causing damage with consequent gliosis.[107]

Ependyma is affected in various infections, and damage to ependymal cells by viruses may result in hydrocephalus (see p. 196). Granular ependymitis can be seen in chronic inflammations, and is a classic feature of neurosyphilis: the small, regular white granulations on the ventricular surface are composed of astrocytes and their processes. This reactive proliferation of subependymal astrocytes may break through the ventricular lining; the ependyma reacts to this by forming rosettes or small clefts.

The astrocyte response, mainly in the form of fibrillary gliosis, which often follows damage to ependymal cells, does not cause any complication around the lateral ventricles, but the consequences are grave when gliosis develops in the wall of the cerebral aqueduct. Obliteration of what is already the narrowest point of the cerebrospinal pathway will result in obstructive hydrocephalus.

That ependymal cells themselves are capable of responding to changes in the cerebrospinal fluid

(CSF) has been recently demonstrated. Loss of CSF, caused by transection of the lumbar spinal cord in rats, results in increased absorption and secretion by ependyma.[108] Moreover, following spinal cord transection, displaced ependymal cells form large clusters, apparently resulting from proliferation, and frequently envelop sprouting axons.[109] Focal mechanical disruption of the ependymal lining in experimental animals may produce hyperplasia, particularly at the wound margins.[110]

MICROGLIA AND MACROPHAGES IN THE CENTRAL NERVOUS SYSTEM

Following various injuries to the central nervous system (CNS), resting microglial cells become activated: they migrate to the site of the lesion, assume different shapes, undergo mitosis and engulf foreign material (Fig. 2.18). In addition, circulating mononuclear cells enter the central nervous system and perform a phagocytic function.[111-113] Thus macrophages in the central nervous system appear to have a dual derivation: they can arise from microglial cells of the central nervous system and from monocytes of the blood; their origin depends on the type of lesions involved. In Wallerian degeneration, and in the retrograde reaction involving neurons of the damaged axons, macrophages appear to be chiefly derived from microglia, whilst in traumatic lesions and infarcts they also arise from haematogenous monocytes. The entry of monocytes into the CNS occurs in those conditions in which there is a breakdown of the blood-brain barrier with the consequent escape of macromolecules from the vascular lumen.[114] In experimental stab wounds, in cold lesions and in herpes encephalitis, the macrophage population of rat and rabbit brains

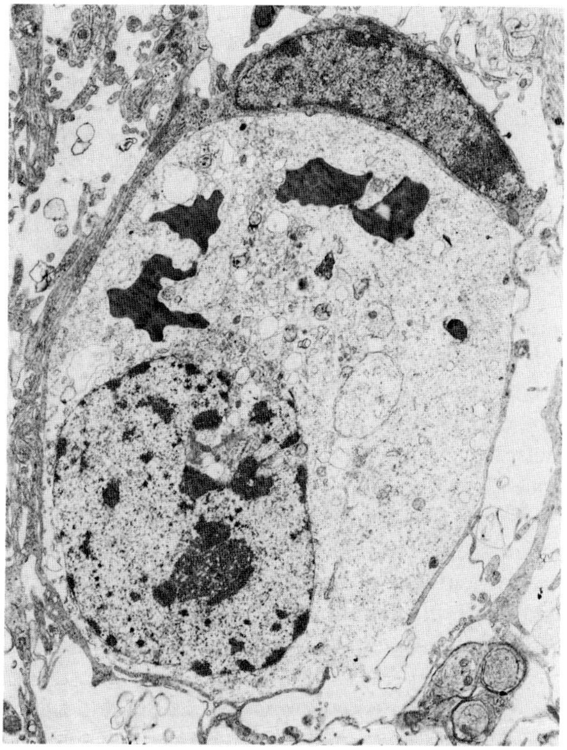

Fig. 2.18 Electron micrograph of a macrophage engulfing a dead cell.
× 5600
Reproduced by permission of the editor from: Lantos PL. J Pathol 1975; 116: 107 (Fig. 8).

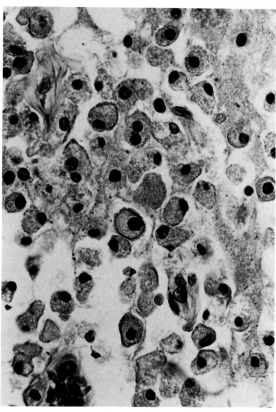

Fig. 2.19 Macrophages in a cerebral infarct. The round nuclei are eccentric in the foamy cytoplasm. Haematoxylin-eosin × 720

increases both by the local proliferation of micro-glial cells and by the infiltration of blood monocytes.[115] In experimental stab injuries of the mouse spinal cord, monocytes become macro-phages, but they do not develop into microglial cells.[116]

The origin of the phagocytic cells is, however, difficult to establish because of the radical morphological changes they may undergo. Macro-phages of microglial and monocytic origin cannot be distinguished by morphological criteria after the third day of experimental thermal necrosis, even by electron microscopy.[117] The macrophage system thus has an intrinsic (microglial) and extrinsic (monocyte) component, and the phago-cytic activity in the central nervous system is a graded response by cells from different sources: it is influenced by the severity, extent and type of the injury.

The microglial response to a wide variety of pathological conditions involves hypertrophy and hyperplasia. Active microglial cells become larger and more rounded, and the small, dark, round nucleus occupies a peripheral position in the abundant cytoplasm which may contain an assort-ment of inclusions: protein-like material in oedema, remnants of erythrocytes in haem-orrhages, and myelin breakdown products, including lipid droplets, in demyelination (Fig. 2.19). In an ultrastructural study around brain tumours, various stages of activity could be dis-tinguished, depending on the number of lysosomes and cytoplasmic inclusions. In the early stage of activation, there is an increase of lysosomes and mitotic activity, while during phagocytosis the cells become replete with engulfed material, chiefly lipid droplets.[118] These cells correspond to the compound granular corpuscles of the old nomenclature or to *Gitterzellen* of the German literature (Fig. 2.20).[119]

Whilst most destructive lesions induce these dramatic microglial changes, another type of response is seen in chronic degenerative disorders (Fig. 2.21). Selective neuronal necrosis caused by hypoxia or ischaemia elicits a transformation of microglia into rod-shaped cells which, although endowed with phagocytic activity, rarely become typical lipid-containing macrophages.[120,121] These rod-shaped microglial cells are also seen in

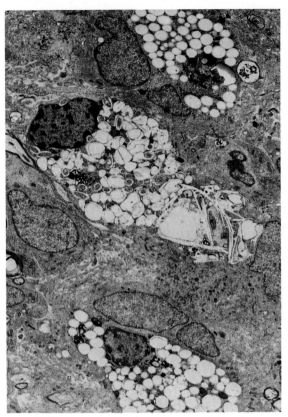

Fig. 2.20 Electron micrograph of macrophages similar to those shown in Figure 2.19: the foamy cytoplasm is replete with lipid droplets which have been dissolved during processing leaving what appear as empty vacuoles. × 3200

encephalitis: they are bipolar cells with tapering processes and an elongated nucleus. In the general paralysis of the insane (GPI) of tertiary syphilis, these cells contain iron pigments. Clusters of activated microglial cells, so-called *microglial stars* (see p. 215; Fig. 9.11) are often associated with neuronal damage and death. Focal accumulation of microglial cells and macrophages, often with multinucleate giant cells, is the histological hallmark of encephalitis found in the acquired immune deficiency syndrome (AIDS; see p. 214).

The microglial response to brain damage is rapid: striking morphological changes develop 24 hours after experimental thermal injury[117] and infarction, and increased microglial mitotic activity is observed in the spinal cord 48 hours after transection of the sciatic nerve.[122] At the end

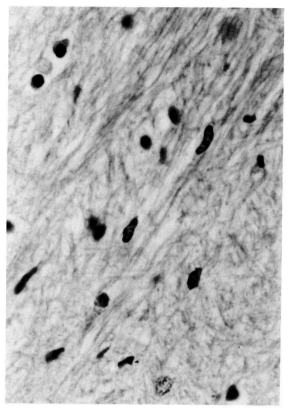

Fig. 2.21 Rod cells in the medulla.
Haematoxylin-eosin × 640

alterations in their enzyme histochemistry. They show an increased activity of acid phosphatase and oxidoreductases;[123] the former, which is a marker enzyme for macrophages, has been demonstrated ultrastructurally in both primary and secondary lysosomes.[126] A high level of 5-nucleotidase activity is also present in the plasma membrane of these cells. The increase of this enzyme, which produces adenosine, a potent intercellular communication molecule, may be of functional importance in the regeneration of motor neurons following nerve transection.[127]

The histological demonstration of microglia has been discussed in Chapter 1 (see p. 29). Recent work[128] has compared the macrophage markers—non-specific esterase, α_1-antitrypsin, α_1-antichymotrypsin and lysozyme—with conventional microglial and macrophage stains in the human nervous system. In cases of head injury the modified Weil–Davenport stain gives superior results for demonstrating activated microglia, whilst α_1-antichymotrypsin is best for showing macrophages in inflammatory, neoplastic and demyelinating diseases of the brain. Non-specific esterase stains macrophages in frozen sections, but is less satisfactory for demonstrating lipid-bearing phagocytes in multiple sclerosis than oil red O.

of the response, lipid-filled macrophages tend to survive in the tissue for a long time, particularly around blood vessels. The route by which macrophages leave the brain has not been convincingly demonstrated. It has been only recently recognised that macrophages in the brain are capable of both immunological and non-immunological phagocytosis. The former requires the presence of surface receptors for the Fc component of the IgG molecule or for C3b, the activated complement component.[123] Furthermore, in the white matter of multiple sclerosis there is an increase of microglial cells which express class II major histocompatibility-complex antigens, indicating their function as antigen-presenting cells in the development of inflammatory lesions.[124] Macrophages also play a rôle in the regeneration of blood vessels after injury: they influence the migration of endothelial cells.[125] The morphological changes of activated microglial cells are complemented by

HISTOLOGICAL ARTEFACTS

Some of the pathological changes in neurons are subtle or non-specific and it is important to distinguish genuine lesions from artefacts caused by delayed fixation, physical trauma, post-mortem delay or treatment on a respirator. The histological artefacts most frequently encountered can be classified as *biopsy artefacts, post-mortem changes* and *'respirator brain'*. There are, however, certain criteria which can be applied to all material prepared for light microscopy. Normal tissue can be regarded as well preserved if there are no perineuronal spaces and no false perivascular spaces and if the size and staining of nuclei of various cell types are normal, the Nissl bodies remain intact, the even calibre of myelinated fibres is maintained and the general integrity of neural tissue is preserved (there should be no separation of cell layers from each other).[10] Similarly, in material preserved for ultrastructural examination, there are features which should be recognised as artefacts: disruption of the cell membrane and the membranes of organelles, swelling of mitochondria, dilatation and vesiculation of the cisternae of the rough and agranular endoplasmic reticulum and of Golgi complexes, rough clumping of chromatin in neuronal and astrocytic nuclei, splitting of myelin lamellae, enlargement of the extracellular space, irregularities of the capillary basement membrane and swelling of astrocyte foot processes.

Biopsy material often shows more severe damage than post-mortem tissue: the physical trauma of surgical intervention coupled with the subsequent handling of freshly removed, unfixed brain and its immersion fixation result in a variety of artefacts. The most notorious of these is the *dark neuron* which can mimic the effects of severe hypoxia. These cells appear pyknotic: the

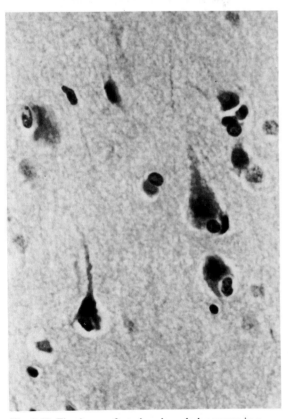

Fig. 2.22 Fixation artefact: shrunken, dark neurons in a biopsy of cerebral cortex.
Haematoxylin-eosin × 800

shrunken dark cytoplasm contains a dense, featureless nucleus and the apical dendrite is corkscrew-like (Fig. 2.22).[129] In contrast, other cells may be swollen and their cytoplasm stains more lightly than usual: this is the *'hydropic'* or *'watery'* cell change. The distribution of these artefacts does not follow the pattern of selective vulnerability (see p. 36); moreover they tend to be more numerous in the crests of gyri, whereas ischaemic cell damage is more severe in the depths of sulci.[1] Similar artefactual changes can also occur in post-mortem brains and in experimental material fixed by immersion or inadequately perfused. The severity of post-mortem change is influenced by the original illness, the agonal state, the environment in which the body is kept and the length of interval between death and autopsy. Advanced autolytic change may obliterate the cytoarchitecture of the cortex and result in softening of the white matter.

The brains of those patients who have been kept alive by artificial ventilation may display severe and extensive damage which has become known by the term *'respirator brain'*.[130] The sequence of events leading to respirator brain remains controversial, but failure of blood flow, hypoxia, cerebral acidosis, endothelial swelling and herniation have all been implicated. Two distinct mechanisms are suggested to explain the pathophysiology of respirator brains: the first is massive swelling, characterised by initial severe hypoxia, whilst the second follows a loss of critical perfusion pressure.[131] The gross features of a respirator brain include congested cerebral cortex, generalised swelling, greatly softened brain, macerated cerebellum (fragments of which may be found along the spinal cord), and swelling and discoloration of the pituitary gland with focal haemorrhage. In contrast to the macroscopic appearances, the histological findings may show little abnormality: a negligible inflammatory cell response compared to the amount of tissue destruction; pyknosis of neuronal nuclei unaccompanied by striking astrocytic and microglial reactions; diffuse or patchy loss of neurons from the cerebral and cerebellar cortices and, often, preferential necrosis of Purkinje and granule cells of the cerebellum.[130-132]

In brains which have been well fixed in buffered

formol-saline, occasional pink patches up to 1·0 cm in diameter are seen; they are not poorly fixed areas, but result from post-mortem, intravascular growth of mainly Gram-negative bacteria.[133]

Some of the artefacts observed in human brains fixed by immersion are unavoidable due to the delays inherent in autopsy practices. In order to prevent the formation of such artefacts in experimental animals the brain is fixed by controlled intravascular perfusion and not removed from the skull until a few hours after the completion of perfusion.

REFERENCES

Pathology of neurons

1. Brown AW. J Clin Pathol 1977; 30 (suppl 11): 155.
2. Brierley JB. J Clin Pathol 1977; 30 (suppl 11): 181.
3. Brierley JB, Graham DI. In: Adams JH, Corsellis JAN, Duchen LW, eds. Greenfield's Neuropathology. 4th ed. London: Arnold, 1984: 125.
4. Graham DI. J Clin Pathol 1977; 30 (suppl 11): 170.
5. Auer RN, Wieloch T, Olsson Y, Siesjö BK. Acta Neuropathol (Berl) 1984; 64: 177.
6. Tomlinson BE. In: Smith WT, Cavanagh JB, eds. Recent advances in neuropathology. Edinburgh: Churchill Livingstone, 1979; 1: 129.
7. Burns BD. The mammalian cerebral cortex. London: Edward Arnold, 1958.
8. Miller AKH, Alston RL, Corsellis JAN. In: Smith WT, Cavanagh JB, eds. Recent advances in neuropathology. Edinburgh: Churchill Livingstone, 1979; 1: 113.
9. Price DL, Porter KR. J Cell Biol 1972; 53: 24.
10. Adams RD, Lee JC. In: Haymaker W, Adams RD, eds. Histology and histopathology of the nervous system. Springfield: Thomas, 1982: 174.
11. Torvik A, Skjörten F. Acta Neuropathol (Berl) 1971; 17: 248.
12. Bisby MA. In: Fedoroff S, Hertz L, eds. Advances in cellular neurobiology. New York: Academic Press, 1980; 1: 69.
13. Simon RP, Schmidley JW, Swan JH, Meldrum BS. Neuropathol Appl Neurobiol 1986; 12: 11.
14. Petito CK, Pulsinelli WA. J Cereb Blood Flow Metab 1984; 4: 194.
15. Petito CK, Pulsinelli WA. J Neuropathol Exp Neurol 1984; 43: 141.
16. Hossmann K-A. In: Smith WT, Cavanagh JB, eds. Recent advances in neuropathology. Edinburgh: Churchill Livingstone, 1982; 2: 191.
17. Beck E, Daniel PM. In: Prusiner SB, Hadlow WJ, eds. Slow transmissible diseases of the nervous system. New York: Academic Press, 1979; 1: 253.
18. Maslinska D, Boellard JW, Schlote W. Acta Neuropathol (Berl) 1984; 64: 222.
19. Ivy GO, Schottler F, Wenzel J, Baudry M, Lynch G. Science 1984; 226: 985.
20. Reichel W, Hollander J, Clark JH, Strehler BL. J Gerontol 1968; 23: 71.
21. Honavar M, Lantos PL. Mech Ageing Dev 1987; 41: 161.
22. Dolman CL, Macleod PM. In: Fedoroff S, Hertz L, eds. Advances in cellular neurobiology. New York: Academic Press, 1981; 2: 205.
23. Blinzinger K. Acta Neuropathol (Berl) 1968; (suppl 4): 146.
24. Leestma JE, Martin E. Arch Pathol 1968; 86: 597.
25. Wade CR, Ohara PT, Lieberman AR. J Anat 1980; 130: 641.
26. Huttenlocher PR, Heydemann PT. Ann Neurol 1984; 16: 595.
27. Kidd M. Nature 1963; 197: 192.
28. Wisniewski HM, Merz GS, Merz PA, Wen GY, Iqbal K. In: Zimmerman HM, ed. Progress in neuropathology. New York: Raven Press, 1983; 5: 139.
29. Wisniewski HM, Merz PA, Iqbal K. J Neuropathol Exp Neurol 1984; 43: 643.
30. Tomlinson BE, Corsellis JAN. In: Adams JH, Corsellis JAN, Duchen LW, eds. Greenfield's Neuropathology. 4th ed. London: Arnold 1984: 951.
31. Gibson PH, Tomlinson BE. J Neurol Sci 1977; 33: 199.
32. Takeuchi S, Hosomi M, Marasigan S, Sato M, Hayashi S, Miyoshi K. Acta Neuropathol (Berl) 1984; 64: 344.
33. Kosaka K, Yoshimura M, Ikeda K, Budka H. Clin Neuropathol 1984; 3: 185.
34. Gibb WRG. Neuropathol Appl Neurobiol 1986; 12: 223.
35. Yoshimura M. J Neurol 1983; 229: 17.
36. Kuzuhara S, Mori H, Izumiyama N, Yoshimura M, Ihara Y. Acta Neuropathol (Berl) 1988; 75: 345.
37. Lafora GR. Virchows Archiv Pathol Anat 1911; 205: 295.
38. Toga M, Dubois D, Hassoun J. Acta Neuropathol (Berl) 1968; 10: 132.
39. Marinesco J. C R Acad Sci (Paris) 1902; 135: 1000.
40. Janota I. Neuropathol Appl Neurobiol 1979; 5: 311.
41. Bunina TL. Korsakov J. J Neuropathol Psychiatry 1962; 62: 1293.
42. Iwata M, Hirano A. In: Zimmerman HM, ed. Progress in neuropathology. New York: Raven Press, 1979; 4: 277.
43. Peters A, Palay SL, Webster HdeF. The fine structure of the nervous system: the neurons and supporting cells. 2nd ed. Philadelphia: Saunders, 1976.
44. Lantos PL. Acta Neuropathol (Berl) 1974; 29: 211.
45. Butts JD, Bouldin TW, Walker DH. Acta Neuropathol (Berl) 1984; 62: 345.
46. Waller A. Philos Trans R Soc Lond 1850; 140: 423.
47. Schlaepfer WW. J Neuropathol Exp Neurol 1987; 46: 117.
48. Brodal A. In: Haymaker W, Adams RD, eds. Histology and histopathology of the nervous system. Springfield: Thomas, 1982: 276.
49. Griffin JW, Watson DF. Ann Neurol 1988; 23: 3.
50. Torvik A. J Neuropathol Exp Neurol 1956; 15: 119.
51. Blakemore WF. In: Smith WT, Cavanagh JB, eds. Recent advances in neuropathology. Edinburgh: Churchill Livingstone, 1982; 2: 53.
52. Seil FJ. In: Fedoroff S, Hertz L, eds. Advances in cellular neurobiology. New York: Academic Press, 1982; 3: 235.

53. Glees P. Acta Anat (Basel) 1948; 6: 447.
54. Strich SJ. J Neurol Neurosurg Psychiatry 1968; 31: 110.
55. Smith MC. J Neurol Neurosurg Psychiatry 1956; 19: 74.
56. Berry M. In: Smith WT, Cavanagh JB, eds. Recent advances in neuropathology. Edinburgh: Churchill Livingstone, 1979; 1: 67.
57. Berry M, Riches AC. Br Med Bull 1974; 30: 135.
58. Kiernan JA. Med Hypotheses 1978; 4: 15.
59. Cotman CW, Nieto-Sampedro M. Annu Rev Psychol 1982; 33: 371.
60. Björklund A, Stenevi U, Schmidt RH, Dunnett SB, Gage FH. Acta Physiol Scand 1983; (suppl 522): 1.
61. Björklund A, Stenevi U. Annu Rev Neurosci 1984; 7: 279.
62. Stanfield BB, O'Leary DDM. Nature 1985; 313: 135.
63. Isaacson O, Brundin P, Kelly PAT, Gage FH, Björklund A. Nature 1984; 311: 458.
64. Gage FH, Björklund A, Stenevi U, Dunnett SB, Kelly PAT. Science 1984; 225: 533.
65. Arendt T, Allen Y, Sinden J, Schugens MM, Marchbanks RM, Lantos PL, Gray JA. Nature 1988; 332: 448.
66. McGeer EG, McGeer PL. In: Fedoroff S, Hertz L, eds. Advances in cellular neurobiology. New York: Academic Press, 1980; 1: 347.

Pathology of astrocytes

67. Mori S, Leblond CP. J Comp Neurol 1969; 137: 197.
68. Cavanagh JB. J Anat 1970; 106: 471.
69. Mathewson AJ, Berry M. Brain Res 1985; 327: 61.
70. Duffy PE. Astrocytes: normal, reactive and neoplastic. New York: Raven Press, 1983.
71. Pilkington GJ, Lantos PL. Neuropathol Appl Neurobiol 1982; 8: 227.
72. Rubinstein LJ, Klatzo I, Miquel J. J Neuropathol Exp Neurol 1962; 21: 116.
73. Nathaniel EJH, Nathaniel DR. In: Fedoroff S, Hertz L, eds. Advances in cellular neurobiology. New York: Academic Press, 1981; 2: 249.
74. Blakemore WF. In: Smith WT, Cavanagh JB, eds. Recent advances in neuropathology. Edinburgh: Churchill Livingstone, 1982; 2: 53.
75. Lantos PL. Acta Neuropathol (Berl) 1974; 30: 175.
76. Vaughn JE, Pease DC. J Comp Neurol 1970; 140: 207.
77. Toshniwal PK, Firestone SL, Barlow GH, Tiku ML. J Neurol Sci 1987; 80: 277.
78. Massa PT, Dörries R, ter Meulen V. Nature 1986; 320: 543.
79. Hansen LA, Armstrong DM, Terry RD. Neurobiol Aging 1987; 8: 1.
80. Mancardi GL, Liwnicz BH, Mandybur TI. Acta Neuropathol (Berl) 1983; 61: 76.
81. Vacca LL, Nelson SR. In: Fedoroff S, ed. Advances in cellular neurobiology. Orlando: Academic Press, 1984; 5: 221.
82. Miquel IJ, Haymaker W. Prog Brain Res 1965; 15: 89.
83. Reisert I, Wildemann G, Grab D, Pilgrim C. J Comp Neurol 1984; 229: 121.
84. Barrett C, Donati EJ, Guth L. Exp Neurol 1984; 84: 374.
85. Bernstein JJ, Getz R, Jefferson M, Kelemen M. Brain Res 1985; 327: 135.
86. Brown AW, Brierley JB. J Neurol Sci 1972; 16: 59.
87. Blakemore WF. J Neurol Sci 1971; 12: 319.
88. Norenberg MD. In: Fedoroff S, Hertz L, eds. Advances in cellular neurobiology. New York: Academic Press, 1981; 2: 303.
89. Cavanagh JB, Kyu MH. J Neurol Sci 1971; 12: 63.
90. Taylor P, Schoene WC, Reid WA Jr, von Lichtenberg F. Arch Pathol Lab Med 1979; 103: 82.
91. Polak M, Haymaker W, Johnson JE Jr, D'Amelio F. In: Haymaker W, Adams RD, eds. Histology and histopathology of the nervous system. Springfield: Thomas, 1982: 363.
92. Opalski A. Z Ges Neurol Psychiatrie 1930; 124: 420.
93. Herndon RM, Rubinstein LJ, Freeman JM, Mathieson G. J Neuropathol Exp Neurol 1970; 29: 524.
94. Smith DA, Lantos PL. Acta Neuropathol (Berl) 1985; 66: 155.
95. Stam FC, Roukema PA. Acta Neuropathol (Berl) 1973; 25: 95.
96. Ramsey HJ. J Neuropathol Exp Neurol 1965; 24: 25.

Pathology of oligodendrocytes

97. Triarhou LC, Del Cerro M, Herndon RM. Neurosci Lett 1985; 53: 185.
98. Blakemore WF. Acta Neurol Scand 1984; 70 (suppl 100): 33.
99. Suzumura A, Silberberg DH, Lisak RP. J Neuroimmunol 1986; 11: 179.
100. Cavanagh JB, Blakemore WF, Kyu MH. J Neurol Sci 1971; 14: 143.
101. Maxwell DS, Kruger L. Am J Anat 1966; 118: 437.
102. Haymaker W. In: Proceedings of the Sixth International Congress of Neuropathology. Paris: Masson, 1970: 211.
103. Ludwin SK. Nature 1984; 308: 274.
104. Bologa L, Z'Graggen A, Rossi E, Herschkowitz N. J Neurol Sci 1982; 57: 419.
105. Manuelidis L, Manuelidis EE. Lab Invest 1985; 52: 1.

Pathology of ependyma

106. Dooling EC, Chi JG, Gilles FH. Ann Neurol 1977; 1: 535.
107. Weller RO, Wisniewski H, Shulman K, Terry RD. J Neuropathol Exp Neurol 1971; 30: 613.
108. Ray PK, Choudhury SR. J Anat 1984; 138: 513.
109. Matthews MA, Onge MFS, Faciane CL. Acta Neuropathol (Berl) 1979; 45: 27.
110. Bruni JE, Del Bigio MR, Clattenburg RE. Brain Res Rev 1985; 9: 1.

Microglia and macrophages

111. Adrian EK Jr, Walker BE. J Neuropathol Exp Neurol 1962; 21: 597.
112. Konigsmark BW, Sidman RL. J Neuropathol Exp Neurol 1963; 22: 643.
113. Huntington HW, Terry RD. J Neuropathol Exp Neurol 1966; 25: 646.
114. Stenwig AE. J Neuropathol Exp Neurol 1972; 31: 696.
115. Oehmichen M, Grüninger H, Saebisch R, Narita Y. Acta Neuropathol (Berl) 1973; 23: 200.
116. Schelper RL, Adrian EK Jr. J Neuropathol Exp Neurol 1986; 45: 1.
117. Blakemore WF. Acta Neuropathol (Berl) 1972; 21: 11.
118. Lantos PL. J Pathol 1975; 116: 107.

119. Russell GV. Tex Rep Biol Med 1962; 20: 338.
120. Brierley JB, Brown AW. J Comp Neurol 1982; 211: 397.
121. Brierley JB, Brown AW. J Comp Neurol 1982; 211: 407.
122. Kerns JM, Hinsman EJ. J Comp Neurol 1973; 151: 237.
123. Oehmichen M. In: Smith WT, Cavanagh JB, eds. Recent advances in neuropathology. Edinburgh: Churchill Livingstone, 1982; 2: 83.
124. Hayes GM, Woodroofe MN, Cuzner ML. J Neurol Sci 1987; 80: 25.
125. Beck DW, Hart MN, Cancilla PA. J Neuropathol Exp Neurol 1983; 42: 601.
126. Lantos PL. Acta Neuropathol (Berl) 1974; 29: 45.
127. Kreutzberg GW, Barron KD. J Neurocytol 1978; 7: 601.
128. Esiri MM, Booss J. J Clin Pathol 1984; 37: 150.

Histological artefacts

129. Cammermeyer J. In: Bourne GH, ed. The structure and function of the nervous tissue. New York: Academic Press, 1972; 6: 131.
130. Towbin A. Hum Pathol 1973; 4: 583.
131. Walker AE. Ann NY Acad Sci 1978; 315: 272.
132. Black PMcL. N Engl J Med 1978; 299: 338.
133. Hedley-Whyte ET. Acta Neuropathol (Berl) 1985; 65: 344.

The pathophysiology of raised intracranial pressure[1]

INTRODUCTION

Although certain diffuse intracranial diseases, e.g. meningitis and subarachnoid haemorrhage, may cause raised intracranial pressure without any marked shift of the brain, most lesions are localised, e.g. tumour, haematoma and infarcts, and may produce shift and herniation of the brain. This frequently leads to differences in pressure (i.e. pressure gradients) between the supratentorial and infratentorial compartments of the skull, or between the intracranial compartment and the subarachnoid space of the spine, and eventually to an increase in the intracranial pressure. The effects of any space-occupying lesion are more often proportional to the rapidity of the growth of the mass rather than to its size. Thus, the brain can sometimes accommodate a large but slowly growing lesion with surprisingly little evidence of raised intracranial pressure, while more rapidly growing, but less bulky, lesions may suddenly become symptomatic or life-threatening.[2,3] Some rapidly enlarging lesions are also associated with swelling of the brain which effectively increases the size of the expanding mass; other features, such as cyst formation, haemorrhage and hydrocephalus, can have the same effect. The age of the patient is another important factor; the older the patient the greater is the capacity to accommodate a space-occupying lesion as there is some degree of pre-existing brain atrophy.

Intracranial pressure

Intracranial pressure (ICP) is the pressure of the

cerebrospinal fluid (CSF) within the cranial cavity; it has a *normal* range in the adult of between 0 and 1·3 kPa (approximately 0–10 mmHg: 10–15 cm H_2O) with an upper limit of 2 kPa (15 mmHg). Although the ICP is transiently raised in the normal individual who coughs or strains, an elevated ICP only becomes important clinically when the increase is sustained for several minutes. Baseline ICP may be raised with intermittent periodic pathological rises in ICP that may take three main forms—pressure waves 'A', 'B' and 'C'. The 'A' or plateau wave is particularly important as it consists of a sudden rise in ICP to over 6 kPa (60 mmHg) that is maintained at this level for 5–20 minutes before falling rapidly to near normal levels.[4] 'B' waves are sharply peaked and occur once or twice per minute, reaching a height of between 4 and 8 kPa: they may be present even when baseline ICP is not significantly raised, as in benign intracranial hypertension (see p. 73). As a result of the introduction of monitoring of ICP into clinical practice in the early 1950s, it is now known that ICP is raised in a variety of conditions that include severe head injury,[5,6] subarachnoid haemorrhage immediately following the bleeding, Reye's syndrome, hepatic coma and post-hypoxic encephalopathy.

Current reviews on the pathophysiology of raised ICP have emphasised the importance of intracranial pressure–volume relationships (Fig. 3.1). As a space-occupying lesion develops, there is

no significant increase in the ICP as long as there is an equivalent reduction in the volume of the intracranial contents. Such *spatial compensation* is largely brought about by a reduction in the intracranial blood volume and the displacement of CSF. When these compensatory mechanisms have been exhausted, a critical point is reached at which any small increase in the volume of the intracranial contents will cause a dramatic rise in the ICP and the development of pressure waves. *Progressive decompensation* then occurs and there is increasing distortion of the brain and herniation of parts of the brain through the opening in the tentorium cerebelli or into the foramen magnum. Initially, displacement of the brain can occur without any elevation in the ICP, but as the expanding lesion becomes larger there is eventually impaction of the brain at either the tentorial opening or the foramen magnum. The loss of communication of pressure between the various intracranial compartments results in a pressure gradient developing across the point of impaction. Eventually the ICP approaches the systemic arterial pressure and there is a reduction in cerebral blood flow.

Cerebral blood flow

The relationships between intracranial pressure (ICP) and cerebral blood flow (CBF) are complex, but it now seems likely that the maintenance of a constant CBF, despite a rising ICP, is similar to the process of autoregulation (see p. 97). Because of the compensating increases in arterial pressure that can occur during intracranial hypertension, CBF may be maintained when the ICP is greater than 8 kPa (60 mmHg). This is because the cerebral perfusion pressure (the difference between arterial and intracranial pressures) is not reduced to any great extent. If autoregulation is impaired, however, as for example after severe head injury or subarachnoid haemorrhage, *vasomotor paralysis* occurs. In this state, there is a linear relationship between pressure and flow, with the consequence that small increases in ICP within the autoregulatory range of perfusion pressure may now cause a reduction in CBF. Thereafter there is usually progression to an irreversible state when ICP attains the level of the arterial pressure.[1,7,8] Complete cessation of brain

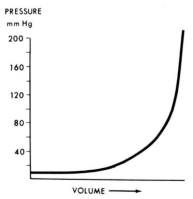

Fig. 3.1 Raised intracranial pressure. Relationship between intracranial pressure and volume of intracranial contents. The time scale may be from minutes to months, but once compensating mechanisms have been exhausted, a small increase in volume will produce a large increase in pressure.

function, 'brain death', is brought about by the arrest of the cerebral circulation, and this may be confirmed by the failure of contrast medium to enter the skull during angiography (pseudo-occlusion).[9,10]

Normal cerebral blood flow (CBF) is 50 ml/100 g/min, and it has been shown that there is an association between levels of CBF and disturbances in cerebral function. Experimental studies in subhuman primates following acute occlusion of the middle cerebral artery have shown that dysfunction becomes evident after 50% reduction in CBF. At levels of about 30% of normal, the electroencephalogram (EEG) becomes isoelectric and the evoked potential is lost.[11,12] At CBF values of about 12–15% of normal there is an efflux of potassium and an influx of calcium, but it is not until CBF has been reduced to levels of about 10% of normal that irreversible brain damage occurs.[13]

Clinical features of raised intracranial pressure

Experience has shown that the association between certain clinical features and the presence of raised ICP is loose, and that some of the signs of raised ICP may be related to brain distortion and others to cerebral ischaemia. A classical symptom of a slowly growing mass lesion is *headache*, which is probably due to tension on the pain-sensitive dura and/or distortion of pain-sensitive cerebral vessels. *Vomiting* is most likely to be due to distortion or ischaemia of the lower brainstem. An important sign is *papilloedema* which is now thought to be due to the accumulation of axoplasm in the optic papilla due to blockage of axoplasmic flow from the ganglion cells of the retina along the optic nerve.[14] The usefulness of papilloedema, however, as a sign of raised ICP is limited; for example, in chronically raised ICP papilloedema is present in only about 60% of cases, and in acute severe head injury papilloedema is present in only some 5%, although the ICP is high in 50%.[15]

The principal clinical signs of tentorial herniation are well known, with *impairment of conscious level* due to distortion or ischaemia of the upper part of the reticular formation, *ipsilateral hemiparesis* due to midbrain compression and damage to the contralateral cerebral peduncle (see

p. 68), and *dilatation of the ipsilateral pupil* due to compression of the oculomotor nerve. The clinical picture of tonsillar herniation on the other hand is *neck stiffness*, followed by *irregularity of respiration* or *apnoea*.

In addition to the cardiovascular and respiratory changes referred to already, systemic effects of raised ICP may include subendocardial haemorrhage and widespread foci of myocardial cell necrosis,[16] and haemorrhagic ulceration in the proximal part of the small bowel[17] and in the urinary bladder.

THE PATHOLOGY OF INTRACRANIAL EXPANDING LESIONS

Expanding lesions inside the skull result in a sequence of pathological complications of increasing severity. Initially, there is deformation or destruction of brain tissue around or within the lesion and a reduction in the volume of CSF within the skull as the mass enlarges. Shift and distortion

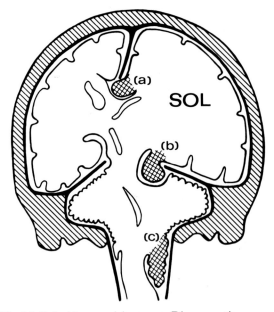

Fig. 3.2 Raised intracranial pressure. Diagrammatic representation of distension and herniation of the brain caused by a space occupying lesion (SOL) in one cerebral hemisphere. There is displacement of the midline structures and ventricles, and supracallosal (a), tentorial (b) and tonsillar (c) herniae have developed.

of the brain occur and, in an intact skull, internal herniae eventually form. Such herniae are the result of the anatomical arrangement of sheets of dura mater within the skull and presence of the foramen magnum at the base of the skull. Figure 3.2 shows how sheets of dura forming the falx cerebri (a), and the tentorium cerebelli (b), divide the intracranial cavity into two supratentorial compartments and a single infratentorial posterior fossa. A space-occupying lesion (SOL) in one cerebral hemisphere may result in herniation of the cingulate gyrus under the free edge of the falx, or herniation of the parahippocampal gyrus of the medial part of the temporal lobe through the opening (or incisura) of the tentorium cerebelli. Space-occupying lesions in the cerebellum may result in herniation of the cerebellar tonsils through the foramen magnum (Fig. 3.2). As internal herniae form and the subarachnoid space and cisterns are obliterated, pressure gradients between the various intracranial compartments develop. In addition, vascular lesions such as haemorrhage and ischaemic necrosis of the brain (see Ch. 5) are significant secondary complications of internal herniae.

Supratentorial expanding lesions

In unilateral supratentorial space-occupying lesions, e.g. tumour, haematoma or abscess, one cerebral hemisphere expands and the surface of the brain is thus pressed against the unyielding dura. The dura becomes tight, cerebral sulci are narrowed, gyri are flattened and CSF is displaced from the surface of the brain. The ipsilateral ventricle and third ventricle become smaller, and there is displacement of the midline structures away from the lesion. In some cases, the contralateral ventricle becomes enlarged due to obstruction of the interventricular foramen (of Monro) (Fig. 3.3). Other external features may include a groove on the undersurface of the frontal lobe as an impression of the lesser wing of the sphenoid bone, and downward displacement of the mamillary bodies into a narrowed interpeduncular fossa. These features are followed by the development of internal herniae as certain parts of the brain are displaced from one intracranial compartment to another.

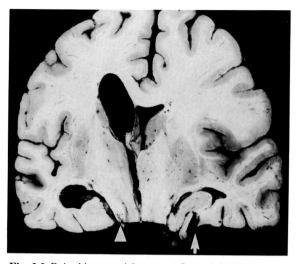

Fig. 3.3 Raised intracranial pressure. Lateral shift due to mass lesion on the right. There is displacement of the midline structures to the left, a supracallosal hernia, enlargement of the contralateral lateral ventricle, a wedge of haemorrhagic necrosis in relation to a tentorial hernia on the right (white arrow), and haemorrhagic necrosis in the contralateral cerebral peduncle (white triangle).

Supracallosal hernia. Known also as a *subfalcine* or *cingulate hernia*, supracallosal herniation occurs when the cingulate gyrus on the same side as a mass lesion herniates under the free edge of the falx cerebri (Fig. 3.3). If the displacement is sufficiently severe, the circulation through the pericallosal artery may be reduced and *infarction* of the medial surfaces of the frontal and parietal lobes, together with the corpus callosum, may ensue.

Tentorial hernia. Known also as an *uncal* or *lateral transtentorial hernia*, tentorial herniation (Fig. 3.4) occurs when the uncus and medial part of the parahippocampal gyrus are displaced downwards and medially through the tentorial incisura.[18] This type of hernia is most pronounced when there is an expanding lesion in one temporal lobe. As the hernia develops, the ipsilateral oculomotor nerve becomes compressed (initially angulated and then focally haemorrhagic) and the midbrain is narrowed in its transverse axis with resulting compression of the aqueduct. As the hernia enlarges, haemorrhagic necrosis occurs in a wedge of tissue along the line of the groove formed in the parahippocampal gyrus. In some cases there

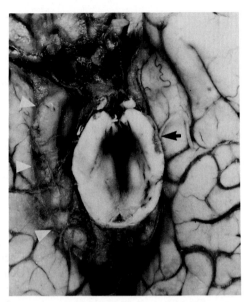

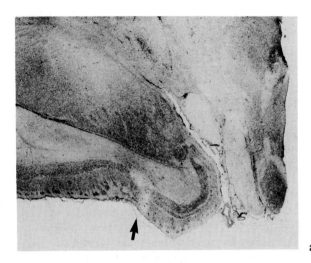

a

Fig. 3.4 Tentorial hernia. There is a tentorial hernia along the full length of the parahippocampal gyrus (white triangles). There is also angulation of the oculomotor nerves, extensive secondary haemorrhage in the midline of the upper brainstem and haemorrhagic necrosis in the contralateral cerebral peduncle (black arrow).

is also a grooved wedge of haemorrhagic necrosis (Kernohan's notch) in the contralateral cerebral peduncle, due to compression of the peduncle against the free edge of the tentorium.[19] This lesion may damage the corticospinal tract within the peduncle and result in hemiparesis.

Because some degree of shift and herniation of the brain can occur during the period of spatial compensation before a rise in ICP has occurred, it may be difficult to establish post mortem whether the intracranial pressure has been high during life. The best indication of high ICP due to a supratentorial expanding lesion is the presence of a wedge of pressure necrosis in one or both of the parahippocampal gyri.[20] Such lesions are only

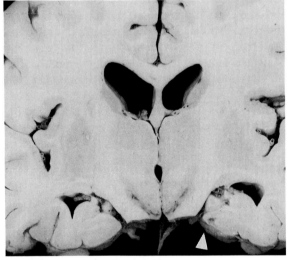

b

Fig. 3.5a, b, c Tentorial hernia. Wedge of pressure necrosis in the parahippocampal gyrus indicative of tentorial herniation. (**a**) Pressure necrosis (pale and not seen macroscopically) in the left parahippocampal gyrus (black arrow). (**b**) Small cystic lesion (white triangle) in the right parahippocampal gyrus indicative of previous tentorial herniation. (**c**) Old wedge of pressure necrosis in the left parahippocampal gyrus (arrow) indicative of previous tentorial herniation.
Cresyl violet × 3
Reproduced by permission of the editor from: Adams JH, Graham DI. Neuropathol Appl Neurobiol 1976; 2: 323.

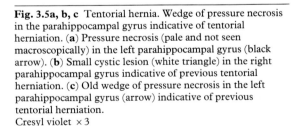

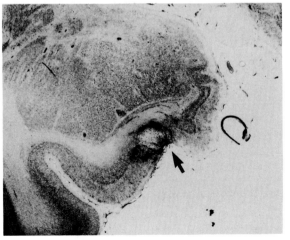

c

present in patients in whom the recorded ICP is greater than 5·3 kPa (40 mmHg) during life.[20] Significant tentorial herniation can, therefore, be recognised by the presence of a wedge of pressure necrosis in the parahippocampal gyrus. Not all such lesions are identifiable macroscopically and some are not haemorrhagic; a past episode of herniation can be recognised by the presence of a small, organised gliotic wedge of pressure necrosis (Fig. 3.5). A tentorial hernia will eventually cause obliteration of the subarachnoid space and of the tentorial incisura, leading to a CSF pressure gradient between the supratentorial compartment and the posterior fossa.

Various factors may exacerbate a rise in ICP and subsequent tentorial herniation; these include the development of hydrocephalus due to blockage of the foramina of Monro or the third ventricle, or following narrowing of the aqueduct by lateral midline shift and midbrain compression. Evidence of a tentorial hernia may not be obvious, either macroscopically or histologically if there has been a very rapid rise in supratentorial ICP[18] and, of course, it will not be seen if the mass lesion is in the posterior fossa.

The ICP may be raised in *subarachnoid*

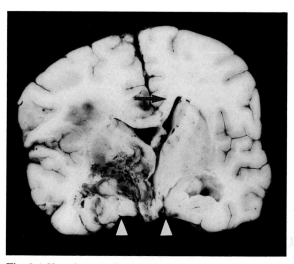

Fig. 3.6 Vascular complication of internal hernia. Infarction in territory supplied by left anterior choroidal artery—medial segment of globus pallidus, lower part of anterior limb of internal capsule, paraventricular structures and pes hippocampi. There is also bilateral tentorial herniation (white triangles), a supracallosal hernia (black arrow) and haemorrhagic necrosis of the upper brainstem.

haemorrhage and *meningitis* but because the disease process is diffuse and does not, at least initially, generate pressure gradients there will usually be no evidence of internal herniation.

Tentorial herniae may obstruct the circulation through the anterior choroidal artery, leading to infarction, particularly in the caudate and amygdaloid nuclei, the medial segment of the globus pallidus, the subthalamic region and the anterior half of the hippocampus (Fig. 3.6). Compression of the posterior cerebral artery and its branches results in necrosis in the thalamus, the posterior part of the hippocampus, the cortex of the undersurface of the temporal lobe and the inferior and medial surfaces of the occipital lobe including the visual cortex (Fig. 3.7). The superior cerebellar artery may be compressed and lead to necrosis of the superomedial portions of the cerebellum. The posterior cerebral artery and its branches are the vessels most commonly affected by tentorial herniation, and the visual cortex is frequently infarcted.

Central transtentorial hernia. This develops particularly when ICP increases rapidly due to either frontal or parietal lobe lesions or to bilateral expanding lesions. Herniation of both parahippocampal gyri occurs through the tentorial incisura to form a *circular* or *ring hernia*.

Haemorrhage and infarction in the midbrain and pons. These features are common and are often terminal events in patients with supratentorial expanding lesions, high intracranial pressure and tentorial herniation.[21] They are found mainly in the midline of the midbrain and upper pons (Figs 3.4 and 3.8), and are thought to be due to displacement and elongation of the upper brainstem.[22] The pathogenesis of the haemorrhage and infarction is uncertain but important contributory factors include caudal displacement and antero-posterior elongation of the rostral brainstem, and relative immobility of the basilar artery. The presence of these factors results in obstruction of venous drainage and stretching of arteries.

The sequence of events noted above is seen also in association with supratentorial extracerebral expanding lesions, such as extradural or subdural haematomas or meningiomas. When there is either

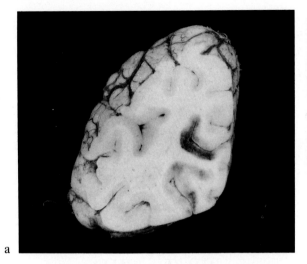

a

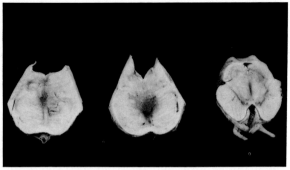

Fig. 3.8 Secondary damage in the brainstem. Compare with the acute changes seen in Fig. 3.4. If the patient survives the acute stage the affected tissue becomes discoloured and partly cystic.

Infratentorial expanding lesions

Tonsillar hernia. Because of the considerable variation in the normal configuration of the cerebellar tonsils, a significant hernia may be difficult to recognise post mortem. Incontrovertible evidence of a hernia is seen, however, when the tonsils become *impacted* and their tips undergo *necrosis,* which is sometimes haemorrhagic. A transverse groove may also be present on the ventral aspect of the medulla where it has become compressed against the anterior edge of the foramen magnum (Fig. 3.9). Though most commonly found in association with a mass lesion

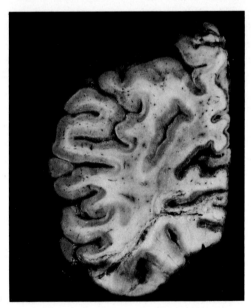

b

Fig. 3.7a, b Vascular complications of internal herniae. Infarction in the territory supplied by the posterior cerebral artery.
(**a**) Recent haemorrhagic necrosis including the medial and inferior surfaces of the left occipital lobe. (**b**) Previous infarction of the medial and inferior surfaces of the left ocipital lobe: the cortex is now shrunken and granular.

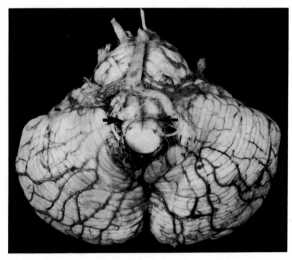

Fig. 3.9 Tonsillar hernia. The tips of the tonsils are haemorrhagic and there is a groove (black arrows) on the ventral surface of the medulla oblongata.

diffuse brain swelling or a bilateral space-occupying lesion, the ventricles may become reduced symmetrically without a lateral shift of the midline structures; bilateral tentorial herniae may then develop.

in the posterior fossa, a tonsillar hernia may also develop as a result of an expanding mass above the tentorium.

Expanding lesions in the posterior fossa characteristically produce obstructive *hydrocephalus*. Tonsillar herniation may be severe, and occasionally one or both posterior inferior cerebellar arteries may be compressed, resulting in extensive infarction and necrosis of the under-surfaces of the cerebellar hemispheres. There may also be upward herniation of the cerebellum through the tentorial opening to produce a so-called *reversed tentorial hernia*.

In a patient with an intracranial expanding lesion, lumbar puncture can precipitate tonsillar or tentorial herniation with serious consequences and even death of the patient. Even if only a small amount of CSF is withdrawn, more may leak into the spinal extradural space via the puncture wound in the meninges. Lumbar puncture is, therefore, contra-indicated in a patient with suspected increased ICP until the presence of an intracranial expanding lesion has been excluded. An exception to the rule is a suspected case of bacterial meningitis without focal signs, when lumbar puncture is an essential step in establishing a rapid diagnosis.

Other features of the pathology of intracranial expanding lesions

If the ICP remains high after a neurosurgical operation, an external hernia may develop through a defect in the skull. This may amount simply to protrusion of small pieces of cortex through burr holes, but if an external decompression has been undertaken, a large part of the cerebral hemisphere may herniate as an *external hernia cerebri* through a craniotomy or craniectomy defect in the calvaria.

Bony changes may be recognisable radiologically in adults with a longstanding moderate increase in ICP; they include erosion of the posterior clinoid processes and enlargement of the pituitary fossa. Pressure effects on the floor of the sella turcica may be accentuated when the subarachnoid space extends into the sella—the so-called *empty sella syndrome*. An empty sella, however, is not necessarily an indication of raised ICP as it is a feature in some 25% of normal adults. In a small number of cases there may be sufficient erosion of the base of the skull to allow small pieces of brain to extrude through the dura mater in the middle cranial fossae. In infants and young children, an elevation of the ICP may be recognised by enlargement of the skull, separation of the sutures of the vault and thinning of the bones of the vault, with an increase in the prominence of the convolutional pattern on the inside of the skull. In CT scans of patients with early post-traumatic brain swelling, reliable indicators of raised ICP include obliteration of the third ventricle and basal cisterns and, when the pathology is unilateral, dilatation of the contralateral ventricle.[23,24]

HYDROCEPHALUS[1]

INTRODUCTION

Hydrocephalus is an increased amount of cerebrospinal fluid (CSF) within the skull. Various types of hydrocephalus have been described. In *external hydrocephalus* there is an excessive amount of CSF in the subarachnoid space over the surface of the brain, whereas in *internal hydrocephalus* there is an increased volume of CSF within the ventricles. If CSF can pass freely from the ventricles into the subarachnoid space, the hydrocephalus is said to be *communicating*. *Non-communicating* hydrocephalus is when the flow of CSF from the ventricles to the subarachnoid space is blocked. Whenever there is diffuse or focal loss of brain tissue (cerebral atrophy), there is a compensatory increase in the volume of CSF to produce *hydrocephalus ex vacuo*. Hydrocephalus may be *progressive* and associated with a rise in ICP, but sometimes the intraventricular pressure returns to normal, in which event the hydrocephalus is in an unstable *arrested* state.

Formation and absorption of cerebrospinal fluid

The normal volume of cerebrospinal fluid (CSF) in the adult is about 140 ml, of which some 20 ml is formed and absorbed per hour. CSF is produced by the specialised epithelium of the choroid plexus by mechanisms that include filtration and active secretion.[25,26] After formation, the CSF becomes distributed throughout the ventricular system, eventually passing into the subarachnoid space via the exit foramina of the fourth ventricle—the midline foramen of Magendie and the lateral foramina of Luschka. Thereafter it flows over the surface of the brain and spinal cord to be absorbed in the arachnoid granulations associated with the major intracranial venous sinuses and the sleeves of the spinal roots respectively.[27] The arachnoid granulations[28] constitute one-way valves that respond to the pressure difference between CSF and the dural venous sinuses.[29-31] Such a mechanism allows for the rapid absorption of CSF in patients with intracranial expanding lesions, thereby making a major contribution to spatial compensation.

If the flow of CSF is obstructed acutely, the ventricles quickly dilate (see p. 323; Fig. 12.11) and the surface of the brain becomes flattened against the dura. As the ventricles enlarge, the ependyma is disrupted and CSF flows into the periventricular white matter causing interstitial oedema (see p. 324; Fig. 12.12) and axonal degeneration. With the passage of time there is loss of axons, and the periventricular white matter becomes gliotic.[32-34] In these circumstances absorption of CSF probably occurs through the periventricular blood vessels.[35] Eventually the hydrocephalus becomes arrested and a new equilibrium between the formation and absorption of CSF is attained, the interstitial oedema is reduced and the ventricle becomes lined by flattened ependyma and a layer of subependymal gliosis.[33,35] Interstitial oedema can be recognised in computerised tomographic (CT) scans of patients with acute hydrocephalus as reduced attenuation of the periventricular white matter (Fig. 3.10).

Causes of hydrocephalus

By far the most common cause of hydrocephalus is obstruction to the free flow of CSF.[36] Obstruction may be *congenital* or *acquired*, and it is the site of the pathological lesion rather than its nature or size which determines the consequences. Thus, a small lesion at a critical point, e.g. near the aqueduct, may cause extensive dilatation of the cerebral ventricles. Hydrocephalus may be the result of focal disease, such as tumour, abscess or haematoma, or

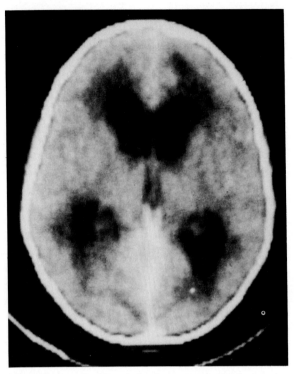

Fig. 3.10 Acute hydrocephalus due to mass lesion in posterior fossa. CT scan showing enlarged ventricles and reduced attenuation in the periventricular white matter—interstitial oedema.
Reproduced by permission of Dr Evelyn Teasdale, Institute of Neurological Sciences, Glasgow, UK.

diffuse disease of the meninges, e.g. tuberculous or carcinomatous meningitis, or subarachnoid haemorrhage.

Enlargement of the ventricular system occurs in that part which lies above the obstruction. Thus, only one lateral ventricle will be enlarged if the block is at the foramen of Monro (Figs 3.3 and 3.11), whereas if there is obstruction in the hindbrain, the third ventricle will also be dilated (Fig. 3.10). If the obstruction is at the exit foramina of the fourth ventricle, or in the subarachnoid space, the entire ventricular system will be enlarged.

Infantile hydrocephalus is commonly due to developmental abnormalities such as the Chiari malformations and forking and gliosis of the aqueduct (see p. 324). Other causes include obliteration of the subarachnoid space due to perinatal haemorrhage or infection. By contrast,

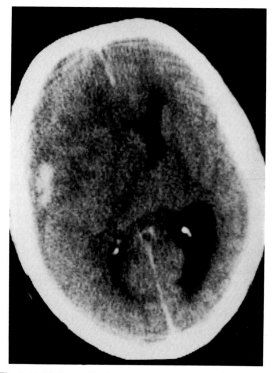

Fig. 3.11 Unilateral hydrocephalus. CT scan shows reduced attenuation in the left cerebral hemisphere due to subdural haematoma with underlying surface contusions. There is displacement of the midline structures with dilatation of the contralateral ventricle.
Reproduced by permission of Dr P. Macpherson, Institute of Neurological Sciences, Glasgow, UK.

the commonest cause of hydrocephalus in older children and adults is a space-occupying lesion in the posterior fossa which causes distortion and compression of the fourth ventricle and the aqueduct.

Hydrocephalus may also be caused either by an *increased production* or by a *decreased absorption* of CSF. The former may occur in association with a papillary tumour of the choroid plexus[37] and the latter may possibly result from blood or tumour in the arachnoid granulations,[36] although this is unproven (see p. 324).

Another common cause of hydrocephalus is focal loss of brain tissue as, for example, after long-standing infarction in the distribution of the middle cerebral artery (Fig. 5.5). If the loss of tissue is diffuse as, for example, when there has been long survival after cardiac arrest, then there

will be generalised enlargement of the ventricular system (Fig. 5.33). Similar *hydrocephalus ex vacuo* occurs in dementia (see Ch. 13).

Normal pressure hydrocephalus

This term is used to describe a condition characterised by chronic hydrocephalus, progressive dementia, gait disturbance and urinary incontinence or urgency.[38-40]

Patients with this condition have episodic moderate increases in ICP, particularly during sleep. A more appropriate term for the condition is therefore *intermittently raised pressure hydrocephalus*. It is thought to be due to an impairment of CSF absorption. Antecedent causes include head injury[39] or subarachnoid haemorrhage,[40,41] but often no known cause can be found. The importance of this condition is that a proportion of patients improve clinically following insertion of a ventricular shunt.[40]

Benign intracranial hypertension

This term is used when patients present with raised ICP without demonstrable cause and with ventricles that are smaller than normal.[42,43] The condition may be related to a failure of CSF absorption,[44] but it has been suggested that it is due to an increase in cerebral blood volume or brain water content.[45] Yet other cases appear to be due to specific causes of diffuse elevation of ICP, such as occlusion of one or more major dural sinuses (otitic hydrocephalus),[46] Reye's syndrome (see p. 210), encephalitis and hepatitis.[47,48]

BRAIN SWELLING AND OEDEMA[1-3]

INTRODUCTION

An increase in the volume of all or part of the brain is a potential complication of many intracranial pathological lesions, such as contusions, tumours and abscesses. It may also occur, however, in the form of diffuse swelling of one or both cerebral hemispheres, particularly after head injury. Whether localised or generalised, brain swelling and oedema can be recognised post mortem by an increase in the weight of the brain, by narrowing of sulci, flattening of gyri and a reduction in the size of the ventricles; it may be of sufficient severity to raise the ICP and cause death from brain shift and herniation and secondary damage to the brainstem. The cause of the swelling of the brain is not always clear, but in general it is due either to an increase in the cerebral blood volume—*congestive brain swelling*—or to an increase in the water content of brain tissue itself—*cerebral oedema*.

Congestive brain swelling

This appears to be due to a rapid increase in the blood volume of one or both cerebral hemispheres. When only one hemisphere is involved, swelling is commonly associated with a traumatic acute subdural haematoma (Fig. 6.17). Both cerebral hemispheres may swell, particularly in children who have sustained a head injury (Fig. 6.18). The pathophysiology of the process remains uncertain but, as implied in the appellation, there is dilatation of the smaller cerebral vessels, possibly as a result of hypoxaemia or hypercapnia, or due to a marked increase in the intraluminal arterial pressure. At post-mortem, the brain is diffusely swollen and the ventricles are small and symmetrical.[49,50] The pathogenesis of this type of brain swelling is not clear, but in children it seems to be associated with a loss of vasomotor tone which leads to vasodilatation.[50,51] The process is dynamic and if the vasodilatation persists, the blood-brain barrier may become defective, and true vasogenic oedema ensues (see below). Experimental evidence suggests that lesions in, or stimulation of, the hypothalamus and the brainstem produce marked cerebral vasodilatation which, when combined with a high intraluminal arterial pressure, raises the ICP to levels that make the brain ischaemic.[52] The end point of this state of generalised cerebral vasomotor paralysis occurs when perfusion of the brain ceases and brain death supervenes.[8]

Cerebral oedema[53]

This means an increase in the tissue water content of the brain. The normal water content of grey matter is 80% of the wet weight, while that of white matter is much lower at 68% of wet weight. In brain oedema, water accumulates preferentially in white matter, through which it can spread more freely than through grey matter.

Breakdown of the blood-brain barrier

The integrity of the blood-brain barrier is vital to the maintenance of a normal brain volume. The barrier has both anatomical components (tight junctions between capillary endothelial cells, the vessel basement membrane and foot processes of perivascular astrocytes) and physicochemical components that together regulate the passage of substances into and out of the brain. The passage of any substance will depend on the permeability of the barrier to that substance, the surface area of the capillary bed involved and other factors such as local blood flow and hydrostatic pressures. Solutes may cross the barrier by vesicular transport, carrier mechanisms which allow passage against a diffusion gradient, and diffusion, bulk flow and cytoplasmic channels that allow the passage of water and electrolytes.[54,55]

Breakdown of the blood-brain barrier, with resultant cerebral oedema, is due to an increase in intravascular pressure, damage to and increased permeability of the cerebral blood vessels, or a decrease in plasma colloid osmotic pressure.[56-58]

Five main types of oedema[58]

Vasogenic oedema. As a result of damage to the blood-brain barrier, water, electrolytes and proteins accumulate in the extracellular space. While some of the fluid may accumulate due to physical disruption of the blood vessels in the damaged tissue, there is increasing evidence that, in some conditions, vasogenic oedema is due to enhanced pinocytotic activity by endothelial cells.[56] This type of oedema is frequently seen in the neighbourhood of malignant brain tumours (Fig. 3.12), cerebral abscesses, contusions and brain infarction: it can most easily be produced experimentally by the application of intense cold to the surface of the brain.[59,60]

Cytotoxic oedema. This occurs in two principal forms. *Ischaemic brain oedema* follows an acute

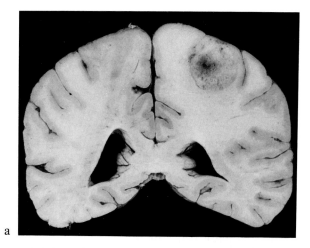

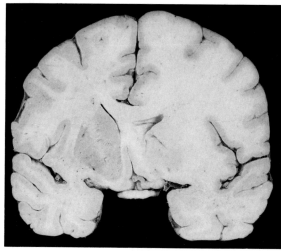

Fig. 3.12a, b Cerebral oedema. (**a**) Metastatic carcinoma in right parietal lobe. (**b**) Diffuse swelling of the same cerebral hemisphere anterior to the metastasis.

matter of the nervous system by the separation of the lamellae of myelin sheaths at the intraperiod line; such agents include triethyltin compounds,[62-64] cuprizone,[65] and hexachlorophane[66] (see Ch. 11).

Hydrostatic oedema. This may develop when the intravascular pressure rises to high levels. There is forced vasodilation with congestive brain swelling, followed by the outflow of water from the vascular bed into the extracellular space. It is seen in patients with hypertensive encephalopathy,[67,68] after craniotomy if the arterial pressure has been high, and following the removal of an intracranial mass that has been inducing a high ICP,[69] e.g. a large meningioma.

Interstitial CSF oedema. An increase in the water content of the periventricular tissues is observed in patients with acute obstructive hydrocephalus (Fig. 12.12).[32-35] It is now possible to identify this condition by CT scanning (Fig. 3.10).

Hypo-osmotic oedema. This is seen in some patients with head injury in whom there is a severe reduction in serum osmolality. It is thought to be due either to excessive replacement of fluid loss by intravenous dextrose water solutions, or to development of the syndrome of inappropriate secretion of antidiuretic hormone (SIADH). A similar condition can be induced experimentally by the infusion of distilled water into the peritoneal cavity or intravenously, so reducing the serum osmolality; such a procedure may produce diffuse swelling of the brain with a raised ICP, an increased tissue water content and reduced cerebral blood flow.[70]

Spread, resolution and effects of cerebral oedema

Factors that regulate the rate and extent of the spread of oedema fluid through the brain have been extensively studied.[58,60,71,72] The rate of formation of oedema can be accelerated by agents that cause cerebral arterial or arteriolar vasodilatation, while any factor that causes cerebral vasoconstriction or elevation of the ICP tends to reduce oedema formation. Once formed, protein, water and other constituents of the oedema fluid

episode of hypoxia,[61] and there is initially an intracellular accumulation of water. There is a basic disturbance of the cellular osmoregulation, which depends mainly on the Na^+–K^+ exchange pump with ATP as its energy source. Within a few hours, this type of cytotoxic oedema is followed by a vasogenic component, particularly at the margins of an infarct.

In *oedema due to noxious agents*, the main feature is swelling of brain parenchymal cells. The best studied examples of this type of oedema are those caused by toxic agents which induce widespread intramyelinic vacuole formation within the white

move at different rates through the extracellular space. Ultimately, the oedema fluid either drains into the ventricular CSF or is absorbed into the bloodstream through brain blood vessels.

It is generally thought that cerebral oedema is an important cause of brain dysfunction, but recent evidence suggests that this is only true when the oedema is sufficiently severe to cause cerebral ischaemia or distortion and herniation of the brain.[73]

Whether localised or generalised, swelling of the brain is manifest by flattened gyri and narrowed sulci. Upon sectioning the brain, an increase in the volume of the affected brain tissue is seen. After fixation, even in colourless formalin, the oedematous region acquires a yellowish–green tinge. In haematoxylin and eosin or Klüver–Barrera (myelin) stained sections, the oedematous tissue appears paler than normal. In the cortex, the extracellular space remains small, much of the oedema fluid being taken up by astrocytes and their processes. However, a different appearance is seen in the white matter, in which oedema fluid spreads in the extracellular space between the myelinated fibres. As white matter can accommodate the most oedema fluid, it is usually more swollen than grey matter (Fig. 3.12). Reactive astrocytes appear and serum proteins may be demonstrated within them by immunohistochemistry.[61] The oligodendrocytes, too, are swollen, and their enlarged nuclei are surrounded by halo-like clear areas. Perfusion fixation, the combined use of tracer materials and electron microscopy have confirmed that, during the first 48 hours, oedema fluid follows the path of least resistance and spreads relatively freely along the extracellular pathways in white matter, whereas in grey matter the extracellular spread of the tracer is limited by the various adhesions between cells.[74]

REFERENCES

Introduction

1. Miller JD, Adams JH. In: Adams JH, Corsellis JAN, Duchen LW, eds. Greenfield's Neuropathology. 4th ed. London: Arnold, 1984: 53.
2. Miller JD. In: Crockard A, Hayward R, Hoff JT, eds. Neurosurgery: the scientific basis of clinical practice. London: Blackwell, 1985: 266.
3. Crockard A. In: Crockard A, Hayward R, Hoff JT, eds. Neurosurgery: the scientific basis of clinical practice. London: Blackwell, 1985: 333.
4. Lundberg N. Acta Psychiatr Neurol Scand 1960; 36 (suppl 149): 1.
5. Miller JD, Becker DP, Ward JD, Sullivan HG, Adams WE, Rosner MJ. J Neurosurg 1977; 47: 503.
6. Miller JD, Butterworth JF, Gudeman SK, Faulkner JE, Choi SC, Selhorst JB. J Neurosurg 1981; 54: 289.
7. Langfitt TW, Kassell NF, Weinstein JD. Neurology (Minneap) 1965; 15: 761.
8. Langfitt TW, Weinstein JD, Kassell NF. Neurology (Minneap) 1965; 15: 622.
9. Heiskanen O. Acta Neurol Scand 1964; 40 (suppl 17): 1.
10. Langfitt TW, Kassell NF. Acta Neurochir 1966; 14: 96.
11. Branston NM, Symon L, Crockard HA, Pasztor E. Exp Neurol 1974; 45: 195.
12. Astrup J, Symon L, Branston NM, Lassen NA. Stroke 1977; 8: 51.
13. Astrup J. J Neurosurg 1982; 56: 482.
14. Tso Mom, Hayreh SS. Arch Ophthalmol 1977; 95: 1148.
15. Selhorst JB, Gudeman SK, Butterworth JF, Harbison JW, Miller JD, Becker DP. Neurosurgery 1985; 16: 357.
16. Connor RCR. Br Med J 1968; 3: 29.
17. Gudeman SK, Wheeler CB, Miller JD, Halloran LG, Becker DP. Neurosurgery 1983; 12: 175.

Intracranial expanding lesions

18. Graham DI, Lawrence AE, Adams JH, Doyle D, McLellan DR. Neuropathol Appl Neurobiol 1987; 13: 209.
19. Kernohan JW, Woltman HW. Arch Neurol Psychiatry 1929; 21: 274.
20. Adams JH, Graham DI. Neuropathol Appl Neurobiol 1976; 2: 323.
21. Duret H. Etudes experimentales et cliniques sur les traumatismes cérébraux. Paris: Publ. du Progrès Med. 1878.
22. Hassler O. Neurology (Minneap) 1967; 17: 368.
23. Robertson FC, Kishore PRS, Miller JD, Lipper MH, Becker JD. Surg Neurol 1979; 12: 161.
24. Teasdale E, Cardosa E, Galbraith S, Teasdale G. J Neurol Neurosurg Psychiatry 1984; 47: 600.

Hydrocephalus

25. Davson H. Physiology of the cerebrospinal fluid. London: Churchill, 1972.
26. Milhorat TH. J Neurosurg 1975; 42: 628.
27. Fishman RA. Cerebrospinal fluid in diseases of the nervous system. Philadelphia: Saunders, 1980.
28. Upton ML, Weller RO. J Neurosurg 1985; 63: 867.
29. Welch K, Friedman V. Brain 1960; 83: 454.
30. Cutler RWP, Page LK, Galicich J, Watters GV. Brain 1968; 91: 707.
31. Davson H, Hollingsworth G, Segal MB. Brain 1970; 93: 665.

32. Weller RO, Wisniewski H. Brain 1969; 92: 819.
33. Weller RO, Wisniewski H, Shulman K, Terry RD. J Neuropathol Exp Neurol 1971; 30: 613.
34. Weller RO, Shulman K. J Neurosurg 1972; 36: 255.
35. Weller RO, Mitchell J. In: Cervos-Navarro J, Ferszt R, eds. Brain edema. Advances in neurology, vol. 28. New York: Raven Press, 1980: 111.
36. Russell DS. Observations on the pathology of hydrocephalus. Special report series of the Medical Research Council. London: HMSO, 1949; no. 265.
37. Eisenberg HM, McComb JG, Lorenzo AV. J Neurosurg 1974; 40: 381.
38. Adams RD, Fisher CM, Hakim S, Ojemann RG, Sweet WH. N Engl J Med 1965; 273: 117.
39. Hakim S, Adams RD. J Neurol Sci 1965; 2: 307.
40. Thomsen AM, Børgesen SE, Bruhn P, Gjerris F. Ann Neurol 1986; 20: 304.
41. Symon L, Dorsch NWC. J Neurosurg 1975; 42: 258.
42. Foley J. Brain 1955; 78: 1.
43. Johnston I, Paterson A. Brain 1974; 97: 301.
44. Johnston I. Lancet 1973; 2: 418.
45. Reid AC, Matheson MS, Teasdale G. Lancet 1980; 2: 7.
46. Janny P, Flori B, Jovan JD, Janny L. In: Lundberg N, Ponten U, Brock M, eds. Intracranial pressure II. Berlin: Springer, 1975: 512.
47. Chandler WF, Kindt GW. Surg Neurol 1976; 5: 311.
48. Mickell JJ, Cook DR, Reigel DH, Painter MJ, Safar P. Crit Care Med 1976; 4: 1.

Brain swelling and oedema

49. Snoek J, Jennett B, Adams JH, Graham DI, Doyle D. J Neurol Neurosurg Psychiatry 1979; 42: 215.
50. Zimmerman RA, Bilaniuk LT, Gennarelli TA. Radiology 1978; 127: 393.
51. Kuhl DE et al. J Neurosurg 1980; 52: 309.
52. Shalit MN, Reinmuth OM, Shimojyo S, Scheinberg P. Arch Neurol (Chic) 1967; 17: 342.
53. Klatzo I. J Neuropathol Exp Neurol 1967; 26: 1.
54. Rapoport SI. Blood-brain barrier in physiology and medicine. New York: Raven Press, 1976.
55. Bradbury M. The concept of a blood-brain barrier. Chichester: Wiley, 1979.
56. Westergaard E. In: Cervos-Navarro J, Ferszt R, eds. Brain edema. Advances in neurology, vol. 28. New York: Raven Press, 1980: 55.
57. Blasberg RG, Fenstermacher JD, Patlak CS. J Cereb Blood Flow Metab 1983; 3: 8.
58. Miller JD. Br J Hosp Med 1979; 20: 152.
59. Clasen RA, Cooke PM, Pandolfi S, Boyd D, Raimondi AJ. J Neuropathol Exp Neurol 1962; 21: 579.
60. Bakay L, Hague I. J Neuropathol Exp Neurol 1964; 23: 393.
61. Klatzo I. Br J Anaesth 1985; 57: 18.
62. Magee PN, Stoner HB, Barnes JM. J Pathol Bacteriol 1957; 73: 107.
63. Torack RM, Terry RD, Zimmerman HM. Am J Pathol 1960; 36: 273.
64. Graham DI, Kim SU, Gonatas NK, Guyotte L. J Neuropathol Exp Neurol 1975; 34: 401.
65. Suzuki K, Kikkawa Y. Am J Pathol 1969; 54: 307.
66. Lampert PW, O'Brien J, Garrett R. Acta Neuropathol (Berl) 1973; 23: 326.
67. Lassen NA, Agnoli A. Scand J Clin Lab Invest 1973; 30: 113.
68. MacKenzie ET, Strandgaard S, Graham DI, Jones JV, Harper AM, Farrar JK. Circ Res 1976; 39: 33.
69. Schutta HG, Kassell NF, Langfitt TW. Brain 1968; 91: 281.
70. Meinig G, Reulen HJ, Magavly C. Acta Neurochir 1973; 29: 1.
71. Hochwald GM, Marlin AE, Wald A, Malhan C. In: Pappius HM, Feindel W, eds. Dynamics of brain edema. Berlin: Springer, 1976: 129.
72. Reulen HJ, Tsuyumu M, Tack A, Fenske AR, Prioleau GR. J Neurosurg 1978; 48: 754.
73. Penn RD. In: Cervos-Navarro J, Ferszt R, eds. Brain edema. Advances in neurology, vol. 28. New York: Raven Press, 1980: 383.
74. Hirano A. In: Cervos-Navarro J, Ferszt R, eds. Brain edema. Advances in neurology, vol. 28. New York: Raven Press, 1980: 83.

Pathological examination of the central nervous system

In this chapter, techniques for the gross and microscopic investigation of neural tissue are described, together with clinico-pathological correlative aspects of neurological disease.

CLINICAL DATA AS A GUIDE TO NEUROPATHOLOGY

Neuropathology originated over a century ago from clinical neurology, and it has remained closely linked to its parent clinical discipline. Most diagnostic pathologists maintain a professional liaison with their physician and surgeon colleagues, but clinico-pathological bonds are of special importance in the study of brain disease— and not simply because of history. The complexity of neuroanatomy, the multiplicity of clinical features in disorders of the nervous system, and the changing picture in a slowly evolving disease present peculiar problems of interpretation. The relationship of clinical features to tissue changes in defined areas of the nervous system is the problem which confronts the pathologist, and is one which cannot be adequately tackled without familiarity with the methods of clinical neurology as well as with the anatomy and pathology of the nervous system. Critical interpretation of case records and evaluation of a patient's medical history and the physical signs found at examination guide the pathologist in making correlative inferences prior to the performance of an autopsy or the dissection of a fixed brain and the viewing of microscope slides.

In the study of brain disease, an accurate and detailed clinical history is of the greatest importance. Very often a precise diagnosis can be made from the history; physical examination—particularly the long, exhaustive examination of classical academic neurology—is then supererogatory. It is not appropriate here to describe different symptoms and signs and their significance, but a few very general points can be made. Thus, the patient's description of the *tempo of the illness*, whether acute or chronic, coming on slowly or abruptly, steadily progressive or remitting, often suggests the type of pathological process. *Vascular problems* are generally of acute onset, *tumour symptoms* tend steadily to progress, *demyelinating diseases* may remit. The characterisation of symptoms needs to be achieved wherever possible. The analysis of such frequent symptoms as headache, giddiness, visual disturbance, epileptic attacks, and deficits of sensory or motor function may provide information of diagnostic or localising value. The methodology of clinical diagnosis in neurology, including the interpretation of symptoms and physical signs, is well described.[1,3]

Clinical diagnosis aims to localise any lesion present and to predict its pathology on the basis of its site and tempo of evolution. In many cases, confirmation of the diagnosis comes from visualising the nervous system by techniques of neuroradiology.

IMAGING TECHNIQUES AND PATHOLOGICAL LESIONS

As investigative techniques for producing images of the living brain have developed, so the capability of the pathologist for clinico-pathological correlation has increased. Skull X-rays, in wide diagnostic use from early in the century, could show only calcified structures (e.g. the pineal gland, some aneurysms, some tumours), local erosive changes and major effects of raised intracranial pressure or brain swelling (e.g. widened sutures, eroded posterior clinoid processes, widened internal auditory meatuses).

Ventriculography, lumbar air encephalography, arteriography and contrast myelography, developed in the 1920s and 1930s, enabled abnormal structures in the brain and spinal canal to be visualised as abnormal contours, distorted anatomy or vascular changes, but remained deficient in showing brain or cord parenchyma. Arteriography and contrast myelography, with sophisticated modern developments, are still indispensible in many cases.

However, computerised tomographic (CT) scanning of the brain has greatly altered the approach to neurological diagnosis over the past two decades through its ability to show alterations in the substance of the brain. It has contributed significantly to the understanding of many diseases of the nervous system and has produced a corresponding increase in interest in neuropathological findings. Pathologists may now be required to carry out brain dissections that match the appearances seen on CT scans, and to evaluate scan abnormalities at the microscopic level.

More recently, the development of magnetic resonance imaging (MRI) for clinical diagnosis has provided an even more sophisticated tool for showing the substance of the CNS, providing diagnostic information with pathological content which can be related to gross and microscopic anatomical changes. The ways in which CT scans and MRI may cast light on neuropathological problems will be briefly examined below.

Positron emission tomographic (PET) scanning gives information about metabolic as well as structural changes in the living brain. At present, PET technology does not produce pictures with sufficient resolution for detailed pathological correlations to be made, but improvements are awaited with interest.

Computerised tomographic scanning

CT scans appear very similar to cut brain sections, and radiological interpretation of scan abnormalities is based on consideration of morbid anatomy; by placing CT scans in the context of the natural history of disease, the clinician has a firm base for diagnosis.[4] CT scanning enables small variations in the physical density of tissue to be recognised radiographically. Plain X-rays demonstrate soft tissues poorly, and are of value mainly in showing calcified structures. CT scans will give an image of the brain and show variable tissue density as the content of water and protein varies. Thus, abnormal density in a CT image may be due to oedema, haemorrhage, necrosis or cyst formation, as well as an abnormal cellular mass. *Blood clots* have a high protein content and appear white on a scan. The clinical recognition of subdural and subarachnoid bleeding has been aided by the use of CT, and intracerebral haematomas can be well visualised. *Serous exudates and oedema fluid* are of lower physical density than the adjacent brain parenchyma and appear hypodense (black) in CT scans. An encysted subdural hygroma is of low scan density; at a certain stage during its evolution from a subdural haematoma (perhaps a month from its onset), this lesion will be of the same density as the underlying cerebral tissue and invisible on a plain scan. Brain oedema produces low density images. The oedema associated with areas of necrosis is readily shown. The CT appearances of *infarcts* can be roughly correlated with the age of the lesion. In the first few hours after infarction occurs the scan is usually normal, but within 24 hours about 50% of infarcts will show as areas of low density. During the next week this figure increases to about 75%. Low density areas are initially ill-defined, but later become more clearly demarcated, often showing localisation to classical territories of arterial supply or to their watershed regions. *Tumours* may be seen in plain scans as localised areas of increased or reduced density, depending on tissue density, haemorrhage, cyst formation or oedema. In tumours, and many other lesions, *abnormalities of blood-brain barrier function* will be present, permitting better visualisation by contrast enhancement. This is the production of change in CT density by the administration of contrast medium, usually iodine-containing compounds. When given intravenously, the contrast medium causes increased scan density (white) in areas of the brain where blood vessels are abnormally permeable. Various patterns of increased density may be seen. Peripheral (ring) enhancement is often observed around abscesses, tumours and haematomas, and is related to local oedema. Irregular or partial enhancement is most common with gliomas, while homogeneous enhancement may occur with many lesions, neoplastic or vascular.

Magnetic resonance imaging

Following the first report[5] of cerebral pathology being demonstrable by nuclear magnetic resonance (NMR: or magnetic resonance imaging, MRI), great advances have been seen in the application of this non-invasive and apparently harmless means of visualising the nervous system for the study of brain disease. MRI is superior to X-ray CT scanning in some respects. It is free of artefacts due to bone images, and has given excellent pictures of posterior fossa structures. The contrast between grey matter and white matter is also excellent, and the visualisation of white matter is so good that small areas of demyelination can be easily demonstrated. This property is of diagnostic value in multiple sclerosis.[6,7] The spinal cord can be well studied. The cord at foramen magnum level is clearly shown, as it is at all levels, without contrast media being required. In MRI imaging, contrast can be enhanced when necessary by the use of gadolinium compounds,[8] though even without these it is easy to show small tumours and early infarcts[9] in the cerebrum. The capacity of MRI to show myelin has enabled the normal developmental process of myelination to be visualised in vivo.[10] With increasing use of this technology, which can supply very fine images of cerebral parenchymal disease, there has been renewed interest on the part of clinicians in correlative neuropathology. While, at the macroscopic level, brain slices may show a strikingly similar picture to MRI scans, rewarding new data are likely to come from microscopic evaluation of MRI scan abnormalities.

HISTOLOGICAL METHODS IN SURGICAL AND AUTOPSY NEUROPATHOLOGY

The methods of the well-equipped histopathology department are appropriate for neuropathological diagnosis and research, though older neuropathological methods,[11] including celloidin embedding and metallic impregnation, are still of specialised use.

Tissue preparation

Surgical neuropathological diagnostic methods, in

the main, are today identical to those of general histopathology. The requirements for paraffin sectioning of autopsy brain tissue do, however, differ from those for other tissues. Cerebral parenchyma is soft and unsupported by collagenous connective tissue. During dehydration it is thus more prone than many tissues to shrinkage artefact. A slow processing schedule, with passage of samples through graded alcohols over a longer than usual period (48 hours is satisfactory for medium-sized brain samples) is desirable if good results are to be assured.

Another special requirement is the capacity to cut large and relatively thick sections. Large sections, on slides of 10 × 8 cm or even more, are occasionally needed to display the anatomy of an abnormal hemisphere or lobe, while thick sections, in the range of 15 to 30 μm, show myelin and cerebral cortical nerve cell layers to advantage. Celloidin formerly met these needs; they are now satisfied by the use of special flexible embedding wax mixtures (e.g. one composed of equal parts of ordinary paraffin wax, beeswax and pink dental wax).

Staining

The stain which is of most general use in neuropathology, as in general histopathology, is *haematoxylin-eosin*. This enables the nuclei of nerve cells and of the different types of neuroglia to be distinguished (Fig. 4.1), highlights myelin

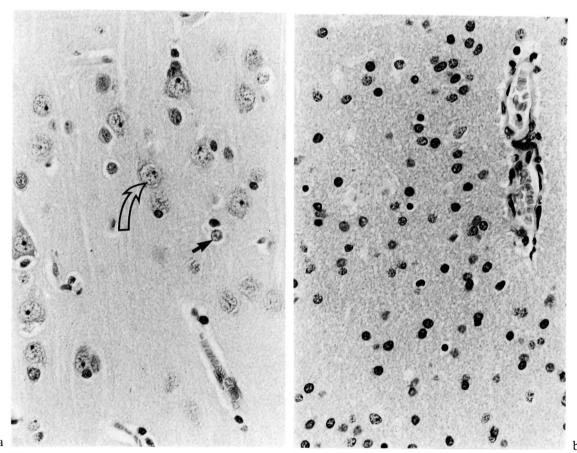

a

b

Fig. 4.1a, b Histology of normal brain. (**a**) Cerebral cortex showing neurons with large vesicular nuclei and prominent nucleoli (open arrow). Astrocyte nucleus (closed arrow). Oligodendrocyte nuclei are smaller and denser than the astrocyte nuclei. Large amounts of neuropil separate the nuclei. (**b**) Cerebral white matter showing the granular appearance of myelin and the well-separated oligodendrocyte and astrocyte nuclei.
Haematoxylin-eosin × 385

because of its eosinophilia, and shows connective tissue and blood vessels clearly. Some neuronal perikarya are well shown, but axons, dendrites and glial processes are poorly differentiated.

Next in value for the neuropathologist is the *Luxol fast blue-cresyl violet* stain (Klüver–Barrera method). On its own, Luxol fast blue gives myelin a rather watery colour, but this is much intensified by the cresyl violet counterstain, which also demonstrates nuclei. The chemical composition of histologically processed central myelin is different from that of peripheral myelin, producing a different affinity for PAS;[12] it may sometimes be advantageous to combine the Klüver–Barrera method with PAS, staining peripheral myelin royal blue and central myelin turquoise.

The *Bodian* method stains nerve processes well, and is used on paraffin brain sections to show axons and dendrites and the senile plaques and neurofibrillary degeneration of Alzheimer's disease. In peripheral nerve sections, a Bodian counterstain to Luxol fast blue-cresyl violet can show axons inside myelin sheaths. Some neuropathologists prefer alternative silver impregnation methods for paraffin sections, notably the Palmgren, Holmes, and Glees and Marsland techniques.

To show astrocytes, most neuropathologists relied, until comparatively recently, on the *Holzer* crystal violet dye impregnation method, which was smelly and capricious. Although it could show astrocyte processes clearly, and produced beautiful birefringence under crossed polarizers to indicate ultrastructural periodicity, it could not be combined with other stains. This method has been largely superseded by *immunoperoxidase staining* using antisera to glial fibrillary acidic protein (GFAP). Staining for GFAP is more sensitive and reliable a technique for showing astrocytes than Holzer or other dye techniques. It is fair to say that GFAP immunostaining is of unique value, and that no other antibody technique has made a comparable contribution to the microscopic study of brain tissue.

Antibodies to neurofilaments, to myelin basic protein and to carbonic anhydrase (present in oligodendroglia and choroid plexus), to lymphoid cells, to endothelial cells, and to non-specific proteins present in the nervous system, such as S100 and enolase, may all be of diagnostic use in neuropathology. The list can be extended to include peptide hormone antibodies (of great importance in the diagnosis of pituitary tumours and occasionally of value in studying neural lesions) and epithelial intermediate filament markers (useful—but not infallible[13]—in helping to distinguish secondary carcinoma from malignant glioma).

Special Techniques

The areas where special techniques remain indispensible to neuropathologists are limited, but important. On the surgical side, expertise in the diagnostic use of brain smears is desirable, while special methods are required for the examination of biopsy specimens of peripheral nerve and of muscle. A few other techniques for brain tissue also deserve mention.

Frozen sections and smears

Frozen section diagnosis is demanded of all surgical neuropathology services. Some pathologists like to prepare smears of a small sample of fresh tumour tissue and make a cytological diagnosis. In experienced hands, this approach gives rapid and accurate results, and avoidable diagnostic errors are rare.[14,15] The technique, first used in Harvey Cushing's service,[16] was developed 50 years ago by Dorothy Russell[17,18] and has survived in an era in which cryostat sections have become the routine means of rapid diagnosis. Smears give better cytology, but lack most of the architectural features of the parent tumour. Small tissue samples are squashed between two microscope slides which are then steadily drawn apart so as to produce an even smear. Preparations are fixed immediately, while still moist, in alcohol, and can then be stained by a variety of methods, the use of 1% toluidine blue for one minute being generally preferred. Under the microscope, normal cellular constituents of the nervous system can be readily identified, and the experienced observer can use distinctive cytological characteristics to diagnose astrocytomas and other classes of glial tumours, medulloblastoma, meningioma, schwannoma (neurilemmoma), metastases and indeed most types of brain neoplasms (see Ch. 16).

Peripheral nerves

Special handling of peripheral nerves is necessary both because of their fragility and because of the need for specialised clinicopathological correlation. Fresh nerves are easily damaged, and in order to avoid artefacts, it is essential that biopsy samples are handled as little as possible before fixation, which preferably is carried out with the specimen aligned on a piece of card. Nerves may be fixed in formalin and/or osmium tetroxide for paraffin embedding and sectioning, or in glutaraldehyde for electron microscopy. For routine histological evaluation resin-embedded glutaraldehyde-fixed sections of transversely cut nerve are recommended, stained by toluidine blue or other methods.[19] Electron microscopy can be carried out if required. Formalin fixation does not give as detailed a picture, but enables whole nerves to be examined, is better for the assessment of inflammatory or vascular changes, and—after osmication—allows maceration in glycerine and teasing for single fibre examination. The full evaluation of a peripheral nerve may include quantitation of fibre diameters and internodal lengths in whole cross-sections and teased fibres respectively. Nerves taken at autopsy require similar handling. It is sometimes necessary at autopsy to take extensive peripheral nerve samples, and if a neuropathy affects autonomic function clinically, it is important that sympathetic nerves and ganglia, and sometimes parasympathetic ganglia, are also sampled, with recourse to anatomy books if needed.

Muscle

Muscle biopsy histological technique is still strongly influenced by enzyme histochemistry,[20] for which cryostat sectioning is required. Open biopsy is generally preferred, although the value of percutaneous needle biopsy of muscle in pathological diagnosis is well established.[21] Surgical biopsy samples are generally 'rested' on card for 15 minutes before fixation or freezing, so as to avoid contraction artefacts. Formalin fixation enables inflammatory and vascular changes to be well seen, but usually produces some distortion of architecture, evident even in perfectly orientated transverse and longitudinal sections. Standard stains such as haematoxylin and eosin are used; a diagnostic immunocytochemical approach to the evaluation of muscle disease has not yet been developed. Frozen sections contain less artefact, and permit fibre typing through the use of myosin ATPase at varying pH, NADH-tetrazolium reductase, myophosphorylase and other enzyme histochemical markers of oxidative or glycolytic activity. Autopsy samples of muscle may also give satisfactory results with cryostat sectioning and enzyme histochemistry, provided they are taken within 24 hours of death.

Degenerating myelin

Finally, the need in neurohistology for identifying degenerate myelin should be noted. The recognition of myelin breakdown products in Wallerian (axonal) degeneration is of some importance since it may enable fibre tracts to be mapped out and neural connections to be demonstrated. The change in chemical composition of myelin involves the release of fatty acids from degraded phospholipid nerve sheaths and the esterification of cholesterol; the cholesterol esters can be demonstrated in frozen sections by fat stains. The classical though uncertain Marchi technique[22] is based on the fact that, after oxidation with potassium dichromate, normal myelin lipids will not react with osmium tetroxide, whereas fatty acids in the cholesterol esters are unaffected by prior dichromate treatment and will still reduce osmium tetroxide. The use of specially selected tissue blocks is necessary, and abnormal myelin products are optimally shown over a rather narrow period of months after the physical breakdown of degenerating nerves. Moreover, only low-power microscopic information can be obtained from Marchi slides. For these reasons, some pathologists prefer alternative means of showing degenerate nerve fibres, and the silver technique of Nauta has its advocates.[23]

AUTOPSY TECHNIQUES IN NEUROPATHOLOGY

Careful autopsy technique is necessary for optimal preservation and comprehensive sampling of the nervous system post mortem. Brain tissue is so soft that it can easily be damaged to a degree which prevents full diagnostic assessment. Some parts of the nervous system are relatively inaccessible and need particularly careful dissection.

Removal of the brain

Removal of the brain from the adult skull is straightforward, with practice. Following reflection of the scalp and cutting of the temporal muscles, a saw cut is made through the frontal bones and backwards through the squamous temporal bones to a point above and behind the ears. Another saw cut is then made at an angle of about 160°, starting at the occiput and joining up with the first cut. The operator must avoid cutting the dura and lacerating the brain. The dura is separated from the inside of the calvarium, which is then removed to expose the superior longitudinal sinus and dural surface of the brain. After the dura is incised and reflected, the cerebral convolutions can be examined for superficial abnormality. By gentle retraction of the frontal lobes, the cranial nerves down to the facial nerve can be exposed and cut, together with the internal carotid arteries. Next the tentorium is cut, on either side, along its line of attachment to the petrous temporal and occipital bones, freeing the contents of the posterior fossa. The lower cranial nerves and vertebral arteries can then be divided, and the cervical cord can be cut at or close to the level of the foramen magnum. It is now possible to remove the entire brain from the backward tilted skull. It is essential at this stage to avoid traction on the brainstem. Disruption of midbrain and adjacent structures is only too easy. 'Rupture of the cerebral peduncles', once a popular forensic pathologists' diagnosis in head injury cases, is a frequent outcome of careless removal of the brain. The appearances of the cerebrospinal fluid should be noted during this procedure, and the base of the skull should be inspected, the venous sinuses examined, and, where necessary, the dura stripped off the base in the search for a fracture. Trigeminal ganglia and internal auditory meatuses may require special examination.

The external state of the brain should be described, and any meningeal abnormality, and any asymmetry, swelling, softening, atrophy or focal lesions of the brain itself recorded as a preliminary to post-fixation study. The brain is weighed, and fixed (see below). In cases of subarachnoid haemorrhage due to rupture of an arterial aneurysm, dissection of the circle of Willis in the fresh state may be preferred.

Removal of the spinal cord

Removal of the spinal cord is preferably done from the front. After thoracic and abdominal evisceration, an anterior wedge of the vertebral column from high cervical to low lumbar region is taken out by sawing through the pedicles so as to expose the spinal canal. Nerve roots and dural sleeves are divided, and the cord can be removed in its entirety, down to and including the cauda equina. Occasionally, it may be necessary to preserve continuity of brain and cord, in which case spinal dissection should precede removal of the brain, which can then be extracted with cord attached. Spinal ganglia are often required for study, and it should be remembered that, apart from sacral ones, which are in the spinal canal, they are situated in the intervertebral foramina, just beyond the point where the nerve roots perforate the dura, and require specific dissection.

Alternative procedure for removal and fixation of the spinal cord. The spine, with the cord in situ, can be removed in its entirety and fixed in formalin for two to three weeks before sawing through bone and extracting the cord.[23] Although damage to the soft and vulnerable unfixed cord is avoided in this way, the need to reconstitute the backbone of the corpse with a wooden support makes this an unattractive method.

Fractures of the cervical spine. It may be desirable to remove just the cervical spine for the examination of fractures (see p. 144).

Examination of other parts

Removal of the pituitary is easy after the circumference of the diaphragma sellae is cut, and should be carried out in all cases. Examination of the inner ears necessitates chiselling into the petrous temporal bones. Dissection of the orbits and paranasal sinuses may be necessary in some cases.

DISSECTION OF THE BRAIN AND SPINAL CORD

Dissection of the brain

Dissection of the brain is sometimes carried out in the fresh, unfixed state. This may be expedient in some routine non-neurological and Coroner's autopsies, and is necessary where tissue samples are needed for biochemical or microbiological study. The softness of the unfixed brain precludes detailed naked eye examination. Only major structures can be seen with certainty, and it is clear that small lesions may be missed. Whenever possible, therefore, the brain should be fixed to facilitate careful study. Fixation is reliably achieved by suspension in 10% neutral buffered formalin in a vessel of several litres capacity. If a piece of string is passed between the pons and basilar artery, and its ends are tied to the sides of the container, the brain can be suspended above the bottom of the vessel. It may be necessary to renew the formalin after a few days. Within a week, the brain may be adequately fixed and hardened, though many neuropathologists prefer to wait for 10 days to 4 weeks before cutting it. The spinal cord is fixed for a similar length of time, either suspended vertically in a tank, or laid horizontally in a tray.

The fixed brain should be carefully re-examined externally before it is dissected. Lack of symmetry of the cerebral hemispheres should be noted. Minor asymmetry is normal, but localised swelling, as occurs over a small tumour or recent infarct, and areas of cortical loss, as seen with old infarcts or with contusions (especially subfrontal and anterior temporal ones) can be overlooked. Generalised hemispheric swelling produces flat gyri and shallow sulci, and should prompt the pathologist to look externally for evidence of tentorial (uncal) herniation and occipital infarction, resulting from compression of the posterior cerebral artery by the herniated temporal tissue. Cortical atrophy, with deep sulci and blade-like gyri, is also readily recognisable.

The meninges should be examined for the presence of subarachnoid blood or purulent exudate. While examining the base of the brain, the basal meninges, cerebral vessels, cranial nerves and cerebellum can all be inspected.

There are a number of methods of dissection, the purpose of which should be to display the internal anatomy of the brain in a standardised manner in a thorough search for lesions and preparatory to taking photographs and tissue sampling for histology. Clinicopathological correlation is the basic purpose of sophisticated brain dissection. In the past it has been customary to slice the cerebral hemispheres in a coronal plane. This is technically simple, and anatomical structures and relations are well displayed. Coronal slices, being the traditional means of showing the internal anatomy of the brain, are easy to understand. However, correlation of brain pathology with CT scans may now necessitate horizontal sectioning. While correlation of scan appearances with horizontal brain slices is often gratifyingly successful, it must be said that with much important brain anatomy crowded into the lower half of the cerebrum, adequate display of basal structures may be hard to achieve. Nevertheless, the pathologist should familiarise himself with dissection of the cerebrum in a horizontal plane.

An easy way to dissect the fixed brain for coronal display is as follows. First the brain is held vertex downwards, and the meninges and basilar artery over the upper pons are cut so as to expose the isthmus of the pons. The oculomotor nerves are pushed down, towards the floor of the third ventricle, and then a horizontal scalpel cut is made from the interpeduncular fossa through the isthmus, separating pons, medulla and cerebellum from midbrain and cerebrum. Posterior fossa structures are put aside, and a second horizontal scalpel cut, starting at the corpora quadrigemina, is made, producing a 3–4 mm thick block of midbrain, with attached oculomotor nerves. With the cerebrum still held vertex down, a vertical cut is made with a large flat-bladed knife just anterior to the mamillary bodies, dividing the cerebral hemisphere into anterior and posterior halves. The flat surface of one half is placed on the cutting board, and the lowest 1·5 cm sliced off by a knife stroke parallel to the board. The remainder of the brain is cut in this way. Slices can be made at a slight angle if necessary to compensate for minor asymmetry. They are then laid out in a standard manner, with posterior surfaces uppermost so that the right side is on the examiner's right. Systematic examination of the cut surface of the slices involves: further general inspection for major lesions and herniations, followed by examination of the meninges; scrutiny of the cortical ribbon for such lesions as small infarcts or scars; examination of white matter for oedema, lacunae, or—particularly around ventricles—plaques of demyelination; inspection of central grey structures; and inspection of the ventricles, for marked asymmetry or abnormal size. Arteries can be well seen in these slices.

Dissection of the contents of the posterior fossa can be done in one of two ways, depending on whether brainstem or fourth ventricular anatomy is more important in the case under study. If good anatomical preparations of pons and medulla are required, angled vertical cuts should be made through the cerebellar peduncles to separate brainstem from cerebellum. The main axis of the brainstem is curved, and the best tissue blocks can be obtained only by cutting at right angles to this axis. To achieve this, the brainstem is held with its concavity upwards, and slightly wedged cuts, 3–4 mm apart, are made. The cerebellum is then bisected through the vermis. Cerebellar tissue blocks for microscopy can be taken from the exposed vermis, and from the hemispheres by cutting vertically at right angles to the folia, so as to present the Purkinje cell dendritic trees en face in sections. When display of the fourth ventricle, surrounded by cerebellar white matter, deep nuclei and cortex, is more important, it is achieved simply by bisecting the cerebellum horizontally at its broadest point rather than by separating the brainstem from the cerebellum, which disrupts ventricular anatomy.

The general techniques of dissection outlined here will be applicable in most cases. However, it may be necessary to modify the approach in some instances, so as to display tumours or normal structures to best advantage and in the context of clinico-pathological or radiological correlation.

Dissection of the fixed spinal cord

This is a comparatively simple matter. The dura is cut with scissors in mid-dorsal and mid-ventral lines. It is necessary to identify the upper end of the specimen (the roots slope downwards), and the front and back of the cord; the single grey–pink anterior spinal artery contrasts with the venous plexus and the longitudinal ridges of the dorsal columns on the posterior aspect of the cord. Segmental levels can be identified as the lowest anterior root emerging from the cervical enlargement, C8, contrasts in its substantial breadth at its origin with the thin adjacent T1 anterior root. The cord can then be transected serially at segmental levels, cutting between the origins of the roots and avoiding cutting the roots themselves.

GROSS EXAMINATION OF THE BRAIN AND SPINAL CORD—SUMMARY GUIDE

It is convenient at this point to summarise what should be sought in the gross examination of the brain and spinal cord.

Brain

1. Weight and size: are these within normal limits?
2. External surface
   a. Symmetry: is one hemisphere abnormally large or small, or flattened?
   b. Swelling or atrophy: are gyri and sulci normal?
   c. Herniation: if swelling is present, is there uncal or parahippocampal grooving?
   d. Softening: check suspicious areas for palpable softening.
   e. Focal abnormality: tumours, infarcts, contusions, subfrontal plaques jaunes, etc.?
   f. Meninges: pus in sulci, haemorrhage?
   g. Blood vessels at base: atheroma, haemorrhage? Dissect off circle of Willis if subarachnoid haemorrhage due to rupture of an aneurysm is present.
3. Cut surface
   a. In all cases, systematically inspect coronal cerebral slices for state of: meninges, cortical ribbon, white matter, central grey matter, and ventricles. Small lesions are often detected in this way. Check symmetry: swelling may be associated with ventricular compression and cingulate

herniation and be due to a relatively small lesion. Note the state of the cut arteries in sulci.

b. Where a gross lesion is present, note appearance, dimensions, and structures affected.

Spinal Cord

1. External surface
   a. Swelling or atrophy of cord: is a localised abnormality visible? Are dorsal columns normal?
   b. Softening or induration: is a localised lesion palpable?
   c. State of roots: are anterior roots brown and shrunken compared with posterior roots? Are any of the roots swollen? Check cauda equina.
   d. Meninges: is meningitis or haemorrhage present?
   e. Blood vessels.
2. Cut surface
   Check for normal appearances of white matter surrounding H-shaped grey matter. Degenerating fibre tracts appear chalky white against a creamy background. Note site, appearance and dimensions of any localised lesion.

TISSUE SAMPLING FOR MICROSCOPY

The minimum requirements in post mortem brain microscopy are samples of a lesion, with a rim of normal tissue; or—when no lesion is evident—a tissue block that will include all normal neural structures. An indispensible block is that taken from the mid-temporal region, which in coronal slices includes the hippocampus and the lower part of the lobe. This block contains cortex and white matter, large and small neurons, and includes the Sommer sector—selectively vulnerable to hypoxia—and a neuronal population that readily shows senile and viral changes.

Proper investigative sampling requires much more tissue. If a brain is to be fully evaluated, it is necessary to take a minimum of 13 samples, namely: frontal lobe, basal ganglia, temporal lobe (as above), thalamus, occipital lobe, midbrain, three levels of pons, cerebellum, two levels of medulla, and cervical cord. Samples from a cerebral hemisphere for paraffin processing can be of generous size, so as to fit onto slides wider than the standard 7.5×2.5 cm. In order to prevent distortion of the large blocks during processing, they should be approximately 1 cm thick rather than the more normal $0.2-0.3$ cm. Thick blocks need modification of the timing of steps in the embedding procedure.

For spinal cord microscopy, slices from representative cervical, dorsal, lumbar and sacral segments should be sampled for sectioning, preferably after the left or right side has been identified by writing on the block with waterproof ink or producing a needle hole. Sampling of spinal roots and ganglia is desirable in most cases. The need for comprehensive examination of nerve and muscle in appropriate cases, already referred to, is self-evident.

REFERENCES

1. Bannister R, ed. Brain's Clinical neurology. 6th ed. Oxford: Oxford University Press, 1984.
2. Matthews WB. Practical neurology. 3rd ed. Oxford: Blackwell, 1975.
3. Patten J. Neurological differential diagnosis. London: Starke, 1977.
4. Kendall B. In: Swash M, Kennard C, eds. Scientific basis of clinical neurology. Edinburgh: Churchill Livingstone, 1985: 739.
5. Hawkes RC, Holland GN, Moore WS, Worthington BS. J Comput Assist Tomogr 1980; 4: 577.
6. Doyle FH, Gore JC, Pennock JM et al. Lancet 1981; ii: 53.
7. Young IR, Hall AS, Pallis CA, Bydder GM, Legg NJ, Steiner RE. Lancet 1981; ii: 1063.
8. Carr DH, Brown J, Bydder GM et al. Lancet 1984; i: 484.
9. Sipponen JT, Kaste M, Ketonen L, Sepponen RE, Katevuo K, Sivula A. J Comput Assist Tomogr 1983; 7: 585.
10. Johnson MA, Pennock JM, Bydder GM. Am J Roentgenol 1983; 141: 1005.
11. Russell DS. Histological technique for intracranial tumours. London: Oxford University Press, 1939.
12. Feigin L, Cravioto H. J Neuropath Exp Neurol 1961; 20: 245.
13. Rubinstein LJ. Neuropathol Appl Neurobiol 1986; 12: 523.

14. Adams JH, Graham DI, Doyle D. Brain biopsy. London: Chapman and Hall, 1981.
15. Barnard RO. In: Koss LG, Coleman DV, eds. Advances in clinical cytology. London: Butterworth, 1981: 254.
16. Eisenhardt L, Cushing H. Am J Pathol 1930; 6: 541.
17. Russell DS, Krayenbuhl H, Cairns H. J Pathol Bacteriol 1937; 45: 501.
18. Russell DS. In: Dyke SC. Recent advances in clinical pathology. London: Churchill, 1947: 418.
19. Weller RO, Cervós-Navarro J. Pathology of peripheral nerves. London: Butterworth, 1977.
20. Dubowitz V. Muscle biopsy: a practical approach. 2nd ed. Eastbourne: Baillière Tindall, 1985.
21. Edwards RHT, Lewis PD, Maunder C, Pearse AGE. Lancet 1973; ii: 1070.
22. Smith MC. J Neurol Neurosurg Psychiatry 1956; 19: 74.
23. Hughes JT. Pathology of the spinal cord. 2nd ed. London: Lloyd-Luke, 1978.

Vascular disease and hypoxic brain damage

INTRODUCTION

'*Stroke*' is the clinical term that describes the sudden onset of a focal neurological deficit which is due to vascular disease and lasts for more than 24 hours. Whereas in clinical practice the cause of stroke is often uncertain, it is usually attributed by the pathologist to either *infarction* or *haemorrhage*. Despite the difficulties of comparing clinical and pathological material, prospective epidemiological studies such as that at Framingham, Massachusetts, USA,[1] have provided much useful information about the morbidity, mortality and pathogenesis of cerebrovascular disease. In the United Kingdom, as in other developed countries, it is now clear that cerebrovascular disease constitutes a major health problem, accounting for some 10% of all deaths, being surpassed only by heart disease and cancer. It has been estimated that about 500 000 new strokes occur annually in the USA, about half of which result in death. In those patients who survive, about 50% are permanently disabled and only 10% return to normal activity. Although strokes are more common in the elderly, it has been shown that some 30% of the estimated two million cases of disability following stroke in the USA are between the ages of 35 and 65 years.

Indeed 'strokes' occur in patients of all ages— including neonates, infants, children and young adults.

Estimates of the major causes of cerebrovascular disease are uncertain and vary depending upon the source of the information. However, data from the Framingham study suggest that some 84% are due to infarction (53% thrombotic and 31% embolic), leaving some 16% due to haemorrhage (10% with intracerebral haemorrhage and 6% with subarachnoid haemorrhage from a ruptured intracranial aneurysm).[1] The epidemiology of stroke, however, is complex, depending upon secular trends, accuracy of death certificate data, incidence, and regional differences in mortality and incidence.[2] Estimates of the various causes of stroke are therefore somewhat variable.

There is general agreement that reductions in death and disability from cerebrovascular disease will be due largely to prevention rather than to more effective medical or surgical treatment. Hence considerable resources have been used in the identification of factors that increase the *risk* of stroke. In this respect atheroma and hypertension have been shown to play dominant rôles, with lesser contributions from raised serum lipids and diabetes mellitus. Other important risk factors include coronary heart disease, cardiac failure and atrial fibrillation, with lesser contributions from a raised haematocrit, which increases viscosity and reduces cerebral blood flow. Open surgery on the heart and great vessels of the neck, and certain medications such as oral contraceptives also increase the risk of a stroke. Various environmental factors have also been incriminated and include cigarette smoking, diet, obesity, whether the drinking water is hard or soft, coffee drinking, alcohol consumption, stress, physical activity and the climate. Factors that predispose to spontaneous intracranial haemorrhage include congenital anomalies, vascular malformations, hypertension, arteritis and bleeding diatheses.

STRUCTURAL CHANGES RESULTING FROM VASCULAR DISEASE AND HYPOXIA

Histological changes may be limited to neurons (selective neuronal necrosis) or may extend to involve glia and blood vessels (infarction).

Neuronal necrosis

Studies in experimental animals and human material have shown that the *ischaemic cell process* is the neuropathological common denominator in all types of vascular disease (see Ch. 2).[3,4]

The time course of the ischaemic cell process is relatively constant for individual groups of neurons but varies according to their size and site, so that the interval between the hypoxic episode and death, if between 2 and 24 hours, can be assessed with reasonable accuracy. The ischaemic cell process is a vital process and can only develop, therefore, in the event of re-oxygenation and/or the restoration of some blood flow, viz. through the collateral circulation or by the disintegration of an embolus, or after successful resuscitation following cardiac arrest. The identification of neuronal changes which are attributable unequivocally to hypoxia, however, is difficult in the human brain because of post-mortem *histological artefact*. Such artefact results partly from autolysis, which takes place between death and the post-mortem examination, partly from slow penetration of the fixative in which the brain is immersed and partly from defects in the processing of the tissue. The commonest artefacts are 'dark cells', 'hydropic cells', 'perineuronal' and 'perivascular' spaces[4,5] and the features of 'respirator brain' (see p. 59–60).[6,7]

The frequency of post-mortem artefacts in the human brain after hypoxia is not proportional to the intensity of the hypoxic stress; furthermore, the distribution of artefacts does not coincide with the selectively vulnerable regions.[8] Artefacts tend to be more numerous on the surface of the brain, while neurons undergoing the ischaemic cell process are more numerous beneath the surface. Artefacts moreover do not change with time. It must be emphasised that any evidence of the ischaemic cell process or of a vital reaction in a specimen showing the features of 'respirator brain' must be interpreted as having preceded the onset of clinical brain death.

If there is only a minimal amount of neuronal damage, there will not be any associated changes in the other tissue elements of the brain. Greater amounts of neuronal damage will be accompanied by reactive changes that may continue for weeks or months after the hypoxic episode. For example, the amount of astrocyte proliferation is usually proportional to the degree of neuronal loss, whereas the changes in oligodendrocytes are slight and may amount to no more than 'acute swelling'. On the other hand, proliferation and hypertrophy of microglia are common and often it is an awareness of the increased numbers of these cells, rather than the neuronal changes, that indicates irreversible damage. Microglia may develop into macrophages within the original locus of tissue destruction. In selective neuronal necrosis the blood vessels appear normal. Changes in white matter are limited if neuronal damage is minimal.

Cerebral infarction[9,10]

Infarcts range in size from a few millimetres to those affecting an entire arterial territory. The *macroscopic* appearances depend upon the size of the lesion and the survival time of the patient. Recent infarcts (1–2 days old) are slightly soft and swollen: indeed a large infarct may swell sufficiently to act as an intracranial expanding

lesion (Fig. 5.1). The lesion may be *anaemic* or *haemorrhagic*, depending upon whether or not some blood flow through the infarct has been restored and upon whether necrosis of vessel walls has occurred, thus allowing extravasation of blood into the necrotic tissue (Fig. 5.1). An intensely haemorrhagic infarct may superficially resemble a haematoma but the distinctive feature of a haemorrhagic infarct is the preservation of intrinsic brain architecture within it.

Microscopic abnormalities by 4–6 hours consist of irregular blotchy pallor of histological staining. Within grey matter the outlines of dead neurons are easily recognisable (Fig. 5.2). Thereafter there is loss of cytoplasmic basophilia until a barely detectable ghost cell remains. Incrustations are not seen in the central region of the infarct but frequently occur at its edges. By about 12–15 hours the neuropil is spongy, due to a combination of swelling of astrocytic processes and axons. A sharp and often irregular line of demarcation between normal and abnormal myelin appears in the white matter between 18 and 24 hours (Fig. 5.3). In a haemorrhagic infarct there is a variable amount of haemorrhage. Polymorphs may be numerous at the edge of an infarct by 24 hours, but macrophages first appear in infarcts in the human brain after 4–5 days and are thought to be derived from circulating blood monocytes and indigenous microglia. As survival time increases, the infarcted tissue becomes rarified due to oedema and loss of

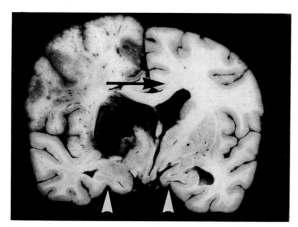

Fig. 5.1 Cerebral infarction. Large 3-day-old swollen infarct in territories of left middle and anterior cerebral arteries. Part of the infarct is 'anaemic' and part is 'haemorrhagic'. Note the asymmetry of the lateral ventricles, the displacement of the midline structures to the right, the supracallosal hernia to the right (black arrow) and deep grooving (white arrows) along the line of tentorial hernia.
Reproduced by permission of the editor from: Graham DI. J Clin Pathol 1977; 30 suppl (R Coll Pathol) 11: 170.

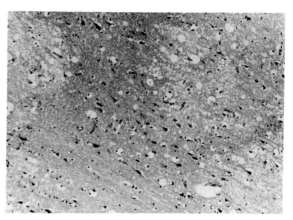

Fig. 5.2 Cerebral infarction. 15-hour-old infarct in cerebral cortex. There is irregular pallor (infarction) of staining of the affected areas.
Haematoxylin-eosin × 330

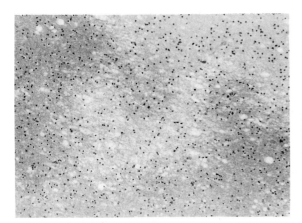

Fig. 5.3 Cerebral infarction. 24-hour-old infarct in white matter. There is a sharply defined border between the abnormal (pale) and normal white matter. Haematoxylin-eosin × 85

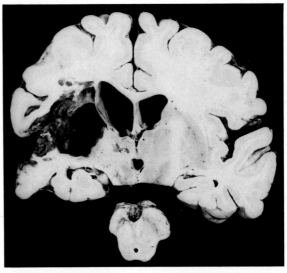

Fig. 5.5 Cerebral infarction. 18-month-old infarct in the distribution of the middle cerebral artery of the left cerebral hemisphere. The necrotic tissue has been removed and there is ipsilateral enlargement of the lateral ventricle.

myelin; after about 7 days destruction of myelin can be recognised by the presence of Sudan-positive lipid droplets. There is an associated reactive astrocytosis and within 1–2 weeks the infarct becomes extremely soft and swelling resolves. Affected grey matter may already be slightly shrunken and granular. Large numbers of macrophages by this time are present throughout the infarct (Fig. 5.4). If the patient survives for several months or more, the necrotic tissue is removed and the lesion ultimately becomes shrunken and cystic (Fig. 5.5). The cysts are often traversed by small vessels and glial processes; some macrophages are usually present for years. If the infarct is in a cerebral hemisphere, the loss of

tissue is usually accompanied by dilatation of the adjacent lateral ventricle. The walls of some cysts are orange–brown in colour because of blood pigments. The outer wall of a cyst or slit in the cerebral cortex may consist only of pia and the heavily gliotic first layer of the cortex. Tissue shrinkage may occur without cyst formation when there is retention of the overall architecture of the tissue as is commonly seen, for example, in lobular sclerosis of the cerebellum (Fig. 5.6), in certain laminae of the cerebral cortex and in the hippo-campus.

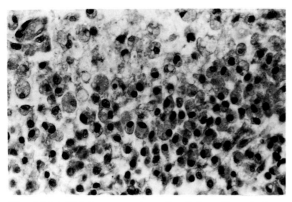

Fig. 5.4 Lipid-laden macrophages in a 5-day-old cerebral infarct. Haematoxylin-eosin × 330

VASCULAR DISORDERS

Arterial blood supply to the brain

Blood reaches the brain through four large arteries—the paired internal carotid arteries which supply most of the cerebral hemispheres, and the paired vertebral arteries which supply the brainstem and cerebellum. At the base of the brain the carotid and vertebral arteries are connected by the anterior and posterior communicating arteries to form the circle of Willis. The circle of Willis ensures, through its communicating arteries, a well-distributed flow of blood to the brain. The

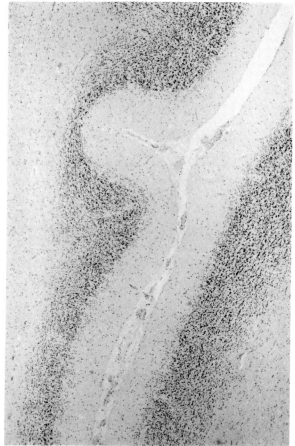

Fig. 5.6 Lobular atrophy of cerebellum. In the affected folia there is widespread loss of Purkinje cells, almost complete loss of the granular layer and gliosis. Haematoxylin-eosin × 70

configuration of the circle of Willis is an important determinant of both the size and location of any ischaemic damage: in only some 50% of adults is the circle of Willis said to be anatomically 'normal';[11] there is an even higher incidence of variation in patients with cerebral infarcts post mortem.[12] An important variant is found in some 10% of patients, in whom the circulation through the posterior cerebral arteries is derived from the internal carotid arteries via the posterior communicating arteries rather than from the basilar artery.

The superficial branches of the cerebral arteries spread over the surface of the brain in the subarachnoid space before entering the brain as the cortical arteries. The traditional teaching is that the cortical vessels carry with them a pial investment, the space between this sheath and the wall of the vessel—the Virchow–Robin space—being continuous with the subarachnoid space. Recent work, using scanning and transmission electron microscopy, has shown that the pia mater forms a continuous sheet which separates the cerebrospinal fluid (CSF) in the subarachnoid space from the subpial and perivascular spaces of the cortex.[13,14] The cortical arteries supply the outer portions of the brain including the cortical mantle and the outer portions of white matter. The deeper portions of the cerebral hemispheres are supplied by perforating arteries that arise directly from the circle of Willis and its branches.

The study of occlusive vascular disease has emphasised the rôle of the collateral circulation, but it should be noted that although anastomotic channels link the internal and external carotid territories and the carotid and vertebro-basilar circulations, they are not sufficiently well developed to prevent infarction in the event of occlusion of any one of these vessels. Dependence on adequate cortical perfusion via a collateral circulation arises in the important clinical situations where a major vessel in the neck is severely stenosed or occluded.

Venous drainage of the brain

The superficial veins of the cerebral hemispheres drain into the superior sagittal and transverse sinuses, and thence to the internal jugular veins. Veins from deep within the cerebral hemispheres enter the internal cerebral veins which join to form the great cerebral vein of Galen which drains into the straight sinus. Emissary veins connect the dural venous sinuses with extracranial veins.

The veins of the brain are similar in structure to veins elsewhere, but the dural venous sinuses are unusual in that their endothelial lining abuts directly onto the fibrous tissue of the dural folds. The dural wall of certain sinuses is penetrated by small projections of the arachnoid called arachnoid villi (see p. 32), through which CSF returns to the bloodstream.

Arterial blood supply and venous drainage of the spinal cord

The spinal cord is supplied by three main arterial

trunks—the anterior spinal artery, which is formed inside the skull by the union of the anterior spinal branches of the right and left vertebral arteries, and the paired posterior spinal arteries, each of which is a branch of the corresponding posterior inferior cerebellar artery or of the vertebral artery itself. As these vessels run the length of the spinal cord they are joined at intervals by 7–10 branches of the intercostal and lumbar arteries, prominent among which is the artery of Adamkiewicz at the level of the tenth thoracic vertebra (T10). In the cervical region of the cord, blood flow is downward in the anterior spinal artery, whereas below this level the blood supply to the cord is largely maintained through the intercostal and lumbar vessels.

The venous drainage of the spinal cord corresponds mainly to the arterial supply and there are many anastomoses.

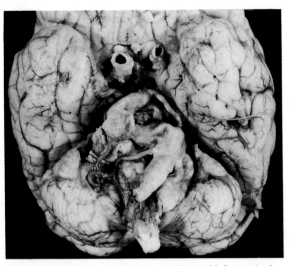

Fig. 5.7 Fusiform aneurysm. The basilar and left vertebral arteries are atheromatous, dilated and tortuous. The right vertebral artery is small.

Practical considerations

In any given patient the causes of a stroke are often complex and multiple, so that the pathologist should be aware that the cerebral circulation may have been adversely affected by disease elsewhere in the body. The respiratory system, the heart and the blood should all, therefore, be assessed. But it is particularly important that the carotid and vertebral arterial trees are examined fully at post mortem. This can best be achieved by post-mortem angiography, but if this facility is not available then the vessels can be examined by extending the usual midline approach into a collar incision which allows dissection of the arch of the aorta and the examination of the full extent of the extra-osseous portions of the carotid and vertebral arteries. The patency of the intra-osseous portions of these vessels can be determined by injecting fluid with a syringe. Removal of the spinal cord from the front greatly facilitates access to the cervical portions of the vertebral arteries in the cervical portion of the spine (see p. 84).

TYPES OF VASCULAR DISEASE

Atheroma (atherosclerosis)

Atheroma is the most common and important arterial disease in adults in developed countries.

As the atheromatous plaques gradually enlarge, they become confluent and encroach upon the lumen of the vessel and may be complicated by calcification, ulceration and thrombus formation.

The cervical and intracranial vessels most commonly affected are the internal carotid and vertebral arteries, followed by the basilar and middle cerebral arteries and then by the posterior inferior cerebellar arteries (Fig. 5.7).[15] Post-mortem studies have established that cerebral atheroma is more common in males than in females between the ages of 40 and 60 years, but after the age of 65 years the incidence is about equal. Geographical studies have shown less atheroma of the cerebral arteries in less developed countries as compared with the population of North America and Europe. Atheroma of the cerebral arteries is usually associated with atheroma in other parts of the body, including the arteries of the limbs. Correlation between the occurrence of coronary artery atheroma and that of cerebral atheroma is usually close, although coronary atheroma tends to be more severe. Occasionally, however, a person with marked atheroma in the aorta and coronary arteries may have little or no disease in the cerebral arteries; the reverse may also be found.

It is important to note that extensive atheroma is not necessarily associated with 'stroke'. It is now recognised that at normal blood pressure the internal cross-sectional area of an artery must be reduced by up to 90% before blood flow is impaired.[16,17] If, however, there is a fall in blood pressure, as may occur with blood loss and as a complication of general anaesthesia or myocardial infarction, flow may be reduced sufficiently to cause ischaemic damage.

Stenosis and occlusion of the extracranial cervical arteries

Atheroma of the internal carotid arteries in the neck[18] and of the cervical vertebral arteries[19,20] is of paramount importance as a cause of strokes. For example, thrombo-embolic occlusion of the *internal carotid artery* may be found in as many as 5% of unselected autopsies.[21,22] Occlusion due to atheroma occurs most commonly in the carotid sinus (Fig. 5.8). The size of any resulting cerebral infarct will be dependent upon a number of factors such as the blood pressure, the efficiency of the

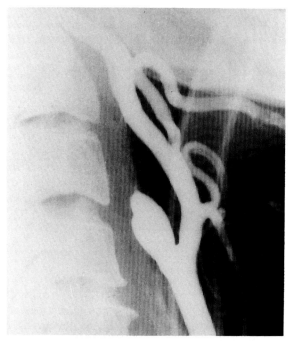

Fig. 5.8 Carotid occlusion. Common carotid arteriogram demonstrating occlusion of the internal carotid artery 1.5 cm above its origin.
Reproduced by permission of Drs Evelyn Teasdale and P. Macpherson, Department of Neuroradiology, Institute of Neurological Sciences, Glasgow, UK.

collateral circulation, and whether the thrombus extends beyond the circle of Willis. Other causes of carotid artery occlusion include embolism, dissecting aneurysm, trauma, blood dyscrasias, the aortic arch syndrome and abscess formation at the base of the skull.[23,24]

Occlusion of an internal carotid artery may be without symptoms or signs, may reveal itself by episodic attacks of transient motor or sensory impairment, or present with a gradual or sudden onset of permanent hemiplegia. Sometimes there is spread of thrombus into one or more of the branches of the circle of Willis; sometimes emboli arise from a thrombus in the internal carotid artery or its branches. Fragmentation and disimpaction of such emboli may explain the transitory character of some symptoms such as transient monocular blindness.[25]

There are five patterns of readily identifiable infarction associated with occlusion or severe stenosis of a carotid artery:

1. There may be massive infarction within the full distribution of the middle cerebral artery and sometimes involving that of the anterior cerebral artery as well (Fig. 5.1). Infarcts of this type were found in 55% of the cases in one series.[26]
2. Infarction of the cortex around the Sylvian (lateral) fissure, with or without involvement of the basal ganglia and the internal capsule.
3. Infarction restricted to the internal capsule (so-called 'capsular infarct').
4. Small infarcts distributed throughout the white matter.
5. Infarction along the boundary zones between the territories of the anterior and middle cerebral arteries (see p. 119).[27]

There may, of course, be no structural brain damage at all in some patients with either severe stenosis or occlusion of one or both carotid arteries.

Obstruction of the *subclavian* and *brachiocephalic arteries* is an insignificant cause of cerebral infarction but is of some clinical importance as a causative factor in *subclavian steal syndrome*.[28] In this condition clinical evidence of cerebral ischaemia may be precipitated by exercise of the upper limbs, thus 'stealing' blood from the basilar artery and the circle of Willis to the subclavian artery distal to an occlusion.

Occlusion of intracranial arteries

The anatomical distribution of arteries in the brain is remarkably constant, and the functional disturbances that result from occlusion of individual branches may be so well defined that one can say with confidence which vessel is affected.

The major portion of the cerebral hemisphere is supplied by the *middle cerebral artery*. This vessel is more often occluded than any other cerebral artery; embolism from the internal carotid artery[29] or the heart is the most frequent cause.

The *anterior cerebral artery* supplies the pole and orbital surface of the frontal lobe, the medial surface of the hemisphere as far back as the parieto-occipital fissure, much of the corpus callosum and part of the striatum. In addition to thrombus formation, the vessel may become occluded by an embolus. There may be a critical reduction in blood flow resulting from arterial spasm in patients with subarachnoid haemorrhage following rupture of an aneurysm of the anterior cerebral or anterior communicating arteries.

The *posterior cerebral artery* supplies the inferior and medial surfaces of the occipital lobe, the posterior half of the thalamus and hippocampal formation, and structures in the upper brainstem and mesencephalon. Infarction within the distribution of this vessel is a common incidental finding post mortem in the elderly. Although this vessel may be occluded by local thrombus formation, infarction within its territory may be secondary either to propagated thrombus or to emboli from the vertebro-basilar system.

Autopsy studies have established that occlusion of one *vertebral artery* may be asymptomatic:[30,31] the most common cause of occlusion, however, is thrombus forming upon atheroma.[32] The vertebral arteries may also be distorted by osteoarthrosis of the cervical spine which, together with atheroma, may be sufficient to cause obstruction following some movements of the neck.[19,33] Other causes of occlusion include subluxation of the atlanto-axial joint in rheumatoid arthritis and as a birth injury following assisted cephalic and breech presentations.

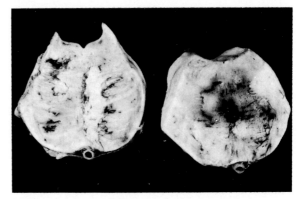

Fig. 5.9 Infarct in brainstem. Transverse section of brainstem from patient who survived 'locked-in' for 22 days after 'stroke'. There is extensive focally haemorrhagic infarction of the pons.

Occlusion of the *basilar artery* is usually due to atheroma.[34,35] Most of the clinical syndromes associated with vertebro-basilar disease are due to ischaemia, either of the hindbrain or of the medial portions of the occipital lobes. In some patients there is extensive infarction of the brainstem and the patient dies, whilst others develop the 'locked-in' syndrome in which a conscious mute patient is completely paralysed apart from eye movements (Fig. 5.9).[36,37]

Another common cause of infarction is compression of vessels by internal herniae in the presence of raised intracranial pressure. For example, it is common for the pericallosal arteries to be compressed, singly or in combination, by a supracallosal hernia; for the anterior choroidal, the posterior cerebral and the superior cerebellar arteries to be compressed by a tentorial hernia; and for the posterior inferior cerebellar arteries to be compressed by a tonsillar hernia (see Figs 3.2, 3.6 and 3.7, pages 66, 69 and 70).

Occlusion of the spinal arteries[38]

This is a common complication of a dissecting aneurysm of the aorta: the pattern of damage is determined by the location of the dissection. The mid and lower thoracic region of the cord is the most vulnerable due to interference of blood flow through the intercostal arteries. Sometimes the whole cord is involved, whilst in other cases the damage is limited to the central grey matter.

Occlusion of the *anterior spinal artery* causes infarction of the ventral half of the upper segments of the cord and is more common than occlusion of a *posterior spinal artery*. Infarction in either or both of these vascular territories may occur without occlusion when it is precipitated by changes in spinal blood flow, as may occur after prolonged hypotension, disease of the aortic ostia of the intercostal or lumbar arteries, embolism following surgery and in association with coarctation of the aorta. There are two principal vascular boundary zones in the cord. One is in the upper thoracic cord between T4 and T7, i.e. between the cervical and radicular circulations, and the other is in the upper lumbar segments where infarction may follow occlusion of the artery of Adamkiewicz at T10.

HYPERTENSION AND THE BRAIN

The pathophysiology of the cerebral circulation in hypertension

The absolute level of cerebral blood flow in the hypertensive patient is the same as in normal individuals, i.e. about 50 ml/100 g/min. During periods of hypotension, however, hypertensive patients develop symptoms of cerebral ischaemia at a higher level of blood pressure than normotensives. This is due to the relative inability of hypertensives to compensate fully for the fall in blood pressure as a result of a 'shift to the right' of the lower limit of autoregulation of cerebral blood flow (Fig. 5.10). This alteration in the pattern of autoregulation is thought to be due to structural changes that occur in hypertension, in which the small arteries and arterioles adapt to the chronically elevated blood pressure and cannot dilate as effectively as those of normotensive individuals. With long-term antihypertensive therapy, however, autoregulation may in some cases re-adapt to normal.[39,40] It has already been noted that hypertensive patients are more vulnerable to cerebral hypoxia during periods of hypotension, as may occur, for example, when they are being treated for accelerated hypertension.[41,42] There is also a 'shift to the right' of the upper limit of autoregulation which is raised to between 160 and 180 mmHg. This is thought to be an adaptation in chronically hypertensive patients

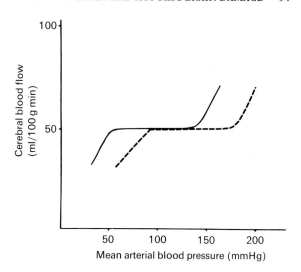

Fig. 5.10 Relationship between cerebral blood flow and mean arterial pressure in normotensive and hypertensive individuals. Note the 'shift to the right' of the autoregulatory curve in hypertensives (unbroken line = normotensive people; broken line = hypertensive patients).
Reproduced by permission of the editors from: Graham DI, Jones JV. In: Robertson JIS, Pickering GW, Caldwell ADS, eds. R Soc Med Int Symposium Series 26. London: Royal Society of Medicine, 1979; 105.

and in animals[43] that can tolerate very high blood pressure without developing hypertensive encephalopathy.

Pathological changes in hypertension[44]

In addition to abnormal cerebrovascular physiology, there are various pathological changes associated with hypertension. For example, there is considerable evidence that *atheroma* of the larger cerebral vessels, in particular, is aggravated by hypertension. In chronic severe hypertension, atheroma can, in addition, be found in the penetrating arteries of the internal capsule, basal ganglia and pons. Hypertension also produces changes in the walls of arteries and arterioles, the latter undergoing *hyaline arteriolosclerosis*. Similar changes are seen in the elderly and in diabetics. Other lesions, such as *lipohyalinosis*—a term indicating acute arterial distension with atheroma—have also been described.[45]

The incidences of stroke and myocardial infarction are increased in hypertension, and modern anti-hypertensive therapy protects patients

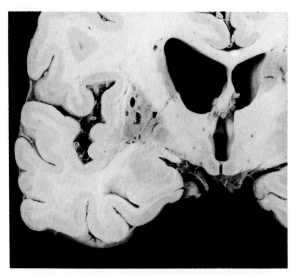

Fig. 5.11 Lacunes and lacunar infarcts. There are several lesions in the basal ganglia. There is also ventricular enlargement.

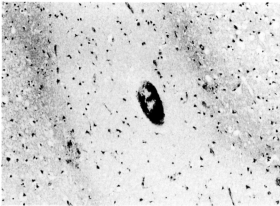

Fig. 5.12 Hypertensive encephalopathy. Arteriolar change in the brain of a patient who died from malignant-phase hypertension. There is necrosis of the vessel wall which is also permeated by constituents of plasma. The perivascular tissue is pale and 'oedematous'.
Martius scarlet blue × 210.

against stroke but not against coronary heart disease associated with hypertension. It has been suggested that the reason for this paradox can be found in differences in blood-flow regulation and metabolic reserve in the brain and heart in hypertension and during anti-hypertensive treatment.[46]

Lacunes. These small cavities, measuring up to some 20 mm in diameter, are commonly found in the basal ganglia and pons in the brains of elderly people (Fig. 5.11). Some 90% are associated with hypertension.[47] Some appear as expanded perivascular spaces, others appear as small infarcts or resolving haemorrhages. When lacunes are numerous in grey and white matter the terms '*état lacunaire*' and '*état criblé*', respectively, are used. According to one school of thought, lacunes are 'the result of spiralled elongations of small intracerebral arteries under the effects of raised blood pressure'.[48] They are also found in the brains of elderly normotensive subjects. Others, however, have attributed them to occlusion of deep perforating arteries by lipohyalinosis,[45,49] atheroma,[47,49] or emboli. The association between lacunes and lacunar infarcts in stroke patients has been reviewed.[50]

Multi-infarct dementia. This is also associated with hypertension and is a condition that is due to multiple areas of infarction: it is discussed more fully elsewhere under 'dementia associated with vascular disease' (see Ch. 13).

Hypertensive encephalopathy. Now a rare condition in developed countries, hypertensive encephalopathy may complicate acute glomerulonephritis, hypertension,[51] and toxaemia of pregnancy.[52] From a study of 20 cases,[53] it was concluded that hypertensive encephalopathy is characterised by *multiple petechial haemorrhages, fibrinoid necrosis* of the walls of arterioles and small arteries, some of which may be occluded by fibrin thrombi, and *micro-infarcts* (Fig. 5.12). These changes are particularly common in the basis pontis.

Although severe hypertension is accepted as the underlying cause of hypertensive encephalopathy, the exact pathogenesis remains uncertain. It has been attributed both to 'spasm' of the cerebral vessels[54] and to excessive vasodilatation, damage to the blood-brain barrier and cerebral hyperaemia.[55] Evidence is increasing that hypertensive encephalopathy is a disorder in which the upper limit of autoregulation is exceeded because of forced cerebral hyperperfusion induced by hypertension (Fig. 5.13).[56] The hypertension may be naturally occurring (e.g. eclampsia, malignant phase hypertension) or may be induced pharmacologically in animals.[56]

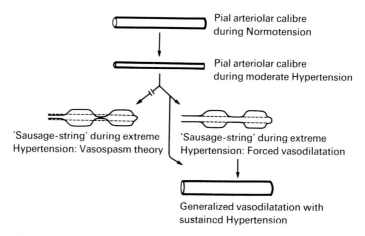

Fig. 5.13 Changes in pial arteriolar calibre in response to induced (experimental) hypertension.
Reproduced by permission of the editor from: MacKenzie ET, Strandgaard S, Graham DI, Jones JV, Harper AM, Farrar JK. Circ Res 1976; 39: 33.

Subcortical arteriosclerotic encephalopathy (Binswanger's disease). This is characterised by slowly developing dementia, focal neurological deficits including pseudo-bulbar palsy, and psychiatric disturbances in patients between the ages of 50 and 60 years.[57] Pathologically, there is both focal and diffuse loss of myelin in the deep white matter of each cerebral hemisphere. This has been ascribed to a reduction in blood flow due to a combination of hyaline arteriolosclerosis and atheroma, which in turn have been interpreted as forms of hypertensive vascular disease. The condition has also been described in normotensive individuals.[58]

Spontaneous intracerebral haemorrhage. There is also a close association between hypertension and various types of intracranial haemorrhage (see p. 105).

CEREBRAL EMBOLISM

According to the Framingham Study, some 31% of strokes are due to embolism, but other studies have estimated that between 50 and 60% of acute strokes are of embolic origin.[59]

Thrombotic and atheromatous embolism

Rheumatic heart disease, particularly mitral stenosis complicated by thrombus formation in the left atrium, is now less commonly a cause of cerebral embolism in adults. A more frequent source of emboli arising from the heart is mural thrombus formed on the endocardium overlying a myocardial infarct; two-thirds of the infarcts caused by emboli from this source occur within the first three weeks of acute myocardial infarction. Other cardiac sources of emboli include infective endocarditis, calcific aortic stenosis (particularly in older patients), prolapsing mitral valve, myxoma of the left atrium, non-bacterial thrombotic endocarditis found in association with the cachexia of advanced chronic illness,[60] cardiomyopathy and arrhythmias. Rarely, a thrombotic embolus reaching the heart from the systemic veins may pass through a patent foramen ovale to enter the systemic arterial circulation (*paradoxical embolism*). Brain damage due to embolism may also complicate cardiac surgery;[61,62] open heart surgery with cardio-pulmonary bypass created new sources of cerebral embolism that included air, fat, particles of silicone and platelet/fibrin emboli from the pump oxygenator.[63] The occurrence, however, of severe CNS complications has diminished, markedly commensurate with developments in surgical technique, anaesthesia and cardio-pulmonary bypass,[64] although there is increasing evidence that diffuse dysfunction of the CNS rather than focal damage is now the most important factor determining both the immediate and long-term outcome.[65]

The treatment of angina by aorto-coronary bypass surgery is well established and is increasingly being carried out in regions with a high incidence of coronary artery disease. Several studies have shown a low incidence of major neurological complications associated with the procedure, although in a recent study 191 out of 312 patients (61%) developed early postoperative neurological abnormalities, of which 4 (2%) were severely incapacitated, 48 (25%) were mildly disabled and 138 (72%) had no important disability.[66] A six-month follow-up study of 165 of the original 191 patients showed that 85 still had detectable neurological signs but these were often minor and of little functional significance.[67] It was therefore concluded that the long-term prognosis for early neurological disorders after coronary artery bypass surgery is favourable in most cases. The pathogenesis of the disorders is uncertain but it has been found that the duration of the bypass procedure relates significantly to the occurrence of neurological damage.

If the fibrous intimal covering of an atheromatous plaque in the carotid or cerebral artery breaks down, excavation of the soft central part of the lesion by the bloodstream may dislodge fatty and crystalline debris as emboli into the cerebral circulation. Thrombi formed on ulcerated atheromatous lesions in the aorta and in the cervical arteries supplying the brain are also a very common source of embolism.

Fat embolism

The syndrome of cerebral fat embolism is rare, as most of the fat is trapped in the lungs, giving rise to pulmonary complications. When it does occur, however, it is usually associated with major fractures,[68] though it has also been noted in the brains of patients after open heart surgery[67] and after the use of methyl methacrylate bone cement.[69] If death occurs within 3 to 4 days, the white matter of the brain is diffusely studded with petechial haemorrhages (Fig. 5.14). There are many fat globules in small arterioles, and the walls of the small vessels are often necrotic.

Air embolism

If a large amount (300–500 ml) of air enters the circulation, then death is likely to ensue, probably due to a combination of pulmonary and cardiac dysfunction. However, cerebral air embolism may develop during abortion, cardiac, brain and pulmonary surgery, catheterisation procedures and sub-atmospheric decompression.[70] When death occurs within a few minutes there is an excess of air in the veins[71] and the brain appears structurally normal. In patients surviving accidental air embolism, the principal changes have been ischaemic damage accentuated along the arterial boundary zones of the cerebral hemispheres; the appearances are indistinguishable from those due to a combination of reduced cerebral blood flow and hypoxaemia.[72]

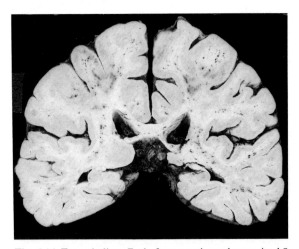

Fig. 5.14 Fat embolism. Brain from a patient who survived 5 days after sustaining fracture of femur. There are multiple petechial haemorrhages in the white matter of the cerebral hemispheres.

Nitrogen embolism

Nitrogen embolism is found in two circumstances. First, in *hyperbaric decompression*, there is a reduction of atmospheric pressure from an elevated level to normal, as encountered by underwater divers and workers in caissons. In these conditions, dissolved gases in the blood come out of solution and nitrogen forms small bubbles that cause the 'bends' and the 'chokes' (caisson disease). At autopsy, if survival is short, the central nervous system may be congested, whereas after longer survival the main finding is that of multiple small infarcts in the posterior columns of the thoracic spinal cord.[73,74] Secondly, in *hypobaric decompression*, there is a reduction of atmospheric pressure from normal to a lower level, as at high altitude or in a hypobaric decompression chamber.[75,76] The principal neuropathological findings are multiple foci of hypoxic damage, seen particularly in the grey matter of the cerebral hemispheres or in the spinal cord. The lesions have been attributed to a mixture of gaseous and fat embolism combined with hypotension.

Other forms of embolism

Among the less common forms of emboli that may obstruct cerebral blood vessels are aggregates of tumour cells, larvae of parasites, clumps of meconium and epidermal squamous cells in cases of amniotic fluid embolism, and fragments of tissue that become detached during various catheterisation procedures.

The site of lodgement of an embolus depends upon its size. Large fragments, as from a chamber of the heart, are likely to become impacted in one of the major intracranial arteries, particularly the middle cerebral artery or one of its larger branches. Small emboli detached from the heart valves or atheromatous plaques in the aorta or extracranial vessels will become lodged in the smaller branches of the main cerebral arteries. The signs and symptoms tend to be of sudden onset, viz. *transient ischaemic attack*, or stroke. Often there is clinical improvement, which has been ascribed to re-establishment of some circulation due to shrinkage of the embolus, relaxation of local arterial spasm or fragmentation of the embolus by fibrinolysis. Full recovery is only possible if the interval between the obstruction and restoration of the circulation has been sufficiently short to avoid permanent neuronal damage. Often, however, the time interval is long enough for necrosis and infarction to occur, so that when the circulation is re-established the tissue becomes haemorrhagic with, in some instances, formation of a haematoma.

CEREBRAL ARTERITIS

There are many types of vasculitis which result in thrombotic occlusion of the affected vessel and cerebral infarction. These include bacterial, fungal and viral diseases, collagen diseases and a miscellaneous group of disorders that includes temporal (giant cell) arteritis, Takayasu's disease, granulomatous angiitis and radiation arteritis.

Arteritis due to infection

In the pre-antibiotic era, acute carotid arteritis sometimes developed in children and young adults with tonsillitis, retropharyngeal inflammation and septic thrombosis of the cavernous sinus. Acute purulent meningitis, particularly due to *Streptococcus pneumoniae* and *Neisseria meningitidis*, was and still is complicated by an acute arteritis and thrombotic occlusion of the vessels on the pial surface of the brain where they are surrounded by inflammatory exudate (see p. 154). In subacute or chronic meningitis, due to *Mycobacterium tuberculosis* or *Treponema pallidum*, it is common to find chronic inflammation and fibrosis of the pial arteries and veins. The intima becomes greatly thickened, the vessels acquiring the appearance of endarteritis obliterans (Fig. 5.15). It is thought

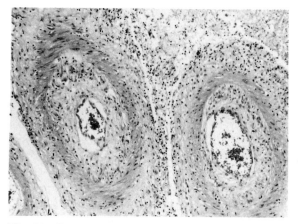

Fig. 5.15 Endarteritis obliterans. Arteries at base of brain from a case of tuberculous meningitis. There is fibrinous exudate in the subarachnoid space and the adventitia is thickened and infiltrated by chronic inflammatory cells. The media is normal and there is marked concentric thickening of the intima.
Haematoxylin-eosin × 80

that the arteritis is due to irritants acting on the vessels from without and does not constitute a primary arterial disease. Support for this view is found in cases of chronic arachnoiditis occurring as a delayed sequel in some cases of spinal anaesthesia in which the pial vessels show end-arteritis obliterans.[77]

Arteritis may be due to invasion by various fungi such as *Aspergillus fumigatus*, *Cryptococcus neoformans* and *Coccidioides immitis* (see Ch. 7). In cases of cerebral malaria, due almost exclusively to infections by *Plasmodium falciparum*, there are multiple petechial haemorrhages in white matter with associated brain swelling. The histological appearances are those of disseminated small vessel occlusion (see p. 181).

Acute vasculitis affecting small vessels is seen in some cases of *typhus* and *scrub typhus*.[78] It is also seen in certain *viral* diseases, as for example in the medial parts of the temporal lobes in herpes simplex encephalitis. More recently it has been suggested that the uncommon condition of *granulomatous angiitis* may have a viral aetiology. A case of granulomatous angiitis following varicella zoster infection has been reported.[79] The exact pathogenesis of this condition, however, remains uncertain as mycoplasma-like structures have been described in it.

Collagen diseases

Polyarteritis nodosa. The vascular lesions of polyarteritis nodosa are multiple and are most commonly seen in the kidneys, heart, gastrointestinal tract, nervous system (Fig. 5.16) and muscle. The arteritis is thought to be a hypersensitivity reaction to a variety of antigenic stimuli. Polyarteritis nodosa affects the CNS in 10–20% of cases; the intracranial arteries may have a beaded appearance due to multiple aneurysms.[80] Rupture of these aneurysms is uncommon but subarachnoid haemorrhage may be a rare presenting feature. More commonly patients present with multiple infarcts. Many of the patients are severely hypertensive and so some of the terminal features may be due to hypertensive encephalopathy. There is a similarity between granulomatous and arteritic diseases, including polyarteritis nodosa on the one hand, and Wegener's granulomatosis on

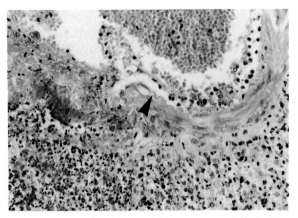

Fig. 5.16 Polyarteritis nodosa. There is segmental fibrinoid necrosis of the full thickness of a leptomeningeal artery. In an adjacent segment the internal elastic lamina is still visible (arrow). There is focal destruction of the muscularis and infiltration by polymorphs.
Haematoxylin-eosin × 210

the other.[81] It has also been suggested that the midline granuloma (Stewart syndrome) is a localised form of Wegener's granulomatosis.[82]

Systemic lupus erythematosus. Clinical evidence of central nervous involvement in systemic lupus erythematosus is said to occur in some 50% of patients,[83] with involvement of the vessels in some three-quarters of fatal cases.[84] Microscopy shows that changes are most marked in small vessels, and consist of acute fibrinoid necrosis and marked thickening with minimal inflammatory cell infiltration. Some of the vessels may be occluded by thrombi, resulting in micro-infarction.[84] The pathogenesis of the condition is not clear.

Giant cell arteritis. In giant cell arteritis (temporal arteritis) there is a granulomatous reaction involving arteries of all sizes, including the aorta.[85] Of the medium- and smaller-sized arteries that may be affected, involvement of the coronary and ophthalmic arteries, including the ciliary arteries and the central artery of the retina, has particularly important consequences. The disease often involves the superficial temporal arteries, which become swollen, tender, tortuous and nodular; pulsation is usually diminished or lost and the artery may eventually shrink and become hard. Because of their accessibility, temporal vessels have remained the most popular choice for biopsy: a negative biopsy, however, does

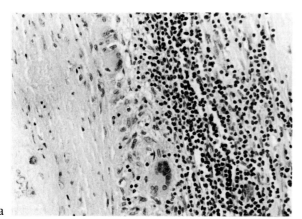
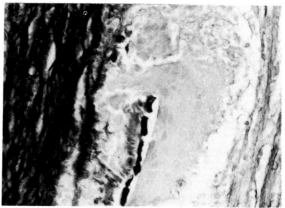

a   b

Fig. 5.17a, b Giant cell arteritis. Vertebral artery showing (**a**) intimal proliferation and cellular infiltration, including multi-nucleated giant cells close to the (**b**) irregularly damaged internal elastic lamina. There is mononuclear infiltration of the media and, to a lesser extent, of the adventitia. (**a**) Haematoxylin-eosin ×210 (**b**) Miller's elastic ×330

not exclude a diagnosis of giant cell arteritis. Histologically there is a panarteritis that may be multi-focal or involve the whole length of the vessel. The internal elastic lamina is severely and irregularly fragmented. Giant cells of Langhans and/or foreign body type are almost invariably associated with the elastic lamina fragmentation (Figs 5.17a and b), and there is lymphocyte infiltration of the intima and media.

Other vasculitides. Other varieties of vasculitis classified as collagen disorders include *Behçet's disease, rheumatic fever* and *rheumatoid arthritis.*

Thrombotic thrombocytopenic purpura (Moschcowitz's disease). This rare disease is characterised by fever, purpura, haemolytic anaemia and thrombocytopenia. The nervous system is involved in some 90% of cases.[86] The lesions are virtually confined to the grey matter; histology shows hyperplasia of endothelium and widespread occlusion of small blood vessels by granular or hyaline eosinophilic material which may be undergoing organisation.

Other causes of cerebral arteritis

Aortic arch syndrome. The aortic arch syndrome (pulseless disease, aortic arch arteritis, Takayasu's arteritis) is a constellation of clinical signs and symptoms which arise following a progressive reduction in blood flow in the territories of the brachiocephalic, left common carotid and left subclavian arteries. There are many causes of this condition but when it occurs in young patients there is often evidence of more generalised disease and features of a 'collagenosis'. The early cases were described in young Japanese women but it is now appreciated that it occurs in older women and in men throughout the world. Various types of arterial disease have been responsible for the syndrome including polyarteritis nodosa, giant cell arteritis, syphilitic aortitis, tuberculosis and thrombo-angiitis obliterans (Winiwarter–Buerger disease). In other cases the underlying cause has been attributed to congenital anomalies of the vessels, to thrombo-embolism and to atheroma.

X-irradiation. The brain and spinal cord may be damaged by X-rays. The immediate response (within weeks) may be an acute inflammatory vasculitis but more characteristically there is a delayed response (between 1 and 4 years) in which the small vessels undergo marked proliferative changes with hyaline degeneration of their walls and necrosis of surrounding brain substance. Such changes may be found in patients given radiotherapy for glioma and less commonly in children given neuraxis irradiation for medulloblastoma or leukaemic infiltration of the meninges, in patients irradiated for pituitary tumour or tumours of the neck, including the parotid and thyroid glands, and after irradiation for ankylosing spondylitis.[87,88] It has been shown that both vascular and glial (see p. 147) damage may occur in the pathogenesis of delayed radiation injury to the CNS and that the relative importance of these two pathological changes is related to radiation dosage.[89]

Miscellaneous causes. Cerebral arteritis has also been ascribed to *drug hypersensitivity*,[90] *sarcoidosis*[91] (see p. 163) and *lymphomatoid granulomatosis*.[92]

LESS COMMON CAUSES OF CEREBRAL INFARCTION

Moya moya disease. The Japanese term *moya moya* refers to a radiological appearance predominant in young women in whom cerebral angiography shows an unusual network of small blood vessels at the base of the brain. The condition was at first thought to be confined to Japan but has now been reported from other parts of the world. Pathological reports have been few but have described marked proliferation of the small pial arteries over the surface of the brain.[93] The aetiology of moya moya disease is unclear; cases occurring in childhood may be a true congenital vascular malformation, whereas those occurring in adulthood may be due to thrombo-embolic disease, tuberculous meningitis, sickle cell disease, X-irradiation, or associated with some cases of neurofibromatosis.

Blood diseases. There is also an association between cerebral infarction and various blood diseases. For example, transient ischaemic attacks, cerebral infarction and cerebral haemorrhage are all recognised complications of *polycythaemia rubra vera*. It has been shown that cerebral blood flow is reduced when high viscosity occurs in poly-cythaemia and in patients with a high normal haematocrit.[94] The nervous system is involved in some 25% of patients with *sickle cell disease*,[95] and in other types of *haemoglobinopathy*, including *thalassaemia*. Neurological complications are also common in patients with *Waldenström's macro-globulinaemia*.

Oral contraceptives. In the early 1960s, attention was drawn to the apparent association between oral contraceptive agents and cerebral infarction in young women.[96] Further evidence indicates that there is a six- to nine-fold increased risk of cerebral infarction in these women.[97,98] The thrombotic tendency appears to be related to the oestrogen content of the preparation, which produces a hypercoagulable state and increases platelet adhesiveness.

Pregnancy. There is also an association between cerebral infarction and pregnancy and the puerperium. Until recently this was regarded as usually due to cerebral venous thrombosis but it is now appreciated that the majority of cases are arterial in origin.[99] Many factors may combine to cause stroke in this group of patients. In some there are features of hypertensive encephalopathy, in others arterial occlusion is due to thrombo-embolism, and in yet others there are various forms of arteritis such as systemic lupus erythematosus. Some cases can be attributed to paradoxical embolism, but it is thought likely that the hormonal changes associated with pregnancy and the puerperium contribute to an increased thrombotic tendency, including an enhanced platelet adhesiveness.

Miscellaneous. Occlusive vascular disease has also been recorded[100] in cases of addiction to *heroin* and *LSD* (lysergide), as a complication of *inflammatory bowel disease*, in association with *migraine*, and in patients with *inherited disorders of connective tissue* (e.g. pseudoxanthoma elasticum, Ehlers–Danlos syndrome and Marfan's syndrome).

THROMBOSIS OF THE VEINS AND VENOUS SINUSES

There are two principal types of venous thrombosis, namely primary (non-infectious) and secondary (due to pyogenic infection).

Primary or aseptic thrombosis of the cortical veins and superior sagittal sinus may complicate pregnancy and the puerperium, various haematological disorders such as sickle cell anaemia, leukaemia and polycythaemia rubra vera, and the use of oral contraceptives. Extreme dehydration in children with, for example, severe

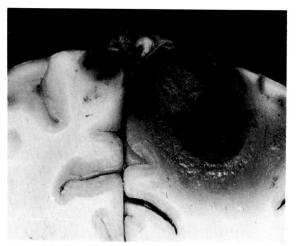

Fig. 5.18 Thrombotic occlusion of the superior sagittal sinus (top centre). There is swelling and intensely haemorrhagic necrosis of the dorsomedial quadrants of the cerebral hemispheres.
Reproduced by permission of the editors and publishers from: Brierley JB, Graham DI. In: Adams JH, Corsellis JAN, Duchen LW, eds. Greenfield's Neuropathology, 4th ed. London: Arnold, 1984: 125–207 (Fig. 4.57)

diarrhoea may result in cortical vein or sinus thrombosis. The aetiology is often uncertain but in some cases it is associated with conditions of hypercoagulability of the blood, such as in pregnancy, the puerperium and some post-operative states. If a number of the cortical veins or the sagittal sinus is obstructed by thrombus, there is interference with venous drainage, and the affected cortex and white matter become markedly congested and haemorrhagic (Fig. 5.18).[10]

Secondary thrombosis is most often found as a complication of pyogenic infection. For example, the superior sagittal sinus may become occluded if infection spreads from the frontal sinuses or a compound fracture of the skull. Likewise the lateral and the cavernous sinus may become occluded if infection spreads from the middle ear or the central part of the face respectively. If the thrombus fragments and is carried into the bloodstream, then pyaemia and systemic abscesses develop.

Acute venous infarction of the spinal cord is rare[38] and is usually due to acute thrombophlebitis, either of the plexus of veins in the spinal canal or of the pelvic veins. Haemorrhage into the deep grey matter is conspicuous and there may be formation of a frank haematoma.

SPONTANEOUS INTRACRANIAL HAEMORRHAGE[101]

Figures from the Framingham Study suggest that some 16% of 'strokes' are due to haemorrhage (10% due to *intracerebral haemorrhage* and 6% to *subarachnoid haemorrhage* from rupture of an intracranial saccular aneurysm).[1] Other causes of spontaneous intracranial haemorrhage, such as vascular malformation and mycotic aneurysms, are uncommon. Traumatic haemorrhages (extradural, subdural and some intracerebral haemorrhages) are considered elsewhere (see Ch. 6).

INTRACEREBRAL HAEMORRHAGE

There are two principal types of intracerebral haemorrhage: primary haemorrhage, which occurs most frequently in individuals with hypertension, and secondary haemorrhage, which complicates systemic or local disease, such as rupture of a saccular aneurysm, and bleeding into a tumour or from a vascular malformation.

Primary intracerebral haemorrhage

Massive haemorrhage into the substance of the brain is a disease principally of late middle age. In four-fifths of cases the haematoma appears to arise in the region of the lentiform nucleus—the so-called capsular haemorrhage (Fig. 5.19). In the remaining one-fifth of cases the haematoma is either in the pons or in the white matter of the cerebellum (Fig. 5.20).[102] The haematoma causes deformation and some destruction of related brain tissue, and once bleeding begins it tends to track along the paths of least resistance. Thus a haemorrhage may extend in any direction by separating the fibres of the white matter; alternatively it may rupture into one of the lateral ventricles or into the subarachnoid space. A large haematoma acts as a rapidly-expanding space occupying lesion, patients rarely surviving more than 24–36 hours.

It is important to distinguish *primary* midbrain or pontine haemorrhage from haemorrhage into the brainstem *secondary* to raised intracranial

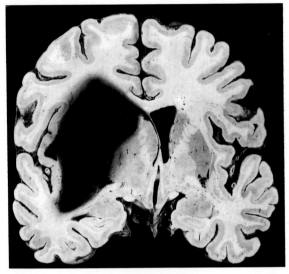

Fig. 5.19 Hypertensive haematoma. There is a large recently formed haemorrhage in the basal ganglia of the left cerebral hemisphere that has ruptured into the lateral ventricle. The midline structures are displaced to the right.

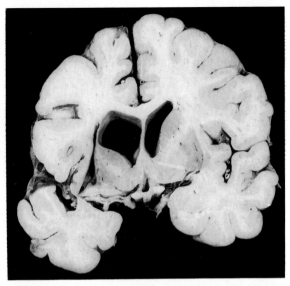

Fig. 5.21 'Apoplectic cyst'. A very old haemorrhage in the basal ganglia of the left cerebral hemisphere. The walls of the lesion were orange–brown in colour. Compare with Figure 5.19.

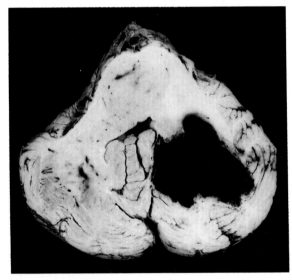

Fig. 5.20 Hypertensive haematoma. There is extensive haemorrhage into one cerebellar hemisphere.

pressure and internal herniation (see p. 69). Fortunately, this is usually not difficult, although a large primary supratentorial haematoma may track downwards into the upper brainstem. In most cases of primary brainstem haemorrhage the haematoma is limited to the hindbrain and does not extend into the cerebral hemispheres to any great extent.

Some patients survive the initial ictus without severe neurological deficit. With time, the haematoma becomes brown in colour and is gradually absorbed. Eventually all that remains is a cavity, the walls of which are often orange–brown in colour—the so-called apoplectic cyst (Fig. 5.21). Smaller slit-like haemorrhages are also commonly found in the basal ganglia and subcortical white matter where they extend along fibre tracts. Around many small haemorrhages there is histological evidence of earlier bleeding with large numbers of haemosiderin-laden macrophages and gliosis.

The pathogenesis of primary intracerebral haemorrhage remains uncertain. It is commonly stated that most primary intracerebral haematomas develop in hypertensive people,[103,104] due to the rupture of miliary aneurysms.[105] These studies have shown that miliary aneurysms (microaneurysms) measure between 1 and 2 mm in diameter and occur most frequently in those areas of the brain in which primary intracerebral haemorrhage is found. The miliary aneurysms, however, are likely to be destroyed by the haemorrhage and are therefore very difficult to demonstrate in ordinary histological preparations; they are best demonstrated in their unruptured state by post-mortem angiographic techniques which use radio-opaque material. By such methods it has been shown that miliary aneurysms are present in about 50% of hypertensive patients, compared with about 5% of those who are normotensive.[103,106,107] More than 90% of patients who die as a result of hypertensive cerebral haemorrhage have miliary aneurysms. The size and number of miliary aneurysms can be related to the severity and duration of hypertension. There is also a relation-ship to age: 70% of hypertensive patients aged between 60 and 65 years have aneurysms, compared with only 5% of those under 50 years. The aneurysms are thought to form following localised degeneration and fibrosis of the tunica media, with loss of muscle and elastic tissue; these changes are commonly found in older hyper-tensive patients. Lipohyalinosis[45] and vessel damage characteristic of malignant hypertension may be superimposed upon the focal fibrosis.[53]

Intracranial haemorrhage, both intracerebral and subarachnoid, has been associated with the use of various monoamine oxidase inhibitors.[108] The bleeding in such cases is believed to result from a hypertensive crisis which may be precipitated by taking sympathomimetic drugs, such as ephedrine and amphetamine, and by tyramine-rich foods such as cheese, bean pods, yeast extracts, and chocolate.

Secondary intracerebral haemorrhage

This is categorised according to cause.[109]

Abnormalities of blood coagulation. The most important factor in the genesis of the often multi-focal white matter haemorrhages in this group of patients is *thrombocytopenia* (Fig. 5.22). Such patients fall into two main categories, those with and those without leukaemia. Although at one stage it was considered that leukaemic infiltration of the brain was the principal cause of the haemorrhage in cases of leukaemia, it is now generally appreciated that thrombocytopenia per se is the most important factor.

Thrombocytopenia is also probably the most

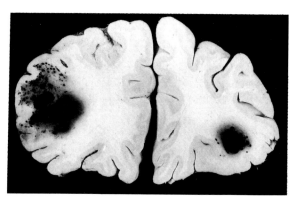

Fig. 5.22 Multiple intracerebral haematomas. Brain from patient with thrombocytopenia due to acute leukaemia.

important factor in the bleeding tendency sometimes seen in alcoholics and patients with aplastic anaemia or disseminated intravascular coagulation. Patients on anticoagulant therapy or those with various clotting factor deficiencies, such as in haemophilia, more often suffer from subdural haemorrhage than from bleeding into the brain parenchyma.

Cerebral amyloid angiopathy. There has been increasing awareness of the clinico-pathological entity of cerebral congophilic or amyloid angiopathy as the probable cause of non-traumatic cerebral haemorrhage in a large proportion of patients who are normotensive and elderly. This condition has a close relationship with the histological features of Alzheimer's disease (see p. 376).[110]

Brain tumours. Massive bleeding may take place in either primary or metastatic brain tumours. In the primary group, haemorrhage is most likely to occur in patients with anaplastic astrocytoma, glioblastoma multiforme and oligodendroglioma. In our experience, bleeding into metastatic tumours may be massive and occurs most often in deposits from primary carcinoma of the bronchus and from cutaneous malignant melanoma.

Miscellaneous. Occasionally, massive brain haemorrhage is due to *cortical vein and venous sinus thrombosis* (see p. 104), to *vasculitis* (see p. 101), particularly in patients with collagen diseases, and following rupture of a *mycotic aneurysm* (see

p. 111), *saccular aneurysm* (see p. 110) or *vascular malformation* (see p. 113). In some instances, however, the cause remains uncertain in spite of careful examination of the specimen. In these circumstances the haematoma is probably due to rupture of a small hidden haemangioma (see pages 114 and 479).

Bleeding into the spinal cord (*haematomyelia*) is uncommon. It is most often due to trauma, though it may develop in patients with thrombocytopenia, haemophilia or vascular malformations.

SUBARACHNOID HAEMORRHAGE

In about 65% of cases, spontaneous subarachnoid haemorrhage is due to rupture of a saccular aneurysm of one of the major cerebral arteries, in another 5% it is due to bleeding from an arteriovenous malformation. In a further 5% the haemorrhage is due to some other disease such as a blood dyscrasia or the extension of either an intra-cerebral or an intraventricular haemorrhage into the subarachnoid space.[111] No cause for the haemorrhage is found in up to 25% of patients, even after complete angiography.

Saccular aneurysms[109,112]

Known also as berry or congenital aneurysms, these occur on the arteries at the base of the brain in between 1 and 2% of the adult population. They are found more often in women than in men and may be found incidentally at autopsy. Multiple aneurysms are found in 10–15% of patients with subarachnoid haemorrhage: in such patients there are usually two or three, but sometimes five or more.[113,114]

Aneurysms are rare in children, and the term congenital is therefore inappropriate. They develop almost invariably at the bifurcation of arteries, and it is at such sites that the develop-mental abnormality of a defective or deficient tunica media is most commonly found. However, aneurysms are rare in comparison with the great frequency of such structural defects,[115] indicating that additional acquired factors may determine the development of the aneurysms.[116,117] Atheroma may be one of the most important of these acquired factors as the plaque can cause degeneration of the internal elastic lamina.[118] Another important factor is the formation of fibrous intimal pads which probably alter the stress upon the bifurcations of cerebral arteries[119] which, together with fenestration of the elastic lamina and the defect in the tunica media, predisposes to the development of a fibrous pouch (early aneurysm).[120] Support for the rôle of haemodynamic stress in the formation of saccular aneurysms is provided by the coincidence of their occurrence on vessels supplying arteriovenous malformations.[121] The contribution of elevated blood pressure to the development of an aneurysm is unclear, for although more than half of the patients have high blood pressure when measure-ments are made shortly after a haemorrhage, in many cases this is a 'reactive' phenomenon and pressure returns to normal within a few days. It seems possible, however, that the relative importance of these factors varies at different ages. For example, subarachnoid haemorrhage from a ruptured saccular aneurysm may occur in adolescents and young children in the absence of local atheroma. The possible importance of transient arterial hypertension is indicated by the frequency with which rupture of an aneurysm takes place during physical exertion or at a time of emotion, especially in young adults.[122] The failure to find any association between hypertension and multiple aneurysms, the age at which they present clinically and the time at which they rupture[123] emphasises the difficulty in establishing any con-clusive proof of a causal relationship with high blood pressure. Many inter-related factors are probably involved. It does seem likely, however, that the prognosis in hypertensive patients following rupture of a saccular aneurysm is worse than that in normotensives.[124] The age at which aneurysms are found also favours an acquired origin: the mean age is 50 years, and only 20% of the patients are under 40 and very few under 20.

About 40% of saccular aneurysms are located at the junction between the internal carotid and the posterior communicating arteries, 30% at the junction between the anterior communicating and anterior cerebral arteries within the inter-hemispheric fissure (Fig. 5.23) and 20% at the bifurcation of the middle cerebral artery within the

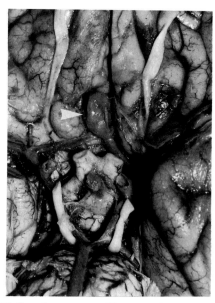

Fig. 5.23 Saccular aneurysm. Unruptured aneurysm (arrow) arising from the anterior communicating artery.

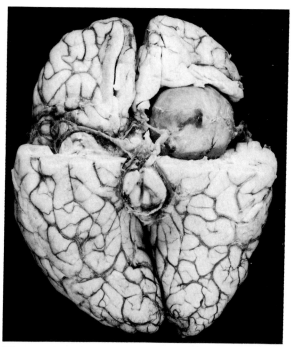

Fig. 5.24 'Giant' unruptured aneurysm. Origin from the left middle cerebral artery. The aneurysm was sufficiently large to cause shift, displacement, internal herniation and death from secondary damage to the brainstem.

Sylvian (lateral) fissure.[113,114] The commonest sites of the remaining 10% are: on the pericallosal artery as it winds round the anterior part of the corpus callosum, the junction between the internal carotid and middle cerebral arteries, at the upper end of the basilar artery, at the junction between the vertebral and posterior inferior cerebellar arteries and at the junction between the internal carotid and ophthalmic arteries within the cavernous sinus. Approximately 85% of aneurysms arise from the upper end of the internal carotid artery and from the major branches of the anterior portion of the circle of Willis. Rupture of an aneurysm occurs when its wall is no longer strong enough to withstand the stress, and it has been calculated to occur when its diameter is about 8 mm with a wall thickness of 40 μm.[125] In general, unruptured aneurysms are smaller than those that have ruptured, and they increase in size over time. Histologically there is no elastic lamina or tunica media, and the aneurysm wall consists of fibrous tissue lined by endothelium. As the aneurysm enlarges, its connective tissue wall becomes stretched and it ruptures, most commonly at the fundus.[126] Some aneurysms measure as much as 20–30 mm in diameter and may be almost filled by laminated mural thrombus. These *giant*

aneurysms[127] are less likely to rupture than the smaller ones, but they may act as space occupying lesions and patients may present with raised intracranial pressure (Fig. 5.24), temporal lobe epilepsy or compression of the third cranial nerve.

Immediate intracranial complications. Subarachnoid haemorrhage from a ruptured saccular aneurysm is a serious but not a common disorder (Fig. 5.25). It has been estimated that in the USA the peak age for rupture of a saccular aneurysm is between 55 and 60 years, the incidence of aneurysmal rupture is 26 000 cases per year,[128] and the incidence of subarachnoid haemorrhage is 11–12 per 100 000 per year.[129] In some cases blood is limited to the immediate vicinity of the aneurysm but more commonly it spreads throughout the subarachnoid space into the cisterns at the base of the brain, over the ventral aspect of the brainstem and along the spinal subarachnoid space. Sometimes quite a large haematoma may develop in the subarachnoid space, usually within the Sylvian (lateral) fissure in association with an

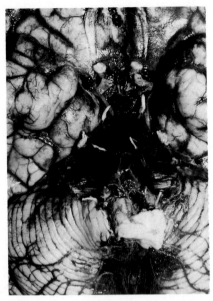

Fig. 5.25 Subarachnoid haemorrhage. There is a large amount of recent haemorrhage in the subarachnoid space due to rupture of a saccular aneurysm arising from the anterior communicating artery. See Fig. 5.26.

aneurysm on the middle cerebral artery or between the medial surfaces of the frontal lobes in association with an aneurysm on the anterior communicating artery. A ruptured aneurysm is not always easy to identify post mortem, not only because of the amount of blood in the subarachnoid space, but also because the walls of the aneurysm often collapse following haemorrhage. A search for the site of haemorrhage should be made at the time of autopsy by washing the blood gently from the subarachnoid space with saline. The process is much more difficult once the blood has been hardened by fixation of the brain in formalin. With survival the blood is phagocytosed and removed: a considerable amount of blood is still present in the subarachnoid space at one week. Often the origin of a previous haemorrhage is indicated by fibrosis and residual orange–brown pigmentation of the meninges. In some of these cases the sac of the aneurysm is occluded by recently formed thrombus.

Many patients die within the first day of the haemorrhage, and the mortality rate during the first week after subarachnoid haemorrhage is 27%:[130] about 45% die within the first 3 months. The risk of a further haemorrhage within one

month is about 33% and carries a 42% mortality.[130] This risk is greatest between the fifth and ninth days. After this time the risk decreases considerably, but remains appreciable, and patients alive at 6 weeks have a 10% risk of a fresh haemorrhage within the next year; thereafter in each year up to 5% have a recurrence of bleeding and about half will die as a result.[131] The cause of death following a ruptured saccular aneurysm varies. In patients who die within an hour or so, massive intraventricular haemorrhage is often found; in others there is usually a combination of subarachnoid haemorrhage, intracerebral haematoma and cerebral infarction.

Another consequence of rupture of saccular aneurysms is bleeding into the brain or ventricles.[132–134] If the fundus of an aneurysm is embedded in the adjacent brain, an *intracerebral haematoma* may result. This is seen most frequently with recurrent haemorrhages; the bleeding occurs directly into the brain as scarring and adhesions between the aneurysm and adjacent brain prevent bleeding into the subarachnoid space. Anterior communicating artery aneurysms tend to rupture into the inferomedial portion of one or both frontal lobes (Fig. 5.26), while posterior communicating and middle cerebral aneurysms commonly rupture into the temporal lobe. The mass effect of the haematoma may be sufficient to cause raised intracranial pressure,

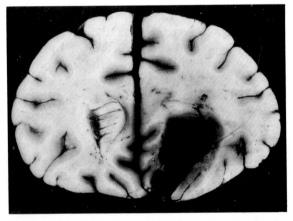

Fig. 5.26 Intracerebral haematoma. Coronal section of brain shown in Figure 5.25. There is an acute haematoma in the inferomedial quadrant of the right frontal lobe following rupture of a saccular aneurysm arising from the anterior communicating artery.

internal herniation and secondary brainstem damage (see p. 66). The intracerebral haematoma may rupture into the ventricles. Aneurysms on the anterior communicating artery may rupture directly through the lamina terminalis into the third ventricle to produce massive *intraventricular haemorrhage*. Occasionally, rupture of an aneurysm on the middle cerebral artery may produce an *acute subdural haematoma*. Whenever, therefore, an acute subdural haematoma is found unexpectedly post mortem, the basal vessels of the brain should be examined carefully in case there has been rupture of a saccular aneurysm. This is particularly important in medico-legal cases when trauma is suspected. Occasionally an aneurysm may rupture into the cavernous sinus causing a *carotico-cavernous fistula*.

Late intracranial complications. These include cerebral infarction and hydrocephalus. *Cerebral infarction* is commonly found in patients who die as a result of a ruptured saccular aneurysm.[132,135-137] While operation for clipping the aneurysm may contribute to the infarction, the condition is also found in patients who have not been subjected to surgery. The lesions are often patchy and easily escape recognition in the unfixed brain. They are most numerous in the territory of the aneurysm-bearing artery but may occur elsewhere, even in the opposite hemisphere. The cause of the infarction may be due to multiple factors including vasospasm, arterial compression by haematomas, the effects of raised intracranial pressure, surgical retraction and resection, and systemic hypotension during operations for clipping the aneurysm.[138] *Hydrocephalus* occurs in two phases after subarachnoid haemorrhage: acute ventricular dilatation is seen within the first few days, and chronic hydrocephalus at about the second week.[139,140] Both are probably the result of blockage of CSF pathways by blood.

Disorders associated with the formation of saccular aneurysms

An association between the occurrence of multiple saccular aneurysms and diseases such as coarctation of the aorta,[141] adult type III polycystic disease of the kidney,[142] and fibro-

muscular hyperplasia of the renal arteries[143] has been suggested, the common denominator being hypertension. However, saccular aneurysms may occur in polycystic disease in the absence of hypertension and in moya moya disease.[144] They are also found in association with connective tissue disorders, such as Ehlers–Danlos syndrome,[145] in which hypertension is not a feature. The increased incidence in conditions such as aortic coarctation may therefore be due to a mesodermal abnormality rather than to elevated blood pressure per se.[146]

Fusiform aneurysms

In patients with severe atheroma there is a tendency for the basilar artery and upper ends of the internal carotid artery to undergo fusiform dilatation (ectasia). In severe cases the basilar artery becomes elongated and S-shaped, with the formation of a fusiform aneurysm (Fig. 5.7).[147] A similar change may affect the supraclinoid segment of the internal carotid artery.[148] This type of dilatation predisposes to transient ischaemic attacks in the appropriate vascular territories, thrombus formation, and occasionally rupture, the latter presenting as subarachnoid haemorrhage.

Mycotic aneurysms

A mycotic aneurysm results from infection of the arterial wall. The name is an old one, dating from the time when 'mycotic' was used of any form of microbic infection and not, as now, confined to fungal and actinomycetic infections.

Between 3 and 10% of all patients with bacterial endocarditis are said to develop intracranial aneurysms of infective inflammatory origin.[149,150] Such mycotic aneurysms are found more commonly in adults than in children. They are situated on the peripheral branches of the intracranial arteries and are said to be multiple in 20% of cases.[151] Bacterial mycotic aneurysms are most commonly due to *Streptococcus pyogenes* and *Staphylococcus aureus*; the organisms spread rapidly from an impacted septic embolus into the vessel wall which then undergoes necrosis, acute inflammatory change and aneurysmal dilatation (see p. 177). About 65% of such aneurysms rupture within the first 5 weeks of the endocarditis.

Fungal mycotic aneurysms are also encountered, most often due to *Aspergillus fumigatus* and *Candida albicans*.[152,153] They tend to be larger than bacterial aneurysms and are found most commonly in the major arteries at the base of the brain. They are often multiple, and the nasal sinuses or heart are frequent sources of infection.

Rupture of a mycotic aneurysm results in haemorrhage, which is often fatal.

Dissecting aneurysms

Dissecting aneurysms of the intracranial arteries are rare and result from haemorrhage between the tunica media and the intima, or between the media and the adventitia, with extension of the bleeding along the tissue plane. Young adults and children account for a considerable proportion of patients, in whom the vessels most commonly affected are the basilar, vertebral and middle cerebral arteries, together with intracranial portions of the carotid arteries. Dissecting aneurysms are readily overlooked, so a careful histological study of occluded cerebral arteries should be made in all cases of young patients dying with cerebral infarction. The causes of dissection include trauma (Fig. 5.27),[154] syphilis, Erdheim's cystic medionecrosis and various forms of angiitis.[155] Following dissection, the aneurysms may rupture and cause subarachnoid haemorrhage, or produce thrombotic occlusion of the vessel with infarction of the tissues supplied by the affected artery.

In some cases a dissecting aneurysm of the aorta may spread distally to involve the carotid and vertebral arteries in the neck. Furthermore, dissecting aneurysms of the vertebral artery in the neck may extend to involve the intracranial portion of the artery.

VASCULAR MALFORMATIONS OF THE BRAIN AND SPINAL CORD

These are hamartomas of blood vessels that are probably the result of faults in the embryonic development of the vasculature of the meninges and brain. There are three main types: arteriovenous malformations (AVM), cavernous angiomas and capillary telangiectases.

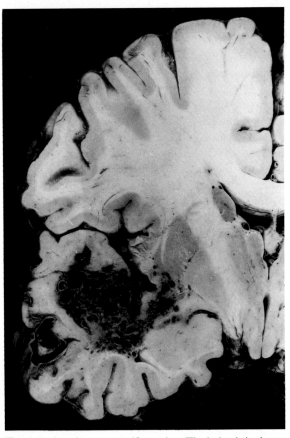

Fig. 5.28 Arteriovenous malformation. The lesion is in the left temporal lobe.

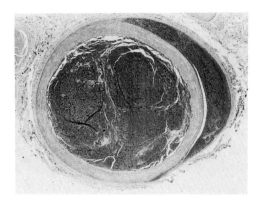

Fig. 5.27 Traumatic thrombosis of an internal carotid artery. Note the dissection in the wall of the artery.
Reproduced by permission of the editor from: Adams JH, Graham DI. J Neurol Neurosurg Psychiatry 1967; 30: 479.

Arteriovenous malformations

These are the most frequent, representing about 90% of vascular malformations. They most commonly present in young adults as recurrent subarachnoid or intracerebral haemorrhage.[156,157] Between 80 and 90% of AVMs are found in the cerebral hemispheres, and more than half of them lie within the distribution of the middle cerebral arteries. They range in size from small, well-circumscribed lesions to malformations that involve much of one hemisphere. Typically the lesion lies in the subarachnoid space and extends through the cortex to the deeper parts of the hemi-sphere in the shape of a cone or wedge (Fig. 5.28). The vessels forming the malformation vary in size, shape and configuration. Usually they are dilated and thin-walled, though some are thick-walled, containing smooth muscle but with only a limited amount of elastic tissue; secondary changes such as thrombosis and calcification are common. Histologically these 'angiomas' consist of arteries, arterialised veins, and veins separated by abnormal gliotic brain tissue containing corpora amylacea, foci of calcification, and evidence of previous haemorrhage.

Spinal AVMs are much less common than those in the brain. They consist of one or more

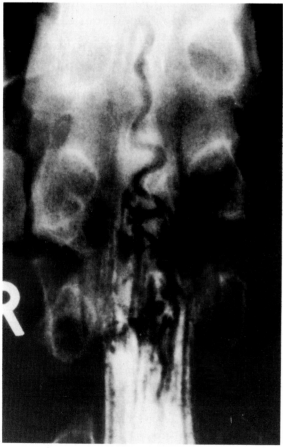

a

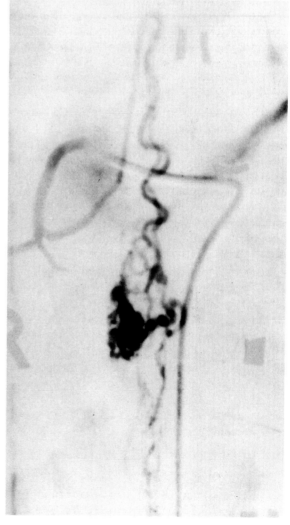

b

Fig. 5.29a, b Spinal vascular malformation. (**a**) Myelogram showing a filling defect of feeding arteries of arteriovenous malformation at L1. (**b**) Selective arteriogram of same lesion. *Reproduced by permission of Drs Evelyn Teasdale and P. Macpherson, Department of Neuroradiology, Institute of Neurological Sciences, Glasgow, UK.*

longitudinal, anomalous, tortuous vessels over the dorsal aspect of the thoracic or lumbar cord (Figs 5.29a and b). Occasionally they exist within the cord. Histologically, they are similar to the cerebral lesions and are subject to the same complications of thrombosis, calcification and haemorrhage. It is now generally recognised that the *subacute necrotic myelitis of Foix and Alajouanine* is due to a spinal AVM involving the lower cord.[38]

Cavernous angiomas

These are composed of a compact purple mass of sinusoidal vessels without any intervening parenchyma. They vary in size and can be found in all parts of the nervous system. There is often marked hyalinisation and thickening of the vessels, in some of which there is evidence of calcification and occasional ossification. There may also be gliosis and evidence of previous haemorrhage in adjacent brain tissue.

Capillary angiomas (telangiectases)

These consist of small spongy areas most commonly in, but not restricted to, the pons. They may be multiple, reach a diameter of 10 mm and consist histologically of small capillary-like vessels separated from each other by more or less normal brain tissue. Gliosis, calcification and haemorrhage are uncommon. These lesions are generally silent until they rupture, leading to spontaneous haemorrhage and haematoma. Many such lesions are destroyed by the haemorrhage itself and are therefore presumed to account for some cases of apparently spontaneous intracerebral or subarachnoid haemorrhage. In such circumstances they are termed *cryptic angiomas*.

Transitional forms of angioma are seen and are called *capillary-venous malformations*. A type frequently recognised at autopsy is that of the *venous angioma* in which the constituent veins are separated by normal brain tissue. The walls of these vessels may become thick and hyalinised but rarely become calcified.

Other forms of vascular malformation

In the *Sturge–Kalischer–Weber syndrome*[158] there is a vascular hamartoma on the face and an underlying intracranial vascular malformation. The skin lesion is usually a port wine naevus on the face or scalp in the distribution of the fifth cranial nerve. The intracranial lesion is a developmental anomaly which usually takes the form of a superficial capillary or venous malformation confined to the meninges and most frequently sited over the posterior half of the cerebral hemisphere on the same side as the skin lesion. Calcification is common. Haemorrhage is rare. *Cobb's syndrome*[159] is a condition comparable to Sturge–Kalischer–Weber syndrome but involving the spinal cord. The vascular malformation is in the pia-arachnoid over part of the cord and the accompanying cutaneous naevus is in the territory innervated by one or more of the corresponding spinal nerves.

A rare lesion is that of *aneurysmal dilatation of the great cerebral vein (of Galen)* which may be associated with high output cardiac failure in newborn children.

In *von Hippel–Lindau disease* (see p. 355) there is an association between haemangioblastomas of the brain and angiomas of other tissues, specially the retina, lungs, liver and kidneys. The disorder, one of the phacomatoses, is often familial and shows a dominant pattern of inheritance.

PURPURIC CONDITIONS AFFECTING THE BRAIN

This is a non-specific descriptive term applicable to any condition of the brain characterised by the occurrence of petechial haemorrhages. The petechiae vary considerably in number but are usually confined to white matter. There are many causes: notable examples include *cerebral malaria* (see p. 180), *acute haemorrhagic encephalomyelitis* (see p. 210) and *thrombotic thrombocytopenic purpura* (see p. 103). They are also seen in fatal cases of *hypertensive encephalopathy* (see p. 98) and of *fat embolism* (see p. 100). Petechiae are often present in cases of *severe head injury* (see p. 127), when they may be a manifestation either of primary injury or secondary complications, such as fat embolism.

Petechial haemorrhages are also seen in cases of *viral meningoencephalitis* (see p. 198), particularly where there is an associated vasculitis, as in acute necrotising encephalitis due to herpes simplex. They are also seen in cases of *septicaemia* and *endotoxic shock*. Brain purpura may result from *poisoning*, for example by carbon monoxide or phosphorus. Another important cause is an *allergic sensitivity to drugs*, penicillin being the best known to have such an effect. This type of drug-induced encephalopathy has always been rare; it was once most frequently seen as a complication of organic arsenicals, such as neoarsphenamine which was widely used in the treatment of syphilis. As in haemorrhagic leucoencephalitis, the underlying lesion is necrosis of the walls of small blood vessels, particularly venules.

Brain purpura may also be a manifestation of *asphyxia*, but in such cases petechiae are less frequent in the brain than in the epicardium and pleurae. They may also be present in some cases when death has occurred during electroconvulsive therapy.[160] Petechiae are also present in the primary and secondary forms of *thrombocytopenic purpura* and in other disorders of blood, notably *leukaemia*. In some of these cases the features are those of *disseminated intravascular coagulation* and *consumptive coagulopathy*.

HYPOXIC BRAIN DAMAGE[10,161]

INTRODUCTION

Irreversible hypoxic brain damage can occur whenever there is insufficient oxygen in the blood or a reduced blood flow to the brain, or both. The supply of oxygen depends on the cerebral blood flow (CBF) and the oxygen content of the blood. Cerebral blood flow, in turn, depends on the cerebral perfusion pressure (CPP), that is, the difference between the mean systemic arterial pressure and the intracranial pressure (ICP). Since the most important factor in maintaining an adequate supply of oxygen to the brain is its blood flow, there are protective mechanisms to preserve it.

Preservation of CBF when systemic arterial pressure is low is brought about by autoregulation, which is defined as the maintenance of a relatively constant blood flow in the face of changes in CPP. As the systemic arterial pressure falls, the cerebrovascular resistance also falls because of autoregulatory dilatation of cerebral arterioles, with

the result that CBF remains within normal limits over a wide range of systemic arterial pressure. When cerebral vasodilatation is maximal at about 50 mmHg (the lower limit), cerebrovascular resistance cannot fall further, so that when systemic arterial pressure falls below this level, CBF also falls. An upper limit of autoregulation has also been recognised (about 160 mmHg), beyond which vasoconstriction is inadequate, CBF increases, dysfunction of the blood-brain barrier develops and hypertensive encephalopathy is induced (see p. 98).

Cerebral arterioles also respond to changes in the blood gases when systemic arterial pressure is within the normal limits; an increase in arterial carbon dioxide or a decrease in arterial oxygen produces arteriolar vasodilatation and hence a fall in cerebrovascular resistance and an increase in CBF. Thus, if arteriolar vasodilatation resulting from hypoxia or, in particular, hypercapnia exists prior to any reduction in systemic arterial pressure, maximal vasodilatation will be maintained at a higher systemic arterial pressure than in the normocapnic state. Such patients, however, are particularly vulnerable to a fall in systemic arterial pressure since the autoregulatory preservation of CBF is impaired. Autoregulation may be impaired, for example, during and following anaesthesia, in patients with acute head injury and after a 'stroke'.

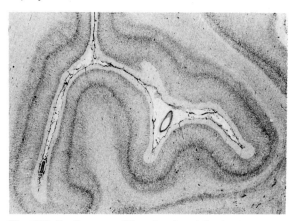

Fig. 5.30 Cardiac arrest. There is subtotal (laminar) recent necrosis of the third, fifth and sixth cortical layers with selective sparing of the second and fourth layers (darker staining) in brain of patient who survived 48 hours after cardiac arrest.
Reproduced by permission. Please see acknowledgement after caption of Fig. 5.1 (page 91).

Brain damage due to cardiac arrest

Complete clinical recovery is unlikely if cardiac arrest of abrupt onset and at normal body temperature exceeds 5–7 minutes. However, there is increasing evidence from clinical and experimental work that the ischaemic threshold of the brain may be extended to approximately 15 minutes.

If death occurs within 24–36 hours of the cardiac arrest, the brain may appear normal externally and on section. By 36–48 hours it is sometimes possible to identify laminar or patchy discoloration in the depths of sulci, particularly in the posterior halves of the cerebral hemispheres, and selective necrosis in region CA1 (Sommer sector) of the hippocampus. Microscopy reveals diffuse neuronal necrosis with a characteristic pattern of selective vulnerability (see p. 36), the changes being accentuated within the depths of sulci rather than at the crests of gyri, and maximal in layers III, V and VI (Fig. 5.30) in the parietal and occipital lobe cortex. In the hippocampus, region CA1 is commonly affected (Figs 5.31a, b, c

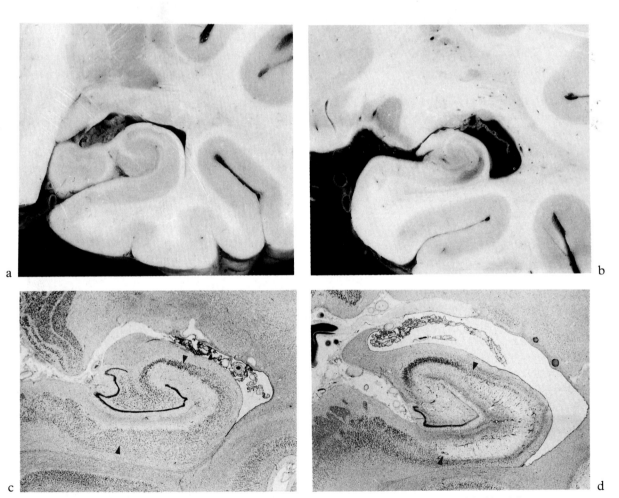

Fig. 5.31a, b, c, d Hypoxic necrosis of hippocampus. (**a**) Normal right hippocampus to compare with (**b**) a right hippocampus in which there is necrosis of the CA1 sector (discoloured region). (**c**) Normal right hippocampus to compare with (**d**). The arrows delineate the CA1 sector. (**d**) Right hippocampus showing recent selective neuronal necrosis of CA1 sector (between arrows) and in CA4.
Cresyl violet (**c, d**) × 3
Reproduced by permission. Please see acknowledgement after caption of Fig. 5.1 (page 91).

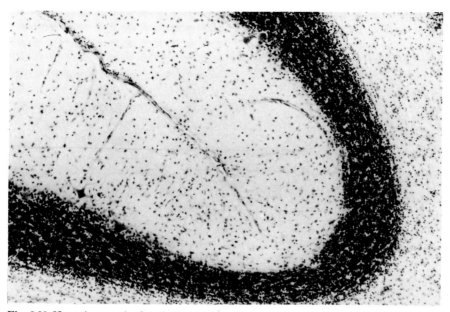

Fig. 5.32 Hypoxic necrosis of cerebellum. The Purkinje cells have undergone selective necrosis and as a result there is an astrocytosis and proliferation of microglia.
Celloidin; cresyl violet × 170

and d) and these changes are sometimes associated with necrosis in the amygdala. The pattern of damage in the basal ganglia and thalamus is more variable and, in the cerebellum, there is characteristically diffuse necrosis of Purkinje cells (Fig. 5.32). Damage to the nuclei of the brainstem tends to be more severe in infants and young children than in adults.

Patients with severe diffuse brain damage due to cardiac arrest rarely survive for more than a few days but occasionally they may remain alive in a persistent vegetative state[162] for several months or longer.[163] In such cases there is an appreciable reduction in the weight of the brain and evidence of atrophy of both the cortical gyri and cerebellar folia. In coronal slices, considerable ventricular enlargement may be seen (Fig. 5.33). The cortex of the parietal and occipital lobes is reduced to a thin band of discoloured tissue, but that of the frontal and temporal lobes may appear normal. The hippocampi may show CA1 sclerosis (Ammon's horn sclerosis). Even when cortical necrosis is severe and survival is for only a few weeks, the thalami may appear grossly normal. Eventually, evidence of retrograde degeneration (see p. 46) is seen in the thalamic projection nuclei.

Brain damage due to hypotension

Brain damage due to a generalised reduction in CBF occurs characteristically in association with an episode of severe systemic hypotension. Brain

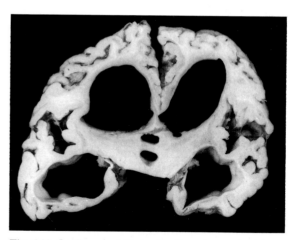

Fig. 5.33 Cardiac arrest. Brain of patient who survived 4 years in a vegetative state after cardiac arrest. The cortex is greatly narrowed and there is gross, but essentially symmetrical, enlargement of the ventricles. The hippocampus and the thalami are also atrophic.
Reproduced by permission. Please see acknowledgement after caption of Fig. 5.1 (page 91).

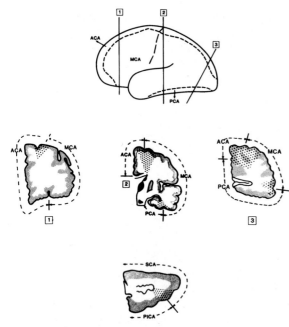

Fig. 5.34 Arterial boundary zones in cerebral and cerebellar hemispheres. The right cerebral hemisphere is shown at three levels, viz. 1 = frontal, 2 = mid-temporal and 3 = occipital. Each boundary zone is stippled. ACA = anterior cerebral artery, MCA = middle cerebral artery, PCA = posterior cerebral artery, SCA = superior cerebellar artery and PICA = posterior inferior cerebellar artery. *Reproduced by permission. Please see acknowledgement after caption of Fig. 5.1 (page 91).*

damage may take several forms, but in the commonest type hypoxic damage is concentrated in the arterial boundary zones ('watershed areas') between the main cerebral and cerebellar arterial territories (Fig. 5.34).[164]

This pattern of brain damage has been described in neurosurgical patients operated on in a sitting position,[165] following a sudden decrease in arterial pressure,[166] after occlusion of one carotid artery,[27] after dental anaesthesia in the semi-recumbent position,[167] after the over-zealous treatment of malignant hypertension by anti-hypertensive agents,[41,42] and in the brains of patients dying from 'non-missile' head injuries.[168] In these circumstances, once the capacity for autoregulation of blood flow is lost as a result of a combination of reduced perfusion pressure and hypoxaemia, oxygenation decreases to a critical level in those parts of the brain at the periphery of the arterial supply and furthest removed from the main trunk

of the vessel, i.e. in the boundary zones, and infarction ensues.[169] This pattern of brain damage has also been described in cases of cerebral embolism.[170]

If the lesions are several days old, they may be recognised macroscopically, provided the brain is cut in the coronal plane (Fig. 5.35a). They vary in size from small foci of necrosis in the cortex to large wedge-shaped lesions extending from the cortex almost to the angle of the lateral ventricle. Cortical damage is most frequent and most severe in the parieto-occipital regions, that is in the common boundary zone between the territories of the anterior, middle and posterior cerebral arteries. Less commonly, there may be lesions between the middle and anterior cerebral artery territories, or between regions supplied by the middle and posterior cerebral arteries. The lesions are usually asymmetrical and may be unilateral. In the cerebellum, the boundary zone between the territories of the superior and posterior inferior cerebellar arteries lies just below the dorsal angle of each hemisphere (Fig. 5.35b). There is variable involvement of the basal ganglia, and the hippocampus and brainstem are usually not involved. In other cases, the ischaemic damage is generalised in the cortex of the cerebrum and cerebellum, is minor or absent in the hippocampi and is often severe in the thalami. Yet other cases show generalised damage in the cortex of the cerebral and cerebellar hemispheres with accentuation along the arterial boundary zones. The hippocampi are usually spared and there is patchy damage in the basal ganglia.

Brain damage due to carbon monoxide poisoning

Carbon monoxide (CO) poisoning may be accidental or associated with attempted suicide. Most accidental cases are due to an escape of domestic gas, but CO is also a component of fumes from solid fuel heaters and of exhaust gases of internal combustion engines. Examples from industry are fewer and include accidents in blast furnaces and in mines. In a non-anaemic subject 15–20% of haemoglobin may combine with CO before symptoms appear. When the level of the carboxy-haemoglobin exceeds 20%, there is dyspnoea on

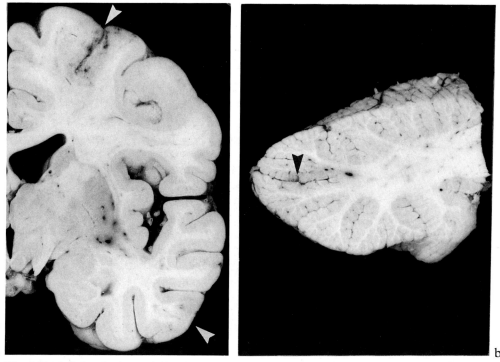

Fig. 5.35a, b Infarction in arterial boundary zones. (**a**) Hemi-section of brain from patient who survived for 17 days after a myocardial infarct. Note focally haemorrhagic infarcts (arrows) in the boundary zones between the anterior and middle cerebral arterial territories, and between the middle and posterior cerebral arterial territories. Compare distribution with Figure 5.34. (**b**) Same case as (a). Slice of left cerebellar hemisphere to show duskily haemorrhagic infarct at dorsal angle of hemisphere, i.e. in the boundary zone between the superior and posterior inferior cerebellar arterial territories. Compare with Figure 5.34.

Reproduced by permission. Please see acknowledgement after caption of Fig. 5.1 (page 91).

exertion and slight headache. At a level of 30% there is severe headache, fatigue and impaired judgement. Consciousness is lost at a level of 60–70% carboxyhaemoglobin, and a concentration of 70% or more is rapidly fatal.

The clinical symptoms of CO poisoning may be monophasic, in which survival may range from hours to years but without remission of symptoms, or biphasic, in which an interval of apparent normality lasting 2–30 days is followed by neurological deficit. While this biphasic pattern of symptoms has often been regarded as a specific feature of CO intoxication, it can also be a sequel of quite different types of hypoxia such as result from cardiac arrest and exposure to nitrogen.[171]

When death occurs within a few hours of CO poisoning the brain may display the pink–red colour characteristic of carboxyhaemoglobin.

When survival is for 36–48 hours, the brain shows evidence of congestion, and petechiae are frequently seen in the corpus callosum and elsewhere in the white matter. Although it is often said there is a particular predilection for necrosis of the globus pallidus (Fig. 5.36) in CO poisoning, neuronal necrosis may also be seen in other selectively vulnerable regions, such as the hippocampus, and the cerebral and cerebellar cortex. It should be noted that ischaemic necrosis of the pallidum can also be a sequel to cyanide intoxication and anaesthetic accidents. It should also be noted that after CO intoxication the globus pallidus may be normal.

Changes in the white matter are a common, and often conspicuous, consequence of CO poisoning. Damage to white matter tends to occur particularly in patients who develop delayed signs of

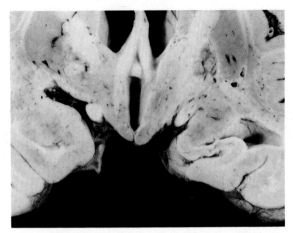

Fig. 5.36 Carbon monoxide poisoning. Brain of patient who survived in coma for 9 months after poisoning by carbon monoxide. There is cystic infarction of the medial segments of each globus pallidus.

intoxication after the period of relative clinical normality which may follow acute poisoning. The changes in white matter, however, are not necessarily proportional to damage in grey matter, and the latter may appear normal even in the presence of extensive myelin breakdown. White matter damage usually takes one or more of three forms:

1. Discrete and usually perivascular foci of myelin destruction occur throughout the white matter, including the optic tracts.
2. Diffuse and widespread destruction of myelinated fibres occurs throughout the brain.
3. Foci of demyelination occur that may or may not be confluent in the more posterior and deeper portions of the central white matter.

The *pathogenesis* of CO encephalopathy has been reviewed.[172] In addition to the high affinity of CO for oxygen and its binding to brain cytochromes, various studies have underlined the importance of systemic circulatory factors, raising the possibility that the concentration of damage in the white matter may be due to a local cytotoxic effect of CO together with a reduction in blood flow.

Selective vulnerability[173]

In its most classical form this is seen after an episode of cardiac arrest (see p. 36). While it is accepted that the more recently evolved regions of the brain are most vulnerable to hypoxia, damage is never total, and even in patients in the vegetative state large numbers of normal nerve cells may be present.

Two major hypotheses have been advanced to explain the characteristic distribution of hypoxic brain damage. That advocated by Speilmeyer[174] is known as the vascular theory and invokes anatomical factors, such as the length and course of a particular artery, in addition to physiological variables as the basis for local vulnerability. The other hypothesis, known as the 'concept of pathoclisis',[175] postulated particular physicochemical properties as a basis of vulnerability. It is difficult to explain the pattern of involvement by anatomical vascular factors alone, and increasing attention has been paid to metabolic events in the search for a common mechanism of cell damage.[176] It has been suggested recently that selectively vulnerable neurons are those in which the entry of calcium is favoured by neuronal depolarisation or "burst" firing during a period of re-oxygenation or recirculation. Thus, in the selectively vulnerable areas the capacity of the nerve cells to sequester or extrude calcium is exceeded, mitochondria swell, calcium is not released into the cytoplasm, and the ischaemic cell process is initiated.[177] Increasing attention is being paid to a possible imbalance between excitation and inhibition of neurons as a factor in the development of neuronal necrosis.[178]

Perinatal hypoxia[179]

The pattern of hypoxic damage varies with the gestational maturity of the brain (see Ch. 12). *Periventricular leucomalacia* (PVL) is the commonest hypoxic lesion in the premature infant's brain; it may also occur in the full-term infant.[180] Periventricular leucomalacia may be the only lesion in the brain of a premature infant, but in infants at term it is usually associated with lesions in the grey matter. It is now widely accepted that PVL is due to failure of cerebral perfusion.[181] It therefore seems likely that prolonged apnoea or peripheral circulatory failure in a pre-term infant may lead to severe hypotension; autoregulation of cerebral blood flow then becomes deranged and hypoxic brain damage ensues.

Epilepsy and hypoxia[182]

The pathogenesis of 'epileptic' brain damage is described in Chapter 14. Discrete seizures are unlikely to produce irreversible brain damage, whereas *status epilepticus* has long been recognised as a serious danger to life at any age, but particularly during childhood. The basic neuropathological changes are widespread necrosis of the cortex, hippocampus, basal ganglia, thalamus, cerebellum and parts of the brainstem.

Experimental studies in primates have emphasised that systemic changes, such as arterial hypotension, hypoglycaemia and hyperpyrexia, contribute to the brain damage caused by epilepsy.[183–185] Thus, status epilepticus, particularly in children, constitutes a medical emergency.

Hypoglycaemia[10]

The respiratory quotient of the brain is almost unity, and glucose is the principal source of energy. Energy is required for the synthesis of large molecules, transport mechanisms, maintenance of membrane potentials and neurotransmitter turnover.

The level of blood glucose can fall from normal (5·5 mmol/l: about 100 mg/100 ml) to less than 3 mmol/l (about 55 mg/100ml) without symptoms. Below this level, however, there is a succession of symptoms ranging from inability to concentrate, irritability and hunger, to loss of memory and disorientation. At a level of about 1·1 mmol/l

(20 mg/100 ml), consciousness is lost and cardio-respiratory dysfunction and epileptic seizures may occur. This sequence of events may be seen in patients who die after insulin shock therapy for the treatment of psychosis, diabetic patients treated with insulin, those with insulin-secreting tumours, and in infants with idiopathic hypoglycaemia. The macroscopic features of the brain depend upon the survival time so that in cases of short survival the CNS may appear normal. Microscopy shows the changes of the *ischaemic cell process* (see p. 39)[186] and a pattern of damage that is similar to that found in other categories of hypoxia.[161] For example, within the cerebral cortex there is often laminar involvement of layers III and V, and typical hypoxic necrosis of the hippocampi is almost invariably present. The small cells of the striatum are often involved, though usually there is sparing of the globus pallidus. There is variable involvement of the thalamus and often there is complete sparing of the cerebellum (this is in marked contrast to other types of hypoxia). With increasing survival there is cortical atrophy and shrinkage of the medial parts of the temporal lobes with compensatory enlargement of the ventricles.[187]

Neuronal changes have been described in hypoglycaemia in newborn human infants[188] and in experimental animals,[189,190] but they are difficult to distinguish from artefact.[161,191] The neuronal changes in experimental hypoglycaemia do, however, appear to differ from those seen in hypotension and status epilepticus.[192]

REFERENCES

Introduction

1. Kannel WB, Wolf PA. In: Russell RWR, ed. Vascular disease of the central nervous system. Edinburgh: Churchill Livingstone, 1983: 1.
2. Wolf PA, Kannel WB, McGee DL. In: Barnett HJM, Mohr JP, Stein BM, Yatsu FM, eds. Stroke. Pathophysiology, diagnosis and management, vol. 1. Edinburgh: Churchill Livingstone, 1986: 19.

Structural changes

3. Brown AW, Brierley JB. Br J Exp Pathol 1968; 49: 87.
4. Brown AW. J Clin Pathol 1977; 30 suppl (Roy Coll Path) 11: 155.
5. Cammermeyer J. Acta Neuropathol (Berl) 1961; 1: 245.
6. Matakas F, Cervos-Navarro J, Schneider H. J Neurol

Neurosurg Psychiatry 1973; 36: 497.
7. Adams H. Arch Neurol (Chic) 1976; 33: 589.
8. Brierley JB, Meldrum BS, Brown AW. Arch Neurol (Chic) 1973; 29: 367.
9. Graham DI. J Clin Pathol 1977; 30 suppl (Roy Coll Pathol) 11: 170.
10. Brierley JB, Graham DI. In: Adams JH, Corsellis JAN, Duchen LW, eds. Greenfield's Neuropathology. 4th ed. London: Arnold, 1984: 125.

Vascular disorders

11. Alpers BJ, Berry RG, Paddison RM. Arch Neurol Psychiatry (Chic) 1959; 81: 409.
12. Alpers BJ, Berry RG. Arch Neurol (Chic) 1963; 8: 398.
13. Hutchings BM, Weller RO. J Neurosurg 1986; 65: 316.
14. Alcalado R, Weller RO, Parrish EP, Garrod D.

Neuropathol Appl Neurobiol 1988; 14: 1.
15. Moossy J. Neurology (Minneap) 1959; 9: 569.
16. Tindall GT, Odom GL, Cupp HB, Dillon ML. J Neurosurg 1962; 19: 917.
17. Brice TG, Dowsett DJ, Lowe RD. Lancet 1964; 1: 84.
18. Fisher M. Arch Neurol Psychiatry (Chic) 1951; 65: 346.
19. Hutchinson EC, Yates PO. Brain 1956; 79: 319.
20. Hutchinson EC, Yates PO. Lancet 1957; i: 2.
21. Torvik A, Jorgensen L. J Neurol Sci 1964; 1: 24.
22. Castaigne P, Lhermitte F, Gautier J-C, Escourolle R, Derouesne C. Brain 1970; 93: 231.
23. Humphrey JG, Newton TH. Brain 1960; 83: 565.
24. Adams JH, Graham DI. J Neurol Neurosurg Psychiatry 1967; 30: 479.
25. Russell RWR. Lancet 1961; ii: 1422.
26. Torvik A, Jorgensen L. J Neurol Sci 1966; 3: 410.
27. Romanul FCA, Abramowicz A. Arch Neurol (Chic) 1964; 11: 40.
28. Reivich M, Holling HE, Roberts B, Toole JF. N Engl J Med 1961; 265: 878.
29. Lhermitte F, Gautier J-C, Derouesne C. Neurology (Minneap) 1970; 20: 82.
30. Fisher CM, Gore I, Okabe N, White PD. J Neuropathol Exp Neurol 1965; 24: 455.
31. Battacharji SK, Hutchinson EC, McCall AJ. Br Med J 1967; 2: 270.
32. Castaigne P et al. Brain 1973; 96: 133.
33. Sherman DG, Hart RG, Easton JD. Stroke 1981; 12: 2.
34. Kubik CS, Adams RD. Brain 1946; 69: 73.
35. Biemond A. Brain 1951; 74: 300.
36. Nordgren RE, Markesbery WR, Fukuda K, Reeves AG. Neurology (Minneap) 1971; 21: 1140.
37. Hawkes CH. Br Med J 1974; 4: 379.
38. Hughes JT. In: Adams JH, Corsellis JAN, Duchen LW, eds. Greenfield's Neuropathology. 4th ed. London: Arnold, 1984: 779.

Hypertension and the brain

39. Strandgaard S. Circulation 1976; 53: 720.
40. Graham DI, Jones JV. In: Robertson JIS, Pickering GW, Caldwell ADS, eds. R Soc Med Internat Symp Series 26. London: Royal Society of Medicine, 1979: 105.
41. Graham DI. Br Med J 1975; 4: 739.
42. Ledingham JGG, Rajagopalan B. Q J Med 1979; 48: 25.
43. Graham DI, McGeorge A, Fitch W, Jones JV, MacKenzie ET. J. Hypertension 1984; 2: 297.
44. Gautier JC. In: Russell RWR, ed. Vascular disease of the central nervous system. 2nd ed. Edinburgh: Churchill Livingstone, 1983: 224.
45. Fisher CM. Am J Pathol 1972; 66: 313.
46. Strandgaard S, Haunso S. Lancet 1987; 11: 658.
47. Fisher CM. Neurology (Minneap) 1965; 15: 774.
48. Cole FM, Yates PO. Neurology (Minneap) 1968; 18: 255.
49. Fisher CM. Acta Neuropathol (Berl) 1969; 12: 1.
50. Mohr J. Stroke 1982; 13: 3.
51. Rosenberg EF. Arch Intern Med 1940; 65: 545.
52. Richards A, Graham D, Bullock R. J Neurol Neurosurg Psychiatry 1988; 51: 416.
53. Chester EM, Agamanolis DP, Banker BQ, Victor M. Neurology (Minneap) 1978; 28: 928.
54. Byrom FB. Lancet 1954; ii: 201.
55. MacKenzie ET, Strandgaard S, Graham DI, Jones JV, Harper AM, Farrar JK. Circ Res 1976; 39: 33.
56. Skinhoj E, Strandgaard S. Lancet 1973; i: 461.
57. Janota I. Psychol Med 1981; 11: 39.
58. Loizou LA, Jefferson JM, Smith WT. J Neurol Neurosurg Psychiatry 1982; 45: 409.

Cerebral embolism

59. Meyer JS. In: Meyer JS, Shaw T, eds. Diagnosis and management of stroke and TIA's. London: Addison-Wesley, 1982: 155.
60. MacDonald RA, Robbins SL. Ann Intern Med 1957; 46: 255.
61. Bjork VO, Hultquist G. Thorax 1960; 15: 284.
62. Branthwaite MA. Thorax 1972; 27: 748.
63. Brierley JB. Proc R Soc Med 1967; 60: 858.
64. Editorial. Lancet 1982; i: 1161.
65. Sotaniemi KA, Mononen H, Hokkanen TE. Stroke 1986; 17: 410.
66. Shaw PJ, Shaw DA et al. Br Med J 1985; 291: 1384.
67. Shaw PJ et al. Br Med J 1986; 293: 165.
68. Szabo G. J Clin Pathol 1970; 23 (suppl 4): 123.
69. Adams JH, Graham DI, Mills E, Sprunt TG. Br Med J 1972; 3: 740.
70. Menkin M, Schwartzman RJ. Arch Neurol (Chic) 1977; 34: 168.
71. Taylor JED. Br Med J 1952; 1: 890.
72. Brion S, Psimaras A, Gallissot MC. In: Arfel G, Naquet R, eds. L'Embolie gazeuse du système carotidien. Paris: Doin, 1974: 194.
73. Haymaker W. In: Lubarsch O, Henke F, Rössle R, eds. Handbuch der speziellen pathologischen Anatomie und Histologie. Berlin: Springer 1957: 1600.
74. Palmer AC, Calder IM, McCallum RI, Mastaglia FL. Br Med J 1981; 283: 888.
75. Haymaker W, Johnston AD. Milit Med 1955; 117: 285.
76. Haymaker W, Davison C. J Neuropathol Exp Neurol 1950; 9: 29.

Cerebral arteritis

77. Hurst EW. J Pathol Bacteriol 1955; 70: 167.
78. Stebhens WE. Pathology of the cerebral blood vessels. St Louis: Mosby, 1972.
79. Rosenblum WI, Hadfield MG, Young HF. Ann Neurol 1978; 3: 374.
80. Ford RG, Siekert RG. Neurology (Minneap) 1965; 15: 114.
81. Drachman DA. Neurology (Minneap) 1963; 8: 145.
82. Anderson JM, Jamieson DG, Jefferson JM. Q J Med 1975; 44: 309.
83. Appenzeller O, Williams RC. Ann Intern Med 1979; 90: 430.
84. Johnson RT, Richardson EP. Medicine (Baltimore) 1968; 47: 337.
85. Crompton MR. Brain 1959; 82: 377.
86. Silverstein A. Arch Neurol (Chic) 1968; 18: 358.
87. Wright TL, Bresnan MJ. Neurology (Minneap) 1976; 26: 540.
88. Peck FC, McGovern FR. J Neurosurg 1966; 25: 536.
89. Hopewell JW. Neuropathol Appl Neurobiol 1979; 5: 329.
90. Lee DK, Andrews JM. JAMA 1967; 200: 720.
91. Douglas AC, Maloney AFJ. J Neurol Neurosurg Psychiatry 1973; 36: 1024.

92. Katzenstein A-LA, Carrington CB, Leibow AA. Cancer 1979; 43: 360.

Less common causes of infarction

93. Coakham HB, Duchen LW, Scaravilli F. J Neurol Neurosurg Psychiatry 1979; 42: 289.
94. Thomas DJ et al. Lancet 1977; ii: 941.
95. Boros L, Weiner WJ. In: Vinken PJ, Bruyn GW, eds. Handbook of clinical neurology, vol. 38, Part I. Amsterdam: North Holland, 1979: 33.
96. Illis L, Kocen RS, McDonald WI, Mondkar VP. Br Med J 1965; 2: 1164.
97. Vessey MP, Doll R. Br Med J 1969; 2: 651.
98. Collaborative Group for the Study of Stroke in Young Women. N Engl J Med 1973; 288: 871.
99. Cross JN, Castro PO, Jennett WB. Br Med J 1968; 2: 214.
100. Russell RWR, ed. Vascular disease of the central nervous system. 2nd ed. Edinburgh: Churchill Livingstone, 1983.

Spontaneous intracranial haemorrhage

101. Weller RO. In: Adams JH, Corsellis JAN, Duchen LW, eds. Greenfield's Neuropathology. 4th ed. London: Arnold, 1984: 208.
102. Russell DS. Proc R Soc Med 1954; 47: 689.
103. Cole FM, Yates PO. Brain 1967; 90: 759.
104. Nakajima K. Stroke 1983; 14: 485.
105. Charcot J-M, Bouchard C. Arch Physiol Norm Pathol 1868; 1: 110, 643.
106. Cole FM, Yates PO. J Pathol Bacteriol 1967; 93: 393.
107. Cole FM, Yates PO. Neurology (Minneap) 1968; 18: 255.
108. De Villiers JC. Br J Psychiatry 1966; 112: 109.
109. McCormick WF. In: Rosenberg RN, Schochet SS, eds. The clinical neurosciences: neuropathology. Edinburgh: Churchill Livingstone, 1983: 35.
110. Vinters HV. Stroke 1987; 18: 311.
111. Pakarinen S. Acta Neurol Scand 1967; 43 (suppl 29): 1.
112. Sekhar LN, Heros RC. Neurosurgery 1981; 8: 248.
113. Locksley HB. J Neurosurg 1966; 25: 219.
114. McKissock W, Richardson A, Walsh L, Owen E. Lancet 1964; i: 623.
115. Glynn LE. J Path Bacteriol 1940; 51: 213.
116. Stehbens WE. Arch Neurol (Chic) 1963; 8: 272.
117. Stehbens WE. Arch Pathol 1963; 75: 45.
118. Crawford T. J Neurol Neurosurg Psychiatry 1959; 22: 259.
119. Sheffield EA, Weller RO. J Neurol Sci 1980; 46: 341.
120. MacFarlane TWR, Canham PB, Roach MR. Stroke 1983; 14: 70.
121. Tognetti F, Limoni P, Testa C. Surg Neurol 1983; 20: 74.
122. Fearnsides EG. Brain 1916; 39: 224.
123. McCormick WF, Schmalstieg EJ. Arch Neurol (Chic) 1977; 34: 285.
124. Franks AJ. Neuropathol Appl Neurobiol 1978; 4: 61.
125. Canham PB, Ferguson GG. Neurosurgery 1985; 17: 291.
126. Suzuki J, Ohara H. J Neurosurg 1978; 48: 505.
127. Whittle IR, Dorsch NW, Besser M. J Neurol Neurosurg Psychiatry 1982; 45: 1040.
128. Sahs AL. In: Sahs AL, Nibbelink DW, eds.

Aneurysmal subarachnoid hemorrhage. Baltimore: Urban and Schwarzenberg, 1981.
129. Drake CG. Stroke 1981; 12: 273.
130. Locksley HB. In: Sahs AL, Perret GE, Locksley HB, Nishioka H, eds. Intracranial aneurysms and subarachnoid hemorrhage. A cooperative study. Philadelphia: Lippincott, 1969.
131. Winn HR, Richardson AE, Jane JA. Ann Neurol 1977; 1: 358.
132. Tomlinson BE. J Clin Pathol 1959; 12: 391.
133. Crompton MR. J Neurol Neurosurg Psychiatry 1963; 26: 535.
134. Mohr G et al. J Neurosurg 1983; 58: 482.
135. Schneck SA. Neurology (Minneap) 1964; 14: 691.
136. Crompton MR. Brain 1964; 87: 263.
137. Crompton MR. Brain 1964; 87: 491.
138. Graham DI, Macpherson P, Pitts LH. J Neurosurg 1983; 59: 223.
139. Foltz EL, Ward AA. J Neurosurg 1956; 13: 546.
140. Kibler RF, Couch RSC, Crompton MR. Brain 1961; 84: 45.
141. Robinson RG. J Neurosurg 1967; 26: 527.
142. Hatfield MP, Pfister RC. JAMA 1972; 222: 1527.
143. Belber CJ, Hoffman RB. J Neurosurg 1968; 28: 556.
144. Yabumoto M, Funahashi K, Fujii T, Hayashi S, Komai N. Surg Neurol 1983; 20: 20.
145. Bannerman RM, Ingall GB, Graff CJ. Neurology 1970; 20: 283.
146. Neil-Dwyer G, Bartlett JR, Nicholls AC, Narcisi P, Pope FM. J Neurosurg 1983; 59: 16.
147. Steel JG, Thomas HA, Strollo PJ. Stroke 1982; 13: 712.
148. Little JR, St Louis P, Weinstein M, Dohn DF. Stroke 1982; 12: 183.
149. Schold C, Earnest MP. Stroke 1978; 9: 267.
150. Frazee JG, Cahan LD, Winter J. J Neurosurg 1980; 53: 633.
151. Bohmfalk GL, Story JL, Wissinger JP, Brown WE. J Neurosurg 1978; 48: 369.
152. Davidson P, Robertson DM. J Neurosurg 1971; 35: 71.
153. Horten BC, Abbott GF, Porro RS. Arch Neurol (Chic) 1976; 33: 577.
154. Adams JH, Graham DI. J Neurol Neurosurg Psychiatry 1967; 30: 479.
155. Alexander CB, Burger PC, Goree JA. Stroke 1979; 10: 294.
156. McCormick WF. J Neurosurg 1966; 24: 807.
157. Graf CJ, Perret GE, Torner JC. J Neurosurg 1983; 58: 331.
158. Weber FP. Proc R Soc Med 1928/29; 22: 431.
159. Cobb S. Ann Surg 1915; 62: 641.
160. Allen IM. NZ Med J 1959; 58: 369.

Hypoxic brain damage

161. Graham DI. Br J Anaesth 1985; 57: 3.
162. Jennett B, Plum F. Lancet 1972; 1: 734.
163. Brierley JB, Adams JH, Graham DI, Simpson JA. Lancet 1971; 2: 560.
164. Brierley JB. In: Rose FC, Behan PO, eds. Animal models of neurological disease. Tunbridge Wells: Pitman Medical, 1980: 338.
165. Wolf A, Siris J. Bull Neurol Inst NY 1937; 6: 42.
166. Zulch KJ, Behrend RCH. In: Gastaut H, Meyer JS, eds. Cerebral anoxia and the electroencephalogram. Springfield, Illinois: Thomas, 1961: 144.

167. Brierley JB, Miller AA. Lancet 1966; 2: 869.
168. Graham DI, Adams JH, Doyle D. J Neurol Sci 1978; 39: 213.
169. Adams JH, Brierley JB, Connor RCR, Treip CS. Brain 1966; 89: 235.
170. Torvik A, Skullerud K. Clin Neuropathol 1982; 1: 99.
171. Plum F, Posner JB, Hain RF. Arch Intern Med 1962; 110: 18.
172. Ginsberg MD. In: Fahn S, Davis JN, Rowland LP, eds. Cerebral hypoxia and its consequences. Advances in neurology, vol. 26. New York: Raven Press, 1979: 21.
173. Kogure K, Hossmann K-A, Siesjo BK, Welsh FA, eds. Progress in Brain Research 1985: 63.
174. Spielmeyer W. Z Gesamte Neurol Psychiatrie 1925; 99: 756.
175. Vogt C, Vogt O. J Psychol Neurol (Leipz) 1937; 47: 237.
176. Siesjo BK. J Cereb Blood Flow Metab 1981; 1: 155.
177. Simon RP, Griffiths R, Evans MC, Swan JH, Meldrum BS. J Cereb Blood Flow Metab 1984; 4: 350.
178. Wieloch T. In: Kogure K, Hossmann KA, Siesjo BK, Welsh FA, eds. Progress in brain research, vol. 63. Amsterdam: Elsevier, 1985.
179. Wigglesworth JS, Pape KE. Early Hum Dev 1978; 2: 179.
180. Banker B, Larroche JC. Arch Neurol (Chic) 1962; 7: 386.
181. Takashima S, Tanaka K. Arch Neurol (Chic) 1978; 35: 11.
182. Meldrum BS, Corsellis JAN. In: Adams JH, Corsellis JAN, Duchen LW, eds. Greenfield's Neuropathology. 4th ed. London: Arnold, 1984: 921.
183. Meldrum BS, Brierley JB. Arch Neurol (Chic) 1973; 28: 10.
184. Meldrum BS, Horton RW. Arch Neurol (Chic) 1973; 28: 1.
185. Meldrum BS, Vigouroux RA, Brierley JB. Arch Neurol (Chic) 1973; 29: 82.
186. Brierley JB, Brown AW, Meldrum BS. Brain Res 1971; 25: 483.
187. Myers RE, Kahn KJ. In: Brierley JB, Meldrum BS, eds. Brain hypoxia. Clinics in developmental medicine, no. 39/40. London: Spastics International/Heinemann, 1971: 195.
188. Anderson JM, Milner RDG, Strich SJ. J Neurol Neurosurg Psychiatry 1967; 30: 295.
189. Agardh C-D, Kalimo H, Olsson Y, Siesjo BK. Acta Neuropathol (Berl) 1980; 50: 31.
190. Kalimo H, Agardh C-D, Olsson Y, Siesjo BK. Acta Neuropathol (Berl) 1980; 50: 43.
191. Brierley JB, Brown AW. Acta Neuropathol (Berl) 1981; 55: 319.
192. Auer RN, Wieloch T, Olsson Y, Siesjo BK. Acta Neuropathol (Berl) 1984; 64: 177.

Trauma[1-3]

INTRODUCTION

Structural damage to the brain is irreversible, and therefore the most important factor governing the outcome in a patient who sustains a head injury is the damage sustained by the brain. Some damage may occur at the moment of injury and be so severe that the patient remains in coma. Fortunately, many patients make varying degrees of clinical recovery from coma; the underlying mechanism of this recovery remains uncertain, and there is little doubt that traumatic coma may be attributed to many different types of brain damage.

There have been many studies on the classification of brain damage in patients who die from a head injury.[4-9] Any classification of fatal traumatic brain damage must include patients who demonstrate a lucid interval prior to fatal coma as well as those who remain in coma from injury until death. In the past, the existence of *primary* and *secondary* damage[10-13] has been emphasised in an attempt to provide clinico-pathological correlations. This approach helps to identify potentially preventable complications in patients with a head injury who 'talk and die'.[14] The trend now, however, is for clinicians[15] and pathologists[1,16] to classify brain damage as *focal* or *diffuse*. Nevertheless, from a pathological point of view it is suggested that there are two main stages in the development of brain damage following injury to the head:

1. *Primary damage.* Damage occurring at the moment of injury in the form of cerebral contusions, lacerations of scalp, fracture of skull, diffuse axonal injury and intracranial haemorrhage.

2. *Secondary damage.* Complications of the original injury that include brain damage due to raised intracranial pressure, hypoxia, swelling and infection.

It may be very difficult at post-mortem to define the nature of any brain damage following a head injury unless the brain has been properly fixed prior to dissection and appropriate histological studies are undertaken (see Ch. 4). This applies both to non-missile (blunt) injuries, which are by far the most common in civilian practice, and to missile (penetrating) injuries. Singly or in combination, both types of injury may affect either the brain or the spinal cord.

NON-MISSILE HEAD INJURY

Brain damage as a cause of death or persistent disability after head injury remains a major health problem. Thus, in the United Kingdom (population about 55 million), it has been estimated that some 1500 patients per 100 000 population per year report to accident and emergency departments, of whom between 200 and 300 per 100 000 are admitted to hospital because of head injury. There are about 9 deaths from head injury per 100 000 population per year,[12] or 1% of all deaths. A quarter of deaths from trauma and almost half of those caused by road traffic accidents are due to head injury. Multi-centre studies have shown that between 1 and 5% of patients with severe head injury remain vegetative, and between 5 and 18% are severely disabled 6 months after their injury.[17] The accumulating population of disabled survivors after head injury is so large now that one family in 300 has a member with such a disability.[18] Given this high prevalence, it is not surprising that the economic and social consequences[19] of head injury have stimulated much research in many countries into its incidence and causes, the nature of the injury sustained, and how the morbidity and mortality may be prevented by improved methods of clinical management. One important result of these studies has been the identification of avoidable factors in the causation of brain damage, such as the early recognition of intracranial haematoma[20,21] and the recognition of

hazards of inter-hospital transfer of comatose head-injured patients.[22]

Mechanisms of brain damage due to non-missile injury

It has been shown that concussion can be reproduced in the laboratory by delivering controlled blows to the freely movable head by a calibrated pendulum (acceleration concussion), and that it is much more difficult to produce concussion if the head is fixed (compression concussion).[23] The forces acting on the brain during head injury produce complex movements and deformations. When the unsecured head is struck by a blunt object, an *acceleration* occurs whereas if the moving head suddenly strikes a blunt object a *deceleration* injury occurs. Sharp blows, in contrast, usually produce open brain injuries as a result of penetrating wounds of the skull. Contributions made by various analytical and physical models to the understanding of the mechanism involved in head injury have been reviewed extensively.[24-26]

A considerable amount of experimental work has been concerned with the *translational* (linear) and *rotational* (angular) movements of the skull which occur following a blow to the head. If the blow is sufficient to produce brain damage, it usually causes the head to accelerate. If the impact is directed at the centre of the head and the head moves forward in a straight line, a translational acceleration injury results. If the blow is directed eccentrically, the result is a combined translational and rotational acceleration type injury. Pure translational acceleration creates intracranial pressure gradients, while pure rotational acceleration produces rotation of the skull relative to the brain.

Two principal hypotheses have been advanced to account for brain damage incurred at the moment of injury, viz. the *skull distortion/head rotation* hypothesis and the *head translation/cavitation* hypothesis. Holbourn,[27,28] in his studies of the mechanisms of head injury, explained *coup* lesions (contusions that occur directly below the site of injury) and *contrecoup* lesions (contusions located on the side of the brain diametrically opposite to the point of injury) on physical principles elaborated by experiments on gelatine models. He postulated that brain damage was due to *rotational acceleration forces*. The main requisite for contrecoup damage was rotational movement of the head in the coronal, sagittal or horizontal plane, or a combination of these, the movement being transmitted to the brain which glided in its dural compartment. The gliding motion was said to be relatively free, except where the brain was confined by bony structures, particularly in the anterior and middle cranial fossae; here *'shear' strains* developed which caused *contusion* of the brain and tearing of blood vessels. The theory was supported by direct observations of brain movement in monkeys fitted with transparent lucite calvaria.[29] It was found that when the head was free to move, blows on the head caused swirling rotational movements of the brain within the cranial cavity. With respect to the head translation/cavitation hypothesis, it was established from a purely theoretical point of view that brain damage due to cavitation (bubble formation due to negative pressure) is possible during changes in intracranial pressure of short duration.[30]

The two main hypotheses for brain injury have been re-examined and it has been concluded that distortion of the skull and rotation of the head are more important in the production of coup and contrecoup injuries than either rotation alone or translation/cavitation and, also, that concussion is produced much more readily by angular acceleration than by translational acceleration.[24,25] Even though various experimental models have provided a substantial body of knowledge about the immediate physiology of cerebral concussion, many of the animals in these experiments were either only briefly unconscious or died rapidly;[31] the very common clinical condition of prolonged traumatic unconsciousness due to diffuse injury was notably absent. In the last few years, attempts have been made to produce prolonged traumatic coma in the absence of intracranial expanding lesions.[13] Initial studies showed that, at low and moderate acceleration levels, cerebral concussion with and without contusions in the frontal and temporal lobes was readily produced, but that, at high acceleration, the animals died rapidly from massive subdural haematomas. It is now possible to reproduce, experimentally, all the types of brain damage which occur in man as a result of a non-

missile head injury. Such experiments are on non-human primates using the Penn I and Penn II devices, which are based on inertial, that is, *non-impact*,[32] controlled angular acceleration of the head through 60° in the sagittal/lateral plane.[33]

There are remarkably close similarities in the principal neuropathological findings in patients who die as a result of a non-missile head injury (with and without diffuse axonal injury)[34] and in non-human primates subjected to angular acceleration by the Penn I[35] and Penn II[36] devices. These studies may be interpreted as reducing all the principal mechanisms of head injury to two phenomena—*contact* and *acceleration*.[24,36] *Contact phenomena* result from an object striking the head, and consist of local effects such as laceration of the scalp, fracture of the skull, extradural haematoma, some types of cerebral contusion and intracerebral haemorrhage. *Acceleration*, in contrast, results from head movement in the instant after an injury and leads to intracranial and intracerebral pressure gradients as well as shear, tensile and compressive strains.[37] Such acceleration or inertial (that is, non-impact) phenomena are responsible for the two most important types of damage encountered in non-missile head injury in man—*acute subdural haematoma* resulting from tearing of subdural bridging veins, and *diffuse damage to axons* which may be attributed mainly to shear or tensile strains generated in the brain at the moment of injury.

NON-MISSILE HEAD INJURIES IN MAN

Primary damage

Lacerations of scalp

These can be of considerable importance as sources of blood loss and as indications of the site of injury. Associated fractures of the skull are potential routes for intracranial infection.

Fracture of skull

The frequency of fracture of the skull varies according to the head injury population studied: the more severe the injury, the more fractures are found. For example, the frequency is 3% among accident/emergency attenders, whereas 65% of patients admitted to a neurosurgical unit have a fracture of the skull.[12] The incidence is 80% in fatal cases of head injury.[11] The vault is involved three times more often than the base, but there may be fractures in both sites. Thus, although it usually means that the blow has been moderately severe, skull fracture is by no means an invariable finding in fatal head injuries. A patient may die as a direct result of a head injury without any evidence of damage to the scalp and without a fracture of the skull. On the other hand, a patient with a fracture may appear to have little or no clinical evidence of brain damage. The importance, however, of a skull fracture cannot be over-emphasised because patients with such a fracture have a much higher incidence of intracranial haematoma. It has been calculated that with radiological evidence of skull fracture and any impairment of consciousness (including disorientation), 1 patient in 4 in an accident and emergency department or primary surgical ward will develop an intracranial haematoma. With no skull fracture and preserved orientation the risk is one in 6000.[38]

Some 62% of patients with severe head injury have a *linear fracture* of the vault, extending into the base of the skull in 17% . In only 4% of cases is the fracture limited to the base of the skull. In 11% of patients the fracture of the vault is *depressed*, that is, the fragments of the inner table of the skull are depressed by at least the thickness of the diploe. A depressed fracture is said to be *compound* if there is an associated laceration of the scalp, and *penetrating* if there is also a tear of the dura. Both of these are important as potential routes for intra-cranial infection; depressed fracture is also associated with an increased incidence of post-traumatic epilepsy. Fractures of the base of the skull may be complicated by intracranial infection, due to spread of organisms from the air sinuses or the middle ear; hence the clinical importance of CSF rhinorrhoea and otorrhoea and of intracranial aerocele. When the injury is particularly severe, there may be a *hinge fracture* extending across the base of the skull, usually in the region of the posterior part of the pituitary fossa and the adjacent squamous parts of the temporal bones. A fall on the occiput may be associated with a *contrecoup fracture* in the orbital roofs and ethmoid plates and, particularly in childhood, a 'growing

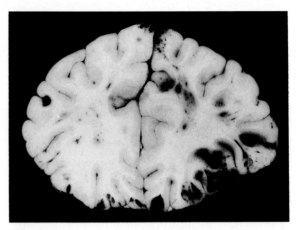

Fig. 6.1 Recent contusions on the orbital surfaces of the frontal lobes extending into the adjacent white matter.

fracture' may develop if brain tissue protrudes into the fracture and not only prevents it from healing but even causes it to enlarge.

Cerebral contusions and lacerations

The pia-arachnoid is intact over contusions but torn in lacerations. Considered to be the hallmark of brain damage due to head injury, these lesions are characteristically haemorrhagic and affect the crests of gyri, though they may extend into sulci and gyral white matter (Fig. 6.1). They are not always visible on the surface of the brain and may develop very rapidly, as they are present in patients said to have died 'instantaneously'. When healed they present as golden-brown shrunken scars, characteristic of a head injury in the past. Healed contusions have been reported as incidental findings in 2·5% of autopsies in general hospitals.[39] Typical contusions are rare in young infants. The characteristic features of a non-missile head injury in this age group are *contusional tears* in the subcortical white matter and in the outer layers of the cortex, particularly in the frontal and temporal lobes.[40]

Contusions in non-missile head injury have a very characteristic distribution affecting the frontal poles, orbital gyri (Figs 6.2a and b), the cortex above and below the Sylvian fissure where the brain is in close contact with the lesser wings of the sphenoid bones (Fig. 6.3), the temporal poles, and the lateral and inferior aspects of the temporal

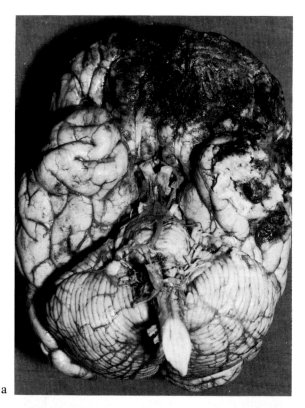

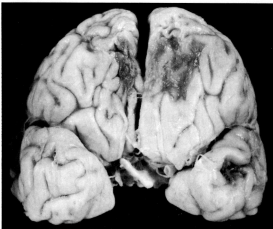

Fig. 6.2a, b Contusions on base of brain. (**a**) Recent contusions in the frontal and temporal gyri. (**b**) Old contusions in the frontal and temporal lobes of a patient who made an apparently complete recovery from a head injury sustained many years previously.

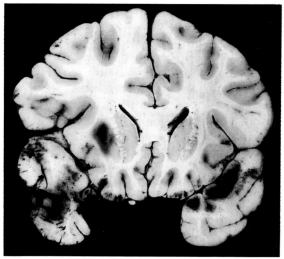

Fig. 6.3 Recent contusions affecting the cortex above and below the Sylvian (lateral) fissures.

lobes. Less frequently, the undersurfaces of the cerebellar hemispheres are affected.[41] Various categories of contusion have been defined. For example, *fracture contusions* occur at the site of a fracture and are particularly severe in the frontal lobes in association with fractures in the anterior fossa; *coup contusions* occur at the site of impact in the absence of a fracture; *contrecoup contusions* occur in the brain diametrically opposite the point of impact; *herniation contusions* occur where the medial parts of the temporal lobe are impacted against the edge of the tentorium, or where the cerebellar tonsils are impacted in the foramen magnum at the time of injury. The term *gliding contusions* describes focal haemorrhage in the cortex and subjacent white matter at the superior margins of the cerebral hemispheres. Gliding contusions are often asymmetrical and they range in size from microscopic to macroscopic haematomas. The term *intermediary coup contusions* refers to single or multiple 'contusion haemorrhages' in the deeper structures of the brain such as the white matter, the corpus callosum, the basal ganglia, the hypothalamus and the brainstem.[8]

In an attempt to assess contusions more precisely, a *contusion index* has been developed which allows the depth and extent of contusions in various parts of the brain to be expressed quantitatively.[42] Not surprisingly, contusions have been found to be most severe in the frontal and in the temporal lobes and to be more severe in patients with a fracture of the skull than in those without. There is no difference in the severity of contusions between patients who had or did not have a lucid interval, but contusions are less severe in patients with diffuse axonal injury (see below).

Lacerations (severe contusions) of the frontal and temporal lobes are often associated with acute subdural and intracerebral haemorrhage. The terms 'burst frontal lobe' and 'burst temporal lobe' are then appropriate.

Contusion is a type of focal brain damage caused mainly by contact phenomena when the surface of the brain impacts on bony protuberances in the base of the skull.[37] In contrast, gliding contusions are considered to be due to rotation.[43] These findings in man have been supported by studies in the non-human primate when impact phenomena, such as fracture of the skull and contusion of the brain, occur at short duration/high acceleration levels with the Penn I device (see p. 127).[35] As in man, the contusions occur particularly at the frontal and temporal poles. It has also been possible to reproduce gliding contusions in non-human primates subjected to specific loading conditions, such as lateral acceleration of the head with a relatively long pulse duration.[36]

Diffuse axonal injury

Recent clinical studies have emphasised that immediate prolonged unconsciousness which is not accompanied by an intracranial mass lesion, and is thus diffuse head injury, occurs in almost 50% of patients with severe head injury and is a cause of some 35% of all deaths from head injury. There are various forms of diffuse brain damage in head injury, but it is likely that in the majority of patients many nerve fibres are torn at the moment of injury.[1] This type of brain damage was first clearly defined as 'diffuse degeneration of white matter' in a series of patients with post-traumatic dementia;[44] it is now widely recognised and has a variety of synonyms including 'shearing injury',[45,46] 'diffuse damage of immediate impact type',[47] 'diffuse white matter shearing injury',[48] 'inner cerebral trauma'[49] and, more recently, 'diffuse axonal injury'.[34] From the outset, Strich[44] attributed the degeneration of white matter to shearing injury affecting nerve fibres at the time of injury. The concept of diffuse axonal injury as a form of primary brain damage, however, has not

remained unchallenged. Some workers have suggested that damage to white matter is often due to hypoxia or oedema, or is secondary to brainstem damage following an intracranial expanding lesion.[50-52] The situation has now been clarified in favour of Strich's views, and structural abnormalities identical to those seen in man have been produced in non-human primates subjected to non-impact controlled angular acceleration of the head without any concomitant increase in intracranial pressure or hypoxia.[36] This type of brain damage is referred to as diffuse axonal injury.

There are three distinctive features in the pathology of diffuse axonal injury (DAI) and it is not difficult to make this diagnosis at post-mortem, provided the brain has been properly fixed prior to dissection, since two of the lesions may be identified macroscopically. In the severe form of DAI there are:

1. a focal lesion in the corpus callosum which usually extends over an antero-posterior distance of several centimetres, lies to one side of

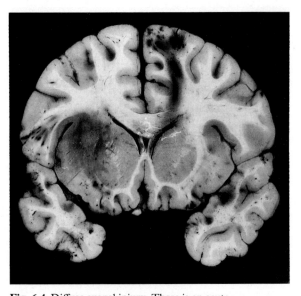

Fig. 6.4 Diffuse axonal injury. There is an acute haemorrhagic lesion in the corpus callosum to the right of the midline almost in continuity with parasagittal 'gliding' contusions in the superomedial quadrant of the right cerebral hemisphere in a patient who survived 32 hours after head injury. There is also an ill-defined haematoma in the left basal ganglia. Conventional surface contusions are seen in the cortex above and below the Sylvian (lateral) fissures.

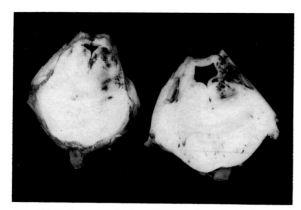

Fig. 6.5 Diffuse axonal injury. Haemorrhagic lesion in the dorsolateral quadrant of the rostral brainstem in a patient who survived 6 days after a head injury.

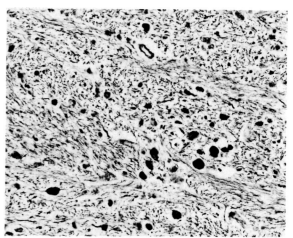

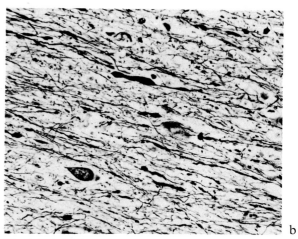

Fig. 6.6a, b Diffuse axonal injury. (**a**) Many black, oval or circular axonal swellings ('retraction bulbs') in the brainstem of a patient who survived 5 days after a head injury. (**b**) In addition to typical axonal swellings, coarse varicosities were also seen on some axons.
Palmgren (**a**) × 190; (**b**) × 190

the midline, often involving the interventricular septum, and is associated with intraventricular haemorrhage (Fig. 6.4);
2. focal lesions of various sizes in the dorsolateral quadrant(s) of the rostral brainstem adjacent to the superior cerebellar peduncles (Fig. 6.5); and
3. microscopical evidence of widespread damage to axons.

The appearances of the individual lesions depend on the length of survival after injury. In the patient surviving for only a few days, the lesions in the corpus callosum and brainstem are usually haemorrhagic, although they may be pale and difficult to detect. Indeed they may only be identified by microscopy.

Histological evidence of DAI also depends upon the length of survival after injury. If survival is short (days), there are numerous axonal swellings ('retraction' bulbs) which may be seen as eosinophilic swellings on nerve fibres in sections stained by haematoxylin and eosin, or as argyrophilic swellings in silver stained preparations (Fig. 6.6a). Their distribution is not uniform or symmetrical, but axon swellings occur particularly in the parasagittal white matter, in the corpus callosum (both adjacent to and remote from the focal lesions noted above), in the internal capsule, in deep grey matter and in various tracts in the brainstem including the medial lemnisci, the medial longitudinal bundles, the central tegmental tracts and the corticospinal tracts. In addition to typical axonal swellings, coarse varicosities may occur on axons (Fig. 6.6b).

If the patient survives for some weeks, the most striking histological finding is the presence of multiple clusters of microglia (Fig. 6.7) throughout the white matter of the brain; in addition there are reactive astrocytes and lipid-filled macrophages. If the patient survives for 2–3 months, myelin breakdown products may be detected by the Marchi technique in the white matter of the cerebral hemispheres, cerebellum, ascending and descending fibre tracts of the brainstem (Fig. 6.8) and in the descending tracts of the spinal cord.

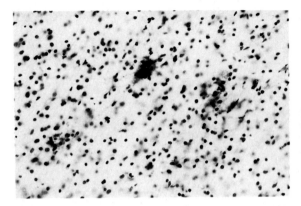

Fig. 6.7 Diffuse axonal injury. Clusters of microglia in white matter of a patient who survived in a vegetative state for 6 weeks after head injury.
Cresyl violet × 76

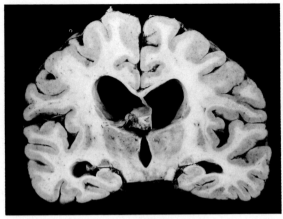

Fig. 6.9 Diffuse axonal injury. Marked enlargement of the ventricular system in a patient who survived in a vegetative state for 21 months after head injury.

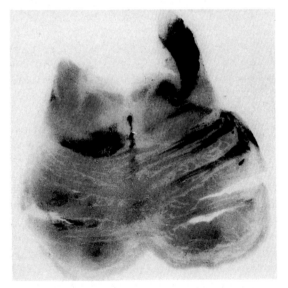

Fig. 6.8 Diffuse axonal injury. Degeneration (seen as black staining) in the superior cerebellar peduncle, medial lemniscus and corticospinal tracts in a case surviving 7 months after head injury.
Marchi × 2.5
Reproduced by permission of the editor from: Adams JH, Mitchell DE, Graham DI, Doyle D. Brain 1977; 100: 489.

In patients who survive for months or years, external abnormalities at post-mortem may be limited to small healed contusions. In coronal section the ventricles are enlarged because of reduction in the white matter. Characteristically, there are small cystic lesions in the corpus callosum (Fig. 6.9) and in, or adjacent to, one or both superior cerebellar peduncles. Macroscopic abnormalities may be so difficult to identify that pathologists unaware of the syndrome may find it hard to reconcile the apparently normal appearances of the brain with the persistent post-traumatic vegetative state.[12,53] Nevertheless, patients with DAI form a distinct group, characterised clinically by a high incidence of head injury due to road traffic accidents and a low incidence of lucid interval, and characterised pathologically by a low incidence of fracture of the skull, cerebral contusions, intracranial haematoma and evidence of high intracranial pressure.[34] Gliding contusions also feature in these cases (Fig. 6.4),[54] as do haematomas in the deep grey matter of the cerebral hemispheres[55] and in the hippocampus. Typical diffuse axonal injury has also been described in a small number of patients who have fallen from a height.[56] A CT scan may be normal in patients with DAI,[57] but eccentric haemorrhages in the corpus callosum have been observed in some cases.[48]

It is of interest that microglial stars have been identified in the white matter of patients who die from some unrelated cause a few weeks after a minor head injury.[58,59] There is increasing evidence that DAI is probably the most important single prognostic factor in non-missile head injury. It is also possible that delayed recovery of intellectual function after a minor head injury is a consequence of DAI.[60-63]

The experimental production of coma in the

absence of an intracranial mass lesion has now been achieved in non-human primates, using the Penn II device (see p. 127).[36] On the basis of the clinical findings and on the physiological data recorded, there seems no doubt that DAI occurs as a primary event at the moment of injury and that it is not secondary to some other process such as hypoxic brain damage, brain swelling or high intracranial pressure.

These experimental results indicate that varying degrees of DAI should occur in man and that there is a continuum of axonal injury without necessarily selective involvement of the corpus callosum or rostral brainstem.[64] Support for this idea has also come from the production of coarse varicosities on axons and of axonal swellings following minor head injury in cats.[65] A suggested mechanism for the varicosities is that minor damage to axons, or possibly to axonal membranes, at the time of injury, may alter axonal transport, thus leading to axonal swellings at the point of injury.[66]

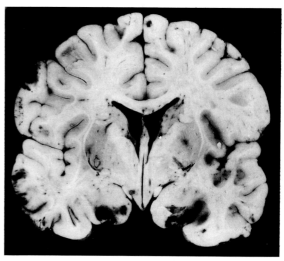

Fig. 6.10 Multiple haemorrhages in the cerebral hemispheres of a patient who died 'instantaneously' after head injury. The distribution of the lesions is reminiscent of the pattern seen in diffuse axonal injury, with 'gliding' contusions and haemorrhagic foci in basal ganglia, the corpus callosum and in the medial parts of the temporal lobes.

Primary damage to the brainstem in head injury

This term is often applied clinically to patients who are in coma from the moment of injury and who do not have an intracranial expanding lesion. By definition the term implies that the patient's clinical condition is due to focal primary damage to the brainstem. Although pontomedullary tears are recognised,[9,67] both in patients who have died 'instantaneously' and in those who have survived, the structural damage in the brainstem in patients who have died as a result of a head injury is often secondary to raised intracranial pressure, distortion and herniation of the brain. Focal lesions in the dorsolateral quadrant(s) of the rostral brainstem are also a feature of diffuse axonal injury, and in some cases of fatal head injury there may be lesions of both primary and secondary type.

Other types of primary damage in head injury

These are many and varied and include *callosal lesions*,[68,69] some of which are due to diffuse axonal injury and others to fat embolism and ischaemic damage in the territory supplied by the anterior cerebral arteries. In patients who die 'instantaneously' or within a few hours of head injury, there are often multiple petechial haemorrhages throughout the cortex, white matter and cerebral hemispheres and in the rostral part of the brainstem. These lesions are thought to be 'indicative of an injury which is incompatible with survival',[70] but it is also possible that they are a manifestation of unusually severe diffuse injury (Fig. 6.10). *Cranial nerves*, particularly the olfactory, optic and acoustic nerves, may suffer contusion directly or may be torn at the time of injury. The cavernous part of the carotid artery may be damaged, resulting in a *carotico-cavernous fistula*. Injury to the dura may lead to thrombosis of meningeal arteries and veins and, in rare instances, *traumatic intracranial aneurysms*[71] or a *dural arteriovenous fistula* may develop. The hypothalamus and pituitary gland may also be damaged.[72] There is no doubt that the pituitary stalk can occasionally be torn at the time of head injury, and massive infarction in the anterior lobe of the pituitary gland[73] inevitably results. However, most of the damage sustained by the hypothalamus and pituitary stalk is probably secondary to raised intracranial pressure and to shift and distortion of the brain.

Some injuries to the neck are of particular importance. For example, after a blow to the side of the upper neck death may ensue rapidly as a result of massive subarachnoid haemorrhage due to traumatic rupture of a vertebral artery.[74,75] Another rare complication of an injury to the neck is thrombosis of the internal carotid artery.[9,13] The pathogenesis of the thrombosis is not always clear but it is due sometimes to dissection in the wall of the artery.

Intracranial haemorrhage

This is a common complication of a head injury, particularly in patients with a fracture of the skull,[76] and there is evidence from CT scans that intracranial haematomas may be present very soon after injury though they may not be apparent clinically. Traumatic intracranial haemorrhage is classified as follows:

a. extradural haematoma
b. intradural haematoma
   (i) subdural haematoma
   (ii) discrete intracerebral or intracerebellar haematomas not in continuity with the surface of the brain
   (iii) 'burst lobe', that is, an intracerebral or intracerebellar haematoma in continuity with a related subdural haematoma.

Some degree of subarachnoid haemorrhage invariably occurs as a result of cerebral contusions in any serious head injury. If the subarachnoid haemorrhage is large, it may be a causative factor of the vasospasm which is frequently seen in the carotid angiograms of patients with acute head injury.[77] If recovery is slower than expected, or if there is late clinical deterioration, this may be due to the development of hydrocephalus following the subarachnoid haemorrhage (see p. 111).

Routine investigation of head-injured patients with CT scanning has shown that intracranial haematomas are often present long before they produce clinical deterioration.[76] Although some haematomas undoubtedly enlarge, the main effects of an intracranial haematoma are delayed because it is the associated swelling of the brain that is largely responsible for subsequent events. Haemorrhage is a primary event, but the clinical presentation is often that of a complication because of the interval between injury and the appearance of the clinical features of an intracranial expanding lesion. The importance of intracranial haema-tomas as a source of secondary brain damage is emphasised by a study of patients who died although they had been able to talk following their head injuries.[14] The fact that they had talked shows that these patients did not have severe diffuse primary brain damage, yet these cases account for many of the deaths caused by head injury. Some of these deaths may be prevented by earlier diagnosis.[20-22,78,79] Thus a patient may be lucid after the injury only to deteriorate and become comatose later as a result of an expanding intracranial mass. This sequence of events is particularly characteristic of *extradural haematoma*, but some patients with acute subdural haematoma also pursue a similar clinical course. On the other hand, *acute subdural* and *intracerebral haematomas* frequently develop while a patient is still in coma as a result of brain damage sustained at the time of injury.[80]

Most intracranial haematomas are present within the first 48 hours after injury, but subdural haemorrhage may also be subacute (developing 2-14 days after injury), or chronic (developing more than 14 days after injury). It has been suggested that the term acute traumatic haematoma should be limited to lesions diagnosed within 2 weeks of injury.[76] Sometimes, an intracerebral haemorrhage is considered to relate to an injury weeks or even years before it is discovered (the delayed traumatic haematoma of Bollinger).[81] The diagnosis is sometimes the subject of medico-legal claims but can probably be supported only when the antecedent injury is of some severity and when the interval is no more than a few weeks, during which there have been persisting symptoms.

The proportional distribution of different types of haematoma varies according to local demo-graphic/geographic influences. At all stages after injury an intradural haematoma is the most common finding and about a third of all haematomas are mixed intradural lesions—a 'burst lobe' (see p. 137).[76] In patients dying as a result of a non-missile head injury there is a correl-ation between intracranial haematoma and hypoxic damage in the ipsilateral cerebral cortex.[77]

Extradural haematoma. This has been found in between 5%[6] and 15%[5] of fatal head injuries.

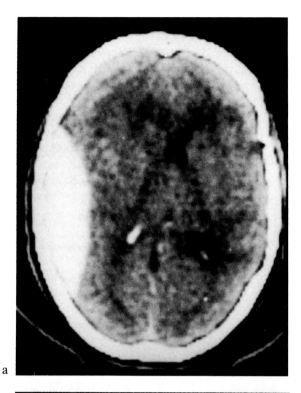

a

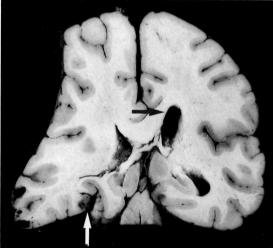

b

Fig. 6.11a, b Extradural haematoma. (**a**) CT scan showing a lens-shaped region of increased attenuation (white) typical of an extradural haematoma over left hemisphere. (**b**) Coronal slice of fixed brain showing distortion by the extradural haematoma (left), a shift of the midline structures, asymmetry of the lateral ventricles, a supracallosal hernia (black arrow) and a tentorial hernia (white arrow). Evidence of primary damage is limited to contusions at the crest of the left inferior temporal gyrus.
(**a**) *Reproduced by permission of Drs Evelyn Teasdale and P. Macpherson, Department of Neuroradiology, Institute of Neurological Sciences, Glasgow, UK.*

Extradural haematoma results most often from haemorrhage from the middle meningeal artery, and although the initial injury is often mild, some 85% of adult patients with extradural haematoma have a fracture of the skull;[82] the incidence of fracture is lower in children. As the haematoma develops, it separates the dura from the skull to form a large ovoid mass that progressively distorts the adjacent brain (Figs 6.11a and b). After a *lucid interval* of some hours the patient becomes drowsy, and the speed of clinical deterioration depends upon the rapidity with which the haematoma forms, the development of brain swelling and the ability of the intracranial contents to compensate for the expanding lesion. In many cases, there is little evidence of brain tissue damage, and therefore swelling tends to play a less important rôle than it does in patients with intradural haematoma.

Extradural haematomas occur most commonly in the temporal region, but in 20–30% of cases the haematoma occurs at other sites,[83,84] such as the frontal and parietal regions or within the posterior fossa; occasionally haematomas are multiple. With time, small haematomas become completely organised, whereas large haematomas may undergo partial organisation, the centre remaining cystic and filled with dark viscous fluid.

In cases of medico-legal interest, especially in fire-related deaths where the head has been exposed to intense heat, there may be fissure fractures of the skull and 'heat haematomas' in the extradural space. These artefactual haematomas have a pink spongy appearance, which is said to be characteristic of thermal injury, and they differ from the dark red appearance of the blood in an ordinary extradural haematoma: they also follow closely the distribution of the charring on the outer surface of the skull. The pathogenesis of this type of haematoma is uncertain, although it has been presumed that the victim must have been alive in order for it to develop. The combination of extradural haematoma and fracture of the skull in fire victims may therefore pose difficulties in interpretation.[85]

Intradural haematoma: (i) *Subdural haematoma.* Thin bilateral films of blood in the subdural space are common in acute fatal head injuries.

Haematomas thought to be large enough to act as significant intracranial expanding lesions have been reported in between 26%[6] and 63%[5] of non-missile head injuries. The initial injury is often severe, and the clinical syndrome is that of an already comatose patient who deteriorates further. Some patients with very little underlying brain damage recover after evacuation of a subdural haematoma, but in general the mortality and morbidity are much greater in subdural haematoma than in extradural haematoma because of the severity of associated brain damage (Figs 6.12a and b).

At operation, subdural haematomas are considered to be *acute* when the haematoma is composed of dark red semi-liquid blood, *subacute* when there is a mixture of clotted and fluid blood, and *chronic* when the contents consist of dark, turbid fluid and varying amounts of apparently fresh blood.[76] As the processes of reabsorption and organisation of the haematoma follow a fairly constant pattern and time course, at least in the early phases, the histological appearances of the 'membranes' developing on dural and arachnoid aspects of the haematoma have been used to estimate its age.[8,9] Despite the presence of an acute or subacute haematoma and distortion of the brain, the cortical gyral and sulcal pattern underlying the haematoma is well preserved, whilst there is a marked flattening of the convolutions in the contralateral hemisphere. This is because the subdural blood is in contact with both gyri and sulci and therefore exerts uniform compression on the subjacent brain.[31] When a haematoma is evacuated the brain simply swells to occupy the available intracranial space.[11]

Clinical studies have shown that in 72% of patients with an *acute subdural haematoma*, the head injury is produced by a fall or an assault, whereas in only 24% is the cause a road traffic accident. This is in marked contrast to patients without mass lesions who are unconscious for more than 24 hours mainly as a result of diffuse axonal injury (see p. 130); 89% of these cases are due to road traffic accidents and only 10% are caused by falls and assaults.[86] The pathogenesis of

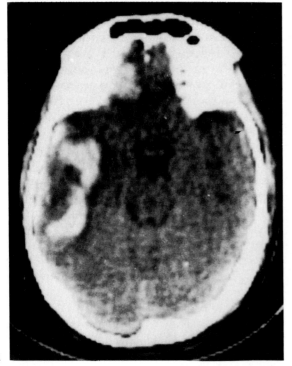

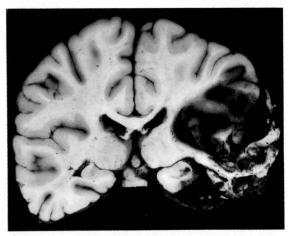

Fig. 6.12a, b Subdural haematoma. (**a**) CT scan showing crescentic region of increased attenuation (white) in the left temporal region typical of subdural haematoma. There is an associated, larger, intracerebral haematoma. The combination of subdural haematoma and intracerebral haematoma is called a 'burst lobe'. (**b**) 'Burst lobe'. The haematoma in the right temporal lobe was in continuity with an acute subdural haematoma.
(**a**) *Reproduced by permission of Drs Evelyn Teasdale and P. Macpherson, Department of Neuroradiology, Institute of Neurological Sciences, Glasgow, UK.*

a

b

the subdural haematoma has been clarified in the Penn series of experiments, in which it was recognised that bridging veins are more liable to tear when acceleration is applied rapidly than when acceleration occurs more slowly.[86] This explains the high incidence of acute subdural haematoma in patients who fall or who are assaulted because these types of injury are associated with a high rate of acceleration or deceleration. In contrast, acute subdural haematomas are much less common in road traffic accidents in which the rate of deceleration is slower.

Chronic subdural haematoma presents weeks or months after what may have appeared to be a trivial head injury. The precise aetiology is not clear but there is an association with long-term anticoagulant therapy and with coagulation defects, such as haemophilia. The haematoma increases in size slowly, probably as a result of repeated small haemorrhages, and ultimately becomes encapsulated in a fibrous membrane. Eventually it becomes large enough to produce distortion and herniation of the brain. Chronic subdural haematoma is particularly common in older patients in whom there is already some cerebral atrophy. As the haematoma expands slowly, the period of spatial compensation may be so long that there may be considerable distortion of the brain before there is any significant rise in the intracranial pressure. Death is usually due to brain damage secondary to increased intracranial pressure in the untreated case (see Ch. 3).

Subdural haematoma is found in a proportion of *battered babies*. Diagnosis is confirmed by needling the fontanelle, which yields yellow fluid with a high protein content; the chronic haematoma also consists of encapsulated xanthochromic fluid. When such a haematoma is found at post-mortem in a child, it is advisable to look for other types of brain injury, e.g. contusional tears and other white matter lesions, including diffuse gliosis.[87]

(ii) *Intracerebral haematoma.* This is found in some 15% of fatal head injuries.[5] These haematomas may be single or multiple and occur principally in the subfrontal and temporal regions (Fig. 6.13) or, less commonly, in the cerebellum. The pathogenesis is obscure, but it seems likely that they are caused by the direct rupture of

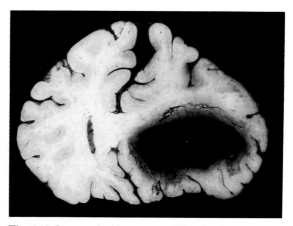

Fig. 6.13 Intracerebral haematoma. There is a large haematoma in the subfrontal region of a patient who survived 8 days after head injury. The haematoma was considered to be traumatic in the absence of other known causes, such as saccular aneurysm, hypertension, vascular malformation.

intrinsic cerebral vessels at the time of the injury. Occasionally, development of intracerebral haematoma appears to be delayed for several days (post-traumatic apoplexy). Correct interpretation of delayed haematomas may have important medico-legal implications if the patient subsequently dies.

If a solitary haematoma is found in the brain of a patient who has suffered a head injury, the possibility that it was due to hypertension or ruptured intracranial aneurysm and hence precipitated the injury should be considered. Interpretation of the findings at post-mortem can be difficult, or even impossible, and much depends on the site of the haematoma. If the haemorrhage is in the subfrontal or temporal region, however, it is more likely that the intracranial haematoma is traumatic rather than spontaneous.[20]

(iii) *'Burst lobe'.* This term describes an intracerebral or intracerebellar haematoma in continuity with a subdural haematoma. The association is found most commonly in the frontal and temporal poles.

Secondary complications

These include brain damage caused by raised intracranial pressure, hypoxia, swelling and infection.

Raised intracranial pressure

This is a common complication. Emphasis has been placed already on the rôle played by intracranial haematoma in fatal head injuries and the fact that in a large proportion of such patients death is attributable ultimately to distortion and herniation of the brain and secondary haemorrhage into the brainstem from raised intracranial pressure (see p. 66). Post-traumatic brain swelling and widespread hypoxic brain damage may also initiate a similar sequence of events. Using the neuropathological criteria of pressure necrosis in one or both parahippocampal gyri (Fig. 3.5, p. 68),[88] evidence of a significantly high intracranial pressure in life was found in 83% of a series of fatal head injuries;[11] brain damage, usually haemorrhage or infarction of the brainstem secondary to a high intracranial pressure, with shift and herniation of the brain, was the most common factor contributing to death in the entire series. On the other hand, some patients in whom the monitored intracranial pressure does not increase during life may die or remain in a vegetative state.[89,90] Thus, the brain may be severely injured without the intracranial pressure becoming elevated.[91] A normal intracranial pressure cannot, therefore, be regarded as necessarily indicative of a favourable outcome. Furthermore, although it is widely accepted that brain damage secondary to an intracranial expanding lesion is a common cause of early deterioration and coma in patients who have sustained a non-missile head injury, it is not a common cause of the persistent vegetative state or severe disability after head injury. The two most common causes of these clinical states are diffuse axonal injury (see p. 130) and diffuse hypoxic damage (see below).[92,93]

Hypoxic brain damage

Hypoxic brain damage is common in patients dying as a result of a non-missile head injury.[5,6,51,94-96] An incidence of 91% was found in one study;[97] it was assessed as severe in 27%, moderately severe in 43% and mild in 30%, and it was found more frequently in the hippocampus and in the basal ganglia than in the cerebral cortex

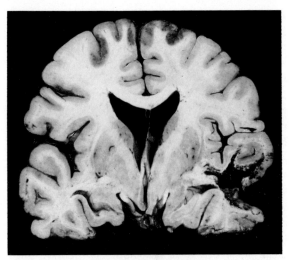

Fig. 6.14 Hypoxic brain damage. Bilateral haemorrhagic infarction in the boundary zones between the territories supplied by the anterior and middle cerebral arteries in a patient who survived for 48 hours after head injury. There is also a 'burst' right temporal lobe.
Reproduced by permission of the editor from: Graham DI, Adams JH, Doyle D. J Neurol Sci 1978; 39: 213.

and cerebellum. In the cases with cortical damage, the lesions were frequently centred on or accentuated in the boundary zones, particularly between the anterior and middle cerebral arterial territories (Figs 5.34, 6.14), but also occurred diffusely throughout the cortex and in the territories supplied by the anterior and/or middle cerebral arteries (Figs 6.15a and b). The evidence suggests that this type of brain damage occurs soon after injury, although it is always possible that an infarct in the brain of a head-injured patient is primary and hence could have precipitated the injury.

Hypoxic brain damage is more common in patients who have sustained a known clinical episode of hypoxia with a systolic blood pressure of less than 80 mmHg for at least 15 minutes or an oxygen partial pressure (PaO_2) in arterial blood of less than 50 mmHg at some time after their injury. It is also more common in patients who have experienced a high intracranial pressure as defined by a wedge of pressure necrosis in one or both parahippocampal gyri (Fig. 3.5).[88] Hypoxic brain damage following non-missile head injury also occurs due to arterial spasm.[77] Although some of the hypoxic damage can be attributed to either an episode of cardiac arrest or status epilepticus,

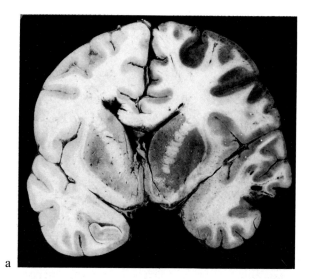

a

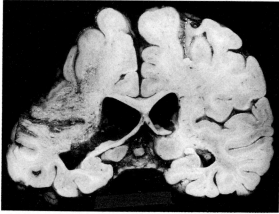

b

Fig. 6.15a, b Hypoxic brain damage. (**a**) There is a swollen, focally haemorrhagic infarct of the right cerebral hemisphere within the distribution of the middle cerebral artery in a patient who survived 7 days after head injury. A contusion is also seen on the lateral aspect of the right temporal lobe. (**b**) There is infarction of the left cerebral hemisphere within the distribution of the middle cerebral artery and in the boundary zone of the right hemisphere between the distributions of the anterior and middle cerebral arteries in a patient who survived in a vegetative state for 12 months after head injury.

cranial occlusive vascular disease may be a factor contributing to the hypoxic damage, it seems more likely that failure of cerebral perfusion results from variations in intracranial perfusion pressure and is therefore related to intracranial pressure. It should be emphasised that extensive brain damage can occur in the absence of high intracranial pressure, as in cases of diffuse axonal injury[34] and of hypoxic damage secondary to status epilepticus or cardiorespiratory arrest.[91,99] Furthermore, hypoxic brain damage is a cause of coma following head injury in the absence of an intracranial mass lesion; such hypoxic damage is frequently found in patients who remain in a vegetative state or severely disabled after head injury.[92,93]

Hypoxic brain damage is therefore common and is clearly a factor contributing to the mortality and persisting disability associated with severe head injury. There is, however, an increasing awareness that at least some of the hypoxia is avoidable,[78,100] e.g. poorly controlled epilepsy, hypotension and delay in the treatment of intracranial haematoma.

Brain swelling

An increase in the volume of all or part of the brain is common in patients who sustain a non-missile head injury. Whether localised or generalised, brain swelling may be severe enough to raise the intracranial pressure and cause death from brain shift and herniation and secondary damage to the brainstem. The cause of a swollen brain is not always clear, but in general it is due either to an increase in the cerebral blood volume (*congestive brain swelling*) or to an increase in the water content of the brain tissue itself (*cerebral oedema*). Swelling and oedema are discussed in greater detail on pages 73–76, but the three main types of brain swelling encountered in patients who sustain a head injury should be described here: (i) swelling adjacent to contusions, (ii) diffuse swelling of one cerebral hemisphere, and (iii) diffuse swelling of both cerebral hemispheres.

Swelling adjacent to contusions. This is common and is due to physical disruption of the tissue with damage to the blood-brain barrier. Water and electrolytes leak into the brain tissue and spread into the adjacent white matter; this type of oedema

many of the lesions appear to be due to a critical reduction in the regional cerebral blood flow. Cerebral perfusion may be altered not only by systemic hypotension, but also by an increase in intracranial pressure. A reduced perfusion pressure due to systemic arterial hypotension is frequently a contributing factor, as shown by the high incidence of lesions in the arterial boundary zones.[98,99] Although extracranial and/or intra-

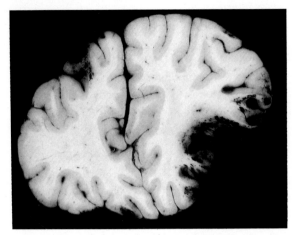

Fig. 6.16 Brain swelling in relation to contusions.

is, therefore, best classified as vasogenic in nature (Fig. 6.16).[101] A similar sequence of events may occur around an intracerebral haematoma.

Diffuse swelling of one cerebral hemisphere. This is most often seen in association with an ipsilateral acute subdural haematoma,[11] and when the haematoma is evacuated the brain simply expands to fill the space so created. A similar situation is seen in experimental studies and attributed to engorgement of a non-reactive vascular bed secondary to cerebral ischaemia produced by a high intracranial pressure (Fig. 6.17).[102] Such a

sequence of events has been seen in non-human primates with the Penn I device (see p. 127).[33] It has been suggested that in patients in whom subdural haematoma does not declare itself clinically until two or three days after the injury, the progressive development of brain swelling is more likely to be the cause of the increase in intracranial pressure and the clinical deterioration than is enlargement of the haematoma itself.[76]

Diffuse swelling of both cerebral hemispheres. This may occur following head injury, particularly in young patients.[11,13] At post-mortem, the brain is swollen diffusely and the ventricles are small and symmetrical (Fig. 6.18).[56] The pathogenesis of this type of brain swelling is not clear, but in children it is possible that the loss of vasomotor tone and consequent vasodilatation contribute to the swelling.[48,103,104] It seems likely that if the vasodilatation persists, the blood-brain barrier may become defective, leading to true vasogenic oedema. In a study of 63 children following head injury, diffuse brain swelling was found to be common after acceleration/deceleration injury to the brain, and swelling was produced mainly by an increase in the cerebral blood volume.[105] In a few cases, swelling may be associated with widespread hypoxic brain

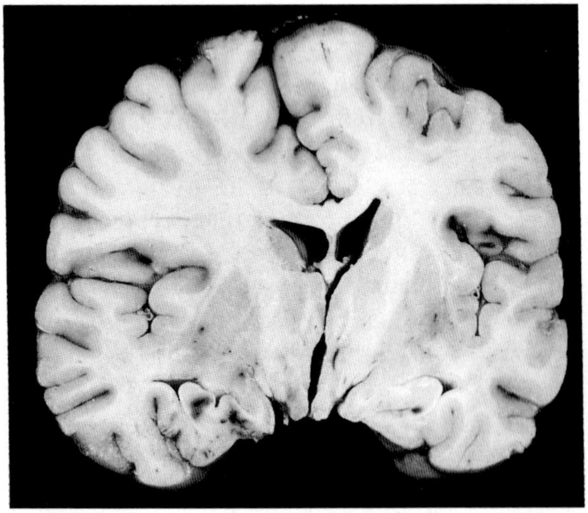

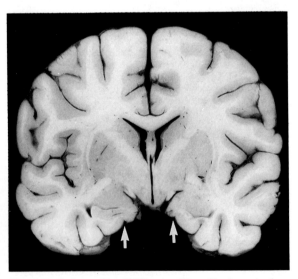

Fig. 6.17 Brain swelling. There is diffuse swelling of the left hemisphere, i.e. on the same side from which an acute subdural haematoma had been evacuated.

Fig. 6.18 Brain swelling. Diffuse swelling of both cerebral hemispheres in a child who survived for 30 hours after head injury. Note the absence of contusions and the presence of bilateral tentorial herniae (white arrows).

damage secondary to post-traumatic status epileptics and/or cardiorespiratory arrest. But, whether the swelling is due to the associated structural damage or simply the addition of further insult to an already damaged brain is not clear. It is often quite difficult at post-mortem to assess the presence of diffuse brain swelling as there is a tendency for the convolutions to become flattened and the ventricles to become reduced in size after death.[106]

Infection

Meningitis is a well-recognised complication after head injury and is usually associated with a basal fracture of the skull. If there is also a dural tear, CSF rhinorrhoea or otorrhoea may develop. In such cases meningitis is not necessarily restricted to the early post-traumatic period, but may be delayed many months; a small traumatic fistula may also be a cause of recurrent episodes of meningitis. Subdural or intracerebral abscesses are uncommon complications of non-missile head injuries but are common after penetrating injuries.

Outcome after head injury

Fortunately, most patients who sustain a head injury make a good recovery. Others, however, remain moderately or severely disabled or in a vegetative state.[12,53,107] Altered consciousness is the most reliable clinical guide to the function of the brain after non-missile injuries, and the duration of this alteration is the best measure of the degree of brain damage. The interval between the injury and the return of continuous memory (*post-traumatic amnesia*) is now considered to be a useful guide to the severity of a head injury.[2,3,12,108]

From the preceding account it is clear that there are many causes of residual neurological deficit after a head injury, e.g. contusions, hypoxic brain damage and diffuse axonal injury. Some authors[51] have emphasised the frequency of damage to the rostral brainstem, intracranial haematoma, brain swelling and cardiorespiratory complications and associated neurological deficit. They consider that this type of *post-traumatic encephalopathy* is, on the whole, dominated by secondary traumatic lesions and their sequelae. Others[7,92,93] have placed

particular emphasis on diffuse axonal injury and diffuse hypoxic brain damage. Persisting disability after head injury is probably due to diffuse rather than to focal brain damage, and even *concussion* may be due to minor degrees of diffuse axonal injury.

About 10% of patients admitted to hospital after non-missile head injury develop *epilepsy*, compared with 45% after missile injuries.[12] Most fits occur either in the first week after injury (*early epilepsy*) or are delayed by two or three months (*late epilepsy*). Early epilepsy is usually associated with severe or complicated injuries, though children under 5 may develop early epilepsy which may progress rapidly to status epilepticus even after trivial injuries. Early epilepsy increases greatly the risk of late epilepsy, which is by far the most frequent delayed complication of a non-missile head injury.[12] The three most important factors predisposing to late epilepsy are the occurrence of early epilepsy, the presence of a depressed fracture and the development of an acute intracranial haematoma.

There is a group of patients who make a reasonably good recovery after a head injury but who subsequently develop a progressive neurological illness with features of *organic dementia*.[7] Alzheimer's disease, Pick's disease and motor neuron disease have been reported, though a direct correlation between these conditions and a previous head injury remains to be established.

Another delayed complication of head injury is *intermittently raised pressure hydrocephalus (normal pressure hydrocephalus)* (see p. 73). This is thought to be a sequel of subarachnoid haemorrhage which obliterates the subarachnoid space as the blood becomes organised.

There is increasing concern about the cumulative effects of repeated concussive or subconcussive blows sustained by boxers,[109-111] jockeys,[112] and players of American or rugby football. Clinical studies have shown that boxers in particular develop a stereotyped syndrome. Ex-boxers with *'punch-drunk syndrome'*[113] show a characteristic pattern of brain damage, with a large and fenestrated septal cavum, scarring of the folia around the groove formed by the sloping edge of the foramen magnum on the undersurface of the cerebellum, degeneration of the substantia nigra, and the presence of numerous neurofibrillary tangles diffusely through the cerebral cortex and the brainstem. Although vast numbers of tangles are seen in the medial portions of the temporal lobes (cf. Alzheimer's disease, see p. 374), senile plaques are sparse or absent. These features vary in severity and appear to correlate with the clinical disorder, which ranges from a mild clumsiness of speech and movement (with or without some loss of memory) to ataxic, dysarthric and perhaps Parkinsonian dementia. As far as is known, the neuropathological features of the punch-drunk syndrome do not include either diffuse axonal injury or hypoxic brain damage, features so commonly found following a non-missile head injury.

MISSILE HEAD INJURIES[8]

These are usually much less common than non-missile head injuries in a civilian population, and they are caused by various types of object. They produce considerable local damage but little rotational injury because there is little movement of the head. The injury may be classified as depressed, penetrating or perforating. In *depressed injuries*, the missile fails to penetrate the skull but produces a depressed skull fracture with contusional injury of the underlying brain. The brain damage is therefore focal and consciousness is rarely altered for long. In *penetrating injuries*, the missile enters the cranial cavity but does not leave it. If the object is small and sharp, there may be very little direct injury to the skull or the brain. The brain damage is focal and there is often no loss of consciousness. The missile, however, may penetrate deeply enough to damage some vital structures. There is a risk of infection in penetrating head injuries, with abscess formation or meningitis. In *perforating injuries*, if the missile—usually a bullet—passes completely through the brain but does not leave the skull, the result is said to be a *perforating brain wound*; if the bullet leaves the head, it is called a *perforating head wound*. The exit wound in the skull is characteristically larger than the entry wound. The number and location of fragments of bone and metal carried into the skull by the missile can be determined by X-rays. Missiles of low velocity rarely leave the skull, though they often ricochet within the cranial cavity and produce multiple destructive tracks through the brain[5,18,114] in which there may be fragments of bone, soft tissue and clothing.[115] Although occasionally a high velocity bullet may pass through the head without causing impairment of consciousness, brain damage in these circumstances tends to be severe, probably because of shock waves generated by the missile.

Three fairly distinct zones have been described in a cross-section of a *wound canal* produced by a missile entering the brain.[8] The central area consists of a cavity containing variable, sometimes large, amounts of blood. Surrounding this cavity is an intermediate band of haemorrhagic tissue necrosis which, in turn, is surrounded by a marginal layer of pinkish-grey discoloured tissue (Fig. 6.19). Radial forces generated by the passage of the missile cause remote *contusions* affecting the frontal and temporal poles and the undersurface of the cerebrum, with herniation contusions and *contrecoup fractures*, especially of the orbital plates of the frontal bone. If the patient survives, death from *infection* may occur months or years later because of fistulae and secondary infections. There is also a high incidence of *post-traumatic epilepsy*.

Recent studies of high velocity penetrating head

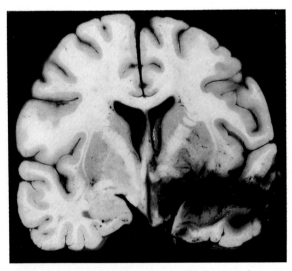

Fig. 6.19 Missile head injury. Track of bullet wound through the right side of the brain.

injuries in non-human primates[116,117] have shown extensive subarachnoid, intraventricular and subependymal haemorrhage. Lesions were found not only in the wound track but also remotely in the hypothalamus, brainstem and cerebellum. Widespread swelling of perivascular astrocytes was also noted within 30 minutes of injury, and this was considered to be a specific abnormality.

Bullet wounds to the head are usually rapidly fatal, and only 10% of patients survive for more than 24 hours.[5]

TRAUMA TO THE SPINAL CORD

Although less often fatal than head injury, trauma to the spinal cord often results in severe neurological deficit. It has been estimated[118] that, each year, from 13 to 27 per million population of the United Kingdom are likely to suffer from serious paralysis following injury of the spinal cord,[119–121] and that the incidence of cord injury is even higher if cases of sudden death after accident are included. Over half of the cases in large hospitals for paraplegic and tetraplegic patients are due to trauma of the spinal cord.[122] In civilian practice about 45% of all new cases of spinal injury result from motor-car or motor-cycle accidents, 30% are due to falls and the remainder are due to sporting injuries and occasionally to gunshot wounds.[120,123] 70% of the patients are less than 40 years of age and nearly 90% are men. The cervical and thoracic spine are injured most commonly in road traffic accidents, whereas the lumbar spine is damaged most commonly in crush injuries of the type seen in mining accidents. Head injury is associated with spinal injury much less frequently in children than in adults.[6,124,125]

As with head injuries, trauma to the spinal cord may be closed or open (penetrating).[126] The mechanisms are various and include a combination of flexion, rotation, extension and compression. In extension injuries, hyperextension of the midcervical vertebrae causes separation and dislocation of intervertebral discs, which in turn cause local haemorrhage and possible rupture of the longitudinal ligaments. Such an injury in patients with cervical spondylosis or ankylosing spondylitis may cause severe cord damage. If there is excessive flexion of the cervical spine, there is compression on the vertebral bodies, parts of which may be displaced posteriorly and cause damage to the spinal cord. The spinal canal may be narrowed by fracture dislocation due to rotation. In patients with compressive fractures, fragments of bone may be displaced backwards into the spinal canal or, if the spinal column is angulated acutely, stretching and compression of the theca and cord may result. Open injuries to the cord may result from missiles such as bullets and associated bony fragments. These may lodge in the cord or, in the case of high velocity missiles, may cause severe damage to the cord by pressure changes resulting from shock waves. The cord may be injured by a stab wound, especially if the knife enters the spinal canal anterolaterally.

As with head injuries, trauma to the spinal cord may be associated with complicating factors such as swelling, hypoxia and infection.

PATHOLOGY OF SPINAL CORD TRAUMA

Where possible, X-rays should be available to the pathologist at the time of autopsy to allow an accurate assessment of bony lesions and location of any missiles. Careful dissection of the relevant part

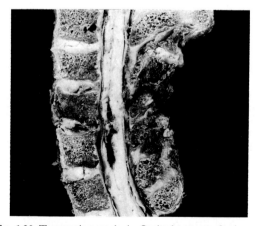

Fig. 6.20 Traumatic paraplegia. Sagittal saw cut of spine. There is a fracture dislocation with angulation. The intervertebral disc between C4 and 5 has prolapsed backwards into the spinal canal. There is contusion of the adjacent spinal cord, the central portions of which have undergone haemorrhagic necrosis.

will then reveal the degree and type of injury, though in many cases it is advisable to remove the entire spine, fix it, and then either dissect the column and cord or section it in the sagittal plane with a band saw (Fig. 6.20) (see p. 84).[122]

If there is only temporary neurological dysfunction, then the term *concussion* is used, and it is presumed that structural abnormalities are minimal, though by analogy with cerebral concussion there may be irreversible changes in myelinated axons due either to the trauma per se or to temporary circulatory abnormalities. In more severe injuries there is *contusion* of the cord, the extent and severity of which will vary from case to case. In many cases there is *extradural, subdural*, or *subarachnoid haemorrhage*. Bleeding may also occur into the spinal cord to form a discrete haematoma or *haematomyelia*, an appearance that may be confused with the haemorrhage associated with a severe contusion.

In cases of mild injury, the external surface of the cord may be normal, whereas in severe injury with incomplete or complete transection, there is an area of *haemorrhagic necrosis* at the site of trauma.[126] Transverse sections reveal a centrally placed fusiform mass of haemorrhagic necrosis which tapers to end one or more segments above and below the point of cord injury. Changes in this area include swelling, necrosis and petechial haemorrhages. Silver impregnation techniques reveal disrupted axons which terminate in axonal swellings; other axons are not disrupted and have a beaded appearance. Myelin sheaths become swollen and disintegrate. In the first few days after injury, there may be an infiltration by polymorphonuclear leucocytes. Over the course of the next few weeks, the swelling of the cord subsides and the small haemorrhages are absorbed. The necrotic tissue is gradually removed by large numbers of macrophages and a cavity is formed. Iron pigment is often seen at the margins of the lesion and there is reactive astrocytosis. In cases of severe injury with survival for many months or years, a predominantly astrocytic scar develops at the site of injury. If the injury has involved root entry zones, then regenerating axons and Schwann cells may invade the cord. Effective axonal regeneration does not appear to occur, though in some cases appearances similar to those of an *amputation*

neuroma may be seen.[127] A late result is *degeneration of ascending and descending tracts*. Sometimes the longitudinally disposed cavity that forms after the removal of the centrally placed necrotic tissue may track upwards to the medulla, or downwards. Unlike a true syrinx (see p. 325), the fluid in this *post-traumatic syringomyelic cavity* has a high protein content. The anatomical extent of these lesions is best demonstrated by the examination of sections from serial blocks of cord.

The nature of the lesions developing in the spinal cord following concussive or contusional injuries has been studied in the rat,[128,129] in the dog,[130] in the cat,[131] and in the non-human primate,[132,133] and is similar to the findings in man.

INJURY TO THE SPINAL CORD AND ROOTS CAUSED BY DISORDERS OF THE SPINE

Malformation or disease of the spine may cause local or widespread pressure, either on the blood supply to the cord or on the cord itself. The presentation may be acute or chronic, and the histological changes in the cord depend upon the duration of the compression. In acute cases, abnormalities may be limited to a wedge-shaped area of spongy degeneration comprising vacuolated myelin and swollen axons in the posterior parts of one or both lateral columns. In more advanced cases, vacuolation is also seen in the deeper parts of the posterior columns, and areas of frank necrosis may become apparent in both white and grey matter; a cavity eventually forms at the site of the lesion with a mixture of astrocytes and capillaries in the walls. Often there is atrophy of the anterior horns due to loss of nerve cells, and some hyaline thickening of the small blood vessels. This progressive type of change is particularly common in cases of subacute or chronic compression, whereas the lesions tend to be more extensive and obviously ischaemic if the cord is compressed acutely.

Tumours are a common cause of compression of both the spinal cord and its nerve roots. Most commonly these are metastatic carcinomas, lymphomas and myelomas, but primary bone tumours, meningiomas, schwannomas and neuro-fibromas also may present in this way (see Ch. 16).

Various *inflammatory diseases* of the spine may present with cord compression. One of the more common organisms involved is *Staphylococcus aureus*, which may cause either a localised abscess or suppuration which may track through the epidural or subdural space. *Tuberculosis* of the spine (Pott's disease) presents most frequently in the cervical and thoracic vertebrae. The disease invariably starts as tuberculous osteitis of the vertebral bodies before spreading into the para-vertebral tissues and into the adjacent epidural and subdural spaces. If kyphosis develops, the cord is likely to be damaged due to compression by gran-ulation tissue or through angulation of the spine or by interference with the vascular supply; these factors may act singly or in combination. Other inflammatory causes of cord compression include *Brucella abortus* abscess and metastatic abscess due to *Escherichia coli* in association with chronic urinary tract infection.

Osteitis deformans (Paget's disease of bone) may also produce cord compression. So also may rheumatoid arthritis, which produces a myelo-pathy by either atlanto-axial (between C1 and C2) or subaxial (below C2) dislocation. *Bony abnor-malities in the region of the foramen magnum* may also present with neurological symptoms due to cord compression. The three most common abnormalities presenting in this way are *occipital-isation of the atlas*, in which there is partial or complete bony fusion of the atlas with the bone around the foramen magnum, *basilar invagination (basilar impression)*, an abnormality that is usually developmental in origin but more rarely may result from osteitis deformans, rickets or osteogenesis imperfecta, and *anomalies or fractures of the odontoid process*.[134] *Achondroplasia* may be associated with compression of the cauda equina due to associated narrowing of the spinal canal.

Prolapse of an intervertebral disc may cause cord compression, but presents more commonly as sciatica due to acute pressure on a lumbar or sacral nerve root. The condition is due to herniation of the nucleus pulposus of an intervertebral disc through part of the annulus fibrosus. The nucleus pulposus develops from the notochord and forms the central portion of the disc. As a result of injury

or of lifting a heavy weight, part of the nucleus pulposus may be forced through the annulus and compress a nerve root, particularly in the lower spine between L5 and S1 and less commonly in the neck between C5 and 6. Most disc prolapses are laterally placed so that only the nerve root is at risk. In the cervical and thoracic regions, however, the cord is also at risk, particularly if there is a centrally placed disc prolapse. Histologically the prolapsed fragments of the disc often show mucoid degeneration, and the tissue appears devitalised with only a few normal cells remaining. Sometimes there is evidence of vascularisation, and macro-phages containing haemosiderin may be seen in the biopsy material. Tissue removed at surgery should always be examined histologically for unexpected lesions such as granulomas and tumours, both of which may simulate prolapse of the nucleus pulposus, both clinically and at operation.

Spondylosis is a condition in which there is pro-gressive degeneration of intervertebral discs in the cervical and lumbar regions of the spine. The condition is common, with radiological evidence of its presence in 50% of people over the age of 50 and 75% over the age of 65.[135] The condition is characterised by calcification at the margins of the vertebral bodies in relation to a thickened annulus fibrosus. *Osteophytes* develop laterally, where they may encroach sufficiently on the lateral recess of the spinal canal or on the intervertebral foramen to compress nerve roots (Figs 6.21a and b). The affected nerve roots become thickened and there may be interference with the blood supply of the root entry zones. There is also a risk of cord com-pression, but the pathogenesis of this *myelopathy* is complex and involves factors such as interference with the blood supply, trauma and protrusion of disc material.[136] An important factor in the production of myelopathy is *congenital narrowing of the cervical spinal canal*:[137] the average antero-posterior diameter of the spinal canal in controls is 17 mm, and in cases with myelopathy due to cervical spondylosis the average measurement is 14 mm. It is thought that while spondylotic changes may reduce the canal size, myelopathy is more likely to occur if the original dimensions of the canal are smaller than average. Under these conditions cord compression is unlikely when the

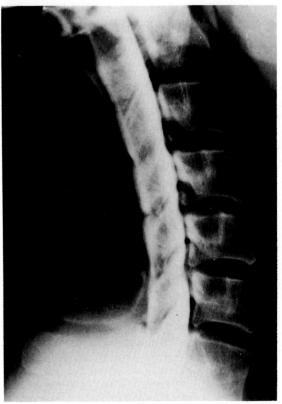 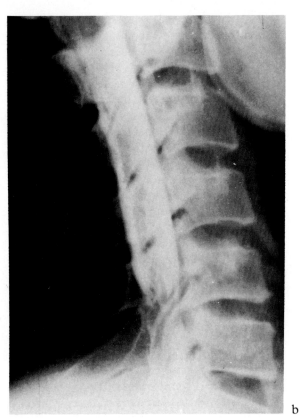

a   b

Fig. 6.21a, b Cervical myelogram by direct puncture. (**a**) Normal apart from minimal impingement on the white column of contrast at level of C5/6. (**b**) There is appreciable impingement on spinal cord by posterior ligaments at C5/6 (bottom of picture).

head is erect but on neck extension the ligamentum flavum becomes buckled sufficiently to compress the cord against the bulging intervertebral disc.[138] A similar condition of spondylotic compression in the lumbosacral region is thought to be the cause of *claudication of the cauda equina*, with root pain.

TRAUMA TO THE NERVOUS SYSTEM IN THE PERINATAL PERIOD

Intracranial and intracerebral haemorrhage are common in the perinatal period, especially in association with prematurity (see p. 327) and a number of other factors that include thrombo-cytopenia, haemolytic disease and vitamin K deficiency. Some haemorrhages, however, are probably traumatic in nature. For example, there may be bleeding accompanied by *tears* of the falx cerebri and of the tentorium in full-term infants. These may be associated with tearing of bridging veins and subdural haemorrhage. Their patho-genesis is uncertain, but the most likely explanation is that they result from deformation of the fetal head during birth. They are particularly common in the full-term infant when the skull is well ossified and the birth is complicated by cephalopelvic disproportion, a high forceps delivery or breech presentation. In premature infants, subdural haemorrhage has been ascribed to the marked deformability of the cranial bones, which readily become distorted and overlap and expand after passage through the birth canal.

In 12% of a series of 48 perinatal post-mortems there was traumatic damage to the cervical spine, and in 4% there was injury to the cervical spinal cord.[139]

INJURY TO THE NERVOUS SYSTEM BY IRRADIATION AND OTHER PHYSICAL AGENTS

X-irradiation. As the principal sequel to irradiation is its effect on cell division, the nervous system with a low rate of cell turnover is relatively resistant to injury by ionising radiation. The doses used in radiotherapy, however, are in the range at which radiation damage to the nervous system may occur even though the dosage is fractionated to minimise tissue damage. Many cases of damage due to X-irradiation have been reported.[140-143]

The delayed effects of irradiation on the central nervous system may be divided into early and late types. The *early* changes may develop up to 13 weeks after irradiation.[142] The principal histological abnormality is damage to white matter. In the *late* delayed cases, coagulation necrosis with minimal tissue reaction (radionecrosis) develops months or years later. Marked changes may also be seen in the walls of vessels, varying from fibrinoid necrosis with marked endothelial proliferation to hyaline thickening. There is perivascular fibrosis, and the nuclei of the fibroblasts are often greatly enlarged and bizarre in character. Likewise, there may be giant reactive astrocytes with bizarre nuclei.

Experimental studies have shown that the effects of X-irradiation on the spinal cord vary depending upon the strain and age of the animal, the dose of radiation and the level of cord irradiated.[144] The principal changes in the cervical cord are demyelination and necrosis of white matter, changes that have been attributed to the effects of irradiation upon the slow natural turnover of neuroglial cells (both astrocytes and oligodendrocytes) in the cervical spinal cord.[145] Another possibility is that the late delayed effects of radiation are vascular in nature and account for the development of telangiectases, haemorrhage and haemorrhagic infarction. These changes are particularly likely to develop in the spinal cord with doses in excess of 3500 rad (35 Gy), but similar doses applied to the brain seem to be less damaging.

Intracranial tumours may occur after a period of several years at sites of ionising irradiation.[146-148] In general a low dose (less than 800 rad, 8 Gy) appears to induce meningiomas, whereas fibrosarcomas do not develop until doses of 1000 rad (10 Gy) or more are given.

Fast neutron irradiation. This has been shown to induce late delayed radionecrosis.[149]

Laser irradiation. Studies in animals have shown that the effects of focused laser radiation depend upon the amount of energy absorbed. If sufficiently great, a focused laser light may cause fracture of the skull, herniation of the brain through the suture lines and instantaneous death. Lesser amounts of energy cause coagulation necrosis and haemorrhage in the brain surrounded by oedema.[150]

Alpha particle radiation. Tissue is damaged according to the amount of energy absorbed. This form of radiation damage appears to be associated with marked nerve fibre regeneration.[151,152]

Ultrasound. Ultrasonic radiation, when directed through a trephine in the skull, produces considerable heat and secondary damage to surrounding tissues. This is particularly marked in white matter where necrosis may ensue, surrounded by a zone of oedema and astrocytosis. Such changes have been described in post-mortem material following the therapeutic use of ultrasound as an alternative to surgical lobotomy.[153]

Heat. In heatstroke,[154] the brain is swollen and there may be petechial haemorrhages in the white matter and in the vicinity of the third ventricle. The neurons swell and some, especially the Purkinje cells, may undergo lysis.

Electricity and lightning. When death is due to electrocution the only abnormality visible in the brain may be hyperaemia, possibly with petechial haemorrhages. If the discharge has been directed through the brain, as in death due to lightning, there may be charring or widespread fissuring of its surface.

REFERENCES

Introduction

1. Adams JH. In: Adams JH, Corsellis JAN, Duchen LW, eds. Greenfield's Neuropathology. 4th ed. London: Arnold, 1984: 85.
2. Becker DP, Povlishock JT, eds. Central nervous system trauma status report, 1985. Washington, DC: National Institutes of Health, 1985.
3. Cooper PR, ed. Head injury. 2nd ed. Baltimore: Williams and Wilkins, 1987.
4. Lindenberg R, Freytag E. Arch Pathol (Chic) 1960; 69: 440.
5. Freytag E. Arch Pathol (Chic) 1963; 75: 402.
6. Maloney AFJ, Whatmore WJ. Br J Surg 1969; 56: 23.
7. Strich SJ. In: Walker AE, Caveness WF, Critchley M, eds. The late effects of head injury. Springfield, Ill: Thomas, 1969: 501.
8. Lindenberg R. In: Minckler J, ed. Pathology of the nervous system. New York: McGraw-Hill, 1971; 2: 1705.
9. Hardman JM. In: Thompson RA, Green JR, eds. Advances in neurology. New York: Raven Press, 1979; 22: 15.
10. Adams JH. In: Vinken PJ, Bruyn GW, eds. Handbook of clinical neurology. Amsterdam: North Holland, 1975; 23: 35.
11. Adams JH, Graham DI, Scott G, Parker L, Doyle D. J Clin Pathol 1980; 33: 1132.
12. Jennett B, Teasdale G. Management of head injuries. Philadelphia: Davis, 1981.
13. Adams JH, Gennarelli TA, Graham DI. In: Smith WT, Cavanagh JB, eds. Recent advances in neuropathology. Edinburgh: Churchill Livingstone, 1982: 165.
14. Reilly PL, Graham DI, Adams JH, Jennett B. Lancet 1975; 2: 375.
15. Gennarelli TA, Spielman GM et al. J Neurosurg 1982; 56: 26.
16. Adams JH, Graham DI. In: Anthony PP, MacSween RNM, eds. Recent advances in histopathology. Edinburgh: Churchill Livingstone, 1984; 12: 241.

Non-missile head injury

17. Jennett B, Teasdale G, Galbraith S et al. J Neurol Neurosurg Psychiatry 1977; 40: 291.
18. Editorial. Lancet 1983; 2: 948.
19. Brooks DN, McKinlay W. J Neurol Neurosurg Psychiatry 1983; 46: 336.
20. Galbraith S. Br Med J 1976; 1: 1438.
21. Seelig JM, Becker DP, Miller JD, Greenberg RP, Ward JD, Choi SC. N Engl J Med 1981; 304: 1511.
22. Gentleman D, Jennett B. Lancet 1981; 2: 853.
23. Denny-Brown JP, Russell WR. Brain 1941; 64: 93.
24. Ommaya AK, Gennarelli TA. Brain 1974; 97: 633.
25. Nusholtz GS, Melvin JW, Alem NM. In: Proceedings of 23rd Stapp Car Crash Conference. New York: Society of Automotive Engineers, 1979: 499.
26. Thibault LE, Gennarelli TA. In: Becker DP, Povlishock JT, eds. Central nervous system trauma status report 1985. Washington, DC: National Institutes of Health, 1985.
27. Holbourn AHS. Lancet 1943; 2: 438.
28. Holbourn AHS. Br Med Bull 1945; 3: 147.
29. Pudenz RH, Shelden CH. J Neurosurg 1946; 3: 487.
30. Unterharnscheidt F, Higgins LS. Texas Report Biol Med 1969; 27: 127.
31. Gennarelli TA, Thibault LE. In: Becker DP, Povlishock JT, eds. Central nervous system trauma status report 1985. Washington, DC: National Institutes of Health, 1985.
32. Ommaya AK, Hirsch AE. J Biomechanics 1971; 4: 13.
33. Adams JH, Graham DI, Gennarelli TA. Acta Neurochir 1983; (suppl 32): 15.
34. Adams JH, Graham DI, Murray LS, Scott G. Ann Neurol 1982; 12: 557.
35. Adams JH, Graham DI, Gennarelli TA. In: Grossman RG, Gildenberg PL, eds. Head injury: basic and clinical aspects. New York: Raven Press, 1982: 141.
36. Gennarelli TA, Thibault LE. Ann Neurol 1982; 12: 564.
37. Dawson SL, Hirsch CS, Lucas FV, Sebek BA. Human Pathol 1980; 11: 155.
38. Mendelow AD, Teasdale G, Jennett B, Bryden J, Hessett C, Murray G. Br Med J 1983; 287: 1173.
39. Welte E. Arch Psychiatr Nervenkr 1948; 179: 243.
40. Lindenberg R, Freytag E. Arch Pathol 1969; 87: 298.
41. Adams JH, Graham DI. In: Critchley M, O'Leary JL, Jennett B, eds. Scientific foundations of neurology. London: Heinemann, 1972: 478.
42. Adams JH, Doyle D, Graham DI, et al. Neuropathol Appl Neurobiol 1985; 11: 299.
43. Voigt GE, Lowenheilm P, Ljung CBA. Acta Neuropathol (Berl) 1977; 39: 201.
44. Strich SJ. J Neurol Neurosurg Psychiatry 1956; 19: 163.
45. Strich SJ. Lancet 1961; 2: 443.
46. Peerless SJ, Rewcastle NB. Canad Med Assoc J 1967; 96: 577.
47. Adams JH, Mitchell DE, Graham DI, Doyle D. Brain 1977; 100: 489.
48. Zimmerman RA, Bilaniuk LT, Gennarelli TA. Radiology 1978; 127: 393.
49. Grcevic N. Rad Jugosl Akad Znan Umjet Odjel Med Nauke 1982;Nr4018: 265.
50. Adams RD. In: Walker AE, Caveness WF, Critchley M, eds. The late effects of head injury. Springfield, Ill: Thomas, 1969: 524.
51. Jellinger K, Seitelberger F. J Neurol Sci 1970; 10: 51.
52. Peters G, Rothemund E. In: Ore GD, Gerstenbrand F, Lucking CH, eds. The apallic syndrome. Berlin: Springer, 1977: 78.
53. Jennett B, Plum F. Lancet 1972; 1: 734.
54. Adams JH, Doyle D, Graham DI, Lawrence AE, McLellan DR. Arch Pathol Lab Med 1986; 110: 485.
55. Adams JH, Doyle D, Graham DI et al. J Neurol Neurosurg Psychiatry 1986; 49: 1039.
56. Adams JH, Doyle D, Graham DI, Lawrence AE, McLellan DR. Lancet 1984; 2: 1420.
57. Snoek J, Jennett B, Adams JH, Graham DI, Doyle D. J Neurol Neurosurg Psychiatry 1979; 42: 215.
58. Oppenheimer DR. J Neurol Neurosurg Psychiatry 1968; 31: 299.
59. Clark JM. J Neurol Neurosurg Psychiatry 1974; 37: 463.
60. Gronwall D, Wrightson P. Lancet 1974; 2: 605.
61. Ewing R, McCarthy D, Gronwall D, Wrightson P. J Clin Neuropsychiatry 1980; 2: 147.
62. Gennarelli TA, Adams JH, Graham DI. In: Baethmann

A, Go KG, Unterberg A, eds. Mechanisms of secondary brain damage. New York: Plenum, 1986: 15.
63. Dacey RG, Dikmen SS. In: Cooper PR, ed. Head injury. 2nd ed. Baltimore: Williams and Wilkins, 1987: 125.
64. Pilz P. Acta Neurochir 1983; (suppl 32): 119.
65. Povlishock JT, Becker DP, Cheng CLY, Vaughan CW. J Neuropathol Exp Neurol 1983; 42: 225.
66. Povlishock JT, Becker DP, Miller JD, Jenkins LW, Dietrich WD. Acta Neuropathol (Berl) 1979; 47: 1.
67. Pilz P, Strohecker J, Grobovschek M. J Neurol Neurosurg Psychiatry 1982; 45: 422.
68. Lindenberg R, Fisher R, Durlacher SH, Lovitt WV, Freytag E. Am J Pathol 1955; 31: 297.
69. Komatsu S, Sato T, Kagawa S, Mori T, Hamiki T. Neurosurgery 1979; 5: 32.
70. Tomlinson BE. In: Sevitt S, Stoner HB, eds. The pathology of trauma. J Clin Pathol 1970; 23 (suppl Roy Coll Path) 4: 154.
71. Parkinson D, West M. J Neurosurg 1980; 52: 11.
72. Treip CS. In: Sevitt S, Stoner HB, eds. The pathology of trauma. J Clin Pathol 1970; 23 (suppl Roy Coll Path) 4: 178.
73. Adams JH, Daniel PM, Pritchard MML. J Neurol Neurosurg Psychiat 1966; 29: 545.
74. Cameron JM, Mant AK. Med Sci Law 1972; 12: 66.
75. Harland WA, Pitts JF, Watson AA. J Clin Pathol 1983; 36: 1335.
76. Teasdale G, Galbraith S. In: Krayenbuhl H, Maspes PE, Sweet WH, eds. Progress in neurological surgery. Basel: Karger, 1981; 10: 252.
77. Macpherson P, Graham DI. J Neurol Neurosurg Psychiatry 1978; 41: 122.
78. Rose J, Valtonen S, Jennett B. Br Med J 1977; 2: 615.
79. Jennett B, Carlin J. Injury 1978; 10: 31.
80. Rodda RA, Adams JH, Graham DI, Doyle D. Clin Neuropathol 1987; 6: 179.
81. Bollinger O. Internationale Beiträge zur wissenschaftlichen Medizin. Festschrift-Rudolf Virchow gewidmet zur Vollendung seines 70. Lebensjahres. Berlin: Hirschwald, 1891; 2: 457.
82. Jamieson KG, Yelland JDN. J Neurosurg 1968; 29: 13.
83. Lewin W. Ann Roy Coll Surg Engl 1949; 5: 240.
84. McKissock W, Taylor JC, Bloom WH, Till K. Lancet 1960; 2: 167.
85. Polson CJ, Gee DJ. The essentials of forensic medicine. 3rd ed. Oxford: Pergamon, 1973: 338.
86. Gennarelli TA, Thibault LE. J Trauma 1982; 22: 680.
87. Calder IM, Hill I, Scholtz CL. J Clin Pathol 1984; 37: 1095.
88. Adams JH, Graham DI. Neuropathol Appl Neurobiol 1976; 2: 323.
89. Johnston IH, Jennett B. Acta Neurochir 1973; 29: 53.
90. Miller JD, Becker DP, Ward JD, Sullivan HG, Adams WE, Rosner MJ. J Neurosurg 1977; 47: 503.
91. Graham DI, Adams JH, Doyle D. In: Schulman K, Marmarou A, Miller JD, Becker DP, Hochwald GM, Brock M, eds. Intracranial pressure IV. Berlin: Springer, 1980: 20.
92. Graham DI, McLellan D, Adams JH, Doyle D, Kerr A, Murray LS. Acta Neurochir 1983; (suppl 32): 65.
93. McLellan DR, Adams JH, Graham DI, Kerr AE, Teasdale GM. In: Papo I, Cohadon F, Massarotti M, eds. Le Coma traumatique. Padova: Liviana Editrice, 1986: 165.
94. Helfand M. J Nerv Ment Dis 1939; 90: 157.
95. Evans JP, Scheinker IM. Arch Neurol Psychiatry (Chic) 1943; 50: 258.
96. Evans JP, Scheinker IM. Res Publ Assoc Res Nerv Ment Dis 1945; 24: 254.
97. Graham DI, Adams JH, Doyle D. J Neurol Sci 1978; 39: 213.
98. Adams JH, Brierley JB, Connor RCR, Treip CS. Brain 1966; 89: 235.
99. Brierley JB, Graham DI. In: Adams JH, Corsellis JAN, Duchen LW, eds. Greenfield's Neuropathology. 4th ed. London: Arnold, 1984: 125.
100. Miller JD, Sweet RC, Narayan R, Becker DP. JAMA 1978; 240: 439.
101. Tornheim PA, McLaurin RL. J Neurosurg 1978; 48: 220.
102. Langfitt TW, Weinstein JD, Kassell NF. Neurology 1965; 15: 622.
103. Kuhl DE, Alavi A, Hoffman EJ et al. J Neurosurg 1980; 52: 309.
104. Obrist WD, Langfitt TW, Jaggi JL, Cruz J, Gennarelli TA. J Neurosurg 1984; 61: 241.
105. Bruce DA, Alavi A, Bilaniuk L, Kolinskas C, Obrist W, Uzzell B. J Neurosurg 1981; 54: 170.
106. Sarwar M, McCormick WF. Radiology 1978; 127: 409.
107. Jennett B, Bond M. Lancet 1975; 1: 480.
108. Russell WR. The traumatic amnesias. Oxford: Oxford University Press, 1961.
109. Martland HS. JAMA 1928; 91: 1103.
110. Critchley M. Br Med J 1957; 1: 357.
111. Mawdsley C, Ferguson FR. Lancet 1963; 2: 795.
112. Foster JB, Leiguarda R, Tilley PJB. Lancet 1976; 1: 981.
113. Corsellis JAN, Bruton CJ, Freeman-Browne D. Psychol Med 1973; 3: 270.

Missile head injuries

114. Kirkpatrick JB, DiMaio V. J Neurosurg 1978; 49: 185.
115. Sights WP. J Neurosurg 1969; 31: 25.
116. Allen IV, Scott R, Tanner JA. Injury 1982; 14: 183.
117. Allen IV, Kirk J, Maynard RL, Cooper GK, Scott R, Crockard A. Acta Neuropathol 1983; 59: 277.

Trauma to the spinal cord

118. Ravichandran G, Silver JR. Br Med J 1982; 284: 953.
119. Fine PR, Kuhlemeier KV, De Vivo MJ, Stover SL. Paraplegia 1979/80; 17: 237.
120. Minaire P, Castanier M, Girard R, Berard E, Deidier C, Bourret J. Paraplegia 1978/79; 16: 76.
121. Kurtzke JF. Exp Neurol 1975; 48: 163.
122. Weller RO, Swash M, McLellan DL, Scholtz CL. Clinical neuropathology. Berlin: Springer, 1983; 85.
123. Frankel HL, Hancock DO, Hyslop G. et al. Paraplegia 1969; 7: 179.
124. Hendrick EB, Harwood-Hash DC, Hudson AR. Clin Neurosurg 1964; 11: 46.
125. Sevitt S. Br J Surg 1968; 55: 481.
126. Hughes JT. In: Adams JH, Corsellis JAN, Duchen LW, eds. Greenfield's Neuropathology. 4th ed. London: Arnold, 1984: 779.
127. Hughes JT, Brownell B. J Neurol Neurosurg Psychiatry 1963; 26: 528.
128. Balentine JD. Lab Invest 1978; 39: 236.

129. Balentine JD. Lab Invest 1978; 39: 254.
130. Griffiths IR, Miller R. J Neurol Sci 1974; 22: 291.
131. Griffiths IR, McCulloch MC. J Neurol Sci 1983; 58: 335.
132. Bresnahan JC, King JS, Martin GF, Yashon D. J Neurol Sci 1976; 28: 521.
133. Bresnahan JC. J Neurol Sci 1978; 37: 59.
134. McRae DL. Acta Radiol 1953; 40: 335.
135. Pallis C, Jones AM, Spillane JD. Brain 1954; 77: 274.
136. Wilkinson M. Brain 1960; 83: 589.
137. Payne EE, Spillane JD. Brain 1957; 80: 571.
138. Stoltmann HF, Blackwood W. Brain 1964; 87: 45.

Trauma in the perinatal period

139. Reid H. Acta Neurochir 1983; (suppl 32): 87.

Injury by irradiation and other physical agents

140. Pallis CA, Louis S, Morgan RL. Brain 1961; 84: 460.
141. Crompton MR, Layton DD. Brain 1961; 84: 85.
142. Lampert PW, Davis RL. Neurology 1964; 14: 912.

143. Kristensson K, Molin B, Sourander P. Acta Neuropathol (Berl) 1967; 9: 34.
144. Hopewell JW. Neuropathol Appl Neurobiol 1979; 5: 329.
145. Hubbard BM, Hopewell JW. Br J Radiol 1979; 52: 816.
146. Goldberg MB, Sheline GE, Malamud N. Radiology 1963; 80: 465.
147. Munk J, Peyser E, Gruszkiewicz J. Clin Radiol 1969; 20: 90.
148. Powell HC, Marshall LF, Ignelz RJ. Acta Neuropathol (Berl) 1977; 39: 165.
149. Manz HJ, Woolley PV, Ornitz RD. Cancer 1979; 44: 473.
150. Hayes JR, Fox JL, Stein MN. J Neuropathol Exp Neurol 1967; 26: 250.
151. Rose JE, Malis LI, Kruger L, Baker CP. J Comp Neurol 1960; 115: 243.
152. Estable-Puig JF, de Estable RF, Tobias C, Haymaker W. Acta Neuropathol (Berl) 1965; 4: 175.
153. Nelson E, Lindstrom PL, Haymaker W. J Neuropathol Exp Neurol 1959; 18: 489.
154. Malamud N, Haymaker W, Custer RP. Milit Surg 1946; 99: 397.

Bacterial and fungal infections and granulomatous diseases

INTRODUCTION

Most bacterial and fungal infections of the central nervous system occur through *haematogenous* spread of organisms to the brain and meninges. However, the frontal, ethmoid and mastoid air sinuses and the middle ear cavities are in close proximity to the brain, and *direct* spread of infection may occur from these sites. Similarly, penetrating injuries of the brain or spinal cord may allow organisms to enter, and osteomyelitis of the cranium and spine may also be a source of infection.

Pachymeningitis, which is inflammation of the dura mater, usually results from the spread of bacterial infection from an epidural abscess or from cranial and spinal osteomyelitis, or it may occur in syphilis. In *leptomeningitis* (meningitis), the arachnoid and pia mater are inflamed; in pyogenic infections of the leptomeninges, pus accumulates in the cerebrospinal fluid in the subarachnoid space between the arachnoid and pia. Spread of infection to the cerebral ventricles (*ventriculitis*) is a severe complication of leptomeningitis. Widespread generalised infection and inflammation of the brain and spinal cord (*encephalomyelitis*) is not usually a feature of bacterial or fungal infections except those caused by *Listeria monocytogenes*. Encephalomyelitis is usually due to viral infections (see Ch. 9). Focal *abscess* formation within the parenchyma of the brain may occur due to spread of bacteria or fungi by the blood. Such abscesses may be multiple. Initially, there is an area of brain necrosis, infection and inflammation (*cerebritis*) which then develops into an abscess. Frontal lobe abscesses may be due to spread of infection from frontal sinuses, and temporal lobe abscesses to the spread of infection from the middle ear or mastoid. Complications arise due either to brain displacement from the abscess and surrounding oedema, or to rupture of the abscess causing meningitis and ventriculitis.

Infection of the subdural space usually spreads from the air sinuses within the skull and may cause *subdural empyema*, in which pus lies as a layer over the surface of the brain between the arachnoid and the dura. Localised *epidural abscesses* within the skull or the spine cause symptoms due to compression of neural tissues.

Rapid spread of infecting bacteria and fungi through the central nervous system occurs most easily via the cerebrospinal fluid (CSF). Normally, there are few leucocytes in the cerebrospinal fluid and the level of immunoglobulin is much lower than in the blood. In pyogenic infections, numerous polymorphonuclear leucocytes are found in the cerebrospinal fluid, whereas in virus infections and in tuberculosis the inflammatory cells are mainly lymphocytes. CSF antibody titres rise during infection, and the normal serum:CSF antibody ratio of more than 200 is lowered in central nervous system infections[1,2] due to local production of antibodies. Cell-mediated immunity is a major defence against viruses, fungi, *Mycobacterium tuberculosis*, *Listeria monocytogenes* and *Toxoplasma gondii*. It is these infections which commonly complicate immunodeficiency in patients with lymphoma and acquired immune deficiency syndrome (AIDS), and those under treatment with chemotherapeutic agents. Complement also plays a rôle in the lysis of invading organisms and of cells containing viruses.[3]

The effects of infection upon the brain differ widely according to the infecting organism and the type of inflammatory lesion. Extensive cerebral *oedema* and focal *necrosis* may be seen in encephalitis due to virus infections (see Ch. 9). The presence of organisms and inflammation in the leptomeninges in bacterial and fungal leptomeningitis may block the cerebrospinal fluid pathways and result in *hydrocephalus*. *Infarction* of brain, spinal cord, and nerve roots may occur in leptomeningitis, due to inflammation of the vessels

on the surface of the brain and thrombotic occlusion of their lumina. Similar vascular damage to the central nervous system may complicate subdural empyema, mainly because of *venous infarction*. The space-occupying nature of cerebral abscesses and their surrounding oedema may cause *brain shift* and transtentorial herniation with brainstem compression. Epidural abscesses, especially in the spine, may cause neurological signs due to *compression* of the long tracts of the spinal cord.

The organisms responsible for intracranial infections differ with the age of the patient, the origin of the infection and the site in the brain affected. Virulent aerobic organisms are often the causative agents of pyogenic leptomeningitis, whereas anaerobic or micro-aerophilic organisms predominate in the causation of cerebral and subdural abscesses.

BACTERIAL INFECTIONS
PYOGENIC LEPTOMENINGITIS

When pyogenic bacteria invade the leptomeninges, the resulting inflammation of the arachnoid and pia leads to the accumulation of pus in the cerebrospinal fluid of the subarachnoid spaces.

Clinical aspects

Patients with acute purulent meningitis appear ill and may be comatose or stuporose, with fever and sweating. The patient is irritable and photophobic and exhibits marked neck rigidity. Signs of raised intracranial pressure may be present, with papilloedema, alteration in consciousness and venous engorgement of the retina. Clinical signs of a source of infection in the lungs, ears or other sites in the body may be present, or there may be evidence of a penetrating head injury. In some cases meningitis follows the rupture of a cerebral abscess. Hemiplegia or focal seizures may occur following infarction due to inflammation and thrombosis of meningeal blood vessels. The mortality rate of leptomeningitis may be as high as 30% even with treatment, but it is reduced by the early recognition of the infection, rapid determination of the causative agent and prompt initiation of antimicrobial therapy. Meningitis may be a complication of septicaemia, which will also require energetic treatment.

Bacteriology and routes of infection

The organisms involved vary with the age of the patient and the source of the infection. *Streptococcus pneumoniae* (the pneumococcus) is the most frequent cause of primary meningitis, and particularly affects the very young and the very old. Pneumococcal meningitis can, however, occur at any age, particularly if there is a source of infection such as pneumonia, sinusitis or endocarditis. Entry of the bacteria may follow a head injury, particularly if there is leakage of cerebrospinal fluid.[4] Alcoholics and patients who have had a splenectomy are also prone to pneumococcal meningitis.

Meningococcal meningitis is caused by *Neisseria meningitidis* in an epidemic form (Groups A and C)[5] or as localised outbreaks of sporadic meningitis with Group B meningococci. Although commonest in children under 5, Group B infections are increasing in prevalence in the 10–20 year age group.[5] Less than 10% of cases of meningococcal meningitis occur over the age of 45 years.[6] The epidemic form usually occurs in the winter and spring, and the serogroups A and C can be controlled by vaccination. Group B infections have become the commonest cause of meningococcal meningitis in Europe during the 1970s and 1980s, and the Group B polysaccharide is not sufficiently immunogenic for use in vaccines. Other antigens in the outer membranes of the meningococcus may be suitable antigens for vaccines but this requires that the subtype and serotype of the organism are known before vaccination is commenced.[5,7] Meningococcal septicaemia may be fatal in 50% of treated cases[5] and is characterised by petechial haemorrhages or purpura in the skin;[8] intravascular coagulation may cause infarction of the adrenals (Waterhouse–Friderichsen syndrome), renal cortical necrosis, pulmonary microvascular thrombosis and shock.

Haemophilus influenzae (type b) is the most common bacterial cause of meningitis between the neonatal period and 6 years of age[8] but it can occur at other ages. The organisms reach the meninges mainly from the pharynx or from middle ear infections. Although the mortality rate is only 3–8%, *H. influenzae* meningitis is a major cause of subsequent mental defect.[9]

Although *Str. pneumoniae*, *N. meningitidis* and *H. influenzae* account for 40% of cases of meningitis in adults, infections by Gram-negative bacilli are becoming more important as a cause of meningitis. This is mainly due to the successful treatment of meningitis caused by the other organisms and the acquisition in hospitals of infections by Gram-negative bacilli.[10] 30% of infections by Gram-negative bacilli follow head trauma, especially if the skull is fractured through the cranial sinuses and there is cerebrospinal liquorrhoea. 50% of cases of meningitis caused by Gram-negative bacilli complicate neurosurgical manoeuvres, and 20% complicate medical conditions such as septicaemia, ruptured abscesses and immunosuppression. After the neonatal period, 40% of infections by Gram-negative bacilli are due to *Klebsiella* species, 15–30% due to *Escherichia coli* and 10–20% due to *Pseudomonas* species, but the incidence varies from hospital to hospital. Symptoms arising from head injuries may mask the onset of meningitis.[10]

Haematogenous spread is the most common mode of infection for leptomeningitis, although rupture of an abscess into the subarachnoid space, or spread from cranial sinuses, an infected myelomeningocele, or a penetrating wound may also allow infection to enter. *Str. pneumoniae*, *N. meningitidis* and *H. influenzae* all colonise the nasopharynx; if meningitis occurs, it usually follows recent colonisation. New strains occur in individuals each year and they spread by close contact in the family or in hostels, camps and prisons; defects in the immune response may result in increased susceptibility to meningitis. *H. influenzae* and *N. meningitidis* have pili that enable them to become attached to the epithelial cells of the nasopharynx or oropharynx.[11]

The bacteria are ingested by phagocytic cells and pass into the blood where they survive due to the presence of antiphagocytic capsules.[12] Gram-negative bacteria avoid destruction by the presence of lipopolysaccharide or membrane

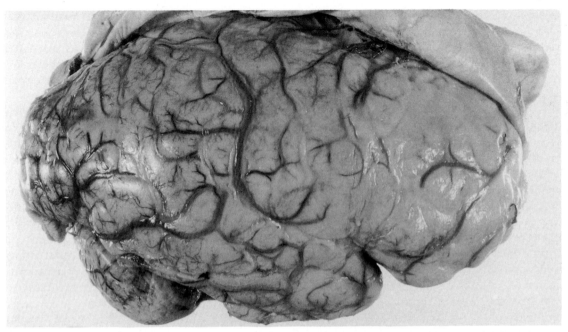

Fig. 7.1 Pyogenic leptomeningitis. The dura has been reflected to reveal pus in the subarachnoid space, mainly over the frontal lobes (right).

proteins which deter bacteriolysis.[13] The mechanism by which bacteria enter the CSF is unknown, but it may be through the choroid plexus. Many bacteria from the oropharynx cause bacteraemia but not meningitis. Small parameningeal septic foci in the spine or related to the ear may also be sources of bacterial infection of the meninges.

Pathology

Macroscopic inspection of the brain in a patient with leptomeningitis (Fig. 7.1) reveals yellow or greenish pus within the subarachnoid space over the vertex or base of the brain and in the basal cisterns. The pus is bounded by the outer arachnoid and bathes the arteries and veins in the subarachnoid space. Bacteriological swabs taken post-mortem may be useful for correlating the organisms causing the meningitis with primary sources of infection in the pharynx, or in septic foci in the lungs, skin or intracranial sites.

Histologically, pus is seen permeating to the depths of sulci (Fig. 7.2) and filling the subarachnoid space over the surface of the cerebral and cerebellar gyri (Fig. 7.3). In the early stages of leptomeningitis, the inflammatory cells are polymorphonuclear leucocytes (Fig. 7.4) but they are replaced by macrophages in the later stages of meningitis. Inflammatory cells may also extend into the perivascular spaces near the surface of the brain and a few small foci of inflammation may also

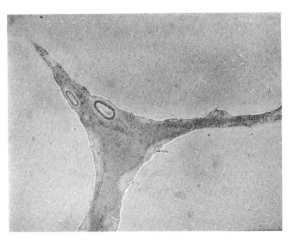

Fig. 7.2 Pyogenic leptomeningitis. The cerebral sulcus is filled with pus.
Haematoxylin-eosin × 8

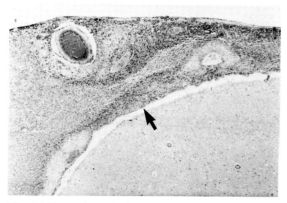

Fig. 7.3 Pyogenic meningitis. Pus is confined within the subarachnoid space by the arachnoid (top) and the pia mater (arrow). Cortex at bottom, right.
Haematoxylin-eosin × 20

be seen around vessels deeper in the brain (Fig. 7.5).

The pus in leptomeningitis is almost totally confined to the cerebrospinal fluid spaces in the subarachnoid space and rarely extends directly into the brain tissue.

The cerebrospinal fluid is produced by the choroid plexuses in the cerebral and fourth ventricles, drains into the subarachnoid space and passes over the surface of the brain to enter the blood through the arachnoid granulations in the walls of the superior sagittal sinus and other venous sinuses.[14] There is free communication between spinal and cranial cerebrospinal fluid in normal individuals. Over the surface of the brain, arachnoid mater forms the outer boundary of the subarachnoid space, and the pia mater forms its

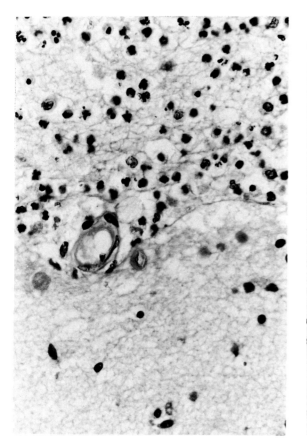

Fig. 7.4 Pyogenic leptomeningitis. Polymorphonuclear leucocytes and fibrin in the subarachnoid space (top) do not extend into the brain (bottom).
Haematoxylin-eosin × 430

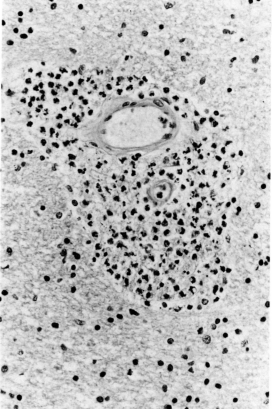

Fig. 7.5 Pyogenic leptomeningitis. Polymorphonuclear leucocytes in the perivascular space around blood vessels in the white matter.
Haematoxylin-eosin × 270

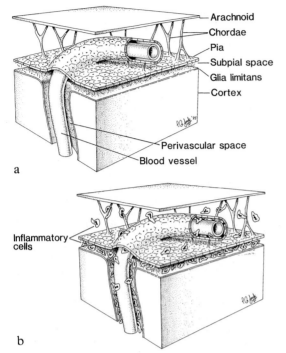

a

b

Fig. 7.6a, b Relationship of the pia mater and subarachnoid space to blood vessels in the cerebral cortex: (**a**) in the normal brain, (**b**) in leptomeningitis.
Reproduced by permission of the editor from: Hutchings M, Weller RO. J Neurosurg 1986; 65: 316 [Fig. 9].

inner boundary, separating the brain surface from the cerebrospinal fluid. It was long considered that there was a direct communication between the perivascular spaces (Virchow–Robin spaces) in the brain and the subarachnoid space, but recent studies suggest that this is incorrect (Fig. 7.6).[15]

In order to enter the CSF in the subarachnoid space, inflammatory cells must penetrate the pia mater as they pass from the perivascular spaces into the CSF.[15] Close histological examination of brain sections reveals inflammatory cells in the perivascular spaces of the cerebral vessels near the surface of the brain, in the subpial space, in the perivascular spaces of the subarachnoid vessels and in the subarachnoid space (Fig. 7.7).[15,16] The lack of antibodies in the CSF and the comparatively large amount of fluid in the subarachnoid space may facilitate the spread of organisms in this compartment.[17]

Complications. Cerebral oedema may compli-

cate meningitis, but due to the diffuse nature of the inflammation, there is little brain shift even though the intracranial pressure may be raised. Another major complication of meningitis is inflammation of the walls of the blood vessels within the subarachnoid space. Thrombotic occlusion of these vessels may result in small areas of infarction on the surface of the brain together with petechial haemorrhages, or, if large vessels are involved, more extensive areas of infarction deep within the cerebral hemispheres are seen. The cranial nerves, which pass through the subarachnoid space, may be affected by the inflammatory exudate, resulting in cranial nerve palsies. The 6th cranial nerve is particularly prone to damage in this way, probably because of its long course through the subarachnoid space. Incompletely treated leptomeningitis may result in extensive fibrosis of the leptomeninges as the inflammatory exudate becomes organised; *hydrocephalus* may ensue with dilatation of the lateral ventricles (Fig. 7.8), third ventricle, aqueduct and fourth ventricle.

Ventriculitis, due to spread of infection and inflammation to the cerebral ventricles, is a severe and usually fatal complication of meningitis. However, ventriculitis more commonly occurs following rupture of an abscess into a ventricle. Macroscopically, there is roughening and opacity of the ventricular lining with a varying amount of pus adherent to the ependymal surfaces and to the choroid plexus. Ventricular dilatation may occur. Histologically, polymorphonuclear leucocytes and macrophages adhere to the ependymal wall and there is perivascular accumulation of inflammatory cells in the periventricular tissue and in the choroid plexus.

Spinal leptomeningitis usually results from direct spread of infection from the blood or from the intracranial subarachnoid space (Fig. 7.9). Isolated spinal leptomeningitis, however, is usually due to the introduction of bacteria at lumbar puncture or due to spread from an infected myelomeningocele or focus of spinal osteomyelitis. Purulent inflammatory exudate surrounds the nerve roots and expands the spinal subarachnoid space (Fig. 7.9). In the normal spinal cord, delicate ligaments and trabeculae traverse the subarachnoid space;[18] inflammation of the

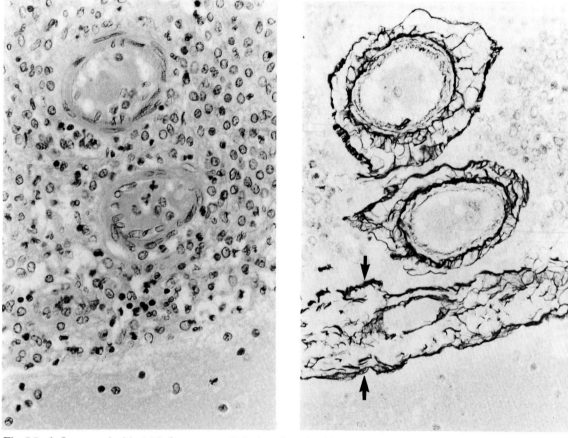

a   b

Fig. 7.7a, b Leptomeningitis. (**a**) Inflammatory cells in the subarachnoid space around two arteries. Cerebral cortex (bottom). (**b**) Same field as (a). Black-stained reticulin marks the leptomeningeal coat of two blood vessels in the subarachnoid space and shows how the perivascular space is expanded by inflammatory cells. The pia mater (top arrow) is separated from the basement membrane of the glia limitans (bottom arrow) by the subpial space, which contains inflammatory cells and a small blood vessel. Subarachnoid space at top. Cortex at bottom.
(**a**) Haematoxylin-eosin × 380; (**b**) Gordon and Sweet × 380

spinal leptomeninges may cause adhesions and loculation of CSF.

Sterile arachnoiditis may follow the injection of foreign materials into the subarachnoid space. This was particularly well recorded with the injection of oil-based myelography fluid, following which some patients developed arachnoid adhesions, loculation of the cerebrospinal fluid, tethering of nerve roots and back pain.

Cerebrospinal fluid in leptomeningitis

There is an increase in the total white cell count in the CSF in purulent meningitis, due to the presence of polymorphonuclear leucocytes. Gram stains may reveal the presence of the infecting bacteria (Fig. 7.10), particularly if the patient has not already been treated with antibiotics. Specific capsular polysaccharide antigens can be detected in the CSF using appropriate antisera; agglutination assays are available for *N. meningitidis*, *Str. pneumoniae*, and *H. influenzae* type b.[19] Gram staining and agglutination assays can be used as an initial screen and the identity of the infecting organisms confirmed by bacteriological culture. CSF protein is greatly increased in leptomeningitis to levels higher than 5 g per litre, and a reduction of the CSF glucose level is seen. Normally, the glucose level in the cerebrospinal fluid is some two-thirds of that in the blood, but in

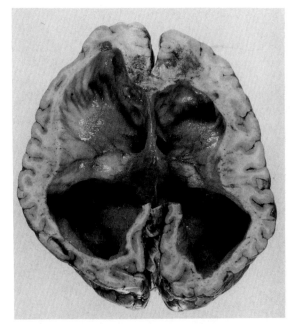

Fig. 7.8 Hydrocephalus. Horizontal section of the brain viewed from above. From a 54-year-old man who had meningitis in childhood. The lateral ventricles are grossly dilated.

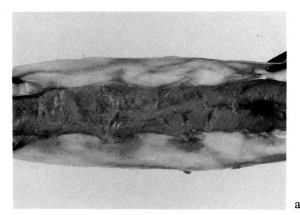

a

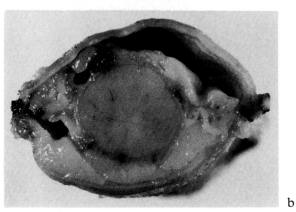

b

bacterial and fungal meningitis the glucose is reduced to less than one-half of the blood level.

Fig. 7.9a, b Spinal leptomeningitis. (**a**) The dura has been reflected from the spinal cord to reveal opacity of the leptomeninges due to pus in the subarachnoid space. (**b**) Transverse section of spinal cord (centre) showing pus filling the subarachnoid space.

Neonatal meningitis (see p. 340)

(see p. 340)

Leptomeningitis in the perinatal period occurs more commonly in low birth weight premature infants and in children with congenital malformations or whose birth has been complicated. *Escherichia coli* is the most common organism, but *Listeria monocytogenes*[20] and *Streptococcus agalactiae* are also common causes of meningitis in the neonatal period and up to the age of 5 years.

Meningitis in the neonatal period may be associated with widespread cerebral infarction. If the infant survives, the infarcts evolve into cystic, softened areas (cystic malacia) within the cerebral hemispheres.

Less common organisms causing meningitis

A wide variety of bacteria, in addition to those mentioned above, can cause leptomeningitis.[21] *Staphylococcus aureus* may spread from cerebral

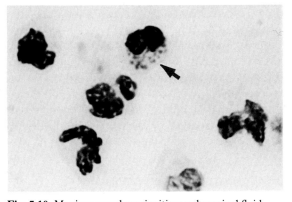

Fig. 7.10 Meningococcal meningitis; cerebrospinal fluid. Inflammatory cells contain Gram-negative intracellular diplococci (arrow). Gram × 1500

abscesses, paranasal sinuses or endocarditis to involve the meninges. *Staphylococcus epidermidis* may infect ventriculo-atrial shunts inserted for the treatment of hydrocephalus;[22] ventriculitis and meningitis may develop, and effective treatment usually requires removal of the shunt.

Listeria monocytogenes may cause meningitis in normal adults but more commonly causes leptomeningitis in the neonatal period following infection by organisms in the maternal genital tract. Immunosuppressed patients are also prone to listeria leptomeningitis. The organism is a Gram-positive bacterium which is commonly found in water, soil and plant material. It causes abortion, encephalitis, septicaemia and mastitis in cattle and sheep and may be transmitted to man either directly or through food, especially cheese and milk.[23] Most infections in adults are symptomless, and the bacteria reside in the intestine, vagina or cervix; it is from these sources that neonatal meningeal infection arises. The organism is intracellular and continues to multiply even when engulfed by macrophages. A fulminating encephalitis may be caused by *L. monocytogenes* in which large areas of the brain and spinal cord become necrotic following invasion by the bacteria; polymorphonuclear leucocytes and microglia[24] are abundant in the necrotic inflamed area (Fig. 7.11).[24]

Anthrax may cause a haemorrhagic meningitis.

Lyme disease (Garin–Bujadoux–Bannwarth syndrome). This disease, first described in 1977 in Lyme County, Connecticut, USA, is caused by the spirochaete *Borrelia burgdorferi*.[25,26] The organism is spread by *Ixodes dammini* and other ticks in the USA[21,27] and by *Ixodes ricinus* in Europe. Following the tick bite, patients may initially present with expanding annular skin lesions (erythema chronicum migrans)[28] and some weeks or months later develop neurological, cardiac and musculoskeletal complications and, even later, arthritis. Meningoradiculoneuritis is the commonest neurological complication.[29] Patients present with painful mononeuritis multiplex or a Guillain–Barré-like syndrome and have high titres of antibodies against *Borrelia burgdorferi*.[29] Sural nerve biopsies in such cases have shown

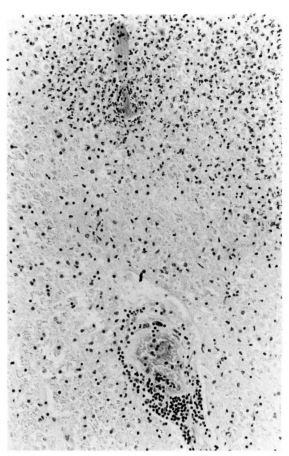

Fig. 7.11 *Listeria monocytogenes* infection. A thrombosed blood vessel (top) in the spinal cord is surrounded by polymorphonuclear leucocytes and necrotic tissue. Rod-shaped microglia (centre) and perivascular lymphocytes (bottom) are seen in the adjacent white matter. Haematoxylin-eosin × 150

axonal degeneration and perivascular cuffing by lymphocytes and plasma cells around epineurial and sometimes endoneurial blood vessels.[29] It is thought that the peripheral nerve damage is due to ischaemia secondary to immunologically mediated blood vessel disease.

Meningoencephalopathy occurs in a minority of patients and is superimposed upon a radiculitis.[28] Patients may present with dementia or evidence of multiple infarcts. Transverse myelitis has also been reported.[28,29] CT scans reveal lesions which resemble small infarcts or large low-density lesions resembling those of multiple sclerosis.[28,30] No detailed pathological studies of the acute central nervous system lesions are available but it is thought that they may be due to inflammation of vessel walls and thrombosis similar to that seen in the peripheral nervous system.[29]

The cerebrospinal fluid in affected patients shows an increase in lymphocytes in about 50% of cases, and the spirochaete may be isolated from the CSF.[28] Treatment by penicillin and steroids may result in improvement of the peripheral nerve lesions but the central nervous system symptomatology may remain unchanged.[28]

TUBERCULOUS INFECTIONS OF THE CENTRAL NERVOUS SYSTEM

The central nervous system may be affected by tuberculosis in a number of different ways. In *tuberculous meningitis* there are caseating granulomas involving the pia and arachnoid mater and the walls of blood vessels in the subarachnoid space. *Subdural tuberculosis* (tuberculoma en plaque) and *tuberculosis of the spine* may secondarily affect the central nervous system. For example, tuberculosis of the vertebral bodies may cause collapse of a vertebra and paraplegia due to spinal cord compression (Pott's paraplegia). Localised *tuberculomas* may also occur within the parenchyma of the brain.

Tuberculous leptomeningitis

Patients with tuberculous leptomeningitis usually present with a prodromal illness lasting 2 or 3 weeks and characterised by lassitude, anorexia, loss of weight and intermittent vomiting and confusion.[31] The onset of neck stiffness may be accompanied by headache, vomiting and convulsions but the symptoms may be less marked than in pyogenic meningitis. Involvement of cranial nerves may result in ptosis, diplopia, facial weakness, deafness and dysphagia. Signs of cerebral infarction may be detected. Most patients have evidence of tuberculosis elsewhere in the body. Examination of the CSF may point to the diagnosis of tuberculous meningitis; the fluid is usually clear but protein clots may form on standing. Between 10 and $1000 \times 10^6/l$ mononuclear cells are present in the fluid and there is a moderate to marked rise in the protein level.

Glucose and chloride levels in the CSF are reduced.[32] There may be very few mycobacteria in the CSF and their presence may only be substantiated on culture, although the detection of tuberculostearic acid may be used as a test in the future. The mortality rate of tuberculous meningitis has been considerably reduced since the introduction of anti-tuberculous agents, and the prognosis is more favourable if patients are treated early.

Meningitis is a complication of tuberculosis in other parts of the body. *Miliary spread* may occur from a lung lesion or from cervical lymph nodes, and the organisms are usually human *Mycobacterium tuberculosis* rather than bovine. *Direct spread* of the disease from a cold abscess in the spine may result in tuberculous meningitis. It is thought that in the majority of cases of miliary tuberculosis, a small tuberculoma in the subependymal or subpial region ruptures into the cerebrospinal fluid and results in spread of the mycobacteria. Most cases of tuberculous meningitis are seen in young children between 6 months and 5 years of age but the elderly are also prone to develop the disease. Tuberculous meningitis also occurs as a complication in immunosuppressed patients of any age—typically, for example, in lymphoma, in which there may be an overwhelming meningeal infection but few direct clinical signs.[33]

Pathology

Macroscopically, the brain from a patient with tuberculous meningitis shows thickening, opacity and granularity of the arachnoid covering the surface of the cerebral hemispheres. The changes are, however, usually most extensive at the base of the brain where the subarachnoid space may be filled by yellow–green gelatinous material in which the cerebral vessels and emerging cranial nerves are embedded. Examination of the sliced brain may reveal widespread infarction, particularly of the basal ganglia; such infarction is due to inflammation of the walls of perforating arteries and thrombosis in their lumina.

Histologically, affected areas of the meninges contain caseating granulomas (Fig. 7.12a) which, in the early stages of tuberculous meningitis, are

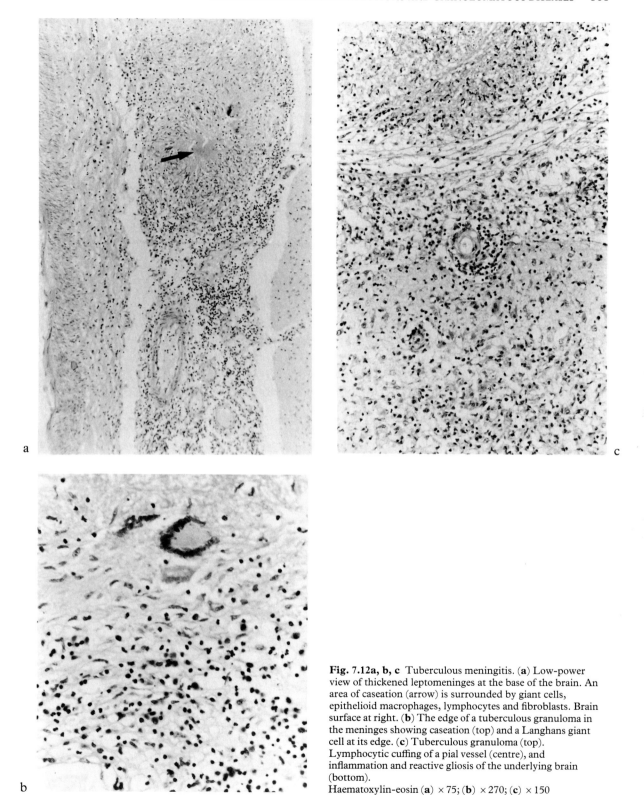

Fig. 7.12a, b, c Tuberculous meningitis. (**a**) Low-power view of thickened leptomeninges at the base of the brain. An area of caseation (arrow) is surrounded by giant cells, epithelioid macrophages, lymphocytes and fibroblasts. Brain surface at right. (**b**) The edge of a tuberculous granuloma in the meninges showing caseation (top) and a Langhans giant cell at its edge. (**c**) Tuberculous granuloma (top). Lymphocytic cuffing of a pial vessel (centre), and inflammation and reactive gliosis of the underlying brain (bottom).
Haematoxylin-eosin (**a**) ×75; (**b**) ×270; (**c**) ×150

small discrete miliary tubercles, but in the later stages consist of large areas of caseation and fibrosis. Langhans giant cells, epithelioid macrophages and lymphocytes (Fig. 7.12b) are seen within the granulomas although there may be few acid-fast mycobacteria identifiable in the Ziehl–Nielsen stained preparations. Lymphocytic infiltration, reactive astrocytes and microglial proliferation are seen under the pial surface of the brain (Fig. 7.12c) and the walls of the subarach-

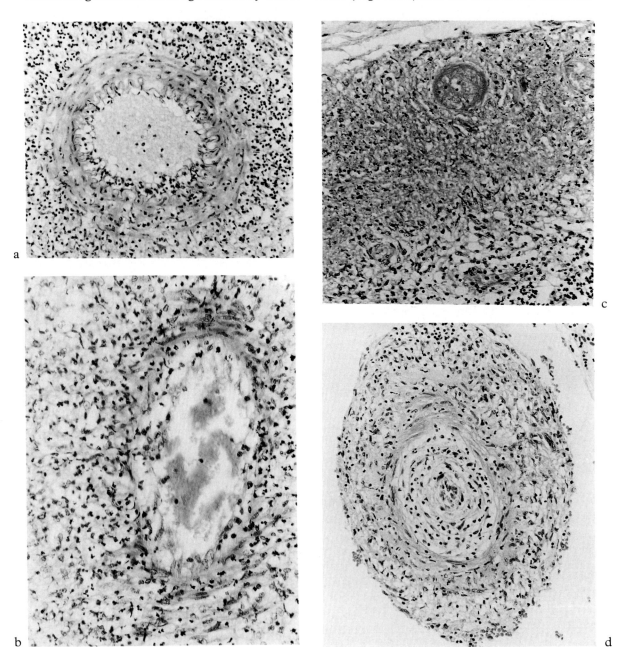

Fig. 7.13a, b, c, d Blood vessel damage in tuberculous meningitis. Subarachnoid vessels showing: (**a**) lymphocytic infiltration of the wall of an artery, (**b**) inflammation and destruction of the arterial media and intima, (**c**) thrombotic occlusion of a vessel (top) in an area of caseation, (**d**) perivascular fibrosis, endarteritis obliterans and fibrosis of the arterial media. Haematoxylin-eosin (**a**) ×150; (**b**) ×240; (**c, d**) ×150

noid vessels may be inflamed (Fig. 7.13). Thrombotic occlusion of affected vessels causing cerebral infarction is one of the major complications of tuberculous meningitis. Not only is the brain itself involved in the infection but cranial nerves crossing the subarachnoid space are affected by the granulomatous inflammation at the base of the brain with destruction of axons and the development of cranial nerve palsies.

Late complications of tuberculous meningitis include hydrocephalus with dilatation of the lateral, third and fourth ventricles due to organisation and fibrosis of the caseating granulomas in the subarachnoid space and impedance of cerebrospinal fluid flow. Residual cranial nerve damage and infarction may be seen at post-mortem.

Tuberculomas

Tuberculous granulomas (tuberculomas) are seen mainly in areas of the world in which tuberculosis is still common. They usually occur in the cerebellum in children.[32] Clinically, patients present with fever, a high erythrocyte sedimentation rate, and evidence of tuberculosis elsewhere in the body. More specifically, tuberculomas may cause epilepsy or present as space-occupying lesions with raised intracranial pressure.[34]

In the cerebral hemispheres, tuberculomas are usually multiple and appear as solid or ring-enhancing lesions on CT scan; they may be confused with metastatic tumour deposits.[34] Macroscopically, tuberculomas in fixed brains appear as cream-coloured, firm, well-circumscribed nodules with necrotic centres and thick, grey, tough capsules 1–3 mm thick. Microscopically, the capsule is composed of collagenous tissue containing caseating granulomas with giant cells. A varying degree of lymphocytic infiltration is seen in the capsule and there may be some calcification.

SARCOIDOSIS

Approximately 5% of patients with sarcoidosis have neurological features—most commonly mononeuritis multiplex. A proportion of those affected have abnormalities of the central nervous system due either to leptomeningeal sarcoidosis or to localised tumour-like masses of sarcoid granulomas. Skeletal muscle is also involved in sarcoidosis (see p. 634).

Clinically, sarcoidosis of the nervous system presents with a monophasic, a chronic relapsing or a progressive course.[35] Transient, sometimes fluctuating, cranial nerve palsies are the most common manifestation; the facial nerves are most frequently involved. Peripheral mononeuritis multiplex involving the limbs is also seen. Due to the wide variation of diffuse or focal involvement of the leptomeninges, neurosarcoidosis may present with a very variable pattern of central nervous system signs.[36] Epilepsy, with focal or generalised fits, is a common presentation of sarcoidosis and patients may die with intractable epilepsy. Symptoms of space-occupying lesions may be present, and diffuse involvement of the meninges may cause dementia and hydrocephalus. When the base of the brain is involved, visual impairment due to optic nerve damage may occur. Hypothalamic syndromes, including diabetes insipidus, somnolence and loss of temperature control, may also be seen. Examination of the cerebrospinal fluid frequently reveals an increase in lymphocytes and CSF protein. CT scans show dilatation of the ventricular system in 50% of cases[35] and areas of enhancement may be seen in the meninges following the intravenous injection of contrast medium, indicating focal breakdown of the blood-brain barrier probably associated with sarcoid granulomata.

Pathology

It may be difficult to distinguish sarcoidosis from tuberculosis. Macroscopically, the brain may exhibit thickening and fibrosis of the meninges and small white granulomas on the surface. The optic nerves, the hypothalamus and pituitary may be involved, as may the cranial nerves. Obliteration of the subarachnoid space may result in hydrocephalus.

Microscopically, non-caseating granulomas are seen involving the leptomeninges on the surface of the brain and in the depths of the sulci (Fig. 7.14). The walls of arteries in the subarachnoid space

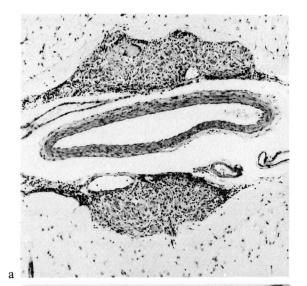

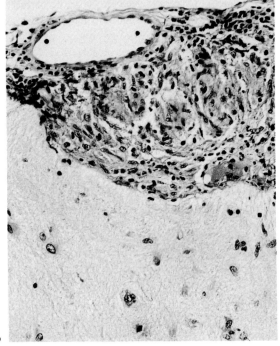

Fig. 7.14a, b Sarcoidosis. (a) Non-caseating giant cell granulomas involving the pia and subpial blood vessels either side of a cerebral sulcus. The blood vessel in the subarachnoid space is hardly affected. (b) High-power view of the lower sarcoid granuloma in (a) showing involvement of a subpial blood vessel and reactive astrocytes in the underlying brain tissue (bottom).
Haematoxylin-eosin (a) ×75; (b) ×210

may be involved and the granulomas may extend along perforating cortical arteries. Multinucleate giant cells and epithelioid macrophages are present, together with a moderate number of lymphocytes. Fibroblasts and collagen are seen within the granulomas, and reactive astrocytes and microglia are present in the surrounding brain. Small areas of infarction may occur as a result of involvement of arteries in the granulomatous process. Cranial nerves are frequently involved, with resulting axonal degeneration. Tuberculosis should be excluded by culture, particularly of biopsy material, and by a search for acid-fast bacilli in Ziehl–Nielsen stained preparations.

Other granulomatous lesions

Other causes of granulomatous lesions in the meninges and parenchyma of the brain include giant cell granulomatous arteritis (see p. 102)[37] and fungal infections (see p. 173).

SYPHILIS

The incidence and progress of neurosyphilis, due to infection by *Treponema pallidum*,[38] have changed dramatically since the introduction of effective antibiotic treatment. Classically, the disease is spread by sexual transmission and, following an incubation period of about three weeks, a non-painful *primary* skin lesion (chancre) occurs at the point of infection (usually on the genitalia) and is accompanied by regional lymphadenopathy. *T. pallidum* can be isolated from the chancre and identified under dark ground illumination microscopy or by Levatidi staining. The organism cannot be cultured in vitro by ordinary methods but it readily infects rabbits. After a variable interval, the chancre disappears and a *secondary* bacteraemic phase with generalised mucocutaneous lesions and lymphadenopathy occurs. The disease passes into a period of subclinical or latent infection after approximately four years, when the patient is not infectious and the disease is only detectable by serology. A small number of inadequately treated or untreated patients enter the late or *tertiary* stage, which is a progressive disease involving principally the ascending aorta or the central nervous system, but any organ can be involved.

Congenital syphilis occurs due to the spread of

treponemas to the fetus in utero or by infection during passage through the birth canal.

It is estimated that 21 000–29 000 cases of syphilis occur in the United States each year.[38]

The basic pathology of neurosyphilis is swelling of endothelial cells, endarteritis obliterans, proliferation of blood vessels and the perivascular accumulation of lymphocytes and plasma cells (see Fig. 7.16) as a direct response to spirochaetal antigens. Tissue necrosis and scarring may be extensive. Several major syndromes[39] of neurosyphilis are recognised:

1. acute lymphocytic meningitis (syphilitic meningitis)
2. stroke-like syndromes due to meningovascular syphilis
3. dementia (general paralysis of the insane) due to parenchymal involvement by neurosyphilis
4. myeloneuropathy (tabes dorsalis)
5. gummas in the central nervous system.

Syphilitic meningitis

This is an early manifestation of syphilis and may be confused with pyogenic meningitis. However, the Wassermann and VDRL reactions are usually positive in CSF and also in blood.

Meningovascular syphilis

Clinically, meningovascular syphilis presents with diffuse signs and symptoms due to widespread involvement of the meninges and focal destruction of brain and spinal cord tissue. Impairment of memory and intellect may occur, and epilepsy may develop. Alternatively, there may be focal neurological deficits such as cranial nerve palsies and, in general, the symptomatology will depend upon the distribution of the meningeal involvement. If the basal meninges are affected, cranial nerve palsies are common and the pupillary reflexes are almost always impaired. Hydrocephalus occasionally occurs and there may be damage to the hypothalamus.

Pathologically, meningovascular syphilis is characterised by endarteritis obliterans in the meningeal vessels with crescentic thickening of the intima and destruction of the media.[40] The arterial elastic lamina usually remains intact but there is lymphocyte and plasma cell infiltration in the adventitia and in the media. In the healed stage, the vessels remain scarred and thickened but cannot be specifically identified as syphilitic. The eventual effect on the meninges is chronic inflammation and fibrous thickening; miliary gummas may occur and resemble miliary tubercles. In the spine, arachnoiditis may be the main manifestation but vessels within the cord may also be affected. It is usually the medium-sized arteries that are involved.

Meningovascular syphilis may affect predominantly the spinal meninges, resulting in *pachymeningitis cervicalis hypertrophica*. This disorder is characterised by thickening of the dura and its adherence to the arachnoid and pia; damage to the long tracts in the spinal cord results. Endarteritis of spinal vessels may also cause damage to the cord and spinal roots.

Parenchymatous neurosyphilis

When it affects the brain, parenchymatous neurosyphilis causes the dementia associated with *general paralysis of the insane* (GPI). Clinically, patients present with a change in personality and affect, hyper-reflexia, small irregular pupils which do not react to light (Argyll Robertson pupils), intellectual deterioration and difficulties with speech. Patients dying in the active stage of GPI may show extensive cerebral atrophy with thickening of the leptomeninges and a granular surface to the underlying brain. Granular ependymitis due to subependymal gliosis may be seen macroscopically, particularly in the fourth ventricle.

Histologically, there is extensive microglial proliferation, neuronal loss and gliosis throughout the cerebral cortex. Perivascular cuffing by lymphocytes and plasma cells is seen in the meninges and in the parenchyma of the brain. Spirochaetes may be visualised within the tissue by silver stains or by immunoperoxidase techniques.[41] In treated cases, cerebral atrophy and scarring may be the only evidence of the disease.

Myeloneuropathy (tabes dorsalis)

Like GPI, tabes dorsalis tends to present many

years after the initial infection. Clinically, patients develop ataxia, shooting pains in the legs, bladder disturbances and impotence. Loss of joint position sense, deep pain and temperature are accompanied by degenerative joint disease (Charcot joints) and foot ulceration.

The pathology of tabes is characterised by axonal degeneration and gliosis of the dorsal columns of the spinal cord (Fig. 7.15). Microscopically, there is meningeal thickening and although it is thought that the meningeal changes may be the cause of the posterior column degeneration, this is not absolutely certain.

Gummas

Gummas are areas of necrosis resembling

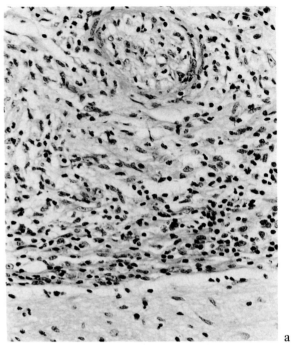

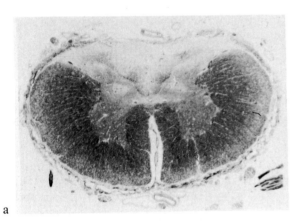

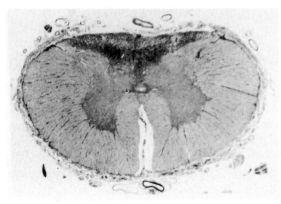

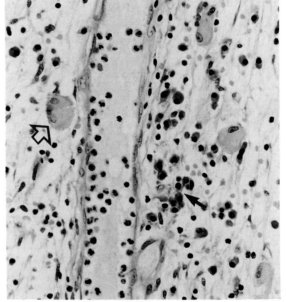

Fig. 7.15a, b Tabes dorsalis—lumbar spinal cord. (**a**) There is loss of axons and myelin from the dorsal columns as shown by the lack of myelin staining (top). (**b**) Same level as (a) showing intense gliosis in the dorsal columns (dark staining at top).
(**a**) Klüver–Barrera × 6.5; (**b**) Holzer × 6.5

Fig. 7.16a, b Gumma in the brain. (**a**) Edge showing an occluded blood vessel (top) and dense fibrous tissue sharply demarcated from the brain tissue (bottom). (**b**) Within the gumma, a blood vessel (centre) is surrounded by plasma cells (solid arrow) and globular, reactive astrocytes (open arrow) trapped in the fibrous tissue of the gumma.
Haematoxylin-eosin (**a**) × 190; (**b**) × 310

tuberculomas, and result from endarteritis obliterans of the supplying arteries. In the brain, gummas are rare; they may be associated with meningovascular syphilis. Occasionally gummas present as space-occupying lesions with areas of decreased density on CT scan and focal enhancement. Histologically, a gumma has a central area of necrosis and extensive fibrosis, with lymphocyte and plasma cell infiltration at the periphery (Fig. 7.16).

Serological tests for syphilis. These include fluorescent treponemal antibody absorption (FTA-ABS), Wassermann reaction and the

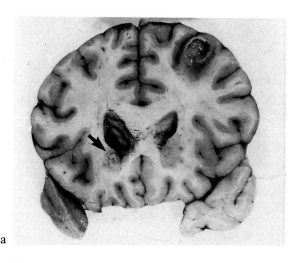

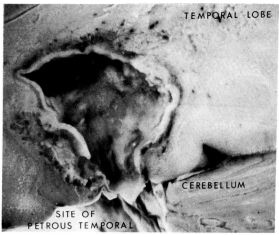

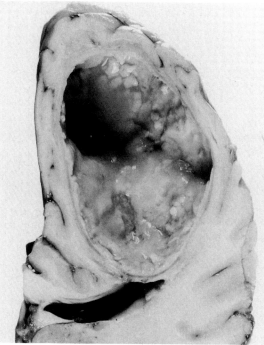

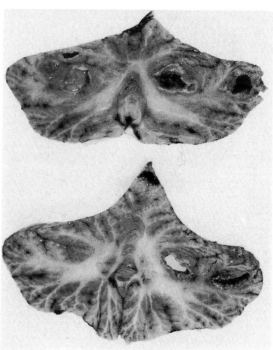

a

b

c

d

Fig. 7.17 a, b, c, d Cerebral abscess. (**a**) An abscess cavity in the frontal gyrus (top right) and a further area of septic softening in the head of the left caudate nucleus (arrow). (**b**) Horizontal section of an occipital lobe showing a huge abscess (8 × 5 cm). The pus has been evacuated but some still adheres to the wall. (**c**) A temporal lobe abscess showing a thick, white, fibrous capsule. (**d**) Multiple abscesses in the cerebellum.

Treponema pallidum haemagglutination assay (TPHA-TP).[42]

BRAIN ABSCESS

Despite the introduction of antibiotics, the incidence of brain abscess has altered little. However, early CT scan diagnosis has reduced the mortality rate from 40–60% in the pre-antibiotic era to the present 15–20%.[43] The median age of incidence of brain abscess is 30–40 years; under the age of 15 years, 25% of abscesses occur in patients with congenital heart disease.[44] The frontal and temporal lobes are the commonest sites for abscess formation, followed by the fronto-parietal, parietal, cerebellar and occipital regions (Fig. 7.17);[44] other sites are rare.

Origins of the infection and modes of entry of the bacteria into the brain are varied. Trauma or surgical operations may introduce bacteria, or the organisms may spread from adjacent structures. In older series, 40% of abscesses were temporal or cerebellar and were associated with otitis media or mastoiditis. Frontal, ethmoid and sphenoid air sinuses are also sources of infection[45] and facial sepsis may result in cavernous sinus suppuration and cerebral abscess.[46]

Although in 20% of cases the source of infection cannot be identified,[47] many cases of brain abscess are due to metastatic haematogenous spread of infection from a distant focus. Chronic pyogenic lung disease remains an important source of infection, and patients with cyanotic heart disease, especially Fallot's tetralogy and transposition, account for 5–10% of brain abscesses.[48] Subacute

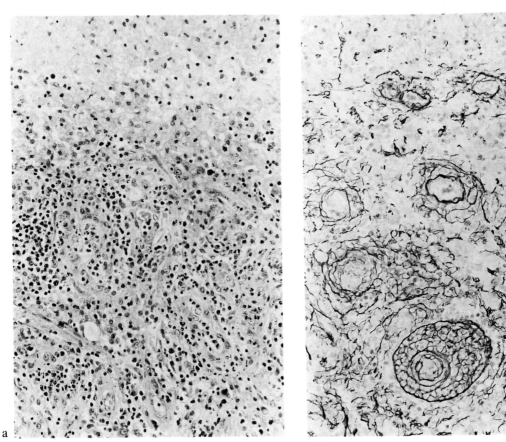

a   b

Fig. 7.18a, b Early abscess formation. (**a**) Dead tissue (top) and adjacent inflamed granulation tissue (bottom). (**b**) Similar field to (a) showing black-stained reticulin in the walls of blood vessels and within inflamed granulation tissue. Necrotic tissue (top). Expansion of perivascular spaces by inflammatory cells (bottom).
(**a**) Haematoxylin-eosin × 150; (**b**) Gordon and Sweet × 150

bacterial endocarditis is an uncommon cause of cerebral abscess,[49] perhaps because the organisms involved are not pyogenic. In contrast, abscess formation results from septic embolism in the course of acute bacterial endocarditis, caused by pyogenic organisms such as *Staphylococcus aureus*. Most commonly, metastatic abscesses develop in areas of the brain supplied by the middle cerebral arteries. The initial location of the abscess is thought to be at the junction of the white matter and cortex.[50] The abscesses are often multiple or multiloculated, and initially they are poorly encapsulated.

Clinical aspects

75% of patients who present with cerebral abscess have a history of symptoms for 2 weeks or less. In about 50% of cases, there is a classical presentation of fever, headache and focal neurological deficit, but in many the predominant clinical picture is that of an expanding lesion with a change in mental state. Epilepsy occurs in 25–35% of cases.

CT scan has greatly facilitated the early diagnosis of cerebral abscess. In the very early stages of cerebritis there may be an area of low density and some focal enhancement. However, in the later stages, when the fibrous capsule has formed, there is typically a ring of enhancement representing the fibrous capsule; an area of low density brain oedema usually surrounds the abscess. Although such an appearance is often typical of an abscess, it may be confused with metastatic carcinoma or even glioma.

Treatment with antibiotics during the stage of cerebritis may prevent an abscess forming. Late diagnosis, multiplicity of abscesses, and fungal infection as a cause give a poor prognosis. Epilepsy develops in some 35% of patients who survive.[44]

Pathology

The macroscopic and microscopic appearances of cerebral abscesses depend partly upon the age of the abscess and partly upon the infecting organism. Initially, an abscess develops as a focal, softened and often haemorrhagic area of cerebritis (Fig. 7.17a).[51–53] Microscopically, such an area appears as a mixture of infarction and acute

inflammation and granulation tissue (Fig. 7.18). As the central area of the abscess becomes further softened and pus forms, there is proliferation of fibroblasts around blood vessels at the periphery of the damaged area, and polymorphonuclear leucocytes, lymphocytes and plasma cells accumulate around the vessels. Reactive hypertrophic astrocytes are seen in the surrounding brain tissue and there is microglial proliferation. Gradually a capsule of granulation tissue forms around the abscess, thickens, and becomes fibrous (Fig. 7.17). It may be 3 weeks or more before a 1 mm thick fibrous capsule develops around an abscess.[53] Once a capsule has developed, the abscess and capsule have a distinct histological organisation (Fig. 7.19). The pus in the centre of the abscess is surrounded by a layer of inflamed granulation tissue with numerous macrophages and varying numbers of polymorphonuclear leucocytes, lymphocytes and plasma cells. Capillaries in the

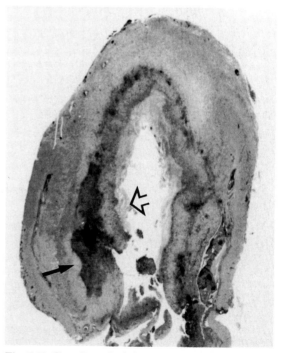

Fig. 7.19 Chronic cerebral abscess—removed surgically. A low-power view to show the various layers. The necrotic contents of the abscess (open arrow) are surrounded by a layer of granulation tissue. The darkly stained region adjacent to this contains large numbers of lymphocytes and plasma cells. The pale-stained fibrous capsule (solid arrow) is surrounded by inflamed, gliotic brain tissue. Haematoxylin-eosin × 4

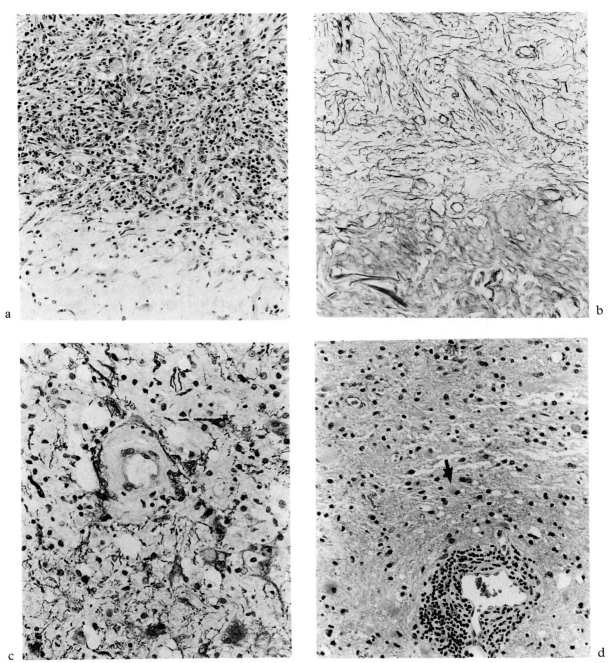

Fig. 7.20a, b, c, d Chronic cerebral abscess. Histology of the wall. (**a**) Junction of granulation tissue (top) and dense fibrous capsule of the abscess (bottom). (**b**) Same field as (a) showing a loose reticulin pattern in the granulation tissue (top) and dense fibrous tissue (bottom). (**c**) Outer wall of the abscess; densely stained astrocytes with a few thick processes are seen in the fibrous capsule (top). Reactive astrocytes with many delicate processes are seen in the gliotic brain tissue (bottom). (**d**) Gliotic brain surrounding an abscess. Reactive astrocytes (arrow). There is lymphocyte cuffing of blood vessels (bottom).
(**a, d**) Haematoxylin-eosin × 150; (**b**) Gordon and Sweet × 150; (**c**) immunoperoxidase for glial fibrillary acidic protein (GFAP) × 150

granulation tissue are often arranged in a radial pattern, whereas plump fibroblasts surrounded by reticulin and collagen fibres form circumferential layers in the inner wall of the abscess. As the capsule matures, a dense layer of fibrous tissue is seen on its outer aspect, often with focal accumulation of lymphocytes and plasma cells within it (Fig. 7.20a and b). Astrocytes may become entrapped within the fibrous capsule of the abscess (Fig. 7.20c) and appear as globular, rounded cells, extension of the fine astrocytic processes being restricted by the fibrous tissue, as in Fig. 7.16b. Outside the capsule, there is reactive astrocytosis and oedema of the brain tissue with perivascular cuffing by lymphocytes and plasma cells (Fig. 7.20d).

Stains for bacteria and fungi may reveal the presence of organisms within the abscess and in the abscess wall, but in cases treated with antibiotics the organisms may no longer be detectable.

Major complications of brain abscesses result from the space-occupying nature of the lesion with its surrounding oedema, and from rupture of the abscess.[32,47] Brain shift, with herniation of the parahippocampal gyrus and midbrain compression and haemorrhage (see p. 67), may result from displacement due to the combined mass of the abscess and the surrounding oedema. Rupture of an abscess may occur, with the release of pus and organisms into a ventricle, causing a fatal ventriculitis. Alternatively, pus may burst from the meningeal aspect of the abscess and cause secondary leptomeningitis. In some cases, abscesses are multilocular and there may be satellite abscesses adjoining them.

Bacteriology

In the pre-antibiotic era, it was estimated that *Staphylococcus aureus* accounted for 25–30% of brain abscesses, *Streptococcus pyogenes* for 30% and *Escherichia coli* for 12%. In 50% of cases, the abscesses were thought to be sterile[54] but at least some of them may have been caused by anaerobic organisms (streptococci and bacteroides). Staphylococci are now decreasing in frequency as a cause, while Enterobacteriaceae are increasing.[44] Anaerobic organisms are found especially when the infection is derived from the mastoid or ear cavities.[55] Recent surveys of the bacteriology of brain abscesses[56] have shown that *Staph. aureus* is a pure culture in 10–15% of abscesses, especially those following trauma. Enterobacteriaceae are isolated in 23–33%, usually in mixed culture of *Proteus* species, *Escherichia coli*, and *Pseudomonas* species. The bacteria usually associated with meningitis (e.g. *Str. pneumoniae* and *H. influenzae*) are responsible for less than 1% of brain abscesses. Micro-aerophilic streptococci, e.g. *Str. milleri*, are found in 60–70% of cases and *Bacteroides* species, including *B. fragilis*, are isolated from 20–40% of brain abscesses, usually mixed with other organisms. Many other bacteria have been cultured from cerebral abscesses.[57]

Fungi, including *Aspergillus* species, *Candida* species, *Cryptococcus neoformans* and *Coccidioides immitis*, and actinomycetes, including *Nocardia* species and *Actinomyces israelii*, have been isolated from 10–15% of brain abscesses in Western populations.

There is regional variation in the organisms causing infective space-occupying lesions in the brain. A survey in Mexico City, for example, revealed that *cysticercosis* accounted for 85% of such lesions, *tuberculomas* for 11% and pyogenic abscesses for only 3%.[43]

SUBDURAL ABSCESS (SUBDURAL EMPYEMA)

Infection of the subdural space occurs mainly over the cerebral hemispheres (Fig. 7.21) and constitutes a neurosurgical emergency.[58] In 50% of cases, organisms spread from paranasal sinuses, usually frontal or ethmoid sinuses,[59] but in 10–20% the middle ear or mastoid cavities are the source of infection. Organisms coming from the lung are seen in 5% of cases.[60] Infection may spread by emissary veins from osteomyelitis in the skull or from an epidural abscess.

Clinical aspects

Subdural empyema develops most commonly in the second and third decades, with males four times more commonly affected than females.[61]

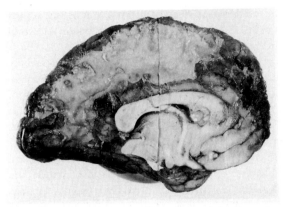

Fig. 7.21 Subdural abscess (empyema) showing a layer of light-coloured pus overlying the brain in the subdural space on the medial aspect of the cerebral hemisphere just above the corpus callosum.

Patients present with fever and focal or generalised headaches, vomiting and meningeal irritation; sinusitis or otitis media is present in 60–90% of cases. Spread of the pus to cover the whole cerebral hemisphere may occur in 24–48 hours. The cerebrospinal fluid may contain polymorpho-nuclear leucocytes but this is not diagnostic of subdural empyema; CT scan may visualise subdural inflammation as a thin enhancing layer on the surface of the brain.[62] The mortality rate is 75% in patients who are comatose and 9% in alert patients. 42% of patients develop focal or general-ised epilepsy following recovery. Treatment is by surgical craniotomy and irrigation of the subdural space, isolation of the organism responsible and antibiotic treatment.

Pathology

Macroscopic inspection of the brain reveals pus distributed as a thin layer between the dura and the arachnoid, covering the convexity of the cerebral hemispheres and extending into the sagittal fissure (Fig. 7.21). The precise distribution depends upon whether the source of infection is the frontal or mastoid sinuses. Subdural infection is rarely seen in the posterior fossa. The main effects upon the brain are due to inflammation and thrombosis of the veins on the surface of the brain, especially those draining into the superior sagittal sinus. Thrombotic occlusion of the veins leads to venous infarction, with flame-shaped haemorrhages orientated superiomedially in the white matter and cortex of the cerebral hemispheres. Severe cerebral oedema may result in the death of the patient.

Bacteriology

Anaerobic streptococci are found in 35% of cases of subdural abscess and staphylococci in 17%. *Streptococcus pneumoniae* or Gram-negative bacteria, including *Haemophilus influenzae*, are present in 14%,[63] and anaerobic and micro-aerophilic streptococci, or *Bacteroides fragilis*, are isolated from 12% of cases. Often, the infection is polymicrobial.[63]

Spinal subdural abscess is uncommon and is usually due to metastatic *Staphylococcus aureus* infection. The abscess is usually posterior to the cord and causes cord compression.[64]

EPIDURAL ABSCESS

Localised collections of pus accumulate as epidural abscesses between the dura and bone in the cranium and in the spine. The sources of the oganisms are similar to those in subdural empyema, and most epidural abscesses are near the frontal sinuses or associated with osteomyelitis of the skull. An associated subdural empyema is present in a high proportion of cases of epidural abscess, and leptomeningitis or brain abscess may also occur.[65]

Intracranial epidural abscess

Clinically, patients with intracranial epidural abscess present with headache, fever, localised neurological signs and cranial nerve palsies. CT scan or skull X-ray may reveal the abscess and cranial osteomyelitis.[66] Treatment is by surgical drainage and antibiotics.

Spinal epidural abscess

Epidural abscesses in the spine may be associated with haematogenous spread of infection, osteo-myelitis of the spine, penetrating injuries or spinal surgery. Sinuses opening on the skin of the back and associated with spina bifida may also be a source of infection.[67] As the spinal dura is separated from the bone by a compartment containing adipose tissue, infection may spread extensively up and down the spine in this compartment. The most frequent site for epidural abscess is the thoracic spine, followed by the lumbar and cervical spine. Most abscesses are posterior to the spinal cord, and the majority are due to *Staph. aureus*[68] although anaerobic streptococci, *Esch. coli* and *Pseudomonas* species may also be a cause. Spread of tuberculous pus from osteomyelitis in the body of a vertebra may cause an epidural abscess anteriorly.

Pathology.   At surgery or post-mortem, pus and granulation tissue may be present over four or five segments of the spine, causing cord compression. Histological examination of tissue taken at laminectomy for drainage of an epidural abscess reveals inflamed granulation tissue and fibrosis. The organisms are identified by bacteriological culture of the pus.

RICKETTSIAL INFECTIONS

Rocky Mountain spotted fever occurs in the USA, Canada, and Central and South America. It is transmitted by ticks from mammalian hosts and can present with a fulminating illness which is fatal in 4–5 days. Most commonly, however, children develop an acute severe febrile illness with myalgia, malaise and a late rash. The disease is caused by *Rickettsia rickettsii*, which may invade in small numbers initially, enter endothelial cells of small capillaries and venules by induced phagocytosis, and multiply within the cells. As the cells burst and release the organisms, there is increased permeability of the blood vessels and vasculitis in the brain and other organs. Ring haemorrhages around the vessels are seen in the brain, together with infarction and oedema. Pulmonary oedema is a major cause of death.[69]

MYCOPLASMA INFECTION

Patients with atypical pneumonia due to *Myco-plasma pneumoniae* may develop neurological syndromes which include meningoencephalitis and transverse myelitis.[70]

MYCOTIC (FUNGAL) INFECTIONS OF THE CENTRAL NERVOUS SYSTEM

Mycotic infections of the central nervous system are much more common in immunosuppressed patients than in immunologically competent individuals. Cell mediated immunity plays a major part in defence against fungal infections, so that patients with lymphomas, on immunosuppressant drugs or suffering from AIDS are particularly prone to opportunistic mycotic infections (see p. 216). Spread of the organisms is usually by blood from a primary site in the lungs or gut, although spread from air sinuses within the skull to the central nervous system also occurs. Fungi may cause subacute or chronic meningitis[4] and are a causative organism in 10–15% of cerebral abscesses in the USA.[43] Characteristically, fungi invade vessel walls causing thrombotic occlusion of the lumen and brain infarction, or haemorrhage due to rupture of the vessel.[71] In most cases, the inflammatory lesion associated with fungal infection is granulomatous, with many macrophages and, in some cases, multinucleate giant cells. There are moderate numbers of lymphocytes in the lesions and surrounding fibrosis. Organisms in the form of hyphae, pseudohyphae or yeasts are usually detectable within the lesions by haematoxylin and eosin staining, by periodic acid Schiff (PAS) and Grocott silver techniques[72,73] or by immunocytochemical techniques.[74] Firm identification of the fungus involved in the lesion is by in vitro culture.

Candidosis

This is the most common fungal infection of the central nervous system[75] and is caused by *Candida* species, which have a wide geographical distribution as part of the human flora. Spread to the brain occurs in immunosuppressed patients treated with broad spectrum antibiotics and in newborn infants who acquire the infection from their mothers. Widespread granulomas may be

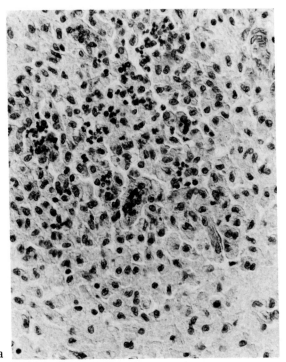
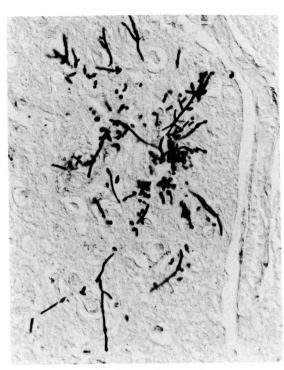

a   b

Fig. 7.22a, b *Candida albicans* infection. (**a**) Candida granuloma in the brain consisting of macrophages and some multinucleate giant cells (centre). (**b**) Pseudohyphae of *Candida albicans*.
(**a**) Haematoxylin-eosin × 300; (**b**) Grocott × 300

seen in the brains of patients dying with candida infection (Fig. 7.22a); there is usually necrosis with macrophages, giant cells and lymphocytes within the granulomas. Pseudohyphae and hyphae (Fig. 7.22b), consisting of chains of elongated cylindrical cells and oval budding cells (blastospores) 3–4 μm diameter,[76] are present in the granulomas and within giant cells. Abscesses may also form.

Aspergillosis

Infection is by one of the few pathological species of *Aspergillus*.[72] The fungi spread by blood to the brain in debilitated or immunosuppressed patients from primary sites in the lung or directly from the ear or paranasal sinuses.[77,78] Colonisation by the fungus of valve prostheses in the heart may also result in spread to the brain.[77] Softened regions of haemorrhagic infarction are found in the brain[79] due to the propensity of *Aspergillus* to infect arterial walls, with resulting necrosis and thrombotic occlusion of the vessel lumen. Histologically,

polymorphonuclear leucocytes are seen in the early lesions, but later granulomatous inflammation is seen with macrophages, multinucleate giant cells and lymphocytes at the site of infection (Fig. 7.23). *Aspergillus* hyphae are septate and branching; they are basophilic in haematoxylin and eosin stained sections[73] and are well demonstrated in Grocott and PAS stains (Fig. 7.23). An area of overlying aspergillus meningitis may be seen adjacent to deeper lesions.

Nocardiosis

The actinomycete *Nocardia asteroides* is found in soil and water and is a cause of cerebral abscess, not only in immunosuppressed individuals but also in apparently normal patients. Although often considered among the fungi, *Nocardia* species are Gram-positive non-motile, non-encapsulated filamentous bacteria which usually range from 7 to 20 μm in length by 0.5 to 1 μm in diameter. Their walls are made of peptidoglycans and not chitin or cellulose as in fungi.[80] The organisms do not stain

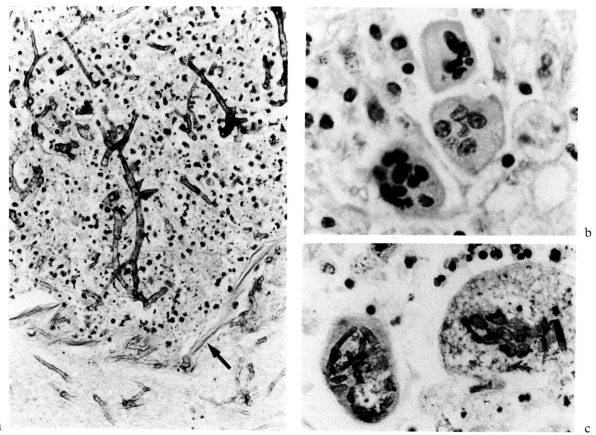

Fig. 7.23a, b, c *Aspergillus* infection. (**a**) Septate hyphae of *Aspergillus fumigatus* in the wall of a cerebral artery. Hyphae (top), internal elastic lamina of the vessel (arrow) at bottom. (**b**) Multinucleate giant cells in *Aspergillus* infection. (**c**) Giant cells containing *Aspergillus* hyphae.
(**a**) PAS × 310; (**b**) haematoxylin-eosin × 600; (**c**) Grocott × 600

consistently with PAS. In vitro testing shows that they are sensitive to some antibacterial antibiotics, but not to antifungal agents.

Spread of nocardiae from the lung can involve any organ. Brain abscesses may arise even though the lung lesion is inconspicuous. Macroscopically, abscesses caused by nocardia resemble pyogenic bacterial abscesses. Pus is present in the centre and there is a firm fibrous capsule with granulation tissue on the inner aspect and fibrous tissue surrounding it.[81] The organisms can be identified histologically in the wall of the abscess as Gram-positive filaments (Fig. 7.24)[73] but can also be stained by a long incubation in Grocott silver solutions. They are often well-stained in Ziehl–Nielsen preparations and they are liable to be mistaken for mycobacteria.

Other actinomycetous infections

Other species of *Nocardia* and, less rarely, *Actinomyces israelii* may cause meningitis and brain abscess.

Cryptococcosis

Cryptococcus neoformans (*Torula histolytica*) is a widely distributed saprophyte in soil, fruit, bird excreta and milk. Most cases of *cryptococcal meningitis* (Fig. 7.25) occur in patients who are immuno-suppressed or on steroids, or who have lymphoma, sarcoidosis[82] or AIDS.[4] Spread of organisms to the central nervous system is usually secondary to lung infection, and the mortality rate is high. The cerebrospinal fluid may contain organisms mixed with polymorphonuclear leucocytes. By adding a

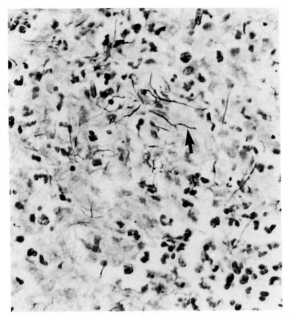

Fig. 7.24 *Nocardia asteroides* seen here as Gram-positive filaments (arrow) in the wall of an abscess. Gram × 600

few drops of India ink or nigrosin to the CSF the organisms are visualised against a dark background as oval yeasts 10 μm in diameter (Fig. 7.25). The yeasts are also PAS-positive. As the organisms are often scarce diagnosis may depend on the demonstration of a high cryptococcal antigen titre in the CSF and serum.

Cryptococcal meningitis is usually most severe at the base of the brain, with the formation of small tubercles but little inflammation in the early stages. Later, cystic lesions with necrosis and infiltration by lymphocytes, plasma cells and eosinophils are seen within the brain and on the surface of the cortex. Cryptococci, 4–7 μm in diameter with a thick mucoid capsule, may be seen within multinucleate giant cells within the lesions (Fig. 7.25).[76] Hydrocephalus may occur as a late complication due to leptomeningeal fibrosis.

Coccidioidomycosis

Coccidioides immitis is found particularly in the semi-arid regions of the south-western states of the USA but also in Mexico and in parts of Central and South America.[83,84] Infection is not usually opportunistic and the fungus generally spreads from the lung to the brain as a terminal event to cause meningitis, which is most severe at the base of the brain. The CSF from affected patients shows elevated coccidioidal complement fixation.[84] Thickening and fibrosis of the meninges may result in hydrocephalus. Histologically, there are granulomas in the meninges with caseous necrosis and giant cells. Occasionally, granulomas are seen in the brain. The fungi are spherical and often within the range of 10–35 μm in diameter; they are commonly seen within giant cells.[73]

Blastomycosis

Blastomycosis may occur as a primary infection or as an opportunistic infection. The organism, *Blastomyces dermatitidis*, is present in the soil and in decaying wood in North America and in parts of Africa.[85]

There may be extradural infection with associated leptomeningitis; such a lesion carries a poor prognosis. Abscesses within the brain result from the spread of the blastomyces from the lungs; they contain caseous material, and a thick capsule may develop in longstanding lesions.

Histologically, polymorphonuclear leucocytes and lymphocytes are seen in the lesion, and the yeasts may be identified in haematoxylin and eosin stained sections as they have a central cell body surrounded by a clear zone adjoining the cell wall. The cell is usually from 5–15 μm in diameter but may be up to 30 μm. The yeast multiplies by the formation of a single bud.[76]

Mucormycosis (zygomycosis)

Zygomycetous fungi are present in soil and manure. Diabetics, drug abusers and immunosuppressed patients are susceptible to infection by this group of fungi.[86] Infection may be centred on one area such as the orbit or paranasal sinuses, stomach, lung or skin, or it may be widespread.[87] Invasion of the meninges and brain probably occurs from the nasal sinuses. Hyphae invade blood vessels causing thrombotic occlusion and infarction in tissues.

Zygomycete hyphae are non-septate, 3–12 μm in width, and characteristically produce right angle branching. Such fungi are found in necrotic,

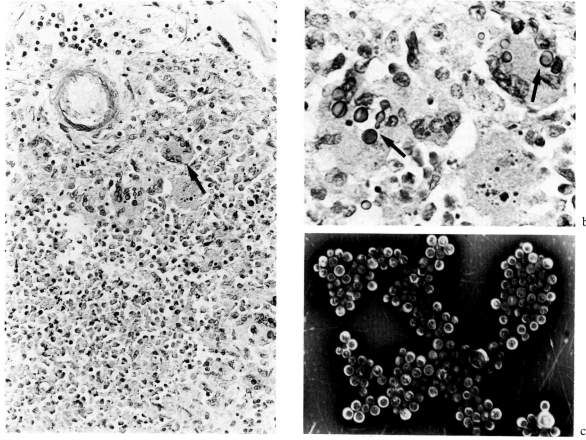

Fig. 7.25 Cryptococcal meningitis in a patient with AIDS. (**a**) Granulomas in the subarachnoid space with multinucleate giant cells (arrow) just below the blood vessel (top). Necrosis and macrophages (bottom left). (**b**) Same giant cells as those indicated in (a) showing circular and budding profiles of intracellular cryptococci (arrows). (**c**) *Cryptococcus neoformans* in the CSF. The unstained capsule of the yeast is shown against the black background.
(**a**) PAS × 240; (**b**) PAS × 600; (**c**) Nigrosin × 600
(**a**) and (**b**) *from material supplied by Dr E. Gessega, Aarau, Switzerland.*

infarcted tissue or in the walls of blood vessels; the hyphae are colourless or, sometimes, brown. They can be stained by immunocytochemical techniques or by the use of cresyl-fast violet which stains zygomycete hyphae red and other mycelial fungi blue or purple.[88]

Other fungi

Rarely, *Histoplasma capsulatum* may invade the central nervous system.[89]

Cladosporium bantianum (*C. trichoides*) may spread from the lungs or paranasal sinuses to infect the CNS;[90] this fungus is recognised by its brown yeast-like forms and hyphae 3–5 μm in diameter with septa marked by indentations at 5–15 μm intervals.

Various other fungi infect the central nervous system less commonly.[76]

ANEURYSMS DUE TO INFECTION OF ARTERIAL WALLS (MYCOTIC ANEURYSMS)

Invasion of the walls of the small arteries by bacteria or fungi causes local weakening, aneurysm formation, rupture of the vessel and haemorrhage. Although, theoretically, the term 'mycotic aneurysm' should be restricted to aneurysms caused by fungal invasion of a vessel wall, it now usually also embraces aneurysms resulting from bacterial infections.

Experimental studies[91] suggest that a small cerebral vessel becomes occluded by an infected embolus and the organisms invade the wall of the artery in the region of the occlusion. With dilatation and weakening of the wall, the aneurysm may then burst.

In man (see p. 111), *Streptococcus* species and *Staphylococcus aureus* are the main bacteria involved in aneurysm formation and *Aspergillus* is the main fungus. Rupture of the aneurysm results in intracranial haemorrhage.

REFERENCES

Introduction

1. Tourtellotte W. J Neurol Sci 1970; 10: 279.
2. Levine DP, Lauter CB, Lerner M. JAMA 1978; 240: 356.
3. Hirsch RL, Griffin DE, Winkelstein JA. J Immunol 1978; 121: 1276.

Bacterial infections

4. Sande MA, Smith AL, Root RK, eds. Bacterial meningitis. New York: Churchill Livingstone, 1985.
5. Leading article. Lancet 1985; 2: 929.
6. Carpenter RR, Petersdorf RG. Am J Med 1962; 33: 262.
7. Poolman JT, Lind I, Jonsdottir K et al. Lancet 1986; 2: 555.
8. Swartz MN, Dodge PR. N Engl J Med 1965; 272: 725.
9. Robbins JB, Schneerson R, Argamon M et al. Ann Intern Med 1973; 78: 259.
10. Mangi RJ, Quintiliani R, Andriole VT. Am J Med 1975; 59: 829.
11. Stevens DS, McGee ZA. J Infect Dis 1981; 143: 525.
12. Robbins JB, McCraken GH Jr, Gotschlich EC et al. N Engl J Med 1974; 290: 1216.
13. Stephens DS, McGee ZA. J Infect Dis 1983; 147: 282.
14. Upton ML, Weller RO. J Neurosurg 1985; 63: 867.
15. Hutchings M, Weller RO. J Neurosurg 1986; 65: 316.
16. Berman PH, Banker BQ. Pediatrics 1966; 38: 6.
17. Rahal JJ, Simberkoff MS. Ann Intern Med 1982; 96: 468.
18. Nicholas DS, Weller RO. J Neurosurg 1988; 69: 276.
19. Sanborn WR, Toure IM. WHO Bull 1984; 62: 293.
20. Bortolussi R. Clin Invest Med 1984; 7: 213.
21. McGee ZA, Kaiser AB. In: Mandell GL, Douglas RG, Bennett JE, eds. Principles and practice of infectious diseases. 2nd ed. New York: Wiley, 1985: 560.
22. Schoenbaum SC, Gardner P, Shillito J. J Infect Dis 1975; 131: 543.
23. Leading article. Lancet 1985; 2: 364.
24. Heck AR. Listeria monocytogenes. In: Vinken PJ, Bruyn GW, eds. Handbook of clinical neurology. Amsterdam: North Holland, 1978; 33: 77.
25. Steere AC, Malawista SE. Lyme disease. In: Mandell GL, Douglas RG, Bennett JE, eds. Principles and practice of infectious diseases. 2nd ed. New York: Wiley, 1985: 1343.
26. Hansen K, Madsen JK. Lancet 1986; 1: 1323.
27. Burgdorfer W, Barbour AG, Hayes SF et al. Science 1982; 216: 1317.
28. Reik L, Smith L, Khan A, Nelson W. Neurology 1985; 113: 135.
29. Meier C, Grehl H. Dtsch med Wochenschr 1988; 113: 135.
30. Kohler J, Kasper J, Kern U et al. Lancet 1986; 2: 35.
31. Walton JN. Brain's Diseases of the nervous system. Oxford: Oxford University Press, 1985.
32. Dastur HM, Desai AD. Brain 1965; 88: 375.
33. Heath PD, Grant JW. Br Med J 1984; 1: 465.
34. Vengsarkar US, Pisipaty RP, Parekh B et al. J Neurosurg 1986; 64: 568.
35. Pentland B, Mitchell JD, Cull RE, Ford MJ. Q J Med 1985; 56: 457.
36. Stern BJ, Krumholz A, Johns C et al. Arch Neurol 1985; 42: 909.
37. Nurick S. Brain 1972; 95: 133.
38. Tramont EC. Treponema pallidum (syphilis). In: Mandell GL, Douglas RG, Bennett JE, eds. Principles and practice of infectious diseases. 2nd ed. New York: Wiley, 1985: 1323.
39. Symon RP. Arch Neurol 1985; 42: 606.
40. Harriman DGF. In: Adams JH, Corsellis JAN, Duchen LW, eds. Greenfield's Neuropathology. 4th ed. London: Arnold, 1984: 236.
41. Beckett JH, Bigbee MA. Arch Pathol Lab Med 1979; 103: 135.
42. Felman YM, Nilcitas MA. Arch Dermatol 1980; 116: 84.
43. Scheld WM, Winn HR. In: Mandell GL, Douglas RG, Bennett JE, eds. Principles and practice of infectious diseases. 2nd ed. New York: Wiley, 1985: 585.
44. Nielsen H. Glydensted C, Harmsen A. Acta Neurol Scand 1982; 65: 609.
45. Lew D, Southwick FS, Montgomery WW. N Engl J Med 1983; 309: 1149.
46. Garvey G. J Neurosurg 1983; 59: 735.
47. Garfield JS. Br Med J 1969; 2: 7.
48. Fischer EG, McLennan JE, Suzuki Y. Am J Dis Child 1981; 135: 746.
49. Morgan H, Wood M, Murphey F. J Neurosurg 1973; 38: 698.
50. Waggener JD. Adv Neurol 1974; 6: 1.
51. Winn HR, Mendes M, Moore P et al. J Neurosurg 1979; 51: 685.
52. Enzmann DR, Britt RH, Yeager AS. Radiology 1979; 133: 113.
53. Britt RH, Enzmann DR, Yeager AS. J Neurosurg 1981; 55: 590.
54. de Louvois J, Gortvai P, Hurley R. Br Med J 1977; 2: 981.
55. Ingham HR, Selkon JB, Roxby CM. Br Med J 1977; 2: 991.
56. de Louvrais J. J Antimicrob Chemother 1983; 11: 205.
57. de Louvrais J. J Clin Pathol 1980; 33: 66.
58. LeBeau J, Creissard P, Harispe L, Redondo A. J Neurosurg 1973; 38: 198.
59. Stephanov S, Joubert MJ, Welchman JM. Surg Neurol 1979; 11: 147.

60. Kaufman DM, Miller MH, Steigbigel NH. Medicine 1975; 54: 485.
61. Kaufman DM, Litman N, Miller MH. Neurology 1983; 33: 123.
62. Weisberg L. Arch Neurol 1986; 43: 497.
63. Yoshikawa TT, Chow AW, Guze LB. Am J Med 1975; 58: 99.
64. Fraser RAR, Ratzan K, Wolpert SM, Weinstein L. Arch Neurol 1973; 28: 235.
65. Handel SF, Klein WC, Kim YW. Radiology 1974; 111: 117.
66. Kaufman DMA, Leeds NE. Neurology 1977; 27: 1069.
67. Baker AS, Ojemann RG, Swartz MN et al. N Engl J Med 1975; 293: 463.
68. Kaufman DM, Kaplan JG, Litman N. Neurology 1980; 30: 844.
69. Walker DH, Hawkins HK, Hudson P. Arch Pathol Lab Med 1983; 107: 121.
70. Clyde WA Jnr. Arch Neurol 1980; 37: 65.

Mycotic infections

71. Duma RJ. In: Sande MA, Smith AL, Root RK, eds. Bacterial meningitis. New York: Churchill Livingstone, 1985: 219.
72. Scaravilli F. In: Adams JH, Corsellis JAN, Duchen LW, eds. Greenfield's Neuropathology. 4th ed. London: Arnold, 1984: 304.
73. Weller RO. Colour atlas of neuropathology. Oxford: Harvey Miller and Oxford University Press, 1984.
74. Saeed EIN, Hay RJ. Histopathology 1981; 5: 437.
75. Parker JC Jr, McCloskey JJ, Lee RS. Hum Pathol 1981; 12: 23.
76. Emmons CW, Binford CH, Utz JP, Kwon-Chung KJ. Medical mycology. 3rd ed. Philadelphia: Lea & Febiger, 1977.
77. Ingwer I, McLeish KR, Tight RR, White AC. Arch Intern Med 1978; 138: 153.
78. Warder FR, Chikes PG, Hudson WR. Acta Otolaryngol 1975; 101: 683.
79. Walsh TJ, Hier DB, Caplan LR. Ann Neurol 1985; 18: 574.
80. Hoeprich PD, Brandt D, Parker RH. Amer J Med Sci 1968; 255: 208.
81. Jacobs SI, Gibson RM. J Neurol Neurosurg Psychiatry 1963; 26: 363.
82. Stocksill MT, Kauffman CA. Arch Neurol 1983; 40: 81.
83. Bouza E, Dreyer JS, Hewitt WL, Meyer RD. Medicine 1981; 60: 139.
84. Caudill RG, Smith CE, Reinarz JA. Am J Med 1970; 49: 360.
85. Chick EW, Sutliff WD, Rakich JH, Furcolow ML. Am J Med Sci 1956; 231: 253.
86. Pierce PF, Solomon SL, Kaufman L. et al. JAMA 1982; 248: 2881.
87. Leading article. Lancet 1986; 1: 1362.
88. Rolph L, Austwick PKC. J Sci Tech 1973; 17: 22.
89. Cooper RA Jr, Goldstein E. Am J Med 1963; 35: 45.
90. Sandhyamani S, Bhatia R, Mohapatra LN, Roy S. Surg Neurol 1981; 15: 431.
91. Molinari GF, Smith L, Goldstein MN, Satran R. Neurology 1973; 23: 325.

Protozoal infections and metazoal infestations

INTRODUCTION

A large volume of data concerning parasitic infection and infestation of the human nervous system is readily available to specialists in tropical medicine and related fields. Such material is much less familiar to pathologists practising in temperate regions of the world. However, in an era of rapid transport, it is clear that virtually any parasitic disease of tropical or subtropical zones may be seen in almost any country. Outline knowledge of a wide range of such diseases should therefore be regarded as essential, and is presented here. Further impetus to the study of protozoal infections of the nervous system comes from their occurrence in immunocompromised patients, including those with the acquired immune deficiency syndrome (AIDS).

PROTOZOAL INFECTIONS

MALARIA

Cerebral malaria is a lethal complication of infection with *Plasmodium falciparum*, the organism that causes malignant tertian malaria.[1] Cases are by no means restricted to the malarial parts of the world, and the incubation period of one to three weeks (or longer) allows clinical manifestations to appear for the first time after the return of exposed individuals to non-endemic countries. The lesions in the brain are essentially ischaemic, and are due to the blockage of capillaries by masses of parasite-containing red blood cells and pigment derived from their

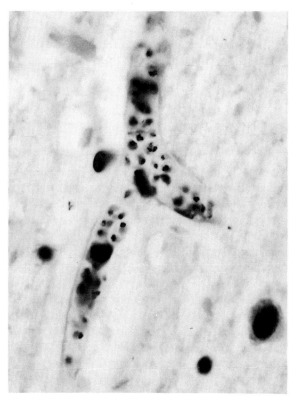

Fig. 8.1 Cerebral malaria. The lumen of this capillary blood vessel in a tertiary lamina of the white matter of the cerebellum is filled with parasitized red cells (*Plasmodium falciparum* infection). The presence in the cytoplasm of the plasmodial trophozoites of the malarial pigment, haemazoin, a breakdown product of haemoglobin, accentuates their appearance in stained preparations. The patient was a business man whose flight from southern Africa to Europe made an unscheduled overnight stop in a malarial region. Although warned of the danger of not taking a prophylactic course of an antimalarial drug, he refused the protection offered. When the symptoms of his illness began he suspected that they were due to malaria and went to a general hospital. He was referred, without investigation or treatment, to a fever hospital, where he had a convulsion while waiting to be seen by a doctor. The latter sent him on the 20 km drive by ambulance back to the general hospital for treatment as a case of cerebral malaria. The patient died half an hour after admission while the doctors were still considering how to treat his infection. *The patient with cerebral malaria will die unless appropriate treatment is given without delay*, and without waiting for the result of laboratory investigations.
Haematoxylin-eosin × 950
Provided by W. St C. Symmers.

breakdown.[2] At autopsy, the brain is swollen and the cortex of the cerebrum and cerebellum is very congested. On dissection, the cut surface of the brain has a dull grey appearance, and the lepto-meninges are clouded. Petechial haemorrhages may be seen, especially at the junction of grey and white matter.

Microscopically, perivascular and diffuse oedema is present. Necrosis of vein walls may be found. Malarial parasites are seen in red blood cells (Fig. 8.1); many are schizonts and other mature forms. Granules of malarial pigment are also seen. In larger vessels, affected red blood cells marginate along the vascular endothelium. By electron microscopy, villous endothelial projections closely related to the surface of parasitised red blood cells have been reported,[3] as have electron-dense knobs protruding from the surface of erythrocytes to form focal junctions with endothelium. Occlusion of small vessels by red cells and fibrin is the cause of haemorrhage and multiple foci of parenchymal necrosis. *P. falciparum* antigens and IgG are reported to be present on capillary basement membrane, implicating immune mechanisms in vascular damage and blockage.[4] Lesions of nerve cells, myelin and perivascular astrocyte end-feet are seen. More chronic lesions arc associated with a degree of proliferation and aggregation of astrocytes, together with pigment-laden macrophages—the so-called malarial nodules (granulomas) of Dürck. Acute perivascular inflammatory changes are not seen. Evidence of hypoxic damage is present in cerebellar Purkinje cells, which show ischaemic change (see p. 90).

INFECTIONS CAUSED BY AMOEBAE

Primary amoebic meningoencephalitis[5]

This term has been applied to infections of the brain by species of free-living amoebae of the genera *Naegleria* and *Acanthamoeba*. These organisms live in the soil, multiply in warm water, and are resistant to standard means of water purification by chlorine. Under adverse circumstances, amoebic trophozoites form resistant cysts.

Infection by Naegleria

Numerous cases of meningoencephalitis caused by *Naegleria fowleri* have been recognised since the disease was first described in 1965.[6,7] Those affected are generally previously healthy children or young adults with a history of swimming or playing in brackish or stagnant fresh water. The incubation period lasts from a few days to two weeks. The disease is almost always rapidly fatal.

At autopsy, the brain is swollen and congested, and the appearances may resemble those of acute suppurative meningitis macroscopically. The olfactory bulbs and adjacent frontal cortical tissue are particularly severely affected, with extensive necrosis and haemorrhage as a conspicuous feature. This reflects the pathway of infection, for

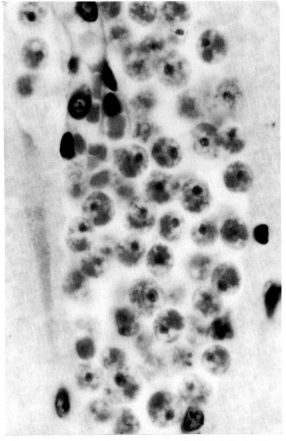

Fig. 8.2 Primary amoebic meningoencephalitis (infection by *Naegleria* species). The amoebae are massed in the circumvascular space and have invaded the adjoining substance of the cerebral cortex. The characteristic appearance of the nucleus, with relatively large nucleolus, fine nuclear membrane and surrounding halo of vacuolate cytoplasm, is seen in several of the parasites. There is an occasional leucocyte in the field but otherwise no evident reaction. From an unpublished case in the south-east of England (1975).
Haematoxylin-eosin × 1100
Provided by W. St C. Symmers.

experimental studies suggest that the organisms enter the body through the nasal mucosa, cross the cribriform plate, and ascend the fibres of the olfactory nerves to invade the brain from the olfactory bulbs.[8] The amoebic form of *Naegleria* (this organism exists also in a flagellate form which is capable of wide dispersal in water) is not as large as *Entamoeba histolytica*; its dimensions range from 7 to 20 μm in hanging-drop preparations and from 5 to 12 μm in histological sections of fixed tissues. In the infected brain the organisms are most numerous in perivascular spaces (Fig. 8.2) where, despite their large, pale, nucleolated nuclei, they may be mistaken for macrophages. Often there is little or no cellular reaction to their presence, particularly when they have invaded the cerebral parenchyma; a lack of inflammatory response to their presence often indicates continued proliferation of the organisms and further invasion of the tissues after the death of a patient. Lymphocytes are sometimes present among the amoebae in the perivascular spaces, but are outnumbered by the organisms. Polymorphs are generally scanty. The rapid development of the disease and the extent of tissue destruction are related to a poor prognosis. Nearly all the patients die within seven days; a few survive with systemic and intrathecal amphotericin,[9] although with serious disabilities from the destruction of brain tissue.

Infection by Acanthamoeba

The clinical features of infection of the brain by *Acanthamoeba culbertsoni* are rather different from those of naegleria meningoencephalitis. The acanthamoebae were formerly regarded as species of the common free-living *Hartmanella* genus; they now have independent generic status. Acanthamoebae are significantly larger than naegleria: in hanging drops they range from 10 to 45 μm in diameter (average 30 μm); in sections of fixed tissues they appear smaller (average 20 to 25 μm), but their indistinct outline obscures their true size. Acanthamoeba infection generally occurs opportunistically in immune-deficient or chronically ill patients, of any age, and is not related to recreational exposure to stagnant water.[10] The organisms may enter the body through ulcerated surfaces and possibly through the lungs. In some cases the interval between exposure of a broken skin surface to the risk of infection and the eventual development of clinical disease has been as much as a year. Though also fatal, the evolution of this brain infection is slower than that of naegleria infection; the clinical course may be as long as four months.

At autopsy, diffuse meningitis and foci of brain tissue necrosis are seen. Microscopically, chronic inflammatory changes with vasculitis are observed in affected areas of brain; the amoebae can be found both in vessel walls and in areas showing no evidence of inflammation. As in cases of naegleria infection, lack of inflammatory reaction is in part explained by post-mortem extension of the infecting organisms into the tissues.

Infection by *Entamoeba* histolytica

Secondary cerebral involvement by *Entamoeba histolytica* may occur in patients with amoebic abscesses of lung and liver, and is almost always fatal.

AFRICAN TRYPANOSOMIASIS[11,12]

The parasites *Trypanosoma rhodesiense* and *T. gambiense* infect a variety of wild and domestic animals as well as man, transmission occurring by the bite of a tsetse fly. Parasitic invasion of the bloodstream develops several days after the bite and causes fever and systemic symptoms. There are major differences between diseases caused by these two species of trypanosome.

T. rhodesiense has a natural reservoir in game (especially the bushbuck) and is spread to man by the bite of the savanna fly, *Glossina morsitans*.[13] An acute or subacute meningoencephalitis develops; this may be fatal within a period of weeks, though patients may die at a relatively early stage if there is severe cardiac involvement. Organisms are readily found in the CSF (Fig. 8.3), where they appear as thin flagellates, 10 to 30 μm long. Trypanosomiasis caused by *T. gambiense* is primarily a human disease, being spread from man to man by the riverine tsetse flies, *Glossina palpalis* and *G. tachinoides*.[13] It is believed that occasionally

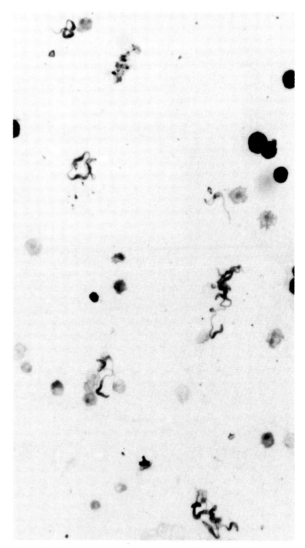

Fig. 8.3 *Trypanosoma rhodesiense* in cerebrospinal fluid. Giemsa × 450

domestic animals may act as a reservoir of the disease. *T. gambiense* produces a more chronic and progressive neurological disease (West African sleeping sickness) with somnolence and restlessness, fits, abnormal movements and paralysis.

In cases of both types of African trypanosomiasis, autopsy shows features of a chronic meningoencephalitis with involvement of the brainstem and spinal cord also. There is a diffuse thickening of the leptomeninges, and many lymphocytes and plasma cells are found both in the pia-arachnoid and around the blood vessels of the cortex and white matter. Typical though by no means pathognomonic of this disease are *morular bodies*, which have a diameter between twice and three times that of an erythrocyte: they are thought to be derived from plasma cells. They are most characteristic of infection by *T. gambiense*, and are present in the leptomeninges and in the perivascular spaces. There may be degenerative changes in the neurons, and microglial rod cells may be plentiful. The microglia should not be mistaken for trypanosomes, which are difficult, if not impossible, to demonstrate in tissues. Iron pigment is also found in the tissues.

AMERICAN TRYPANOSOMIASIS[14]

American trypanosomiasis (Chagas' disease) is caused by *Trypanosoma cruzi*. This disease is important in tropical parts of South America, particularly Brazil; it is also seen, though less frequently, in Central America and Mexico and very rarely in the USA (Texas). It is spread by triatomine bugs of the family Reduviidae.[15] Three of the important species in South America, going from north to south in the worst affected areas, are *Rhodnius prolixus*, *Panstrongylus megistus* and *Triatoma infestans*.[15] These bugs, which infest the poor housing of rural communities, convey the infection to man from mammalian reservoirs, including rats, dogs, bats and armadillos.

There are acute and chronic forms of the disease. Fever, facial swelling, hepatomegaly, splenomegaly and lymphadenopathy characterise the acute form of the disease, which occurs almost exclusively in children; sometimes encephalitis develops. The chronic form of the disease affects older children and adults and is comparatively seldom complicated by encephalitis; in contrast, it causes severe damage to the conduction system and to the muscle fibres of the heart and to the muscle and nerve plexuses of the alimentary tract, resulting in cardiac dysfunction and dilatation of oesophagus, stomach or colon. The abnormalities produced in these organs by *T. cruzi* are described in other volumes of this series. Involvement of the central nervous system produces congestion of the leptomeninges and, sometimes, small parenchymal haemorrhages in the brain. Inflammatory

infiltration of the meninges is evident microscopically. There is nodular proliferation of microglia in relation to small blood vessels. Parasites, when demonstrable, are in the cytoplasm of astrocytes; they are less often seen in microglia or capillary endothelial cells.

TOXOPLASMOSIS

In 1937, Wolf and Cowen[16] isolated *Toxoplasma gondii* from a fatal case of encephalitis in a child. Their observation initiated medical interest in the rôle of toxoplasma as a cause of cerebral disease; after 50 years this interest has developed considerably because of current concern about the acquired immune deficiency syndrome (AIDS) (see p. 214).

Toxoplasmosis is worldwide in distribution. The rate of infection rises through adult life.[17] When pregnant women are infected, parasitaemia may lead to placental involvement with consequent transmission of infection to the fetus. If infection occurs early in pregnancy, abortion may result. Infection later in pregnancy may produce a variety of severe fetal abnormalities, including hydrocephalus, microcephaly and chorioretinitis. Lesions in the cerebral hemispheres are concentrated around the ventricles, where there are foci of necrosis with chronic inflammation and eventually focal calcification. The organisms may be seen both in the form of tachyzoites (trophozoites), which are free in the tissues, and as cysts (Fig. 8.4). The tachyzoites are crescentic, 4 to 8 μm long by 2 to 3 μm wide. The cysts are rounded, up to 200 μm in their longest dimension, and filled with rounded or ovoid bradyzoites (merozoites) which range from 2 to 4 μm in diameter. Where infection occurs in peri-aqueductal tissue, chronic inflammation is associated with tissue changes which may produce obstruction of CSF flow, with resultant hydrocephalus.

Systemic toxoplasma infection may occur as a result of eating undercooked meat or from exposure to encysted organisms in faecally contaminated material. Infection may be manifested clinically as a mild systemic disturbance with macular rash, malaise, myalgia and lymphadenopathy. It seems certain that many

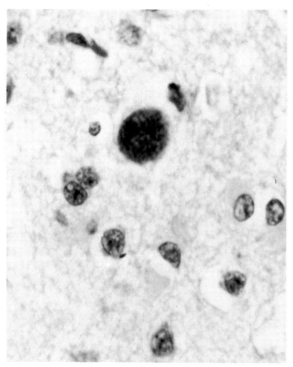

Fig. 8.4 Toxoplasmosis. Cysts are seen in this section of the brain of a stillborn microcephalic baby. See Fig. 12.23, p. 339. Haematoxylin-eosin × 700

infections are subclinical. By the fourth decade of life, about half of all individuals in large cities appear to have been infected.[18] The development of host resistance does not necessarily destroy the parasites, which can encyst and remain dormant for years in a variety of tissues, including the brain. It is the reactivation of previous infection in immunocompromised patients that may be the mechanism underlying fulminant cerebral toxoplasmosis in patients with AIDS.

Toxoplasmic encephalitis associated with AIDS

At least 10% of patients with AIDS develop cerebral lesions of toxoplasmosis, which thus has about half the frequency of cytomegalovirus infection of the brain (see p. 214) and of the subacute encephalitis with multinucleated cells attributed to HIV infection itself (see p. 215).[19] The brain lesions of toxoplasmosis are abscess-like and measure from a few millimetres to several centimetres in diameter.[20,21] They have been divided into three histological types according to

the degree of organisation. *Necrotising abscesses* are poorly defined zones of coagulative or haemorrhagic necrosis infiltrated or surrounded by variable numbers of acute and chronic inflammatory cells and lipid-laden macrophages. Both free and encysted organisms can be found at the periphery of these lesions. *Organising abscesses* are well-defined areas of necrosis surrounded by a dense rim of lipid-laden macrophages. Organisms are infrequently found in these lesions. *Chronic abscesses* are well-demarcated cystic spaces containing variable numbers of lipid-laden macrophages. Rarely the cysts of toxoplasmosis can be found. Abscesses are most numerous in cerebral and cerebellar cortex, and may be connected to the subarachnoid space. Organisms are often more readily detectable by immunohistochemical means than by standard stains.

The clinical presentation of toxoplasmosis in immunosuppressed patients is with headache, fever and coma, and the subacute onset of focal neurological signs. Computerised tomography (CT) scans show the appearances of abscesses with ring-shaped contrast enhancement related to vascular proliferation and inflammation at the periphery of the lesion. Prompt therapy with pyrimethamine, sulphadiazine and clindamycin will produce clinical improvement with evidence of healing on CT scan.

INFECTIONS BY OTHER PROTOZOA

Rare cases of human infection by *Babesia* species have been recorded, mainly in Eastern Europe but also in parts of North America and in Ireland. The infection is carried by ticks from cattle or rodents to man. A systemic illness resembling malaria may occur. In otherwise normal patients the febrile haemolytic illness resolves without specific treatment, but in splenectomised individuals an overwhelming intra-erythrocytic infection may develop and may be fatal.[22] Parasites in red blood cells may be found in all parts of the body, including the brain, and patients may have neurological symptoms. Polyneuritis has been reported following treatment of human *Babesia* infection with diminazene.[23]

METAZOAL INFESTATIONS

CYSTICERCOSIS[24,25]

Man is the only definitive host of the cestodes *Taenia solium* and *Taenia saginata*. Ripe proglottids are shed in human faeces and the released ova are consumed by an intermediate host. The pig (occasionally sheep, bears, cats, dogs and monkeys) has this role in the *T. solium* cycle, whereas various cattle are involved in the life cycle of *T. saginata*.

The embryos, freed in the gut of the intermediate host, burrow through the intestinal mucosa and gain access to the bloodstream, in which some are carried eventually to skeletal and cardiac muscle, the nervous system, eyes, lungs, liver and subcutaneous tissue, where, within two

to three months, they develop into their infective stage, the bladder worms or cysticerci. The larval forms of *T. solium* and *T. saginata* are known respectively as *Cysticercus cellulosae* and *C. bovis*. These forms were recognised and named before their relationship to their parent worms was recognised. The pseudo-generic names have no taxonomic significance. When parasitised undercooked pork or beef is eaten by man, the scolex (head) of the cysticercus evaginates like the finger of a glove and becomes attached by its suckers and hooklets to the gut wall. The adult tapeworm then develops in the human host within 5 to 12 weeks. Cysticercosis develops in man only when ova of *T. solium* or *T. saginata* are swallowed. Usually this results from faecal contamination of food or drink. The source of this contamination may be the patient himself, when host to an adult taenia.

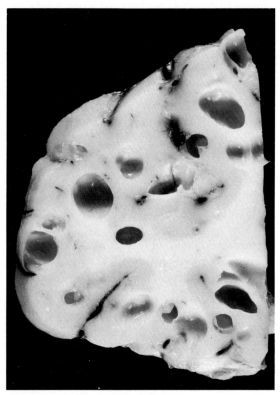

a

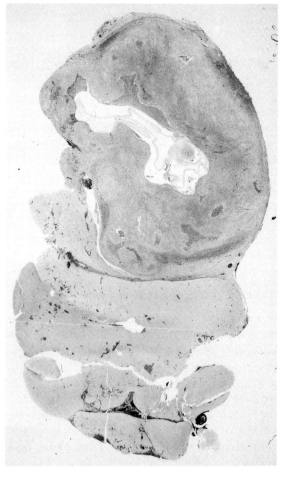

b

Fig. 8.5a, b Cerebral cysticercosis. (**a**) Gross appearance, with mainly subcortical lesions. (**b**) Sections to show granulomatous rim encasing parasite (top). Brain tissue (bottom).
(**b**) Haematoxylin-eosin × 6

Rarely, auto-infestation results from failure to follow anthelmintic treatment with an adequate purge to clear the bowel of ova released by the partial digestion of the adult worm that is effected by some modern anthelmintics. Cysticercosis in man is almost always the result of ingesting ova of *T. solium*; ingestion of the ova of *T. saginata* hardly ever produces cysticercosis.

Infestation by *Taenia solium* has virtually disappeared from Europe and many other areas. In the Middle East, Muslim Africa and Indonesia it was always very rare or non-existent because of religious practices which forbid the consumption of pork. Human cysticercosis continues to occur in many parts of India, Mongolia, Korea, China, Central and South America and South Africa. It is uncommon in the USA.

Involvement of the central nervous system by cysticerci may be asymptomatic or may produce focal neurological deficits or seizures. Cysticerci most commonly involve the cerebral hemispheres, where they are often situated subcortically in the situation classically associated with the development of metastatic tumours. They may also expand within the ventricular system, causing hydrocephalus.[26] Spinal cord compression may occur[27,28] due to cysticerci within the spinal canal.

The early cysticercal lesion contains an apparently intact parasite, identifiable by the presence of suckers and hooklets on the rostellum of the scolex (Fig. 8.5), evaginating the wall of its cyst. Surrounding this is a sharply demarcated granulomatous zone containing fibrous tissue, an often dense lymphocytic and plasma cell infiltrate, many histiocytes and foci of polymorphs and eosinophils. Giant cells may be present but are inconspicuous in the early cellular lesion.

HYDATID DISEASE[29]

Two dog tapeworms (*Echinococcus granulosus* and *Echinococcus multilocularis*) may cause hydatid disease in man.

Ova of *E. granulosus*, discharged in canine faeces, are ingested by the intermediate host (usually sheep but occasionally goats, cattle, pigs, wild herbivores or man). After hatching, the embryos penetrate the venules of the intestinal wall and become established in the liver. If they can get beyond the hepatic circulation, they lodge in the lungs. A small proportion may reach other tissues, including muscle and the brain; cerebral hydatids occur in only a small percentage of all cases of hydatidosis. The natural cycle is completed when dogs eat infested offal.

In echinococcosis due to *E. multilocularis*, the natural reservoir is the fox; dogs and cats may also harbour the parent tapeworm. The usual intermediate hosts are wild rodents. Man may become the intermediate host through swallowing ova in uncooked food contaminated by the excreta of dogs or foxes.

Hydatid cysts due to *E. granulosus* are unilocular and show a featureless eosinophilic capsule and an inner germinal epithelium; they may contain many daughter cysts. In contrast, the larval stage of *E. multilocularis* consists of a honeycomb-like aggregate of innumerable small cysts with no proper limiting capsule. This lesion may have a necrotic centre, resembling an abscess. It behaves locally like an invasive tumour; rarely, metastatic cysts may develop elsewhere in the body as a result of dissemination through the bloodstream.

In sheep-rearing countries, where hydatidosis in man is most frequent, skeletal muscle is involved in over 5% of human cases. Muscle is in fact the third most frequent site (after liver and lung) of the cysts.

Hydatid disease of the brain[30,31] may cause local pressure effects (including hydrocephalus). The cysts may rupture, seeding the infestation locally and causing a local inflammatory response resembling that seen with cerebral cysticercosis. Where skull bones are the site of infestation a meningeal reaction and local cerebral damage may occur.

SCHISTOSOMIASIS[32]

The ova of three blood flukes may be carried in the bloodstream to the meninges, brain and spinal cord, where they excite a granulomatous reaction. The cells of the granuloma include lymphocytes, plasma cells and multinucleate giant cells; eosinophils may be plentiful at first. In the earlier stages of infestation, necrosis may occur in the

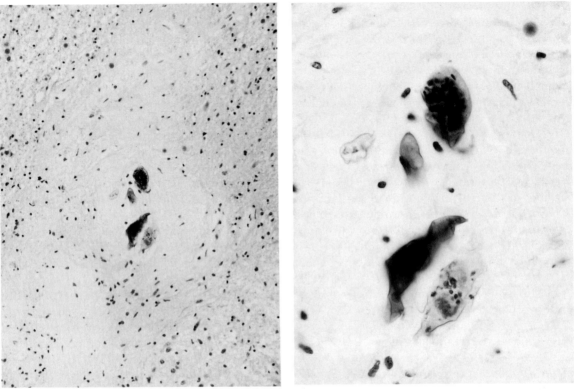

a

b

Fig. 8.6 Schistosomiasis of the spinal cord. Cluster of distorted ova of *Schistosoma haematobium* in glial scar in vicinity of a posterior grey column in the lumbar region of the spinal cord. The patient had long suffered from a condition mimicking tabes dorsalis, without history or serological evidence of syphilis. He eventually developed paraplegia and died of acute bacterial infection of the urinary tract. Although he had last visited a country where schistosomiasis is endemic 25 years before his death, living adult schistosomes were found in the vertebral venous plexuses at necropsy.
Haematoxylin-eosin (**a**) × 130; (**b**) × 400
Provided by W. St C. Symmers.

tissue round the ova; later, fibrosis (Fig. 8.6) and calcification develop. *Schistosoma japonicum* has been found in the central nervous system more often than *S. mansoni* and *S. haematobium*. This may be because *S. japonicum* has the smallest eggs and an inconspicuous terminal spine, which could favour venous spread. Although the lesions are frequently distributed widely through the brain, as is consistent with blood-borne dissemination of the ova from a distant source in the body, they are sometimes very localised: it has been suggested that in such cases the female fluke may produce eggs while lying in a cerebral vein or venous sinus.[33]

Neurological signs may develop from months to years after initial exposure to schistosomes. The brain is involved three times as often as the spinal cord.[34] A non-specific chronic inflammatory response with giant cells is seen in the nervous tissue around the parasites.

PARAGONIMIASIS[35]

The lung flukes *Paragonimus westermani* and *P. skryabini* are endemic in the Far East; the latter is found only in China. Adult worms mainly parasitise the lungs, but can invade other organs, of which the brain is the most frequently involved. The first case of cerebral paragonimiasis was reported as long ago as 1887. Infection occurs as a result of eating uncooked crustacea, the second intermediate hosts (snails are the first). Encysted larval metacercariae are released in the human gastrointestinal tract, pass through viscera to reach the lungs, and develop there over six weeks into adult worms in an abscess cavity. Ova in sputum (or faeces) become free-swimming miracidia, and will eventually develop into sporocysts in suitable snails. Occasionally, this cycle is disrupted due to the migration of metacercariae to brain rather than lung. Any part of the brain may be affected, though involvement of the spinal cord, brainstem and cerebellum is rare. A granulomatous mass develops, which is generally superficial and accompanied by meningeal adhesion. Eggs are found in necrotic granulomatous tissue, around which collagenous connective tissue, reactive astrocytosis and iron-laden macrophages are seen. Longstanding lesions undergo calcification. Intact mature worms are rarely seen, even in apparently recent lesions.

and slugs, and in South East Asia these may be eaten uncooked by man. Parasitisation of the nervous system occurs via the bloodstream and produces a severe meningitis with encephalopathic manifestations. Lumbar puncture reveals a large increase in the number of cells in the CSF; almost all the cells are eosinophils. Rarely, adult worms may be found in the CSF (Fig. 8.7). Histopathological features are those of chronic inflammation of the meninges with necrosis and thrombosis of blood vessels. Granulomas are found around dead larvae.

In contrast to cerebral gnathostomiasis (see below), angiostrongylus infestation follows a benign and self-limiting course, with a mortality rate of less than 1%.

EOSINOPHILIC MENINGITIS DUE TO *ANGIOSTRONGYLUS*[36]

The nematode *Angiostrongylus cantonensis*, a parasite of the rat lung, may involve human brain, meninges and eyes. Larvae of the worm are harboured by several species of terrestrial snails

GNATHOSTOMIASIS[37]

Another nematode capable of causing eosinophilic meningitis in man is *Gnathostoma spinigerum*, which is found in South East Asia, especially in Thailand. The adult worm is harboured by cats and dogs. Excreted ova begin their development in small crustacea and continue to grow in freshwater fish and other aquatic vertebrates. Human infestation occurs when raw or undercooked fish is eaten. Involvement of brain and spinal cord by sexually immature adult gnathostomes produces meningeal and focal neurological signs. The spinal cord manifestations, which include paraplegia, are commoner than cerebral disease. Eosinophils can be found in the CSF. Parenchymal foci of haemorrhage and necrosis occur, with a macrophage and eosinophil tissue response but no granulomas. Migration of worms through the nervous system may be seen: in one patient who died of respiratory failure, a living gnathostome was seen moving near the medulla, and multiple haemorrhagic tracks were found in cord and brainstem (Fig. 8.8).[37]

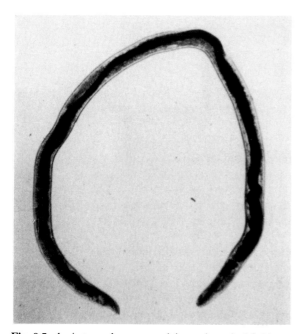

Fig. 8.7 *Angiostrongylus cantonensis* in cerebrospinal fluid. × 80
Reproduced by permission of Prof. A. Vejjajiva, Bangkok.

TOXOCARIASIS[38]

Toxocara cati and *T. canis* are nematodes, 4 to 12 cm long, which are normally resident in the

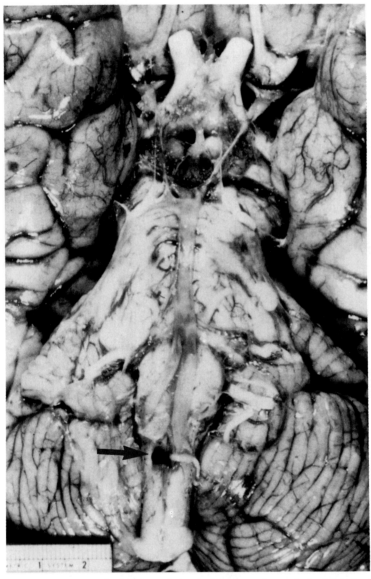

a

Fig. 8.8a, b Gnathostomiasis. (**a**) A parasite is visible as a dark coiled lesion on the cervical cord to the right of the midline at the level of the foramen magnum (arrow). (**b**) On section, multiple haemorrhagic tracks are seen in the brainstem and spinal cord (see opposite page).
Reproduced by permission of Prof. A. Vejjajiva, Bangkok.

intestine of cats and dogs. Excreted ova may be ingested by other animals. Larvae hatch in stomach and intestines and penetrate the intestinal wall to reach the portal vein and lymphatics, then migrating to liver, lungs and other organs. Re-entry into the alimentary tract completes the life cycle of toxocara in its normal hosts. In man, completion of the life cycle cannot occur and adult worms do not exist in the intestines, but larvae can migrate and lodge in a variety of organs, including brain and eyes as well as liver and lungs. Puppies and young children are infected disproportionately often. Intra-ocular granulomas can be mistaken clinically for retinoblastoma.[39] Clinical neurological disorders are minor, but fits and meningism sometimes occur. Toxocaral brain lesions are granulomatous and may include larval remnants (Fig. 8.9).

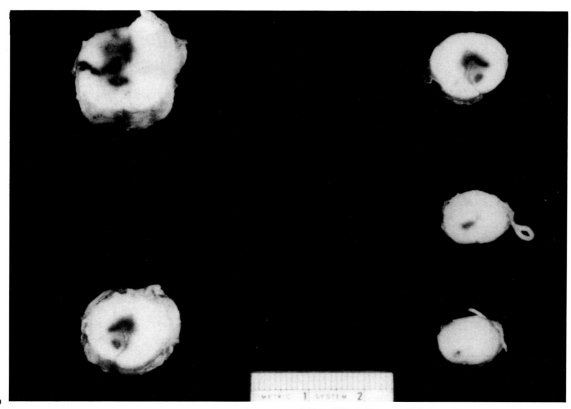

b

FILARIASIS

Several species of filariae are capable of invading the brain and meninges. *Loa loa* is widespread in equatorial West Africa, and is the most frequent cause of cerebral filariasis. After introduction through the skin as a result of insect bites, the parasites enter the circulation and may reach cerebral vessels. Occlusion of brain capillaries by the organisms produces petechiae and oedema. Histologically, perivascular granulomatous nodules can be found throughout the brain, often with a central necrotic region and sometimes containing identifiable microfilariae. These lesions

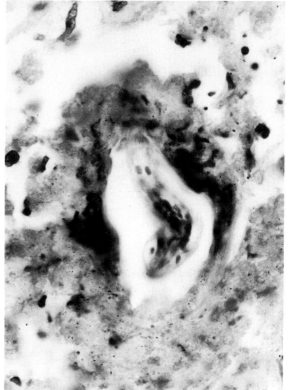

Fig. 8.9 Larva of *Toxocara* species in a necrotic focus in the brain of a boy, aged four years, the only child of parents who had brought him up in constant close association with large numbers of ill-cared-for dogs and cats. The child died of an obscure encephalitis-like illness accompanied by blindness. Larvae, identified as those of toxocara, were found in the retina of each eye and in multiple minute foci of necrosis in the brain.
Haematoxylin-eosin × 750
Provided by W. St C. Symmers.

are accompanied by cerebral cortical astrocytosis and microglial infiltration.[40] Clinically, *Loa loa* parasitisation of the nervous system causes meningitic and encephalitic symptoms. Focal cerebrovascular lesions may be recognised clinically. Microfilariae may be present in the lumbar CSF.

INFESTATIONS BY OTHER METAZOA

Sparganosis

Cerebral involvement is sometimes seen in *sparganosis*, which is due to extra-intestinal infection by the plerocercoid larvae (spargana) of diphyllobothriid tapeworms of the genus *Spirometra*. Man is not a normal host, but can be infected in a variety of ways, including the accidental ingestion of crustacean intermediate hosts, eating pork, fish or other infected flesh, or from the use of raw frog flesh (infected by plerocercoids) as poultices. Most sparganotic lesions are cystic soft tissue masses containing a worm surrounded by a granulomatous rim. Occasional brain lesions, causing raised intracranial pressure, focal neurological features and haemorrhage, have been described[41].

Miscellaneous infestations

Hyperinfestation with *Strongyloides stercoralis* may be associated with meningitis, cerebral microinfarcts and brain abscesses.[42]

A single case of fatal meningoencephalitis due to the free-living nematode *Micronema deletrix* has been reported. The patient was a 5-year-old boy who had been severely injured by a manure-spreading machine.[43]

MUSCLE INVOLVEMENT BY PARASITES[44]

Clinically important involvement of skeletal muscle in man (see p. 631) is seen in some protozoal infections, including sarcocystis infection, toxoplasmosis, and African and American trypanosomiasis. It also occurs in cestode infestations (cysticercosis, coenurosis, hydatidosis, and sparganosis) and in cases of infestation by certain nematodes (trichinosis and toxocariasis).

REFERENCES

Protozoal infections

1. Bruce-Chwatt LJ. Essential malariology. 2nd ed. London: Heinemann, 1975.
2. Toro G, Román G. Arch Neurol 1978; 35: 271.
3. MacPherson GG, Warrell MJ, White NJ, Looareesuwan S, Warrell DA. Am J Pathol 1985; 119: 385.
4. Maung Maung Oo, Aikawa M, Than Than et al. J. Neuropath Exp Neurol 1987; 46: 223.
5. Duma RJ. In: Vinken PL, Bruyn GW, eds. Handbook of clinical neurology, vol. 35. Infections of the nervous system, part III. Amsterdam: North Holland, 1978: 25.
6. Fowler M, Carter RF. Br Med J 1965; 2: 740.
7. Carter RF. Trans R Soc Trop Med Hyg 1972; 66: 193.
8. Martinez AJ, Duma RJ, Nelson EC, Moretta FL. Lab Invest 1973; 29: 121.
9. Seidel JS, Harmatz P, Visvesvara GS, Cohen A, Edwards J, Turner J. N Engl J Med 1982; 306: 346.
10. Martinez AJ. J Neuropath Exp Neurol 1982; 41: 548.
11. Dumas M, Girard PL. In: Vinken PL, Bruyn GW, eds. Handbook of clinical neurology, vol 35. Infections of the nervous system, part III. Amsterdam: North Holland, 1978: 67.
12. Poltera AA. Br Med Bull 1985; 41: 169.
13. Potts WH. In: Smith KGV, ed. Insects and other arthropods of medical importance. London: British Museum (Natural History), 1973: 209.
14. Spina-França A, Mattosinho-França LC. In: Vinken PL, Bruyn GW, eds. Handbook of clinical neurology, vol 35. Infections of the nervous system, part III. Amsterdam: North Holland, 1978: 85.
15. Ghauri MSK. In: Smith KGV, ed. Insects and other arthropods of medical importance. London: British Museum (Natural History), 1973: 373.
16. Wolf A, Cowen D. Bull Neurol Inst N Y 1937; 6: 306.
17. Fleck DG. Proc R Soc Med 1975; 68: 368.
18. Remington JS, Desmonts G. In: Remington JS, Klein JO, eds. Infectious diseases of the fetus and newborn infant. 2nd ed. Philadelphia: Saunders, 1983: 144.
19. Navia BA, Petito CK, Gold JMW, Cho E-S, Jordan BD, Price RW. Ann Neurol 1986; 19: 224.
20. Bamford CR. Neurology 1975; 25: 343.
21. Petito CK, Cho E-S, Lemann W, Navia RA, Price RW. J Neuropath Exp Neurol 1986; 45: 635.
22. Teutsch SM et al. Am J Trop Med Hyg 1980; 29: 738.
23. Ruebush TK II, Rubin RH, Wolpow ER, Cassaday PB, Schultz MG. Am J Trop Med Hyg 1979; 28: 184.

Metazoal infestations

24. Dixon HBF, Lipscomb EM. Spec Rep Ser Med Res Counc (London), 1961: 229.
25. Trelles JO, Trelles L. In: Vinken PJ, Bruyn GW, eds. Handbook of clinical neurology, vol 35. Infections of the

nervous system, part III. Amsterdam: North Holland, 1978: 291.

26. Bickerstaff ER, Small JM, Woolf AL. Brain 1956; 79: 622.
27. De Souza Queiroz L, Filho AP, Callegarro D, Lopez de Faria L. J Neurol Sci 1975; 26: 61.
28. Stern WE. J Neurosurg 1981; 55: 382.
29. Arana-Iñiguez R. In: Vinken PL, Bruyn GW, eds. Handbook of clinical neurology, vol. 35. Infections of the nervous system, part III. Amsterdam: North Holland, 1978: 175.
30. Phillips G. J Neurol Neurosurg Psychiatry 1948; 11: 44.
31. Samiy E, Zadeh FA. J Neurosurg 1965; 22: 425.
32. Bird AV. In: Vinken PL, Bruyn GW, eds. Handbook of clinical neurology, vol 35. Infections of the nervous system, part III. Amsterdam: North-Holland, 1978: 231.
33. Greenfield JG, Pritchard EAB. Brain 1937; 60: 361.
34. Herskowitz A. J Neurosurg 1972; 36: 494.
35. Oh SJ. In: Vinken PL, Bruyn GW, eds. Handbook of

clinical neurology, vol 35. Amsterdam: North Holland, 1975: 243.

36. Vejjajiva A. Clin Exp Neurol 1978; 15: 92.
37. Boongird P, Phuapradit P, Siridej N, Chirachaviyavej T, Chuahirun S, Vejjajiva A. J Neurol Sci 1977; 31: 279.
38. Woodruff AW. Br Med J 1970; 3: 663.
39. Ashton N. Brit J Ophthalmol 1960; 44: 129.
40. Van Bogaert L, Dubois A, Janssens PG, Radermecker J, Tverdy A, Wanson M. J Neurol Neurosurg Psychiatry 1955; 18: 103.
41. Anders K, Foley K, Stern WE, Brown WJ. J. Neurosurg 1984; 60: 1282.
42. Masdeu JC, Tantulavanich S, Gorelick PP et al. Arch Neurol 1982; 39: 62.
43. Hoogstraten J, Young WG. Can J Neurol Sci 1975; 2: 121.
44. Pallis CA, Lewis PD. In: Walton J, ed. Disorders of voluntary muscle. 5th ed. Edinburgh: Churchill Livingstone, 1988: 611.

Viral infections

INTRODUCTION

Viruses cause a variety of neurological syndromes with infection of the leptomeninges (*meningitis*) or of the brain (*encephalitis*). The spinal cord may be the main area of the nervous system involved (*myelitis*), or the brain and cord (*encephalomyelitis*), or all three sites may be infected (*meningoencephalomyelitis*). Different viruses affect different parts of the brain with corresponding variation in clinical presentation. The neurological syndrome may run an acute, subacute or chronic course.

Quite apart from direct invasion of the nervous system by viruses, *post-infectious encephalomyelitis*, *neuritis* or *radiculitis* occurs as a complication of a number of common viral infections.

VIRUSES CAUSING ENCEPHALITIS AND MYELITIS

A wide variety of viruses cause encephalomyelitis;[1-3] their worldwide distribution and seasonal occurrence often depend upon the mode of transmission. With the mosquito-borne *togaviruses* (Eastern and Western equine encephalitis viruses and St Louis encephalitis virus) and *bunyaviruses*, encephalitis tends to occur in spring and summer,[4] whereas the tick-borne togavirus encephalitides are seen in early summer.[5,6] Infection by *paramyxoviruses*, including the mumps and measles viruses, tends to occur in the winter and spring, whereas lymphocytic choriomeningitis, which is caused by an *arenavirus*, is spread by rodents[2] and has a peak incidence in the winter. Infection by *enteroviruses* (*Picornaviridae*), which include poliovirus, the Coxsackieviruses and echoviruses, generally cause encephalomyelitis in the late summer and autumn. Geographical restriction of encephalitides, such as Eastern and Western equine encephalitis, depends upon the distribution of the arthropod vector. The *Rhabdoviridae* include members of the lyssavirus group (rabies, Ebola, Marburg and Mokola viruses). Rabies, in particular, is spread by mammalian vectors. Herpes simplex virus encephalitis occurs throughout the year and is the most common cause of severe sporadic encephalitis. Varicella-zoster may cause a localised necrotising myelitis.[7]

Post-infectious encephalomyelitis occurs in a minority of individuals infected by common viruses such as rubella, influenza A and B, mumps, measles, vaccinia, varicella-zoster and Epstein–Barr virus.[8]

ROUTES OF VIRAL INFECTION

The blood is the most common route by which viruses invade the central nervous system.[9] But, apart from Eastern equine encephalitis,[10] in which a very high proportion of infected individuals develop encephalitis, involvement of the central nervous system is an infrequent complication of common viral infections.[8] Viruses enter the blood via lymphatic drainage pathways from the respiratory tract, as in measles, mumps, influenza and varicella-zoster infections, or from the gastro-intestinal tract, as with enteroviruses (e.g. poliovirus). Insect bites on the skin allow mosquito-borne and tick-borne viruses to enter the blood. The peripheral nerves may be an important site of entry into the nervous system for rabies virus[11,12] and occasionally for poliovirus.[13] Retrograde transport of herpes simplex virus along nerves has been well demonstrated experimentally,[14] and both anterograde and retrograde

transport along nerves almost certainly occurs in man. The olfactory nerves have also been shown to be a portal of entry in experimental viral infections.[15]

ENTRY OF VIRUSES INTO CELLS

During the stage of viraemia, viruses cross capillary endothelial cells either by pinocytosis or by infecting the endothelial cells themselves. Once the virus is in the central nervous system, it attaches to cell membranes using a variety of receptors, some of which are part of the major histocompatibility complex;[16] in the case of rabies, the receptor appears to be associated with the acetylcholine receptor.[17] Internalisation of the virus is effected in most cases by receptor-mediated endocytosis,[18] although in some instances the outer envelope of the virus fuses directly with the cell membrane. Viral glycoprotein remaining on the cell surface following penetration of the virus may induce an immune attack upon the cell prior to the replication of the virus,[19] but only in the immune host. Once inside the cell, the protein coat of the virus is removed, probably by host cell lysosomal enzymes. Transcription and translation of the viral nucleic acid coding for virus-specific macromolecules is then initiated, sometimes by redirecting cell metabolism towards the synthesis of viral components. Multiplication of the virus depends upon transcription of specific messenger RNA from viral nucleic acid. The mechanism of such transcription and replication depends upon whether the nucleic acid is DNA or RNA and whether it is single or double stranded and of negative or positive polarity;[20] both DNA and RNA viruses invade the central nervous system.[19] The formation of new viral nucleic acid generally involves viral enzymes.

Assembly of the mature virus particle or *virion* occurs as the protein shell (*capsid*) coats the core of interwoven nucleic acid and protein (Fig. 9.4). Such viral particles can be observed inside cells by electron microscopy (Figs 9.5, 9.10, 9.17). Many viruses acquire an outer envelope by budding from host cell membranes, a phenomenon that is particularly well demonstrated by herpes simplex virus.[21] Viral glycoproteins are inserted into the membranes of infected cells and into the coat of the mature virion.

EFFECTS OF VIRAL INFECTION UPON CELLS OF THE NERVOUS SYSTEM

Neurons

The physiological effects of viral infection of neurons include seizure activity and neurological deficit due to death of infected cells. Lysis of neurons occurs particularly with non-enveloped viruses such as poliovirus; the cells burst and release mature viruses.[22] Other viruses, such as herpes simplex virus, bud from the surface of neurons, and cell death occurs as a result of inhibition of synthesis of macromolecules within the cell. Infected cells show many of the characteristics of hypoxic change, with brightly eosinophilic cytoplasm and shrunken pyknotic nuclei. *Neuronophagia* (see p. 40) subsequently occurs with phagocytosis of dead neurons—either by polymorphonuclear leucocytes, as in poliomyelitis, or more usually by microglia. Neuronophagia is seen in necrotic or oedematous, inflamed areas of the brain in acute viral encephalitides. In more chronic viral infections of the brain, more selective destruction of neurons occurs and neuronophagia is seen in otherwise intact or mildly inflamed grey matter; it is recognised by the small clusters of microglia (microglial stars) around the dead neurons (Figs 9.8 and 9.11).

Viruses can be identified within the infected cells by immunocytochemistry (Fig. 9.3), using appropriate antibodies, or by electron microscopy, relying upon ultrastructural features for identification of the virus.[23] Viral inclusion bodies may be seen in the nucleus or in the cytoplasm; they may be eosinophilic or basophilic, with or without a clear surrounding halo. Inclusion bodies are particularly well seen in herpes simplex encephalitis and in progressive multifocal leuco-encephalopathy. Both nuclear and cytoplasmic inclusions are seen in subacute sclerosing panencephalitis (Fig. 9.9). The presence of viral particles within a nucleus may produce change in the chromatin pattern and hyperchromasia (Figs 9.16 and 9.17).

Viral infection of a cell may be latent, particularly in neurons. The virus may not be isolated by usual laboratory methods during asymptomatic periods and neither viral particles nor antigen can be detected within the cells, although viral genome is present. Non-specific triggers can activate the virus and cause acute disease, as in the recurrent skin lesions of herpes simplex.[24]

Unconventional agents causing the spongiform encephalopathies of Creutzfeldt–Jakob disease and kuru[25] are associated with fine microvacuolar (spongiform) change in the cortical and subcortical neuronal dendrites and axons.[26,27] There is no ultrastructural evidence of virus invasion and rarely any evidence of inflammation.

Oligodendrocytes

Oligodendrocytes may be selectively damaged in post-infectious encephalomyelitis, resulting in demyelination which is frequently perivascular (Fig. 9.6); the myelin sheaths are destroyed and the axons are preserved. Direct viral invasion of oligodendrocytes occurs in progressive multifocal leucoencephalopathy and to some extent in subacute sclerosing panencephalitis; nuclear hyperchromasia, viral inclusions and change in chromatin distribution in oligodendrocytes are seen in both these diseases.

Astrocytes

Astrocytes respond to virus infections by proliferation and hypertrophy. Death of astrocytes occurs in severe acute viral encephalitides. Occasionally, as in progressive multifocal leucoencephalopathy, astrocytes become large and bizarre and show hyperchromasia of their nuclei.

Ependyma

Viral infection may cause death of ependymal cells in the fetus; if the ependyma of the aqueduct is involved, scarring and aqueductal stenosis may follow, resulting in hydrocephalus. This sequence has been demonstrated in experimental animals and may also occur in man.[28]

HOST RESPONSES TO VIRAL INFECTIONS OF THE NERVOUS SYSTEM

The absence of specific receptors on nerve cells may prevent a particular virus from infecting the nervous system. Even if infection does occur, host defence mechanisms may limit the degree of damage to the cell, and immunological responses may eliminate infected cells and virus. Interferon is produced rapidly by any cell in response to virus infection, and particularly by lymphocytes and macrophages. Although the interferon may have no effect upon the already infected cell, it mediates the production in other cells of antiviral proteins which interfere with subsequent viral replication in these cells.

Immunological defences against virus infections involve B and T lymphocytes and macrophages. Specific IgA is present in secretions on the mucosal surfaces and may be effective in controlling infection. IgM is produced initially following virus infections, and persistent IgG virus-specific antibodies may confer lifelong immunity. Antibodies interact with surface antigens on viruses and not only prevent attachment to susceptible cells but also agglutinate the viruses and facilitate phagocytosis. Antibody-antigen complexes may activate the complement system and cause an inflammatory response, producing lysis of enveloped viruses and of host cells bearing viral antigens on their surfaces. However, there is some evidence that in some situations antibody may alter the expression of viral proteins on cell surfaces and induce persistent infections, as in subacute sclerosing panencephalitis.[29]

Cells infected with virus and expressing viral antigen on their surfaces are destroyed by specific cytotoxic T-cells. The interaction between antigen-presenting cells, such as macrophages, and T-cells is only possible when both cell types share major histocompatibility antigens.[30] Similarly, the interaction of cytotoxic T-cells with cells expressing viral antigens is also restricted by major histocompatibility antigens.[31] Thus cytotoxic T-cells will only kill virally infected cells if the target cells have the same Class I histocompatibility complex as the T-cell itself.

T-cells, B-cells, plasma cells and macrophages invade the virus-infected brain via the post-capillary venules and accumulate within the perivascular spaces around arteries and veins. One of the characteristics of encephalomyelitis, therefore, is the perivascular cuffing by lymphocytes and monocytes and, in the acute encephalitides, the widespread invasion of damaged neural tissue by these inflammatory cells. Although the brain has no well-recognised lymphatic system, fluid does drain along perivascular spaces and probably enters the cerebrospinal fluid before some, at least, drains into the lymphatics of the neck.[32,33] Such a connection with the lymphatic system may be important in the immunological response to viral infections of the central nervous system.

VIRAL DISEASES OF THE NERVOUS SYSTEM

VIRAL (ASEPTIC) MENINGITIS

Generally, the clinical presentation of viral meningitis is acute—with fever, drowsiness, neck stiffness, nausea and vomiting. There may be an associated systemic illness with diarrhoea, pneumonia, fever or diffuse myalgia. Patients usually recover completely within a few days.

Enteroviruses are the commonest cause of viral meningitis. This group includes Coxsackieviruses and echoviruses, and most cases of meningitis occur in late summer and autumn.[34] Poliovirus infection may also present as meningitis in areas of the world not controlled by vaccination. Mumps virus infection, with or without parotitis,[35] is the second most common cause of viral meningitis. Less common viruses causing meningitis include herpes simplex type 2, varicella-zoster, and the arenavirus which causes lymphocytic choriomeningitis.

Examination of the cerebrospinal fluid (CSF) in viral meningitis reveals up to $100 \times 10^6/l$ polymorphonuclear leucocytes initially; later, more than $1000 \times 10^6/l$ lymphocytes are found. Protein is slightly raised at $0.5-1.5\,g/l$ (normal $0.15-0.40\,g/l$); glucose levels are usually normal. Virus may be isolated from the CSF, throat swabs or faeces. The identity of the viral infection may also be obtained from the rise in blood antibody levels when serum is taken at the beginning of the illness and some two weeks later, although the number of enterovirus serotypes causing meningitis may make exact diagnosis impractical by this method.

Pathologically, in the few fatal cases of viral meningitis reported, infiltration of the leptomeninges by lymphocytes and a few monocytes has been observed, together with some perivascular cuffing of vessels in the superficial layers of the cerebral cortex.[36]

ACUTE SPORADIC VIRAL ENCEPHALITIS

In addition to signs and symptoms of meningeal inflammation, patients with acute viral encephalitis develop headache, fever and an alteration in the level of consciousness. Initially there may be mild lethargy which progresses to confusion, stupor and coma within a few days.[37] Focal neurological signs are frequently seen and epilepsy is common. The specific pattern of signs and symptoms and the progression of the encephalitis varies with the infecting virus.

Enteroviruses (especially Coxsackieviruses and echoviruses), respiratory viruses, herpes simplex type 1 virus, and measles and mumps viruses are the commonest causes of acute encephalitis in Britain.[36,38] Viruses that are spread by insect vectors cause acute viral encephalitis which varies from region to region in the United States and elsewhere.[2] Epstein–Barr virus and adenoviruses are less common causes of encephalitis. The occurrence of encephalitis due to the rabies virus depends upon the distribution of the infection. Diagnosis of viral encephalitis is confirmed by virus culture from blood, brain tissue, nose and throat swabs, urine and faeces, and from the detection of specific antibodies in blood and CSF.[38,39] Interferon levels can also be measured in the serum and CSF.[38] In a minority of cases, brain biopsy may be the only sure technique for diagnosis.

Herpes simplex encephalitis

Herpes simplex virus type 1 is the commonest

cause of severe acute sporadic encephalitis in Western Europe and the USA. Some 50 cases are reported per year in England and Wales,[40] and 1000–2000 cases each year in the USA.[2]

Clinical features

The patient develops a headache with drowsiness and personality change over a few days and may then lose consciousness. Focal neurological signs such as hemiparesis may be seen, and seizures may occur.[42] One or both temporal lobes are the most severely affected regions of the brain and the oedema accompanying the encephalitis may be seen as low attenuation areas on CT scan.

Laboratory diagnosis can be achieved by showing rising titres of specific herpes simplex virus antibody in serum and CSF. If the rise of antibody is significantly higher in the CSF than in the blood, it indicates antibody production within the central nervous system.[39] Cerebrospinal fluid may not be available for examination as lumbar puncture is a dangerous procedure because of the brain swelling that usually accompanies severe herpes simplex encephalitis. If CSF is available, there is usually a moderate rise in lymphocytes $(100-400 \times 10^6/l)$ and protein level $(0.5-1.5\,g/l)$, with a normal glucose level.[41,42] Virus is rarely found in the CSF. Isolation of the virus is most satisfactorily achieved from brain biopsy,[43] but this procedure is now less common since the introduction of acyclovir as an effective non-toxic treatment for herpes simplex encephalitis.[44]

Therapy is usually initiated without prior isolation of the virus. Untreated, the mortality rate of herpes simplex encephalitis approaches 70%, and only 10% of patients are subsequently able to lead a normal life.[45,46] Patients die with severe cerebral oedema and necrosis of the temporal lobes. Those who survive may suffer gross loss of recent memory due to bilateral destruction of the hippocampus.

Treatment

Intravenous acyclovir is the treatment of choice. Acyclovir is a purine nucleoside analogue which binds more avidly to viral thymidine kinase than to the host enzyme. Acyclovir is phosphorylated within the cell to form a potent inhibitor of herpes simplex virus DNA-polymerase.[47] The drug has a low toxicity and is effective against herpes simplex types 1 and 2 and against varicella-zoster virus. The use of acyclovir administered early in the illness has reduced the mortality of herpes simplex encephalitis to 19% and allowed 56% of treated individuals to return to a normal life.[48] These results are significantly better than those with the antiviral agent vidarabine.

Pathology

Herpes simplex type 1 virus infects sensory ganglion cells in the dorsal spinal roots or in the trigeminal ganglion. It is responsible for recurrent cold sores. The exact route of entry of the virus into the central nervous system is unclear, but it may pass through the cribriform plate of the ethmoid and along olfactory nerves to the temporal lobe.[49]

Macroscopic examination of the brain of a patient who has died in the acute stages of herpes simplex encephalitis reveals cerebral oedema and swelling, particularly of one or both temporal lobes. The secondary effects of brain swelling, with shift of the midline, subfalcine herniation and trans-

tentorial herniation (see p. 67), midbrain compression and haemorrhage, may cause the patient's death. Necrosis involves the cortex of the anterior portion of the temporal lobe, the white matter of the temporal lobe, the hippocampus, the amygdala and the putamen.[50] The cingulate gyrus may also be involved. In patients who die some weeks after the onset of herpes encephalitis, the brain shows disintegration of the temporal lobes (Fig. 9.1), which is often asymmetrical. There may also be infarction of the occipital lobe on the more severely affected side due to compression of branches of the posterior cerebral artery during transtentorial herniation in the acute stages. Those patients who survive 5–10 years after a severe episode of herpes simplex encephalitis show extensive shrinkage and cystic change in the temporal lobes with destruction of the hippocampus and atrophy of the fornices (Fig. 9.2). If

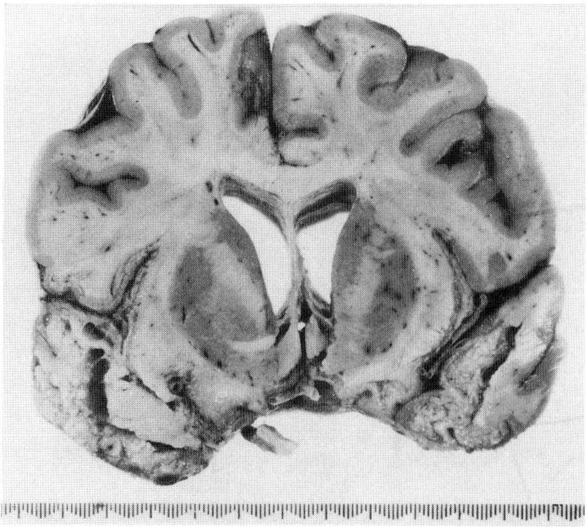

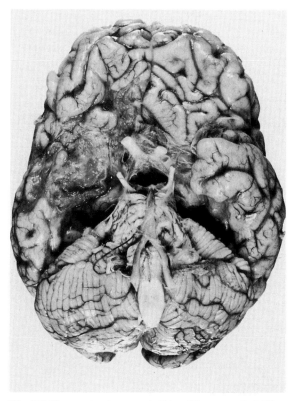

Fig. 9.1 Herpes simplex encephalitis—3 months survival. There is softening and disintegration of both temporal lobes, the insular cortex and part of the frontal cortex on the left. The cingulate gyri, just above the corpus callosum, are also necrotic.

Fig. 9.2 Herpes simplex encephalitis—10 year survival. The right temporal lobe (left of picture) is necrotic and shrunken; there is less damage to the left temporal lobe. The patient suffered severe loss of recent memory.

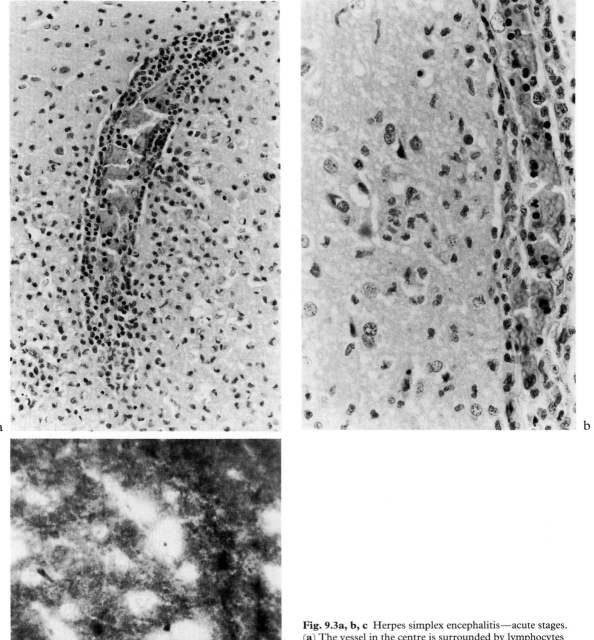

Fig. 9.3a, b, c Herpes simplex encephalitis—acute stages.
(**a**) The vessel in the centre is surrounded by lymphocytes
and plasma cells. Inflammatory cells have migrated into the
surrounding necrotic tissue. Rod-shaped microglial cells can
also be seen. (**b**) At higher magnification, an eosinophilic
damaged neuron with a pyknotic nucleus is seen (centre left),
together with microglial cells and lymphocytes. (**c**) Bright
immunofluorescence is seen in cells infected with virus.
(**a**) Haematoxylin-eosin ×210; (**b**) Haematoxylin-eosin
×360; (**c**) Immunofluorescence for herpes simplex virus
×480
(**c**) *Reproduced by permission of Dr M. Ogilvie, Microbiology,
Southampton, UK.*

the corticospinal tracts in the internal capsule are involved, there may be shrinkage of the pyramidal tracts in the medulla.

Histological examination of the brain in the acute stage of herpes encephalitis shows a generalised meningoencephalitis with extensive tissue necrosis and widespread perivascular cuffing by T and B lymphocytes and plasma cells. In very severely affected areas, the basement membrane of the glia limitans surrounding the perivascular spaces[51] breaks and inflammatory cells stream into the necrotic tissue (Fig. 9.3a). Initially there is microglial proliferation with many rod-shaped cells in the tissue (Fig. 9.3b), but after a few days many foamy macrophages are seen. Neurons with eosinophilic cytoplasm and pyknotic nuclei are seen in the affected areas, and eosinophilic nuclear inclusions composed of viral particles may be detected in the neurons. Phagocytosis of neurons (neuronophagia) by microglial cells is also prominent in the areas of necrosis. Herpes simplex antigen can be detected by immunocytochemistry using anti-herpes antibodies (Fig. 9.3c); it is most abundant in the first weeks after the onset of the encephalitis but can be detected in tissue for up to three weeks.[52] In some cases the vessels are necrotic and polymorphonuclear leucocytes are present in the walls and in the perivascular spaces.

If the patient survives, the dead tissue is removed by macrophages and the necrotic area becomes converted to a cyst lined by reactive astrocytes and eventually by atrophic gliotic tissue. Lymphocytes and macrophages may persist for months or years in the tissue although the virus is no longer present.

When a *biopsy* is taken in the acute stages of herpes simplex encephalitis, either through a burr hole or during a decompressive craniotomy, the tissue can be used for histological diagnosis of encephalitis and for the isolation of the virus. Similar techniques can be used on autopsy tissue. Fresh, unfixed brain tissue can be examined in smear preparations, which show perivascular cuffing by lymphocytes, plasma cells and numerous rod-shaped microglia.[53] Cryostat sections are ideal for detecting inflammatory exudates, the eosinophilic change in neurons and the viral inclusions. Furthermore, cryostat sections can be used for the immunocytochemical

detection of herpes antigen.[52] The diagnosis may therefore be made within a few hours, either by immunofluorescence or by detection of herpes virus particles by electron microscopy in negatively stained disrupted cell preparations (Fig. 9.4).[39] The virus can be isolated by inoculation into tissue culture, although this may be difficult if antibodies are present. Prior trypsinisation of minced brain for some 30 minutes before inoculation improves the chance of successful viral culture.[54]

The detection of virus particles in intact tissue by electron microscopy is most satisfactory on fresh biopsy material fixed in glutaraldehyde (Fig. 9.5). However, viral particles are often well-preserved in post-mortem material and despite the disruption of the tissue by autolysis, it may be possible to detect herpes virus particles some hours after death in acute cases. Examination of toluidine blue-stained 1 µm resin sections will reveal areas of inflammation in which intranuclear inclusions may be found. By light microscopy, the involved nuclei may exhibit clear, unstained areas in the centre or disruption of the chromatin pattern. By electron microscopy, the incomplete viral particles are visible in the nucleus (Fig. 9.5); membrane-bound complete enveloped virus may be seen in the interstitial spaces.

Rabies

Rabies has a worldwide distribution except for its exclusion from Britain, Iceland, Sweden, Spain, Japan, New Zealand and Australia. Repeated epidemics have occurred in foxes in Europe; the latest started in Poland in 1939 and has spread at 30–60 km per year to reach the north coast of France.[55] Various carnivores are the natural hosts for the virus, especially dogs in India and Southeast Asia, foxes in Europe, skunks in the Western USA and racoons in the Eastern USA.[55] The disease is spread by vampire bats in South America, and the mongoose is a reservoir in South Africa.[56] Transmission of rabies to man is principally by dogs.

Rabies virus is an enveloped single-stranded RNA rhabdovirus and a member of the lyssavirus group; it is 150×100 nm in size.[57] The disease is usually transmitted from one infected animal to another through inoculation of saliva as a result of

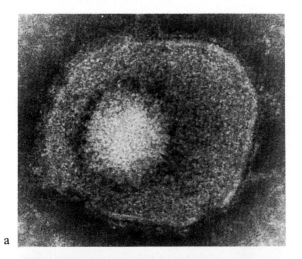

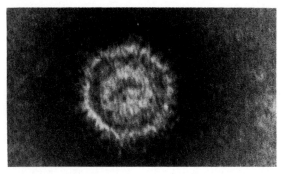

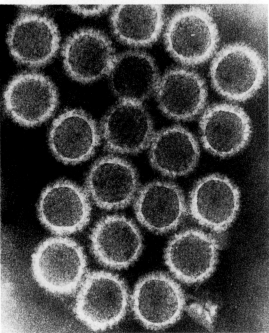

Fig. 9.4a, b, c Herpes simplex virus in negatively stained electron microscope preparations. (**a**) Complete herpes virus showing the central virus capsid and the outer envelope. (**b**) Herpes simplex virus capsids released from disrupted brain tissue. The particles lack outer envelopes. (**c**) Isolated herpes simplex virus showing the central nucleic acid core surrounded by the protein capsid; the virus lacks an outer envelope.
(**a**) ×210 000; (**b**) ×155 000; (**c**) ×275 000

a bite, although the respiratory route has been implicated in infection from bat-infested caves. During the incubation period of 15 days to a year (average 40 days),[58] replication of the virus occurs in striated muscle before the organism enters the peripheral nervous system.[59] Rabies virus has a high affinity for neural cells. Spike glycoprotein on the virus surface has a similar structure to some long neurotoxins in snake venom, and both types of glycoprotein have an affinity for acetylcholine receptors at neuromuscular junctions.[59] It is probable that the virus is taken up by nerve endings and transported by retrograde axoplasmic flow to motor neurons in the spinal cord. From here, infection ascends rapidly by transneuronal spread to the brain. Rabies virus is highly selective for certain groups of neurons, especially the Purkinje cells in the cerebellum and the pyramidal cells of the hippocampus. From the brain, the virus spreads centrifugally into peripheral nerves and

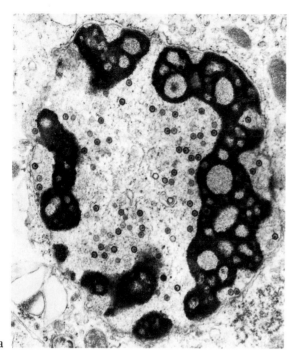 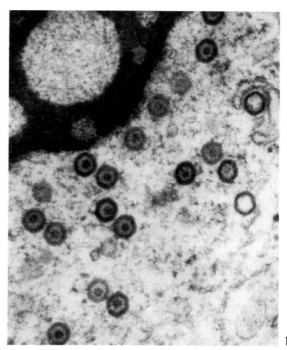

a

b

Fig. 9.5a, b Herpes simplex virus in sections of brain tissue—electron microscopy. (**a**) A nucleus showing disruption of the chromatin pattern and scattered viral particles. (**b**) Details of the intranuclear viral particles showing a central core and a ring-like capsid.
(**a**) × 18 000; (**b**) × 69 000

may be localised in most organs. In the salivary glands, the virus replicates in mucous acinar cells and buds from the apical surfaces of the cells into the ducts carrying saliva.[60] Although the selective infection of neurons appears to depend largely upon the attachment of the virus to acetylcholine receptors, rabies virus does infect cells which do not bear acetylcholine receptors.

Clinical features

The *incubation period* of the disease is shorter when bites from infected dogs are on the head and neck; it is also shorter in children than in adults. After an initial prodromal stage of malaise, headaches, fever, nausea and diarrhoea, the patient may develop the *furious type* of rabies with convulsions, meningism, fasciculation of skeletal muscles and cerebellar signs, and death in 3–5 days. Pharyngeal spasm in 50% of patients is the cause of the *hydrophobia*.[61] In approximately 20% of patients, there is a *paralytic disease* (dumb rabies) resembling the Guillain–Barré syndrome; death usually

occurs in 11 days. Rabies is usually fatal, although the cases of two patients who survived have been reported.[62,63]

Pathology

Macroscopically, the brain at post-mortem shows little abnormality. Histological examination of the brain shows features of acute encephalitis with perivascular cuffing by lymphocytes and plasma cells, microglial invasion and proliferation in the surrounding tissue and, in severely inflamed areas, astrocytic proliferation and hypertrophy. These changes are mainly seen in the grey matter. The pathognomonic change in rabies is the presence of *Negri bodies*, which are round or oval eosinophilic cytoplasmic inclusions 1–7 μm in diameter.[36,53] Negri bodies may be seen in the cell bodies of neurons or in the dendrites, and they may be single or multiple. They are largest in the pyramidal cells of the hippocampus, in Purkinje cells and in anterior horn cells of the spinal cord. Virus antigen and viral particles have been identified within

Negri bodies[64] and in the more eosinophilic *lyssa bodies*.[65]

In the paralytic form of rabies, the anterior horn cells of the spinal cord are severely affected, with lymphocyte and plasma cell infiltration and destruction of anterior horn cells.[61] Similar changes are seen in the brainstem of patients with bulbar involvement.

Myocarditis may be found at post-mortem and is a well-recognised complication of rabies.[66] Histologically, there is necrosis of myocardial muscle fibres and infiltration by lymphocytes, histiocytes and occasionally neutrophils.

Diagnosis. The diagnosis of rabies can be made by detecting viral antigen in epithelial cells from corneal smears by immunofluorescence in 50% of cases or, less effectively, in skin and buccal mucosa biopsies.[67] Tissue from infected human or animal brain can be inoculated into mice, and the animals become positive for viral antigen 3–4 days after inoculation. Virus can also be isolated from the saliva. At post mortem, Negri bodies should be sought.[68]

There are strict codes of practice for dealing with suspected rabies tissue in most countries.

Treatment

Preventative measures against exposure to rabies are very strict in those countries free of the disease, with stringent restrictions on the importation of animals and long periods of quarantine.

Treatment of suspected cases of rabies should be prompt, with cleansing of the wounds and the administration of rabies vaccine. Until recently, rabies vaccines were prepared from adult rabbit, sheep or goat brain by a method similar to that used by Pasteur. Approximately 0·1% of those receiving the vaccine developed an *allergic encephalomyelitis*.[69] Subsequent vaccines produced in suckling mice resulted in an allergic neuritis in 1:8000 patients.[70] Complications also occur with duck embryo vaccine, and the preferred vaccine is human diploid cell rabies vaccine.[19] A course of vaccine should be initiated as soon after exposure to rabies as possible, and penetrating wounds should be infiltrated by human immune serum.

Other causes of sporadic acute viral encephalitis

Acute encephalitis is an uncommon consequence of a number of common viral infections.[3] Enteroviruses such as Coxsackievirus, poliovirus and echoviruses can cause encephalitis,[69] as also can measles, mumps, rubella and a variety of other viruses.[37] Clinically, acute encephalitis caused by viruses such as measles virus may be indistinguishable from post-infectious encephalomyelitis (see p. 207). Pathologically, the brain is swollen and the histological characteristics are similar to those seen in herpes simplex encephalitis except that viral inclusions are not usually seen and the temporal lobes are not preferentially involved. Virus may be isolated from throat swabs, faeces or blood mononuclear cells, or from biopsy or autopsy brain tissue. A rise in titres in serum and CSF may be detected during the course of the illness. Despite these methods of investigation, however, the aetiology of encephalitis is usually only confirmed in some 30% of cases.[39] This is mainly due to the very large number of different viruses and their subgroups which can cause encephalitis and the difficulty of distinguishing viral encephalitis from post-infectious encephalitis clinically.

ACUTE EPIDEMIC VIRAL ENCEPHALITIS

The majority of cases of epidemic viral encephalitis are caused by *arboviruses*, viruses spread by arthropods. Although there are some 500 different viruses which are known to circulate between vertebrates and arthropods, only 18 species infect man regularly and all are RNA viruses. The primary hosts are wild birds, horses and small mammals, and the arthropod vectors are mosquitoes and ticks. Cases of epidemic encephalitis due to arboviruses are not usually seen in the winter as the number of vectors is diminished.[3]

Virus is introduced by the insect vector and is spread by the blood to the central nervous system. The viraemic phase is short-lived and it may be difficult to isolate the virus during this period, but virus can usually be isolated from post-mortem brain in fatal cases. Diagnosis is more usually made by showing a progressive rise in antibody levels in CSF and serum.[70]

Several types of arthropod-borne encephalitis are seen in North and South America, in the USSR and in Asia.[3] Some of the viruses circulate between mosquitoes and birds, and others are tick-borne with small mammals and birds as the main hosts.

St Louis encephalitis

The commonest acute epidemic viral encephalitis in the USA is due to the St Louis encephalitis virus, in the flavivirus group. St Louis encephalitis occurs throughout the USA but is most common in Mississippi and Ohio. Most infections are sub-clinical and only about 1 in 300 of those infected develops overt encephalitis. Clinically,[71] patients develop headache, fever, neck stiffness and mild lethargy which may progress to confusion, stupor and coma, with death in 10–20% of cases. Focal neurological signs may develop, with seizures.

Pathologically, the brain shows similar changes to other forms of acute encephalitis[72] with wide-spread perivascular cuffing by lymphocytes, plasma cells, monocytes and macrophages. The cerebral hemispheres are most severely affected. Microglial proliferation is seen throughout the brain, and microglial cells accumulate in nodules. Inflammation is seen in the meninges but no virus is usually detectable by immunocytochemistry. Neuritic plaques (see p. 362) may be present.[72]

Eastern and Western equine encephalitis

These diseases are both caused by alphaviruses which, like the St Louis virus, are togaviruses. Spread by mosquitoes which have birds as their principal host, Eastern equine encephalitis usually occurs along the Atlantic coast of the USA, and clinically evident encephalitis occurs with a high frequency among those infected.[10] The mortality rate is high.

Western equine encephalitis is distributed in the Western and Central parts of North America, but the incidence of overt disease is low and the mortality rate is 3–7%. The clinical disease is more fulminant in Eastern equine fever and the pathological changes are more severe.[73]

Pathologically, the brain is swollen and congested, and histologically there is severe meningoencephalitis with polymorphonuclear leucocyte infiltration. Acute vasculitis with deposition of fibrin in necrotic vessels is seen, and there are large areas of tissue necrosis, neuronal loss and neuronophagia. The whole brain is affected, but in some cases the cerebrum is more severely involved and in other cases the disease is concentrated in the brainstem. The spinal cord is usually spared although the upper cervical region may be affected. In comparison with St Louis encephalitis, there is much more extensive necrosis in Western equine fever, although the inflammation is more widespread in St Louis encephalitis.[74]

Other forms of acute epidemic viral encephalitis

The *Venezuelan type of equine encephalitis* is also due to an alphavirus, spread by mosquitoes from horses and small mammals. There is a mild encephalomyelitis and most of the fatal cases are in children under the age of five years.[3]

Viruses in the bunyavirus group also cause encephalitis and are spread by mosquitoes, whereas the encephalitogenic reoviruses are spread by ticks. The pathological changes in these encephalitides bear no specific features but show the general inflammatory changes of acute viral encephalitis (Fig. 9.3).[3]

POLIOMYELITIS

Endemic poliomyelitis has been largely eradicated in several countries, including Britain, the USA and Sweden, by the use of oral attenuated polio-virus or by intramuscular injection of inactivated poliovirus vaccines. However, even in countries with a high level of vaccination, sporadic out-breaks of paralytic poliomyelitis may occur. Such an outbreak occurred in Finland in the autumn and winter of 1984 and was due to an epidemic strain of poliovirus type 3 which differed from the type 3 vaccine strain.[75] An outbreak due to type 1 polio-virus occurred in Taiwan in 1982.[76] Rare cases (0·5–3·4 per million) of paralytic disease associated with poliomyelitis vaccine strains also occur.[77] Furthermore, disease indistinguishable from classical poliomyelitis can be due to infection by other enteroviruses.[78] Poliomyelitis still occurs in those countries without a comprehensive vaccination programme and in unvaccinated individuals visiting those regions. Infection occurs especially through swimming in non-chlorinated water.

Spread of infection

Poliovirus is an enterovirus which is spread by contamination of water or food by faeces or by flies carrying the virus. The virus multiplies in the oropharynx and then infects the mucosa of the ileum and the Peyer's patches,[13,79] but spread to the central nervous system is infrequent.[80] Infectious virus may be shed in the faeces for 3–12 weeks. Entry of the virus into the central nervous system probably occurs during the viraemic stage of the infection, either directly from the blood or possibly through the autonomic nervous system.[81]

Clinical features

Infection in some individuals may be subclinical, others may exhibit symptoms during the viraemic stage with general malaise but without involvement of the nervous system. As many as 75% of patients who are infected develop fever, headache, malaise and often meningism, but never develop paralysis.[82] In the minority of cases which progress to paralysis, muscle fasciculation may follow a pre-paralytic stage with pain in the limbs and tenderness in the muscles. Paralysis reaches its maximum within the first 24 hours, most commonly affecting the lower limbs but with a variable distribution of involvement; in some cases the disease results in respiratory paralysis. In a small percentage of cases the brainstem is affected, with facial, pharyngeal, laryngeal and lingual paralysis. Only a proportion of the muscles affected remain permanently paralysed, and improvement usually begins at the end of the first week after the onset of paralysis.

The diagnosis is confirmed by examination of the cerebrospinal fluid, which may contain an excess of cells, both polymorphonuclear leuco-cytes and lymphocytes, and an excess of protein. Poliovirus may be isolated from the pharynx or from faeces by culture, but it is seldom possible to isolate it from the cerebrospinal fluid.

The mortality rate of poliomyelitis varies from 5–25%, and death is usually due to respiratory paralysis.

Pathology

Macroscopically, the spinal cord in acute poliomyelitis may show necrosis of the anterior horns, particularly the lumbar regions. Despite the often widespread involvement of the cerebrum, cerebellum, pons and medulla in patients dying in the acute stages of poliomyelitis, these regions of the brain may show little macroscopic abnormality.

Histologically, affected areas of the spinal cord show widespread lymphocytic infiltration together with polymorphonuclear leucocyte accumulation. In severely involved areas there is tissue necrosis. Inclusion bodies may be seen in neurons in the early stages of the disease but they are not usually prominent. Around the necrotic areas, there is microglial invasion and, as the virus-infected cells die, there is *neuronophagia*.[36,53] As the disease progresses, the inflammatory reaction may be so intense that, in patients dying within the first few weeks of the illness, the normal anatomy of the spinal cord may be obscured. Eventually, the inflammatory cell infiltration is reduced, but neuronophagia may continue, and microglial cells persist within the affected areas long after the virally infected neurons have been eliminated. In cases of bulbar poliomyelitis, the cranial nerve nuclei are involved, with invasion by inflammatory cells and neuronophagia. Widespread inflammatory changes are seen in the cerebral hemispheres and cerebellum but they are not as severe as in the spinal cord.

Histological examination of paralysed muscles reveals widespread neurogenic atrophy with small groups of angular denervated fibres.

Late sequelae of poliomyelitis

These include entrapment neuropathies, brachial plexus lesions resulting from the use of crutches or wheelchairs, and spinal deformity predisposing to cervical or lumbar spondylitic radiculopathy or myelopathy. Such complications mainly result from the severe and often asymmetrical muscle paralysis and wasting.

An uncommon cause of neurological deterioration is *post-poliomyelitis muscular atrophy*, a syndrome that has been recognised in a small minority of the estimated 300 000 individuals in the USA with a history of poliomyelitis.[83] New muscle weakness and wasting develop some 15 years or more after a period of neurological stability following poliomyelitis. There is progressive muscular atrophy without definite pyramidal signs. The cause is unclear. Small angulated fibres indicating recent denervation are seen in muscle biopsy specimens, but large group atrophy suggesting loss of neurons is not seen.[84] It is possible that, at this late stage, nerve terminals, which originally sprouted to reinnervate denervated muscle, degenerate with consequent progressive denervation.

Examination of the spinal cord in patients dying some years after severe poliomyelitis may reveal cavitation in previously necrotic areas of the spinal cord and atrophy of the anterior spinal roots. There is gliosis and neuronal loss from the affected areas of the spinal cord. Poliovirus can only be isolated from the cord in acute cases. Wasted muscles show extensive group atrophy and fibre type grouping, indicating widespread reinnervation.

VARICELLA-ZOSTER

Varicella-zoster virus remains latent in the neurons of dorsal root and trigeminal ganglia following the primary attack of varicella (chicken pox).[85] During reactivation of the virus, often following immunosuppression, the vesicular rash of herpes zoster (shingles) develops in the distribution of the cutaneous nerves arising from the involved sensory ganglia. An eye may be involved, resulting in corneal damage. In patients dying in the *acute stage*, the dorsal root or trigeminal ganglia may be swollen with an intense lymphocytic infiltration. Virus has been identified by electron microscopy and by immunofluorescence within acutely involved ganglia.[86] *Transverse myelitis* with inflammation and necrosis of the spinal cord may occur due to direct invasion by varicella-zoster virus.[7] Generalised varicella encephalitis is rare but may occur in immunosuppressed patients with leukaemia and lymphoma[87] and in neonatal varicella.

POST-INFECTIOUS ENCEPHALOMYELITIS

In as many as 70% of cases of acute encephalitis, a viral aetiology cannot be proved.[39] This may be due partly to an inability to detect the virus; the detection rate may improve in the future by the use of in situ hybridisation techniques with cDNA probes to parts of viral genomes.[88] However, many cases of acute encephalitis may be *allergic* rather than due to direct invasion of the nervous system by the virus.

Clinical features

Post-infectious encephalomyelitis may be clinically indistinguishable from encephalitis caused by direct invasion of the brain by a virus. The illness begins a few days to three weeks after a viral infection or an influenza-like illness. Fever and confusion may be followed by seizures and focal neurological disturbances.[82] A classical cerebellar syndrome may be associated with post-varicella encephalomyelitis.[89] The majority of patients are not particularly ill and recover in 3–6 weeks with little or no residual neurological deficit. In a few patients, however, the disease follows a rapidly fatal course. Investigation of patients with post-infectious encephalomyelitis may show a rise in CSF pressure and an increase in the number of lymphocytes and monocytes within the fluid; no virus can be isolated.

In the past, the majority of cases of post-infectious encephalomyelitis followed childhood viral infection such as measles (1·2 per 1000)[90] and mumps,[91] with rubella and varicella (chicken pox) as less frequent antecedent infections. The mortality rate of post-infectious encephalomyelitis associated with mumps and varicella is less than 5%, but that associated with measles may be as high as 40%.[19] Post-infectious encephalomyelitis has also been recorded after successful treatment of herpes simplex encephalitis.[92]

With the decline in other childhood virus infections in Europe and the USA which followed widespread vaccination, varicella is now the most common antecedent infection, but in many cases of post-infectious encephalomyelitis the specific identity of the original virus infection remains obscure.

Post-vaccination encephalomyelitis also occurs.

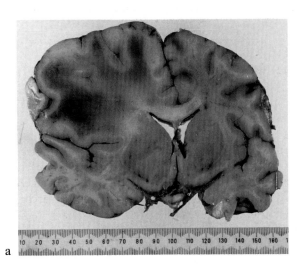

a

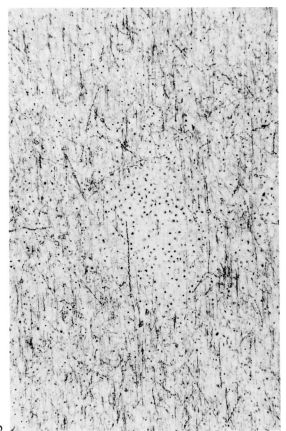

b

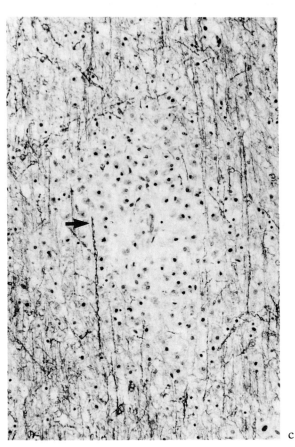

c

Fig. 9.6a, b, c Post-infectious encephalomyelitis. (**a**) The brain from a patient who died 7 days after the onset of clinical symptoms. The left cerebral hemisphere shows swelling and discoloration of the white matter but no obvious disintegration. (**b**) The affected cerebral white matter from the same case showing focal perivascular loss of myelin staining (centre). (**c**) Detail from (**b**) showing macrophages around a vessel; demyelination is indicated by the loss of myelin as nerve fibres (arrow) enter the perivascular lesion. (**b**) Klüver–Barrera × 75; (**c**) Klüver–Barrera × 150

Quite typical is the post-rabies vaccination encephalitis induced by the classical Pasteur preparations containing rabbit or other mammalian central nervous system myelin.[69] The pathology in these lesions resembles experimental allergic encephalomyelitis, which is also produced by the injection of central nervous system myelin.[92] Encephalitis may follow vaccination against measles[93] or smallpox vaccination (vaccinia).[94] Rabies and pertussis vaccines contain killed organisms, but vaccinia and measles vaccines contain live virus. The association between pertussis vaccine and typical post-infectious encephalomyelitis is doubtful.[95]

Post-infectious encephalomyelitis may recur.

There is no specific investigation for the diagnosis of post-infectious encephalomyelitis. CT scan may show areas of oedema in the white matter or may be normal. CSF pressures may be raised, and an increased number of lymphocytes and monocytes may be seen in the fluid.

Pathology

Patients dying with acute post-infectious encephalomyelitis may show congestion of the brain and oedema of the white matter. The affected areas of the white matter often exhibit grey discoloration and may be granular and soft (Fig. 9.6a). In some cases, however, little abnormality is seen on macroscopic inspection of the brain and the only guide to abnormal areas may be from CT scan findings and in the clinical features of the disease.

Histologically, the disease is characterised by areas of demyelination, particularly around small veins (Figs 9.6b and c), giving the alternative name of acute *disseminated perivenous encephalomyelitis*. Myelin sheaths are destroyed and axons are relatively well-preserved within the demyelinated areas. Myelin stains such as Luxol fast blue and its modification, the Klüver–Barrera stain, show the perivenous areas of demyelination well. In some cases these areas are confluent, and large expanses of cerebral white matter show loss of myelin. Smaller punctate areas of myelin loss are seen in the cerebellum, brainstem and spinal cord. Preserved axons within the demyelinated areas can be stained by silver techniques (e.g. Palmgren—Fig.

10.6) or by immunocytochemistry for neuro-filament proteins. Damaged axons are detected by the presence of axon swellings (see p. 46).

Perivascular and particularly perivenous inflammation is also a characteristic of this disease. In the very early stages, the inflammatory exudate consists mainly of polymorphonuclear leucocytes, but after a few days lymphocytes predominate. However, the degree of inflammation and the number of lymphocytes is not usually as great as in acute viral encephalitis. After one week or ten days most of the inflammatory cells around the vessels and in the surrounding demyelinated areas are microglia and macrophages. Such cells contain neutral fat droplets (cholesterol esters) resulting from myelin breakdown; this feature is best demonstrated in frozen sections using the oil red O stain, or can be well illustrated using the Marchi technique (see p. 83).

Although the white matter of the cerebral hemispheres, brainstem and spinal cord is principally involved, perivascular inflammation may also be seen in grey matter. In patients who survive the acute stages and die some weeks or months later, there is gliosis around blood vessels and the vessel walls show collagenous thickening, particularly in the adventitia.

There are a number of features which suggest that the lesions in the brains of patients dying with acute post-infectious encephalomyelitis are not due to direct viral infection,[96] for example, the failure to recover viruses from the brain, the recognised latent interval between a virus infection and the onset of the illness, and the mild nature of the lymphocytic response. Furthermore, the lesions in the brain are similar to those seen in experimental allergic encephalomyelitis (EAE), which suggests that autoimmune mechanisms may be involved. EAE can be produced in animals by the injection of myelin or certain myelin components.[92] It appears that a humoral reaction to myelin galacto-cerebroside and a T lymphocyte reaction to myelin basic protein combine to cause demyelination in EAE, with the oligodendrocyte and myelin as the targets of the immunological attack. The exact cause of the immunological reaction in post-infectious encephalomyelitis in man has not been established. It has been suggested that brain cell membranes share antigenic determinants with a number of viruses or that there is a release of brain antigens during a viral infection which initiates the immunological reaction. A further suggestion is that tissue damage occurs during immunological attack on a virus or its components and thus that the damage is a 'bystander' effect.[97]

ACUTE HAEMORRHAGIC ENCEPHALOMYELITIS

Some patients with encephalitis present with an abrupt onset of pyrexia and coma, and die within a few days. Such an illness may be preceded by a viral infection. At autopsy, the brain is swollen but the major feature is the widespread distribution of

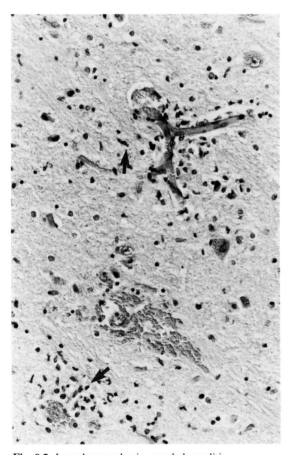

Fig. 9.7 Acute haemorrhagic encephalomyelitis. Extravascular extravasation of red blood cells (bottom) and perivascular inflammation (top). Numerous microglial cells (arrows) are seen within the intervening white matter. Haematoxylin-eosin × 225

numerous *petechial haemorrhages* (brain purpura) in the cerebral white matter, cerebellum, brainstem and spinal cord. The cortex and basal ganglia are relatively spared.

Histologically (Fig. 9.7), there is necrosis of vessel walls with exudation of fluid and fibrin. It is mainly the small vessels that are affected but arteries may show some necrosis. There is extravasation of red blood cells into the perivascular regions[98] and the appearances are very similar to those seen in fat embolism and cerebral malaria.[53] Neutrophil polymorphonuclear leucocytes are seen in the oedematous perivascular tissue, which may also show some degree of demyelination. At a later stage in the disease, there is perivascular accumulation of macrophages. The appearances of acute haemorrhagic leucoencephalitis resemble the hyperacute form of experimental allergic encephalomyelitis and may be due to immune complex disease.[100] Lesions found in other organs support this hypothesis.[101]

REYE'S SYNDROME

An acute encephalopathy with fatty degeneration of the liver was first documented by Reye, Morgan and Baral in 1963.[102] It occurs in children aged 6 months to 16 years, usually when they are recovering from a virus infection. The syndrome presents with persistent vomiting, lethargy, delirium, coma and seizures. Children may die within a few days from raised intracranial pressure. All patients show evidence of liver disease, and the detection of raised serum transaminases and ammonia is important in the diagnosis of the syndrome.

Antecedent viral infections, most notably influenza B, varicella and occasionally gastrointestinal infections, have been implicated in this syndrome. In 1977 it was one of the major causes of death from virally associated central nervous system disease in the United States, with an estimated incidence of 0·7 cases per 100 000 of the population under 18 years.[103] Case control studies have also shown that over 95% of children with the full-blown syndrome have a history of aspirin ingestion.[104] It has been recommended in Britain and the USA that aspirin should not be administered to children and adolescents. More than 80% of affected children died or were left with severe permanent neurological handicap in the 1960s.[102] But with early diagnosis, due to the recognition of raised serum ammonia, and the early treatment of seizures and brain oedema, the mortality and disability rate have been reduced to 25%.[105]

Pathology

The main pathological features in Reye's syndrome are severe fatty change in the liver and severe cerebral oedema without inflammatory change.[106] Microvesicular fat droplets and mitochondrial changes are seen in liver biopsies, which may therefore be helpful in the diagnosis of the syndrome.

In patients dying with the disease, the brain is large, swollen and soft, with oedematous white matter and compressed ventricles. Cerebellar tonsillar herniation is frequently seen. Histological examination of the brain reveals diffuse severe oedema but no inflammatory reaction to suggest direct viral infection. No virus has been isolated from the brain, and although virus infections and aspirin administration have been implicated, the exact cause of the disease is unknown. Ultrastructural studies have shown neuronal, astrocytic and myelin abnormalities and mitochondrial changes in the acute stages.[106] Fatty change is seen not only in the liver but also in renal tubular epithelium.

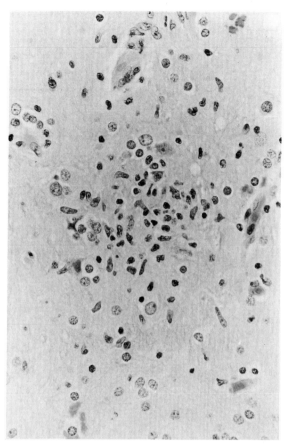

Fig. 9.8 Microglial star in subacute encephalitis. Cerebral cortex showing a collection of rod-shaped microglial cells (centre).
Haematoxylin-eosin × 300

SUBACUTE VIRAL ENCEPHALITIDES

Not all patients with viral encephalitis present with an acute illness. In some cases there is a progressive history lasting many months in which the patient exhibits intellectual deterioration with or without seizures and there is a gradual progression to a fatal outcome. At autopsy, there may be no macroscopic abnormality in the brain. Histological examination of biopsy or autopsy material from the cerebral hemispheres shows scattered groups of microglial cells (microglial stars; Fig. 9.8) in grey and white matter, and

neuronophagia. Small numbers of perivascular lymphocytes are also seen in the affected regions. Virus is rarely isolated from such cases and, due to the large number of viruses that could be implicated, it is rarely possible to identify the organism by immunocytochemistry.

There are also well-recognised subacute viral encephalitides in which the virus can be identified. Progressive multifocal leucoencephalopathy mostly occurs in immunosuppressed patients (see p. 219), as does measles inclusion body encephalitis (see p. 218). Subacute sclerosing panencephalitis and progressive rubella panencephalitis, however, are not so obviously associated with immunosuppression.

Subacute sclerosing panencephalitis (SSPE)

This disease is usually seen in children between the ages of 5 and 17 years, and most patients have had an early exposure to measles infection, generally in the first two years of life. SSPE has always been rare but it has now been almost eliminated in those countries in which live measles vaccination programmes have been introduced.[107]

Clinical features

Children with SSPE present with declining intellectual function, myoclonus, focal and generalised seizures, and severe neurological signs and coma as the disease progresses. Death occurs in most cases, from 6 weeks to as long as 10 years after the onset of the illness. Diagnosis is made on the clinical history, and an abnormal electroencephalogram with a burst-suppression pattern. High levels of measles antibody, including measles-specific IgM, are present in serum and particularly in CSF.[108]

Pathology

Macroscopically, the brain at post-mortem may appear almost normal in early cases but shows severe cortical atrophy and gliosis (sclerosis) of the white matter in patients who survive for 6 months or a year.

Microscopically, the more florid changes are seen in the early cases.[109] There is widespread perivascular cuffing by lymphocytes and plasma cells

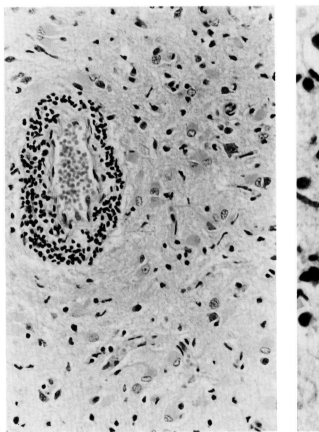
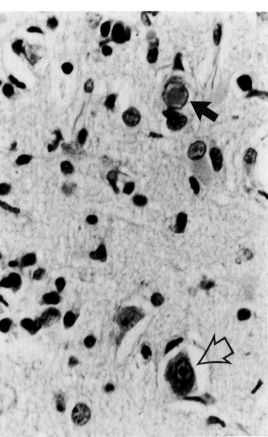

a   b

Fig. 9.9a, b Subacute sclerosing panencephalitis. (**a**) Perivascular cuffing by lymphocytes, with large numbers of rod-shaped microglial cells and plump reactive astrocytes in the cortex. (**b**) Viral inclusions in the nucleus of an oligodendrocyte (solid arrow) and in the nucleus and the cytoplasm of a neuron (open arrow).
Haematoxylin-eosin (**a**) ×240; (**b**) ×600

throughout grey and white matter with microglial infiltration, particularly in the grey matter areas (Fig. 9.9a). Irregular eosinophilic inclusion bodies are seen in the nuclei of neurons and oligodendroglia and also in the cytoplasm of neurons (Fig. 9.9b). Electron microscopy shows the presence of 16 nm helical profiles of viral nucleocapsid within the inclusions (Fig. 9.10). Immunocytochemistry of early cases shows abundant measles virus antigen distributed throughout the brainstem, basal ganglia, cerebral white matter and cortex, but not in the cerebellum.[110] Histological changes in the white matter are mainly extensive astrocyte hypertrophy and proliferation with varying degrees of demyelination and relative sparing of the axons. In longstanding cases of SSPE there is less inflammation, fewer inclusion bodies, extensive cortical atrophy with loss of neurons, and widespread gliosis of the white matter. Degeneration of the pyramidal tracts within the spinal cord reflects the widespread neuronal and white matter damage in the cerebral hemispheres.

Measles virus has been isolated from brains in SSPE, but only by co-cultivation techniques.[111]

The exact mechanisms involved in SSPE are unclear. Measles virus is an RNA virus which usually replicates in the cytoplasm and buds from the cell surface. Entry of virus into the nucleus does occur in tissue culture following administration of large doses of the virus. The virus associated with SSPE does not seem to differ from measles virus.[112]

There is no evidence of significant cellular immunodeficiency.[107] It has, however, been suggested that low levels of maternal antibodies to the matrix (M) protein of the measles virus may inhibit virus release from the cells and cause accumulation of immature virus within the cells.[112] Cell to cell spread of virus may thus occur, rather than release of intact infectious virus into the extracellular compartments.

Progressive rubella panencephalitis

This disease presents with intellectual deterio-

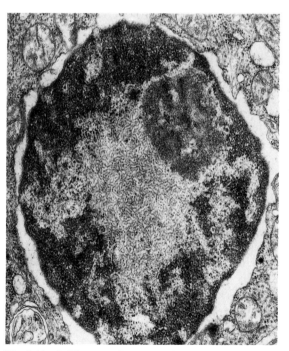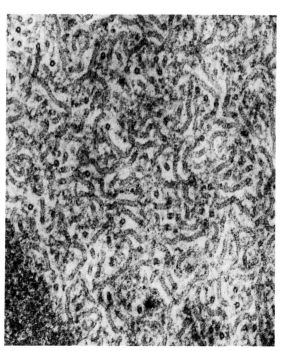

a   b

Fig. 9.10a, b Electron microscopy of viral inclusions in subacute sclerosing panencephalitis. (**a**) The nucleus of a neuron containing viral nuclear capsid (centre). Nucleolus upper right. (**b**) Detail from (a) showing 16 nm diameter helical profiles of viral nuclear capsid. They resemble paramyxovirus nuclear capsid.
(**a**) × 24 000; (**b**) × 102 000

ration, epilepsy and ataxia and is seen in patients between the ages of 8 and 19 years. It has been recorded as a late complication of congenital rubella infection and following non-congenital rubella.[113] The disease resembles subacute sclerosing panencephalitis and lasts from 4–10 years. Antibodies to rubella are present in the CSF and serum. It is a rare disease which pathologically shows panencephalitis with neuronal destruction in the cerebrum, cerebellum and brainstem. Perivascular lymphocytic infiltration is seen and there is vasculitis and fibrinoid necrosis of the vessels. Viral antigen has not been demonstrated within the brain of patients with this disease, and the vasculitic element suggests that it is a result of immune complex deposition.[19]

ACQUIRED IMMUNE DEFICIENCY SYNDROME (AIDS)

AIDS in Western Europe and the USA has so far occurred mainly in homosexual men, in bisexual men and in their sexual contacts, in intravenous drug abusers, and in haemophiliacs receiving pooled blood products. In Africa, AIDS affects sexually active adults of both sexes equally.

Often presenting with generalised lymphadenopathy, fever and weight loss, a proportion of patients progress to a full-blown picture of AIDS with opportunistic infections and neoplasms. At the stage of lymphadenopathy, the lymph nodes show a distinctive histopathological picture with exuberant reactive hyperplasia in the follicles and, to a lesser extent, in the interfollicular zones and sinuses. Eventually, there is involution of the follicles and other lymphoid elements.[114] The tumours associated with AIDS include Kaposi's sarcoma and B-cell lymphomas, which frequently present in the brain (see Ch. 16).[115]

The AIDS virus (human immunodeficiency virus—HIV) was first isolated in 1983 in France as the lymphadenopathy-associated virus (LAV)[116] and in the USA as the human T-cell lymphotrophic virus III (HTLV-III).[117] HIV is a member of the retrovirus family which includes *oncoviruses* such as HTLV-I, which causes adult T-cell leukaemia and is also associated with a myelopathy.[118] HIV belongs to the subfamily

Lentivirinae.[119] Other members of the lentivirus group cause encephalitis in animals. Maedi-visna has a long incubation period in sheep, causes cell lysis and inhabits blood cells in the bone marrow. It appears that the virus survives through genetic shift; thus proteins in the virus coat change, and antibodies against the virus are often ineffective.[120]

HIV selectively infects and destroys T-helper-inducer (T4) lymphocytes and ultimately causes a profound defect in cell-mediated immune responses, resulting in opportunistic infections.

Neurological features

Patients with AIDS may develop neurological signs and symptoms due either to opportunistic infections causing mass lesions within the brain and meningitis, or to a primary effect of HIV upon brain cells. In some series[119] there is a progressive dementia in more than half the patients. The dementia is accompanied by motor and behavioural dysfunction with loss of memory and concentration and with psychomotor slowing. The neurological disease may be steadily progressive but may also show abrupt accelerations. In 20% of cases[119] the course is indolent. In the advanced stages of the disease, the patients show severe dementia, mutism, incontinence and paraparesis; some exhibit myoclonus. CT scans may show cerebral atrophy and ventricular enlargement or evidence of focal necrosis due to opportunistic infections (see p. 175).

Central nervous system pathology

Complications in the central nervous system are seen in over 50% of AIDS patients and are related either to the direct invasion of the brain by HIV or to opportunistic infections or primary cerebral lymphoma similar to those seen in patients with immunosuppression due to other causes (see p. 472).

Macroscopically, areas of softening may be seen within the brain and represent sites of localised opportunistic infection.[121] Identification of the nature of these infections usually requires microscopic examination.

The lesions due to *cytomegalovirus* infection show several characteristic features.[122] Microglial

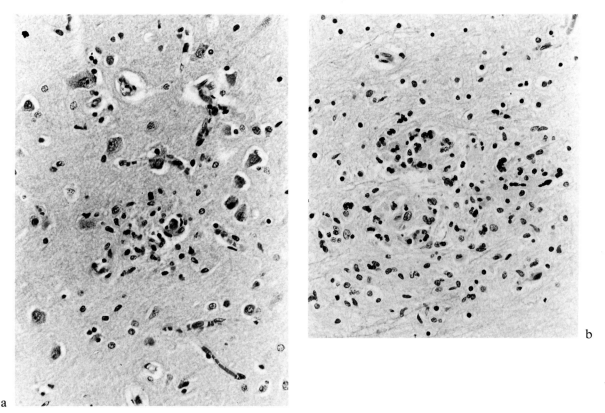

Fig. 9.11a, b Acquired immune deficiency syndrome (cytomegalovirus infection). Microglial nodules or stars are seen in (**a**) the cerebral cortex and (**b**) the white matter. They consist of rod-shaped microglial cells and reactive astrocytes. At higher power the typical intranuclear inclusions of cytomegalovirus were seen (as in Fig. 12.21, p. 338). Haematoxylin-eosin × 210

nodules (Fig. 9.11) are seen, particularly in the subcortical grey matter, and are present in all cytomegalovirus-infected brains, together with isolated inclusion-bearing cells which are usually astrocytes, endothelial cells or neurons. Microglial nodules and inclusions are often independent of each other. Focal necrosis may be present in some brains, and a necrotising ventriculoencephalitis may be present with cytomegalovirus inclusions in the ependymal cells (Fig. 12.21, p. 338). A necrotising radiculomyelitis may also be seen.[122]

Immunocytochemistry can be used to localise cytomegalovirus within the brain and also *herpes simplex virus*. *Progressive multifocal leuco-encephalopathy* (see p. 219) also occurs in AIDS patients. *Cryptococcal meningitis* (Fig. 7.25, p. 177) is seen, and in some cases a more localised crypto-coccal lesion is present in the brain. Infections by *mycobacteria* and *toxoplasma* are commonly found

in patients dying from AIDS. A nodular encephal-itis (subacute encephalitis) seen in the brain in AIDS is, in most cases, attributable to cytomegalovirus or toxoplasma infection.[123]

HIV exhibits neurotropism, and in addition to the lesions caused by opportunistic infections, a range of pathological lesions has been described which are almost certainly due to direct invasion of the brain by HIV virus.[123,124] Such changes are often associated with the AIDS dementia complex.[119,124] *Multifocal giant cell encephalitis* is characterised by the perivascular accumulation of microglia, monocytes and macrophages, and by the presence of multinucleated giant cells (Fig. 9.12). Such giant cells are derived from macrophages and contain HIV.[123] *Progressive diffuse leucoencephalopathy* is characterised by diffuse myelin loss from the cerebral white matter and elsewhere in the brain, by astrocytic

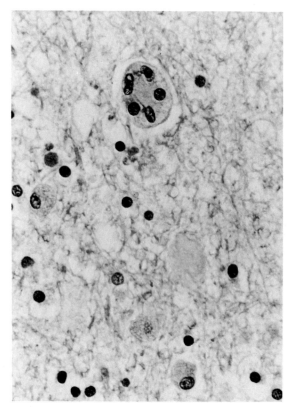

Fig. 9.12 Acquired immune deficiency syndrome. A multinucleate giant cell, typical of multifocal giant cell encephalitis, is seen in the white matter (top); foamy macrophages and reactive astrocytes (bottom). Haematoxylin-eosin × 580
Specimen kindly supplied by Prof. P. Kleihues, University of Zürich, Switzerland.

proliferation, and by infiltration by monocytes and multinucleate giant cells similar to those in Figure 9.12. Such changes are seen in the absence of evidence of opportunistic infections such as those caused by cytomegalovirus, herpes simplex virus, papovavirus, bacteria, fungi and toxoplasma. *Diffuse poliodystrophy* is seen in a high proportion of brains of patients with HIV infection; there is diffuse proliferation of astroglia with swollen nuclei, occasionally minor neuronal loss and microglial proliferation.[123] Such changes have been reported in the brains of patients with gyral atrophy and may be another type of HIV-induced damage.

Children born to mothers with AIDS fail to thrive, brain growth is arrested and there is microcephaly. Microglial nodules and multinucleate cells are seen in the brain, and there is gliosis of the white matter and calcification of blood vessels. Opportunistic infections are not usually seen in newborn patients with AIDS but HIV RNA can be localised within microglial nodules in the brains of children with AIDS.[126]

NEUROLOGICAL COMPLICATIONS OF IMMUNODEFICIENCY

Immunodeficiency may result from genetic disorders or may be a consequence of acquired disease or drug therapy. Neurological complications in these patients are broadly similar, although the incidence differs depending upon the cause of the immunosuppression. The main complications are from infections and from neoplasms. Patients particularly at risk include those who are immunosuppressed following organ transplantation,[127] patients with lymphomas, particularly if they are treated with immunosuppressive agents,[128] and patients with acquired immune deficiency syndrome (see above).[121]

Opportunistic infections by viruses and fungi are the most common complications seen in immunosuppressed patients. Mycotic infections include those caused by *Aspergillus fumigatus*, *Cryptococcus neoformans*, *Nocardia asteroides*, *Candida* species and *Coccidioides immitis* (see Ch. 7, p. 173). Many bacterial infections also occur in immunosuppressed patients but they are usually no different from those in immunocompetent patients, except that they are more severe. Two bacterial infections, however, do seem to have a predilection for immunosuppressed patients— infection by *Listeria monocytogenes* and tuberculosis (see Ch. 7, p. 159). Of the protozoa which infect the central nervous system, *Toxoplasma gondii* (see Ch. 8, p. 184) is most commonly seen in patients with organ transplants and those with lymphomas or AIDS.

There is an increased incidence of malignant tumours in patients who are immunosuppressed. These tumours include skin cancers, Kaposi's sarcoma and lymphomas. Primary B-cell lymphomas of the central nervous system have a markedly increased incidence in immunosuppressed patients (see Ch. 16, p. 472).[129]

Tumours and infections may occur concurrently in the same patient.

Viral diseases of the nervous system in immunodeficiency

Viruses of the herpes group, papovaviruses, and measles virus are the major viruses which infect the central nervous system in immunosuppressed patients, but enterovirus and adenovirus infections may also occur. Syndromes resulting from these infections are dealt with elsewhere in this volume and include encephalitis, meningitis, myelitis, progressive multifocal leucoencephalopathy and polyradiculoneuritis. The disease may have an acute onset or, as in the case of progressive multifocal leucoencephalopathy (see below), a more protracted progressive course.

Varicella-zoster infections occur in organ transplant recipients,[130] including patients who have had bone marrow transplantation,[131] and in patients with Hodgkin's disease.[132] *Herpes simplex* infections of the central nervous system are rare in immunosuppressed patients but *cytomegalovirus* (CMV) is an important member of the herpes group causing neurological complications in immunosuppression. CMV infections are mainly seen in transplant patients[133] and in patients with AIDS.[121] CMV encephalitis is characterised histologically by small groups of microglial cells (Fig.

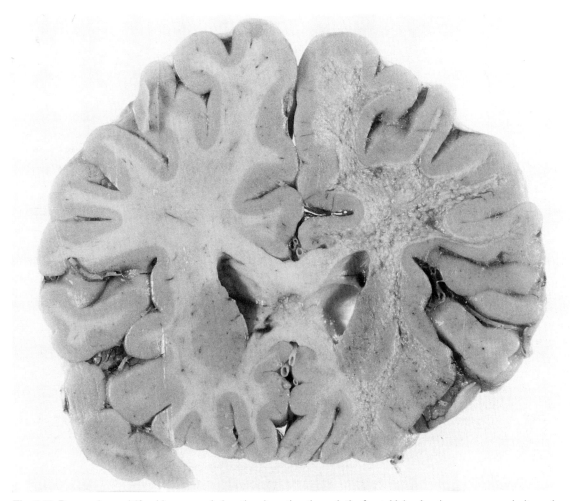

Fig. 9.13 Progressive multifocal leucoencephalopathy. A section through the frontal lobe showing coarse granularity and some cavitation in the white matter of the right cerebral hemisphere.

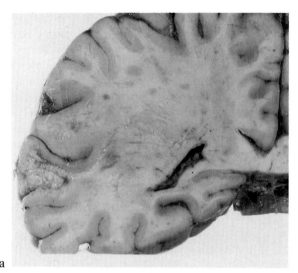

a

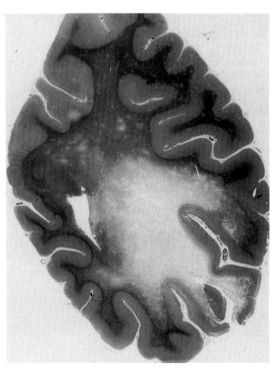

b

Fig. 9.14a, b Progressive multifocal leucoencephalopathy. (**a**) The occipital lobe white matter shows a focus of obvious granularity (left) but only vague discoloration in the periventricular regions. (**b**) Histology of the occipital lobe in (a) (picture reversed) showing extensive demyelination in the periventricular region.
Klüver–Barrera

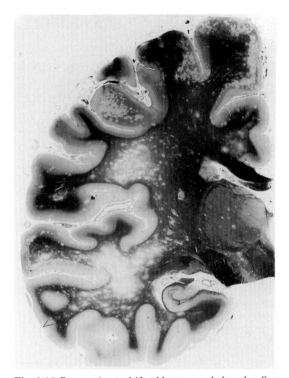

Fig. 9.15 Progressive multifocal leucoencephalopathy. Same case as Figure 9.14, showing multiple 'fluffy' areas of demyelination in the temporal and parietal white matter.
Klüver–Barrera

9.11) within the brain and the presence of typical CMV intranuclear and cytoplasmic inclusions. There is a striking absence of lymphocytic infiltration within the brain in this disease. CMV choroidoretinitis also occurs in AIDS.[134]

Measles inclusion body encephalitis is seen in immunosuppressed patients.[135] It is most commonly associated with acute lymphatic leukaemia.[136] Many of the affected patients have been in contact with measles and they present with confusion, lethargy and myoclonus. Because of their immunodeficiency, leukaemic patients may not make detectable amounts of antibody to the measles virus. They also lack a cytotoxic T-cell response and so they do not produce a measles skin rash. The majority of cases of measles inclusion body encephalitis are fatal, and the survivors have severe neurological damage. Macroscopically the brain may appear normal, and histologically it may show little inflammation. The diagnosis can be confirmed by the detection of eosinophilic intranuclear inclusions in neurons and oligodendroglial cells[36] and by immunocytochemical detection of measles antigen within the brain.[137] Although inclusion bodies may be widespread, they are often uncommon and difficult to find.

Progressive multifocal leucoencephalopathy (PML)

This disease is due to an opportunistic infection of the brain by human polyomavirus. It most commonly affects immunosuppressed patients, particularly those with lymphomas and AIDS, although it is also occasionally seen in patients with no detectable underlying immuno-suppression.

Clinical features

Patients present with progressive dementia and multifocal neurological signs, including hemiplegia, dysphagia, hemianopia, and cerebellar and brainstem features, due to the widespread involvement of the brain, especially in white matter areas. CT scan shows irregular low density non-enhancing lesions of the cerebral white matter. Most patients die within a few months or a year of the onset of the disease although some may survive for 5 years or more; the longer survival is seen in immunocompetent patients.

Pathology

Macroscopically, the fixed brain shows changes ranging from barely perceptible grey, slightly soft patches in the cerebral white matter to extensive softening and even cavitation and cystic change involving the white matter of one or both cerebral

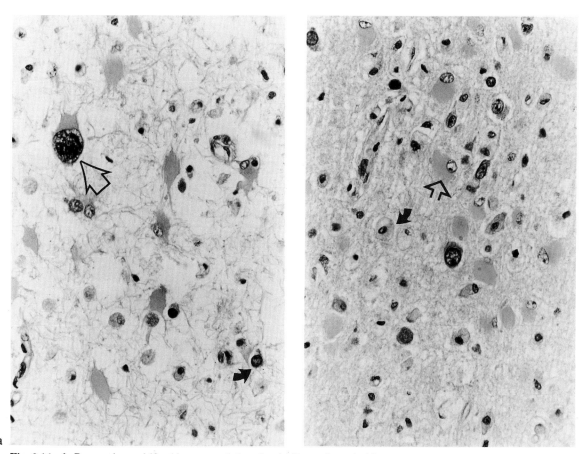

a   b

Fig. 9.16a, b Progressive multifocal leucoencephalopathy. (**a**) Demyelinated white matter showing rarefaction of the tissue with hyperchromatic nuclei of oligodendrocytes (solid arrow) and reactive astrocytes (open arrow). (**b**) Cortex adjacent to the demyelinated area showing hyperchromatic oligodendrocyte nuclei (centre) containing viral inclusions, reactive astrocytes (open arrow) and foamy macrophages (solid arrow).
Haematoxylin-eosin ×285

hemispheres (Figs 9.13 and 9.14). Similar changes may be seen in the cerebellum and brainstem.

Histologically, the affected areas show demyelination in preparations stained for myelin, e.g. by the Klüver–Barrera method. The unstained, demyelinated areas have an irregular fluffy outline. in the cerebral white matter (Figs 9.14b and 9.15)

which distinguishes this disease from multiple sclerosis, in which the demyelinated plaques have a sharply defined border (see Ch. 10, p. 231). Within the affected areas, many of the axons are preserved despite the widespread myelin loss.

The most typical histological changes in progressive multifocal leucoencephalopathy are

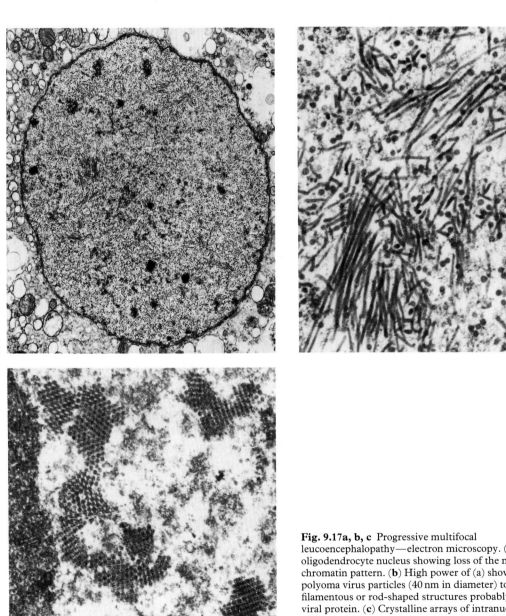

Fig. 9.17a, b, c Progressive multifocal leucoencephalopathy—electron microscopy. (a) An oligodendrocyte nucleus showing loss of the normal chromatin pattern. (b) High power of (a) showing individual polyoma virus particles (40 nm in diameter) together with filamentous or rod-shaped structures probably composed of viral protein. (c) Crystalline arrays of intranuclear polyoma virus particles.
(a) × 8500; (b) × 50 000; (c) × 40 000
(b) *Reproduced by permission of Dr J. W. Grant, Neuropathology, Southampton, UK.*

the large hyperchromatic oligodendrocyte nuclei containing basophilic viral inclusions (Fig. 9.16). In addition, astrocytes are enlarged and bizarre with hyperchromatic nuclei, often resembling those seen in glial tumours. These features are detectable in haematoxylin and eosin stained sections within the demyelinated areas of white matter and in the adjacent grey matter (Fig. 9.16). There is usually little lymphocyte accumulation around vessels, but foamy macrophages containing myelin breakdown products are present throughout the demyelinated areas. In long-standing cases, however, particularly in immuno-competent patients, there may be extensive lymphocytic infiltration, and plasma cells may be prominent in the inflammatory exudate. The large lesions are usually seen in the white matter of the cerebral hemispheres but the cerebellum and brainstem may also be extensively involved.

The distribution of polyomavirus in oligodendrocytes and astrocytes in this disease may be detected by immunocytochemistry[138] or by electron microscopy. The virus particles are usually well preserved in post-mortem tissue. Infected nuclei can be initially located by light microscopy by their abnormal chromatin patterns in 1 μm resin sections stained with toluidine blue. Low-power electron microscopy often shows a diffuse abnormality in oligodendrocyte and astrocyte nuclei (Fig. 9.17). At higher magnification the 40 nm polyomavirus particles can be detected (Fig. 9.17), either mixed with filaments and rods of redundant viral protein or in crystalline arrays.[139]

Viruses causing PML belong to the genus *Polyomavirus* in the papovavirus group. JC virus, named after the first PML patient from whom it was isolated,[140] is the causative organism in the majority of cases.[36] A few cases, however, are due to infection by SV40-like virus.[141] Infection by JC virus is widespread throughout the population; 80% of the adult population have antibodies to it.[141] It appears that infection is acquired early in life and reactivation occurs following immuno-suppression.

UNCONVENTIONAL AGENTS AND TRANSMISSIBLE DEMENTIAS

Two transmissible dementias, Creutzfeldt–Jakob disease and kuru, are discussed and illustrated in Chapter 13 (pp. 385 and 386). These two human diseases are related in their pattern of pathology and in their transmissibility to the disease scrapie in sheep. All three diseases are characterised by spongiform change in the grey matter areas of the brain and by the isolation of scrapie-associated fibrils[142] and their constituent protein PrP_{27-30}[143] from brain tissue. The nature of the transmissible agent is, as yet, unknown, but it appears to be associated with the fibrils.[144] Strict precautions are recommended when handling tissues, fluids and other material from patients with Creutzfeldt–Jakob disease,[145] as the transmissible agent is resistant to many of the conventional sterilisation procedures. Although iatrogenic routes of transmission of Creutzfeldt–Jakob disease, including patients treated with human growth hormone injections, have been recorded[27,146,147] the natural route of infection in most cases is not known.

REFERENCES

Introduction

1. Noah ND, Urquhart AM. J Infect 1980; 2: 379.
2. Griffin DE, Johnson RT. In: Mandell GL, Douglas RG, Bennett JE, eds. Principles and practice of infectious diseases. 2nd ed. New York: Wiley, 1985: 579.
3. Johnson RT. Viral infections in the nervous system. New York: Raven Press, 1982.
4. Lennette EH, Longshore WA. Calif Med 1951; 75: 189.
5. Spruance SL, Bailey A. Arch Intern Med 1973; 131: 288.
6. Hattwick MAW, Peters AH, Gregg MB et al. JAMA

1973; 225: 1338.
7. Hogan EL, Krigman MR. Arch Neurol 1973; 29: 309.
8. Johnson RT, Griffin DE. In: Vinken PJ, Bruyn GW, eds. Handbook of clinical neurology. Amsterdam: North Holland, 1978.
9. Mims CA. The pathogenesis of infectious diseases. 2nd ed. London: Academic Presss, 1982.
10. Goldfield M, Sussman D. Am J Epidemiol 1968; 87: 1.
11. Murphy FA. Arch Virol 1977; 54: 279.
12. Fields BN. Virology. New York: Raven Press, 1985.
13. Bodian D, Howe HA. Bull Johns Hopkins Hosp 1941; 68: 248.
14. Kristensson K, Vahlne A, Persson LA, Lycke E. J

Neurol Sci 1978; 35: 331.
15. Lundh B, Kristensson K, Norrby E. Neuropathol Appl Neurobiol 1987; 13: 111.
16. Helenius A, Morein B, Fries E et al. Proc Natl Acad Sci USA 1978; 75: 3846.
17. Lentz TL, Burrage TG, Smith AL. Science 1982; 215: 182.
18. Howe C, Coward JE, Genger TW. In: Fraenkel-Conrat H, Wagner RR, eds. Virus-host interactions: viral invasion, persistence and disease. New York: Plenum, 1980: 1.
19. Weiner LP, Fleming JO. J Neurosurg 1984; 61: 207.
20. Baltimore D. Bacteriol Rev 1971; 35: 235.
21. Leestma JE, Bornstein MB, Sheppard RD, Feldman LA. Lab Invest 1969; 20: 70.

Effects of viral infection upon cells

22. Bablanian R. Prog Med Virol 1975; 19: 40.
23. Madeley CR. Virus morphology. Edinburgh: Churchill Livingstone, 1972.
24. Robb JA. Prog Med Virol 1977; 23: 51.
25. Adams JH, Corsellis JAN, Duchen LW, eds. Greenfield's Neuropathology. 4th ed. London: Arnold, 1984: 289 & 997.
26. Masters CL, Richardson EP Jr. Brain 1978; 101: 333.
27. Weller RO, Steart PV, Powell-Jackson JD. Neuropathol Appl Neurobiol 1986; 12: 117.
28. Margolis G, Kilham L. Lab Invest 1969; 21: 189.

Host responses

29. Fujinami RS, Oldstone MB. J Immunol 1980; 125: 78.
30. Amos DB, Kostyu DD. Adv Hum Genet 1980; 10: 137.
31. Zinkernagel RM, Doherty PC. Adv Immunol 1979; 27: 51.
32. Bradbury MWB, Cserr HF, Westrop RJ. Am J Physiol 1981; 240: F329.
33. Szentistvanyi I, Patlak CS, Ellis RA, Cserr HF. Am J Physiol 1984; 246: F835.

Viral diseases

34. Melnick JL, Wenner HA, Phillips CA. In: Lennette EH, Schmidt NJ, eds. Diagnostic procedures for viral, rickettsial and chlamydial infections. 5th ed. Washington: American Public Health Association, 1979: 471.
35. Azimi PH, Cramblett HG, Haynes RE. JAMA 1969; 207: 509.
36. Brownell B, Tomlinson AH. In: Adams JH, Corsellis JAN, Duchen LW, eds. Greenfield's Neuropathology. 4th ed. London: Arnold, 1984: 260.
37. Kennard C, Swash M. Brain 1981; 104: 129.
38. Kennedy CR, Chrzanowska K, Robinson RO et al. Lancet 1986; 1: 989.
39. Ogilvie MM, Weller RO. In: Weller RO, Swash M, McLellan DL, Scholtz CL, eds. Clinical neuropathology. Berlin: Springer, 1983: 145.
40. Longston M. In: Heath RB, ed. Virus diseases. Tunbridge Wells: Pitman Medical, 1979: 73.
41. Illis LS, Gosling JVT. Herpes simplex encephalitis. Bristol: Scientechnica, 1972.
42. Klapper PE, Laing I, Longson M. Lancet 1981; 2: 607.
43. Nahmias AJ, Whitley RJ, Visintine AN et al. J Infect

Dis 1982; 145: 829.
44. Leading article. Lancet 1986; 1: 535.
45. Whitley RJ, Soong S-J, Dolin R et al. N Engl J Med 1977; 297: 289.
46. Longson M. J Antimicrob Chemother 1977; 3 (suppl A): 115.
47. Nicholson KG. Lancet 1984; 2: 503.
48. Sköldenberg B, Forsgren M, Alestig K et al. Lancet 1984; 2: 707.
49. Tomlinson AH, Esiri MM. J Neurol Sci 1983; 60: 473.
50. Adams JH, Miller D. Postgrad Med J 1973; 49: 393.
51. Sapsford I, Buontempo J, Weller RO. Neuropathol Appl Neurobiol 1983; 9: 181.
52. Esiri MM. J Neurol Sci 1982; 54: 209.
53. Weller RO. Colour atlas of neuropathology. Oxford: H Miller and Oxford University Press, 1984.
54. Grist NR, Bell EJ, Follett EAC, Urquhart GED. Diagnostic methods in clinical virology. 3rd ed. Oxford: Blackwell, 1979.
55. Murray JD, Stanley EA, Brown DL. Proc R Soc B 1986; 229: 111.
56. Fekadu M. Lancet 1975; 1: 569.
57. Schneider LG. Comp Immunol Microbiol Infect Dis 1982; 5: 101.
58. Nicholson K. In: Pattison JR, ed. Rabies a growing threat. Wokingham: Van Nostrand Reinhold, 1983: 6.
59. Lentz RL. Trends Neurosci 1985; 8: 360.
60. Dierks RE, Murphy FA, Harrison AK. Am J Pathol 1969; 54: 251.
61. Chopra JS, Banerjee AK, Murthy JMK, Pal SR. Brain 1980; 103: 789.
62. Hattwick MAW, Weiss TT, Stechschulte CJ et al. Ann Intern Med 1972; 76: 931.
63. Porras C, Barboza JJ, Fuenzalida E et al. Ann Intern Med 1976; 85: 44.
64. De Brito T, Araujo MD, Tiriba A. J Neurol Sci 1973; 20: 363.
65. Sung JH, Hayano M, Mastri AR, Okagaki T. J Neuropathol Exp Neurol 1976; 35: 541.
66. Cohen SL, Gardner S, Lanyi C et al. Br Med J 1976; 1: 1041.
67. Larghi OP, González L, Held JR. Appl Microbiol 1973; 25: 187.
68. Johnson HN. In: Lennette EH, Schmidt NJ, eds. Diagnostic procedures for viral, rickettsial and chlamydial infections. 5th ed. Washington: American Public Health Association, 1979: 843.
69. Grist NR, Bell EJ, Assaad F. Prog Med Virol 1978; 24: 114.
70. Shope RE, Sather GE. In: Lennette EH, Schmidt NJ, eds. Diagnostic procedures for viral, rickettsial and chlamydial infections. 5th ed. Washington: American Public Health Association, 1979; 767.
71. Monath TP. Bull WHO 1979; 57: 513.
72. Reyes MG, Gardner JJ, Poland JD, Monath TP. Arch Neurol 1981; 38: 329.
73. Lindenberg R, Haymaker W. In: Haymaker W, Adams RD, eds. Histology and histopathology of the nervous system. Springfield: Thomas, 1982: 1037.
74. Leech RW, Harris JC. J Neuropathol Exp Neurol 1977; 36: 611.
75. Hovi T, Cantell K, Huovilainen A et al. Lancet 1986; 1: 1427.
76. Kim-Farley RJ, Rutherford G, Lichfield P et al. Lancet 1984; 2: 1322.

77. WHO consultative group. Bull WHO 1982; 60: 231.
78. Sabin A. Rev Infect Dis 1981; 3: 543.
79. Bodian D. In: Rivers TM, Horsfall FL, eds. Viral and rickettsial infections of man. 3rd ed. 1959: 479.
80. Nathanson N, Martin JR. Am J Epidemiol 1979; 110: 672.
81. Fox JP. Rev Infect Dis 1980; 2: 277.
82. Walton JN. Brain's Diseases of the nervous system. Oxford: Oxford University Press, 1985.
83. Dalakas MC, Elder G, Hallett M et al. N Engl J Med 1986; 314: 959.
84. Dalakas MC. Muscle Nerve 1986; 9 (suppl 5): 117.
85. Hyman RW, Ecker JR, Tenser RB. Lancet 1983; 2: 814.
86. Esiri MM, Tomlinson AH. J Neurol Sci 1972; 15: 35.
87. McCormick WF, Rodnitzky RL, Schochet SS, McKee AP. Arch Neurol 1969; 21: 559.
88. Hallam NF, Eglin RP, Holland P et al. Lancet 1986; 2: 1213.
89. Takashima S, Becker LE. Arch Pathol Lab Med 1979; 103: 209.
90. Miller DL. Br Med J 1964; 2: 75.
91. Hart MN, Earl KM. J Neurol Neurosurg Psychiatry 1975; 38: 585.
92. Raine CS. In: Zimmerman HM, ed. Progress in neuropathology. New York: Grune and Stratton, 1976: 225.
93. Landrigan PJ, Witte JJ. JAMA 1973; 223: 1459.
94. Christie AB. Infectious diseases. 3rd ed. Edinburgh, Churchill Livingstone, 1980: 222.
95. Corsellis JAN, Janota I, Marshall AK. Neuropathol Appl Neurobiol 1983; 9: 261.
96. Allen IV. In: Adams JH, Corsellis JAN, Duchen LW, eds. Greenfield's Neuropathology. 4th ed. London: Arnold, 1984: 338.
97. Dal Canto MC, Rabinowitz SG. Ann Neurol 1982; 11: 109.
98. Crawford T. J Clin Path 1954; 7: 1.
99. Wisniewski HM, Lassmann H, Brosnan CF et al. In: Matthews WB, Glaser GH, eds. Recent advances in clinical neurology. Edinburgh: Churchill Livingstone, 1982; 3: 95.
100. Chou SM. J Neuropathol Exp Neurol 1982; 41: 357.
101. Graham DI, Behan PO, More IAR. J Neurol Neurosurg Psychiatry 1979; 42: 19.
102. Reye BDK, Morgan G, Baral J. Lancet 1963; 2: 749.
103. Trauner A. Ann Neurol 1980; 7: 2.
104. Starko KM, Ray GC, Domingnes LB et al. Pediatrics 1980; 66: 859.
105. Glasgow JFT. Arch Dis Child 1984; 59: 230.
106. Crocker JFS, Renton KW, Lee SH et al. Lab Invest 1986; 54: 32.
107. Agnarsdóttir G. In: Waterson AP, ed. Recent advances in clinical virology. London: Churchill Livingstone, 1977; 1: 21.
108. Kiessling WR, Hall WW, Yung LL, ter Meulen V. Lancet 1977; 1: 324.
109. Ohya T, Martinez AJ, Jabbour JT et al. Neurology 1974; 24: 211.
110. Esiri MM, Oppenheimer DR, Brownell B, Haire M. J Neurol Sci 1981; 53: 29.
111. Payne FE, Baublis JV, Habashi HH. N Engl J Med 1969; 281: 585.
112. Choppin PW. Ann Neurol 1981; 9: 17.
113. Townsend JJ, Stroop WG, Barringer JR et al. Neurology 1982; 32: 185.
114. Millard P. J Pathol 1983; 143: 223.
115. Levine A, Gill P, Meyer P, JAMA 1985; 254: 1921.
116. Barre-Sinoussi F, Chermann JC, Rey F et al. Science 1983; 220: 868.
117. Gallo RC, Saladhuddin SZ, Popovic M et al. Science 1984; 224: 500.
118. Osame M, Usuku K, Izumo S et al. Lancet 1986; 1: 1031.
119. Navia BA, Jordan BD, Price RW. Ann Neurol 1986; 16: 517.
120. Narayan O, Cork LC. Rev Infect Dis 1985; 7: 89.
121. Levy RM, Bredesen DE, Rosenblum ML. J Neurosurg 1985; 62: 475.
122. Morgello S, Chou E-S, Nielsen S et al. Hum Pathol 1987; 18: 289.
123. Budka H, Costanzi G, Cristina S et al. Acta Neuropathol 1987; 75: 185.
124. Navia BA, Chou E-S, Petito CK et al. Ann Neurol 1986; 19: 525.
125. Johnson RT, McArthur JC. Trends Neurosci 1986; 9: 91.
126. Shaw GM, Harper ME, Hahn BH. Science 1985; 227: 177.
127. Hooper DC, Pruitt AA, Rubin RH. Medicine 1982; 61: 166–188.
128. Henson RA, Urich H. Cancer and the nervous system. The neurological manifestations of systemic malignant disease. Oxford: Blackwell, 1982; 487.
129. Penn I. Surgery 1978; 83: 492.
130. Luby JP, Ramivez-Ronda C, Rinner S et al. J Infect Dis 1977; 135: 659.
131. Locksley RM, Flournoy N, Sullivan KM, Meyers JD. J Infect Dis 1985; 152: 1172.
132. Ho M. Arch Virol 1977; 55: 1.
133. Schober R, Herman MM. Lancet 1973; 1: 962.
134. Kennedy PGE, Newsome DA, Mess J. Br Med J 1986; 293: 162.
135. Lyon G. C R Acad Sci (Paris) [D] 1972; 274: 1878.
136. Agamanolis DP, Tan JS, Parker DL. Arch Neurol 1979; 36: 686.
137. Drysdale HC, Jones LF, Oppenheimer DR, Tomlinson AH. J Clin Pathol 1976; 29: 865.
138. Budka H, Shah KV. J Neuropathol Exp Neurol 1982; 41: 366.
139. ZuRhein GM, Chou SM. Science 1965; 148: 1477.
140. Padgett BL, Walker DL, ZuRhein GM et al. Lancet 1971; 1: 1257.
141. Padgett BL, Walker DL. J Infect Dis 1973; 127: 467.
142. Merz PA, Rohwer RG, Kascsak R et al. Science 1984; 225: 437.
143. Prusiner SB. Science 1982; 216: 136.
144. Kimberlin RH. Neuropathol Appl Neurobiol 1986; 12: 131.
145. Rosenberg RN, White CL, Brown P et al. Ann Neurol 1986; 19: 75.
146. Matthews WB. Neuropathol Appl Neurobiol 1986; 12: 111.
147. Weller RO. Psychol Med 1989; 19: 1.

Demyelinating diseases: Multiple sclerosis

INTRODUCTION

By definition, there is destruction of myelin and preservation of axons in demyelinating diseases. If the demyelination is extensive and the disease longstanding, many of the axons may also degenerate. Demyelination is a feature of several central and peripheral nervous system disorders:

1. Central nervous system
   a. Multiple sclerosis (this chapter)
   b. Post-infectious encephalomyelitis (p. 207)
   c. Progressive multifocal leucoencephalopathy (PML) due to papovavirus infection (p. 219)
   d. Toxic and nutritional disorders
      (i) Machiafava–Bignami syndrome (p. 259)
      (ii) Central pontine myelinosis (p. 260)
   e. Leucodystrophies (p. 348)
2. Central and peripheral nervous systems
   Certain leucodystrophies
      (i) Metachromatic leucodystrophies (p. 344)
      (ii) Krabbe's disease (p. 345)
      (iii) Adrenoleucodystrophy (p. 349)
3. Peripheral nervous system
   a. Post-infectious polyradiculoneuropathy (Guillain–Barré syndrome) (p. 551)
   b. Toxic and metabolic neuropathies: Diphtheria (p. 273), diabetes (p. 555)
   c. Hereditary sensorimotor neuropathies (hypertrophic neuropathies) (p. 573).

Many of these disorders are discussed in other chapters; the structure of myelin is reviewed in Chapter 1 and the general pathology of demyelination in Chapter 2. This chapter is mainly devoted to the pathology of multiple sclerosis.

MULTIPLE SCLEROSIS

Originally well documented by Charcot[1] in the mid-nineteenth century, multiple sclerosis (sclérose en plaques, disseminated sclerosis), presents clinically with the onset of focal neurological deficits and usually runs a relapsing and remitting course which may eventually become progressive, or the course may be progressive from the start.[2] The average survival of patients with multiple sclerosis is between 13 and 20 years although some patients die within a few weeks or months of the onset of the disease. Pathologically,[3,4] multiple sclerosis is characterised by the presence of multiple plaques of demyelination throughout the central nervous system, including the spinal cord and optic nerves, but the peripheral nervous system is largely spared. Many of the older plaques are sharply defined, grey and sclerotic due to the absence of myelin and the presence of astrocytic scar tissue.

Although much is known about the epidemiology of multiple sclerosis, its clinical patterns, pathophysiology and pathological features, the exact cause of the disease is unknown. It does appear, however, that multiple sclerosis is caused by an environmental agent or agents which induce damage to the central nervous system in genetically susceptible individuals, probably by auto-immune mechanisms. The identity of the antigens to which the immunological reaction is directed is not known.

Epidemiology

The age of onset of multiple sclerosis shows a consistent pattern, particularly in areas where it is common.[5] Risk of developing the disease rises steeply with age from early adolescence to a peak in the late twenties or early thirties at which age, in Boston, Massachusetts, for example, the annual incidence is 9 per 100 000 of the population. After the age of 30 years, the incidence declines steeply so that the onset of the disease is uncommon after the age of 60 years. Multiple sclerosis is more common in females, but the female to male ratio

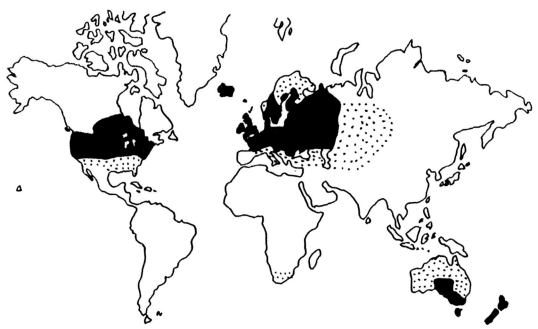

Fig. 10.1 Geographical distribution of multiple sclerosis. High frequency areas: black. Medium frequency areas: dotted. Areas of low frequency or of insufficient data: white.

varies from 1·1 in high incidence areas to 1·8 in the USA and 2·5–2·8 in low incidence areas such as South Africa and Western Australia.

There is a distinct geographical distribution of multiple sclerosis (Fig. 10·1).[5] The frequency of the disease increases with distance from the equator, both in the northern and southern hemispheres. Thus, the annual incidence, i.e. the number of new cases per year divided by the population at risk, is 3·2 per 100 000 in Rochester, Minnesota, and 0·4 per 100 000 in New Orleans in the south of the USA. The highest annual rate of incidence of 9·3 per 100 000 is in the Orkney Islands, north of Scotland. Prevalence rates, i.e. the number of cases living on a particular date divided by the population at risk on that date, vary from 10 per 100 000 in New Orleans to an overall figure for the USA of 62 per 100 000 for whites and 32 for non-whites. The highest prevalence rates are in the North-east of Scotland at 144 per 100 000, and multiple sclerosis is more common in Northern Europe and Switzerland than in the USA.[5] It is less common in the southern hemisphere and is rare in Japan and in the tropics. Emigration from a high risk to a low risk area before the age of 15 years is associated with a reduced risk of multiple sclerosis.[5]

Genetic factors

In addition to the influence of latitude upon the incidence of multiple sclerosis, it is also clear that, for some races, the risk of developing the disease is low and does not depend upon the latitude of their environment. For example, multiple sclerosis is rare in the Bantu and in Eskimos and in oriental races.[5] It appears, therefore, that genetic factors may play a rôle in the aetiology of multiple sclerosis. This is further reinforced by the study of twins, in which it was found that both of a pair of twins more commonly develop multiple sclerosis if they are monozygotic than if they are dizygotic.[6,7]

There is also a relationship between the histocompatibility antigens (HLA) and multiple sclerosis.[5,8] Sited on chromosome 6, the HLA region is concerned with the genetic control of the immune system.[8] In most Northern European populations, there is an association between multiple sclerosis and the gene products DW2 and DR2, but in Japanese the association is with BW22 and DR6.[7,8] The association between HLA and multiple sclerosis is seen as evidence of an auto-immune pathogenesis.[8] Inconsistency of the HLA association is explicable on the basis that there are other genes which also influence the character and persistence of chronic immune responses.[8]

Clinical features

Clinical presentation and the course of the disease are very varied.[2] In the early stages of multiple sclerosis, most patients present with a single focal neurological deficit which is present in the acute stages of the disease and then remits. Such remissions may be long and often complete in the early stages of the disease. With time, however, there is a cumulative effect of earlier lesions and this creates a persistent background of disability upon which the neurological deficit associated with fresh lesions is superimposed. During this time, the patient's neurological state fluctuates as fresh lesions appear and then temporarily regress. Patients with longstanding multiple sclerosis often exhibit ataxia, spasticity, motor weakness and bladder dysfunction. Occasionally, severe cases with the onset in early adult life run a progressive course from the onset, without remission. More indolent, chronic cases occurring in middle age may also run a progressive course.

Focal neurological deficits in multiple sclerosis have a rapid onset, developing over a few hours or 1–2 days. 50% of the patients show limb weakness and some 30% have visual symptoms such as blurring of vision with retrobulbar neuritis, double vision or blindness. Others have sensory symptoms, tremor or vertigo. Some intellectual impairment is not uncommon and there may be dementia in the later stages of the disease. Emotional changes are frequent, with euphoria, depression or irritability. Sphincter control involving the bladder and bowel is frequently impaired.

Although the onset and course of the disease vary considerably between different patients, a number of symptom complexes are recognised.[2,9] Devic's disease, for example, is a rather rare form of multiple sclerosis but is recognised clinically from the presence of retrobulbar neuritis and severe spinal cord involvement (see p. 240).

Investigations

The diagnosis of multiple sclerosis is made primarily on clinical grounds.[2] No test is consistently positive or abnormal in 100% of cases of clinically definite multiple sclerosis, but a number of investigations may be helpful in establishing the diagnosis.

Cerebrospinal fluid (CSF) tests have shown that 90% of patients with multiple sclerosis have abnormal synthesis of immunoglobulins in the central nervous system with oligoclonal IgG bands on electrophoresis of CSF.[10,11]

Electrophysiological investigations are also often used in the assessment of multiple sclerosis. Visual evoked potentials (VEP) are the minute electrical responses of the occipital cortex to visual stimuli. VEPs are abnormal in some 90% of patients with multiple sclerosis,[2,12] with an increase in the time interval between stimulus and response (Fig. 10.2); this is attributed to slowing of conduction through demyelinated segments of the optic nerve. Auditory evoked potentials are abnormal in a high proportion of cases of definite multiple sclerosis, due to the presence of plaques of demyelination in the brainstem. However, lack of correlation between electrophysiological and clinical findings limits the use of this investigation in the diagnosis of multiple sclerosis.[2]

Computerised tomography (CT) scans reveal multiple sclerosis plaques as areas of low attenuation which enhance in the acute stages of the disease.[13] More plaques are visualised by magnetic resonance imaging (MRI) than by CT scans, and their typical periventricular location is emphasised.[14] However, neither CT nor MRI is specific for multiple sclerosis plaques, and with MRI it may be difficult to distinguish the focal lesions of cerebrovascular disease from multiple sclerosis plaques.[14]

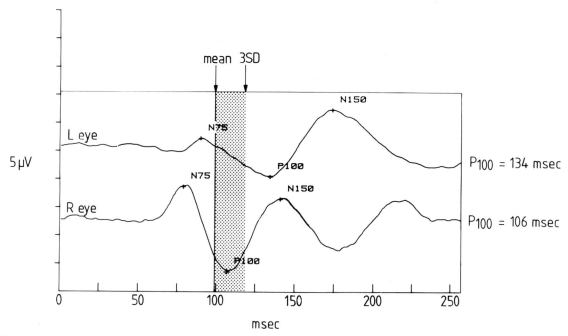

Fig. 10.2 Visual evoked potentials in multiple sclerosis showing the wave form evoked by pattern reversal of a chequerboard screen. Recordings were made from electrodes placed over the occipital lobes. P100 is the positive wave form normally seen at about 100 ms; it is normal in the right eye (100 ms) but significantly delayed in the left eye (134 ms). The delay is attributed to slowing of axon conduction across a demyelinated plaque in the optic nerve.
Illustration kindly supplied by Dr. EM Sedgwick, Clinical Neurophysiology, Southampton, UK.

Pathology

The majority of patients with multiple sclerosis survive for many years with the disease. Thus, most of the cases seen at post-mortem exhibit the classical picture of chronic multiple sclerosis with old, grey, sclerotic plaques distributed throughout the brain and spinal cord. A minority of patients die within a few months of the onset of an acute attack or of a major relapse. These patients may have acute, soft, granular, actively demyelinating plaques in the brain and spinal cord. Less common forms of multiple sclerosis include Schilder's type which is characterised by widespread demyelination throughout the cerebral white matter, with extensive gliosis and shrinkage of the brain (see p. 238). Baló's concentric sclerosis is a rarer form of multiple sclerosis (see p. 240).

One major feature which tends to distinguish most cases of multiple sclerosis from other pathological lesions, such as infarcts, is the presence of sharply defined plaques of demyelination in the brain and spinal cord with relative preservation of axons.

Acute active multiple sclerosis

Death within the first five years of the onset of multiple sclerosis is uncommon,[2] but those patients who do die within the first few months of the disease may have extensive brainstem lesions or transverse myelitis with a large multiple sclerosis plaque in the spinal cord. Respiratory paralysis and bronchopneumonia are commonly the causes of death.

Macroscopic inspection of the brain may reveal

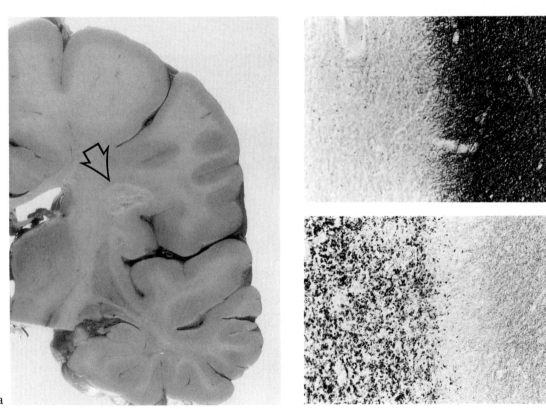

Fig. 10.3a–c Acute multiple sclerosis. (**a**) Coronal section of brain showing a soft granular acute plaque in the white matter (arrow). (**b**) The sharply defined edge of a plaque: normal white matter stained black; plaque (left) is unstained. (**c**) Same field as (b) showing lipid-filled macrophages in the plaque (left).
(**b**) Weil × 50; (**c**) Frozen section, oil red O × 50
(**c**) *Reproduced by permission of the editors and publishers from: Weller RO. In: Matthews WB, Acheson ED, Batchelor JR, Weller RO. McAlpine's Multiple Sclerosis. Edinburgh: Churchill Livingstone, 1985 (Figs. 12.1 & 12.2)*

little external abnormality at post-mortem. When the brain is sliced, acute multiple sclerosis plaques appear as soft pink or yellow granular areas in the cerebral white matter (Fig. 10.3a), brainstem or spinal cord. Such plaques may be difficult to identify macroscopically.

Histologically, frozen sections and paraffin sections of brain and spinal cord stained for myelin show sharply defined demyelinated plaques (Fig. 10.3b) which, despite the loss of myelin from the centre of the plaque, still contain many intact axons. Lipid stains (oil red O) on frozen sections show large amounts of myelin breakdown products in the form of droplets of globular cholesterol esters in macrophages within the

demyelinated area (Fig. 10.3c).[15] There is widespread perivascular cuffing by lymphocytes, plasma cells, monocytes and macrophages in the acute lesions (Fig. 10.4). The inflammatory cells accumulate in the perivascular spaces between the basement membrane of the glia limitans and the vessel wall.[16] Lymphocytes, plasma cells and rod-shaped microglia, together with foamy macrophages, are also abundant within the plaque away from the perivascular regions (Figs 10.4 and 10.5). Most of the lymphocytes are T-cells[17] with mainly T-suppressor-cytotoxic cells in the perivascular regions and T-helper cells at the edges of the plaques and in adjacent white matter. The majority of the plasma cells in the plaques contain

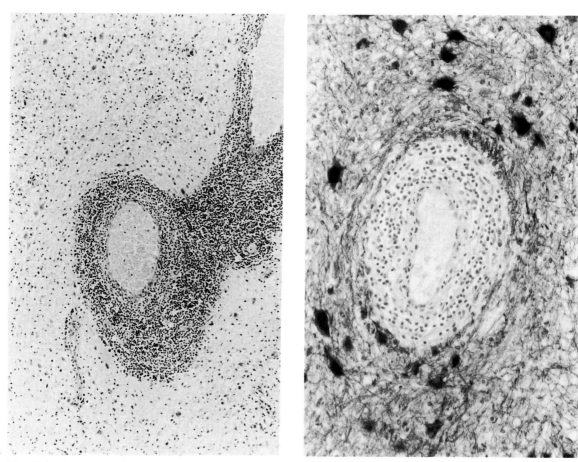

a   b

Fig. 10.4a, b Acute multiple sclerosis. (a) A thick collar of lymphocytes, plasma cells and monocytes around a vein in the centre of a plaque. Inflammatory cells are also seen in the surrounding plaque tissue. (b) A blood vessel in the plaque surrounded by mononuclear inflammatory cells and by darkly stained reactive astrocytes.
(a) Haematoxylin-eosin × 75, (b) Immunocytochemistry for GFAP × 190
(a) *Reproduced by permission of the editors and publishers from: Weller RO. In: Matthews WB, Acheson ED, Batchelor JR, Weller RO. McAlpine's Multiple Sclerosis. Edinburgh: Churchill Livingstone, 1985 (Fig. 12.3).*

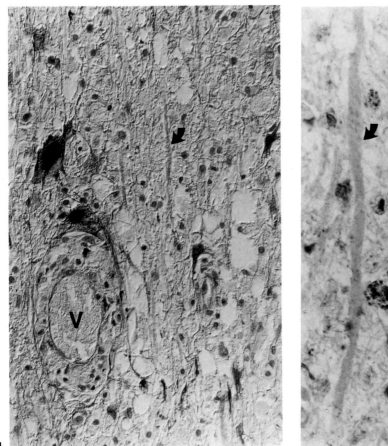

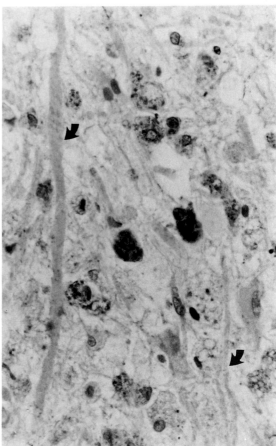

a

b

Fig. 10.5a, b Acute multiple sclerosis: the centre of a demyelinated plaque. (**a**) Darkly stained reactive astrocytes extend processes towards a vessel (V). Demyelinated axons arrowed. Foamy macrophages are seen in the perivascular spaces and between the demyelinated axons. (**b**) Darkly stained macrophages are seen among the demyelinated axons (arrows). (**a**) Immunoperoxidase for GFAP (interference contrast) × 300; (**b**) Immunoperoxidase for α_1-antichymotrypsin × 480

IgG, but small amounts of IgA are also present.[18] Although the thick perivascular inflammatory cuffs are mainly around thin-walled veins within the demyelinated plaques, peri-arterial cuffs of cells are also seen.[4] The perivascular distribution of inflammatory cells probably reflects their usual route of migration from venules into the tissue.

Lymphocytes, microglial cells and macrophages also form a hypercellular border to a demyelinated plaque and inflammatory cells extend into the intact white matter at the edges of acute plaques.

Another major feature of acute active multiple sclerosis plaques is the hypertrophy and proliferation of reactive astrocytes (Figs 10.4b and 10.5a). Processes of the reactive astrocytes stain strongly for glial fibrillary acidic protein (GFAP)

in immunocytochemical preparations; such processes interweave among the demyelinated axons and inflammatory cells (Fig. 10.5a). Astrocyctes also contain serum protein taken up from the oedema fluid in the plaque; the presence of oedema fluid reflects the breakdown of the blood-brain barrier in multiple sclerosis plaques which accompanies the inflammatory reaction and the destruction of myelin.

Axons preserved within a multiple sclerosis plaque can be demonstrated either by silver stains such as the Palmgren technique (Fig. 10.6), by immunocytochemistry for neurofilament proteins, in 1 μm resin sections, or by electron microscopy. As axons enter the plaque, myelin sheaths are lost and the axons are left surrounded only by extra-

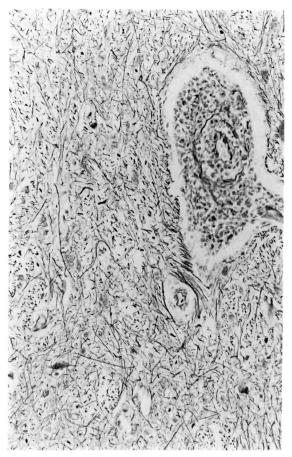

Fig. 10.6 Acute multiple sclerosis. Intact axons within a plaque of demyelination are stained black. Perivascular inflammatory cells (top right).
Palmgren × 240

functionally insignificant. Such remyelinated segments of axons are surounded by very thin myelin sheaths and this may account for the pale myelin staining that occurs around some plaques (shadow plaques).[21]

The presence of large numbers of inflammatory cells in acute multiple sclerosis lesions helps to distinguish these lesions from chronic plaques and from other causes of demyelination. Furthermore, the influx of lymphocytes, plasma cells and macrophages into the brain in these plaques strongly suggests that immune mechanisms are involved in the demyelination.

Chronic multiple sclerosis (classical type)

In more than 50% of patients dying with chronic multiple sclerosis, the cause of death is directly related to multiple sclerosis.[2] Pneumonia, septicaemia, pyelonephritis following bladder dysfunction, and sepsis from bedsores are the usual causes of death.

Macroscopic appearances and distribution of the plaques. Little abnormality may be visible on external inspection of the brain or spinal cord at postmortem. However, in some cases of chronic multiple sclerosis, there is cerebral atrophy with grey gliotic plaques of demyelination visible on the external aspects, particularly of the optic nerves and chiasma and on the anterior surface of the brainstem (see Fig. 10.12a). Removal of the arachnoid and pia mater from the front of the pons and medulla may be necessary to display the sharply defined but irregular shrunken grey plaques.

In the unfixed brain, plaques appear as firm, dark grey, sharply defined areas silhouetted against the white matter or barely discernible in the grey matter. However, the unfixed brain is soft and easily distorted. The distribution of plaques is, therefore, more accurately determined in slices of fixed brain and in large histological sections stained for myelin by the Klüver–Barrera technique.

Multiple sclerosis plaques may occur virtually anywhere in the central nervous system. They are usually asymmetrical in their distribution and the pattern varies widely from case to case.[21] However, the optic nerves, the chiasma, the periventricular

cellular fluid, astrocyte processes and macrophages (Fig. 10.5). Some axonal destruction occurs in acute multiple sclerosis plaques, as seen by the presence of irregular swellings and terminal axon balloons in white matter plaques and chromatolysis of neurons in the adjacent grey matter.

Oligodendrocytes are severely reduced in number in multiple sclerosis plaques but, in the acute plaques, it may be difficult to distinguish oligodendrocytes from other cell types, especially lymphocytes. Immunocytochemical studies, however, suggest that oligodendrocytes may be increased in number at the edges of acute multiple sclerosis plaques.[19] Some remyelination may occur at the edge of the plaque[20] but it is probably

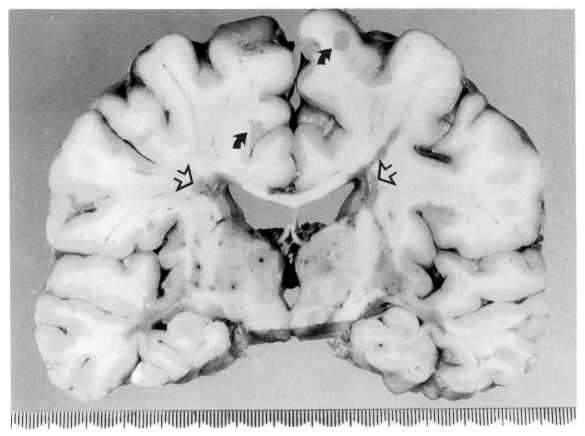

Fig. 10.7 Chronic multiple sclerosis. A coronal slice through the cerebral hemispheres at the level of the thalamus. Grey, slightly shiny opalescent plaques are seen at the corners of both lateral ventricles (open arrows) and adjacent to the temporal horns of the lateral ventricles. Circular plaques in the grey matter (solid arrows).

white matter, the brainstem and the spinal cord are sites of predilection.[21] In one survey[22] 40% of plaques in the cerebral hemispheres abutted on the lateral ventricles, 22% were in the frontal lobes, 15% in the parietal regions, 12% in the temporal lobes and only 1% in the occipital lobes. 74% of plaques involved the white matter and 17% involved the cortex and white matter. Only 5% were restricted to the cortex and 4% to the central grey matter.

In coronal sections of a fixed brain, multiple sclerosis plaques are seen as sharply defined firm grey areas, especially around the lateral corners and the temporal horns of the lateral ventricles (Fig. 10.7). The plaques in the grey matter may be difficult to detect but appear as well-circumscribed areas which are slightly darker than the grey matter itself (Fig. 10.7). Detailed examination of the

plaques reveals in most cases a very sharply defined border between the plaque and the white matter (Fig. 10.8). Horizontal sections of brain allowing a view of the roof of the lateral ventricles show that the plaques extend along the walls of the ventricles and are, in fact, blocks of demyelinated tissue rather than flat plaques.

Multiple sclerosis plaques can be distinguished from areas of infarction, which are either haemorrhagic in the early stages or necrotic and cystic in the later stages.

In large histological sections chronic multiple sclerosis plaques are seen as sharply defined areas devoid of myelin. In Figures 10.9 and 10.10 such plaques are seen in the periventricular regions and in the corpus callosum and as small, well-circumscribed, often circular areas in the cortical grey matter and in the basal ganglia (Fig.

10.9). Small finger-like extensions (Dawson's fingers),[4,23] may be seen where the plaque of demyelination has extended along a blood vessel (Fig. 10.10).

The extensive gliosis which occurs in multiple sclerosis plaques can be well demonstrated by the Holzer stain for astrocytes (Fig. 10.11). Such plaques of gliosis mirror the areas of demyelination.[3]

Although many of the large plaques are seen in the cerebral hemispheres, smaller plaques elsewhere in the brainstem, cerebellum and spinal cord may be responsible for many of the more severe disabilities of the multiple sclerosis patient. As the brainstem has white matter on the surface, multiple sclerosis plaques may be detected on the external aspects (Fig. 10.12a). On horizontal slicing of the brainstem, the distribution of plaques may be random but the peri-aqueductal grey matter (Fig. 10.12b) is frequently involved, producing disorders of eye movement.

The optic nerves are frequently involved in multiple sclerosis—at post-mortem the nerves and chiasma may be shrunken, and plaques may be visible on the external surfaces. Histological sections (Fig. 10.13) show the sharply defined plaques within the optic nerve.

Grey, shrunken plaques of demyelination may be detected on the external surface of the spinal cord in many cases of multiple sclerosis. Serial horizontal sections of the spinal cord reveal plaques as grey, shrunken, often triangular areas of demyelination within the white matter. Although all levels of the spinal cord may contain plaques, they are most commonly seen in the cervical region and a high proportion involve the lateral columns of white matter.[24] In Figure 10.14, there is a large, triangular plaque of demyelination laterally. The secondary effects of multiple sclerosis are also seen in this figure, with loss of myelin staining due to axonal degeneration in the gracile tracts: dorsal column axons passing through a plaque lower down in the cord have been damaged and axons in the tract have degenerated.

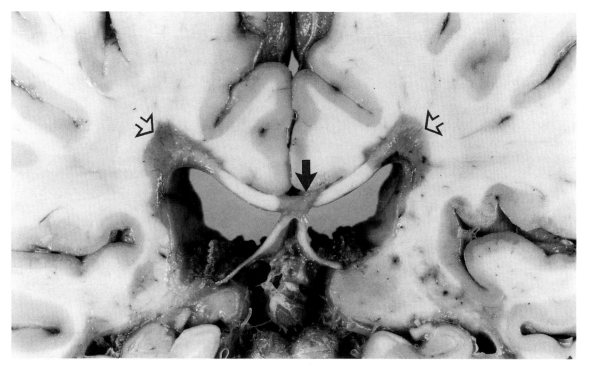

Fig. 10.8 Chronic multiple sclerosis. A close-up view of periventricular plaques (open arrows). A plaque is also present in the centre of the atrophic corpus callosum (solid arrow).

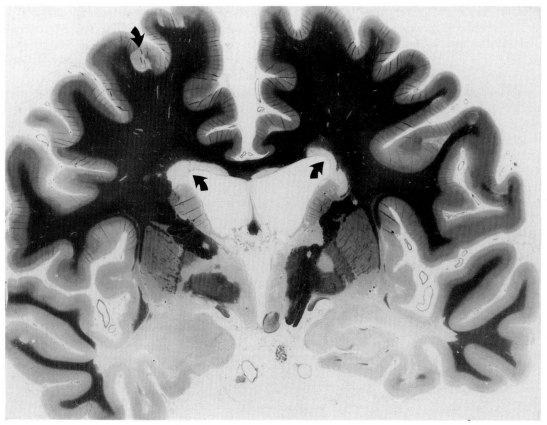

Fig. 10.9 Chronic multiple sclerosis. A histological section of a coronal slice of both cerebral hemispheres through the basal ganglia. Myelin: black; plaques: white. The plaques are distributed around the ventricles (arrows), in the temporal lobes, and around the third ventricle and in the globus pallidus. A circular plaque in the cortex is seen top left (arrow). Klüver–Barrera.
Reproduced by permission of the editors and publishers from: Weller RO. In: Matthews WB, Acheson ED, Batchelor JR, Weller RO. McAlpine's Multiple Sclerosis. Edinburgh: Churchill Livingstone, 1985 (Fig. 12.19)

Histology of chronic multiple sclerosis. A major feature of chronic multiple sclerosis is the wide spatial distribution of plaques. There is also, however, temporal distribution so that some plaques in multiple sclerosis brains are still showing active demyelination where others are completely 'burnt-out' and quiescent. The distinction between *chronic active plaques* and *burnt-out plaques* can usually only be made histologically.

The appearances of the *chronic active* plaque are shown in Figure 10.15. At the centre of the plaque, a few vessels may still be partly surrounded by lymphocytes and macrophages. Within the adjacent plaque tissue (Fig. 10.15a) the histological appearance is intermediate between an acute active plaque and a burnt-out plaque. There are plump,

reactive astrocytes and preserved axons but few macrophages. At the edges of the plaque, however, there are signs of active myelin breakdown (Fig. 10.15b), with foamy macrophages distributed between the preserved axons and reactive astrocytes. The macrophage invasion extends right up to the border with the normal white matter at the edge of the plaque (Fig. 10.15c). Immunocytochemical techniques can be used to identify the cellular elements in these active regions. The axons can be stained for neurofilament protein, the macrophages for α_1-antichymotrypsin or other macrophage markers, and the astrocytes for glial fibrillary acidic protein.

In association with both acute active and chronic active multiple sclerosis, mononuclear inflammatory cells may be seen around vessels in the

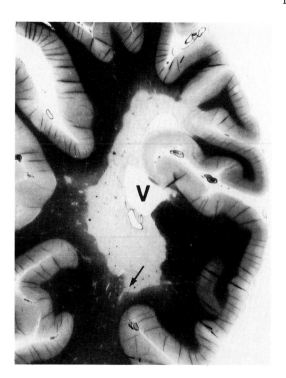

leptomeninges (Fig. 10.15d). Usually the inflammatory cells are around veins.

The histological appearance in *chronic, burnt-out,* multiple sclerosis plaques differs from that in the chronic active plaques. Very few inflammatory cells are present and the astrocytes are no longer plump and reactive but have long, thin processes and smaller, often elongated, nuclei. Many, but by no means all, of the axons are preserved within chronic multiple sclerosis plaques although the myelin has been completely destroyed. Figure 10.16a shows the edge of a chronic multiple sclerosis plaque where the myelinated white matter ends abruptly. Within the plaque, not only is the myelin lost but the number of oligodendrocytes is greatly reduced. This destruction of oligodendrocytes is

Fig. 10.10 Chronic multiple sclerosis. A histological section of the occipital lobe showing a demyelinated area around the temporal horn of the lateral ventricle (V). Myelin: black. Finger-like extensions of the plaque are seen (arrow). Klüver–Barrera

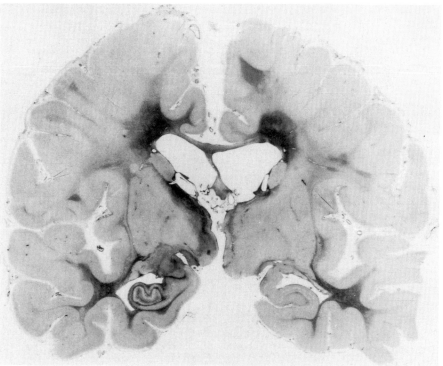

Fig. 10.11 Chronic multiple sclerosis. A histological section of both cerebral hemispheres stained for astrocytes (dark). There is gliosis in periventricular plaques and in the temporal white matter. Holzer

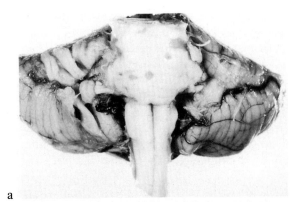

a

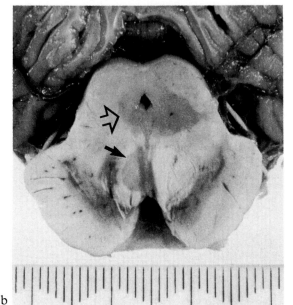

b

Fig. 10.12a, b Chronic multiple sclerosis in the brainstem. (**a**) Anterior surface of the pons from which the leptomeninges have been stripped, showing shrunken grey, multiple sclerosis plaques on the surface. (**b**) Horizontal section of the midbrain showing the peri-aqueductal plaque (open arrow) and another plaque just ventral to it (solid arrow).

thought to be the main reason why remyelination does not occur to any significant extent in multiple sclerosis. Using a combined axon and myelin stain, the loss of myelin sheaths can be observed at the edge of the plaque (Fig. 10.16b); although the myelin is lost, many of the demyelinated axons continue into the plaque.

Burnt-out multiple sclerosis plaques show little or no direct residual evidence of the inflammation that occurred during the active stages of demyelination. However, small blood vessels in

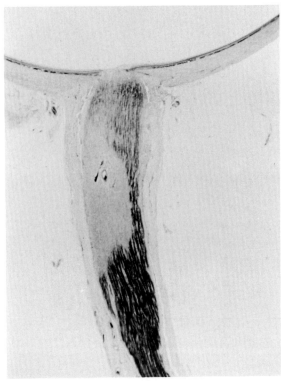

Fig. 10.13 Chronic multiple sclerosis. A demyelinated plaque in the retrobulbar portion of the optic nerve. The back of the eye is at the top of the picture. Loyez × 5

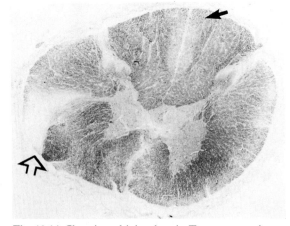

Fig. 10.14 Chronic multiple sclerosis. Transverse section through the cervical spinal cord showing a triangular demyelinated plaque (open arrow) abutting onto the surface of the cord. There is degeneration of the gracile tracts in the posterior columns (solid arrow). Klüver–Barrera × 5

Reproduced by permission of the editors and publishers from: Weller RO. In: Matthews WB, Acheson ED, Batchelor JR, Weller RO. McAlpine's Multiple Sclerosis. Edinburgh: Churchill Livingstone, 1985 (Fig. 12.27)

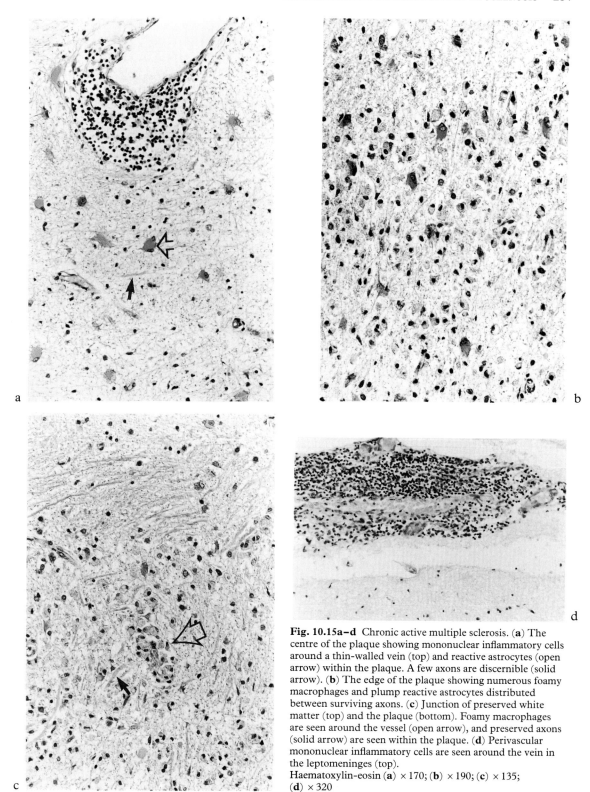

Fig. 10.15a–d Chronic active multiple sclerosis. (**a**) The centre of the plaque showing mononuclear inflammatory cells around a thin-walled vein (top) and reactive astrocytes (open arrow) within the plaque. A few axons are discernible (solid arrow). (**b**) The edge of the plaque showing numerous foamy macrophages and plump reactive astrocytes distributed between surviving axons. (**c**) Junction of preserved white matter (top) and the plaque (bottom). Foamy macrophages are seen around the vessel (open arrow), and preserved axons (solid arrow) are seen within the plaque. (**d**) Perivascular mononuclear inflammatory cells are seen around the vein in the leptomeninges (top).
Haematoxylin-eosin (**a**) × 170; (**b**) × 190; (**c**) × 135; (**d**) × 320

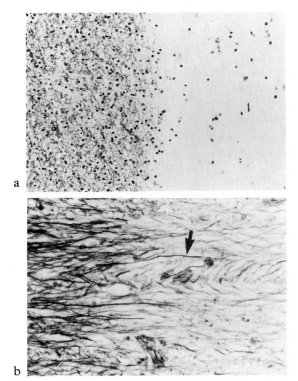

a

b

Fig. 10.16a, b Chronic inactive (burnt-out) multiple
sclerosis. (**a**) The edge of a plaque stained for myelin.
Normal white matter and numerous oligodendrocyte nuclei
are seen on the left. Demyelinated plaque lacking myelin
sheaths and with very few oligodendrocytes at right. (**b**) Edge
of plaque stained for myelin and axons. Myelinated axons
(left) lose their myelin sheaths as they enter the plaque
(right). Demyelinated axon (arrow).
(**a**) Klüver–Barrera × 160. (**b**) Palmgren–Luxol fast blue × 160
(**a**) *Reproduced by permission of the editors and publishers from:
Weller RO. In: Matthews WB, Acheson ED, Batchelor JR,
Weller RO. McAlpine's Multiple Sclerosis. Edinburgh:
Churchill Livingstone, 1985 (Figs 12.34 and 12.35)*

the centre of the plaque and larger vessels in the
periventricular regions are surrounded by a thick
coat of perivascular reticulin (Fig. 10.17). The
reticulin was probably induced and laid down
during the active inflammatory stage of the plaque
when large numbers of lymphocytes and plasma
cells surrounded these vessels.

The summary diagram in Figure 10.18
illustrates the major features in the evolution of the
multiple sclerosis plaque.

Schilder type of multiple sclerosis

In some patients with multiple sclerosis, and
particularly those with a history of progressive
intellectual deterioration and dementia, the brain

is mildly or severely atrophic. The ventricles are
large and much of the cerebral white matter is
shrunken, opalescent and grey, and firm in
consistency; there may even be cavitation of the
affected areas of white matter.[25] Well-defined
multiple sclerosis plaques are also present in the
cerebral hemispheres and throughout the
brainstem, cerebellum and spinal cord in 70% of
cases of Schilder's type of the disease.[26]

Histological sections reveal extensive gliosis and
diffuse, though often incomplete, loss of myelin
from the shrunken cerebral white matter. The loss
of axons from the cerebral white matter may be
more extensive than in classical multiple sclerosis
plaques, and there may be signs of inflammation
with the presence of lymphocytes, microglia and
macrophages within the affected areas.

The term *'Schilder's disease'* is derived from the
original description by Schilder[27] of brains

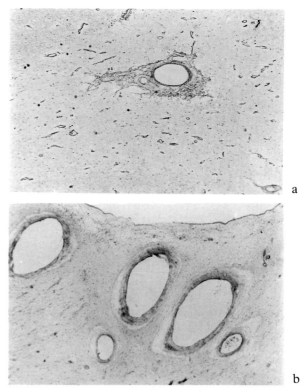

a

b

Fig. 10.17a, b Blood vessels in a chronic inactive (burnt-
out) plaque. (**a**) Centre of the plaque showing a small vein
surrounded by perivascular fibrosis. (**b**) Vessels in the
periventricular portion of a plaque. Ventricle at top. The
vessels are probably veins and have thickened fibrotic walls.
Gordon and Sweet (**a**) × 40; (**b**) × 25

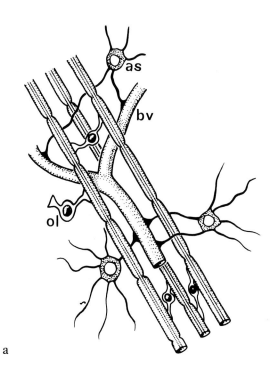

a

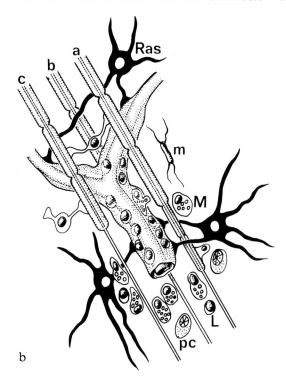

b

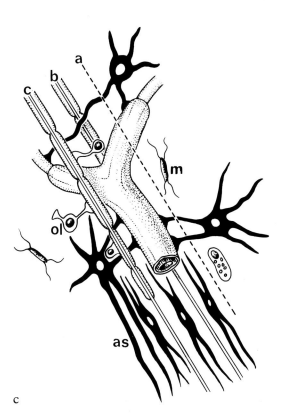

c

Fig. 10.18a–c Diagrammatic summary of the histological features of multiple sclerosis. (**a**) Normal white matter: three axons are myelinated by oligodendrocytes (ol). Fine processes of astrocytes (as) extend towards blood vessel (bv)—an artery or a vein. (**b**) Edge of an active plaque. The three axons are demyelinated as they enter the plaque below. Axon **a** shows some thin, short segments of remyelination. Perivascular lymphocytes and monocytes are seen between the blood vessel wall and the perivascular glial basement membrane. Microglia (m), foamy macrophages (M), lymphocytes (L), and plasma cells (pc) are seen at the edge of the plaque. The astrocytes have become reactive (Ras) and hypertrophied. (**c**) Edge of a chronic inactive plaque. It lacks the cellularity of the active plaque. Axon **a** has degenerated and axons **b** and **c** are demyelinated as they enter the plaque; axon **c** shows some remyelination with short segments of myelin. There is no perivascular inflammation and the blood vessel wall has become thickened and fibrotic. Astrocytes (as) have many long thin processes orientated parallel to the surviving axons. Oligodendrocytes (ol) are not present in the demyelinated plaque region and only occasional microglia cells (m) are seen.
Reproduced by permission of the editors and publishers from: Weller RO. In: Matthews WB, Acheson ED, Batchelor JR, Weller RO, McAlpine's Multiple Sclerosis. Edinburgh: Churchill Livingstone, 1985 (Fig. 12.41)

showing diffuse sclerosis of the cerebral white matter. Poser[26] defined two categories. The first comprises demyelinating diseases, in which there is loss of normally constituted myelin and which include cases of multiple sclerosis as described above. In the second group, there is dysmyelin-ation, i.e. abnormal myelin formation, due to bio-chemical defects in the myelin formation, and there is also subsequent demyelination. This group includes the leucodystrophies with bio-chemical defects in myelin formation (see p. 348). The term 'Schilder's disease' is useful for describing the pathological appearance of the brain but it has no meaning with regard to aetiology.

Balo's concentric sclerosis (encephalitis periaxialis concentrica)

This is a very rare form of multiple sclerosis in which the demyelinated plaques are formed from concentric rings of demyelination separated by zones of myelin preservation.[5] In a typical lesion, the plaque is some 4–5 cm in diameter and appears as if several globes have been placed one inside the other and then sectioned. The demyelinated areas are hypercellular due to the presence of microglia and lipid-filled macrophages.

In a series of 20 cases of concentric sclerosis examined by Courville[28] the age range was 10–51 years, but more than half were aged between 20 and 33 years. All but 5 cases survived for less than one year and the shortest survival was 2 weeks. Most cases had an acute onset of motor and psychiatric symptoms; oedema associated with the areas of demyelination may result in a clinical picture mimicking that of a space-occupying lesion.

Devic's type of multiple sclerosis (neuromyelitis optica)

Despite the well-defined clinical association of visual failure and spinal cord signs in some cases of multiple sclerosis,[2,29] the pathology of Devic's type of the disease is usually indistinguishable from that of the classical form of multiple sclerosis except in the distribution of the plaques. Even so, plaques may be found throughout the brain in cases of this disease, in addition to involvement of the optic nerves and spinal cord. Fulminating cases have been described in which there is necrosis over several segments of the spinal cord, possibly due to ischaemia secondary to swelling of the cord from oedema.

Pathology of multiple sclerosis compared with other demyelinating diseases

There are a number of pathological features in multiple sclerosis which allow it to be dis-tinguished from other demyelinating diseases. Multiple sclerosis plaques are sharply defined areas of demyelination, often sited in the peri-ventricular regions of the cerebral hemispheres, in the brainstem, in the spinal cord and in the optic nerves. The loss of oligodendrocytes is very striking in the chronic multiple sclerosis plaques, and the thick perivascular cuffs of lymphocytes, plasma cells and macrophages are distinctive in the acute stages of the disease.

Areas of demyelination in *progressive multifocal leucoencephalopathy* (PML) (see p. 219) have an irregular 'fluffy' appearance (Fig. 9.15), unlike the sharply defined plaques of multiple sclerosis (Figs 10.9 and 10.10). Abnormal hyperchromatic nuclei are seen within the areas of demyelination in PML, and viral nuclear inclusions, particularly in oligodendrocytes, may be prominent in some cases.

Large plaques of demyelination are not usually seen in *post-infectious encephalomyelitis* (see p. 209), and loss of myelin is usually restricted to the immediate perivascular regions. Although macro-phages may be prominent in the demyelinated perivascular zones and a few lymphocytes may be present, these cells are usually less abundant than in acute multiple sclerosis.

Central pontine myelinolysis (see p. 260) is characterised by moderately well-circumscribed areas of demyelination in the pons (Fig. 10.19) and in extrapontine sites such as the cerebral and cerebellar white matter.[30] The demarcation is not usually as sharp as in multiple sclerosis.[3,15] Although there is some axonal degeneration within the demyelinated area (Fig. 10.19), many axons remain intact. Large numbers of foamy macro-phages containing myelin debris are seen in the affected regions, but perivascular cuffing by lymphocytes and plasma cells is conspicuously absent even in the acute stages of the disease.

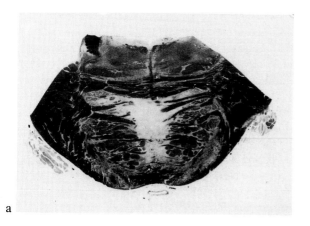

a

Fig. 10.19a, b Central pontine myelinolysis. (a) The pons stained for myelin showing an irregular demyelinated unstained area in the centre. (b) The edge of the demyelinated area showing myelinated fibres (bottom) entering an area of demyelination (top). Although many axons are intact, axon balloons indicating axon degeneration are also seen (arrow).
(a) Klüver–Barrera; (b) Palmgren–Luxol fast blue × 150

b

Myelin loss or dysmyelination in the *leucodystrophies* (see p. 348) often has a symmetrical distribution in the cerebral white matter and could be confused with the Schilder's type of multiple sclerosis. The history and clinical course of the disease, however, are usually helpful in making the distinction. In a number of lipidoses, histochemical techniques can be used to identify abnormal lipids, as in metachromatic leucodystrophy and Krabbe's disease. In addition, histological and electron microscopic studies may reveal the typical globoid cells of Krabbe's disease or the laminar intracellular inclusions of adrenoleucodystrophy.

Clinico-pathological correlations in multiple sclerosis

Although it is clear from the pathological features of multiple sclerosis that there is demyelination in the plaques and little effective remyelination, clinical recovery of neurological deficits occurs. The reasons for such recovery are not fully known. Experimental studies of demyelination in the central nervous system[31] have shown that conduction of impulses along axons is blocked as they pass through large demyelinated plaques, whereas conduction velocity is merely reduced as axons pass through small areas of demyelination. Partial loss of function in multiple sclerosis may result from the asynchronous arrival of impulses due to the passage of axons through demyelinated plaques. Abnormal visual evoked potentials illustrate this feature in many patients with multiple sclerosis (see p. 227, and Fig. 10.2).[12] Neuroelectric blocking factors have been reported in the serum of patients with multiple sclerosis but their significance is unclear.[32]

Saltatory conduction along normal myelinated fibres is associated with the presence of sodium channels at the nodes of Ranvier; such channels are not present in the internodal portions of the normal axons.[33] Following demyelination, however, the continuous conduction that can be demonstrated in demyelinated axons[34] may be due to the development of sodium channels in the internodal axonal membrane. Conduction of impulses along demyelinated axons is slow and precarious and may be completely blocked by a rise in temperature or by an increase in the local extracellular calcium.[35] These features may account for some of the fluctuation in signs and symptoms in multiple sclerosis.

Partial or complete recovery of neurological function following an episode or exacerbation in multiple sclerosis may be partly explained by the subsidence of inflammation and oedema in the plaque, by physiological adaptation to the asynchronous arrival of impulses, and by synaptic re-organisation. Remyelination does not occur to any significant extent in multiple sclerosis, probably due to the widespread destruction of oligodendrocytes in the plaques. This contrasts with the rapid and often complete remyelination that occurs in experimental demyelinating lesions in which oligodendrocytes are preserved.[36]

Correlation between the position of multiple sclerosis plaques seen at autopsy and the clinical course of the disease may be lacking. Lumsden[21] reported from his extensive study of post-mortem brains that in some cases of clinically mild multiple sclerosis there were large numbers of plaques, whereas a small number of plaques might be associated with devastating clinical disease. In some 10–20% of cases in which multiple sclerosis is observed at autopsy, there has been no clinical suspicion of the disease during life,[4] whereas at autopsy some 5% of patients with clinically diagnosed multiple sclerosis do not have demonstrable disease.[37] However, there is usually good clinico-pathological correlation between visual deterioration and optic nerve lesions.[38]

Mechanisms of demyelination and the cause of multiple sclerosis

There are a number of experimental models of demyelination.[36] In some toxic models, remyelination occurs readily except when the intoxication is chronic and persistent.[39] A number of *virus infections* also cause demyelination:[40] these include a relapsing demyelinating disease due to the Theiler murine encephalomyelitis virus. But, despite various reports of virus particles in multiple sclerosis, the disease has not been transmitted to experimental animals nor has direct involvement by viruses in the demyelinating process been substantiated.[7]

The pathology of chronic relapsing *experimental allergic encephalomyelitis* (EAE) closely resembles multiple sclerosis.[41] Sharply defined plaques of demyelination with perivascular cuffing by lymphocytes and monocytes are seen. But the major difference between EAE and multiple sclerosis is that EAE is induced by a combination of cell-mediated immunity to myelin basic protein and an antibody-mediated reaction to lipid haptens such as galactocerebroside.[42] There is no indication that myelin basic protein is the antigen in multiple sclerosis. Even in diseases such as acute post-infectious encephalomyelitis (see p. 209), in which antibodies to myelin basic protein are present in the serum,[43] it is uncertain whether this indicates a primary aetiological factor or a secondary effect of the disease.[7]

It has been suggested that demyelination in multiple sclerosis may be a result of a 'bystander' effect.[42] In this way, myelin damage would result from the immune attack on a non-myelin antigen. Such a mechanism may be responsible for the demyelination that occurs as a secondary phenomenon in experimental viral infections and, in the absence of recoverable virus, as an allergic phenomenon.[44] Although in multiple sclerosis the identity of the antigen or antigens is unknown, it has been shown in vitro that astrocytes could act as the antigen-presenting cells[45] in the induction of an immune response.

Comparison of the pathology of multiple sclerosis with experimental models suggests that the demyelination in multiple sclerosis is due to an immune mechanism. In addition, genetic data indicate that multiple sclerosis is due to an auto-immune process although the triggering agent is still not known.[7]

REFERENCES

1. Charcot J-M. Gazette Hôpital (Paris) 1868; 41: 566.
2. Matthews WB. In: Matthews WB, Acheson ED, Batchelor JR, Weller RO. McAlpine's multiple sclerosis. Edinburgh: Churchill Livingstone, 1985: 49.
3. Weller RO. In: Matthews WB, Acheson ED, Batchelor JR, Weller RO. McAlpine's multiple sclerosis. Edinburgh: Churchill Livingstone, 1985: 301.
4. Allen IV. In: Adams JH, Corsellis JAN, Duchen LW, eds. Greenfield's neuropathology. 4th ed. London: Arnold, 1984: 338.
5. Acheson ED. In: Matthews WB, Acheson ED, Batchelor JR, Weller RO. McAlpine's multiple sclerosis. Edinburgh: Churchill Livingstone, 1985: 3.
6. Spielman RS, Nathanson N. Epidemiol Rev 1982; 4: 45.
7. McDonald WI. J Neurol Psychiatry 1986; 49: 113.
8. Batchelor JR. In: Matthews WB, Acheson ED, Batchelor JR, Weller RO. McAlpine's multiple sclerosis. Edinburgh: Churchill Livingstone, 1985: 281.
9. Tallis RC. Neuropathol Appl Neurobiol 1980; 6: 325.
10. Johnson KP, Nelson BT. Ann Neurol 1977; 2: 425.
11. Walsh MJ, Tourtellotte WW. In: Hallpike JF, Adams CWM, Tourtellotte WW, eds. Multiple sclerosis. London: Chapman Hall, 1983: 275.
12. Halliday AM, McDonald WI, Mushiu J. Br Med J 1973; 4: 661.
13. Weinstein MA, Lederman RJ, Rothner AD et al. Radiology 1978; 129: 689.
14. Ormerod IEC, Roberts RC, du Boulay EPGH et al. Lancet 1984; 2: 1334.
15. Weller RO. Colour atlas of neuropathology. Oxford: Harvey Miller and Oxford University Press, 1984.
16. Sapsford I, Buontempo J, Weller RO. Neuropathol Appl Neurobiol 1983; 9: 181.
17. Traugott U, Reinherz EL, Raine CS. Science 1983; 219: 308.
18. Esiri MM. Neuropathol Appl Neurobiol 1980; 6: 9.
19. Raine CS, Scheinberg LC, Waltz JM. Lab Invest 1981; 45: 534.
20. Prineas JW, Connell F. Ann Neurol 1979; 5: 22.
21. Lumsden CE. In: Vinken PJ, Bruyn GW, eds. Handbook of clinical neurology. Amsterdam: North Holland, 1970; 9: 217.
22. Brownell B, Hughes JT J Neurol Neurosurg Psychiatry 1962; 25: 315.
23. Dawson JW. Trans R Soc Edinburgh 1916; 50: 517.
24. Oppenheimer DR. Neuropathol Appl Neurobiol 1978; 4: 151.
25. Lhermitte F, Escourolle R, Hauw JJ et al. Rev Neurol 1981; 137: 589.
26. Poser CM. In: Vinken PJ, Bruyn GW, eds. Handbook of clinical neurology. Amsterdam: North Holland, 1970; 9: 469.
27. Schilder PF. Z Gesamte Neurol Psychiatr 1912; 10, Orig: 1.
28. Courville CB. In: Vinken PJ, Bruyn GW, eds. Handbook of clinical neurology. Amsterdam: North Holland, 1970; 90: 437.
29. Cloys DE, Netsky MG. In: Vinken PJ, Bruyn GW, eds. Handbook of clinical neurology. Amsterdam: North Holland, 1970; 9: 426.
30. Okeda R, Kitano M, Sawabe M. Acta Neuropathol 1986; 69: 259.
31. McDonald WI, Sears TA. Brain 1970; 93: 583.
32. Schauf CL, Schauf V, Davis FA, Mizen MR. Neurology 1978; 28: 426.
33. Waxman SG. Neurology 1978; 28, 9(2): 27.
34. Sears TA, Bostock H, Sheratt M. Neurology 1978; 28, 9(2): 21.
35. Schauf CL, Davis FA. J Neurol Neurosurg Psychiatry 1974; 37: 152.
36. Blakemore WF. In: Smith WT, Cavanagh JB, eds. Recent advances in neuropathology 2. Edinburgh: Churchill Livingstone, 1982: 53.
37. Adams CWM. In: Hallpike JF, Adam CWM, Tourtollotte WW, eds. Multiple sclerosis. London: Chapman and Hall, 1983: 203.
38. Ulrich J, Groebke-Lorenz W. Neuro-ophthalmology 1983; 3: 149.
39. Ludwin SK. Lab Invest 1980; 43: 382.
40. Dal Canto MC, Rabinovitz SG. Ann Neurol 1982; 11: 109.
41. Raine CS. In: Hallpike JF, Adams CWM, Tourtellotte WW, eds. Multiple sclerosis. London: Chapman and Hall, 1983: 413.
42. Wisniewski HM, Lassmann H, Brosnan CF et al. In: Matthews WB, Glaser GH, eds. Recent advances in clinical neurology 3. Edinburgh: Churchill Livingstone, 1982: 95.
43. Lisak RP, Behan PO, Zweiman B, Shettey T. Neurology 1974; 24: 560.
44. Watanabe R, Wege H, Ter Meulen V. Nature 1983; 305: 150.
45. Fontana A, Fierz W, Werkerle H. Nature 1984; 307: 273.

Toxic and deficiency disorders

PATHOLOGICAL INVESTIGATION OF A CASE OF INTOXICATION

Careful study of the clinical notes, questioning of the clinicians responsible for the case and even interviews with the relatives may be essential to obtain details of occupational history, hobbies and other reasons why the patient might have been poisoned. It is in the manner of the death, as well as in the clinical signs and symptoms, that suspicion may be first aroused. The possibility of 'foul play' may be missed by unsuspecting clinicians: thallium poisoning (see p. 254) is a particular case in point. The cardinal sign of thallium intoxication is loss of hair, but it is a late event in the case history, and, in the early stages, even after the neuropathy has developed, it may be necessary to pull on the hair quite forcibly to show its fragility.

The medicolegal implications of acute intoxication must be considered if there is any suspicion that the toxic agent was self-administered or administered with homicidal intent. It is important to retain samples of tissue from the major organs and body fluids (including urine and hair), in clean containers at $-20°C$, until analysis is completed. If the toxic substance is thought to have been taken by mouth, then samples of the gastric and intestinal contents should also be retained for further study.

The effects of neurointoxication are primarily centred either on the central nervous system or on the peripheral nervous system, and the distribution of the clinical features should guide the way in which the post mortem is conducted. Investigation of the central nervous system in intoxications should include a thorough examination of the brain, both macroscopically and by the histological examination of blocks from major regions of the cerebral hemispheres, cerebellum and brainstem, depending, to some extent, upon the signs and symptoms and the suspected intoxication. The more common medicolegal problems are those of poisoning by carbon monoxide (see p. 118), carbon dioxide and cyanide as well as other acute toxic agents that affect the central nervous system. However, it is also particularly important to examine the spinal cord and the dorsal root sensory ganglia as these regions are frequently affected in toxic disorders. For example, in organophosphorus intoxication, the dorsal columns, the spinocerebellar tracts and the corticospinal tracts show selective degeneration (see p. 269).

Many of the toxic agents which affect the nervous system cause peripheral neuropathy. These agents include therapeutic drugs, and metals such as arsenic, thallium, lead and mercury. It is important, in such cases, that a systematic analysis of the peripheral and central nervous system be performed. The aim of the examination should be to define as accurately as possible which peripheral nerves are affected. Samples should be taken from the autonomic as well as the somatic nerves and include the vagus and phrenic nerves. In many cases, the peripheral neuropathy is a 'dying back' neuropathy (see p. 540). As it is the long nerves that are most severely affected in the 'dying back' process, samples should be taken from the distal parts of the nerves in the hands and feet and from the more proximal portions of these nerves in order to estimate how far the damage has progressed towards the spinal roots. Damage in the long peripheral nerves (e.g. from the limbs) and the short peripheral nerves (e.g. cranial or trunk nerves) should be compared. Most toxic neuropathies are due to *axonal degeneration*, and the damage in the distal motor and sensory nerves, and in the more proximal parts of the spinal nerves, can be estimated using the quantitative techniques outlined by Dyck.[1] If clinical and electrophysiological studies suggest that there is primary *segmental demyelination*, peripheral nerves and spinal roots should be sampled and the nerve fibres teased and stained with Sudan black B or with osmium tetroxide (see p. 536).[1] A good example of such a study is that of Said[2] on nerve biopsies in perhexiline intoxication (see p. 284).

Accurate documentation of the pathological changes in patients dying with toxic disorders is essential not only for confirmation of intoxication in a particular patient, but also for elucidation of the mechanisms of toxicity; patterns of damage in man and in experimental animals are usually very similar.

TOXIC DISORDERS DUE TO CHEMICALS

METAL INTOXICATIONS

Arsenic

Two major forms of arsenic exist. The *pentavalent* forms, such as arsenic pentoxide (As_2O_5), have many chemical similarities to phosphorus compounds and are widely used as a basis for arsenical insecticides in agrochemical industries. They are also the basis for a number of compounds with significant medical uses, especially in the treatment of syphilis in the past, and of certain tropical parasitic diseases, such as trypanosomiasis. While pentavalent arsenic is substantially less toxic than the trivalent form, there have been questions raised as to possible carcinogenic effects.[3] *Trivalent* arsenic has long been known for its toxicity, particularly as an instrument of homicide.[4] Its toxic effects have been noted from medicines, e.g. Fowler's solution, from 'anticancer' pastes,[5] from contaminated beer and confectionery,[6,7] and in Japan from a number of foods including soy sauce.[8] Volatile arseniuretted hydrogen or arsine (AsH_3) has been responsible for a number of outbreaks of poisoning, particularly among submariners and balloonists.[9]

Trivalent arsenic

Chronically administered trivalent arsenic affects actively proliferating tissues, including the gastrointestinal epithelium, the skin and its appendages, and blood cells. This leads to anaemia (usually normocytic), gastroenteritis, loss of hair, and hyperkeratosis of the soles of the feet and the palms of the hands. Hyperpigmentation of the skin, often in the distal regions of the limbs, is particularly prominent and is sometimes spotty or guttate. Transverse white lines or grooves often develop in the nails, and are particularly well seen after an acute attack. These are termed Mees' lines,[10] though they are not specific for arsenic and may be found in any condition where the growth of the nails is temporarily retarded. All these clinical effects result from impairment of energy production within the cell, leading to reduced energy availability for cell proliferation.

Arsenical peripheral neuropathy

Clinical features. About half the cases of chronic arsenical intoxication show a typical symmetrical distal peripheral neuropathy.[11-13] Sensory disturbances and pain in muscles occur early in a glove and stocking distribution. In the more severe cases excruciating splitting and tearing pains may be unbearable. Loss of fine touch and position sense are particularly important but all modalities are involved and reflexes are lost early. Motor weakness in the feet and in the hands follows and may be profound, but proximal nerves, such as the cranial nerves, are never involved. There is mild to moderate slowing of nerve conduction velocity,[14] and arsenic is present in the urine as well as in hair and nails. Excretion of arsenic in the urine is rapid at first with a half time of about three weeks. Pyruvate levels in the blood are raised, particularly in the acute phase of intoxication.

Pathological changes. Post-mortem studies are very few,[15] which is in keeping with the usual good recovery. Radial and peroneal nerves have shown severe axonal degeneration as well as accompanying signs of regeneration. A variable number of anterior horn cells may be lost, and those that remain are chromatolytic. Degeneration of dorsal columns, which might be expected, has not been reported.

Biopsy studies confirm Wallerian degeneration;[16-18] in addition, minor degrees of segmental degeneration have been found in teased nerve fibres from the sural nerve.[17]

Mechanism of toxicity. Inorganic trivalent arsenic is very reactive with a number of radicals, in particular $-SH$ groups.[19] In view of the biological importance of the $-SH$ radicals in so many cell functions, particularly those involving the dehydrogenases, this seems to be the key to the toxicity of trivalent arsenic. The interaction is a stable one.

$$R-As=O+2HSR' \rightarrow R-As\begin{array}{c} SH-R \\ \\ SH-R' \end{array} +H_2O$$

The studies of Peters et al.[20,21] on the mode of

action of the very toxic vesicant war gas, Lewisite, which is dichloro(2-chlorovinyl)arsine,

$$Cl - CH = CH - As \begin{matrix} \diagup Cl \\ \diagdown Cl \end{matrix}$$

provided the first detailed analysis of the metabolic interactions of arsenicals, and recognition of the importance of the formation of a relatively stable ring structure, particularly in combination with the co-factor, lipoate.

$$R - As = O + \begin{matrix} | \\ HS—C— \\ | \\ HS—C— \\ | \end{matrix} \rightarrow R - As \begin{matrix} \diagup S—C— \\ | \\ \diagdown S—C— \\ | \end{matrix} + H_2O$$

From this work stemmed the design of the potent and specific antidote, dimercaptopropanol (dimercaprol, British Anti-Lewisite, BAL). Originally there had been much speculation as to whether arsenite acted on respiration in the manner of cyanide, but now it is generally recognised that the main toxic effects arise because of its interaction with the co-factor lipoate, which is critical for the second step of pyruvate decarboxylation. The main energy-providing pathway of the tricarboxylic acid (TCA) cycle is thus blocked at almost the same point as it is in thiamine deficiency (see p. 289). Tissues with a high and continuous energy requirement are thus seriously at risk, and these, in the clinical context, are proliferating tissues and neurons with very long axons.[22]

Pentavalent arsenic

Paul Ehrlich began the era of chemotherapy, using synthetic compounds for the treatment of syphilis with pentavalent arsenicals in 1909. Subsequently this class of compounds was widely explored for therapeutic purposes and indeed they are still being used for treating tropical parasitic diseases, such as trypanosomiasis.

Toxic reactions to pentavalent arsenic have always shown themselves as clearly quite dissimilar to, and distinct from, those due to trivalent arsenic, suggesting quite different toxic

mechanisms. *Haemorrhagic encephalopathy*[23-26] is the typical neuropathological complication of pentavalent organic arsenicals. Other complications are reported, especially *polyneuropathy*, with or without *exfoliative dermatitis*,[27] *optic neuritis*,[28] *myelitis*[29] and *vestibular disturbances*.[30] However, the polyneuropathy is clinically quite different from that caused by trivalent arsenic. It is predominantly motor with little sensory change, it commonly affects cranial nerves,[31] and it has many similarities to the Guillain–Barré syndrome (see p. 551).

Pathologically, the brain shows purpura; the petechial haemorrhages are scattered in both grey and white matter, forming 'balls' or rings around capillaries (Figs 11.1 and 11.2). Some mild microglial response may be seen, depending upon the duration of the illness, but there is little serious neuronal loss.

Mechanisms of toxicity. Pentavalent forms of arsenic are much less lethal in terms of their LD_{50} than trivalent arsenic. In general, although reduction to the trivalent form is necessary for killing spirochaetes or other parasites, there is relatively little transformation to the trivalent form in the tissues.[32] Experimental studies have shown that haemorrhagic changes in the retina or the brain may occur even after a single dose of pentavalent arsenic, and certainly the average number of doses before a toxic response occurs is two. Several pentavalent forms have produced vascular retinal lesions in animals,[28,33] and Weston Hurst[34]

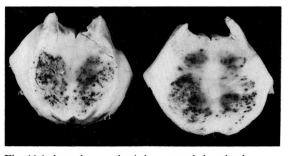

Fig. 11.1 Acute haemorrhagic leucoencephalopathy due to the organic arsenical melarsoprol used in the treatment of trypanosomiasis. Transverse sections of pons. Note that punctate haemorrhages affect white and grey matter. *Reproduced by permission of Professor J. H. Adams, Institute of Neurological Sciences, Glasgow, UK.*

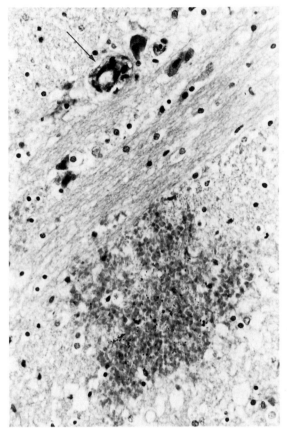

Fig. 11.2 'Ball' haemorrhage in the pons in the case shown in Figure 11.1. Note also fibrinoid necrosis of the vessel (arrow) near the haemorrhage.
Martius yellow–brilliant crystal scarlet–soluble blue × 250
Reproduced by permission of Professor J. H. Adams, Institute of Neurological Sciences, Glasgow, UK.

was able to produce vascular brain lesions in monkeys after a single dose. Credit should be given to Young and Loevenhart[28] for pointing out that pathological changes only occurred with para-substituted organic compounds, and not with ortho- or meta-substituents. This structural feature is well known to be associated with vascular Arthus-type responses in tissues.[35]

Lead

Inorganic lead salts

Because of the world abundance of this metal and its many uses through the ages, lead has been with urban civilisation almost from its outset. In consequence, the toxic effects of lead have long been recognised. Lead mining and smelting in the past

was one of the main sources of serious intoxication. Now, with greater awareness of the dangers, lead is only occasionally encountered, and then in relatively small amounts, from water running through lead pipes in soft water areas, from old lead paint and more often from contamination derived from lead in petrol. It is, thus, now unusual in developed countries to find blood lead levels above 35 µg/dl, although even this level is considered by some to be potentially dangerous to very young children and perhaps to pregnant women.

The question of lead toxicity to the nervous system can be conveniently divided into high and low dose effects—the line being drawn at 80–100 µg/dl in the blood. Above 100 µg/dl there are distinct chances that classical signs of neuro-

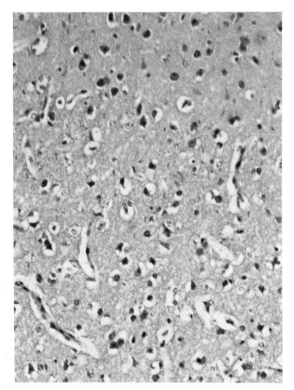

Fig. 11.3 From a region of focal oedema in the cerebral cortex of a Jersey bull calf intoxicated with lead acetate. Note that most of the nerve cells and the vessels are surrounded by oedematous spaces, except at the top beyond the affected area, where the nerve cells are normal.
Haematoxylin-eosin × 135
Reproduced by permission of Professor J. McC. Howell, Murdoch University, Western Australia.

toxicity may develop, particularly in very young children, although whether they appear seems to depend very much on the individual case. Below 80 μg/dl, classical toxic effects are unlikely, but blood levels of 50–80 μg/dl in the pregnant mother and in the very young child could have detrimental effects on the developing brain—that is, if experimental studies on young rats are relevant to man. Such experimental studies, while often difficult to evaluate, do suggest that there may be persistent adverse effects on the catecholaminergic system of the brain, particularly when exposure has been in utero.

Encephalopathy and neuropathy are associated with higher doses of lead and blood levels will often be well above 100 μg/dl in such cases.

Lead encephalopathy

The clinical picture of lead encephalopathy is essentially that of raised intracranial pressure. Headache is dominant, with vomiting, fits, drowsiness, papilloedema, clouding of consciousness and perhaps eventually coma. Focal deficits are uncommon. There may also be a history of general signs of lead poisoning, such as painful abdominal colic, constipation, and anaemia with basophilic stippling of red cells. According to the severity of the condition, recovery may be good, or there may be persistent sequelae. In very young children symptoms may persist in as many as 60%.[36]

Pathology. Post-mortem studies of cases of lead encephalopathy tend to show only a generally swollen brain with a few scattered petechial haemorrhages in the cerebral hemispheres. The best reports are those of Blackman[37] and of Smith et al.[38] These authors described oedema associated with acute neuronal necrosis. Blackman[37] particularly emphasised vascular haemorrhages and protein exudation in and around vessel walls.

Experimental studies with newborn rats[39] and Jersey bull calves (Fig. 11.3) confirm the essentially vascular nature of the changes and the greater sensitivity of the developing brain. In the cerebrum, focal areas of perineuronal and perivascular oedema (Fig. 11.3) can be found, while in

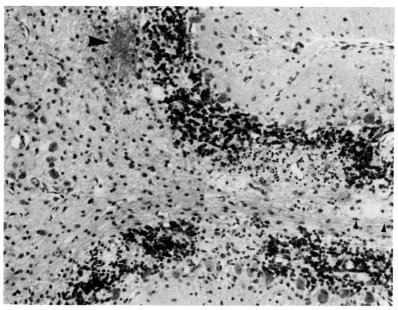

Fig. 11.4 Cerebellum from a young rat whose mother had 4% lead acetate included in the drinking water. Note focal areas of loss of granule cells and a small haemorrhage (arrowhead). There is early white matter oedema at the small arrowheads on the right. Haematoxylin-eosin ×200

the cerebellum of the newborn rat, which is going through a rapid growth phase in the first three weeks of life, there are very severe haemorrhagic changes (Fig. 11.4) with focal loss of neurons. Similar but smaller foci can also be found in the more mature forebrain and spinal cord. After four weeks the animals become resistant to the toxic effects of lead just as the adult human brain is relatively insusceptible.

Peripheral neuropathy

Clinical features.   Lead neuropathy is clinically a mononeuropathy with severe slowing of nerve conduction velocity and signs of motor weakness progressing to paralysis in one or more sets of muscles, particularly those repeatedly used in work or other exercise. Wrist drop or foot drop is, therefore, common and may be unilateral. Muscle wasting is not marked in the early stages of the paresis and sensory changes are either unimportant or absent. Significant slowing of the conduction velocity, even in nerves not apparently involved, implies that the changes are in fact much more widespread than might first be thought.

Pathological changes.   These are unique in that both axonal degeneration and segmental demyelination are present in large numbers of fibres.[40] Post-mortem studies are few,[41] but show that the changes are widespread, well beyond those nerves affected clinically, but confined to the peripheral nervous system.

Experimental studies in rats[42] have emphasised the endoneurial oedema as a major pathological component, in excess of what might be expected from degenerative changes alone. This raises the question whether some of the focal clinical features of lead neuropathy might be due to entrapment of the swollen nerve beneath ligaments, etc.

Mechanisms of lead toxicity.   Lead in the body follows calcium pathways, uses calcium routes of entry, and has a strong tendency thus to sequester in bones. In the blood it is almost entirely bound to red cells, but rather loosely. Lead readily enters the brain but just as readily passes out again, so there is no special accumulation in nervous tissue.

Inside cells, lead is sequestered within mitochondria in the electron-dense calcium phosphate granules by an energy-consuming process, and, when in high concentrations, it forms intranuclear inclusions, best seen in the kidneys. It is doubtful whether lead has any special direct effects upon nerve cells; any neuronal damage is probably secondary to the vascular lesions. The sensitivity of the porphyrin pathways to lead does not appear to have any relevance to the neurological lesions. δ-aminolaevulinic acid dehydratase is inhibited by lead but it readily regenerates, and the neurological changes found in conditions where porphyrin metabolism is disturbed are quite different from those of lead poisoning (see p. 560).

The reason for the selective damage to the vascular bed is obscure, but lead may have some affinity for the endoneurium of peripheral nerve. Dyck et al.[42] found that the concentration of lead in nerve was about ten times higher than blood lead levels; this demonstrates perhaps an affinity of lead for glycoproteins of the endoneurium.

Organic lead intoxication

Clinical features.   Cases of organic lead intoxication are few and have occurred in the industrial context of tetraethyl lead or tetramethyl lead absorption. Saunders[43] lists the sources of these cases as tank cleaning, manufacturing processes involving such compounds, handling them at refineries and in transport, and suicide. The symptoms are irritability, insomnia, excessive dreaming (often of a wild and terrifying nature), emotional instability, anorexia and constipation. It is possible that some components of the state induced by petrol sniffing may come from the organic lead content. There are no stippled red cells in the blood or porphyrins in the urine. In 4 Polish cases[44] there were signs of raised intracranial pressure and a schizophrenia-like syndrome that progressed to coma. Blood tetraethyl lead levels were more than 200 μg/dl. At post-mortem there was cerebral oedema and capillary haemorrhages in the brain and the lungs, but no other changes. There is no evidence for any significant conversion in the tissues to the inorganic form of lead.

Mercury

Inorganic mercurous salts and Pink Disease

At one time a widely used formulation for teething powders for infants contained calomel (mercurous chloride). Infants affected by the powder became whining and fretful, showed excessive perspiration and pink cold extremities; they commonly developed peripheral neuropathy from which some of them died. Wallerian degeneration was present in peripheral nerves at post-mortem, and in the spinal cord there was unexplained 'cuffing' of vessels by inflammatory cells.[45,46] Warkany and Hubbard[47] in 1948 demonstrated mercury in the urine of such infants, and when calomel was removed from the formulation the disease disappeared. Occasional cases of poisoning have been reported in adults taking calomel for constipation over many years. These patients[48] showed intention tremor, ataxia, slight dementia and marked shyness. At post-mortem the brain was small (1150 g) and there was diffuse loss of granule cells from the cerebellum as well as loss of a few Purkinje cells.

Inorganic mercuric salts

The symptomatology of mercury poisoning is epitomised by the phrase 'as mad as a hatter' and the term Hatters' Shakes. Metallic mercury and mercuric salts, particularly mercuric nitrate (once used in the felting of fur in the hat-making trade), are volatile and readily absorbed by inhalation. Today mercury poisoning is still a risk in industry, particularly in chloralkali works, where metallic mercury may be spilled from heavy switch gear.

Clinical features. The symptoms of poisoning constitute a syndrome known as erethism, comprising shyness, timidity, mental confusion, irritability, insomnia and increasing tremor made worse on excitement. Except in the most severe cases, all these symptoms are reversible on removal from the source of poisoning. Available post-mortem records indicate that little or no structural damage can be found in such cases, though persisting mercury has been demonstrated by specific histochemical staining and by X-ray microanalysis within lysosomal dense bodies of many neurons in the CNS as long as 16 years after poisoning.[49]

Organic mercury compounds

Alkylmercury compounds (methyl and ethyl compounds), being relatively stable in the tissues, are cumulative poisons. Arylmercury compounds, on the other hand, readily break down in the tissues; they are much used as diuretics and their effect is caused by the products acting on the proximal convoluted tubules of the kidneys. Any poisoning by aryl compounds will thus be of the inorganic type

Clinical features. Considerable experience of alkylmercury poisoning has been gained as the result of several outbreaks, especially that at Minamata Bay on Kyushu Island, Japan.[50,51] Moreover, because the changes are destructive and irreversible, post-mortem material has been available, though usually months or years after the event. There are three separate major clinical components: those associated with a *sensory neuropathy*, those associated with *cerebellar cortical atrophy*, and those arising from *damage to the granular isocortex*, namely visual, auditory and post-central gyral cortex. Other brain regions are less consistently and less severely affected (Fig. 11.5).

Pathological features. Hunter and Russell,[51] and Takeuchi et al. from Minamata cases,[52] described severe atrophy of the visual, auditory, and post-central gyral cortex as the principal change in the cerebral hemispheres. The cerebellum showed striking cortical atrophy, particularly in the depths of the sulci, suggesting that brain swelling may have introduced a vascular hypoxic component to the lesion. There was also dilatation of the ventricular system due to general atrophy of the brain.

Microscopically, small neurons were strikingly lost from both the cerebral and the cerebellar cortices. In the cerebellum, the granular layer was very thin (Fig. 11.6). Purkinje cells were notably spared, and in Hunter and Russell's[51] case (death 13 years after the event), Purkinje cell dendrites showed remarkable sprouting as though at-

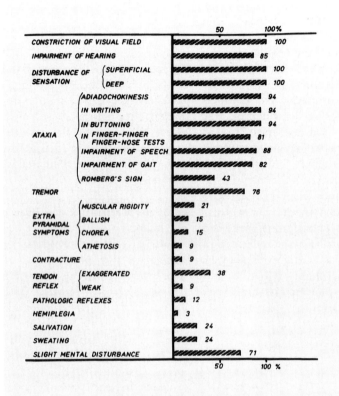

Fig. 11.5 Frequency of signs and symptoms in cases of methyl mercury poisoning from Minamata.
(From T. Tsubaki, quoted by Nordisk Hygienisk Tidskrift 1971; suppl. 4.)

tempting to re-establish contact with surviving granule cell axons. In the cerebral cortex, too, larger neurons tended to be spared, while smaller neurons were widely lost; this explains the restriction of cell loss to the granular isocortex, where there are many small neurons.[52] Where the destruction was severe only gliotic tissue remained; this was seen especially in the visual cortex of Hunter and Russell's case.[51]

Scattered loss of neurons was found in many other regions of the brain and this contributed to the symptomatology of individual cases. Anterior horn cells were intact in the spinal cord, but some loss of spinal sensory ganglion cells occurred and contributed to the sensory loss and loss of peripheral nerve sensory fibres found in the Japanese cases.[52a,53]

Mechanisms of mercury toxicity

Mercurous salts are very insoluble, and it is probably only because of the relatively greater permeability of their gastrointestinal tracts that infants are so susceptible to calomel. Mercuric salts are more water-soluble than alkylmercury salts and are correspondingly more nephrotoxic. But even mercuric salts are also substantially lipid-soluble,[54] which explains their ready entry into brain and other tissues. However, mercuric salts do not have the same cumulative potential as the alkylmercury compounds, which remain in the tissues, probably sequestered in lipid components of membrane systems.

The earliest changes seen in cells after dosing animals with alkylmercury are dissolution of ribo-

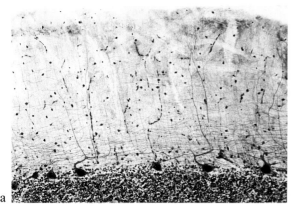
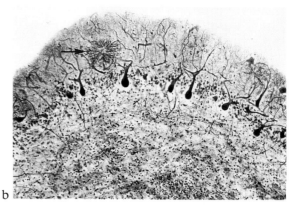

a   b

Fig. 11.6a, b Damage to cerebellum from methyl mercury poisoning. Normal remaining region (**a**) and damaged region (**b**) at the same magnification. Note the severe depletion of the granule cells (bottom) in **b** as well as the very great shrinkage of the molecular layer (top) into which the granule cell axons project. Purkinje cell dendrites are greatly shrunken in **b**, and have occasionally undergone striking hyperplasia (arrow) during the 13 year survival period after intoxication, presumably seeking to re-establish synaptic contacts with surviving granule cell axons.
Hortega's double impregnation method × 175
Reproduced by permission of the late Professor D. S. Russell, London Hospital, UK.

somal complexes in dorsal root ganglion and other cells,[55] followed by either axon degeneration (Fig. 11.7) or, if the dose is high enough, cell death. However, the same kind of intracellular lesion can also be found in early mercuric salt intoxication,[56] and both forms of mercury can also produce focal loss of granule cells from the cerebellum,[57] although this occurs more readily with alkyl-mercury. It should be noted, too, that all three classes of mercury lead to some form of peripheral

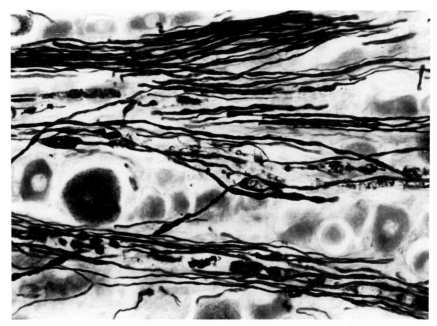

Fig. 11.7 Spinal ganglion from a rat given 8 doses of 5 mg/kg methyl mercury dicyandiamide. At 12 days there are numbers of fragmenting axons present, but the cell bodies are largely intact.
Glees and Marsland × 270

nerve damage. It seems, therefore, that all three types of mercury can produce essentially the same changes in nervous tissue. The effect, however, is greatest, most damaging to the cells and least reversible with alkylmercury; it is least marked with mercurous salts.

The earliest metabolic change described is loss of capacity of tissues to synthesise proteins,[58,59] and this correlates with the observed loss of ribosomes. The greater susceptibility of small neurons in the CNS may reside solely in the very small numbers of polyribosomes that they contain by comparison with large neurons. The larger neurons would also be more capable of sequestering mercury harmlessly within their abundant lysosomes, as noted in inorganic mercury poisoning (see above).[49]

Mercury salts, whether inorganic or organic, avidly combine with sulphydryl groups as well as with other radicals. Divalent inorganic forms produce more stable complexes than do monovalent alkyl forms, and it is possible that even in organic mercury poisoning the relatively small proportion of divalent inorganic mercury, degraded from the organic form in the cell, is the principal proximate toxic agent.

In summary, all three classes of mercury compound damage tissues, probably by destroying ribosomes and impairing protein synthesis. But whether the poisoning is mild, or moderate and reversible, or severe and irreversible, probably depends largely upon the solubility of the chemical form and thus its capacity to enter nervous tissue and remain in cells for prolonged periods in relatively large amounts. Whether cells die or survive depends very much upon their size and their total RNA or ribosomal content as well as their lysosomal content.

Manganese

Intoxication by manganese is little understood, though it causes a striking disease picture. Chronic inhalation of manganese dust in mines is the principal source of poisoning. This occurs in India and in Chile; in the pyrolusite (MnO_2) mines of Chile, the dust may have a manganese content of 40–60%.

Clinical features. Upon chronic inhalation of manganese-containing dust, a remarkable series of signs occurs. They have many features in common both with parkinsonism and Huntington's disease, and are summarised thus:[60,61] languor and sleepiness, mask-like facies, low monotonous voice ('economical speech'), muscular twitching ranging from fine twitching of the hands to gross rhythmic movements of the limbs and trunk, cramps in the calves and muscle stiffness, ankle and patellar clonus, retropulsion and propulsion, a wide-based slapping gait, and uncontrollable laughter and crying. The condition is not life-shortening.

Pathological features. The number of post-mortem studies reported is few. Canavan et al.[60] found slight atrophy of the cerebral cortex and moderate cell loss in the caudate nuclei, the putamen, the globus pallidus and the thalamus; the large cells tended to be lost rather than the small neurons. The subthalamic nuclei were also affected. Gliosis was marked in all these regions.

Mechanisms of toxicity. While many enzymes are manganese-dependent, it is not known whether this fact has any relevance to the process of toxicity. Manganese, when absorbed, is rapidly taken up by cells into mitochondria, but its subsequent fate is unknown.[62,63] Manganese tends also to accumulate in nervous tissue.[64] Dosing monkeys with manganese has led to functional changes somewhat similar to those found in man,[65] and these are associated with marked gliosis of the same basal nuclei, as in man. However, there was a noteworthy absence of nerve cell degeneration in these animals.

Thallium

Thallium exists in two oxidation states, as thallic (trivalent) salts and as thallous (monovalent) salts. Only the thallous salts are responsible for intoxication. Thallium has gained a well-earned notoriety as one of the more potent toxic substances, having an LD_{50} of 12 mg/kg. It is used in specialist industries such as lens making, photographic and firework manufacture, and as a fungicide and ant-killer, but most frequently as a rodenticide. It is still widely used as such in many parts of the world; it is banned for such purposes in Australia, Britain and the United States of America.

Thallium was sometimes administered as a depilatory agent in the treatment of ringworm until it was found that about 10% of patients given the therapeutic dose of 8 mg/kg subsequently developed peripheral neuropathy and other clinical signs.

Thallium has been used for homicide.[66,67]

Clinical features. The signs and symptoms resemble arsenic poisoning, though thallium is more acutely toxic. Like arsenic, it affects the gastrointestinal tract, the skin and its appendages and the longer peripheral nerves. In each of its effects the consequences of thallium poisoning are more severe in manifestation and more destructive than those of arsenic.[68]

Acute poisoning presents with severe vomiting followed by diarrhoea. A few days later, subjective sensory disturbances commence distally in the fingers and toes with numbness and tingling, and ascend more proximally during the next few days. All forms of sensation may ultimately be lost. Weakness also begins distally in the limbs and ascends proximally. Unlike the picture with arsenic, involvement of proximal muscles can be serious, particularly if muscles of respiration and those supplied by cranial nerves are involved. In milder cases there is recovery, but when cranial nerves are involved the prognosis is not good.[69-71] In more *chronic poisoning* from repeated dosing there are sensory disturbances and the patients complain of severe pains, particularly in bones, as well as weakness and wasting and profound general malaise.[67]

Changes in the skin are striking in severe instances of poisoning, with exfoliative desquamation—particularly of the face, axillae, and groin. At the same time the hair begins to be easily pulled away. The alopecia is rarely total; usually it is patchy, with only the head hair and the outer parts of the eyebrows generally affected. Pubic and other body hair is not so involved because, unlike head hair, it is quiescent. On the head, 90% of the hair follicles are in the growth phase (anagen), a fact that is important in understanding the mechanism of hair loss. Hair loss almost always follows the onset of the neurological disturbances by a week or more and is usually of little help in early diagnosis. Mees' lines also commonly occur, as in arsenic intoxication (see p. 246); they are not in any way specific. Clinical recovery begins after the third week or so, and the length of the recovery period depends on the severity of the acute phase and the distribution of the neurological deficit.

Pathological changes. These are confined to the

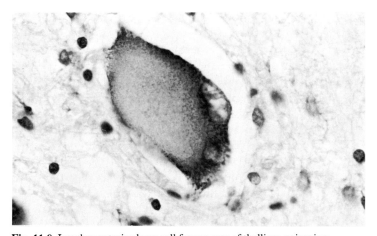

Fig. 11.8 Lumbar anterior horn cell from a case of thallium poisoning showing severe chromatolysis as part of the attempted regenerative response to severe Wallerian degeneration of the axon.
Cresyl fast violet × 440

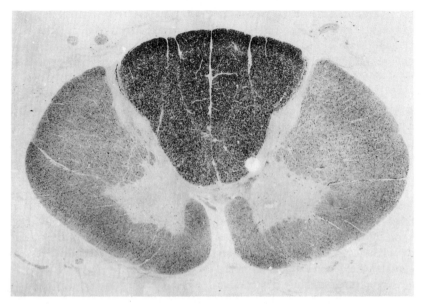

Fig. 11.9 Spinal cord from the case of thallium poisoning reported by Kennedy and Cavanagh,[73] showing marked degenerative changes in the dorsal columns of the cervical region due to extensive and severe degeneration of the peripheral sensory nerves. Marchi × 11

peripheral nervous system. Wallerian degeneration of sensory and motor nerves will be found on biopsy.[72] In severe cases coming to post mortem there is extensive and widespread nerve fibre degeneration, which is always more severe and extensive in the distal parts of the limbs. Indeed, structural changes closely mirror in time and degree the earlier functional disturbances. In severe cases, degeneration of cranial nerves, including the oculomotor nerves, may be more recent than degeneration in limb nerves; this implies that damage is progressive and has continued up to the time of death.[71]

Chromatolysis of the anterior horn cells of the spinal cord is likely to be found and is more marked in the lumbar than in the cervical regions (Fig. 11.8); it may also be seen in cranial nerve motor nuclei.[71] There is little specific damage to be found elsewhere in the CNS, except for the severe axon degeneration described in the dorsal columns, both in a recently poisoned patient[73] and in one who survived for a period of 9 months (Fig. 11.9).[74]

Skin changes. Loss of mitotic activity, hyperkeratosis and oedema of the affected skin all occur.

Each hair shaft is narrowed to a point which breaks, whereas when normal hair is pulled out it shows a bulbous ending. Experimental studies[75] on the young rat have shown that thallium reduces the mitotic activity of the actively growing hair follicle (anagen), so that it may cease altogether, producing a false catagen going on to telegen, with necrosis of the proliferative base of the follicle. The narrow zone in the affected hair shaft is the point of weakness that allows hair to break and fall out. The presence of thallium in the hair is also a useful diagnostic feature.

Mechanisms of toxicity. The tissue responses to thallium strongly imply a general disturbance to the energy supply of the most demanding cells. The mechanism of this is not known, though indirect evidence suggests that there may well be a *disturbance of riboflavin metabolism*. Thallium behaves in the tissues like potassium: it enters cells and is excreted along potassium pathways.[76] The toxic effects of thallium, however, are more likely to be mediated through its ability to combine with riboflavin.[77] Removal of riboflavin from tissues will cause depletion of flavoprotein co-factors and flavine adenine dinucleotide (FAD), essential for the entry of many energy-providing intermediates into the electron transport sequence. It may be no coincidence that thallium intoxication in monkeys causes signs, such as hair loss and skin changes around the face and mouth, which closely resemble changes produced in this species by riboflavin deficiency (see p. 294).[78] The animals also show ataxia and signs of peripheral neuropathy.

Organo-tin

Triethyltin

Inorganic tin compounds have no specific neurotoxic actions. Organic compounds (alkyltins), by contrast, have marked effects on the nervous system, although the mechanisms are not understood.[79] Alkyltins have been used for a number of years as fungicides, molluscicides, and slimicides as well as in the plastics industry. They came into prominence in France when a preparation, Stalinon, containing alkyltin, was used in the treatment of furunculosis and was responsible for more than 200 cases of poisoning from which about 90 people died.[80] The preparation contained mainly diethyltin with a small amount of monoethyltin and about 10% triethyltin. Diethyltin has general inhibitory effects on respiration, similar to arsenic, and is countered by dimercaprol (BAL), but it has no specific action on nervous tissue. Triethyltin is about 10 times more toxic than the diethyl form.

Clinical features. The signs of triethyltin intoxication are those of acute raised intracranial pressure with headache, vomiting, visual disturbances, cranial nerve palsies, mild hemiparesis, and clouding of consciousness. Marked psychiatric signs have been seen. The CSF pressure is increased and electro-encephalogram abnormalities have been noted. Recovery is slow but without residual effects.

Pathological features. Despite the many deaths in the French outbreak only one post-mortem study was reported;[81] it showed only general brain swelling without specific changes.

Experimental studies[82] have shown that a striking diffuse swelling occurs throughout the CNS but is confined to the white matter. Brain water is increased and the fluid has the characteristics of a plasma ultrafiltrate. The fluid lies within the myelin sheaths, and does not expand the general extracellular space. Fluid-filled vacuoles form and lie within the space created by splitting of the lesser dense line of the compacted myelin sheath,[83] implying that it is 'outside' the flattened membranous extension of the oligodendrocyte forming the myelin sheath (see p. 13). Despite the enormous numbers of vacuoles, oligodendrocytes show no morphological changes to suggest intoxication. Astroglia and neurons show only secondary changes.

Mechanism of toxicity. This is not known. Triethyltin has some mild uncoupling action on oxidative phosphorylation, but this is not considered to be enough to cause the changes. Moreover, exactly the same changes may be brought about by hexachlorophane (see p. 282), by the acaricide 2'-chloro,2,4,dinitro-5,6,-di(trifluoromethyl) diphenylamine,[84] by isoniazid (see p. 279) in certain species, and by cuprizone. That four such structurally dissimilar chemicals have such closely similar biological effects suggests that they all affect a particularly important metabolic function of oligodendrocytes. Triethyltin has a marked binding affinity for a protein component in myelin.

Trimethyltin

Trimethyltin has no action upon the myelin sheath, but causes a marked general disturbance to nerve cells in rats, accompanied by the accumulation of lysosomal dense bodies, which displace the other cell organelles.[85-87] Nerve cells die in many parts of the CNS, especially in the hippocampus, where pyramidal cells and dentate fascia cells become severely depleted. Again the mechanism is not known, but preceding the accumulation of intracellular dense bodies there is widespread swelling of the Golgi apparatus of the affected cells, suggesting that the lysosomal accumulations may be a reflection of earlier damage to this important organelle. Human cases of intoxication are fortunately rare,[88] but show essentially the same cellular changes.[89]

Aluminium

Repeated renal dialysis is associated with dementia, in which brain aluminium levels are increased from a normal level of 2–4 µg/g to 12–30 µg/g. However, the brain shows no significant morphological changes to account for the dementing process. Attempts to relate the mental deterioration to neurofibrillary degeneration have been unconvincing, as have been the efforts to identify increased brain levels of aluminium in Alzheimer's disease (see p. 377).[90] The suggested association between aluminium and dementia probably arises because of the abundance of 10 nm filaments which appear within large nerve cells of experimental animals within a few days of local implantation of aluminium salts into the CNS or into the CSF.[91] However, the specific twisted filaments characteristic of Alzheimer's disease (Fig. 13.14, p. 374) do not occur, and although there is gross disorganisation of the neuronal cytoskeleton, nerve cells do not necessarily die. It can be concluded that the relationship between the increased aluminium in the brain and the dementia associated with chronic dialysis is indirect. An association between long-term excessive intake of aluminium and Alzheimer's disease remains to be proved.

SOLVENT TOXICITY

Ethyl alcohol (ethanol)

The consequences of irregular and excessive intake of ethyl alcohol ('alcohol') on the nervous system are manifold, and often it is difficult in any one syndrome to disentangle direct from indirect effects. So far, for most of the syndromes, no experimental animal models have been developed, so that much in our conclusions about underlying mechanisms is conjecture. In the effects of sustained drinking over long periods, alcohol is rarely the sole cause of the changes found. The occurrence either of nutritional effects, from malnutrition or from malabsorption due to associated gastritis, or of actual intoxication by other constituents in the liquor, or indeed even by its contamination with toxic adulterants, must always be considered. Additionally, the frequent occurrence of head injuries during drunken episodes, fighting, etc., may go unreported by the subject and be followed by cerebral oedema or brain hypoxia. In the presence of such an aetiologically complex situation it is not surprising that there are syndromes associated with alcoholism that presently defy explanation.

Wernicke's encephalopathy (see also p. 286)

In any society where alcohol is freely available, Wernicke's encephalopathy,[92] due to a deficiency of thiamine (see p. 286), is probably more common than is often considered. A chronic high alcohol intake, poor diet, associated chronic gastritis, as well as increasing age, all contribute to its occurrence.[93] Harper,[94] in a study from Perth (Western Australia), found an incidence of Wernicke's encephalopathy of 1·7% in 3000 consecutive necropsies: only a small proportion of these cases (about 10%) had been diagnosed during life. Nystagmus, ataxia, cranial nerve palsies, particularly oculomotor, and confusion, with memory loss, whether associated with peripheral neuropathy or not, are the major clinical features of this syndrome. A high sudden intake of glucose, perhaps from a parenteral infusion, could precipitate the encephalopathy by hastening the consumption of the last remaining amounts of thiamine in the tissues.

Pathological features. Haemorrhagic and oedematous foci, with or without necrosis of the involved brain tissue, occur fairly constantly in the mamillary bodies (Fig. 11.10) and less regularly but more or less equally in the walls of the third ventricle, the peri-aqueductal tissue, and the pons, midbrain and thalamus. Table 11.1 shows that there are few nuclear centres that are not at risk, though the medulla tends to show the fewest lesions.[95]

Microscopy of the lesions shows red cells scattered abundantly in the focally oedematous tissues and evidence of capillary thickening and hyperplasia (Fig. 11.11). Neuronal loss is often very slight in the early stages, explaining the relatively rapid reversal of the signs and symptoms

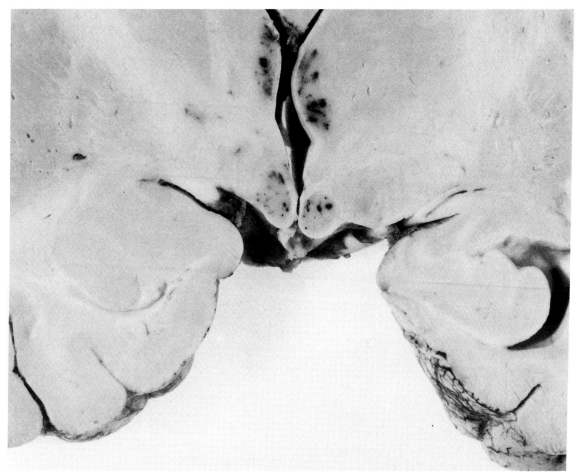

Fig. 11.10 Wernicke's encephalopathy in an alcoholic. Note the haemorrhagic lesions in the mamillary bodies and in the medial walls of the third ventricle.
Reproduced by permission of Professor Clive Harper, University of Sydney, NSW, Australia.

on treatment with thiamine, provided it is administered early in the development of the syndrome. Later the neuronal loss is more severe, and astrogliosis and microglial invasion are both common; in subacute and chronic cases, gliosis may be marked. Atrophy of the mamillary bodies, suggesting recovery from previous attacks, and general cerebral atrophy with ventricular dilatation may be not uncommon associated findings.

Evidence of peripheral neuropathy is also part of the picture of acute-on-chronic alcoholism.

Marchiafava–Bignami syndrome

This rare complication of alcoholism was originally described among Italians drinking coarse red wine. It is seen also in other alcoholics.[96] While the clinical picture contains a variety of disorders of cerebral function—e.g. tremors, rigidity, apraxia, aphasia—pathological changes are mainly restricted to symmetrical demyelination of the corpus callosum and the anterior commissure (Figs 11.12 and 11.13). Other white matter areas are rarely involved. An increase in macrophages is seen in demyelinated areas, but axons remain largely intact.

Alcoholic cerebellar degeneration

Signs of ataxia, and a broad-based gait and stance, even between drinking bouts, may suggest this

Table 11.1   Frequency distribution of lesions in 42 cases of Wernicke's disease. Those regions showing changes in more than half the cases examined are marked in **bold type**. Reproduced by permission of the authors and editor from: Riggs H E, Boles R S. Q J Alcohol Studies 1944; 5: 361.

Region	Number examined	Number present	%
Forebrain			
Cerebral cortex	28	11	39
Septum pellucidum	24	9	37
Fornix	27	3	11
Corpus callosum	28	1	3·6
Caudate nucleus	28	2	7
Hypothalamus			
Dorsomedial nucleus	29	14	48
Ventromedial nucleus	29	23	79
Supraoptic nucleus	26	1	3·8
Mamillary bodies	23	21	91
Thalamus			
Dorsomedial nucleus	27	23	85
Ventromedial nucleus	25	3	12
Pulvinar	14	10	71
Midbrain			
Superior colliculi	18	8	44
IIIrd nerve nucleus	26	6	23
IVth nerve nucleus	14	3	21
Peri-aqueduct grey	14	9	64
Brainstem			
VIth nerve nucleus	13	4	31
Locus ceruleus	10	3	30
Nuclei pontis	18	2	11
Vestibular nucleus	20	12	60
Acoustic nucleus	9	2	22
Xth nerve nucleus	29	20	69
Inferior olive	29	11	38
Cerebellar nucleus	29	3	10

condition. The physical signs change little once established and are related to depletion of Purkinje cells of the superior vermis, more on the surface than in the depths of the sulci. Golgi preparations show 'pruning' of the dendrites and loss of spines from the surviving cells.[97] The occasional occurrence of this condition in non-alcoholic patients suffering from malnutrition suggests that it may not be primarily due to alcohol, but related, as with the neuropathy, to a defect in a vitamin or some other essential dietary factor.

Central pontine myelinolysis

Clinical features. In 1959, Adams, Victor and Mancall[98] described focal demyelinating lesions in the pons of chronic alcoholics; many further cases of this condition have now been reported. It is now clear that alcohol is not essential for inducing central pontine myelinolysis, though a nutritional deficiency may be. The condition has been associated with uraemia, kidney transplantation and other non-alcoholic conditions.[99,100]

Pathological features. The lesions are focal areas (up to 1·0 cm diameter) of oedema and myelin degeneration (see Fig. 10.19, p. 241), usually with loss of some of the axons in the affected regions and the formation of argyrophilic spheroids—'retraction balls' (Fig. 11.14). Microglia and reactive astrocytes are increased within the lesions.

The lesions are reminiscent of the focal pontine damage that can be produced in rats rendered chronically deficient in thiamine,[101] but it is now considered that too rapid a correction of the hyponatraemia present in such cases may be responsible for the lesion.[102] The nature of the

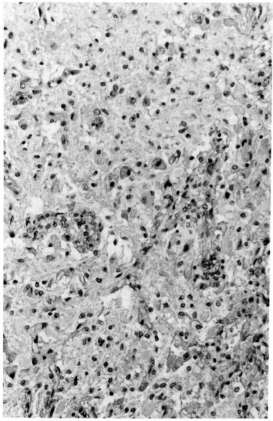

Fig. 11.11 Wernicke's encephalopathy. Endothelial proliferation and increased cellularity of the mamillary body. Note especially the vascular proliferation and the oedematous spaces around these vessels.
Haematoxylin-eosin × 200
Reproduced by permission of Professor A. Torvik, Ullevaal Hospital, Oslo, Norway.

intimate cellular mechanisms involved, and why only this region of the brain is affected, are questions which remain unanswered.

Alcoholic neuropathy

Clinical features. The peripheral neuropathy commonly associated with chronic alcoholism is now almost universally believed to be of nutritional origin, and there is no serious evidence that alcohol has any direct pathological actions on peripheral nerves.[103] There are many close clinical similarities with beri-beri (see p. 288), though there are also many differences, particularly in the circumstances associated with the illness. The alcoholic history is always longstanding; there may

be evidence of chronic gastritis that impairs absorptive processes, and there may well be a history of many previous minor episodes of neuropathy with partial recovery. *Sensory disturbances* dominate the early stages of the illness, with numbness, tingling, dysaesthesias and tenderness in the feet and the hands. The muscles may be exquisitely tender and painful to the touch. Loss of tendon jerks and leg *weakness* follow, with or without associated foot drop; muscular wasting, particularly below the knees, is common in chronic cases. Clumsiness and weakness of the fingers and hands occur later. The cranial nerves are very rarely affected. Evidence of Wernicke's encephalopathy may be found, with characteristic disturbances of oculomotor functions.

Ascites, and oedema of the extremities, may be associated with hepatic cirrhosis, cardiomegaly or protein malnutrition. Blood levels of thiamine and other members of the B group of vitamins will inevitably be low,[104] and indeed, low vitamin blood levels will be found in about 40% of chronic alcoholics, regardless of whether or not they show symptoms of disease. The effects of the polyneuropathy will be reversed in time by administration of B vitamins, and refractory cases will always show evidence of severe liver disease. Except in the more advanced cases, given adequate nutrition, continuing a high alcohol intake need not necessarily impede recovery.[105]

Pathological features. This is characteristically a symmetrical polyneuropathy with Wallerian degeneration, particularly in the distal parts of the limbs, though longer nerves elsewhere, such as the vagus and recurrent laryngeal nerves, will also show degeneration. Biopsy of the sural nerve or other peripheral nerves, particularly distal nerves, shows *loss of axons* and some evidence of *regeneration*, but no segmental demyelination.[106] Evidence of axonal regeneration with clusters of small nerve fibres is seen, particularly where there have been recurrent attacks and active treatment.

Fetal alcohol syndrome

Clinical features. In recent years it has become recognised that infants born of mothers

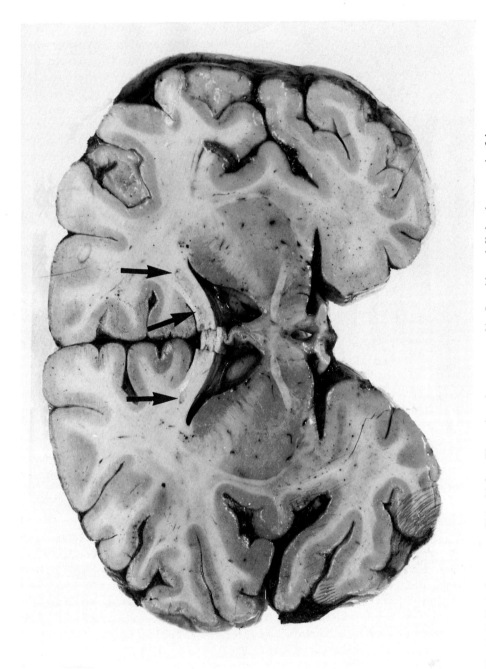

Fig. 11.12 Brain from a case of Marchiafava–Bignami syndrome reported by Ironside et al.,[96] showing necrosis of the corpus callosum (arrows).
Reproduced by permission of Dr R. O. Barnard, Maida Vale Hospital, London, UK.

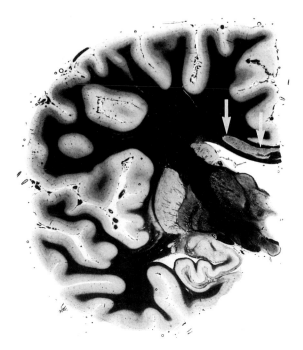

Fig. 11.13 The same brain as in Figure 11.12 stained for myelin. Note the sharp delineation of the damage to the corpus callosum (white arrows).
Reproduced by permission of Dr R. O. Barnard, Maida Vale Hospital, London, UK.

who continue a high alcohol intake during pregnancy will show a number of characteristic deformities and poor mental development.[107,108] While the condition does not appear to be common in England, it is certainly not uncommon in many urban areas in other parts of Europe and in America. In the USA the incidence is estimated to be from 1 to 3 in every thousand live births. Such infants may show microcephaly, hypotonia, poor co-ordination and irritability; they may be hyperactive. There is usually also growth retardation and rather striking craniofacial deformities, such as short palpebral fissures (80%), a short upturned nose, a hypoplastic filtrum (80%), retrognathia or micrognathia. Mental development is usually well behind normal.

Pathological features. There are no post-mortem studies to confirm the conjecture of a brain growth deficiency, but experimental work has shown that ethyl alcohol given to rats during the

first two weeks after birth will lead to smaller brains in the presence of normal body weight.[109] There is some evidence for specific inhibition of hippocampal pyramidal cell growth[110] and of Purkinje cell dendrite growth. Whether this is a direct action of alcohol on growth processes is not known.

Hexacarbon (γ-diketones) Intoxication

n-Hexane and some alkyl substituted analogues are valuable in industry as solvents for rubbers, paints, varnishes, and glues. They are, thus, widely available and have produced many cases of intoxication. In industry, outbreaks of *n*-hexane[111] and methyl *n*-butyl ketone[112] intoxication have been described, while individual cases of poisoning from irregular addictive inhalation of volatile glue solvents are now well documented.[113] Although *glue sniffing* is still widespread, responsible commercial organisations no longer use hexacarbons as solvents for domestic glues, and toluene (itself probably a toxic substance—see p. 267) is now the chief additive. This is not true for many underdeveloped countries, however.

Clinical features. Usually addicts are young persons with grave social problems. Signs of neurotoxicity include a marked general tiredness and weakness of the limbs. *Sensory disturbances*, both subjective and objective, are distal and symmetrical in distribution. *Motor weakness* also occurs in the same distribution; there may be variation from case to case in the extent to which motor or sensory features dominate the clinical picture. Muscle fasciculation is not prominent, but there is distal wasting of muscles, and as the condition becomes more severe, a distal flaccid quadriplegia may develop. Reflexes are depressed or absent. Ataxia is infrequent. Cranial nerves are rarely affected but optic neuritis is occasionally seen. Nerve conduction velocity is decreased.

Pathological features. Muscle biopsy shows denervation atrophy; many nerve fibres present in the biopsy may be swollen and argyrophilic. There may also be some Wallerian degeneration in both sensory and motor fibres.

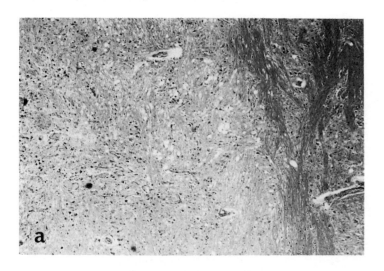

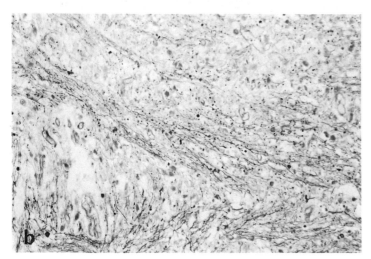

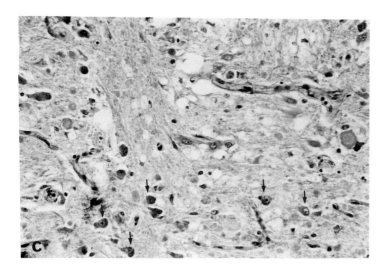

Fig. 11.14a–c Central pontine myelinolysis.
(**a**) Edge of pontine lesion showing loss of
structure. To the right are normal
myelinated bundles. (**b**) Separation and
fragmentation of axons within the lesion
with loss of axons and many black fragments
of axonal debris. (**c**) Surviving pontine
nucleus neurons (arrows) amidst astroglial
and vascular hyperplasia and many lipid-
containing foam cells.
(**a**) Haematoxylin-eosin × 50; (**b**) Glees and
Marsland × 125; (**c**) Haematoxylin-
eosin × 250
*Reproduced by permission of Professor H. H.
Goebel, Neuropathologie, Universität, Mainz,
Federal Republic of Germany.*

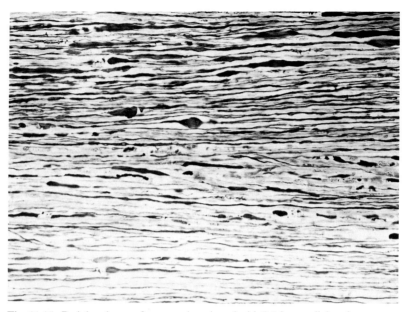

Fig. 11.15. Peripheral nerve from a rat intoxicated with 2,5-hexanediol to show axonal swellings that are often proximal to nodes of Ranvier. Such changes are difficult to see with conventional haematoxylin and eosin stains. The silver stain specifically picks out neurofilaments, and accumulations of these are plainly seen. A few fibres are undergoing degeneration.
Glees and Marsland × 200

Nerve biopsy shows many greatly swollen axons covered by attenuated myelin sheaths. Electron microscopy shows that the swollen axons are filled with 10 nm neurofilaments ('Giant Axonal Neuropathy').[114] Mitochondria, microtubules and other axonal organelles are either displaced to the periphery or lie in clumps among the filaments. Teased preparations of nerve fibres show that the swellings lie predominantly in a zone 30–40 μm proximal to nodes of Ranvier (Fig. 11.15); internodal swellings may also occur. The axon swellings are well demonstrated by silver stains and they often cause gross distortion of the nodes of Ranvier; this is the likely cause for the early slowing of nerve conduction.

Experimental results. Studies of the effects of *n*-hexane and analogues, such as methyl-*n*-butyl ketone, 2,5-hexanediol, and 2,5-hexanedione, show that chronic exposure leads to accumulation of 10 nm filaments within axons in all parts of the nervous system, both peripheral and central.[115] Constriction of axons, caused by binding of the myelin spiral of Schwann or oligodendroglial cells to the axolemma at the normal juxtanodal regions, is a major factor in producing axonal damage (Fig. 11.16).[116] The neurofilamentous masses appear able to pass through the relatively unconstricted nodes of Ranvier of smaller axons with little difficulty, and reach preterminal and terminal axonal regions where they are degraded, probably by Ca^{++} activated proteases. In the larger diameter axons, the filament masses become progressively less able to negotiate these nodal constrictions, and ultimately the flow of axoplasmic materials required to maintain the remainder of the axon is impeded. Axoplasmic flow becomes significantly slowed as the nervous disability increases. Wallerian degeneration occurs, presumably due to the mechanical obstruction to normal mechanisms for axon maintenance.

Mechanism of toxicity. *n*-Hexane and its congeners are lipid-soluble substances metabolised in tissues to water-soluble compounds.[117] Conversion to the diketone, 2,5-hexanedione, is critical (Fig. 11.17) and takes place in all tissues,

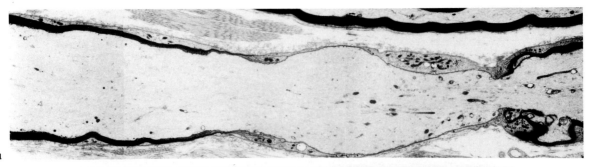

a

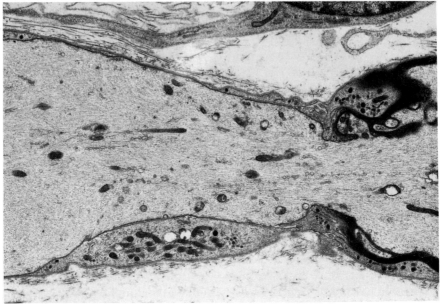

b

Fig. 11.16a, b Electron micrographs of peroneal nerve of a rat intoxicated with 2,5-hexanediol. (**a**) The proximal paranodal region is grossly swollen by neurofilaments, greatly attenuating the myelin sheath and distorting the nodal region. Node of Ranvier at right. (**b**) At higher magnification, the nodal region is seen to be greatly simplified and the myelin severely thinned. Schwann cell cytoplasm covers the partly denuded axon. The distal paranodal region (right) is much less altered. (**a**) × 3300; (**b**) × 7900
Reproduced by permission of the editor from: Jones HB, Cavanagh JB. J Neurocytol 1983; 12: 439.

including the central nervous system. Diketones with this configuration can cross-link proteins at their lysine residues[118] with subsequent effects on the capacity of long fibrous proteins to flow readily along axons, and to negotiate nodal constrictions. Normally, 10 nm filaments formed in the cell body pass slowly (1–3 mm/day) along the axon to the terminals where they are degraded. Their functions are unknown, but one of these must be the purely physical one of helping to maintain the circularity of the larger diameter axons and thus, by minimising volume-to-surface ratio, increase efficiency of axon maintenance. Other γ-diketones

derived from hydrocarbons with varying chain lengths can also produce these effects, so that the term, suggested by O'Donohue and Krasavage, 'γ-diketone intoxication',[119] may be preferable.

Carbon disulphide

Carbon disulphide (CS_2) is widely used in industry in a number of important manufacturing processes, particularly as a solvent in the rubber industry and in the spinning of rayon. Its toxicity may affect many tissues,[120] the three most important being those of the vascular system,

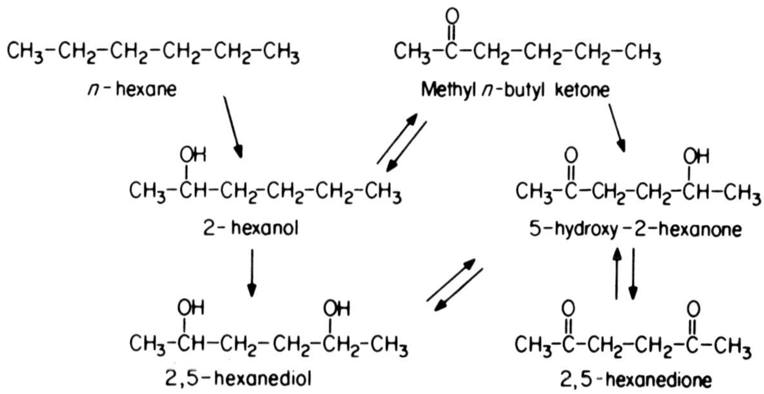

Fig. 11.17 Metabolic conversion pathway of *n*-hexane and some analogues to the proximate toxic chemical, 2,5-hexanedione.
Reproduced by permission of the authors and editor from: DiVincenzo GD, Kaplan CJ, Dedinas J Toxicol Appl Pharmacol 1976; 36: 511.

those subserving higher mental functions, and large diameter long axons in the peripheral and central nervous systems. The first is of particular importance in long-term exposure and may predispose to coronary heart disease and other forms of vascular disease.

Clinical features. Striking psychiatric changes occur in acutely and severely intoxicated patients. Wild dreams, emotional instability, depression, excitation, hallucinations and many other bizarre disturbances have been described, and occasionally have led to suicide. These symptoms are reversible on withdrawal from exposure. They have no structural basis; their origin is in the inhibition of dopamine β-hydroxylase.[121] This enzyme requires copper: carbon disulphide, after conversion in the tissues to dithiocarbamate, chelates with the copper and thus indirectly inhibits the enzyme.

A more slowly developing peripheral neuropathy occurs on chronic exposure to relatively high concentrations of CS_2. Slowing of conduction velocity is often the first change to be detected, and is associated with mild distal sensory or motor neuropathy.[122] However, with modern strict control of the occupational environment, the more marked distal weakness, wasting and paresis is now rarely seen. As with hexacarbon neuropathy (see above), recovery is very slow and may take many months.

Pathological features. Post mortems have been rare. Abe in 1933[123] reported a case showing evidence of spinocerebellar degeneration associated with hypoxic-type brain lesions. Subsequent experimental studies have shown that the changes are identical with those found in hexacarbon intoxication (see above),[124,125] by both light and electron microscopy. In the peripheral nervous system filamentous accumulations, axonal swellings and Wallerian degeneration are found. In the central nervous system, axonal swellings are numerous especially in larger diameter fibres, but axon degeneration is less obvious than in the peripheral nervous system.

Mechanism of toxicity. CS_2 is very reactive and in the tissues is changed both to the highly reactive carbonyl sulphide (COS) as well as to dithiocarbamate. Cross-linking of proteins, particularly 10 nm filaments, as in 2,5-hexanedione toxicity, must be occurring, but direct evidence is lacking.

Toluene

Used as a solvent for paints and varnishes and for many glue formulations, toluene is widely available, having gained, perhaps by default, a reputation for being non-toxic. It has a sweetish odour and narcotising effects, and has been much used by addicted 'sniffers' or 'huffers'.

Clinical features. There are marked mental effects from inhalation of toluene. But appearances on CT scans and the long persistence of clinical signs after ceasing exposure to toluene are evidence for irreversible structural damage in the cerebellum, as well as perhaps cerebral cortical damage.[126-128] The clinical signs of ataxia of cerebellar origin and perhaps also of mental deterioration have been noted, but there are so far no animal studies to substantiate the clinical findings. In the absence of biopsy or post-mortem material it is difficult to judge the significance of the clinical changes.

Trichloroethylene

A curious kind of solvent toxicity occasionally follows heavy exposure to trichloroethylene (Trilene®). This is a valuable degreasing solvent and was used also at one time as a general anaesthetic. It was also recommended some decades ago for the treatment of trigeminal neuralgia. Cranial nerve palsies and attacks of orofacial herpes simplex follow its use and have led to its therapeutic decline.[129]

Clinical features. Reports of polyneuritis cranialis from trichloroethylene exposure, both clinical and industrial, are numerous.[129] The trigeminal nerve is always affected earliest, producing both subjective and objective sensory changes, which may then spread to involve the motor component. In more severe cases other closely related cranial nerves may become involved, the damage apparently moving both up and down the brainstem. Rarely it may extend to involve cervical spinal nerves. Recovery from the paresis and the sensory changes is always slow and often incomplete. The occurrence of circumoral herpes simplex ('cold sores') in such cases has been frequently reported.

Pathological features. The only post-mortem study reported[130] in detail has shown that not only was there severe Wallerian degeneration of the trigeminal nerves, there was also extensive loss of nerve cells in the motor nuclei of these nerves as well as in the oculomotor nuclei and to a lesser degree in the facial, hypoglossal and vagal nuclei.

In addition, there was damage to neurons of the globus pallidus, substantia nigra, hypothalamus and mamillary bodies. These changes were not accompanied by an inflammatory reaction.

Mechanism of toxicity. This curiously local and unique intoxication is inexplicable on the basis of direct toxic damage to neurons, and it is difficult even to suggest how this solvent could selectively and regularly damage these cranial nerve nuclei in the manner described. Local invasion of the nervous system does not occur with any other toxic agent. While it is most probable that dichloroethylene, a breakdown product, may be responsible, in the absence of an experimental animal model there is much uncertainty about this. A strong but untested possibility is that the chemical may activate latent herpes simplex virus locally in the trigeminal nerve ganglion and perhaps the mesencephalic trigeminal nucleus. The frequent occurrence of herpes simplex skin lesions ('cold sores') in this intoxication is in favour of such a mechanism.[130a]

Methyl alcohol (methanol, wood alcohol)

Clinical features. Wood alcohol has been responsible for a number of outbreaks, large and small, of poisoning from contamination of (usually illicit) alcoholic liquors. The symptoms and signs of poisoning are variable in degree and in the timing of their onset; they may be delayed for up to 24 hours or more without regard to the amount of alcohol drunk. Some loss of vision and other, less serious, visual symptoms such as photophobia, are present in all cases, but amaurosis is fortunately complete in only a few. Headache, vomiting, decrease in conscious level, fits and coma occur in severe cases.[131,132]

Pathological features. Retinoscopy shows hyperaemia of the vessels and oedema of the retina. Later, as atrophy of the retinal ganglion cells and their fibres supervenes, pallor of the optic disc will be seen. Except for necrosis of the retinal ganglion cells and secondary degeneration of the optic nerves, other changes in the nervous system are few and probably non-specific.

Mechanism of toxicity. Methanol readily diffuses throughout body water and is present in CSF and aqueous humour in concentrations slightly higher than those in plasma. It is only slowly oxidised by alcohol dehydrogenase, at about one-fifth of the oxidation rate of ethanol, and this may account for the frequently slow onset of symptoms. Indeed, ethanol will competitively inhibit oxidation of methanol, and the amount of ethanol mixed with the drink will thus affect the time of onset of toxic effects. Methanol is broken down in the tissues to formic acid and formaldehyde, and it is the formaldehyde that is considered, on rather slender evidence, to be the proximate toxic agent.

INDUSTRIAL CHEMICALS

Organophosphorus neurotoxicity

Various organophosphorus (O-P) compounds are used in many major industries. The chances of becoming exposed, therefore, to these products are considerable, and cases of neurotoxicity from this cause continue to be reported in the literature.

There are two principal forms of O-P compounds, either with predominantly aryl or predominantly alkyl side chains, and each has markedly different properties.

Aryl organophosphorus compounds, typified by tri-*ortho*-cresyl phosphate, are oily with little or no taste or smell. They are relatively chemically inert and are used, for example, as high or low temperature lubricants and plasticisers, and as 'molecular lubricants' for softening celluloid and polyvinyl chloride (PVC). To become toxic they must be metabolised by the liver via mixed function oxidases. Their relative inertness has been largely responsible for past outbreaks of poisoning, due to their inadvertent mixture with edible salad or cooking oils or with drinks, their use as sunburn oil and in abortifacients, and even at one time in the treatment of tuberculosis.[133] In consequence of all these accidents, many thousands of cases of paralysis have been caused. Most patients have been mildly affected and have recovered completely, but there are many less fortunate showing permanent neurological defects many years later.

Alkyl organophosphorus compounds, in contrast, tend to be highly reactive chemicals, directly inhibitory to many enzymes. They are widely used in agriculture, as pesticides, and in medicine; they are also war gases. They include some of the most potent chemicals made by man, causing paresis with doses of the order of 0·1 μg/kg. This is less than one-thousandth of the amount of an aryl-phosphate producing the same degree of paralysis. A further important feature of all alkyl O-P compounds is that the majority are capable of causing severe acute functional disturbances, often fatal, because of their anti-esterase, particularly anti-cholinesterase, activity, but only a minority are able to produce delayed peripheral neuropathy with structural and irreversible damage to the nervous system. This specific potential of individual chemicals can now be determined experimentally and *in vivo*, as discussed below. But because of the complexities outlined above, predicting the likely effects and outcome in any one case of O-P poisoning is difficult.

Arylphosphate poisoning

Clinical features. The majority of case reports of neuropathy come from poisoning by arylphosphates, usually in the form of tri-*ortho*-cresyl phosphate, although the compound in question is rarely pure. Thus, it may also contain varying amounts of mono-substituted and di-substituted forms, which are toxic, as well as *meta*- and *para*- forms that are not.[134] Clinical experience comes from outbreaks of poisoning in various parts of the world. In some outbreaks many thousands of people have been affected—for example, 'Ginger Jake Paralysis' from illicit liquor in the USA in the 1930s and the epidemic poisoning by contaminated cooking oil in Morocco in 1959. Following ingestion of toxic oil, acute gastrointestinal symptoms are accompanied by pins and needles and burning pains in the palms of the hands and soles of the feet. About 2 weeks after dosing, the feet become clumsy, foot drop appears and with it a high-stepping, flapping gait. Weakness extends proximally in a few and spreads to the hands. Rarely, if ever, does the weakness extend above the knees or the elbows. Sensory symptoms are so infrequently described as to have led to the mistaken belief that this is a pure motor neuropathy. Ataxia, due to denervation of muscle spindle afferents, is a distinct feature, and loss of reflexes is common. Undue sweating of the hands and feet and Raynaud's phenomenon suggest autonomic involvement. Careful examination has revealed glove and stocking anaesthesia in at least half the cases at some time during the illness. Later, signs of spinal tract involvement may be found as recovery of peripheral nerve function takes place. Damage to most cranial nerves is not seen, although laryngeal paralysis from involvement of the very long recurrent laryngeal nerve is not infrequently seen.

Electrophysiologically, evidence of denervation and some mild slowing of nerve conduction velocity, both motor and sensory, is found, but more important are reduction of amplitude of sensory and motor action potentials and increase in excitability thresholds.

Recovery is slow and about 5% of patients may be troubled by increasing spasticity due to the expression of spinal tract damage as the peripheral nerve lesions recover. However, the majority recover well with time and show little residual disability.

Pathological features. Death rarely occurs during the acute phase of the intoxication. In cases dying several years after acute intoxication, there is Wallerian degeneration of axons in the posterior columns of the spinal cord, particularly in the gracile tracts, but not the cuneate tracts. The gracile tract degeneration is marked in the cervical regions and there is degeneration of the distal parts of the corticospinal tracts in the lumbosacral regions of the cord. No significant changes are found elsewhere in the central nervous system (CNS), but in the peripheral nervous system (PNS) there is evidence of earlier peripheral nerve degeneration and muscle denervation.[135]

Experimental studies in many species have produced distal nerve fibre degeneration in longer axons of large diameter in both the PNS and the CNS.[136] Distal axonal degeneration is seen in both motor and sensory nerves, but especially in nerves from primary sensory endings of muscle spindles and from Golgi tendon organs; this pattern of damage is probably the cause of the limb

clumsiness and ataxia. The degeneration is often very distal in distribution and regeneration may, therefore, be relatively rapid during recovery.

Ultrastructural studies have shown that just before nerve fibre degeneration occurs there is abundant accumulation of smooth endoplasmic reticulum in large diameter axons.[137]

Alkylphosphate poisoning

Clinical features. These chemicals strongly inhibit acetylcholinesterase and, therefore, cause all the signs of acetylcholine poisoning. Such signs can often be countered with atropine and oximes. About 10 days later, peripheral nerve signs develop. Earlier reports of such cases arose from the handling of mipafox (dimethyl diamidic fluorophosphate) in the laboratory, but more recently there have been reports of cases of insecticide poisoning from metriphonate (trichlorphon; Chlorophos® or Dipterex®; dimethyl 1-hydroxy-2,2,2-trichloroethyl phosphonate) intoxication that have been well studied clinically.[138] Signs of neuropathy are essentially those of tri-*ortho*-cresyl phosphate (TOCP) poisoning; the changes evolve during the 3–5 weeks after absorption of the chemical. Sensory symptoms in the feet may herald the appearance of severe distal motor weakness of the feet and then of the hands. Objective sensory disturbances tend to be mild or absent, but electrophysiologically a reduction in amplitude of action potentials in both sensory and motor nerves indicates equal involvement of large diameter motor and sensory fibres. Evidence of damage to pyramidal tracts develops in a few subjects.

Mechanisms of organophosphorus toxicity

Arylphosphates are chemically inert and become neurotoxic only after conversion in the liver to a more reactive product. In order to be transformed in this way the arylphosphate must possess at least one *ortho*-substituted ring. Transformation occurs via mixed function oxidases in the liver; the first step is α-hydroxylation of one ring and loss of another ring with cyclisation forming phenyl saligenin phosphate (Fig. 11.18).[139] The product is a potent inhibitor of acetylcholinesterase, pro-

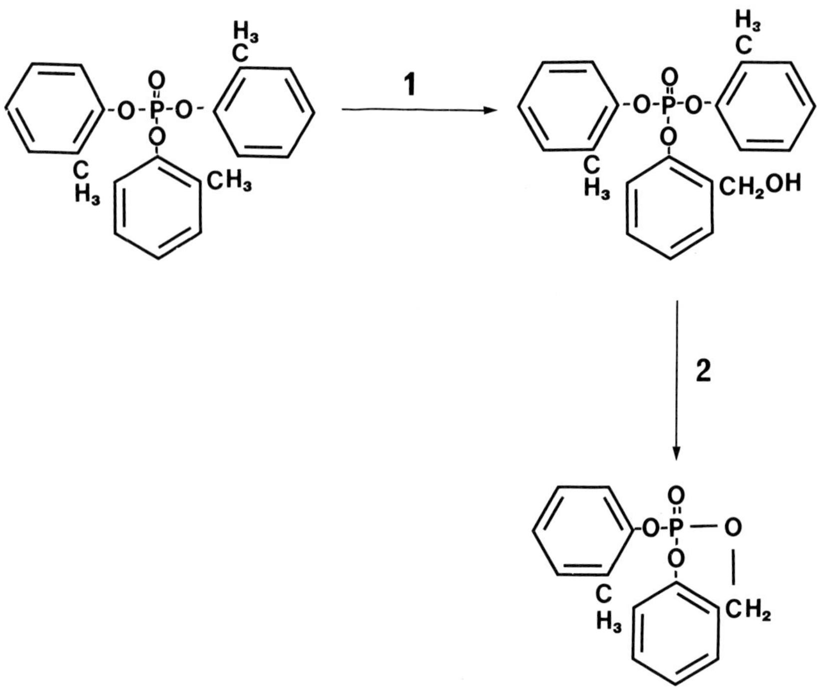

Fig. 11.18 Conversion pathway of tri-*ortho*-cresyl phosphate (TCOP) to phenyl saligenin phosphate, the proximate toxic and anti-cholinesterase product. The toxic dose of TOCP is 500 mg/kg, and that of the conversion product 10 mg/kg. Conversion is effected through the microsomal P 450 enzyme system, and the first step (1) is by α-hydroxylation of one methyl group, which leads (2) to loss of a ring and cyclisation.

ducing ataxia in hens at 2 mg/kg, which is about one-hundredth of the dose needed of the original *ortho*-cresyl phosphate. *Alkylphosphates*, by contrast, are more reactive and are able to inhibit a wide variety of esterases and other enzymes by phosphorylation.

It is now established that neurotoxic O-P compounds can specifically inhibit an enzyme, 'neurotoxic esterase', which is present in nervous and other tissues.[140] In contrast, non-neurotoxic O-P compounds are unable to inhibit this enzyme. The function of this enzyme or protein is unknown, but irreversible phosphorylation of its active site and subsequent 'ageing', in which the R-O-P bond is cleaved to leave an ionised phosphoryl residue, produce what is believed to be the proximate toxic agent. The final result seems to be that axons in most regions of the nervous system are adversely affected, but that the majority are able to overcome these effects. Only the larger diameter and longer fibres with their very much greater work load of membrane maintenance seem unable to cope with this adverse situation. There are recent suggestions that retrograde axoplasmic transport may be selectively inhibited.[141]

Acrylamide intoxication

Acrylamide polymers are widely used in industry as flocculants, grouters, sealants, and water-proofers in building and engineering works, as well as in laboratories. The polymers are non-toxic, but the monomer is a highly reactive chemical, causing neurotoxic effects in both PNS and CNS. Exposure comes either from handling the monomer itself at work or from monomer that contaminates the polymer and becomes leached out from it. Mostly the neurological effects are not serious and may not be long-lasting.

Clinical features. Acute exposure from contamination of drinking water has caused bizarre psychological symptoms, such as hallucinations, disorientation and other behavioural changes, accompanied by slurred speech and nystagmus. Truncal ataxia, disturbances of bladder function and defaecation, and signs of distal sensory neuropathy have followed.[142] Most other reported cases have occurred from industrial handling of the monomer and its absorption through skin. The subjects complain of skin peeling, sweating, bluish and cold extremities, muscle weakness, and abnormal skin sensations in the limbs. There is loss of reflexes and distal sensory loss in the limbs; truncal ataxia and Rombergism are characteristic. Coarse tremor and dysarthria are occasionally noted. Most patients recover slowly, although residual signs have been reported.[143]

Electrophysiological findings are mild slowing of nerve conduction velocity and reduction in amplitude or even absence of the sensory action potentials. The muscle responses to stimulation are often dispersed.[144]

Pathological features. Nerve biopsy shows Wallerian type degeneration of the larger diameter fibres, but 'giant axonal' swellings (see p. 265) containing neurofilaments have been noted.[145] No post-mortem reports are available.

Abundant experimental studies to determine the nature of the axonal lesion have been made, but the mechanism has eluded analysis. In animals, after daily administration of from 10 to 50 mg/kg, functional disturbances commence after 2 to 4 weeks. Distal nerve fibre degeneration occurs in large diameter peripheral sensory axons and less markedly in distal intramuscular motor fibres. Axonal degeneration is seen in the CNS involving the distal regions of the dorsal columns and the spinocerebellar tracts as they enter the cerebellum, as well as the lumbosacral parts of the corticospinal tracts, but CNS changes tend to be mild even in severely poisoned animals.[146] Distal axon degeneration is preceded by accumulations of argyrophilic neurofilaments in axon terminals and preterminals throughout many parts of the PNS and the CNS regardless of axon length and size or whether they will show later degeneration. Neurons in the dorsal root ganglia often show chromatolysis before axon degeneration has occurred, indicating that the whole neuron is affected in acrylamide poisoning even though only the distal regions may degenerate. Acute degenerative changes may be seen in Purkinje cells.[147]

This complex of pathological changes does not resemble any known human disease pattern, but may indicate the presence of a general defect in neuron metabolism and possibly of membrane maintenance, with subsequent failure of axon integrity. Biochemically, acrylamide is highly reactive, binding firmly to sulphydryl groups of proteins. Cell respiration and energy production appear normal, but mitochondrial hypertrophy and hyperplasia in neuron perikarya, often with excess calcium phosphate granules, suggest continuing membrane leakiness to calcium ions and the need to sequester the calcium, a process that is very energy consuming.[148]

BACTERIAL TOXINS

Botulinum intoxication (botulism)

Botulism is rare. The sudden outbreak of the intoxication, the rapid progress of the paralysis and the frequent swiftness of death have sometimes had a profound impact upon human communities.

Clinical features. Outbreaks of botulism more often follow family gatherings and small parties than industrial canning and bottling misadventures. Home-canned vegetables (particularly beans), pickled meats, sausages and similar foods have been common sources of intoxication. If food contaminated by *Clostridium botulinum*, an anaerobic organism widely distributed in nature, is not adequately heated before preservation, the bacilli and particularly their spores are not destroyed. The bacilli then release their toxins into the preserved food in such quantity that, on ingestion, sufficient toxin escapes destruction in the alimentary tract to cause the illness. Symptoms usually begin 12 to 36 hours after ingestion, but are sometimes delayed up to 72 hours. Early signs are vomiting and diarrhoea but, with the onset of paresis, constipation and ileus may follow.

Neurological signs begin with blurred vision and diplopia. Dry mouth and diminished secretions are common and other cranial nerve pareses follow, such as aphonia, dysphagia, ptosis and facial weakness. Marked proximal weakness of the limbs without loss of reflexes steadily increases and leads eventually to respiratory paralysis. Recovery of those who survive is slow and may take several weeks.

Pathological features. Experimental studies have shown that botulinum toxin specifically blocks the release of acetylcholine from motor nerve terminals.[149,150] In response to this action, a vigorous neuritic sprouting occurs at muscle nerve terminals, especially from motor end-plates (ultraterminal sprouting), and large numbers of sprouts seek to form new terminals on the functionally denervated muscle fibres. The new endings ultimately replace the old end-plates.[151] At the same time, a chromatolysis-type response occurs in motor nerve cells[152] in response to the functional denervation. Despite these striking events at the axon terminals, if the tracer protein, horseradish peroxidase, is injected into the region of the motor terminals, it is still actively taken up by endocytosis and transported at normal rates to the nerve cell bodies. The general biological functions of the neuron, therefore, are not lost.[153]

Mechanism of toxicity. The toxin is produced by the bacterium *Clostridium botulinum* when grown under strictly anaerobic conditions. Several types of toxin are produced. They are heat labile. They constitute one of the most lethal groups of poisons known; as little as $10^{-5}\mu g$ of the toxin is capable of killing a 20 g mouse. The common type A toxin is a 150 kd protein. It has been shown to bind to nerve terminals, preventing the release of acetylcholine. The number of toxin molecules which reach the end-plates agrees closely with the number of vesicles released at each nerve impulse and the finite number of active efflux sites on the terminal for the acetylcholine vesicles.[154] There is also said to be close agreement between the size of the botulinum toxin (10–15 nm) and the vesicle size (10–20 nm). The Ca^{++}-mediated exocytosis mechanism involved in the release of acetylcholine is probably a ganglioside generating or unmasking process, and in some unknown manner botulinum toxin interferes with the mechanism of synaptic

vesicle release from the presynaptic membrane.[155] The postsynaptic membrane remains responsive to acetylcholine, however, and venom from the black widow spider, *Latrodectus mactans*, which causes massive release of synaptic vesicles at nerve terminals, can locally overcome the effect of botulinum toxin.

Diphtheria

While diphtheria is now rarely seen in most developed countries, due to adequate control by immunisation procedures, it is still common among children in other parts of the world. Immunity is the key to its control. Thus, in a non-immunised community it is young children who are most at risk, while adults only develop diphtheria if their immunity has waned or they have somehow escaped immunisation by a natural mild infection or by vaccination.

Clinical features. Infection is usually in the upper respiratory tract, and faucial diphtheria is the most common form. Rarely, infection of the skin or the genital tract occurs. Clinical neurological findings, however, are the same whatever the part infected and there is no evidence that local spread of the toxin along the nerves occurs.

The local lesion has a characteristic soft leathery membrane overlying the inflamed and ulcerated mucosa of the throat, tonsils and fauces. Inflammation may spread downwards into the pharynx and trachea causing respiratory embarrassment, which may require tracheotomy. The organism responsible is *Corynebacterium diphtheriae*; it is spread by droplets and the infection has a short incubation period of 1 to 7 days. Toxic complications affect in particular the heart but also the liver and kidneys. The heart shows functional disturbances of the sino-atrial nodes and the conducting system; arrhythmias and heart block are frequent. Sudden death may follow.

Neurological complications are confined to the peripheral nervous system (PNS). The earliest of the neurological clinical signs are paralysis of the palate and of visual accommodation. Paresis of the limbs, if it occurs, always follows the premonitory cranial nerve changes after a variable delay of 3 weeks to 3 months. The paralysis is always motor, with little or no sensory component, and it frequently involves all four limbs. Sensory changes are uncommon but may be noted at the outset as numbness, tinglings and pains in the limbs. Ataxia, sometimes referred to as 'pseudotabes', is frequent, perhaps from loss of function of muscle afferent fibres.

Electrophysiological studies show a gradual reduction in conduction velocity in limb nerves and an increase in distal latencies: these features are characteristic of a demyelination process. The cerebrospinal fluid may show increased protein levels.

Pathological features. Extensive and widespread myelin degeneration (*segmental demyelination*; see p. 541) in peripheral nerves is the cardinal pathological change, with degeneration of axons occurring where myelin changes are most severe. All PNS regions are involved and the dorsal spinal roots are particularly affected, perhaps because of the fenestrated blood vessels in the dorsal root ganglia.

Myelin breakdown is followed by Schwann cell multiplication and macrophage infiltration everywhere in the affected nerves, and remyelination may be found going on side by side with the features of myelin breakdown. Remyelination is active and always complete, although it may take several months for the nerve conduction velocity to return to normal. Permanent sequelae are unknown. There are no significant findings in the CNS, and chromatolysis of the anterior horn cells has not been reported, a negative feature which emphasises the general lack of axonal involvement.[156]

Experimental studies have shown that the earliest myelin degeneration occurs in the adaxonal, paranodal regions,[157,158] that is to say in the part of the Schwann cell furthest from the sites of protein synthesis. It is, thus, a form of 'dying back' process analogous to that more commonly found in nerve fibres in toxic and other conditions (see p. 540). The myelin breakdown is often restricted to the paranodal regions, but because the complex structure of the node of Ranvier is critical to the passage of the nerve impulse, its disorganisation blocks the passage of the action potential, and leads to paralysis. Remyelination and restitution of the node of Ranvier is followed by return of function.

Mechanism of toxicity. Lysogenic strains of *C. diphtheriae* are infected with a phage that under certain rather specific cultural conditions, such as high iron concentration, becomes activated and synthesises the toxin which eventually lyses the bacterium. The toxin is a protein of about 63 kd. On entry into the body it is antigenic and immune responses will, in time, control not only the infection but also the intoxication. The toxin binds to receptors on cell surfaces and the number of these per cell depends upon the species and determines the susceptibility to the toxic effects. While capable of passing into dorsal root and autonomic ganglia and into peripheral nerve, the toxin does not appear able to penetrate the blood-brain barrier.

On entry into the cell, the toxin is broken by protease into two fragments. Fragment 'A' is toxic and catalyses adenine diphosphate ribosylation of peptide elongation factor 2, with resulting release of nicotinamide, even at very low toxin concentrations. The transfer of amino acids from transfer factor 2, which requires reduced nicotinamide adenine dinucleotide (NADH), is thus prevented and protein synthesis ceases.[159] One molecule of diphtheria toxin introduced into a cell may be sufficient to kill it by this means.[160] For the Schwann cell, cessation of protein synthesis must mean that provision of basic protein and other factors necessary to maintain compaction and stability of the myelin sheath begins to fail: the part of the internode furthest from the site of synthesis is first affected by this loss.[161]

Tetanus

Clostridium tetani is a spore-bearing soil organism that may readily infect skin wounds. It is an obligatory anaerobe and produces the toxin, tetanospasmin. When the toxin is produced by bacilli in deep wounds, it is released and gains access to the central nervous system through nerve endings and thence by transportation along axons. Many thousands of cases of tetanus infection occur annually throughout the world. Antitetanus immunisation helps considerably to reduce the incidence of this painful and often fatal condition.

Clinical features. The site of infection may be a deep cut, an ulcer, the birth canal following childbirth, the umbilical stump in a newborn infant, or where an injection of an addictive or therapeutic drug has been given. The incubation period is long and may vary from 7 days to more than a month. Muscle rigidity and spasms are characteristic, and often start with the face and jaw ('lock-jaw'). Usually the disturbances are generalised, but occasionally the infected limb may be principally affected ('local tetanus'), at least at the outset. Muscle spasms occur repeatedly and are very painful. They are easily triggered by minor stimuli, such as a medical examination. The pulse is rapid and the blood pressure can fluctuate markedly.

Pathological features. Background studies have been well reviewed by Payling Wright.[162] There are no specific structural changes on post-mortem examination. Experimental studies have shown that the toxin probably gains access to the nervous system not by the blood stream but by entry into the terminals of motor nerves throughout the body, passing up the axons by retrograde transport. General toxicity is thus the summation of the entry along many axonal routes and, of course, specific therapy is made very difficult for this reason. Once inside the neuronal cell body the fate of the toxin is unknown, but there is evidence that it can act on many different transmitters and synapses by blocking transmitter release; this includes the myoneural junction. The toxin must, therefore, be able to pass from the postsynaptic to the presynaptic cell membrane. There is evidence, too, that tetanus toxin particularly inhibits γ-aminobutyric acid and glycine, major inhibitory transmitters. Most of the major signs of tetanus toxicity arise from effects upon these inhibitory synapses.[163]

PLANT TOXINS

Lathyrism

Clinical features. The neurological syndrome known as lathyrism was first noted in India by General Sleeman in 1844 and has probably existed there from time immemorial. It has remained common in India and has also been observed in other parts of the world, such as Spain and North Africa. Its basis is the consumption, in times of drought and famine, of the drought-resistant pea *Lathyrus sativus* in place of the usual peas and beans.

The clinical syndrome is the relatively sudden onset of spasticity of the lower limbs accompanied by pains in the limbs. There is no evidence of peripheral neuropathy, and therefore no muscle wasting, no fasciculation and no sensory loss.[164,165]

Pathological features. Post-mortem studies are few despite the large number of clinical cases. There have been reports of degeneration of the lateral and anterior corticospinal tracts but very little else.[166-168]

The numerous experimental studies have been inconclusive. A rôle for selenium has been seriously considered[169] and various amino acids have been extracted and postulated as the active principles.[170] However, recent studies[171] suggest that an amino acid, β-N-oxalylamino-L-alanine, extracted from *Lathyrus sativus*, can produce signs of pyramidal tract degeneration in macaque monkeys on chronic feeding. This amino acid has some excitatory properties as it is an agonist of the transmitter glutamate.

The toxic aminonitriles isolated from *L. odoratus*, the sweet pea, have no association with the neurological lesions of lathyrism. They are known to disturb collagen metabolism and thus cause distortion of growing bones, so-called osteolathyrism. Other compounds, such as β,β'-imino-dipropionitrile (IDPN), can induce filament accumulations in large neurons by disturbing the cytoskeleton.[171-173] No human cases of intoxication by IDPN have been reported, however, and it remains an interesting experimental entity unrelated to human lathyrism.

Cycad intoxication and the ALS-Parkinsonism-dementia of Guam

Following World War II, a high incidence of a neurological disease was noticed in the Western Pacific islands of Guam and Rota, in the Marianas Group. The condition is characterised by three main clinical features occurring either alone or in various combinations:

1. amyotrophic lateral sclerosis (ALS; motor neuron disease) with spasticity, muscle fasciculation and atrophy, and bulbar dysfunction,
2. Parkinsonism with rigidity, limitation of movement and tremor, and
3. dementia of the Alzheimer type.

The motor neuron disease component of this triad was the most frequent, and its incidence in the island population was many times greater than in the world as a whole.[174] In addition to the expected degeneration of large motor nerve cells and their axons in the pyramidal and other long motor pathways, a significant pathological feature was the presence of neurofibrillary tangles in many nerve cells both in the cerebral cortex and elsewhere, in all cases, regardless of the clinical type of the disease, and even sometimes in people dying with no obvious signs of this condition.[175]

During the investigations of this illness in the 1950s and 1960s it became apparent that the natives of these islands were in the habit of using the nuts of the cycad trees (*Cycas* species) as food. From these nuts they obtained a kind of flour, and this practice had greatly increased in some areas during the war due to shortages of other food. A similar regular exposure to the nut was also noted amongst the peoples in other areas of the Pacific region where the condition was later found,

namely in the Kii peninsula of Honshu island in Japan, parts of New Guinea (Irian Jaya) and the northern Philippine islands.

Recently, extracts of this plant have been found to contain an amino acid, β-N-methylamino-L-alanine (Fig. 11.19), that has excitotoxic actions on the glutamate/aspartate neurotransmitter system. If this compound is fed regularly for some months to rhesus monkeys, they develop degeneration of the pyramidal tracts with severe chromatolytic changes in the cortical pyramidal neurons. Less marked changes were also present in the anterior horn cells, but such changes do not occur in rats similarly treated.[176]

It has been suggested that chronic intake of this amino acid in some way disturbs neuronal metabolism and that large neurons with long axons may be most particularly at risk from this metabolic lesion. The mechanism is by no means clear, but there appears to be connection with the problem of lathyrism. A closely analogous amino acid, β-N-oxalylamino-L-alanine (Fig. 11.19), can be extracted from the chick pea; it is similarly excitotoxic to the same transmitter system and also seems to be capable of producing damage to the pyramidal pathways. These two conditions together, as with MPTP intoxication (see p. 284), strongly emphasise the possible rôle of environmental agents in the causation of serious neurological disease, but these conjectures are by no means proven.

A.

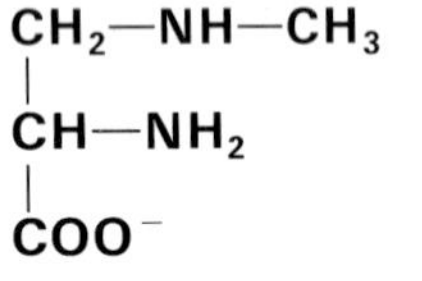

CH$_2$—NH—CH$_3$
|
CH—NH$_2$
|
COO$^-$

α-amino, β-Methylamino proprionic acid.
(β-N-methylamino-L-alanine)

B.

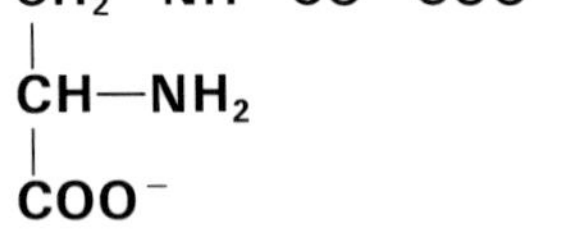

CH$_2$—NH—CO—COO$^-$
|
CH—NH$_2$
|
COO$^-$

α-amino, β-Oxalylamino propionic acid.
(β-N-Oxalylamino-L-alanine)

Fig. 11.19 Note the close similarities between the amino acid extracted from the cycad nut (A) and that extracted from the chick pea (1 B). Both are derivatives of propionic acid but with different substituents. Both have excitotoxic actions in animals.

Buckthorn neuropathy (tullidora)[177]

Clinical features. The shrub coyotillo (*Karwinskia humboldtiana*) grows in Central America, Mexico, Texas and Southern California, and has long been associated with a toxic paralytic syndrome in man and other animals when the fruits are eaten.[177] In man, the condition is predominantly a flaccid ascending motor paralysis with a relatively slight sensory component. Ataxia is also present and when the poisoning is severe, as it may be in children, death may follow.[178,179]

Pathological features. One biopsy from an affected child showed the presence of segmental demyelination.[180] Most of our information about this intoxication has come from animal studies. In goats, segmental demyelination has been stressed,[181] but the presence of chromatolysis in the anterior horn cells indicates a significant degree of axonal damage as well. Whether there are also spinal tract changes is debatable. More recent studies on rats[182] have shown that as well as myelin loss there is distal axonal degeneration, and this is the main lesion. In cats,[183] however, segmental demyelination is pronounced and it affects pre-

dominantly the large diameter, fast conducting fibres (Fig. 11.20). This raises a particularly interesting question as to the mechanism of selective demyelination of axons according to their size, a question not hitherto considered and one for which we do not have the answer.

Mechanism of toxicity. This is unknown. Purified karwinskia toxins injected into rat nerve cause local segmental demyelination.[177,184] In vitro the toxin is an uncoupler of mitochondrial oxidative phosphorylation,[185] but whether this is therefore an energy-deprivation neuropathy is uncertain. It certainly does not resemble beri-beri or arsenical neuropathy, which are typical energy-dependent conditions, so if this observation is relevant to the pathogenesis of the disorder then there must be other factors operating to give such emphasis to the motor component of the neuropathy.

DRUG TOXICITY

Nitrofurans and nitroimidazoles

Derivatives of these two important classes of chemicals (Fig. 11.21) are valuable in the control of

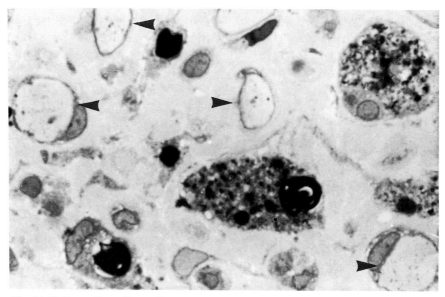

Fig. 11.20 Demyelinated large diameter axons (arrowheads) in cat nerve after a dose of tullidora toxin (toxin of Mexican buckthorn, *Karwinskia humboldtiana*). Note that each nerve has a rim of Schwann cell cytoplasm. Phagocytic cells contain granular dark myelin debris. *Reproduced by permission of Professor E. J. Muños-Martínez, Mexico City, Mexico.*

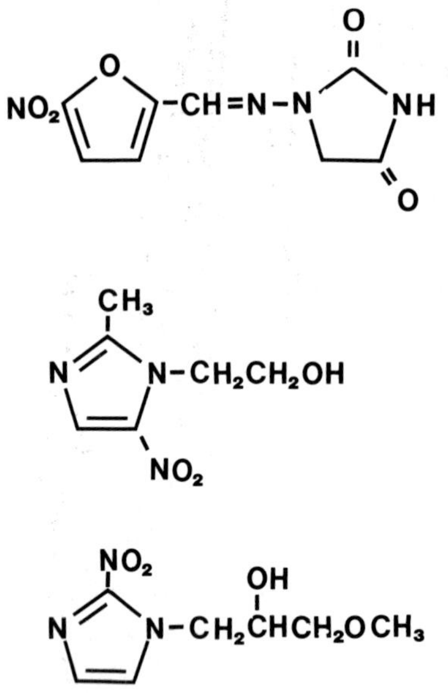

Nitrofurantoin

Metronidazole

Misonidazole

Fig. 11.21 Chemical structure of three principal nitro-aromatics used against bacterial and protozoal infections, and as hypoxic radiation sensitisers. Metronidazole (Flagyl®) is a 5-nitro and misonidazole is a 2-nitro compound.

bacterial and protozoal infections. Of the nitrofurans, nitrofurantoin and nitrofurazone have a place in the therapy of bacterial infections resistant to antibiotics; nitrofurazone has been used also to treat trypanosomiasis not responding to organic arsenicals. Nitrofuran derivatives are also widely used in veterinary medicine and as feed additives. The nitroimidazoles, metronidazole (Flagyl®) and misonidazole (see also p. 291), are used in infections of the gastrointestinal tract, especially against lambliasis and amoebiasis, and also in genital infections with trichomonas. Both types of drug are thought to be valuable in enhancing radiosensitivity ('hypoxic cell sensitisers') in cancer radiotherapy. Unfortunately, they both cause peripheral neuropathy, seriously restricting their therapeutic value.

Clinical features. Both classes of compound produce a distal sensory neuropathy with glove and stocking sensory loss and relatively minor motor denervation and weakness;[186-188] the motor effects may only be detectable electrophysiologically. The neuropathy is persistent, and slow to recover, with both compounds and clinically resembles beri-beri (see p. 288) but treatment with large doses of vitamin B_1 has no effect on either. This is also despite the fact that when large doses of nitrofurantoin are used in the treatment of refractory trypanosomiasis, the patients may show striking cardiovascular signs, with or without neuropathy, resembling those in beri-beri.[189]

Pathologically, the nerves of patients with peripheral neuropathy show Wallerian (axonal) degeneration. Large doses of misonidazole given to rats cause a relatively minor peripheral neuropathy, but induce symmetrical vasculonecrotic changes in the brainstem resembling the lesions of acute thiamine deficiency in that species.[190] No satisfactory animal model of the neuropathy has been produced with the nitrofuran group of drugs, however.

Mechanism of toxicity. This is not exactly known, but both the nitrofurans and the nitroimidazoles are active electron acceptors. They are both potentially toxic, being mutagenic and carcinogenic, probably through reduction of the nitro group under hypoxic conditions, leading to the formation of alkylating products capable of binding to DNA.[191] In the conditions of free oxygen availability that would exist in nervous tissue, however, nitroreduction is reversed ('redox cycling'). The electrons then released may either pass into the electron chain, reducing its efficiency, or lead to the production of an excess of super-oxides. Such 'useless cycling' of the compound will also cause a reduction in available adenosine triphosphate (ATP) in the cell, over-utilisation of reduced nicotinamide adenine dinucleotide phosphate (NADPH) and glutathione and an increase in oxygen and glucose consumption. In addition, there is the potential toxic action of free radicals generated in the process which leads to further detrimental effects. Selective involvement of the largest cells in the nervous system, the primary sensory cells, emphasises once more the risk that these cells are exposed to when cellular energy sources become endangered.

Aminoglycosides

The various aminoglycosides, derived from different species of bacteria of the order Actino-mycetales, are effective against a wide range of bacterial infections. Those principally causing neurotoxicity are neomycin, kanamycin and streptomycin, all of which are obtained from different species of *Streptomyces*, and gentamycin, obtained from a species of *Micromonospora*. These aminoglycosides are potentially ototoxic, and whether this occurs or not depends upon both the plasma levels and the diffusion of the drug from the inner ear back into the plasma. Selective damage occurs to outer hair cells of the organ of Corti and to the vestibular cristae.

How the cell changes come about is not clear, but it may be from interference with transport mechanisms concerned with ionic balance within the endolymph, which has a high potassium content.[192] The final result is selective loss of outer hair cells and subsequently other neural elements, but the early symptoms and signs are likely to be reversible since they represent the effects of the initial ionic imbalance. There is no reason to think that any other regions of the auditory and vestibular pathways are affected.

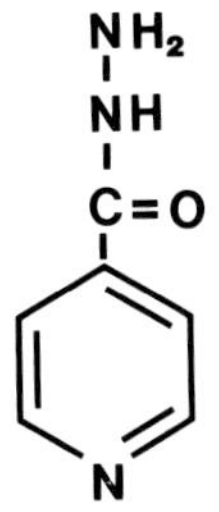

Isoniazid (isonicotinic acid hydrazide: INH)

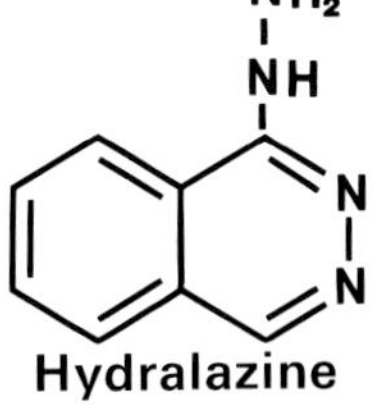

Clinical features. This cheap but very effective anti-tuberculosis drug (Fig. 11.22) may cause a distal sensory neuropathy in some people, with burning pains in the feet and hands and character-istic loss of sensory discrimination. Motor dis-turbances are less noteworthy.[193] Only peripheral nerves are affected, but with the higher doses that may be taken in suicide attempts there may be general irritability, nervousness, insomnia and muscle twitching. These signs probably arise from inhibition of synthesis of γ-aminobutyric acid in the CNS.

Susceptibility to the development of INH neuropathy is genetically determined and depends upon the ability of the individual to acetylate and thus detoxicate the drug.[194] Slow inactivators are genetically recessive, but there are marked racial differences in the frequency of rapid or slow inactivators. Thus, Japanese have a high fre-

Fig. 11.22 Structural formulae of isoniazid and hydralazine. Both compounds will chelate pyridoxal phosphate.

quency of rapid inactivators, whereas Caucasians have a relatively low incidence.

Pathological features. There are few post-mortem or biopsy reports of the structural changes in this condition. Wallerian degeneration is found in many peripheral nerves and this may extend as far proximally as the spinal roots. Anterior horn cells, however, are intact. The dorsal columns of the spinal cord may show degeneration.[195]

The clinical picture in man, as well as the complete recovery that usually occurs, indicates that the distal sensory nerve degeneration and the less severe motor nerve fibre degeneration are repaired by axon regeneration and that CNS changes are probably minor.

In experimental animals, using larger doses than those given to man,[196] Wallerian degeneration occurs in sensory and in motor nerves and in the CNS. Except for the dorsal columns, there is no long tract degeneration. In motor nerves the 'dying back' may progress as far as the spinal roots, but neuronal perikarya remain intact and later show a chromatolytic response as part of the axon regeneration process. Some degeneration of axons occurs in the upper parts of the dorsal columns of the spinal cord as an expression of the involvement of the dorsal root ganglion cells.

A second type of cellular response is seen, in dogs in particular,[197] in which ballooning of the myelin sheath occurs, similar to the changes seen with triethyltin (see p. 257) and hexachlorophane (see p. 282). This perhaps may also occur in man, since 'optic neuritis' has been occasionally reported, and could be caused by swelling of the nerve and its compression in its passage through the optic foramen.

Mechanism of toxicity. Isoniazid (INH) is detoxicated principally by an acetylation reaction and the acetylated product is excreted in the urine. INH chelates strongly with pyridoxal phosphate and in addition the chelate so formed can inhibit the essential enzyme, pyridoxal phosphokinase.[198] The drug thus causes cellular depletion of the co-factor, pyridoxal phosphate (PPO_4). Since PPO_4 is essential to the nervous system in a number of metabolic pathways,[199] particularly trans-aminations and amino-decarboxylations, its

toxicity is not surprising. It is, thus, epileptogenic through inhibition of the synthesis of γ-aminobutyric acid. It also has a lathyrogenic property, preventing collagen polymerisation through inhibition of lysyl oxidase, an enzyme requiring PPO_4. It is, moreover, important for the synthesis of the antioxidant, glutathione, through dependence of cystathionine synthetase and cystathionase upon PPO_4. Red cell survival is affected by this in pyridoxal-deficient anaemia, and xanthurenic acid excretion is increased in INH intoxication.[200]

The mechanism of the neuropathy is still, however, obscure. INH has no actions upon energy pathways, but it has been suggested[201] that there may be depression of glutathione synthesis in neurons. Those neurons with very long axons may particularly require glutathione to protect their very large membrane surfaces against free radical damage. There may thus be similarities with the neuropathy associated with vitamin E (α-tocopherol) deficiency (see p. 297). Similarities also exist with the neuropathy found in acute intermittent porphyria (see p. 560) in which an acute consumptive deficiency of PPO_4 occurs during the attacks.

Hydralazine

Hydralazine (Fig. 11.22) is effective in the treatment of hypertension, increasing the cardiac output and preferentially dilating arterioles. Like isoniazid, it also can produce sensory neuropathy in slow acetylators. The patients show a high xanthurenic acid excretion in the urine as evidence of tissue depletion of pyridoxal phosphate and they respond rapidly to vitamin B_6 medication.[202] Hydralazine is a chelating agent interacting with pyridoxal phosphate.

Ethionamide

Ethionamide has a place in the treatment of pulmonary tuberculosis. Two cases of neuropathy have been reported: the patients showed symptoms identical to those of isoniazid intoxication.[203,204] From its chemical structure, ethionamide would, perhaps, be expected to behave in a similar way in the tissues. There are no pathological or experimental studies. Like hydralazine, ethionamide is a chelating agent and capable of interacting with pyridoxal phosphate.

Vincristine

Clinical features. Vincristine is valuable in the treatment of Hodgkin's disease and other lymphomas as well as of leukaemias. Neuropathy is common, however, particularly when high doses are employed and this limits treatment with this useful drug. The neuropathy is manifested by numbness and tingling in the fingers and toes, weakness of the hands and feet, areflexia, ataxia and muscle cramps. There is electrophysiological evidence of both motor and sensory nerve degeneration.[205]

Pathological features. Nerve biopsies show Wallerian degeneration without any special features. The few post-mortem studies have shown hyaline changes in the nerve cells which ultrastructurally are found to contain accumulations of 10 nm filaments.[206]

Experimental studies have been disappointing and, except by direct injection of vincristine into the CSF or into nerves, it has not been possible to reproduce the neuropathic changes found in man. This difficulty almost certainly arises from the inability of vincristine to penetrate the blood-brain and blood-nerve barriers in the normal animal. Thus, it has been found to have a marked effect on the brain if the barrier is broken by a prior intravascular injection of mannitol.[207] It also has a striking inhibitory effect on the regeneration of nerve, where the blood-nerve barrier has been lowered after a crush injury.[208] This raises the interesting question why neuropathy occurs in man but not in the experimental animals. The answer may be that the presence of the tumour in some way allows the drug access through the blood-nerve barrier, either as the result of local tumour infiltrations into nerve or by some other mechanism.

Mechanism of toxicity. Vincristine and its analogue vinblastine, in common with colchicine and podophyllotoxin, interfere with the stability of microtubules of cells and also prevent their polymerisation.[209] This is the basis of their anti-cancer actions for they arrest cell division by preventing formation of the mitotic spindle. By the same process, depolymerisation of the axonal microtubules blocks axoplasmic transport, leading to nerve fibre degeneration. Vincristine changes are unusual in that not only do accumulations of 10 nm filaments occur in affected nerve cells but large crystal-like lattice formations appear which may represent aggregations of dimeric tubulin forms.[210]

Cisplatin

Clinical features. Cisplatin is a valuable drug in the treatment of many different types of cancer; it is often used in combination with other drugs. Not infrequently, when the dose exceeds a certain amount, a sensory neuropathy develops. The clinical signs are restricted to sensory functions, and motor changes do not seem to occur. Numbness and tingling of the feet occur associated with a broad-based gait and loss of fine control of the fingers.[211] More important is the occurrence of renal toxicity, and ototoxicity affecting the hair cells of the sensory epithelium of the inner ear is also common.

Pathological features. Few cases have been examined post-mortem. In one, a child,[212] there was loss of axons and gliosis in the dorsal columns, but no other changes. The dorsal root ganglion cells were not reported upon. Experimentally, cisplatin has been found to cause segregation of the fibrillar and granular components of the nucleoli of dorsal root ganglion and other cells in the rat. Associated with this, there may be accumulations of 10 nm filaments in the sensory cell bodies and in the initial segment of the emerging axon[213] as well as dispersal of polyribosomes. Degeneration of the Wallerian type may be seen in sensory nerve fibres, but the exact basis for this change is not yet clear.

Metabolic mechanisms. Cisplatin binds to DNA and its cell-killing properties depend upon the number of molecules bound and the amount of inter-strand and intra-strand cross-linking that occurs. This would seem an irreversible process.[214] In addition to inhibition of DNA synthesis, there is also inhibition of RNA and protein synthesis, but the latter two changes are reversible in about 48 hours. Dorsal root ganglion cells are presumably at risk because of the leakiness of their vascular bed, but although the DNA damage may not be a problem to these non-dividing cells, the effects upon RNA and protein synthesis are apparently toxic to these very large nerve cells.

Comparisons might be made with doxorubicin (adriamycin), another antineoplastic agent which is not neurotoxic to man, but can cause nucleolar segregation in rat dorsal root ganglion cells that leads to cell death within a few days of a single dose.[215] Adriamycin also intercalates with the DNA coils but localises particularly in the nucleolar chromatin.[216] While, therefore, cisplatin and adriamycin are both selectively toxic to dorsal root ganglion cells, producing sensory neuropathy, they act on the neuron in distinctly different ways.

Hexachlorophane

Hexachlorophane (UK) (hexachlorophene in the USA) has for many years been incorporated into soaps and cosmetics in low concentrations as a bland antiseptic. It is also a useful fungicide and pesticide. It came into prominence when used to bathe newborn, often premature, infants in maternity units; it was found to be responsible for causing signs of raised intracranial pressure from brain swelling from which the infants not infrequently died. Hexachlorophane has occasionally also produced toxicity when used for cleansing skin burns or ichthyotic skin lesions in adults.

Clinical features. Given by mouth, hexachlorophane causes gastrointestinal disturbances, such as diarrhoea and vomiting. Absorption through the skin has led to generalised weakness, lowering of the level of consciousness, visual disturbances and blurred optic discs, muscle paralysis, and irritability occasionally progressing to convulsions; delirium and coma, and death, may follow. When recovery occurs it is complete.

Pathological features. The essential change is a generalised swelling of the white matter of the brain. In newborn infants, birth weight and maturity are important factors determining the severity of the brain swelling. In a series of 248 infants studied at post-mortem, noticeable brain swelling was found only in premature infants under 1400 g in weight.[217] When the use of hexachlorophane in nurseries was restricted the problem disappeared.

Experimental studies have shown that hexachlorophane causes vacuolation of the myelin sheath in adult rats in the same manner as triethyltin (see p. 257). Thus there is splitting at the minor dense line of the compacted myelin sheath where the two outer surfaces of the plasma membrane come together.[218] As with organic tin compounds, this change is associated with an increase in brain water with the characteristics of a plasma ultrafiltrate. Unlike triethyltin, hexachlorophane causes in addition vacuolation of peripheral nerve myelin, though this is less intense than the vacuolation in myelin in the central nervous system. Vacuolation of the photoreceptor discs of the outer retinal segments of the eye is also seen. Here there are also compacted membranes somewhat similar in form to myelin; the vacuolation may lead to retinal cell degeneration. Swelling of the myelin of the optic nerve as it passes through the optic foramen in the skull can lead to constriction of the nerve with consequent swelling of the optic disc and nerve fibre degeneration.[219]

Mechanism of toxicity. This is unknown, but hexachlorophane actively binds to lipids and to proteins, though not specifically to myelin proteins.[220] How the vacuolation comes about is unknown, and there is no reason to believe that the metabolism of the glial cells is primarily damaged. Whether the basic protein of the myelin is involved, as suggested for triethyltin toxicity, is unknown.

Halogenated hydroxyquinolines (clioquinol and related drugs): subacute myelo-optico-neuropathy (SMON)

Clinical features. For many years clioquinol (iodochlorhydroxyquin) and other halogenated (iodinated and/or chlorinated) 8-hydroxyquinoline compounds (Fig. 11.23) have been used clinically in the prophylaxis and treatment of

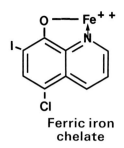

Fig. 11.23 Structural formulae of clioquinol and of the ferric iron chelate probably responsible for the green coloration of the tongue, urine and faeces, and capable of inhibiting cellular respiration.

intestinal infections, despite the paucity of firm evidence for their efficacy. From about 1950 onwards large numbers of cases of poisoning from this drug occurred in Japan (possibly as many as 10 000); neurological complications occurred after heavy dosing over relatively short periods. Because of the distribution of the neurological damage, the condition came to be known as *subacute myelo-optico-neuropathy* or SMON. The persistent signs and symptoms were visual failure (sometimes going on to amblyopia), spasticity (predominantly of the lower limbs), and symmetrical sensory disturbances (usually of the legs and trunk).[221] In addition, a curious green discoloration of the surface fur of the tongue and also sometimes of the urine and the faeces was noted. Similar cases have been observed in smaller numbers in other parts of the world.[222] A number of deaths occurred in Japan, but milder cases showed significant but rarely complete recovery; visual impairment was often permanent. Children were less affected than adults, while the condition was seen in women about twice as frequently as in men. The incidence and severity of the symptoms, it is generally agreed, were related to the dosage of the compound prescribed.

Pathological features. About 150 cases have been studied post mortem.[223] Sensory ganglion cells showed marked degenerative changes with necrosis and the formation of residual nodules of Nageotte (see p. 565). Chromatolysis was present in many of the remaining neurons. Lumbosacral anterior horn cells were often markedly chromatolytic and there was active degeneration of Wallerian type in the peripheral nerves. In the spinal cord severe degeneration was found consistently in the gracile tracts, but rarely if ever in the cuneate tracts, whose fibres originate in the cervical dorsal root ganglia. The lateral and the anterior corticospinal tracts were also consistently involved, but almost exclusively in the lower half of the spinal cord, once more demonstrating the peculiar and striking predilection of the degeneration for long axons.

The retinal ganglion cells, especially in the papillomacular region, and the axons of the optic nerve showed extensive degeneration, although the nerve cells of the lateral geniculate bodies were usually unaffected. In the optic pathway there were many more degenerate fibres in the distal regions (i.e. the optic tract) than in the proximal part of the nerve near the bulb. Thus there was a 'dying back' pattern of degeneration here as well as in the spinal cord. Recovery from an episode of poisoning was in general not good because of CNS involvement.

Experimental studies have confirmed that it is possible to induce a somewhat similar pattern of changes in dogs.[224] However, although long spinal cord and retinal tracts were affected in the same way as in man, peripheral nerves in the dog showed no abnormalities. Nonetheless, the pattern of the nerve fibre degeneration was sufficiently similar to be acceptable as a model of the human disease. However, relatively severe degeneration was found in the proximal component of the primary sensory cells of the dorsal root ganglia (i.e. the ascending fibres of the dorsal column) but not in the distal component that runs in the peripheral nerves. This unusual finding is significantly at variance with the pathological features of the human cases.

Mechanism of toxicity. This is unknown, but the green discoloration of the tongue, etc., was undoubtedly due to the formation of a chelate between the 8-hydroxyquinoline and ferric iron, and this reaction may be very relevant to the toxic effects in neurons with long axons. 8-hydroxyquinolines have long been known to have some bactericidal, protozoocidal and fungicidal activity. Their mechanism of killing organisms is related to the formation within the cell of a chelate with ferric iron or with divalent copper ions. The chelate, when incomplete, binds avidly to sulphydryl groups (Fig. 11.23). The chelate must therefore be in 1:1 or 1:2 ratio of metal to agent for when the ratio is 1:3, metal ion to quinoline, and the quinoline is in excess, the chelate is no longer toxic. In an intracellular environment an excess of quinoline is not likely to occur. Moreover, while the chelate itself cannot penetrate the cell membrane, the hydroxyquinoline can do so; the chelate is ineffective against bacteria for this reason. According to Albert[225] the incomplete metal-hydroxyquinoline complex most probably combines in the cell with lipoate, and cell death results from energy deprivation. If this process also occurs in clioquinol intoxication, then the 'dying back' of the long pathways in peripheral as well as central neurons may well be regarded as analogous to the other energy-deprivation neuropathies discussed earlier. An important difference is, however, the ability of the hydroxyquinoline to readily enter cells and thus to pass the blood-brain barrier. Involvement of the retinal cells and the long spinal tracts may be accounted for in this way.

Perhexiline

Perhexiline maleate, or 2-(2,2-dicyclohexylethyl)-piperidine hydrogen maleate, was introduced for the treatment of angina pectoris. It produces dilatation of the coronary arteries by direct action on the vascular smooth muscle and at the same time has a further action on the sino-atrial node, slowing the heart rate.

Clinical features. Usually, after several months of therapy, the patient develops burning pains in the feet and reduction of sensation in the stocking distribution. Sometimes all four limbs become involved with pain and numbness; the reflexes disappear and motor and sensory nerve conduction velocities in the limbs become slowed.[2]

Pathological features. Biopsy studies have demonstrated both segmental demyelination as well as Wallerian degeneration, but the severity of such changes varies greatly. Thus, it was found that 90% of nerve fibres showed segmental demyelination in one patient and only 16% in another.[2] Again Wallerian degeneration varied from 3% of fibres to 20% in another patient. In general the density of nerve fibres in the nerve biopsies was severely reduced in all groups, with greater loss of the larger diameter fibres.

From these observations, and from the long recovery time on withdrawal of the drug, it must be concluded that there is a 'dying back' type of neuropathy, but the large amount of segmental demyelination also present makes it unusual.

Mechanism of toxicity. This is unknown. However, an increase in ganglioside but not of other lipids has been found in biopsy samples of nerve.[226] Large numbers of dense bodies have also been noted in nerve biopsy samples.[2] The drug tends to accumulate during dosing but, except for some details of the breakdown products, no toxic mechanism has been suggested.[227] It should be noted that quite a significant number of patients may show electrophysiological disturbances in their peripheral nerves during treatment, even in the absence of overt neuropathy.[228]

MPTP toxicity and its simulation of Parkinson's disease

The dramatic selective intoxication by MPTP (1-methyl-4-phenyl-1,2,3,6-tetrahydropyridine) and the rapid unravelling of its metabolic mechanism have been strong incentives to further work on the rôle of environmental agents in causing human disease.

MPTP is a by-product of the synthesis of 1-methyl-propionoxy-pyridine, an analogue of the potent drug pethidine (meperidine), and a narcotic in its own right. The presence of MPTP as a contaminant in this narcotic drug led to cases of severe illness that closely resembled Parkinson's disease, and which also responded to the administration of levodopa. The development of animal models, first in primates and then in other species, showed that the condition was very similar to the natural disease in man (see p. 411) both in its pharmacology and in the topography of the nerve cell damage. Thus, there was degeneration of neurons in the zona compacta of the substantia nigra with associated gliosis; this also occurred in the locus ceruleus. But intraneuronal Lewy bodies (see p. 412) were not found at either anatomical site.[229]

Mechanism of toxicity. Neurochemically, MPTP is a powerful depleter of striatal dopamine; depletion also occurs in the nucleus accumbens and the olfactory tubercle. While the likely steps in the synthesis of the putative toxic metabolite have been worked out, there is still some doubt about exactly how the final product causes cell destruction and why these particular neuronal regions are selectively affected. The process is a classical example of a multi-stage metabolic conversion to a toxic metabolite.[230]

MPTP readily enters the brain and is rapidly converted to 1-methyl-4-phenylpyridine (MPP$^+$) (Fig. 11.24) by mitochondrial enzymes that are inhibited by the drugs pargyline and selegiline (deprenyl), which are inhibitors of monoamine oxidase (MAO) B, but these enzymes are not blocked by inhibitors of MAO A. MAO B is known to be in astrocytes and in serotonin-containing neurons, but not in dopaminergic neurons. Following this transformation, probably taking place in astrocytes, MPP$^+$ is taken up by catecholergic nerve terminals. This step can be prevented by drugs such as maprotiline that block noradrenaline uptake. The selective uptake of MPP$^+$ explains the concentration of this toxic product in catecholergic neurons. The accumulation of MPP$^+$ in neurons containing melanin may well play an important rôle in the selective toxicity, and may also explain the increased susceptibility of older animals whose cells contain more neuromelanin. Melanins have a number of sites that bind with relatively high affinity for a variety of ionic substances,[231] and thus will form a reservoir for the concentration of the toxic product. It is thought that melanin might generate MPP$^-$ and, with the release of an electron, set up a redox cycling system and the resultant formation of free radical species. Thus, the mechanism of toxicity within cells appears to resemble the mechanism of paraquat toxicity in lung.[232] If this is true, then one of the consequences is the reduction of cellular GSH

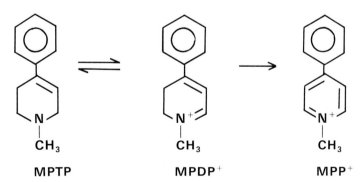

MPTP   **MPDP$^+$**   **MPP$^+$**

Fig. 11.24 MPTP is lipophilic and readily enters astrocytes from the bloodstream where it is acted upon by monoamine oxidase B, becoming converted to MPDP$^+$ (1-methyl-4-phenyl-2,3-dihydropyridinium). This readily disproportionates to MPP$^+$, which enters the neuron where it may accumulate on the neuronal melanin and probably undergoes redox cycling, perhaps with the release of toxic free radicals species.

(glutathione); another consequence is that agents that inhibit superoxide dismutase, such as diethyldithiocarbamate, might be expected to potentiate the toxicity. However, it has recently been shown that MPP$^+$ also irreversibly inhibits mitochondrial respiration and that dopaminergic cells may also die from this cause.[232a]

While, therefore, MPTP toxicity gives rise to selective cell damage that closely mimics Parkinson's disease in man, it does not tell us the cause of Parkinson's disease. It may, however, point the way not only towards discovering this, but also conceivably to the causes of other major human neurological diseases such as motor neuron disease.

DEFICIENCY AND METABOLIC DISEASES

VITAMIN B DEFICIENCY DISEASES

Vitamin deficiency is rarely confined to a single vitamin. When there is a deficiency state it is usual for many, if not all, vitamins of the B group to be seriously reduced. This is well demonstrated in alcoholics with deficiency disorders (see p. 261). Severity of dietary imbalance and rate of deprivation both help to determine the disease pattern expressed. Thus, for example, in *thiamine deficiency*, either Wernicke's disease or peripheral neuropathy, or even both together, may occur according to the circumstances prevailing. In a general state of malnourishment, plasma levels of all B vitamins will be reduced but the type of syndrome that develops often depends upon outside factors, which again may determine the relative demand of a tissue for the co-factor. A heavy loading with carbohydrate such as glucose increases the tissues' needs and is likely to precipitate an acute Wernicke-type syndrome. More chronic deficiency coupled with a predominantly carbohydrate intake and heavy physical labour is the background to the neuropathy of beri-beri.

Similarly, although the circumstances leading to pellagra are less well understood, dietary *deficiency of nicotinic acid* is an essential component of this disease. However, other factors such as the growth of toxogenic moulds in ingested corn and low tryptophan intake may also be important.

The specific pattern of tissue damage in deficiency diseases depends on the relative demand of specific brain regions and on external factors. This is well shown in *pyridoxine deficiency* in which the standard vitamin intake may be insufficient for heavy manual workers, for people with a very high protein intake, or in pregnancy, where protein metabolism is enhanced.[233] The margin between health and deficiency is often surprisingly finely drawn.

Thiamine deficiency syndromes

There are two well-established neurological syndromes, *Wernicke's encephalopathy* and *beri-beri*, which are closely associated with dietary deficiency of thiamine. In addition, there are several other syndromes showing similarities to Wernicke's disease that are now thought to be caused through a similar mechanism, but are not directly related to thiamine metabolism. A number of conditions occur in other species in which thiamine is deficient through its destruction in the gastrointestinal tract by thiaminases in natural diet, as in carnivores such as silver foxes (Chastek paralysis) and cats that have eaten fish containing thiaminase, and in herbivores, particularly horses, that have grazed on bracken and other thiaminase-containing plants.

There are a number of drug-induced conditions that show either a neuropathy very similar to beri-beri or brainstem lesions closely resembling Wernicke's disease. The causes include drugs (see p. 277 et seq.), trivalent arsenic (see p. 246), 6-chloro-6-deoxy-glucose, and 6-amino-nicotin-amide. They interfere directly or indirectly with the energy generating pathways. All can produce vasculonecrotic lesions essentially similar to Wernicke's disease. Alternatively, they may produce a peripheral neuropathy clinically and morphologically indistinguishable from beri-beri.

Wernicke's encephalopathy (polioencephalitis haemorrhagica superioris)

This condition has been discussed among conditions associated with chronic ethyl alcohol intake (see p. 258). The clinical syndrome described by Wernicke is now most commonly seen, at least in Western urbanised communities, as a complication either of chronic alcoholism or in conditions of which malnourishment is an important component, such as carcinoma of the stomach.

Clinical features. There is an acute onset of ocular disturbances and ataxia. Paresis of ocular movements is an essential feature for diagnosis together with weakness of the lateral rectus muscles of the eyes and paralysis of conjugate gaze. Nystagmus, both horizontal and vertical, is usually present, and sixth nerve palsy (when present) is bilateral though unequal. Ataxia, which is always a feature of the condition, may be so severe as to interfere with walking or even standing. Caloric tests reveal absent vestibular responses.

Disturbances of higher mental functions occur in about 90% of cases, usually shown by confusion, disorientation, apathy, poor memory, and indifference. Other evidence of thiamine deficiency may well be present, especially cardiovascular disturbances and polyneuritis. The condition must be regarded as an acute medical emergency and delay in giving thiamine at the early stages could turn an essentially reversible clinical condition into an irreversible pathological process. The outcome, therefore, is dependent upon early diagnosis and treatment.

Pathological features. The changes in the brain have been described in detail in the section on the effects of chronic ethyl alcohol intake (see p. 258).

The essential histological lesion is varying degrees of neuronal cell death accompanied by reactive astrocytosis and striking vascular hypertrophy associated with numerous small petechial haemorrhages. According to Torvik,[234] some regions of the brain may show more neuronal damage while in others the reactive astrocytosis may be more prominent. Less advanced lesions are not well seen in the post-mortem room except when there are petechial haemorrhages. Older lesions, from earlier episodes of the disease

with irreversible tissue damage, are firmer due to astrogliosis and they are stained brown with haemosiderin pigment. Smaller old gliotic lesions may be less easily visible, and naked eye appraisal will tend to understate the extent of the changes.

Experimental studies. It is possible to produce the same type of tissue changes in many species by dietary means with or without the use of thiamine antagonists such as pyrithiamine and amprolium. Apart from the original work in pigeons,[235] experiments have been done in monkeys,[236] cats[237] and foxes.[238] To produce the typical lesions, a certain minimum of usable thiamine must be provided for it is necessary that the cells function in a disadvantaged condition, rather than in a state of complete deprivation. Whether the nerve cell or the astrocyte is the more susceptible to the state of energy deprivation is as yet unresolved. The tissue appearances are essentially the same as in man, namely focal oedema, neuronal necrosis, glial responses and vascular proliferation; the lesions are always confined to grey matter. The topographical distribution, however, varies from one species to another. Thus, pigeons show haemorrhagic lesions in the thalamus, the hypothalamus and the oculomotor nuclei only. Monkeys have a distribution closely similar to man, while cats show few lesions above the upper brainstem, but marked damage to the colliculi, vestibular nuclei, inferior olives and vagal, gracile and cuneate nuclei; silver foxes behave similarly (Chastek paralysis). Lesions are difficult to produce in rats, but they do develop oedematous and mildly haemorrhagic lesions confined to brainstem centres, particularly in the vestibular nuclei, olivary nuclei and roof nuclei of the cerebellum.[239] Cattle, sheep and goats, in contrast, show marked necrotic and vascular lesions in the cerebral cortex (polioencephalomalacia or 'cerebrocortical necrosis'), which suggests that an additional factor is at work in these species; brainstem nuclei, such as the inferior colliculi, are less affected than in other species.[240]

It seems that in all these species, the topography of the damaged grey matter centres covers those regions which are important for maintaining functions vital to the animal. Thus balance, movement, and other sensory and motor activities are especially affected. Auditory functions, critical to some species such as rat and cat, are also affected. These are all areas of the brain with a high uptake of glucose, as shown by studies using the radioactive 2-deoxy-glucose technique.

Beri-beri neuropathy

The disease beri-beri (the Singhalese word *beri* means 'weakness') has been known since the last century to afflict poorer persons. In the Far East it is traditionally associated with the consumption of milled rice. This, the staple diet of a large proportion of the world's inhabitants, is rice from which the germ has been removed to enable it to be more easily stored and transported. The problem lies in the unbalanced as well as the deficient nature of the diet; this results in a high carbohydrate intake but in inadequate supply of cofactor to metabolise it.

Clinical features. No better description of the condition has been given than that of Platt.[241] He defined three types of beri-beri occurring in male patients.

1. The *chronic dry atrophic type*, beginning with wrist and foot drop, is usually found in older adults and shows little response to sustained dietary treatment. Almost certainly this is due to associated high alcohol intake; the two conditions are inextricably mixed.

2. The *subacute or mild form* shows loss of reflexes, paraesthesiae in the limbs, and weakness. The regions affected, Platt stressed, depend upon the length of the nerves, the amount and type of work being done by the patient, and the blood supply. Thus, working men usually show the earliest signs in the legs below the knees, while working women show involvement of the fingers first. Other occupational features are seen, such as early 'thumb drop' in the right hand of tailors' cutters and weakness of the left (knife-holding) arm of hide strippers. When the larynx is affected the left vocal cord is always the one to be affected first, its nerve being the longer. A high proportion of affected women are pregnant and have some complication of pregnancy, such as toxaemia.

Early in this type of the disease the muscles are found on biopsy to be dry, but oedema occurs later and is often first noticed in the evenings. Cardiovascular signs not infrequently precede the onset of peripheral neuropathy. This subacute form of beri-beri may become worse in the presence of a fever, such as from malaria, which increases bodily demands for the vitamin.

3. The third form of the disease is *acute beri-beri* and accounts for only about 5% of cases. Before thiamine was given therapeutically, all these patients died within 48 hours of admission to hospital. The clinical picture is dominated by cardiovascular signs, though it is usually the neuropathy that forces the patients to take to their bed. Platt paints a terrible picture of intense precordial pains, thirst, vomiting, restlessness and mental anxiety in such patients. Oedema is not a feature of the acute form.

In summary, in modern terms, beri-beri produces a predominantly distal sensory neuropathy with later increasing motor weakness. Cranial nerves are little affected although the phrenic and vagal nerves are often involved because of their great length and their constant activity. It is the long nerves of the limbs that are particularly affected, and there is a pronounced work factor evident. In addition, oedema—partly from protein lack and partly from cardiac failure—complicates the picture. Pregnancy, fever and alcohol all exacerbate the condition. The condition is treatable with thiamine although recovery of nerve function may be slow if the condition has been severe, due to the slow regeneration rate (1 mm/day) of damaged axons.

Pathological features. Wallerian degeneration is a constant feature and a necessary finding for the diagnosis. There may be evidence of earlier nerve degeneration in the form of regenerating fibres. More distally lying nerves will show the more severe changes. Sensory ganglion cells and anterior horn cells will show chromatolysis as evidence of their attempts to regenerate the damaged fibres. Degenerative change will be seen in phrenic and vagal nerves, particularly the recurrent laryngeal nerves. Everything mentioned about the nerves in alcoholic neuropathy will apply in beri-beri for the two are essentially identical.

There may also be evidence of Wernicke's disease in the same patient, particularly where alcohol has played an important rôle.

Metabolic mechanism. It is now generally understood that nervous tissue, more than any other tissue except heart muscle, is dependent upon oxidative metabolic mechanisms for providing energy. Pyruvate oxidative decarboxylation is the principal source of intermediates for this.

In man, thiamine must come principally from the diet, for unlike many other species, e.g. rat, we do not rely upon the gut flora to synthesise it. The co-factor, thiamine pyrophosphate or co-carboxylase, is synthesised from the vitamin in the cells and is required in a number of enzyme reactions, particularly α-keto-acid dehydrogenases, pyruvate decarboxylase and transketolase of the pentose phosphate shunt. Oxidation of pyruvate to acetyl coenzyme-A is performed by a multi-enzyme complex, the process requiring coenzyme-A, nicotinamide-adenine dinucleotide (NAD^+), lipoic acid, flavine-adenine dinucleotide (FAD), Mg^{2+}, and thiamine pyrophosphate (TPP).[242] The absence of any of these components, notably TPP and lipoate (as in arsenic intoxication), will seriously reduce the activity of the enzyme complex and ultimately diminish the energy available, in the form of ATP, to neurons. The most active regions of the brain, namely those found to have the highest uptake of 2-deoxy-glucose, are most susceptible to acute deprivation of energy, whereas those neurons with the greatest amount of axon membrane to maintain are the most susceptible to chronic deprivation of energy. In this context, it does not matter at which point along the energy-generating pathway the metabolic lesion occurs.

Subacute necrotising encephalomyelopathy (Leigh's disease)

Although Leigh's disease has not been shown to be due to a defect of thiamine metabolism, there are strong circumstantial reasons for believing that the basic cellular changes that characterise the condition are related to those of Wernicke's disease. It is quite possible, because of the clinical variability in the condition, that the disease may have several causes, but since they all bear upon the same energy-generating metabolic pathways, they lead to the same pathological lesions. There is evidence also for a recessive genetic trait in many cases and, moreover, not all patients are infants when the diagnosis is first made.

Clinical features. The first described case was an infant who failed to thrive, often vomited, and progressed from hypotonia to immobility, with characteristic facial grimaces and eye-rolling.[243] In the many cases that have been reported since then there has been some recovery, but where this occurs development usually remains poor and relapses occur with a gradual decline of neuro-muscular functions. In older children psycho-motor development is retarded, and death from seizures is not uncommon.[244,245]

Pathological features. The histological changes that constitute the disease are characteristically constant even though the clinical presentation and the topographical distribution of the lesions may be variable. As with Wernicke's disease, the process is vasculonecrotic in type, affecting many grey centres of the brainstem, the diencephalon and the basal ganglia. There is loss of nerve cells, reactive astrocytosis and vascular hypertrophy and hyperplasia, with small haemorrhages visible in the more recent lesions. Older lesions are firmer and gliotic with some brown staining from old blood pigment. The centres most frequently affected are the caudate nuclei, the walls of the third ventricle, the peri-aqueductal grey matter, the tegmental plate, the red nuclei, the inferior olivary nuclei and the cerebellar roof nuclei. Other cranial nerve nuclei may be affected as well as the grey matter of the spinal cord in some cases. Occasionally degeneration of the tracts of the spinal cord has been noted. The distinction from Wernicke's disease, stressed by all authors, is the rarity of involvement of the mamillary bodies.

Metabolic background. Fasting plasma levels of pyruvate, lactate and alanine may be raised in this disease, suggesting that energy metabolism is impaired. This conclusion is supported by the finding that pyruvate carboxylase activity may be defective in some cases.[246] There is no certainty that we are dealing with a single metabolic lesion. Other reports have suggested that there may be an inhibiting factor present in some cases that antagonises the enzyme thiamine pyrophosphate transferase found in rat brain.[247] Furthermore, a case has been described in which there was biochemical evidence of cytochrome oxidase deficiency in muscle.[248]

We do not yet know which of these putative biochemical lesions is primary. There is no guarantee that only one primary abnormal metabolic process need necessarily be present, since, in the very complex pathways concerned with energy metabolism, lesions at several sites could all ultimately produce the same basic tissue changes. It is already known from animal experiments that there are several ways of producing analogous patterns of lesions in the grey centres of the brain, and this indicates that there may be several causes for the disease in man.

Analogous experimental energy-deprivation syndromes

Pyrithiamine and amprolium are two thiamine analogues that prevent adequate supplies of thiamine to the brain for the formation of thiamine pyrophosphate; they thereby produce changes that closely mimic Wernicke's encephalopathy. There is, in addition, a number of other chemicals which induce metabolic lesions by acting at other points along the energy-generating pathways; they also are thus capable of causing damage to grey matter centres in different parts of the brain. For completeness these might be briefly mentioned.

1. *6-chloro-6-deoxyglucose.* One member of a family of compounds that have been assayed as possible male contraceptives, this analogue of glucose is converted to 3-chlorolactaldehyde which selectively inhibits the enzymes triose-phosphate and glyceraldehyde-3-phosphate dehydrogenase in the glycolytic pathway. Single or repeated injections into mice and

marmosets cause spongiform necrotic lesions, which are often haemorrhagic and occur in many grey matter areas throughout the brain, including cerebral cortex, thalamic nuclei, amygdala, colliculi, brainstem motor nuclei, vestibular and cochlear nuclei, the nuclei in the cerebellar white matter, and the grey matter of the spinal cord.[249] Astroglial cells are earliest and primarily affected in the lesions and many nerve cells may subsequently die; there is, moreover, significant hyperplasia of vascular elements in the lesions.

2. *6-aminonicotinamide.* This analogue of nicotinic acid readily exchanges with nicotinamide to form analogues of nicotinamide adenine dinucleotide (NAD) and nicotinamide adenine dinucleotide phosphate (NADP), but these products are unable to replace the normal nicotinamide co-factors in cell functions. The principal metabolic lesion is a block in the pentose phosphate shunt where the NADP-requiring enzyme acting on 6-phosphogluconate is strongly inhibited. The consequent 200- to 400-fold increase in concentration of this intermediate leads fortuitously to inhibition of the enzyme glucose-6-phosphate transferase, which is vital in the glycolytic chain. The result is a serious energy impairment due to impairment of glycolysis and also of reduced nicotinamide adenine dinucleotide (NADH) and reduced nicotinamide adenine dinucleotide phosphate (NADPH) dependent pathways, particularly mitochondrial systems associated with oxidative phosphorylation. A drastic decrease in available adenosine triphosphate (ATP) follows. The reason for the remarkably selective effects on glial cells is not clear, but histochemical studies have shown that glial cells contain abundant dehydrogenase enzymes dependent upon NADP. Neurons, on the other hand, contain more such enzymes dependent upon NADH.[250]

Within 24 hours of a single injection of 6-amino nicotinamide focal necrotic and mildly haemorrhagic lesions appear in many grey centres in the CNS. They extend from the lumbar spinal cord grey matter through to many nuclei in the brainstem (Fig. 11.25) and to the thalamus and the cerebral cortex. Many astrocytes in the lesions die, and while there is a lesser degree of damage to

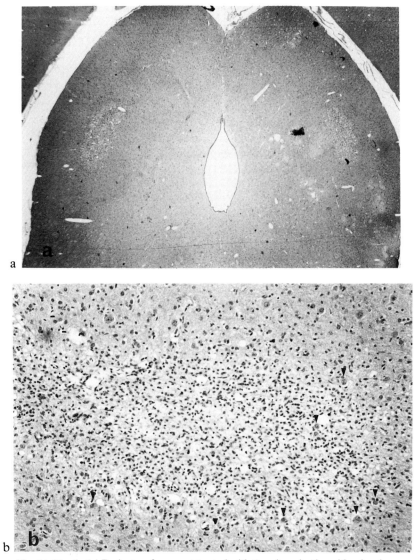

Fig. 11.25a, b (a) Brainstem from a rat treated with 6-amino nicotinamide, showing symmetrical necrotic lesions in the inferior colliculi as part of a symmetrical series of changes in many parts of the grey matter of the brainstem and spinal cord. (b) Higher magnification to show the sharply demarcated lesion containing macrophages and astroglia. Normal neurons remain at the edge of the lesion (arrowheads). Haematoxylin-eosin (a) × 16; (b) × 67

oligodendrocytes, the neurons are only mildly and secondarily affected.[251]

3. *Nitroimidazoles*. Metronidazole (a 5-nitro-imidazole) and misonidazole (a 2-nitroimidazole) (see p. 277) are electron-affinic agents used against certain bacterial and protozoal infections, particularly of the gut and the urinary tract. They have also been employed as radiosensitising agents because of their electron affinity. In man they both can produce an indolent sensory peripheral neuropathy with many clinical features similar to the B_1 deficiency neuropathy (see p. 288). When given to rats in doses of 400 mg/kg daily, they cause acute haemorrhagic lesions in the vestibular, cochlear and cerebellar nuclei and in other brainstem

nuclei. The lesions are haemorrhagic, with neuron loss and reactive astrocytes; the vascular bed becomes markedly hyperplastic. In these respects the lesions fairly closely resemble those of acute vitamin B$_1$ deficiency in this species.[252] The metabolic lesion responsible is not known. But reduction of the nitro-group by nitroreductases, in the presence of oxygen, leads to redox cycling with release of electrons; this causes considerable disturbance to the electron transport chain as well as excessive consumption of tissue NADPH and the generation of excess superoxides and other toxic ion species (see p. 279).

Pellagra (nicotinic acid-tryptophan deficiency)

Clinical features. The term 'pellagra', meaning an unpleasant incapacitating condition of the skin, emphasises the commonest of the three principal features of the disease, which are: light-sensitive skin lesions, gastrointestinal disturbances and mental changes. An early feature is erythema of the parts of the skin exposed to sunlight, especially the hands and wrists, accompanied by severe itching and burning sensations.[253] This may go on to desquamation and exfoliation with later pigmentation and atrophy. In addition, there is glossitis with a fiery-red sore tongue. The gastrointestinal disturbances are anorexia and vomiting with diarrhoea and loss of weight. Disturbances to higher mental functions, including depression, irritability and loss of concentration, are common. There is evidence of involvement of the peripheral nerves shown by burning sensations in the hands and feet, with numbness and increasing weakness of the distal parts of the limbs.[253,254]

Epidemics of this condition were common a few decades ago amongst people whose staple diet was maize (*Zea mays*), particularly around the Mediterranean and in the southern states of North America. In Mexico, however, where the peasants also subsist on a diet largely derived from maize, pellagra is avoided by the way in which the corn is prepared (see below).[255] Pellagra is presently seen among chronic alcoholics with severe nutritional problems, in patients treated with isoniazid for tuberculosis, particularly if they are vegetarians or

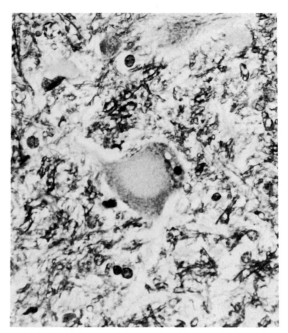

Fig. 11.26 Pellagra. Typical 'chromatolytic' neuron in a pontine nucleus. Klüver–Barrera × 270
Reproduced by permission of Dr I. Ferrer, Hospitalet de Llobregat, Barcelona, Spain.

vegans, and in cases of Hartnup disease (see opposite page).

Pathological features. There have been a number of detailed neuropathological postmortem reports.[254,256–258] These have uniformly shown that almost the only abnormal feature in many cases is a chromatolysis-like change in large nerve cells in various regions of the CNS. The Betz cells of the precentral cortex are affected, but the same change is also seen in many brainstem nuclei, particularly in the pons (Fig. 11.26). The significance of this striking and unique feature of the condition is uncertain, for the expected axonal degeneration that might account for the change in terms of an axon reaction is not found. It is most probably a direct effect, therefore, upon the cell body of the neuron. In addition, degeneration of the dorsal columns has often been described; this is more marked in the funiculus gracilis, and the spinocerebellar tracts have shown less change, which accounts for the sensory disturbances and ataxia that are not infrequently seen.

Experimental studies. Experiments using either dietary means or analogues of nicotinic acid have not helped to clarify the basis of the neuropathological changes in pellagra. The dietary methods have produced an analogous condition termed 'black tongue' in dogs; this is readily reversed by the administration of nicotinic acid. Increasing the tryptophan levels in the diet is found to lower the nicotinic acid requirements in these animals.

Even using the antagonists to nicotinic acid, 6-aminonicotinamide and 3-acetylpyridine, have not reproduced either the same clinical condition as pellagra nor the chromatolysis of nerve cells. This is probably because of the very much more acute nature of the intoxication, despite the fact that the effects of 6-aminonicotinamide are cumulative. As noted on page 290, 6-aminonicotinamide causes acute damage to astrocytes with secondary effects on nerve cells after 24 hours or more. 3-acetylpyridine is also a nicotinic acid antagonist that cannot be metabolised: it causes selective damage to inferior olivary nuclei and other brainstem nuclei,[259,260] but again without producing the features of pellagra. However, the production of pellagra by chronic feeding of these analogues and dietary control of nicotinic acid and tryptophan intake does not appear to have been tried.

Metabolic mechanisms. Nicotinic acid (niacin) is essential for the synthesis of the co-factors NADH and NADPH which are important in a number of metabolic steps critical for the cell. It is normally absorbed from the diet, particularly from meat, liver, rice bran and yeast. It is also synthesised from tryptophan by a multi-step process in which pyridoxal phosphate is required as a co-factor for at least one step and NAD itself for another. Pyridoxal deficiency will cause a block in this important synthetic pathway, whether the deficiency is induced by diet or by a drug antagonist, such as isoniazid, which specifically chelates with and inactivates pyridoxal phosphate. The block is shown by excessive excretion in the urine of the intermediates, xanthurenic acid, kynurenic acid and kynurenin. The tryptophan load test specifically tests for an inadequacy in this pathway. How much the body depends upon this synthetic pathway will depend upon the availability of dietary nicotinic acid and tryptophan. Arising from this, it is not surprising that pellagra has frequently been reported in vegetarians or vegans treated with isoniazid. In these circumstances both sources of the essential co-factor are jeopardised.[261] The particular tendency for maize to produce pellagra is due to the relatively unavailable state of its nicotinic acid content combined with its low tryptophan content; the nicotinic acid can be released by washing in an alkaline solution, and this is part of the culinary process used unwittingly by Mexican Indians that enables them to avoid the deficiency state.

Hartnup disease

Clinical features. Hartnup disease is a familial autosomal recessive condition characterised by cutaneous, neurological and psychiatric disturbances which are very similar to pellagra, but associated with a defect in the transport of neutral amino acids from the intestine. A red scaly cutaneous eruption occurs in regions exposed to light, as in pellagra. A severe but completely reversible cerebellar ataxia occurs in association with the skin rash and may be accompanied by diplopia and attacks of unconsciousness. Mental retardation, behavioural problems and emotional instability are frequent in the reported cases.

The biochemical changes found are related to the inadequately absorbed neutral amino acids.[262] This leads to excessive amino acids being excreted in the faeces, and increased absorption of bacterial breakdown products such as indoles and their excretion in the urine. The failure of tryptophan absorption is responsible for the tissue depletion of nicotinic acid and the pellagra-like signs. The skin and neurological lesions can be adequately treated by nicotinic acid supplementation, but the amino acid absorption defect has not been resolved. There is one published report of a patient who died with Hartnup disease;[263] the post-mortem findings were not described.

Pyridoxine deficiency

Although much is known from experimental studies about the nutritional and metabolic importance of pyridoxine (vitamin B_6) and its metabolites, no clear neurological syndrome has been defined in man. Experimental exclusion of this vitamin from the diet combined with the administration of desoxypyridoxine to 50 volunteers produced a pellagra-like condition with dermatitis, glossitis and cheilitis.[264] Only 3 showed clinical evidence of peripheral neuropathy. A similar syndrome has been produced in monkeys.[265]

However, a condition of inadequate pyridoxine absorption may be found in newborn infants, either as an inborn error of metabolism or from imperfect artificial feeding. Seizures occur which are reversed by giving large doses of pyridoxine.[266] The urine of such infants usually contains a raised concentration of xanthurenic acid as an index of the pyridoxine deficiency.[267] The metabolic basis of the epilepsy lies in the dependence of the synthesis of γ-aminobutyric acid (GABA) on the co-factor, pyridoxal phosphate. Other evidence of pyridoxal deficiency may be found, such as a mild haemolytic anaemia from disturbance of glutathione synthesis, which is also B_6-dependent. Glutathione is an essential agent for the protection and stability of cell membranes.[268]

It is only when pyridoxal phosphorylation and the functions of the co-factor, pyridoxal phosphate, are blocked by agents such as isoniazid that the tissue depletion of the co-factor becomes sufficiently severe to be associated with tissue damage and peripheral neuropathy.

Riboflavine deficiency

The syndrome of amblyopia, painful neuropathy and orogenital dermatitis (Strachan's syndrome) is well recognised in the West Indies and in the Far East.[269] Its cause is deficiency of riboflavine (vitamin B_2). A somewhat similar condition has been studied extensively in Nigeria.[270] There have been few post-mortem studies of the condition, but it appears that the gracile tracts of the dorsal columns of the spinal cord are degenerate and show gliosis; the anterolateral tracts may also show changes.[271,272] It is probable that sensory peripheral nerve fibres also degenerate during the acute phase of the illness, but that later these fibres are able to recover and regenerate, while those in the spinal cord are not.

Experimental studies have produced a somewhat analogous condition in rats,[273] dogs[274] and monkeys.[275] They showed skin lesions, especially of the lips (cheilitis) and around the mouth in the monkeys, and degeneration of peripheral nerves as well as of the dorsal columns with secondary gliosis. There are close similarities between this condition and thallium intoxication (see p. 254).

Metabolic mechanisms. Riboflavine is necessary for the synthesis of flavine-adenine dinucleotides and other flavoproteins that play an important part as hydrogen receptors in many metabolic pathways, especially oxidative phosphorylation and the generation of the high energy phosphates which are so important for such energy-demanding tissues as skin and the nervous system.

Vitamin B_{12} (cyanocobalamin) deficiency

Subacute combined degeneration of the spinal cord

Clinical features. Almost invariably the onset of the neurological condition is heralded by symmetrical sensory disturbances in the feet, with loss of the discriminative modalities of sensation, 'pins and needles' and a feeling of 'walking on cotton wool'. These paraesthesiae may be very distressing. The sensory changes progress to involve the hands and fingers; the legs may become unsteady and the limb movements clumsy. Loss of vibration and joint position sensations is another early feature, while ataxia, Rombergism, spasticity and loss of reflexes will be found in the fully developed case.

The spinal cord signs and symptoms are the usual major and early forms of dysfunction, but occasionally amblyopia may occur, even early in the condition. Mental disturbances are important and identification of cases of the disease in mental institutions is not unknown.

Pathological features. The fully developed case of subacute combined degeneration shows multi-focal vacuolated and demyelinated lesions in the white matter of the spinal cord, particularly in the dorsal and lateral columns, and affecting both motor and sensory pathways. However, in the early stages, vacuolation of white matter related to venules and small veins is seen (Fig. 11.27), particularly in the dorsal columns of the thoracic spinal cord.[276] The vacuolation process spreads to involve large areas of the white matter and is accompanied by the breakdown of myelin, the presence of foamy macrophages and a small amount of lymphocytic perivascular infiltration. As demyelination and vacuolation increase, evidence of axon degeneration appears in the most affected tracts.

It should be stressed that this is not a system degeneration in the normal meaning of the term (see p. 407) and the axon degeneration appears to be entirely secondary to the myelin changes. Early diagnosis and treatment must take these secondary features into account, for the myelin alterations at the outset of the disease are associated with normal looking oligodendroglial cells, while astroglia are not greatly increased until axon degeneration is advanced. The possibility of repair of the early myelin changes is considerable. Later in the disease the increase in astrocytes may be marked.

It is probable that extensive swelling of the myelin within the fibrous dural sheath of the optic nerve and canal leads to increased pressure that is responsible for axon degeneration and the funduscopic appearances of optic atrophy. The white matter of the brain may also show multifocal

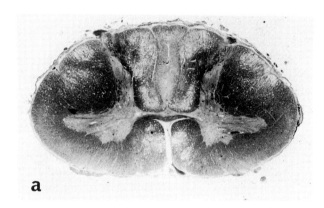

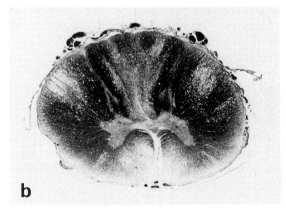

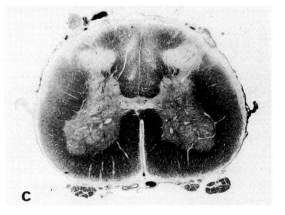

Fig. 11.27a–c Spinal cord from a pre-therapy case (1920) of subacute combined degeneration of the spinal cord. (a) Cervical cord. (b) Thoracic cord. (c) Lumbar cord. Note the abundant vacuolation (pale areas) in the white matter of thoracic and cervical levels with significantly less change in the lumbar level. The smaller lesions are centred upon veins and become confluent as the condition progresses to produce large spongy areas, in which axons become involved. The dorsal columns also show secondary degeneration in the gracile tracts.
Celloidin sections: iron haematoxylin stain for myelin (a) ×5·7; (b) ×8; (c) ×6·7

vacuolation without any particular regional localisation.

Peripheral neuropathy. While signs and symptoms often strongly suggest a definite peripheral neuropathy, specific studies of the peripheral nerves have been remarkably disappointing. Slowing of conduction velocity may be found, especially in distal regions of the limbs,[277] but proximal regions seem unaffected. Early pathological studies reported changes of Wallerian degeneration in a proportion of cases,[278] but by no means all authors have identified these changes. The oft-quoted paper of Greenfield and Carmichael[279] should be taken in the context of its time and the technical methods and concepts then current. It is probable that distal degeneration of axons and perhaps also segmental demyelination would be found in many more cases if examined by the methods now available. While there is no doubt that many of the symptoms and signs could be explained on the basis of the spinal cord changes alone, there is a strong likelihood that a 'dying back' type of axon degeneration also is occurring with, perhaps, additional segmental demyelination.

Experimental studies. Three experimental approaches have shed considerable light on the mechanism underlying the pathological changes in the nervous system.

1. *Cage paralysis in primates.* An unwitting experiment was carried out in many zoos that kept captive primates during the 1920s and 1930s. These animals were kept on the conventional fruit diet and they frequently developed a serious vitamin B_{12} deficiency.[280] The clinical condition associated with this change, 'cage paralysis', is one in which the animals develop evidence of progressive paresis in their hind limbs and, to a lesser degree, in their forelimbs together with ataxia, closely resembling subacute combined degeneration of the spinal cord in man. The pathological changes, too, are similar in almost every way, except for a tendency to show more marked loss of myelin in the white matter of the cerebral hemispheres, especially the corpus callosum.[281] In a more recent study of rhesus monkeys made deficient in vitamin B_{12}, the ultrastructural

changes were shown to begin in the myelin sheath with gross ballooning at the intraperiod line (i.e. the point of compaction of the external surfaces of the oligodendroglial cell membrane). This lesion is closely similar to the vacuolation seen in triethyltin and hexachlorophane intoxication (see p. 257) as well as in many other conditions in which the metabolism of the oligodendrocyte may be embarrassed in some way. In experimental vitamin B_{12} deficiency, the oligodendrocytes are not destroyed while the vacuolation is occurring, though they decrease in number as the lesions mature. The myelin subsequently breaks down and many naked axons can be found; later in the deficiency state these axons undergo Wallerian degeneration.[282] In vitamin-B_{12}-deficient animals, segmental demyelination is present more frequently in peripheral nerves than axon degeneration.[283]

2. *Nitrous oxide intoxication.* It had been noted that people chronically exposed to nitrous oxide (N_2O) sometimes developed evidence of vitamin B_{12} deficiency.[284] Monkeys similarly exposed for 6 or more weeks begin to show signs of paralysis and pathological changes identical to those found in vitamin B_{12} deficiency. Moreover, they can be almost completely protected by the administration of methionine by mouth,[285] a point of considerable aetiological importance.

3. *Cycloleucine intoxication.* The compound cycloleucine, while being tested for anticancer activity, was found to produce myelin vacuolation in mouse spinal cord similar to that occurring in subacute combined degeneration.[286] As in the vitamin B_{12} lesion in the monkey, the vacuolation seen ultrastructurally is due to expansion of the intraperiod line. The importance of this compound is that it competitively inhibits the conversion of methionine to S-adenosylmethionine, a donor of methyl groups in many methylation reactions.

Metabolic background to the tissue changes. Vitamin B_{12} is required for normal growth and maturation, especially of nervous tissues. Dietary deficiency of this vitamin is rare. Absorption of vitamin B_{12} can be reduced in many ways, including absence of the 'intrinsic factor' from gastric mucosa required for its absorption. Tape-worm infestation, and severe gastritis or gastric surgery which removes the region secreting the intrinsic factor, may also reduce absorption of vitamin B_{12}. Vegetarians, particularly vegans, are at risk, if their diet is low in methionine as well as in sources of vitamin.

In the mammalian nervous system two vitamin-B_{12}-requiring enzymes are identified, methionine synthetase and methylmalonyl CoA (coenzyme A) mutase. The first enzyme is probably more important in the genesis of the lesions of B_{12} deficiency than the second. Particularly significant is the finding that methionine alone given by mouth (see experimental study 2, above) will protect against the action of chronic N_2O intoxication. In such intoxication, there is specific inactivation of methionine synthetase through interference with methylation of cobalamin, a step which is essential for action of the vitamin as a cofactor. The finding that cycloleucine blocks the availability of the important methyl donor, *S*-adenosylmethionine, helps to confirm the idea that methyl donation may be at the root of the problem. Small et al[287] have suggested that inhibition of the methylation of myelin basic protein required for the process of myelin compaction may be responsible for the failure of maintenance of normal myelin relationships. The peculiar sensitivity of man, as opposed to other species, to develop the myelin lesion may be due to the higher requirement of man's myelin basic protein for labile methyl groups. Methylation of the basic protein helps to stabilise its insertion into the myelin membrane.

VITAMIN E (α-TOCOPHEROL) DEFICIENCY

Since the discovery of the requirement of the fat-soluble vitamin α-tocopherol for reproduction,[288] there has been considerable controversy over the rôle of this vitamin both in tissues generally and in the nervous system in particular. There is a large body of experimental data regarding its importance in the nutrition of muscle and in the development of muscle disease when it is deficient in the diet.[289] Also, veterinary workers have long recognised the association between its deficiency and the development of encephalomalacia in growing chicks.[290] Its importance in axonal maintenance and the occurrence of serious neurological disease when it is lacking have been recognised only recently. This has come about less from experimental studies on animals than from observations upon patients with defects in fat absorption and transport in which the fat-soluble vitamin became circumstantially involved.

Neuropathy associated with abetalipoproteinaemia

Clinical features. Abetalipoproteinaemia (Bassen–Kornzweig disease) is a rare inherited disorder. The diagnostic signs of steatorrhoea and acanthocytosis (spikiness) of red cells are usually present from birth. Over the next decade signs of peripheral neuropathy develop, with loss of proprioception and of other sensory modalities, and muscle weakness. These signs begin in the distal limb regions and in time are associated with loss of reflexes and ataxia, and perhaps with dysarthria, nystagmus and extensor plantar responses. Treatment with large doses of α-tocopherol (vitamin E) will prevent the onset of the neurological condition and halt its progress.[291]

Laboratory studies in such cases show the absence of low density lipoproteins in the serum, and very low or undetectable levels of vitamin E. Electrophysiologically there is moderate slowing of conduction velocity and reduced sizes of the action potentials with increased latencies; these signs indicate a reduction in numbers of axons distally, particularly those of large diameter.[292]

Pathological features. From biopsy studies,[292] it is apparent that sensory fibres are more affected than motor fibres in peripheral nerves, thus confirming the electrophysiological findings, and that there may be some evidence of regeneration, as shown by increased small fibres and cluster formation. Unmyelinated fibres might also show degeneration, and paranodal myelin degeneration has been described in two advanced cases of the disease. There have been no detailed post-mortem studies, but analogous conditions outlined below tell us the probable state of the nervous system.

Neuropathy of chronic liver disease

Cases of *biliary atresia*, of *cystic fibrosis* (muco-viscidosis)[293,294] and of *chronic malabsorption syndromes*[295] have been reported in which there has developed a neurological illness of gradual onset very closely similar to that occurring in abetalipo-proteinaemia (see above). Loss of sensory functions—particularly of proprioception and vibration sense—and of reflexes, with muscle weakness and ataxia, may be followed by dysarthria, oculomotor disturbances and perhaps extensor plantar responses. Treatment with large does of α-tocopherol is reported to have very beneficial effects on the clinical picture.

Pathological features. Post-mortem studies on cases of biliary atresia[296,297] and of cystic fibrosis[293,294] have demonstrated that there are the changes of axonal dystrophy, namely preterminal argyrophilic axonal swellings, in the gracile nuclei of the medulla accompanied by severe loss of fibres in the dorsal columns of the spinal cord and focal loss of neurons in the dorsal root ganglia. Spino-cerebellar tract degeneration may also be seen and, in the peripheral nerves, there is loss of the larger diameter fibres with a 'dying back' pattern (see p. 540). The process is, thus, very similar to changes in many other neuropathies, but in this instance it is reversible by treatment with α-tocopherol.

Experimental studies. Early studies with rats on vitamin E deficient diets regularly produced myopathic changes with muscle fibre necrosis, mild reactive inflammatory infiltration and evidence of myofibre regeneration which were all reversed or prevented by vitamin E sup-plements.[298] In later studies, several investigators using rats[299–302] and monkeys[303] have shown that more prolonged dietary deprivation of vitamin E will lead to degeneration of both sensory and motor axons in peripheral nerves accompanied by severe loss of fibres in the dorsal columns of the spinal cord. Other spinal tracts have not apparently shown changes and the cerebellum in

these animals is not implicated. Ultrastructurally there is characteristic evidence of preterminal axonal dystrophic changes, namely large amounts of accumulated smooth endoplasmic reticular membranes and lysosomal dense bodies, in the gracile nuclei.[304] Dosing with vitamin E prevents all these changes.

Metabolic basis. α-tocopherol has long been regarded as a compound with important cellular antioxidant properties, although until recently its rôle in this respect in the intracellular economy has been ill understood. It has become apparent, however, that auto-oxidation in tissues is ever present as the result of many oxidative intra-cellular processes. In consequence there is the constant generation of free radicals which, unless they are inactivated, are capable of causing damage to cells, particularly by oxidation of polyun-saturated fatty acids within membranes. It has been suggested that α-tocopherol plays a rôle parallel to that of glutathione in protecting against the action of free radicals, particularly in cell membranes, in which α-tocopherol readily dissolves. It may thus act as a catalytic regulating agent.[305,306]

The metabolic lesion in abetalipoproteinaemia is the absence of the apoprotein B (an essential component of chylomicrons) and of very low density and low density lipoproteins. Failure of production of these lipoprotein carriers results in inadequate absorption and transport of vitamin E, as well as other factors, from the gut to the tissues. Where fat absorption is impaired by the absence of bile a similar defect occurs, although the exact mechanisms involved are obscure.[307]

THE BRAIN IN LIVER DISEASE AND ALLIED CONDITIONS

ACQUIRED HEPATOCEREBRAL ENCEPHALOPATHY (portal-systemic shunt encephalopathy)

Clinical features. Patients with hepatic cirrhosis from any cause may have episodes of con-fusion, forgetfulness, and drowsiness, perhaps progressing to stupor or even coma from which they may recover with treatment.[308] These attacks recur and patients may develop ataxia, dysarthria, flapping tremor of the outstretched arms (asterixis), choreoathetosis and increasing dementia. The clinical syndrome is notoriously variable, but gradual deterioration of the mental and neurological state is inevitable.

Patients submitted to portocaval anastomosis, for portal hypertension or other reasons, may also become severely incapacitated after a few years with the same clinical syndrome as noted above for chronic liver disease.[309]

Neuropathological features. Many patients with chronic liver disease die with few neurological disturbances, and in these cases the only detectable changes to be found in the brain at post-mortem are a general watery swelling and the presence of Alzheimer type II astrocytes (Fig. 11.28). Described by von Hoesslin and Alzheimer in 1912,[310] the type II astrocytes have a watery swollen pale-staining nucleus, often with a tortuous outline and a prominent nucleolus. Glycogen is characteristically present in the nuclear region, but the cytoplasm is pale and structureless without an increase in glial filaments. Such cells are most frequently seen in the corpus striatum, in layers 5 and 6 of the cerebral cortex and in the dentate nuclei of the cerebellum, but they may occur almost anywhere where there are collections of large neurons.[311] While typically present in the brains of patients dying with hyperammonaemia from whatever cause, Alzheimer type II astrocytes are not in fact specific for this condition and may be seen in other conditions in which there is gliosis in the presence of oedema.

The second astroglial change, *Alzheimer type I astrocytes*, is much less common, and also not specific either for liver disease or for hyperammonaemia. The nuclei in these cells are greatly enlarged, often multilobulated, and deeply staining. On Feulgen staining and microdensitometry, they are found to contain more DNA than normal,[312] and it has been shown in experimental animals that the Alzheimer type I astrocytes arise by arrest in mitosis; the cells are unable to pass metaphase and therefore reconstruct as tetraploid cells.[313] Such cells are uncommon, except in

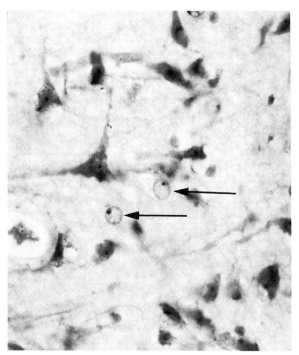

Fig. 11.28 Alzheimer type II astrocytes in the brain of a patient with hyperammonaemia due to ornithine transcarbamylase deficiency. Note the swollen watery astrocyte nuclei (arrows) and prominent nucleoli; very little of the cytoplasm can be distinguished. Haematoxylin-eosin × 575
Reproduced by permission of Dr J. A. N. Corsellis, Runwell Hospital, Wickford, Essex, UK.

regions where there is extensive neuronal damage from the deposition of copper in Wilson's disease (see p. 303). In fact, for Alzheimer type I cells to appear there must also be some stimulus for the astroglia to divide, such as a small infarct or substantial loss of neurons from other causes.

In addition to the presence of Alzheimer type II astrocytes, patients dying with serious neurological disturbances due to liver disease may show patchy widespread loss of nerve cells in the cortex in a laminar or pseudolaminar distribution, frequently associated with areas of microvacuolation. These changes are particularly common in the depths of cerebral sulci as well as in the cerebellum. Neuron loss may also occur to a lesser degree in the lentiform nuclei (basal ganglia) and in other regions of grey matter.[314] Astrogliosis is common in these areas and Alzheimer type I astrocytes may be seen.

Myelopathy of hepatic disease

Occasionally patients with liver disease have been reported in whom myelopathy with spasticity of unusual type ('puppet-like gait'), slurred speech and reduction of vibration sense have developed.[315] In such cases there is degeneration of the corticospinal tracts in the spinal cord, but rarely more rostrally than cervical level. There may also be loss of fibres in the gracile tracts of the dorsal columns but not in the cuneate tracts. Evidence of encephalopathy may be present.[316] From the pattern of pathological change in the cord it seems likely that it is a 'dying back' type of neuronal degeneration, but it is not known whether the peripheral axons are affected to the same extent as the spinal cord tracts.

Experimental studies

It was demonstrated in 1893[317] that dogs fed on a meat diet following an Eck fistula (portocaval anastomosis) develop neurological changes ('meat intoxication'). Since that time there have been numerous studies on both dogs and rats after the Eck operation, the chief result of which is a many-fold rise in the plasma ammonia levels. The only significant structural abnormality visible in the brains of such animals is the presence of Alzheimer type II astrocytes after two or more weeks. There is, however, also a slight increase in brain water, a slight decrease in brain potassium ion concentration and a regular increase in brain glutamine levels by about 2·5 times.[318] After perfusion fixation of the brain, nuclear lobulation but not nuclear swelling is seen in astrocytes, and it is only after immersion fixation that nuclear enlargement takes place and cells come to resemble the Alzheimer type II astrocytes seen in human cases.

The earliest ultrastructural change seen in rat brain following portocaval anastomosis is gross watery swelling of the astroglia without apparent change in cytoplasmic organelles. Later, however, an increasing amount of nerve fibre and neuronal degeneration is seen, and astroglial cells now respond by hypertrophy of their cytoplasmic organelles and an increase in 10 nm glial filaments.[319]

While rarely found in uninjured brains, Alzheimer type I astrocytes can be readily produced by making a brain wound in the presence of hyperammonaemia. As astrocytes begin to divide in response to the injury, many typical type I cells appear that are tetraploid or, rarely, octoploid. It is likely that astrocytes become overhydrated if they divide in the presence of oedema associated with excess ammonia, and mitosis is arrested in metaphase; the nuclei then reconstruct into giant forms.[320] The process is not specific for hyperammonaemia, however, and cells with similar characteristics have been seen in other conditions in which astrocytes divide in the presence of severe oedema, e.g. in venous infarcts of the cerebral cortex.

Animal experiments have not reproduced the laminar and pseudolaminar loss of neurons seen in man in the cerebral cortex, but focal micro-vacuolation with loss of Purkinje cells is seen in the depths of cerebellar sulci in rats, 5 or more weeks after portocaval anastomosis.[321] It is probable that both tissue oedema and anoxia play rôles in this process.

Metabolic basis of the lesions

Ammonium ions behave like potassium (K^+) ions; they enter cells through K^+ channels and may replace K^+ in many functions. With high plasma ammonium levels, muscles form the major 'sink' and up to 40% of the ammonium content of arterial blood passing through muscle may be removed in this way; this is more than twice the amount that is removed by the brain.[322] Ammonia, however, is readily released again on exercise and indeed muscular activity has been known to precipitate hepatic coma. In precoma and coma, levels of ammonia in carotid arterial blood are higher than in jugular venous blood, indicating that ammonia is extracted by the brain; during recovery this process is reversed.[323] The brain, unlike muscle, actively incorporates ammonia into the α-ketoglutarate–glutamate–glutamine pathway; two molecules of ammonia enter for one molecule of α-ketoglutarate. The high glutamine levels in the brain and cerebrospinal fluid of humans in hepatic coma and in animals with portocaval anastomosis result from such an ammonia-trapping mechanism. As glutamine synthetase is restricted solely to the endoplasmic

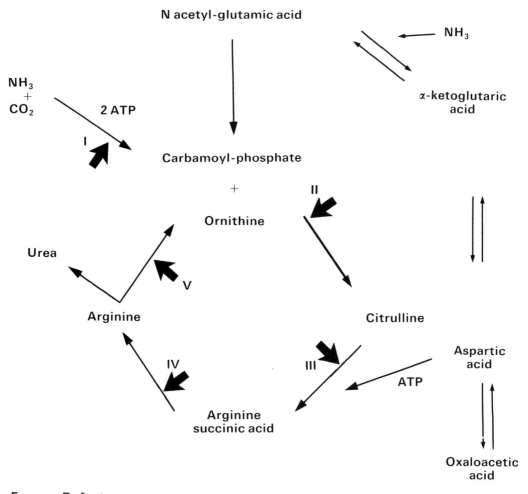

Enzyme Defects

  I Carbamoyl-phosphate Synthetase (cofactor:N-acetylglutamic acid)
     Carbamoyl-phosphate Synthetase Deficiency

 II Ornithine Transcarbamylase
     Ornithine transcarbamylase Deficiency

III Argininosuccinic acid Synthetase
     Citrullinaemia

IV Argininosuccinase
     Argininosuccinic aciduria

 V Argininase
     Hyperargininaemia

Enzyme Defects in the Urea Cycle

(from Sinclair, 1979)

Fig. 11.29 Diagram to show the steps in the urea (Krebs–Henseleit) cycle and the points at which enzyme defects may occur.
Reproduced by permission of Dr L Sinclair, Westminster Hospital, London, UK.

reticulum of astrocytes in the brain, this means that the astrocyte is the major ammonium-trapping cell.[324]

Despite such explanations for the astroglial changes in liver disease, the reasons for the neuronal loss remain obscure, as does the metabolic basis for the development of coma.

HYPERAMMONAEMIC SYNDROMES

A number of genetic conditions with abnormalities in the urea (Krebs–Henseleit) cycle are known; they result from specific enzyme defects at points around the cycle (Fig. 11.29). The effect of each defect is to cause a rise in plasma ammonia as well as the specific accumulation of relevant intermediates in the blood or urine. There are features in some of the clinical syndromes that allow recognition of the condition, as with the dry friable hair characteristic of argininosuccinic aciduria. However, varying degrees of mental defect are seen in all the syndromes, not infrequently complicated by seizures. Radiologically, the brain is usually reported to be atrophic, and varying degrees of cortical atrophy have been described in post-mortem studies. Histologically, sections show an abundance of Alzheimer type II astrocytes associated with severe neuronal loss. It is not certain whether the neuronal loss is the direct result of the hyperammonaemia or secondary to the repeated seizures. Good post-mortem studies are few, but have been reported in ornithine transcarbamylase deficiency[325] and in argininosuccinic aciduria.[326] In citrullinaemia, diffuse cortical atrophy was reported radiologically.[327] Walser[328] discusses the metabolic basis of these disorders in detail.

REYE'S SYNDROME

Reye's syndrome affects young children (see p. 210) and is sometimes referred to as 'white liver, wet brain'.[329,330] Its cause is unknown; many toxic and infective agents have been implicated but none is definitely proven. Salicylates have been suggested as the toxic agent,[331] but there is so far no firm evidence to implicate any drug.

Hypoglycaemia is an important clinical feature and may be associated with seizures. Uraemia, hyponatraemia, and hyperammonaemia are all usually present.

At post-mortem, the liver and kidneys show severe fatty change, but the findings in the brain are non-specific. The brain is oedematous; there is scattered nerve cell loss, and occasional ring haemorrhages may be found. Hypoxic changes occur in the cerebral cortex, the hippocampus, the basal ganglia and the cerebellum.[332] It is not certain what part hyperammonaemia plays in the syndrome.

Ultrastructurally,[333] abnormalities in the mitochondria, swelling of astrocytes and focal ballooning of the myelin sheath, reminiscent of the organic tin lesion (see p. 257), have suggested that there is primary toxic damage to mitochondria.[334]

WILSON'S DISEASE (hepatolenticular degeneration)

Clinical features. The basis of Wilson's disease is a disturbance of copper metabolism which is inherited as an autosomal recessive trait. Signs of liver disease may be present in children at 8 years of age or older, and in young adults. In the younger patients, the signs of liver disease are usually more prominent than the neurological changes; in older patients the reverse is generally true. The liver disease presents with malaise, jaundice, gastrointestinal disorders and vomiting; a haemolytic crisis may be the first sign of Wilson's disease. During the course of the disease evidence of renal disturbances may become apparent, as well as bone and joint disorders. The occurrence of a Kayser–Fleischer ring of yellow–brown pigmentation in the outer part of the cornea is characteristic, but is frequently absent in children.

The neurological disturbances principally involve the extrapyramidal system, with disorders of movement control. Dysarthria, poverty of limb coordination, with or without involuntary movements and dystonias, may be seen, together with deterioration of intelligence. Flapping tremor and spasticity are common. Early diagnosis is important, for the progress of the neurological disease can be arrested by treatment with chelating agents to remove copper, particularly penicillamine.[335]

Pathological features. Liver cirrhosis may be finely, but more usually coarsely, lobular. Brown pigmentation, due to deposition of large amounts of copper, should allow Wilson's disease to be distinguished from other causes of cirrhosis. In the brain the external appearances are usually normal, but on sectioning, symmetrical widening of the lateral ventricles draws attention to atrophy of the lentiform nuclei and other basal ganglia. The putamen is softened with spongy cavitations and stained a yellowish or reddish brown. The globus pallidus is small and discoloured but is not as severely affected as the putamen. In the more severe cases, softening and cavitation may be seen in the cerebral cortex, often at the crests of the gyri, but usually the grey and the white matter away from the basal ganglia show little macroscopic abnormality.

Microscopically, there is loss of nerve cells in the lentiform nuclei, with gliosis and widespread Alzheimer type II astrocytes. Alzheimer type I astrocytes are found less often. Opalski cells, which are said to be grossly enlarged and rounded microglial cells, are distinctive in this condition. Spongy change with loss of nerve cells and astrogliosis may be present in many other basal nuclei, including the thalamus, mamillary bodies, red nucleus, and substantia nigra, but not in the nuclei of the brainstem, where Alzheimer type II astrocytes are the main abnormality.

Metabolic basis of the lesions. The central defect in Wilson's disease is failure of excretion of copper into the biliary tract and failure of binding of copper to ceruloplasmin, the normal transport protein.[336] Accumulation of copper in hepatic cells leads to their damage and to the subsequent development of lobular cirrhosis, with nodules of regeneration and portal-systemic shunting of blood through the altered vascular bed. Failure of binding to ceruloplasmin leads to the attachment of copper to other carrier proteins, such as albumen. Attached to this smaller protein, copper enters the brain more easily and excretion of copper into kidney tubules is facilitated. Copper is also deposited in other tissues, such as Descemet's membrane of the cornea (to give the Kayser–Fleischer ring), and in bones and joints.[337] Copper deposition damages the tissue cells, although the mechanism of such damage is unclear; it is perhaps mediated by the generation of free radical or by the oxidation of membrane lipids. Adequate chelation therapy will usually halt the progress of Wilson's disease. The reason for the localisation of brain damage to the region of the basal ganglia is obscure.

REFERENCES

Pathological investigation

1. Dyck PJ. In: Dyck PJ, Thomas PK, Lambert EH, eds. Peripheral neuropathy. Philadelphia: Saunders, 1975; 1: 15.
2. Said G. Ann Neurol 1978; 3: 259.

Toxic disorders due to chemicals

3. Byron WR, Bierbower GW, Bronwer JB, Hansen WH. Toxicol Appl Pharmacol 1967; 10: 132.
4. Glaister J. The power of poison. London: Christopher Johnson, 1954.
5. Robinson TJ. Br Med J 1975; 2: 139.
6. Reynolds ES. Lancet 1901; 1: 166.
7. First Royal Commission appointed to enquire into arsenical poisoning from the consumption of beer and the articles of food and drink. London: HMSO, 1901.
8. Tsuchiya K. Environ Health Perspect 1977; 19: 35.
9. Dudley SF. J Ind Hyg 1919; 1: 215.
10. Mees RA. JAMA 1919; 72: 1337.
11. Hassin GB. J Nerv Ment Dis 1930; 72: 628.
12. Jenkins RB. Brain 1966; 89: 479.
13. Senanayake N, DeSilva WAS, Solgado MSL. Ceylon Med J 1972; 17: 195.
14. Murphy MJ, Lyon LW, Taylor JW. J Neurol Neurosurg Psychiatry 1981; 44: 896.
15. Erhlicki A, Ribalkin J. Arch Psychiatr Nervenkr 1892; 23: 861.
16. Chhuttani PN, Chawla LS, Sharma TD. Neurology (Minn) 1967; 17: 269.
17. Dyck PJ, Gutrecht JA, Bastrom JA, Karnes WE, Dale AJD. Mayo Clin Proc 1968; 43: 81.
18. Ohta M. Acta Neuropathol (Berl) 1970; 16: 233.
19. Webb JL. Enzyme and metabolic inhibitors. New York: Academic Press, 1966.
20. Peters RA. Symp Soc Exp Biol 1949; 3: 36.
21. Peters RA. Bull Johns Hopkins Hosp 1955; 97: 1.
22. Jacobs JM, Macfarlane RM, Cavanagh JB. J Neurol Sci 1976; 29: 95.

23. Schmorl G. Munch Med Wochenschr 1913; 60: 1685.
24. Alpers BJ. Arch Neurol Psychiatry 1928; 20: 497.
25. Globus JH, Ginsburg SW. Arch Neurol Psychiatry 1933; 30: 1226.
26. Russell DS. J Pathol Bacteriol 1937; 45: 357.
27. Beeson BB. Arch Dermatol Syphilol (Chic) 1920; 2: 337.
28. Young AG, Loevenhart AS. J Pharmacol Exp Ther 1924; 23: 107.
29. Glaser MA, Immerman CP, Immerman SW. Am J Med Sci 1935; 189: 64.
30. Diamant H. Arch Otol 1958; 67: 546.
31. Kellogg F, Epstein NN. Arch Dermatol Syphilol (Chic) 1934; 30: 251.
32. Crecoelius EA. Environ Health Perspect 1977; 19: 147.
33. Longley BJ, Clausen NM, Tatum AL. J Pharmacol Exp Ther 1942; 76: 202.
34. Weston Hurst EW. J Pathol Bacteriol 1959; 77: 523.
35. Cavanagh JB. J Clin Pathol 1953; 6: 128.
36. Perlstein MA, Attala R. Clin Pediatr 1966; 5: 292.
37. Blackman SS. Bull Johns Hopkins Hosp 1933; 61: 1.
38. Smith JF, McLaurin RL, Nichols JB, Astbury A. Brain 1960; 83: 411.
39. Pentschew A, Garro F. Acta Neuropathol (Berl) 1966; 6: 266.
40. Fullerton PM. J Neuropathol Exp Neurol 1966; 25: 214.
41. Cavanagh JB. In: Smith WT, Cavanagh JB, eds. Recent advances in neuropathology. Edinburgh: Churchill Livingstone, 1979; 1: 247.
42. Dyck PJ, Windebank AJ, Low PA, Baumann WJ. J Neuropathol Exp Neurol 1980; 39: 700.
43. Saunders LW. Environ Health 1974; 8: 270.
44. Stasek M, Byckowska Z, Szendzikowski S, Fiedorczuk F. Arch Toxicol 1968; 24: 283.
45. Paterson D, Greenfield JG. Q J Med 1923–24; 17: 6.
46. Wyllie WG, Stern RO. Arch Dis Child 1931; 1: 829.
47. Warkany J, Hubbard DM. Lancet 1948; 1: 829.
48. Davis LE, Wands JR, Weiss SA, Price DL, Girling EF. Arch Neurol Psychiatry 1974; 30: 428.
49. Hargreaves RJ, Evans JG, Janota I, Magos L, Cavanagh JB. Neuropathol Appl Neurobiol 1988; 14: 443.
50. Hunter D, Bomford RR, Russell DS. Q J Med 1940; NS 9: 193.
51. Hunter D, Russell DS. J Neurol Neurosurg Psychiatry 1954; 17: 235.
52. Cavanagh JB. J UOEH 1988; 10 (suppl): 127.
52a. Takeuchi T, Morikawa N, Matsumoto H, Shiraishi Y. Acta Neuropathol (Berl) 1962; 2: 40.
53. Igata A. In: Tsubaki T, Takahashi H, eds. Recent advances in Minamata disease studies. Tokyo: Kodansha, 1986.
54. Magos L. Br Med Bull 1975; 31: 241.
55. Jacobs JM, Carmichael N, Cavanagh JB. Neuropathol Appl Neurobiol 1975; 1: 1.
56. Jacobs JM, Cavanagh JB, Carmichael N. Neuropathol Appl Neurobiol 1975; 1: 321.
57. Enders A, Noetzel H. Arch Exp Pathol Pharmacol 1955; 225: 346.
58. Yoshino Y, Mozai T, Nakao K. J Neurochem 1966; 13: 1223.
59. Cavanagh JB, Chen FC-K. Acta Neuropathol (Berl) 1971; 19: 216.
60. Canavan MM, Cobb S, Drinker CR. Arch Neurol Psychiatry 1934; 32: 501.
61. Pañalver R. Ind Med Surg 1955; 24: 1.
62. Maynard LS, Cotzias GC. J Biol Chem 1955; 214: 489.
63. Cotzias GC. Physiol Rev 1958; 38: 503.
64. Dastur DK, Mangani DK, Raghavendra KV, Jeejebhoy KN. Q J Exp Physiol 1969; 54: 322.
65. Pentschew A, Ebner FF, Korvatch RM. J Neuropathol Exp Neurol 1963; 22: 488.
66. Matthys R. Ann Med Leg 1955; 35: 237.
67. Prick JJG, Smith WGS, Muller L. Thallium poisoning. Amsterdam: Elsevier, 1955.
68. Bertrand-Capella A, Hernandez-Gutierrez F, Corbella J. Collection de médecine légale et de toxicologie. Masson, 1972.
69. Heyroth FF. US Public Health Service Rep 1947; suppl 197.
70. Reed D, Crawley J, Faro SN, Pieper SJ, Kurland LJ. JAMA 1963; 183: 516.
71. Cavanagh JB, Fuller NH, Johnson HRM, Rudge P. Brain 1974; 53: 293.
72. Davis LE, Standefer JC, Kornfeld M, Abercrombie DM, Butler C. Ann Neurol 1981; 10: 38.
73. Kennedy P, Cavanagh JB. J Neurol Sci 1976; 29: 295.
74. Greving R, Gegel O. Z Gesamte Neurol Psychiatrie 1929; 120: 805.
75. Cavanagh JB, Gregson L. J Pathol 1978; 125: 179.
76. Gehring PJ, Hammond PB. J Pharmacol Exp Ther 1967; 155: 187.
77. Kuhn R, Rudy H, Wagner-Jauregg T. Ber Dtsch Chem Ges 1933; 66: 1950.
78. Pentschew A, Garro F. J Neuropathol Exp Neurol 1969; 28: 163.
79. Barnes JM, Stoner H. Pharmacol Rev 1958; 11: 211.
80. Alajouanine Th, Dérobert L, Thieffry S. Rev Neurol 1958; 98: 85.
81. Gruner J-E. Rev Neurol 1958; 98: 109.
82. Magee PM, Stoner HB, Barnes JM. J Pathol Bacteriol 1957; 73: 107.
83. Alea FP, Katzman R, Terry RD. J Neuropathol Exp Neurol 1963; 22: 403.
84. Lock EA, Scales D, Little RA. Br Toxicol Soc Abstr, 1980.
85. Brown AW, Aldridge WN, Street BW, Verschoyle RD. Am J Pathol 1979; 97: 59.
86. Bouldin TW, Goines ND, Bagnell CR, Krigman MR. Am J Pathol 1981; 104: 237.
87. Brown AW, Cavanagh JB, Verschoyle RD, Gysbers MF, Jones HB, Aldridge WN. Neuropathol Appl Neurobiol 1984; 10: 267.
88. Fortemps E, Amand G, Bomboir A, Lauwerys R, Laterre EC. Int Arch Occup Environ Health 1978; 41: 1.
89. Besser R, Krämer G, Thümber R, Bohl J, Gutmann L, Hopf HC. Neurology 1987; 37: 945.
90. Petit TL. In: Dreosti IE, Smith RM, eds. Neurobiology of the trace elements. New Jersey: Humana Press, 1983; 2: 237.
91. Wisniewski HM, Narkiewicz O, Wisniewska K. Acta Neuropathol (Berl) 1967; 9: 127.
92. Wernicke C. In: Lehrbuch der Gehirnkrankheiten. Kassel: Fischer, 1881; 2: 229.
93. Victor M, Adams RD, Collins GH. The Wernicke–Korsakoff syndrome. Philadelphia: Davis, 1971.
94. Harper C. J Neurol Neurosurg Psychiatry 1979; 42: 226.
95. Riggs HE, Boles RS. Q J Alcohol Studies 1944; 5: 361.
96. Ironside R, Bosanquet FD, McMenemy WH. Brain 1961; 84: 212.
97. Ferrer I, Fabregues I, Pineda M, Gracia I, Ribalta T.

Neuropathol Appl Neurobiol 1984; 10: 245.
98. Adams RD, Victor M, Mancall EI. Arch Neurol Psychiatry 1959; 81: 154.
99. Schneck SA. J Neuropathol Exp Neurol 1966; 25: 18.
100. Boon AP, Potter AE. Neuropathol Appl Neurobiol 1987; 13: 1.
101. Collins GH. Am J Pathol 1967; 50: 791.
102. Narins RG. N Engl J Med 1986; 314: 1573.
103. Victor M, Adams RD. Proc Assoc Res Nerv Ment Dis 1953; 28: 526.
104. Fennelly J, Frank O, Baker H, Leery CM. Br Med J 1964; 2: 1290.
105. Strauss MB. Am J Med Sci 1935; 189: 378.
106. Walsh JC, McLeod JG. J Neurol Sci 1970; 10: 457.
107. Jones KL, Smith DW, Ulleland CN, Streissguth AP. Lancet 1973; 1: 1267.
108. Clarren SK, Smith DW. N Engl J Med 1978; 298: 1063.
109. Diaz J, Samson HH. Science 1980; 208: 751.
110. Walker DW, Barnes DE, Zornetzer SF, Hunter BE, Kubains P. Science 1980; 209: 711.
111. Herskowitz A, Isii N, Schaumburg H. N Engl J Med 1971; 285: 82.
112. Mendell JR, Saida K, Ganasia MF et al. Science 1974; 185: 787.
113. Korobkin R, Asbury A, Sumner AJ, Nielson SL. Arch Neurol 1975; 32: 158.
114. Astbury AK, Nielsen SL, Telfer R. J Neuropathol Exp Neurol 1974; 33: 191.
115. Cavanagh JB. Neuropathol Appl Neurobiol 1982; 8: 19.
116. Jones HB, Cavanagh JB. J Neurocytol 1983; 12: 439.
117. Couri D, Abdel-Rahman MS, Hetland LB. Toxicol Appl Pharmacol 1976; 37: 124.
118. Graham DG, Anthony DC, Boekelheide K, Maschmann N, Richards RG, Wolfram JW, Shaw BR. Toxicol Appl Pharmacol 1982; 64: 415.
119. O'Donohue JL, Krasavage WJ. J Neuropathol Exp Neurol 1979; 38: 333.
120. Brieger H. J Occup Med 1961; 3: 302.
121. Magos L. Ann Occup Hyg 1972; 15: 303.
122. Vigliani EC. Br J Ind Med 1954; 11: 235.
123. Abe M. Jpn J Med Sci 1933; 3: 1.
124. Szendzikowski S, Stetkiewicz J, Wronska-Nofer T, Zdrajkowska I. Int Arch Arbeitsmed 1973; 31: 135.
125. Cavanagh JB, De Groot DMG. Unpublished work.
126. Grabski DA. Am J Psychiatry 1961; 118: 461.
127. Boor JW, Hurtig HI. Ann Neurol 1977; 2: 440.
128. Fornazzaro L, Wilkinson DA, Kapur BM, Carlen PL. Acta Neurol Scand 1983; 67: 319.
129. Defalque RJ. Clin Pharmacol Ther 1961; 2: 665.
130. Buxton PH, Haywood M. J Neurol Neurosurg Psychiatry 1967; 30: 511.
130a. Cavanagh JB, Buxton PH. J Neurol Neurosurg Psychiatry 1989; 52: 297.
131. Bennell IL, Cary FH, Mitchell GL, Cooper MN. Medicine (Baltimore) 1953; 32: 431.
132. Røe O. Acta Med Scand [Suppl] 1946; 182: 1.
133. Cavanagh JB. Int Rev Exp Pathol 1964; 3: 219.
134. Cavanagh JB. CRC Crit Rev Toxicol 1975; 2: 365.
135. Aring CD. Brain 1942; 65: 34.
136. Smith HV, Spalding JMK. Lancet 1959; 2: 1019.
137. Bouldin TW, Cavanagh JB. Am J Pathol 1979; 94: 253.
138. Vasilescu C, Alexianu M, Dan A. J Neurol Neurosurg Psychiatry 1984; 47: 543.
139. Eto M, Casida JE, Eto T. Biochem Pharmacol 1962; 11: 337.
140. Johnson MK. Arch Toxicol 1975; 34: 259.
141. Moretto A, Lotti M, Sabri MI, Spencer PS. J Neurochem 1987; 49: 1515.
142. Igisu H, Goto I, Kawamura Y, Kato M, Kumi K, Kuruiwa Y. J Neurol Neurosurg Psychiatry 1975; 38: 581.
143. Garland TD, Patterson MWH. Br Med J 1967; 4: 134.
144. Fullerton PM. J Neurol Neurosurg Psychiatry 1969; 32: 186.
145. Davenport JG, Farrell DF, Simm SM. Neurology 1976; 26: 919.
146. Spencer PS, Schaumburg HH. Can J Neurol Sci 1974; 1: 152.
147. Cavanagh JB. Neuropathol Appl Neurobiol 1982; 8: 315.
148. Jones HB, Cavanagh JB. Neuropathol Appl Neurobiol 1984; 10: 101.
149. Ambache N. J Physiol (Lond) 1949; 108: 127.
150. Wright GP. Pharmacol Rev 1955; 7: 413.
151. Duchen LW, Strich SJ. Q J Exp Physiol 1968; 53: 84.
152. Watson WE. Br Med Bull 1974; 30: 112.
153. Kristensson K, Olsson T. Brain Res 1978; 155: 118.
154. Hanig JP, Lamanna C. J Theor Biol 1979; 77: 107.
155. Hambledon P, Shone CC, Melling J. In: Jenner P, ed. Neurotoxins and their pharmacological implications. New York: Raven Press, 1987.
156. Batten FF. Br Med J 1898; 2: 1540.
157. Cavanagh JB, Jacobs JM. Br J Exp Pathol 1964; 45: 309.
158. Allt G, Cavanagh JB. Brain 1969; 92: 459.
159. Pappenheimer AM Jr. Ann Rev Biochem 1977; 46: 69.
160. Yamaizumi M, Nekada E, Uchida T, Okada Y. Cell 1978; 15: 245.
161. Pleasure DE, Feldman B, Prockop DJ. J Neurochem 1973; 20: 81.
162. Wright GP. Pharmacol Rev 1955; 7: 413.
163. Mellanby J, Green J. Neuroscience 1981; 6: 281.
164. Acton HW. Indian Med Gaz 1922; 57: 241.
165. Denny Brown D. Medicine (Baltimore) 1947; 26: 41.
166. Buzzard EF, Greenfield JG. Pathology of the nervous system. London: Constable, 1921.
167. Filimonoff IN. Z Gesamte Neurol Psychiatrie 1926; 105: 76.
168. Strieflex M, Cohn DF, Hirano A, Schujman E. Neurology 1977; 27: 1176.
169. Rudra MM. Nature 1952; 170: 124.
170. Spencer PS, Schaumburg HH, Cohn DF, Seth PK. In: Rose FC, ed. Res progr in motor neuron disease. London: Pitman, 1984: 312.
171. Spencer PS, Roy DN, Ludolph A, Hugon J, Dwivedi MP, Schaumburg HH. Lancet 1986; 2: 1066.
172. Chou SM, Hartmann HA. Acta Neuropathol (Berl) 1965; 4: 590.
173. Papasozomenos S.Ch, Autilio-Gambetti L, Gambetti P. J Cell Biol 1981; 91: 866.
174. Kurland LT, Mulder DW. Neurology 1954; 4: 355.
175. Malamud N, Hirano A, Kurland LT. Arch Neurol 1961; 5: 401.
176. Spencer PS, Nunn PB, Hugon J, Ludolph AC, Ross SM, Roy DN, Robertson RC. Science 1987; 237: 465.
177. Weller RO, Mitchell J, Daves GD. Buckthorn (Karwinskia humboldtiana) toxins. In: Spencer PS, Schaumburg HH, eds. Experimental and clinical neurotoxicology. Baltimore: Williams & Wilkins, 1980; 336.

178. Padron-Payou F. Gac Med Mex 1951; 8: 299.
179. Marsh CD, Clawson AB, Roe GC. Tech Bull US Dept Agric 1928; 29: 1.
180. Calderon-Gonzales R, Rizzi-Hernandez H. N Engl J Med 1969; 277: 67.
181. Charlton KM, Pierce KR. Pathol Vet 1970; 7: 385, 420.
182. Muñoz-Martinez EJ, Cueva J, Joseph-Nathan P. Neuropathol Appl Neurobiol 1983; 9: 121.
183. Hernandez-Cruz AC, Muñoz-Martinez EJ. Neuropathol Appl Neurobiol 1984; 10: 11.
184. Mitchell J, Weller RO, Evans JI, Daves GD. Neuropathol Appl Neurobiol 1978; 4: 85.
185. Wheeler MH, Camp BJ. Life Sci 1971; 10: 41.
186. Collings H. Arch Neurol (Chic) 1960; 3: 656.
187. Urtasun RC, Chapman JD, Feldstein ML et al. Br J Cancer 1978; 37 (suppl 3): 271.
188. Dische S, Saunders MI, Flockhart IR. Br J Cancer 1977; 35: 567.
189. Robertson DHH. Rep East Africa Trypan Res Org 1959: 41.
190. Griffin JW, Price DL, Kuethe DSO, Goldberg AW. Neurotoxicol 1979; 1: 299.
191. Knight RC, Skolimowski IM, Edwards DI. Biochem Pharmacol 1978; 27: 2089.
192. Neu HC, Bendush CL. J Infect Dis 1976; 134: S 206.
193. Jones WA, Jones GP. Lancet 1953; 1: 1073.
194. Evans DAP, Manley KA, McKusick VA. Br Med J 1960; 2: 485.
195. Ott T, Rabinowicz T, Moraud B. Rev Neurol 1959; 100: 103.
196. Cavanagh JB. J Neurol Neurosurg Psychiatry 1967; 30: 26.
197. Palmer AC, Noel PRB. Nature 1965; 205: 506.
198. McCormick DB, Snell EE. J Biol Chem 1961; 236: 2088.
199. Holz P, Palm D. Pharmacol Rev 1964; 16: 113.
200. Axte F, Bunger P, Lass A. Forsch Neurol Psychiatrie 1956; 24: 369.
201. Cavanagh JB. Lancet 1984; 1: 1284.
202. Raskin NH, Fishman RA. N Engl Med J 1965; 273: 1182.
203. Leggat PO. Tubercle 1962; 43: 95.
204. Poole GW, Schneeweiss J. Amer Rev Respir Dis 1961; 84: 890.
205. Bradley WG, Lassman LP, Pearce GW, Walton JW. J. Neurol Sci 1970; 10: 107.
206. Shelanski ML, Wisniewski H. Arch Neurol (Chic) 1969; 20: 199.
207. Tomiwa K, Hazama F, Mikawa H. Neuropathol Appl Neurobiol 1983; 9: 345.
208. Shiraishi S, LeQuesne PM, Gajree T, Cavanagh JB. J Neurol Sci 1985; 71: 165.
209. Dustin P. Microtubules. Berlin: Springer, 1984.
210. Bensch KG, Marantz R, Wisniewski H, Shelanski M. Science 1969; 165: 495.
211. Hadley D, Herr HW. Cancer 1979; 44: 2026.
212. Hemphill M, Pestronk A, Walsh T, Parhad I, Clark A, Rosenshein N. Neurology 1980; 30: 429.
213. Clark AW, Parhad IM, Griffin JW, Price DL. Neurology 1980; 30: 429.
214. Pasco JM, Roberts JJ. Biochem Pharmacol 1974; 23: 1345.
215. Cho ES. J Neuropathol Exp Neurol 1977; 36: 907.
216. Egorin MJ, Hildebrand RC, Cimino EF, Bachur NR. Cancer Res 1974; 34: 2243.
217. Shuman RM, Leech RW, Alvord EC Jr. Pediatrics 1974; 54: 89.
218. Towfighi J, Gonatas NK, McCree L. Lab Invest 1975; 32: 89.
219. Udall V. Proc R Soc Med 1972; 65: 197.
220. Cammer W, Rose AL, Norton WT. Brain Res 1975; 98: 547.
221. Tsubaki T, Toyokura Y, Tsukoyushi H. Jpn J Med 1965; 4: 181.
222. Baumgartner G, Gawal MJ, Kaeser HE et al. J Neurol Neurosurg Psychiatry 1979; 42: 1073.
223. Shiraki H. In: Roizin L, Shiraki H, Grcević, N, eds. Neurotoxicology. New York: Raven Press, 1977.
224. Worden AN, Heywood R, Prentice D, Chesterman H, Skerrett K, Thomann PE. Toxicology 1978; 9: 227.
225. Albert A. Selective toxicity, 5th ed. London: Chapman and Hall, 1973.
226. Pollet S, Hauw JJ, Escourolle R, Baumann N. Lancet 1977; 1: 1258.
227. Wright GT, Leeson GA, Zeiger AV. Postgrad Med J 1973; 49 (suppl 3): 8.
228. Sebille A. Br Med J 1978; 1: 1321.
229. Burns RS, Chieuh CC, Markey SP, Ebert MH, Jacobowitz DM, Kopin IJ. Proc Natl Acad Sci USA 1983; 80: 4546.
230. Kopin IJ. In: Jenner P, ed. Neurotoxins and their pharmacological implications. New York: Raven Press, 1987.
231. Lyden A, Bondessen U, Larsson BS, Linquist NG. Acta Pharmacol Toxicol 1983; 53: 429.
232. Bus JS, Cogen S, Olgaard M, Gibson JE. Toxicol Appl Pharmacol 1976; 83: 501.
232a. Rollema H, Kuhr WG, Kraumburg G, de Vries J, van der Berg C. J Pharmacol Exp Ther 1988; 245: 858

Deficiency and metabolic diseases

233. Sauberlich HE. Vitam Horm 1964; 22: 807.
234. Torvik A. Neuropathol Appl Neurobiol 1985; 11: 179.
235. Alexander L. Am J Path 1940; 16: 61.
236. Rinehart JF, Friedman M, Greenberg LD. Arch Pathol 1949; 48: 129.
237. Jubb KV, Saunders LZ, Coats H. J Comp Pathol 1956; 66: 21.
238. Evans CA, Carlson NE, Green J. Am J Pathol 1942; 18: 79.
239. Dreyfus PM, Victor M. Am J Clin Pathol 1961; 9: 414.
240. Edwin EE, Jackson R. Nature 1970; 228: 772.
241. Platt BS. Fed Proc 1958; 17: 8.
242. McIlwain H, Batchelard H. Biochemistry of the nervous system, 2nd ed. Edinburgh: Churchill Livingstone, 1984.
243. Leigh D. J Neurol Neurosurg Psychiatry 1951; 14: 216.
244. Pinkus JH. Dev Med Child Neurol 1972; 14: 87.
245. Giroud M, Dumas R. Rev Pediatr (Paris) 1982; 18: 395.
246. Sander J, Packman S, Berg BO, Hutchinson HT, Caswell N. Neurology 1984; 34: 515.
247. Cooper JR, Hokawa Y, Pinkus JH. Science 1969; 164: 74.
248. Willems JL, Monnene LAH, Trijbels JMF, Veerkamp JH, Meijer AEHF, van Dam L, Haelet W. Pediatrics 1977; 60: 850.
249. Ford WCL, Jacobs JM. Neurotoxicology 1981; 2: 405.
250. Sims KL, Kauffman FC, Johnson EC, Pickel VM. J Histochem Cytochem 1974; 22: 7.

251. Schneider H, Cervos-Navarros J. Acta Neuropathol (Berl) 1974; 27: 11.
252. Griffin JW, Price DL, Kuethe DO, Goldberg AM. Neurotoxicology 1980; 1: 229.
253. Roberts SR. Pellagra. London: Kimpton, 1912.
254. Leigh D. J Ment Sci 1952; 98: 130.
255. Carpenter KJ. Fed Proc 1981; 40: 1531.
256. Greenfield JG, Holmes JM. Br Med J 1939; 1: 815.
257. Hsu YK. Arch Neurol Psychiatry 1942; 48: 271.
258. Ishii N, Nishihara Y. J Neurol Neurosurg Psychiatry 1985; 48: 628.
259. Desclin JC, Escubi J. Brain Res 1974; 77: 349.
260. Johnson WJ, McColl JD. Fed Proc 1956; 15: 284.
261. Benda DA, Russell-Jones R. Lancet 1979; 2: 1125.
262. Jepson JB. In: Stanbury JB, Wyngaarden JB, Fredrickson DS, eds. The metabolic basis of inherited disease. New York: McGraw Hill, 1972: 1486.
263. Visakarpi JK, Hjelt, Lahikainen T, Ohman S. Ann Paediatr Fenn 1964; 10: 42.
264. Vilter KLW, Mueller JF, Glazer HS, Jerrold T, Abraham J, Thompson C, Hawkins VR. J Lab Clin Med 1953; 42: 335.
265. Victor M, Adams RD. Am J Clin Nutr 1956; 4: 346.
266. Bessey OA, Adam DJD, Hanson AE. Pediatrics 1957; 20: 33.
267. Scriver CR, Hutchinson JH. Pediatrics 1963; 31: 240.
268. Holtz P, Palm D. Pharmacol Rev 1964; 16: 113.
269. Stannus HS. Br Med J 1944; 2: 103, 140.
270. Osuntokun BO. Trans R Soc Trop Med Hyg 1971; 65: 454.
271. Scott HH. Ann Trop Med Parasitol 1918; 12: 109.
272. Fisher CM. Can Services Med J 1955; 11: 157.
273. Shaw H, Phillips PH. J Nutr 1941; 22: 345.
274. Zimmerman HM, Burack E. J Exp Med 1934; 59: 21.
275. Mann GV, Watson PL, McNally A, Goddard J. J Nutr 1952; 47: 225.
276. Greenfield JG, O'Flynn E. Lancet 1933; 2: 62.
277. Mayer RF. Arch. Neurol 1965; 13: 355.
278. Russell JSR, Batten FE, Collier J. Brain 1900; 23: 39.
279. Greenfield JG, Carmichael EA. Brain 1935; 58: 483.
280. Oxnard CE, Smith WT. Nature 1966; 210: 507.
281. Perdrau JR. J Pathol Bacteriol 1930; 32: 991.
282. Agamanolis DP, Victor M, Harris JW, Hines JD, Chester EM, Kark JA. J Neuropathol Exp Neurol 1978; 37: 273.
283. Torres I, Smith WT, Oxnard CE. Experientia 1969; 25: 273.
284. Amess JC, Burman JF, Rees GM, Nancekievill DJ, Moulin DL. Lancet 1978; 2: 339.
285. Scott JM, Wilson P, Dinn JJ, Weir DG. Lancet 1981; 2: 334.
286. Jacobson W, Gandy G. In: Behan PO, Rose FC, eds. Progress in neurological research. London: Pitman Medical, 1978; 211.
287. Small DH, Carnegie PR, Anderson R McD. Neurosci Lett 1981; 21: 287.
288. Evans HM, Bishop KS. Science 1922; 56: 650.
289. Pappenheimer AM. Proc Assoc Res Nerv Ment Dis 1941; 22: 85.
290. Adamstone FB. Arch Pathol 1941; 31: 613.
291. Muller DPR, Lloyd JK, Wolff OH. Lancet 1983; 1: 225.
292. Wichman A, Buchtal F, Pezeshkpour GH, Gregg RE. Neurology 1985; 35: 1279.
293. Geller A, Gilles F, Schwachman H. Neurology 1977; 27: 185.
294. Sung JH, Park SH, Mastri AR, Warwick WJ. J Neuropathol Exp Neurol 1980; 39: 584.
295. Harding AE, Muller DPR, Thomas PK, Willison HJ. Ann Neurol 1982; 12: 419.
296. Sung JH, Stadlan EM. J Neuropathol Exp Neurol 1966; 25: 341.
297. Rosenblum JL, Keating JP, Prensky Al, Nelson JS. N Engl J Med 1981; 304: 503.
298. Pappenheimer AM. Am J Pathol 1939; 16: 179.
299. Einarsen L, Ringsted A. Effects of chronic vitamin E deficiency on the nervous system and skeletal musculature of the rat. London: Oxford University Press, 1938.
300. Pentshew A, Schwarz K. Acta Neuropathol (Berl) 1962; 1: 313.
301. Machlin LJ, Filipski R, Nelson J, Horn LR, Prin MJ. Nutr 1977; 107: 1200.
302. Towfighi J. Acta Neuropathol 1981; 54: 261.
303. Nelson JS, Fitch CD, Fischer VW, Brown GO, Chou AC. J Neuropathol Exp Neurol 1981; 40: 166.
304. Lampert P, Blumberg JM, Pentschew A. J Neuropathol Exp Neurol 1964; 23: 60.
305. Schwatz K. Ann NY Acad Sci 1972; 203: 45.
306. Diplock AT, Lucy JA. FEBS Lett 1973; 29: 205.
307. Elias E, Muller D PR, Scott J. Lancet 1981; 2: 1319.

Liver disease and allied conditions

308. Editorial. Lancet 1984; 1: 489.
309. Read AE, Laidlaw J, Sherlock S. Lancet 1961; 1: 961.
310. Hoesslin C von, Alzheimer A. Z Neurol Psychiatrie 1912; 8: 183.
311. Waggoner RW, Malamud N. J Nerv Ment Dis 1942; 96: 410.
312. Lapham LW. Am J Path 1962; 41: 1.
313. Cavanagh JB, Kyu MH. J Neurol Sci 1971; 12: 241.
314. Victor M, Adams RD, Cole M. Medicine (Baltimore) 1965; 44: 345.
315. Liversedge L, Ranson MD. Lancet 1966; 1: 277.
316. Leigh AD, Card WI. J Neuropathol Exp Neurol 1949; 8: 338.
317. Hahn M, Massen O, Nencki M, Pawlow J. Arch Exp Path Pharmakol 1893; 32: 161.
318. Cavanagh JB. Res Publ Assoc Res Nerv Ment Dis 1974; 53: 13.
319. Zamora AJ, Cavanagh JB, Kyu MH. J Neurol Sci 1973; 18: 25.
320. Cavanagh JB, Kyu MH. J Neurol Sci 1971; 12: 241.
321. Cavanagh JB, Lewis PD, Blakemore WF, Kyu MH. J Neurol Sci 1972; 15: 13.
322. Bessman SP, Bradley JE. N Engl J Med 1955; 253: 1143.
323. Stahl J. Ann Intern Med 1963; 58: 117.
324. Norenberg MD. In: Federoff S, Herz L, eds. Advances in cell neurobiology. London: Academic Press, 1981; 2: 304.
325. Bruton CJ, Corsellis JAN, Russell A. Brain 1970; 93: 423.
326. Solitaire GB, Shih VE, Nelligan DJ, Dolan TF Jr. J Ment Defic Res 1969; 13: 153.
327. McMurray WC, Rathbon JC, Mohyuddin F, Koegler. Pediatrics 1963; 32: 347.
328. Walser M. In: Stanbury JB, Wyngaarden JB, Goldstein JL, Brown MS, eds. The metabolic basis of inherited disease, 5th edn. New York: McGraw-Hill, 1983.

329. Brain WR, Hunter D, Turnbull HM. Lancet 1929; 1:221.
330. Reye RDK, Mortgan G, Baral J. Lancet 1963; 2: 749.
331. Chu AB, Lata NS, Witsel N et al. Am J Dis Child 1983; 140: 1009.
332. Cullity GJ, Kakulas BA. Brain 1970; 93: 77.
333. Partin JS, McAdams AJ, Partin JC, Schubert WK. J Neuropathol Exp Neurol 1978; 37: 796.
334. De Vivo DC. Neurology 1978; 28: 105.
335. Walshe JM. Q J Med 1973; 42: 441.
336. Walshe JM. Br J Hosp Med 1970; 4: 91.
337. Evans GW, Dubois RS, Hambridge KM. Science 1973; 181: 1175.

Developmental, neonatal and paediatric neuropathology

INTRODUCTION

Disorders of the nervous system in the fetus, newborn infants and children may be the result of genetic factors or exogenous influences. The clinical features and patterns of pathology depend upon the type and severity of the insult sustained and the stage of fetal or childhood development at which the insult is applied to the nervous system. Thus damage to the brain or spinal cord in early fetal life may profoundly affect development of the nervous system and result in gross abnormalities and malformations. In such cases the fetus may be spontaneously aborted or may die soon after birth. Those children who survive with brain damage sustained in fetal life or in the perinatal period are often mentally retarded and may have focal neurological deficits. If the degree of damage is minor, intellectual and neurological development may be within normal limits.

DEVELOPMENT OF THE CENTRAL NERVOUS SYSTEM

The neural tube develops from ectoderm on the dorsal aspect of the embryo at 14 days of gestation and closes between 18 and 26 days.[1] As the tube closes, the neural crests form and their cells separate from the tube to develop mainly into dorsal root ganglia, autonomic ganglion cells, adrenal medulla, Schwann cells and melanocytes. By the 7th week of gestation the primitive cerebral hemispheres have developed. During the first 20 weeks of gestation, developing neurons and glia migrate from germinal sites around the cerebral ventricles and central canal of the spinal cord to form the future cerebral cortex, basal ganglia, brainstem nuclei and grey matter of the spinal cord. By the end of the first half of gestation, i.e. 20 weeks, the major neuronal groups have formed and the brain weighs approximately 60 g. At this time the cerebral hemispheres are almost completely smooth externally, and only the lateral fissures and calcarine fissures have started to form (Fig. 12.1). The meninges develop initially at 20–50 days from mesenchyme derived from several sources, including the neural crest.[2] It is by the ingrowth of vessels from the surrounding meninges that the brain becomes vascularised.

During the second half of gestation, more gyri and sulci form on the surface of the cerebral hemispheres (Fig. 12.1) and neuronal differentiation occurs. Thus by 39 or 40 weeks of gestation the opercula of the lateral fissure are just closing over the insula (Fig. 12.1). In late fetal life, the germinal layers of the cerebral hemispheres become restricted mainly to the subependymal plate regions at the superiolateral corners of the lateral ventricles (Fig. 12.2); by birth, only small groups of immature matrix cells remain in the subependymal layer. Development of the cerebellum occurs mainly in the second half of pregnancy, with Purkinje cells migrating outwards from the periventricular germinal layers and internal granular cells migrating inwards from the external granular layer on the surface of the cerebellar folia (see p. 326).

At birth the brain weighs approximately 400 g. Postnatal development of the brain is characterised by further differentiation and enlargement of neurons and by myelination of the white matter. Growth in thickness of the cerebral cortex continues until about the end of the second postnatal year; the external granular layer of the cerebellar cortex also persists into the second year. Myelination commences in the spinal cord and brainstem in the second half of fetal life but at birth there is still little myelin in the cerebral hemispheres. Because of the lack of myelin it is difficult to distinguish macroscopically the cortex from white matter in the brain of a newborn infant. Myelination begins in the internal capsules of the cerebral hemispheres soon after birth and in the rest of the hemisphere during the first few months of postnatal life. By the age of 6 years, myelination is nearly complete but it continues slowly into the second decade. Between birth and 6 months of postnatal life the brain weight nearly doubles[3] and by the age of 6 years it has reached 90% of the adult weight of 1200 g.

AETIOLOGY OF BRAIN DAMAGE IN THE FETUS AND IN CHILDHOOD

Malformations of the central nervous system are found in 3–4% of early spontaneous abortions[4] and in approximately 0·6% of births in Britain.[5]

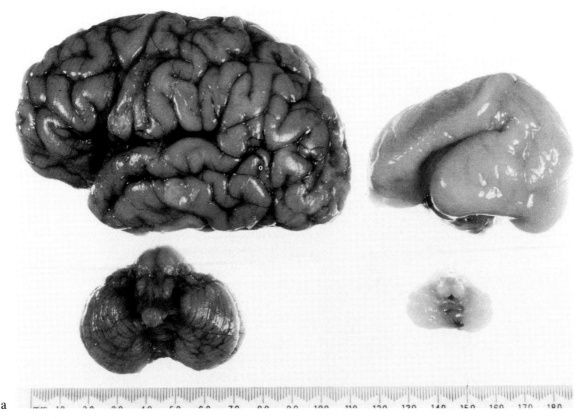

a

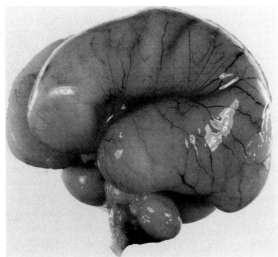

b

Fig. 12.1a, b (**a**) The brain of a 23-week fetus (right) shows development of the lateral fissure (the meninges have been removed). A newborn infant (39 weeks gestation) (left) has a much more complex gyral pattern and the anterior end of the lateral fissure has almost closed. (**b**) Fetal brain at 27 weeks gestation showing a well-marked lateral fissure and a central sulcus above it. Fine arterial branches are seen within the leptomeninges and radiating from the lateral fissure.

13–16% of pre-school children exhibit neuro-developmental disability, although major forms of disability such as severe mental retardation and cerebral palsy occur in less than 1% of children.[6]

Congenital malformations of the brain are present in 20–30% of mentally retarded patients.[7] Some of these brain disorders may be due to genetic abnormalities and thus carry a risk of recurrence in subsequent offspring.[8] Others are due to exogenous factors operating during preg-

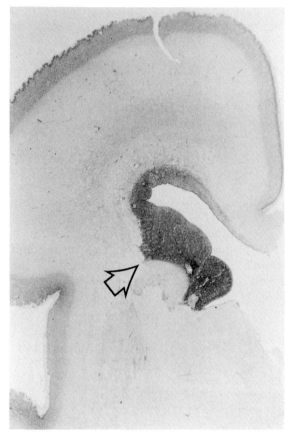

Fig. 12.2 Cerebral hemisphere of a 22-week fetus—histology. In this coronal section, the developing cerebral cortex is seen in the lateral fissure (bottom left) and over the superior surface of the hemisphere. The lateral ventricle is partly surrounded by a mass of cells forming the subependymal plate (arrow).
Haematoxylin-eosin × 5

nancy or at birth and there may be little or no risk of recurrence.[6] Pathological features of the brain observed at autopsy play a major rôle in deciding whether a disorder is due to genetic or non-genetic factors.

GENETIC DISORDERS

There are at least 1000 genetic disorders which affect the nervous system, some 500 of these resulting in microcephaly due to disorders of brain growth or due to destruction of brain tissue in fetal life.[8,9] Some of these disorders present in adult life, e.g. Huntington's disease (see p. 382). In many

disorders, the genetics are complex.[8] The main object of this account is not to give detailed descriptions of individual combinations of malformations, but to describe the patterns of pathology that occur so that a diagnosis can be made by consulting the relevant genetics literature.[8,9]

The factors involved in *malformation* and *maldevelopment* of the central nervous system are unknown in 60% of cases. In a further 20%, the malformations are due to the interaction of hereditary tendencies and non-genetic factors. Maldevelopment is due purely to genetic influences in only 8%. Some 12% of malformations are due to extrinsic factors affecting the mother and fetus. Thus, some malformations of the central nervous system carry a risk of recurrence, although many do not.[10] There is a genetic predisposition for neural tube defects in 60–70% of cases,[8] and agenesis of the corpus callosum may occur in a number of single gene mutations including X-linked recessive disorders.[8] X-linked hydrocephalus has been described.[11] Both megalencephaly and micrencephaly may have a genetic basis.[8] In some cases, malformations of the central nervous system form part of a complex multiple malformation.[12]

Another major group of genetic disorders includes *inborn errors of metabolism*, affecting amino acid, purine, pyrimidine, carbohydrate and trace metal metabolism.[13] These disorders show little specific histological abnormality in the brain. On the other hand, lysosomal disorders, which include lipidoses and leucodystrophies, frequently exhibit characteristic histochemical, histological and ultrastructural abnormalities in the brain (see p. 341).[14]

Phacomatoses are inherited disorders characterised by multiple malformations and tumours.[8] The most prominent of these are neurofibromatosis (von Recklinghausen's disease), tuberous sclerosis and von Hippel–Lindau disease (see p. 353).

CHROMOSOMAL DISORDERS

Chromosomal disorders may be diagnosed prenatally by karyotyping fetal lymphocytes[15] or chorionic villus samples.[16] Cytogenetic techniques or in-situ hybridisation methods using DNA probes are employed for such karyotyping.[17] Cytogenetic analyses of skin fibroblasts can be used for postnatal diagnosis. A number of different types of chromosome disorder are associated with mental retardation and abnormalities of the central nervous system.[18,19] They fall into several distinct patterns. *Trisomies* in chromosome group G (21–22) are associated with mongolism, whereas trisomies in group D (13–15) may be accompanied by multiple congenital abnormalities, including cyclopia, holoprosencephaly, and arhinencephaly. Trisomy E (chromosome 17–18) is associated with cerebellar malformations. Translocation of D/G or G/G is associated with mongolism with 46 chromosomes. *Deletions* entailing loss of part of one chromosome may be seen in conditions such as 'cri du chat' syndrome, in which there is deletion of the short arm of chromosome 5. Abnormalities of sex chromosomes, e.g. XXY-Klinefelter's syndrome or XO-Turner's syndrome, may occasionally be associated with central nervous system malformations. *Mosaicism* may also be found in patients with mental retardation, only a proportion of the cells being affected by the chromosomal abnormality. Apart from the gross disorders mentioned above, patients with chromosomal abnormalities may show microscopic abnormalities including heteropias in the cerebrum or cerebellum (see p. 319).

Down's syndrome (mongolism)

Down's syndrome has an incidence of 1·4 per 1000 live births and accounts for 30% of all cases of developmental abnormality due to chromosomal anomalies.[19] Trisomy G with an additional chromosome 21 occurs in 90% of cases of Down's syndrome and is associated with advanced maternal age. 2–4% of Down's syndrome cases have translocation of D/G or G/G and this occurs in children of younger mothers. Mosaicism occurs in 2–3% of cases of Down's syndrome.[20]

Trisomy 21 is associated with growth deficiency, abnormal morphogenesis and mental retardation, together with an increased risk of auto-immune disease, diabetes mellitus, thyroiditis and malignant disease.[21] The brain in Down's syndrome is usually reduced in weight to about 1000 g in the adult. It is globular in shape, and the gyri show a paucity of secondary gyrus formation. The insula may be visible on the surface of the brain through an incompletely closed lateral fissure, and the superior temporal gyrus may be narrow. A number of microscopic abnormalities may be seen,[19] including irregular grouping of neurons and relatively acellular adjoining areas, but these changes are not specific for Down's syndrome. Patients with Down's syndrome over the age of 40 years show changes of Alzheimer's disease with neurofibrillary tangles and senile plaques[22] (see p. 374); calcification of the basal ganglia may also be present.[23]

The gene coding for the β-amyloid peptide in senile plaques in both Alzheimer's disease and Down's syndrome has been localised to the proximal portion of the q-arm of chromosome 21.[24,25]

EXOGENOUS FACTORS

When damage to the brain occurs early in fetal life, gross malformations may result and it is often difficult to determine whether the damage is due to genetic factors or a result of an exogenous insult. A variety of exogenous factors are known to affect the fetal brain, particularly in the early weeks and months of gestation, and these are discussed below. Much of the damage occurring in later fetal life is due to ischaemia.

Irradiation

Microcephaly (small head) with *micrencephaly* (small brain) and abnormalities of the eyes have been described following deep X-ray therapy to the maternal pelvis during the first 4 months of pregnancy.[26] Similar changes after irradiation from nuclear fission explosions have also been described.[27] Experimental X-irradiation of fetal mice has shown that the pattern of abnormality at birth depends upon the stage of development at which the irradiation is applied;[28] a similar relation may hold in man. Fetuses irradiated on day 9 of the 21-day rat pregnancy, before somites have appeared, developed severe neural tube defects and anencephaly. Irradiation on day 10 (6 somites)

produced eye and optic tract defects whereas irradiation on day 11 (20 somites) produced a ven-
triculocele and defects in the brain, spine, eyes,
viscera and skeleton. Various forebrain abnormalities were produced by irradiation between day
13 and birth at day 21. Cerebellar defects were produced by irradiation in the last third of fetal life
and shortly after birth.

Infections (see also p. 337–340)

Viral, bacterial and protozoal infections of the
fetus may severely damage the brain. Maternal
rubella infection during the first 4 months of pregnancy produces a variety of defects, including
micrencephaly, cardiac defects, deafness and
cataracts. Hydrocephalus, absence of the corpus
callosum and mongolism are among others that
have been described.[29] The incidence of stillbirths,
neonatal deaths and malformation has been
reported as 17% in the children of mothers
infected with rubella during the first 4 months of
pregnancy compared with 6% in controls.[30]
Infections by other viruses, e.g. *cytomegalovirus*,[31]
cause chronic encephalitis, brain tissue destruction and malformations in the fetus, resulting in
microcephaly. *Toxoplasma* infection of the
developing nervous system causes a granulomatous meningoencephalitis, hydrocephalus and
widespread calcifications with thickening of the
meninges.[32] *Syphilitic* infection of the nervous
system causes meningoencephalitis. *Staphylococcal* infections are a rare cause of congenital
hydrocephalus.[33]

Toxins and drugs

A number of drugs have been implicated in the
production of fetal abnormalities of the central
nervous system. Reduction in fetal brain weight is
seen following heavy maternal smoking and
alcohol consumption during pregnancy, and this
abnormality is accompanied by various other
abnormalities throughout the body.[34]

Hypoxia

Hypoxia and ischaemia are major causes of brain
damage in the second half of pregnancy and in the
perinatal period (see p. 333).

POST-MORTEM EXAMINATION OF THE FETUS AND NEWBORN INFANT

Aborted fetuses, stillbirths, and children dying in
infancy or later in childhood should be examined
in a systematic manner so that the maximum
information will be available for assessing the
nature of the lesion, its aetiology and any possible
genetic cause.

Careful examination of the full clinical notes is
essential before starting the examination of a fetus
or newborn infant. Accurate descriptions and
photographs are invaluable for recording abnormalities in fetuses and stillbirths.[35]

Karyotyping can be performed even on stillbirths.[35] Some 50% of spontaneous abortuses in
the first and second trimesters have chromosomal
abnormalities.[36]

Tissue for biochemical analysis should be taken
from organs, including the brain, and stored at
−40°C if an enzyme defect is suspected.[37,38]
Fibroblast culture may also be required as may
material for viral and bacterial culture.

The tissues of the central nervous system are
particularly easily disrupted during pathological
examination in the fetus, especially in the 17–20
week fetuses aborted when CNS malformations,
including neural tube defects, are detected by
ultrasound. If the occipital bone is removed at
post-mortem in these cases, the spinal cord can be
exposed in the midline and the brain and cord can
be fixed in 20% formalin for 48 hours before
removing the hardened tissue. The brain and
spinal cord can be removed in continuity and thus
Arnold–Chiari and Dandy–Walker malformations
are well demonstrated.

Removal of the brain from a newborn infant is
also a very delicate task. The newborn brain is still
very soft and there is little myelination in the cerebral hemispheres. In these cases the brain should
be removed carefully from the skull, either by
making a cruciate incision through the fontanelles
and major sutures or by initial removal of the
occipital bone and exposure of the spinal cord. A
particularly delicate brain may be removed under
formalin or preferably hypertonic (saturated)
saline so that it is allowed to float from the skull.
Following fixation in buffered formalin for 2 to 3
weeks, the brain should be hardened in 70%

alcohol before cutting unless such treatment will interfere with histochemical investigations. The weight and the external appearance of the brain are together a good guide to the age of a premature infant (Fig. 12.1).[39]

Blocks for histological sections should be taken in such a way that they retain anatomical landmarks. They are best embedded in paraffin using a prolonged 12-day dehydration schedule. Much of the cellular detail can be observed in haematoxylin and eosin stained sections[40] but astrocyte stains, e.g. Holzer, or immunoperoxidase preparations for glial fibrillary acidic protein (GFAP), may be required to detect brain tissue damage. The Nissl stain for neurons is useful for identifying abnormalities of neuronal distribution and features such as polymicrogyria (Fig. 12.8).[40] In older children, a combined myelin and neuron stain (Klüver–Barrera) is valuable for detecting focal histological damage.[41]

PATTERNS OF CENTRAL NERVOUS SYSTEM DAMAGE IN THE FETUS AND NEWBORN INFANT

The brain or spinal cord may be damaged in early or late fetal life. In general, damage occurring early in fetal life results in gross abnormalities of the brain, and the affected fetus may be aborted or the child may die soon after birth. If the damage is less severe the infant may appear to be normal at birth, and neurological deficits become evident in childhood or even in adult life. To some extent, the pathological features in the brain can be related to the time in fetal life at which the insult occurred.

EARLY GESTATION: THE FIRST 20 WEEKS

It is during the first half of pregnancy that much of the cell proliferation in the brain occurs; neurons migrate to their future adult positions and the major structures form in the cerebral hemispheres, brainstem and cerebellum. Damage to the brain during this period may result in very gross abnormality of the anatomy and histology of the central nervous system.

Neural tube defects (dysraphic malformations)

The neural tube closes between 18 and 26 days of gestation.[1] Although, in general, the caudal portion closes last, the extreme caudal part of the tube is formed by 'hollowing out' rather than 'rolling up'. Gross abnormality of the formation of the neural tube at the cranial end results in *anencephaly*, whereas abnormalities of the neural tube in the caudal region give rise to lesions ranging from extensive *spina bifida*, and *meningomyelocele*, to the minor defect of *spina bifida occulta*.

The incidence of neural tube defects differs from one geographical area to another. They are particularly common in Ireland and relatively uncommon in Africa and in Japan.[8] Family studies suggest that there is a combination of genetic factors and environmental forces in the causation of neural tube defects. Prenatal diagnosis of a neural tube defect is suspected if there is a high level of α-fetoprotein in the mother's serum. The diagnosis can be confirmed by high α-fetoprotein levels and the presence of an abnormal acetylcholinesterase in the amniotic fluid at 12–16 weeks gestation.[42] Careful external examination of therapeutically aborted fetuses may reveal the neural tube defect, but well-aligned anterior–posterior X-rays of the spine may be necessary to exclude minor degrees of spina bifida. In the more advanced stages of pregnancy, ultrasound may reveal neural tube defects, especially anencephaly.

Anencephaly

Infants born with anencephaly rarely survive more than a few hours. The head is flattened from above and the vault of the skull and brain are replaced by a dark red soft mass of tissue which histologically consists of vascular structures, glial nodules and choroid plexus.[19] The anterior lobe of the pituitary and the trigeminal nerves may be present but the hypothalamus is usually absent. Spina bifida is present in 14–17% of cases of anencephaly, and other abnormalities may include hypoplastic adrenals.[43] The eyes are prominent and almost frog-like in fetuses with anencephaly.

Anencephaly is the most striking malformation of the human fetus and it is associated with polyhydramnios. Incidences vary from 1–6 per 1000 live births in Wales to 0·5–2 per 1000 live births in the USA.[44] Anencephaly may be detected by ultrasound from the 12th week of pregnancy or from high α-fetoprotein levels and an abnormal acetylcholinesterase in the amniotic fluid.[42]

Spina bifida, meningomyelocele and meningocele

A range of abnormalities may be associated with neural tube defects in the spine. In the most severe form of dysraphism, there is a complete failure of fusion of the vertebral spines which extends into the cranial region (*craniorachischisis*). Neural tissue of the spinal cord is exposed throughout the length of the back, presenting a soft jelly-like dark red mass similar in consistency to the tissue on the heads of anencephalics.

Meningomyeloceles are pouch-like structures most commonly seen in the lumbar region but also occurring at other levels (Fig. 12.3). They are covered with a thin membrane or intact skin and contain a clear fluid. There is underlying spina bifida and the spinal cord is often flattened and attached to the deep surface of the meningomyelocele sac.

Children born with meningomyeloceles frequently have gross denervation of the leg musculature and sphincter problems due to the disruption of the lower spinal cord and the cauda equina.[45] Infection entering through a meningomyelocele may cause meningitis. Surgical excision of meningomyelocele sacs after birth, and repair of the defect, often resulted in the extirpation of neural tissue. Such neural tissue is best demonstrated in sections stained with haematoxylin and van Gieson's technique, which highlights the pale yellow spinal cord tissue against the red collagen of the dermis and subcutaneous tissue. There is frequently a collection of dilated blood vessels in the subepidermal region.

Meningoceles are formed by the herniation of dura and arachnoid through a spina bifida defect. The spinal cord may be in the correct position and unaffected. In some cases, the neural tube defect is

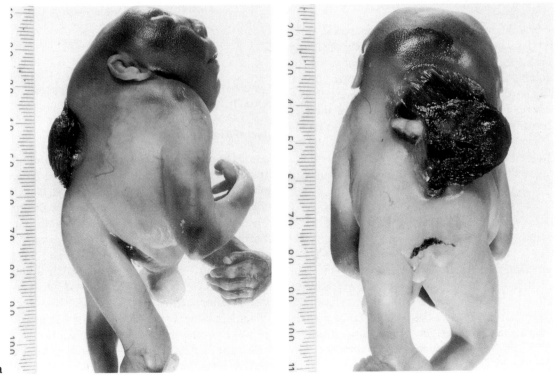

a   b

Fig. 12.3a, b Spina bifida: meningomyelocele and occipital encephalocele in an 18-week fetus.

associated merely with a sinus connecting the spinal canal with the epidermis and partly lined by arachnoid cells.

Hydrocephalus is frequently associated with spina bifida and is most frequently due to the Arnold–Chiari *malformations* (Chiari type II malformation—see below). Other spinal cord malformations may be associated with meningomyeloceles or may be independent of this lesion. They include *hydromyelia* with dilatation of the central canal of the cord, *diastematomyelia* with a double spinal cord in the same dural sac, and *diplomyelia* in which the cord is divided into two, each with its separate meningeal sac and often a bony spur separating the two cords.[19] *Lipomas* may occur at the lower end of the spinal cord, and they are usually associated with spina bifida.[46] They may cause tethering of the roots in the cauda

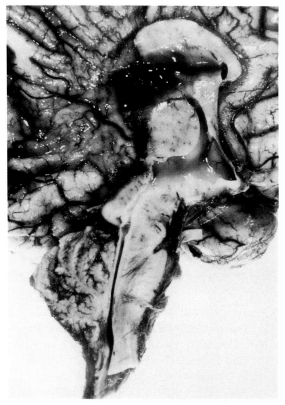

Fig. 12.4 Arnold–Chiari malformation. Sagittal section through the brain showing S-shaped malformation of the brainstem and prolongation of the cerebellar vermis (bottom left). The fourth ventricle is a slit-like cavity leading to the aqueduct (centre) and the third ventricle. There is gross hydrocephalus and a hypoplastic corpus callosum (top).

equina, with bladder paresis and back pain in infancy, childhood or early adulthood. Surgical removal of such lipomas may relieve some of the neurological symptoms.

Arnold–Chiari malformations

There are a number of different malformations under this heading (Chiari's classification).[19] *Chiari type I* malformation is characterised by ectopia of the cerebellar tonsils which may herniate through the foramen magnum and be associated with arachnoiditis and thickening of the leptomeninges. In such cases, *syringomyelia* of the spinal cord may result. *Chiari type II* malformation is the Arnold–Chiari malformation which is associated with *meningomyelocele*. There is elongation of the medulla, with or without an S-shaped deformity, and prolongation and herniation of the cerebellar vermis into the foramen magnum (Fig. 12.4). *Hydrocephalus* develops, especially after closure of the meningomyelocele; the cause of the hydrocephalus is unclear but it may be due to obstruction of the foramina draining CSF from the fourth ventricle. *Chiari type III* malformation is cervical spina bifida in which the cerebellum is herniated through the foramen magnum and forms part of a myelocerebellomeningocele. *Chiari type IV* malformation exhibits cerebellar hypoplasia.

Abnormalities of telencephalic (cerebral) vesicle formation

The cerebral hemispheres (prosencephalon) develop from vesicles arising in the lateral wall of the anterior portion of the neural tube. Development of this part of the brain is thought to be associated with pre-chordal mesoderm which normally migrates into the area anterior to the notochord during the third week of embryonic development.[7] Abnormalities of cerebral vesicle formation are frequently associated with facial abnormalities. In the most severe form there is *cyclopia* with one central eye in the forehead and gross abnormalities of the nose and mouth; the forebrain in these cases may be represented by a globular structure with a single ventricle and broad abnormal gyri (holoprosencephaly).[19]

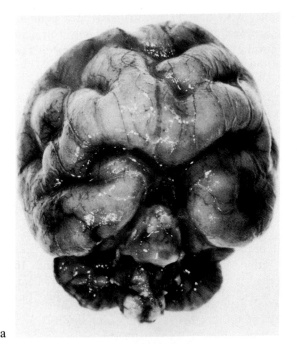

a

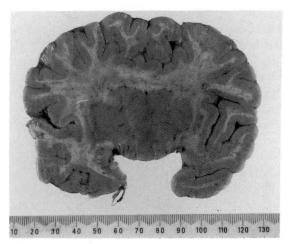

Fig. 12.6 Sporadic holoprosencephaly—7-year-old boy. Coronal section through the cerebrum shows fusion of the central grey matter and lack of an interhemispheric fissure.

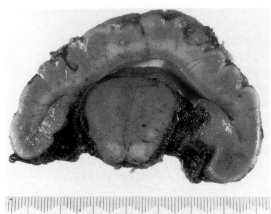

b

Fig. 12.5a, b Alobar holoprosencephaly—newborn infant. (**a**) The brain viewed from the front shows failure of separation of the cerebral hemispheres, with no sagittal fissure and a simplified gyral pattern. (**b**) Coronal section through the posterior aspects of the cerebrum showing gross abnormality with a single ventricle and failure of separation of the cerebral hemispheres.

The name *arhinencephaly* has been applied to this group of abnormalities of forebrain development, as absence of one or both olfactory bulbs is a constant feature. However, the group comprises a wide range of abnormality, with absence of the olfactory bulbs at one end of the spectrum and

holoprosencephaly at the other. In *alobar holo-prosencephaly* (Fig. 12.5), the brain is small and globular, with fusion of the cerebral hemispheres and often a single ventricle and broad abnormal gyri on the surface. In some cases the posterior aspect of the brain shows separation of the cerebral hemispheres. Widespread abnormalities may also be seen throughout the brainstem. Chromosomal abnormalities may be present, e.g. trisomy 13. Some cases are sporadic and some affected patients live for several years (Fig. 12.6). Holopros-encephaly may be detected during prenatal ultrasound examination, which shows the small size of the head (microcephaly) and the single ventricle.

Abnormalities of commissures and midline structures

The corpus callosum develops as a thickening of the lamina terminalis in the midline which starts to extend caudally at 13–14 weeks of gestation;[1] the fornix also extends backwards with the corpus callosum. *Agenesis of the corpus callosum* may be part of holoprosencephaly (Fig. 12.5) or it may be an isolated abnormality, either as complete absence or partial absence. Various other familial and sporadic abnormalities of midline structures have been described which may be associated with neurological defects or mental retardation.[19]

Micrencephaly and megalencephaly

Microcephaly (small head) is seen whenever the brain is reduced in size, either due to severe malformation or due to a destructive lesion of the brain. In some cases the brain itself shows no particularly gross abnormality but is just small; it may appear to be almost perfectly formed[40] and merits the term *micrencephaly*. Such symmetrical failure of growth of the brain may result from exogenous influences such as X-irradiation causing destruction and permanent depletion of neurons during development. Histologically, micrencephalic brains may show normal columns of neurons in the cortex, but the number of neurons is drastically reduced. In many cases the cause of micrencephaly is unknown. Mental retardation is associated not only with micrencephaly but also with *megalencephaly*, in which the brain may weigh 2000 g or more, and again may seem perfectly formed. Some cases show histological abnormalities. *Primary megalencephaly* may be an isolated finding or may be associated with achrondroplasia and endocrine disorders.[19] *Secondary megalencephaly* may be seen particularly in the lipidoses (see p. 341) in which the brain has an increased bulk due to the storage of abnormal amounts of lipid.

Abnormalities of neuronal migration—heterotopias and pachygyria

Centrifugal migration of neurons to the cerebral cortex occurs in two major waves during the first half of pregnancy. The first wave is at 8–10 weeks gestation and the second between 10 and 16 weeks.[1] In cases of cerebral *ectopia* or *heterotopia*, the cerebral cortex is usually well formed but islands of grey matter are found—either around

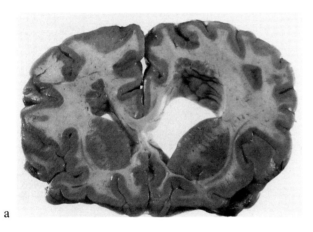
a

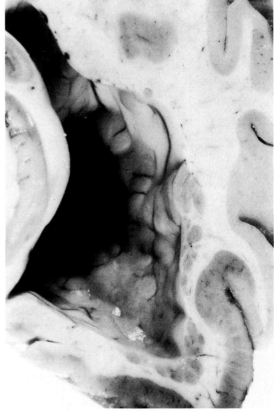
b

Fig. 12.7a, b Cerebral ectopias in an epileptic mentally retarded 26-year-old man. (**a**) Coronal section through the cerebral hemispheres showing ectopic grey matter in the roofs of both lateral ventricles; the right lateral ventricle is dilated. (**b**) Close-up view of ectopic grey matter in the lateral wall of the ventricle, in the right occipital lobe; the ectopias form raised nodules in the lining of the ventricle.

the ventricle or within the subcortical white matter (Fig. 12.7). Such ectopias are thought to be due to disruption of the second wave of neuronal migration. Isolated neurons in the white matter are a common finding in infants and in some adults but they appear to have little pathological significance. Cerebral ectopia and heterotopia may be associated with mental retardation and may form part of Zellweger's syndrome[47] and other multiple malformations. Heterotopic foci in the cerebellum (see p. 327) are much more common than cerebral heterotopias. In some cases heterotopias of the cerebellum are associated with chromosomal abnormalities.

Severe abnormalities of neuronal migration may result in *agyria*, in which the gyri do not form at all, or *pachygyria*, in which there are few but very wide gyri on the surface of the cerebral hemispheres. The term *lissencephaly* is synonymous with agyria and is sometimes applied to pachygyria also; it describes the smooth outer surface of the cerebral hemispheres in the absence of gyri. Histologically, the agyric and pachygyric cerebral hemisphere shows an increased thickness of cortical grey matter, often with cortical heterotopias near the ventricular wall. Agyria and pachygyria may be associated with multiple abnormalities in other organs. Their exact causes are unknown. They occur in genetic and metabolic disorders[9] and it seems likely that they are due to disruption of the waves of neuronal migration during the first 16 weeks of gestation.

Polymicrogyria

In polymicrogyria there is an increase in the number of gyri but the gyri themselves are very small. Such an appearance may be seen macro-

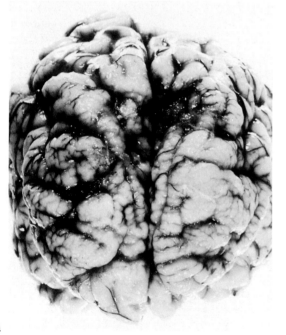

a

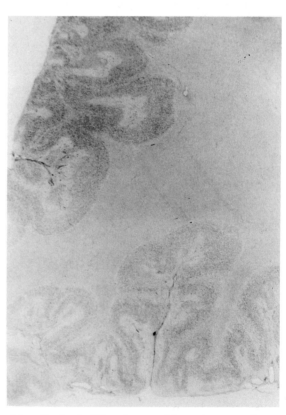

b

Fig. 12.8a, b Polymicrogyria. (**a**) The cerebral hemispheres viewed from the front. Although some of the gyri appear to be normal, the small intricate folds of polymicrogyria are seen on the surface, particularly in the centre on the medial aspects of both hemispheres and on the lateral aspects. (**b**) Histology of polymicrogyria. The cortical layers of neurons are thrown into folds but only two true sulci are present (centre left and centre bottom).
(**b**) Nissl ×5

scopically involving focal areas or wide regions on the surface of the cerebral hemispheres (Fig. 12.8). More often, the appearance of poly-microgyria is detected histologically in areas of macroscopically normal or pachygyric cerebral cortex. A distinctive appearance is seen histo-logically in which the cortical ribbon is thrown into multiple small irregular folds which are not separated by sulci (Fig. 12.8). Although abnormal, the cortical ribbon contains neurons and, in most cases, shows no scarring or cavitation although calcification may be present. Such an appearance must be distinguished from *polygyria*, with many small, true gyri. *Ulegyria* may also be confused with polymicrogyria. However, ulegyria is the result of hypoxic damage to the cortex, usually occurring during the second half of preg-nancy or in the perinatal period and causing infarc-tion and cavitation, particularly in the depths of the sulci, and consequent shrinkage of the gyri (see p. 333).

The exact cause of polymicrogyria is not clear. In some cases it may be due to *disturbance of cell migration* before the third and fourth fetal month, and it may be associated with other evidence of disordered neuronal migration, e.g. Zellweger's syndrome.[47] Polymicrogyria may also be due to *selective destruction* of neurons during the phase of gyrus formation in the second half of pregnancy and is commonly seen in association with poren-cephalic cysts (see below).

Cerebellar polymicrogyria is uncommon and may be associated with other cerebral malformations; it is recognised most easily in histological sections as multiple very small folia.

SECOND HALF OF GESTATION: 20 TO 40 WEEKS

By 20 weeks of gestation, the cerebral hemispheres are recognisable but they are smooth, and although the lateral fissure has formed there are virtually no gyri or sulci. Over the next 20 weeks, the gyri and sulci form, the more prominent sulci appearing first (Fig. 12.1).[39] The brainstem has formed by 20 weeks but the cerebellum is still relatively small and much of the neuronal migration in the cere-bellum occurs during the second half of gestation.

Destructive lesions of the cerebral hemispheres are the major lesions that occur in the brain in the second half of gestation. Such lesions are due to a variety of causes, especially *ischaemia* and *infec-tion*. The mother may suffer asphyxia, cardiac failure or trauma, or severe systemic disease resulting in ischaemic lesions in the fetal brain.[48] Similar lesions may be due to fetal disorders. Emboli from placental veins may occlude cerebral vessels,[49] and ischaemic lesions may be seen in twins. Placental insufficiency has also been impli-cated as a cause of fetal cerebral infarction.

The appearance of the lesion depends upon the time which has elapsed between the ischaemic episode and examination of the brain.[48] Long-standing ischaemic lesions involving the whole hemisphere may leave merely a thin-walled sac (*hydranencephaly*). Less extensive longstanding lesions may result in localised *porencephalic cysts*. Areas of brain softening (*encephalomalacia*) are seen if the infarct is of recent origin. The majority of these lesions can be detected by ultrasound in the fetus;[48] it is thus possible to separate the lesions occurring before birth from those due to birth hypoxia.

Damage to the cerebellum during late fetal life may result in abnormalities of cell migration, cere-bellar ectopia or gross abnormalities of the cere-bellum.[50]

Porencephaly

Porencephalic cysts form in the cerebral hemi-spheres and are often bilateral (*schizencephaly*).[51] Such cysts are seen postnatally in severely mentally retarded children with neurological deficits who fail to speak or walk; epilepsy is common and there is a reduced life expectancy. In some cases fluid accumulates progressively in the cyst and gives rise to raised intracranial pressure. Examination of the brain (Fig. 12.9), reveals circumscribed defects, often in the precentral or postcentral gyri and involving the insula. The cysts are smooth-walled, confluent with the ventricles (Fig. 12.9) and covered by an outer membrane composed of glia and meninges. *Poly-microgyria* is frequently seen around these cysts, but also affects gyri at a distance from them. The presence of polymicrogyria suggests that the

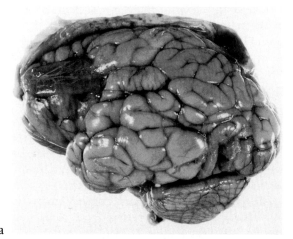

a

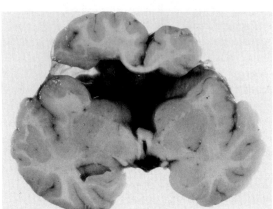

b

Fig. 12.9a, b Porencephaly in a 6-year-old boy. (**a**) Lateral surface of the brain showing a thin-walled porencephalic cyst anteriorly in the frontal lobe. Polymicrogyria is seen on the surface of a gyrus extending back from the posterior limit of the cyst. (**b**) Coronal section through the frontal lobes of (**a**) showing bilateral porencephalic cysts, confluent with the lateral ventricles and covered by a translucent membrane (seen on the left).

damage occurred before or during the fifth month of gestation, prior to the onset of gyrus formation. The cerebellum and brainstem are not usually primarily affected by porencephaly.

Hydranencephaly

This condition should not be confused with hydrocephalus, for, although the head may be enlarged at birth and the ventricles may be distended, hydranencephaly is due to massive destruction of the cerebral hemispheres, probably by vascular occlusion or as a result of

abnormalities of the main branches of the cerebral arteries. One or both cerebral hemispheres remain as thin-walled sacs but the basal grey matter nuclei may be partly or completely preserved (Fig. 12.10).

Histologically, the walls of hydranencephalic cysts are composed of glial tissue and meninges, often with calcification. Any residual cortex may show *polymicrogyria*. Hydranencephaly probably results from ischaemic damage in the fifth month of gestation, usually involving areas of brain supplied by the anterior and middle cerebral

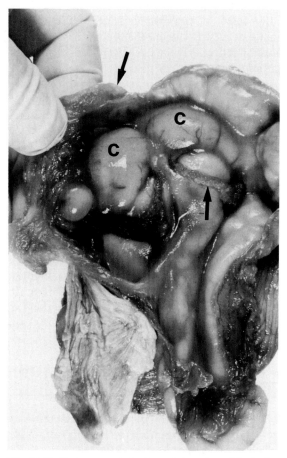

Fig. 12.10 Hydranencephaly. A confusing view of the brain seen from above. All that remains of the superior aspects of the cerebral hemispheres is the thin-walled cyst (upper arrow) which has been reflected to reveal the bulbous caudate nuclei (c) in the basal regions of the brain. The foramina of Monro and a piece of choroid plexus (lower arrow) can also be seen. Some cerebellar folia are seen projecting from the right-hand side of the specimen.

arteries. The cerebellum and brainstem are usually normal but may contain small cystic infarcts. Dating of the episode causing hydranencephaly may be possible from examination of the spinal cord. Agenesis of the lateral corticospinal tracts is seen if damage occurred before the fifth month of gestation; relatively small tracts remain if damage occurred in the 5th–6th month of gestation; normal configuration of the corticospinal tracts is seen if damage occurred later, but there is loss of axons and no myelination within the tracts.[52]

An intermediate stage between the smaller lesions of porencephaly and the very large destructive lesions of hydranencephaly may be seen, large symmetrical hemispheric cysts causing the appearance of 'basket brain'.[53]

Destructive lesions occurring in the brain of infants near term or at birth produce a multilocular cystic encephalopathy and ulegyria (see p. 333).

Hydrocephalus

Pathology

Hydrocephalus results from obstruction to the flow and absorption of cerebrospinal fluid or, more rarely, is associated with excessive production of cerebrospinal fluid by a choroid plexus papilloma.

In children, hydrocephalus may develop before or after birth, largely depending upon the primary cause. Untreated, hydrocephalus causes enlargement of the head and delay in fusion of the sutures of the skull. In severe cases, there is gross thinning of the cranial bones.

At post mortem, the brain may be very large (Fig. 12.11) and the superior and lateral walls of the lateral ventricles may be so thin that they are translucent. Rupture of the ventricles and collapse of the brain may occur during removal from the skull. Meningeal thickening may be seen over the base of the brain in children who develop hydrocephalus secondary to meningitis, or there may be malformations within the brain that are associated with the hydrocephalus. Often the gyri over the surface of the brain are flattened. Coronal slices of the hydrocephalic brain reveal large lateral and third ventricles with dilatation of the temporal horns of the lateral ventricles (Fig. 12.11). The

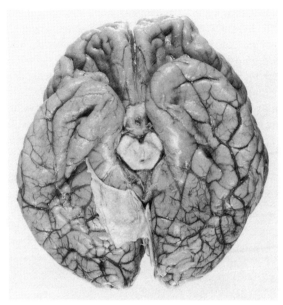

a

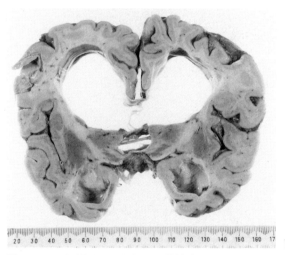

b

Fig. 12.11a, b Hydrocephalus. (**a**) This hydrocephalic brain has a maximum bihemispheric width of 18·4 cm (normal adult is 12 cm). (**b**) Coronal section through a hydrocephalic brain showing gross dilatation of the lateral and third ventricles with thinning of the corpus callosum and periventricular white matter.

periventricular white matter may be very thin although the basal ganglia are often well preserved. In extreme cases, the gyral pattern is destroyed and the cortex and white matter of the cerebral mantle may be compressed to a thin rim of tissue, less than 1 cm in thickness. The septum pellucidum is often ruptured and the basal regions of the brain flattened.

Histologically, the appearances depend upon the stage of hydrocephalus. In the acute stages of ventricular dilatation, there is cerebrospinal fluid oedema of the periventricular white matter. This is particularly well seen by electron microscopy (Fig. 12.12)[54] although it can be detected by light microscopy.[55,56] Such oedema may also be obvious on CT scan in the acute stages of hydrocephalus (Fig. 3.10, p. 72). During the acute stage of white matter oedema there is axonal destruction. In untreated hydrocephalus, the oedematous area gradually becomes gliotic[54–57] and in longstanding cases there is a rim of gliotic tissue around the ventricles. Despite the damage to the periventricular white matter, the central grey matter around the ventricles is relatively well preserved.

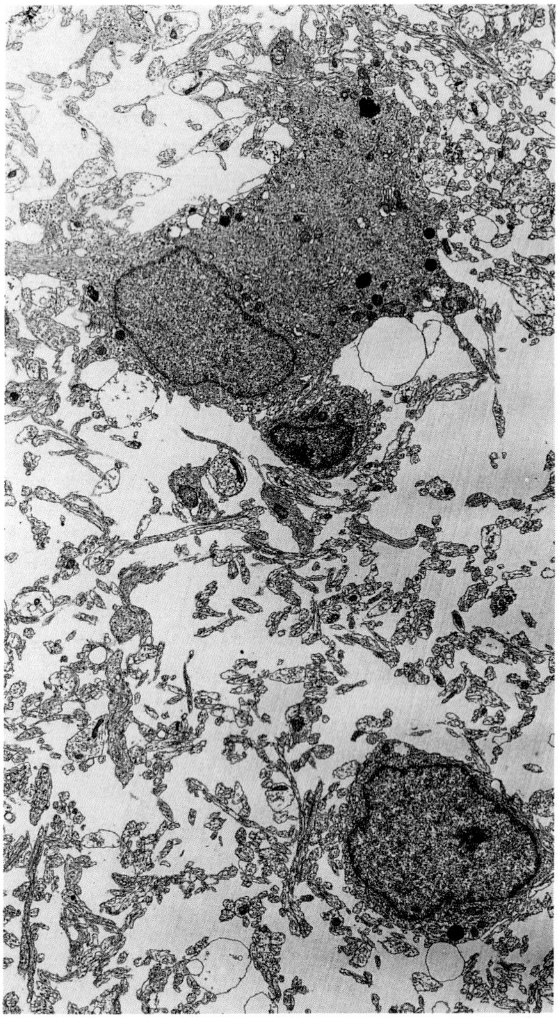

Causes

Stenosis of the aqueduct of Sylvius may occur before or after birth, either as a rare X-linked disorder[11] or associated with other malformations, most often with the Arnold–Chiari malformation. The cause of isolated aqueductal stenosis is unclear. It is improbable that true atresia of the aqueduct occurs. Acquired aqueductal stenosis may be due to damage to the ependymal lining and periaqueductal tissue. Experimental studies have shown that certain viral infections[58] cause destruction of ependyma in fetal and newborn animals and this results in aqueductal stenosis and hydrocephalus. A stenosed aqueduct in a hydrocephalic baby may not be visible macroscopically when the fixed brain is cut at post mortem. Microscopically it may appear to be broken into several channels, giving the impression of 'forking' of the aqueduct.

Acquired stenosis of the aqueduct may also be associated with perinatal intraventricular haemorrhage. Blood and macrophages arising from periventricular infarcts associated with intraventricular haemorrhage may obstruct the aqueduct and cause subsequent gliosis in the periaqueductal region. Brainstem astrocytomas, vascular malformations and tumours in the region of the pineal (see p. 507) may also cause compression and stenosis of the aqueduct.

Obstruction of the foramina of Luschka and Magendie may occur following cerebellar haemorrhage. Obliteration of the subarachnoid space by fibrosis may follow organisation of a subarachnoid haemorrhage or the inflammatory exudate in meningitis. A few cases of complete absence of the arachnoid granulations have been reported but, although often quoted as a cause of hydrocephalus, blockage of the arachnoid granulations by subarachnoid haemorrhage and meningitis is difficult to prove.[59] *Venous sinus thrombosis* or raised cerebrospinal fluid protein

Fig. 12.12 Acute hydrocephalus. An electron micrograph of the periventricular occipital white matter from a 29-day-old child. There is extensive oedema with clear fluid separating the axonal processes and glial cells. Reactive astrocyte (top). Electron micrograph × 3000
Reproduced by permission of the editor from: Weller RO, Shulman K. J Neurosurg 1972; 36: 255 (Fig. 1).

may also result in hydrocephalus. Ventricular dilatation may accompany dysplasia of the cranial bones, as in achondroplasia.

The *Dandy–Walker malformation* is a distinctive abnormality and a cause of hydrocephalus early in life. It is characterised by the triad of malformed vermis, a cystic roof to the expanded fourth ventricle and an elevated tentorium cerebelli. If these features alone are present, the individual may lead a normal life; it is the frequent association of other developmental brain defects which causes problems.[60] At post mortem, the posterior fossa is enlarged, a thin-walled cyst expanding out of the fourth ventricle through the midline of the cerebellum (Fig. 12.13). The malformation is thought to originate before the third fetal month, causing developmental arrest of the hindbrain and persistence of the membranous area of the roof of the fourth ventricle.[61,62] Associated defects may include agenesis of the corpus callosum, aqueduct stenosis and hydrocephalus.

Effects of hydrocephalus

In young infants, hydrocephalus results in head enlargement and, unless the ventricles are drained by the insertion of a shunt, the child may suffer irreparable brain damage and be mentally retarded.[54,55,63] In some cases, the hydrocephalus becomes arrested before significant brain damage has occurred. Complications of the shunting procedure include infection of the shunt and ventriculitis. Further, there is the need for repeated revisions of the shunt as the child grows. Children under 2 months of age have little myelin in the white matter and appear to tolerate gross ventricular dilatation and thinning of the cerebral mantle better than children over 6 months of age with partly myelinated white matter.[54] Although the ventricles may be reduced in size following shunting in older children, the periventricular white matter may be oedematous and show cavitation and spongy change.[54]

Syringomyelia and syringobulbia

In *syringomyelia*, an elongated cavity (syrinx) forms in the spinal cord, usually in the cervical region. The syrinx causes enlargement of the cord and is visible on computerised tomographic (CT) scan or magnetic resonance imaging (MRI) as a fluid-containing cyst. Usually the syrinx collapses on removal of the spinal cord at post mortem and is seen only as a slit-like cavity extending from the centre of the cord along one dorsal horn of grey matter.[40] Histologically, the syrinx is surrounded by a layer of gliosis and there may be some destruction of anterior horn cells. Clinically, patients develop signs and symptoms of syringomyelia in adult life. There is wasting of the small muscles of the hands and of the arms due to local destruction of anterior horn cells. Loss of pain and temperature sensation occurs[64] due to damage to nerve fibres as they cross the cord into the lateral spinothalamic tracts at the level of the syrinx. The patient may suffer burns on his fingers and develop severe arthritis of the shoulder joints due to the abnormal movements allowed by the loss of pain sensation.

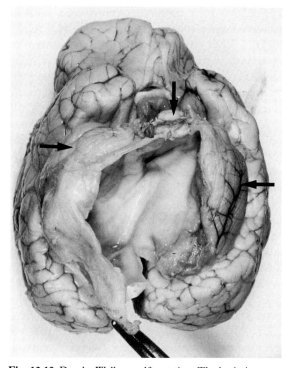

Fig. 12.13 Dandy–Walker malformation. The brain is viewed from below with the frontal poles at the top of the picture. The medulla (top arrow) has been displaced forwards and the cerebellar hemispheres (lateral arrows) have been displaced to the side by an enormous cyst. The membranous covering of the cyst has been incised to reveal an expanded fourth ventricle.

Syringobulbia is the formation of elongated cavities in the medulla and pons. In the medulla, the cavities containing cerebrospinal fluid often connect with the fourth ventricle and extend deep into the long tracts of the medulla. In the pons the syringes usually extend only into the tegmentum in the floor of the fourth ventricle.

In a proportion of cases of syringomyelia, there is elongation of the cerebellar tonsils and fibrosis and thickening of the overlying arachnoid covering the tonsils as they extend down through the foramen magnum. Gardener[65] suggested that this arrangement would interfere with drainage of the cerebrospinal fluid through the foramen of Magendie and with the passage of cerebrospinal fluid through the foramen magnum. Thus CSF would be forced down into the central canal from the fourth ventricle, causing dilatation of the central canal (*hydromyelia*) and ultimately syringomyelia. Although a proportion of cases of syringomyelia do have abnormalities at the foramen magnum which may be treatable, in other cases the exact cause is unknown.

Cavities in the spinal cord may form as a result of destructive lesions of the cord caused by trauma or haemorrhage, or they may form in association with tumours; such *secondary syringomyelia* may be found at all levels of the cord.

Encephalocele and cranial meningocele

75–80% of encephaloceles and cranial meningoceles occur in the occipital region of the skull.[19] Varying proportions of the occipital lobes and cerebellum herniate through the defect in the skull into the sac. These lesions probably do not occur until late in gestation, as the herniated brain tissue is usually well-formed and well-developed. In some cases the thin-walled sac is resected surgically and despite the absence of obvious brain tissue macroscopically, islands of brain tissue may be found histologically in the deep dermal regions of its skin covering. Such islands are most easily detected in sections stained with haematoxylin and van Gieson, in which the light yellow neural tissue is contrasted with the red-stained collagenous dermis.

Encephaloceles also occur in the parietal and frontal regions of the skull. *Anterior encephaloceles* in the frontal region may extend through the ethmoid bone and into the nose and the mouth. Occasionally, anterior encephaloceles are so large that they are incompatible with survival, whereas others present with skeletal abnormalities and small foci of brain tissue in the nasopharynx. Small encephaloceles may take the form of nasal polyps which may be associated with cerebrospinal fluid rhinorrhoea. Histological examination of the polyps reveals islands of central nervous system tissue, composed mainly of glia.

Cerebellar abnormalities

The cerebellum develops later in fetal life than the cerebrum, and much of its development occurs during the second half of gestation and in postnatal life. Thus the weight of the cerebellum is only 5·7% that of the cerebrum in the newborn infant and does not reach the adult proportion of 10·6% until the age of 18 months.[66] The flocculus and vermis (palaeocerebellum) develop earlier than the cerebellar hemispheres (neocerebellum). Early in the development of the cerebellum, the future Purkinje cells migrate from the periventricular regions to their positions in the cerebellar folia, and differentiation occurs in the third trimester. By the 30th–32nd week of gestation the external granular cell layer is well-developed and cells migrate into the folia along glial processes to form the internal granular layer.[50] This development extends into postnatal life and the external granular layer persists for 9–13 months after birth. Thus, although the Purkinje cells are intimately related to the granule cells in the postnatal brain, they differ in their origins and paths of migration. Purkinje cells and neurons of the dentate nucleus and other internal nuclei of the cerebellum migrate outwards from the rhombic lip of the hindbrain at an earlier stage than the inward migration of the granule cells, basket cells and stellate cells from the external granular layer.

Developmental abnormalities of the cerebellum are rare and often complex. *Aplasia* is due to damage to the cerebellar anlage during early embryonic life.[50] Some patients with this uncommon condition may be clinically normal whereas others show motor incoordination with difficulty in walking and also mental retardation. Some cases are familial whilst others are sporadic.

The aplastic cerebellum is represented only by a few nodules of cells and there is secondary aplasia of the pons and parts of the medulla such as the olive.

Dysplasias of the cerebellum include focal cortical dysplasias and diffuse hypertrophy of the cerebellar cortex.[50] Disturbances of migration of the Purkinje cells from the rhombic lip give rise to *heterotopias*, which consist of three main types.

1. Nests of cells with dense elongated nuclei resembling the matrix cells of the external granular layer; such nests are usually found in the dentate nucleus. Minor dysplasias of this type are frequently seen in the neonatal cerebellum.[67]
2. Clumps of larger cells resembling dentate neurons or Purkinje cells, with or without admixed granule cells and glia.
3. Organised but ectopic areas of cerebellar cortex.

Heterotopias are often associated with other nervous system abnormalities and may be seen in chromosomal disorders.[50]

Focal dysplasia of the cortex also occurs, in which there is a derangement of the Purkinje cells and other cell types but at their appropriate sites. This disorder is often referred to as *cerebellar polymicrogyria* but it is not strictly comparable to cerebral polymicrogyria (see p. 320) as there are no false sulci.

Diffuse hypertrophy of the cerebellar cortex,[68] first described by Lhermitte and Duclos, is another rare abnormality in which very large folia are present in portions of the cerebellum and there is a thick layer of abnormal cells underlying the granule cell layer. Some of these cells resemble Purkinje cells and others are smaller.[50]

Experimental studies have shown that damage to the external granular layer of the cerebellum late in gestation prevents the migration of basket, stellate and granule cells into the cortex of the cerebellar hemispheres. Such loss of cells is accompanied by crowding of the Purkinje cells and distortion of their dendrites. It is possible that virus infections could cause such granular layer aplasia in human infants. The outer granular layer in animals has remarkable powers of reconstitution, so that a single insult may not result in detectable cerebellar abnormality.[69]

PERINATAL BRAIN DAMAGE

Improved perinatal care in many parts of the world has reduced perinatal mortality but this has not been accompanied by a reduction in mental handicap.[70] Patterns of pathology responsible for the mental retardation differ, depending upon the maturity of the fetus at birth. In premature infants (i.e. low birth weight infants, under 1500 g), subependymal plate haemorrhage, parenchymal and intraventricular haemorrhages and periventricular leucomalacia are the commonest forms of perinatal brain damage, whereas in full-term infants it is diffuse hypoxic damage to the cerebral cortex, basal ganglia and thalamus that is commonest.

Premature infants

Ultrasound and CT scanning[71] have shown that haemorrhages and periventricular leucomalacia (PVL) occur most commonly on the first day of life, within a few hours of birth, and are associated with respiratory distress syndrome and hyaline membrane disease,[72,73] hypercapnia, acidosis, pneumothorax and coagulation defects.[74] The majority of affected infants are undersized and born prematurely; some 40–60% of infants with birth weight under 1500 g, or under 35 weeks gestation, have subependymal plate haemorrhages with or without intraventricular extension. Similar haemorrhages may occur in utero and are seen in approximately 6% of stillbirths.

In an ultrasound study of 200 low birth weight infants,[75] 53% had intraventricular haemorrhages and 6% true intraparenchymal haemorrhages in the periventricular white matter; 13% showed periventricular leucomalacia. In 13% of cases, prolonged 'flares' were detected by ultrasound which proved (at post mortem) to be areas of spongiosis and micro-infarction in the periventricular white matter.[71,75] 10% developed ventricular dilatation, of whom about half had parenchymal lesions.[75] Haemorrhage and prolonged 'flares' were more common in infants under 30 weeks of gestation; 26% of this group had evidence of periventricular leucomalacia.[75]

Subependymal plate haemorrhages appear to be of little consequence in the absence of posthaemorrhagic ventricular dilatation or inter-

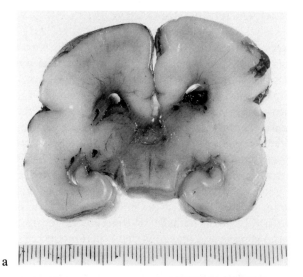

a

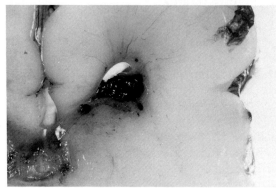

b

Fig. 12.14a, b Subependymal haemorrhage in a 26-week fetus. (**a**) Coronal section through the cerebral hemispheres showing haemorrhage in the wall of the right lateral ventricle. (**b**) Detail of the subependymal haemorrhage in **a** showing that it is localised mainly to the subependymal plate region of the ventricle but with small haemorrhages around it.

parenchymal extension of the haemorrhage.[74] However, intraparenchymal and intraventricular haemorrhages and PVL are important causes of mental handicap and cerebral palsy; the neuro-developmental prognosis for haemorrhages is much better than that for periventricular leuco-malacia.[71,76]

Haemorrhage

Infants with extensive haemorrhage, especially haemorrhage into the ventricles, deteriorate clinically and may pass into coma or develop seizures. A fall in the haematocrit reflects the

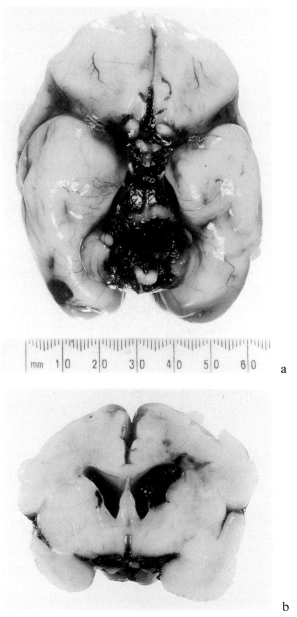

a

b

Fig. 12.15a, b Intraventricular haemorrhage in a 27-week fetus. (**a**) The brain viewed from below showing blood clot in the cisterna magna (bottom) and in the subarachnoid space over the front of the medulla and pons. The blood has followed the CSF pathways from the ventricles. (**b**) Coronal section through the frontal lobes showing a small subependymal haemorrhage in the wall of the left lateral ventricle and a larger subependymal haemorrhage with intraventricular extension on the right. There is also periventricular leucomalacia adjacent to the superior lateral corner of the right lateral ventricle.

amount of bleeding, and ultrasound or CT scanning may be used to estimate the size and extent of the haemorrhage.[77,78]

At post mortem, haemorrhages may be confined to the subependymal plate regions in the lateral corners of the lateral ventricles; they may be unilateral or bilateral (Figs 12.14, 12.15, and 12.16). Haemorrhage may rupture massively from the subependymal plate region or from the choroid plexus into the lateral ventricle, frequently spreading thence through the third and fourth ventricles and into the cisterna magna (Fig. 12.15). In addition to rupturing into the ventricles, haemorrhage may track into the immature unmyelinated white matter of the cerebral hemispheres; such

intraparenchymal haemorrhages usually occur at the level of the foramen of Monro.

With very small haemorrhages, histology of the subependymal plate region shows fresh blood around thin-walled veins and capillaries and disruption of the subependymal cells. Pseudocysts frequently form in the subependymal plate in association with subependymal haemorrhages but their origin is obscure.[19] Small haemorrhages into the periventricular tissue, at the corners of the lateral ventricles, may be seen histologically (Fig. 12.16) and are centred around thin-walled blood vessels.

There are a number of theories regarding the pathogenesis of subependymal plate haemor-

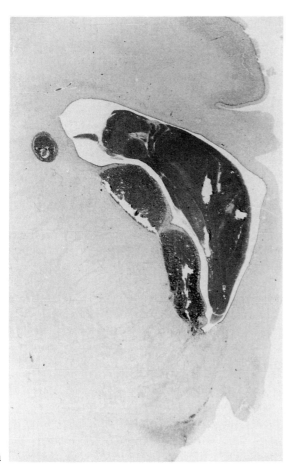
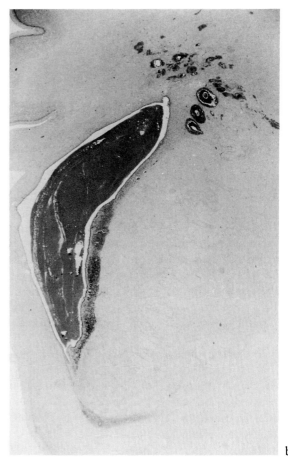

a

b

Fig. 12.16a, b Subependymal, intraventricular, and intraparenchymal haemorrhage—28-week fetuses—histological sections. (a) Haemorrhage has disrupted the subependymal plate in the wall of the lateral ventricle. There is also haemorrhage within the ventricle itself. (b) In addition to the intraventricular haemorrhage, there are small perivascular haemorrhages in the periventricular brain parenchyma (top). Haematoxylin-eosin × 5

rhages and intraventricular haemorrhages.[51] The subependymal plate matrix is the germinal centre for the cerebral hemispheres during fetal life. It has almost disappeared by 24 weeks of gestation but persists until 35 to 36 weeks in the lateral corners of the lateral ventricles between the caudate nucleus and the thalamus (Fig. 12.2) and in the roof of the temporal horns of the lateral ventricles. The association of subependymal plate haemorrhages with the respiratory distress syndrome (hyaline membrane disease) in 95% of cases[79] suggests that hypoxia and changes in cerebral blood flow may result in the rupture of fine vessels in the capillary bed of the subependymal matrix.[80] With the fibrinolytic activity of the matrix, blood may rupture through the ependyma into the ventricles. A further factor in the occurrence of subependymal plate haemorrhages may be the poor development of autoregulation of the blood supply in the brain of the premature infant.

Post-haemorrhagic ventricular dilatation

With resuscitation and supportive measures, infants with intraventricular haemorrhage may survive, but 10–50% develop ventricular dilatation.[75,81] In most cases, the lateral, third and fourth ventricles become dilated. The ventricular dilatation appears to be due to a combination of factors. It is observed in high risk premature infants, with or without haemorrhage, and particularly in those who show some cerebral atrophy.[82] Thus, destruction of brain tissue at birth and blockage of CSF drainage pathways may both contribute to the ventricular dilatation. This point is further emphasised by the observation that the insertion of a ventricular shunt in post-haemorrhagic ventricular dilatation is only effective in preventing severe mental handicap in 18% of cases.[83] In contrast, ventricular shunting in congenital hydrocephalus due to non-haemorrhagic causes results in normal neurological development in 57% of patients.[84]

At post mortem, the brains of infants with post-haemorrhagic ventricular dilatation may show rusty discoloration of the meninges, choroid plexus and ependyma. The hydrocephalus may be partly due to obstruction of the flow of cerebrospinal fluid through the cisterns and subarachnoid space. Necrotic debris in the aqueduct or fourth ventricle may also be a cause of hydrocephalus, in which case only the lateral and third ventricles are dilated. In addition to thinning and gliosis of the cerebral white matter, damage associated with intracerebral extension of the haemorrhage may be seen and probably contributes to the cerebral atrophy observed by ultrasound.[82]

Periventricular leucomalacia (PVL)

Premature infants (under 1500 g birth weight) who suffer prolonged apnoea and hypotension from birth hypoxia frequently sustain infarcts in the unmyelinated cerebral white matter in the centrum semiovale near the lateral corners of the lateral ventricles. This is the boundary zone between the major blood supplies of the white matter, one of which extends centrifugally from the ventricular aspect of the hemisphere and the other centripetally from the cerebral cortex.

Clinically, there may be no specific signs of PVL and, unless the lesions have progressed to a stage of calcification, they may be difficult to detect except at autopsy. Periventricular leucomalacia is found in 26–35% of brains of low birth weight infants post mortem.[75,85]

Ischaemic-hypoxic lesions in the periventricular white matter may occur in patients with congenital heart disease and those suffering circulatory collapse in the course of septicaemia and meningitis.

Periventricular leucomalacia has a poor prognosis for neurodevelopment, and patients who survive have a variety of neurological signs and visual impairment. PVL is a major cause of spastic monoplegia and diplegia in cerebral palsy.[71,75,76,86]

Pathology. Coronal sections of the cerebral hemispheres at post mortem reveal necrotic areas in the various arterial boundary zones, namely, at the corners of the lateral ventricles opposite the foramina of Monro (Fig. 12.17), in the temporal lobes (involving the acoustic radiations) and in the occipital lobes (involving the optic radiations).

Lesions initially may be congested, haemorrhagic spots or more extensive areas of necrosis.

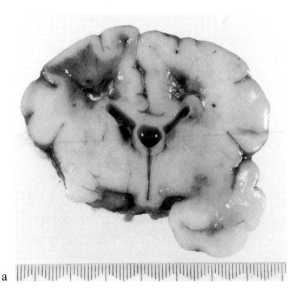

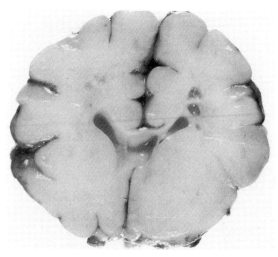

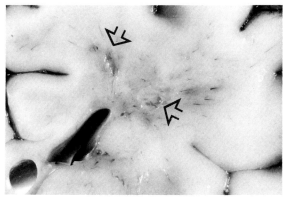

Fig. 12.17a–c Periventricular leucomalacia. (a) Large areas of shrunken discoloured periventricular white matter are seen superiolateral to both lateral ventricles—32-week fetus—still-born. (b) Small areas of periventricular damage (arrows) showing early cavitation. Infant born at 33 weeks gestation who survived for 15 days postnatally. (c) Cystic cavitation in the brain of an infant who was born at 29 weeks gestation and who survived for 45 days postnatally.

Later, they are pale and, within a few days, chalky white. Subsequently, PVL lesions show cavitation and often calcification; they may then form cysts in the periventricular white matter (Fig. 12.17). Such cavities often collapse and may no longer be visible after 6 months,[71] although some persist into adult life.

Histology of the early stages of periventricular leucomalacia reveals coagulation necrosis; the affected area contains material that stains with PAS and with Luxol fast blue. Later there is microglial proliferation and macrophage invasion, and swollen axon balloons (see p. 48) are seen around the edge of the infarcted region. The dead tissue is rapidly removed by macrophages to leave a cystic area surrounded by gliosis (Fig. 12.18),

often with calcium deposition in the walls of blood vessels. Histological evaluation of the newborn infant brain must obviously take into account the absence of myelin in the white matter which means that two of the usual criteria for establishing brain damage—i.e. the loss of myelin and the presence of myelin breakdown products—are of little relevance in these cases. The remnants of the subependymal plate matrix may also cause confusion. The cells of this matrix have small round or oval nuclei with few processes, and they form cuffs around the blood vessels (Fig. 12.18): they should not be confused with lymphocytes.

Those patients who die later in childhood or adult life may exhibit single or multiple cysts in the white matter or merely glial scarring and diffuse

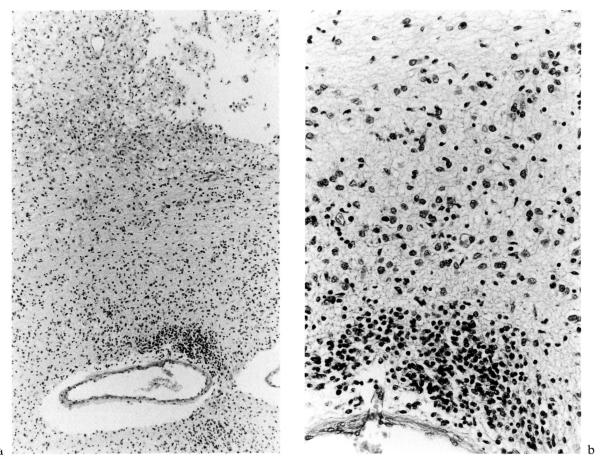

a

b

Fig. 12.18a, b Periventricular leucomalacia. Histology at 4 days after birth. (**a**) Cavitating leucomalacia (top) is surrounded by gliotic brain tissue containing macrophages. A focus of perivascular subependymal plate cells is seen at bottom. (**b**) Detail of **a** showing subependymal plate cells (bottom) and reactive astrocytes in the tissue near the PVL (top). Haematoxylin-eosin (**a**) × 75; (**b**) × 150

loss of myelin in the centrum semiovale. Calcium and iron salts are often deposited around blood vessels and in dead neurons (ferruginated neurons) (see Fig. 12.20d). The loss of brain tissue is reflected in the enlargement of the lateral ventricles (hydrocephalus ex vacuo). In addition to the periventricular leucomalacia, there may be hypoxic damage to the basal ganglia and thalamus resulting in *état marbré* (*status marmoratus*) (see p. 335).

Full-term infant

The pattern of perinatal brain damage that occurs in full-term infants is different from that usually seen in premature infants. Subependymal and intraventricular haemorrhage rarely occurs at term,[87] when the most common type of perinatal brain damage is *hypoxic-ischaemic encephalopathy* with diffuse neuronal destruction involving mainly the cerebral cortex, the basal ganglia and the thalamus. Such brain damage is usually associated with a difficult labour, particularly when there is precipitous delivery in a primiparous mother or when labour lasts longer than 15 hours in primiparous or multiparous women. Prolongation of the second stage of labour beyond two hours may also be associated with brain damage in full-term infants, as may forceps delivery. With improvements in obstetric care, brain damage in full-term neonates has become less common[51] but it still occurs in 1:1000 live births.[19]

Hypoxic-ischaemic encephalopathy

Following severe hypoxic-ischaemic brain damage, infants may be hypotonic at birth with an Apgar score of less than 3 and requiring resuscitation and ventilation. Coma may ensue, and epilepsy in 50% of cases; the child may have a weak cry and be unable to suck. Those children who survive suffer lethargy and may have spastic paraplegia or quadriplegia with choreoathetosis, seizures and mental retardation. After several weeks or months, CT scans reveal cerebral atrophy and enlargement of the cerebral ventricles. In very severe cases, there is microcephaly and a small atrophic brain.

Such children may present diagnostic difficulties during life, and pathological assessment of the brain is frequently essential before deciding whether the brain damage is due to an hereditary defect, damage during early gestation or hypoxia and ischaemia late in pregnancy or at birth.

Pathology. In affected children dying soon after birth, post mortem reveals a swollen brain with compressed ventricles. Coronal sections of the brain reveal friable white matter and brown or red infarcted cortex. The brain damage is usually bilateral and symmetrical. The temporal lobes are often spared. Typically, cortical damage occurs in the depths of the sulci and may show a laminar pattern with necrosis in layers 3 and 5. The hippocampus, basal ganglia, pons and medulla may be damaged although neuronal loss may only be detectable histologically. The cerebellum is often severely affected, with loss of Purkinje cells and granular cells. Boundary zone infarcts (see p. 138) in the cortex between the major areas of supply of the anterior and middle cerebral arteries may occur as a less severe form of damage.

In children dying weeks or months after birth, the brain is shrunken and atrophic (Fig. 12.19). In some cases, the diffuse neuronal damage has resulted in generalised atrophy of the cortex, white matter and central grey matter (Fig. 12.19). The ventricles are enlarged and the sulci are wide. In other cases, there is widespread cavitation within the cortex and within the white matter (*multicystic encephalopathy*) (Fig. 12.20a). Coronal sections of such brains show a pattern of *ulegyria* (see p. 321)

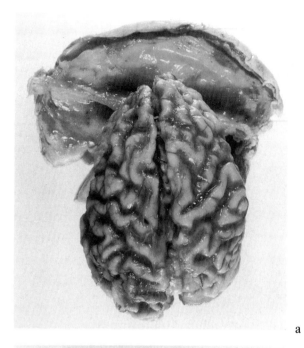

a

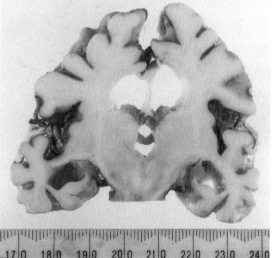

b

Fig. 12.19a, b Hypoxic-ischaemic encephalopathy—full-term infant: 'cot death' at 14 months. (**a**) A view of the brain from above showing extensive cerebral atrophy (walnut brain). (**b**) Coronal section of the brain showing diffuse atrophy of the cortex, white matter and central grey matter with enlargement of the ventricles and cerebral sulci.

(Fig. 12.20b) in which the major cortical damage is in the depths of the sulci and the crests of the gyri may be relatively well preserved.

Histological examination of damaged areas of cortex may reveal diffuse loss of neurons and gliosis. Cavities within the damaged cortex and

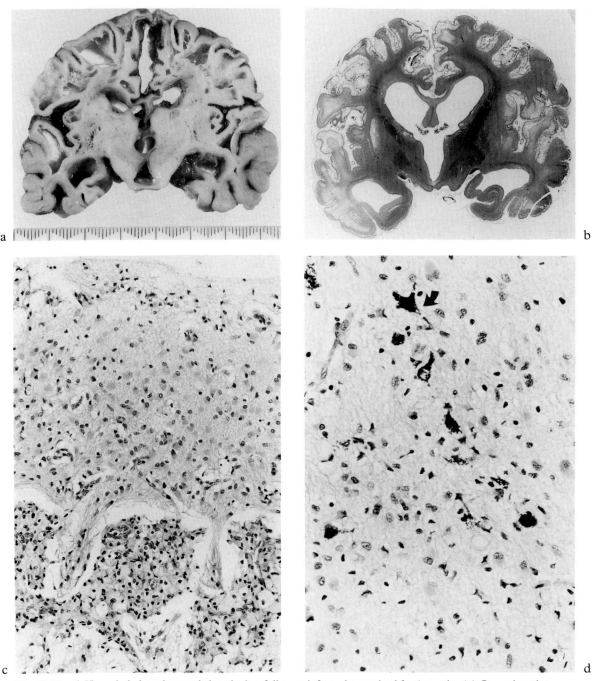

Fig. 12.20a–d Hypoxic-ischaemic encephalopathy in a full-term infant who survived for 4 months. (**a**) Coronal section through the cerebral hemispheres showing extensive cavitation of the white matter. (**b**) Histological section showing cavitation and disintegration of the cerebral cortex, particularly in the depths of the sulci. (**c**) Histology of the cavitated cortex in **b**. Cavities (bottom) are filled with foamy macrophages. The molecular layer of the cortex contains reactive astrocytes. Meningeal surface at top. (**d**) Ferruginated neurons. They are densely stained structures, some of which retain the pyramidal shape of neurons (arrow). The rest of the cortex is gliotic.
(**b–d**) Haematoxylin-eosin (**c**) × 150; (**d**) × 270

white matter contain macrophages and are surrounded by reactive astrocytes (Fig. 12.20c). Encrusted mineralised ferruginated neurons may be seen within the damaged cortex (Fig. 12.20d). Ferruginated neurons are deeply basophilic in haematoxylin and eosin stained sections and can be stained for calcium with the alizarin red technique and for iron with the Perls technique. In addition to the cortical damage, the corpus callosum may be atrophic, and the ventricles widely dilated due to the destruction of neurons and white matter in the hemispheres. Scarring of the basal ganglia produces the effect of *état marbré* (*status marmoratus*), particularly in the putamen and less often in the caudate nucleus and thalamus. The appearance resembles that of marble due to an abnormal distribution of myelinated fibres within the grey matter areas. Status marmoratus may be difficult to detect macroscopically and is best shown by careful examination of histological sections stained for myelin (e.g. Klüver–Barrera) or for astrocytes (e.g. Holzer, or immunoperoxidase for glial fibrillary acidic protein). Proliferation and hypertrophy of astrocytes are seen within the areas of status marmoratus, together with loss of neurons and areas of perivascular hypermyelination. The cerebellum may also show extensive areas of ulegyria.

Although widespread ulegyria and cavitation of the white matter may be seen following birth hypoxia, these changes cannot be distinguished with certainty from widespread brain damage occurring in late fetal life. A history of maternal anaemia, toxaemia, renal disease or seizures in pregnancy with a subsequent normal labour may suggest that the damage occurred in fetal life. Ultrasound imaging can detect cerebral damage in the fetus, thus allowing a more accurate assessment of the timing of brain tissue destruction.[48]

Severe brain damage of the pattern described in perinatal cases does not commonly occur in the postnatal period. However, progressive postnatal degeneration of the grey matter in the cerebral hemispheres has been described; its aetiology is unknown.[88]

Cerebral infarction in the fetus and newborn

Cerebral infarction involving the territories of major cerebral arteries may be seen in newborn infants. If recent, the infarcts are often haemorrhagic. Such infarction appears to be associated with vascular occlusion but the origin of emboli or the cause of thrombosis is not always clear. Infarcts are particularly associated with respiratory distress syndrome, sepsis, meningitis and congenital heart disease, especially with a right to left shunt.[89] In some series,[90] infarcts were seen in 5·4% of autopsies on neonates.

Macroscopically and histologically, recent infarcts resemble those in the adult except that there is more rapid removal of damaged brain tissue in the fetus and the infarct soon progresses to a cystic lesion. In children dying a few months after birth with a cystic unilateral infarct, it may not be possible to determine whether the infarct occurred in the perinatal period or in the late fetal period as the appearances are very similar.

Birth trauma and perinatal intracranial haemorrhage

Tearing of the tentorium cerebelli or the falx cerebri may occur during difficult deliveries, particularly in full-term infants, with the formation of small haematomas. If superficial veins of the cortex are torn, subdural haematomas may form. Clinically, the children may suffer hemiparesis, convulsion and hypoxia. Such lesions have been reduced in recent years due to better obstetric care and the use of Caesarean section rather than forceps deliveries.

Subarachnoid haemorrhages may be seen in children dying soon after birth. They may be focal or diffuse; if focal, they may become green in colour with age and be mistaken for collections of pus. The origin of subarachnoid haemorrhages in the newborn is obscure but they may be due to disorders of coagulation. *Subpial haemorrhage*, in which the blood accumulates between the pia mater and the glia limitans of the surface of the brain, may be seen in newborn children.[91]

The cervical and upper thoracic spinal cord may be injured, particularly during breech deliveries[92] or occasionally during external version in utero.[93] Clinically, the affected neonates are paraplegic and may show spinal shock. Fractures of the spine may be found; the cord may be transected with accompanying haemorrhage and tissue destruction.

VASCULAR MALFORMATIONS IN THE NEWBORN

Vascularisation of the central nervous system is seen in the 24-day fetus[50,94] with the formation of a primitive vascular plexus covering the outer aspect of the developing brain. By 28 days of gestation, arteries and veins have started to differentiate in the superficial regions of the vascular plexus, and sheets of capillaries form in the deeper aspects. As the vasculature divides into three layers to supply the scalp, dura and pia mater, the major cerebral arteries develop. The basilar artery appears at 29 days and the cerebral arteries at 32–40 days; the circle of Willis forms by the 44th day. A pattern resembling the adult arrangement has developed by 52 days.

Vascular abnormalities of the brain which present in the neonate or in childhood appear to be mainly due to disordered development of the cerebral vasculature. The most common severe abnormalities are those in which major arteries feed directly into veins or venous sinuses. The majority of the vascular abnormalities are sporadic. These include diffuse *meningocerebral angiodysplasia*, in which the cerebral surface is covered by dilated tortuous vessels, with associated cortical and subcortical infarcts and mineralisation of the tissue.[95] Persistence of the fetal meningeal vasculature has been described most commonly in association with dysraphic malformations such as anencephaly and encephaloceles.[96] The vessels over these abnormalities are thin-walled and dilated.

Arteriovenous malformations, formed from a convoluted mass of arteries and veins, usually present in adult life (see p. 113); only some 10% present in children. If there is extensive arteriovenous shunting, the child may develop an enlarged head, cranial bruit and cardiac failure.[97] Saccular aneurysms are uncommon in childhood (see p. 108). Gross disorganisation of the major arteries, as in moya moya disease (see p. 104), may be seen.

Arteriovenous aneurysm of the vein of Galen develops due to direct shunting of blood into major cerebral veins.[98] Normally, the great cerebral veins drain blood from the deep aspects of the cerebral hemispheres into the great vein of Galen, which subsequently drains into the straight sinus at the apex of the tentorium cerebelli. The clinical presentation of the aneurysm depends upon the age of the patient and the size of the shunt. Large shunts in the newborn may lead to high output cardiac failure and death within a few weeks unless correction of the shunt is performed. The most dramatic appearances are seen on angiography; the vessels are collapsed when seen at post mortem. The great vein of Galen may be dilated to form a sac several centimetres in diameter which then drains into a dilated straight sinus. Large vessels feed the aneurysm; they most commonly arise from the posterior cerebral artery or from a combination of the anterior and posterior cerebral arteries. Abnormalities such as duplication and hypoplasia of the feeding arteries may be seen, but apart from intimal fibrosis there is little abnormality in the arteries as they gradually change to become veins. In children dying early in life from cardiac failure there may be little change in the underlying brain. In older patients, however, there may be thrombosis of the abnormal vessels with calcification and cortical infarction or intraventricular haemorrhages from rupture of dilated veins. Hydrocephalus develops in 50% of those who survive, due to pressure on the dorsum of the midbrain and occlusion of the aqueduct.

There are a few reports of arteriovenous shunts in which the middle and posterior cerebral arteries drain into the superior sagittal sinus or the sigmoid sinus.[99]

THROMBOSIS OF THE SUPERIOR SAGITTAL SINUS

Thrombotic occlusion of the sinus and the large cerebral veins that drain into it may be seen in children following periods of dehydration or may be associated with meningitis. Haemorrhagic infarction of the underlying brain occurs, particularly in the superior medial aspects of the cerebral hemispheres.

KERNICTERUS (BILIRUBIN ENCEPHALOPATHY)

Blood group incompatibility between fetus and mother, particularly rhesus incompatibility, was a major cause of kernicterus, but with the introduction of anti-D rhesus prophylaxis[100] kernicterus is much less common. It is now mainly seen in low birth weight infants, 6% of babies under 2000 g being affected.[51] Kernicterus is also associated with septicaemia, resorption of large haematomas, certain drug treatments[101] and glucose-6-phosphate dehydrogenase deficiency. The acute phase of bilirubin encephalopathy usually lasts no longer than a week, during which time the child is restless, has an abnormal cry, is hypotonic and shows poor sucking ability. The patient is jaundiced and the indirect serum bilirubin is usually above 340 μmol/l.

At autopsy, children dying with kernicterus may have yellow discoloration of the CSF, meninges and surfaces of the cerebral hemispheres. Central grey matter areas appear yellow, with symmetrical involvement of the globus pallidus, lateral part of the thalamus, subthalamic nuclei, putamen, lateral geniculate bodies, brainstem nuclei, olives and dentate nuclei. The choroid plexus is also yellow. Histologically, yellow pigment is seen within the neurons of the affected areas, but the yellow discoloration may fade with time in formalin-fixed material.

Those children who survive for weeks or months may exhibit extrapyramidal motor disabilities, delayed motor development, athetoid movements and rigidity. Their brains show neuronal loss and gliosis in the areas affected by kernicterus and poor myelination of the white matter.[102]

Jaundice and the high indirect serum bilirubin levels associated with kernicterus result from an insufficient capacity of the neonatal liver to conjugate the overload of bilirubin caused by abnormal haemolysis.[51] 75% of bilirubin in the newborn is derived from the destruction of red cells by the liver and spleen. Bilirubin bound to albumin is conjugated with glucuronic acid by the enzyme uridine diphosphoglucuronyl transferase, and in this form passes out into the bile and into the intestine. With the overload of bilirubin, there is a failure of conjugation and the bile remains in the blood. The exact mechanism of entry of bile into the brain is uncertain but periods of hypoxia may interfere with the blood-brain barrier, allowing entry of bile pigments into areas of grey matter.

VIRUS INFECTIONS IN THE FETUS AND NEWBORN INFANT

Infections, particularly by viruses, may not only result in destructive lesions in the fetal brain but may cause malformations, depending upon the time at which the infection occurs. A number of viruses have been implicated in congenital malformations[50] although causal relationships are often difficult to establish.

Rubella

The highest incidence of fetal malformations in rubella (10–12%) occurs following maternal infection during the first 4 weeks of gestation.[103] The incidence is lower for infections at 4–10 weeks, and there are no subsequent malformations if the infection is after 20 weeks. Viraemia occurs in the initial stages of the maternal disease and the virus crosses the placenta.[104] In one series[105] 52% of affected fetuses had congenital heart disease, particularly a patent ductus arteriosus, with or without pulmonary artery stenosis and ventricular septal defect. 52% had a damaged organ of Corti leading to deafness, and 40% had cataracts, sometimes associated with microphthalmos or buphthalmos and retinopathy. In 40% of cases there was slight or moderate mental retardation, often with microcephaly. Rubella infection may persist after birth[106] so that changes of meningo-encephalitis with areas of necrosis and mineralisation of blood vessels may be seen.[107] Progressive rubella panencephalitis is discussed on p. 213.

Cytomegalovirus infection

Generalised cytomegalovirus infection is virtually restricted to the newborn infant; the fetus is probably infected during a stage of maternal viraemia, the mother usually having no symptoms. Cytomegalovirus may be found in the salivary glands of children without symptoms of disease. In the generalised disease there is hepatosplenomegaly, jaundice, anaemia, thrombocytopenia, petechial haemorrhages and diarrhoea beginning soon after birth; death may ensue within a few days or weeks. Some 10% of cases have central nervous system involvement and in children who survive[108] there may be mental retardation, deafness, diplegia and seizures, with microcephaly and cerebral calcification.

Epithelia and other cells in various affected organs produce the enlarged cells typical of cytomegalovirus infection (Fig. 12.21). The cerebral lesions[109] are most commonly found in the olfactory bulbs and the lining of the lateral ventricles. There is destruction of ependyma and the formation of glial nodules (Fig. 9.11, p. 215). Areas of necrosis with surrounding gliosis and calcification may be seen in the cortex, white matter, cerebellum and spinal cord. The cytomegalovirus inclusions are up to 15 μm in diameter (Fig. 12.21) and appear as acidophilic intranuclear bodies in astrocytes, microglia, ependyma, leptomeninges, vascular endothelium and, occasionally, neurons. Electronmicroscopically, the particles are hexagonal or pentagonal and 93 nm in diameter.[110]

Herpes simplex

Disseminated herpes simplex infection may occur before birth or be due to infection by herpes simplex type 2 (the virus of genital herpes) during birth. Manifestations of the infection include respiratory distress, hepatosplenomegaly, jaundice and skin lesions appearing 5–7 days after birth. Although the generalised systemic involvement is usually the most severe aspect of the disease, disseminated focal meningoencephalitis may be seen with lymphocytic cuffing of blood vessels and areas of necrosis in the brainstem and cerebellum.[51]

MYCOTIC INFECTIONS IN THE NEWBORN INFANT

Candida albicans is the commonest fungus infecting the newborn infant.[33,50] Infection is probably derived from the maternal genital tract during birth. In disseminated candida infection, multiple necrotic granulomatous lesions (Fig. 12.22) containing fungal hyphae (pseudohyphae) are seen throughout the brain and other organs. Other fungal infections such as *cryptococcosis*, *mucormycosis* and *aspergillosis* may occur but are uncommon.

OTHER INFECTIONS

Toxoplasmosis

Transplacental infection of the fetus, at or after the third month, by *Toxoplasma gondii* may occur but is uncommon.[111] Most commonly, toxoplasmosis is connatal (acquired at the time of birth) and symptoms begin at birth or within 6 weeks of birth, with convulsions, opisthotonos, paralysis, general

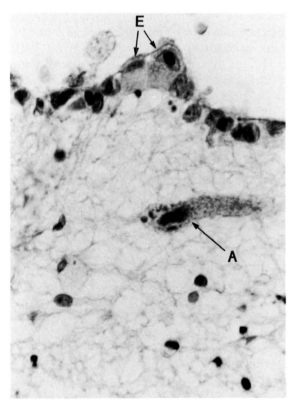

Fig. 12.21 Cytomegalovirus infection in the brain, showing typical intranuclear inclusions in ependymal cells (E) and astrocytes (A).
Haematoxylin-eosin × 675

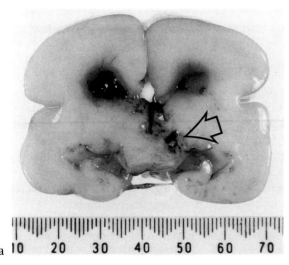

a

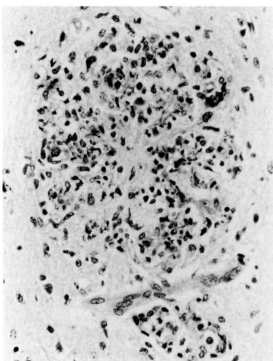

b

survive may be mentally retarded. At post mortem, the brain shows numerous depressed yellow lesions, ranging from a few millimetres to several centimetres in diameter, randomly distributed over the surface of the brain and throughout the hemispheres.[50,112] Hydrocephalus may be a compensatory ('ex vacuo') consequence of destruction of brain tissue or it may be due to obstruction by periventricular inflammatory lesions.

Microscopically,[50] there is chronic focal meningoencephalitis with large areas of necrosis containing macrophages and granulation tissue. Polymorphonuclear leucocytes, lymphocytes and plasma cells, eosinophils and macrophages may also be present. The organisms, $2-3\,\mu m \times 1.5-2\,\mu m$ in size, may be single or

Fig. 12.22a, b Disseminated candida infection in a 2-week-old infant born at 26 weeks gestation. (**a**) Coronal section of the cerebral hemispheres showing an area of necrosis in the right thalamus (arrow). (**b**) Granulomatous lesion in the pons. PAS and Grocott stains revealed fungal hyphae. (**b**) Haematoxylin-eosin × 270

malaise and jaundice. Chorioretinitis may be present, hydrocephalus is common and cerebral calcification may be seen on X-ray. 20% of patients die within the first month and those who

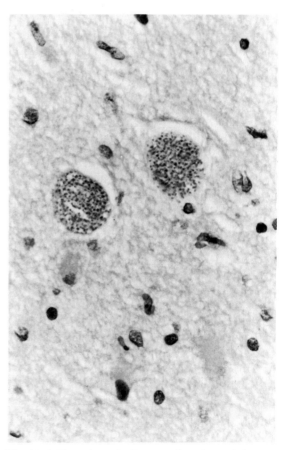

Fig. 12.23 Toxoplasmosis. Two pseudocysts containing many toxoplasmas.
Haematoxylin-eosin × 550

multiple and contained within pseudocysts 20–30 μm in diameter (Fig. 12.23).[40] Such pseudocysts may be present in the brain without any apparent inflammation surrounding them. Coarse and fine mineralisation within the brain is seen and individual cells may be calcified. There is extensive gliosis around the lesions but no giant cells are seen. Similar granulomatous and necrotic lesions are seen in the retina and in other organs, particularly the lung, heart and adrenals. Fetal infections may produce abnormalities such as hydranencephaly (see p. 322) and polymicrogyria (see p. 320).

Syphilis

The fetus may become infected in utero by *Treponema pallidum* during the 4–7th month of pregnancy. Such infections have become uncommon since the introduction of penicillin.[50] Many of the affected fetuses are aborted or still-born; others show exanthema, chronic rhinitis and hepatosplenomegaly. Scattered lymphocyte and plasma cell infiltration of the leptomeninges is seen, with cuffing of vessels in the brain and intimal proliferation. Numerous spirochaetes may be seen. In latent congenital syphilis, keratitis with corneal opacities develops, accompanied by loss of hearing, deformed incisors, saddle nose and some-times the early onset of general paralysis of the insane.

LEPTOMENINGITIS IN THE NEWBORN INFANT

Children are very susceptible to meningitis during the first 28 days of life. In some cases it is due to the spread of organisms from a meningomyelocele (see p. 316). Premature infants are particularly susceptible to infection, especially if the labour or delivery is complicated. The clinical picture is often vague, with lethargy, fever or a subnormal temperature, anorexia, vomiting, coma and bulging of the fontanelles. Septicaemia may ensue, most commonly due to Gram-negative bacilli; enteric organisms are involved in an overall 80%

of cases and *Escherichia coli* accounts for a third of the cases. Streptococci and staphylococci may be responsible for the infection. The organisms are thought to come from the mother. The mortality rate is high (60–75%) and death may occur within 4 days of onset.[113] Up to two-thirds of the survivors develop hydrocephalus or neurological deficit.[114]

Examination of the brain at post mortem[115] shows vascular congestion, with pus in the lepto-meninges over the hemispheres and less extensive involvement of the spinal cord, unless the infection has arisen from a meningomyelocele. In the acute stages the brain is swollen, but later hydro-cephalus may supervene. Polymorphonuclear leucocytes are seen in the initial exudate (see p. 154) but, later, lymphocytes and macrophages appear and there is organisation of the exudate in the subarachnoid space, especially on the pial aspect.

Thrombophlebitis of subarachnoid veins leads to haemorrhagic venous infarction in the cortex and white matter; the basal ganglia may be infarcted if the subependymal veins around the ventricles are also thrombosed following infection and inflam-mation of the ventricular walls. Infarcts occur in 30% of cases of neonatal leptomeningitis.[89]

In children who survive, multiloculated smooth-walled cavities resulting from infarcts may be seen deep in the hemispheres together with old abscess cavities. Diverticula from the ventricles may also be present with extensive gliosis of the subependymal regions. Fibrosis of the meninges is usually most prominent over the base of the brain and may be a major cause of hydrocephalus. The cavitation in these infant brains should not be confused with the encephalo-malacia that occurs following severe hypoxia in late fetal life or at birth (see p. 330).

Although enteric organisms and streptococci are the bacteria that most commonly cause meningitis in infants under the age of 2 months, after this age *Haemophilus influenzae*, *Streptococcus pneumoniae*, and *Neisseria meningitidis* become the more common causes.

Listeria monocytogenes may also cause neonatal meningitis; this organism can infect the fetus and cause abortion or result in destructive lesions in the fetal cerebrum.[116]

BRAIN TRAUMA IN INFANCY
('battered baby')

In addition to accidents, infants may sustain *non-accidental injuries*, usually inflicted by parents or other relatives. Many of the infants suffer repeated injuries to various parts of the body. Violent shaking may result in acute subdural haemorrhage. Blunt injury may cause skull fractures and brain damage. Probably because of the smooth internal surface of the skull, surface contusions on the brain are rare in infants under the age of 2 years. In abused children under 5 months of age, macroscopic contusional tears may be seen in the cerebral white matter,[117] together with diffuse axonal injury[118] similar to that seen in the adult (see p. 130).

SUDDEN INFANT DEATH SYNDROME
(SIDS)

Characteristically, in SIDS, the infant dies quietly during sleep by a mechanism involving a fatal apnoeic episode.[119] Children between 1 and 4 months of age are particularly susceptible: in Scotland in the years 1981–1982, SIDS accounted for nearly half the deaths in this age group.[120] A variety of predisposing factors have been suggested, including abnormal respiratory control mechanisms.[119] Much of the pathology at post mortem is seen in the lungs[121] but in some 20% of cases there are areas of subcortical and periventricular leucomalacia[122] and gliosis in the brainstem, suggesting that previous brain damage may play a rôle in SIDS.

INBORN ERRORS OF METABOLISM

There are many different genetic disorders which result in the deficiency of a single enzyme or co-factor.[8] Each disorder has a low incidence but usually a high morbidity or early mortality. Inherited biochemical defects involve many groups of compounds including amino acids, purines and pyrimidines, carbohydrates, trace metals, lipids and mucopolysaccharides.[13,123,124] A significant number of these diseases cause damage to the central nervous system. Some, such as phenylketonuria, can be treated by a restricted diet if diagnosed early.[13] Disorders due to defects in lysosomal enzymes or their co-factors form an important group of genetic diseases which affect the nervous system.[14,125]

LYSOSOMAL ENZYME DEFECTS— STORAGE DISORDERS

Lysosomes are membrane-bound intra-cytoplasmic bodies containing enzymes which are active at an acid pH in the degradation of the lipids, proteins and nucleotides that are integral parts of normal cell structures.[125] Genetic disorders in which a single enzyme or a co-factor is deficient or inactive may result in the intracellular accumulation of substances that the enzyme normally degrades. These disorders are usually inherited as autosomal recessive traits but they are sometimes dominant.

The nervous system is significantly affected in a number of lysosomal disorders, and the diagnosis depends upon the pattern of clinical onset of the disease, the pathology, and the identification of the enzyme defect. Patients frequently present in infancy or childhood with psychomotor disturbances and epilepsy and die within a short time. In many disorders, the lysosomal enzyme defect is known, so that the diagnosis may be made prenatally from amniotic cells obtained by paracentesis or postnatally from enzyme estimations in leucocytes, serum, cultured fibroblasts and, in some cases, urine.[14,124,125] When the exact identity of the enzyme defect in a family is unknown, it may be necessary to identify the material stored in neurons, white matter or other organs of the body by biochemistry or histochemistry before the enzyme defect is sought in leucocytes.[14]

Lysosomal enzyme disorders affecting the nervous system fall into several groups, namely, lipidoses, mucopolysaccharidoses, mucolipidoses and other disorders of glycoconjugate metabolism.[124]

The lipidoses

The lipid storage diseases (lipidoses) are

characterised by the accumulation of abnormal amounts of lipid in neurons or within macrophages in the central nervous system as well as in other organs of the body. Those which involve the white matter cause demyelination and are termed 'leuco-dystrophies'. All lipidoses in which the storage material has been identified, and in which the enzyme defect is known, are disorders of sphingo-lipid metabolism (sphingolipidoses). Sphingo-lipids are based on sphingosine and are components of cell membranes and myelin.

Gangliosidoses

Gangliosides are water-soluble sphingolipid components of cell membranes and they have been classified, according to their mobility on thin-layer chromatography, into G_{M1}, G_{M2}, G_{M3} etc. They are degraded by the enzymes hexosaminidases A and B; when these enzyme systems are defective, gangliosides accumulate within neurons and cells of other organs.

G_{M1} and the more common G_{M2} gangliosidoses have an autosomal recessive inheritance pattern[8] and present clinically with psychomotor retard-ation and fits. Dysmorphic features may be seen and hepatosplenomegaly is a feature of G_{M1} gangliosidosis. Cherry red spots are seen in the ocular fundi as loss of neurons from the macula reveals the vascular choroid.

The deficient enzyme in G_{M1} gangliosidosis is β-galactosidase which converts G_{M1} to G_{M2}.[125]

In *infantile* G_{M2} gangliosidosis type I (*Tay–Sachs disease*) there is a deficiency of β-hexosaminidase A which converts G_{M2} to G_{M3}, whereas in G_{M2} gangliosidosis type II (*Sandhoff's disease*) there is a deficiency of β-hexosaminidase A and B. The children are normal at birth but show psychomotor retardation and fits at 4–5 months; they are blind and decerebrate by the age of 3 years. In the *juvenile* forms the onset is at 4–6 years and the patients are dead by 10 years. An *adult* form[126] is characterised by neurogenic muscular atrophy.

Post mortem may reveal a large brain due to swollen neurons and astrocytes containing gangliosides. In the later stages of the disease, the brain may be shrunken due to the loss of white matter, especially in the infantile forms. The histo-

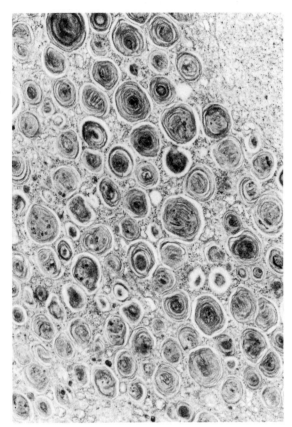

Fig. 12.24 G_{M2} gangliosidosis showing membranous cytoplasmic bodies in the cytoplasm of an affected neuron. Electron micrograph × 7200
Reproduced by permission of the authors and editor from: Purpura DP, Suzuki K. Brain Res 1976; 116: 1 (Fig. 11).

logical appearances are similar for all types of gangliosidosis, with ballooning of neuronal cyto-plasm and eccentricity of the nucleus due to the accumulation of intra-cytoplasmic ganglio-side.[14,125] Neurons throughout the brain, spinal cord and adrenal medulla are affected and contain Luxol-fast-blue positive granular material which, in frozen sections of formalin-fixed tissue, stains with PAS for ganglioside and is lysosomal acid phosphatase positive. Electron microscopy reveals membranous cytoplasmic bodies composed of concentric whorls of membrane in neurons and glia (Fig.12.24).[14,127,128] Examinations of fetal brains in this disorder shows little storage of lipid until 20 weeks of gestation.

Diagnosis is made by detecting the enzyme defects in leucocytes, serum, cultured fibroblasts, tears and tissue samples, and in cells in amniotic fluid, obtained by amniocentesis.[14] Rectal biopsy reveals accumulation of ganglioside within neurons in the gut wall. Extraction of the stored lipid from biopsy tissue and its identification by thin-layer chromatography may then allow the appropriate enzyme defect to be sought.[14]

Niemann–Pick disease

This is a heterogeneous group of disorders with an autosomal recessive pattern of inheritance. Sphingomyelin accumulates in the spleen and liver and in foam cells; the central nervous system is involved to a variable degree in different types of the disease. In types A and D[129] there is a central nervous system defect, in type C the central nervous system is only moderately involved and in type B the central nervous system is normal. A deficiency of sphingomyelinase activity has been demonstrated in types A and B.[125,130]

The *neurovisceral* form of the disease[131] includes the severe infantile form in which there is hepatosplenomegaly, failure to thrive and mental retardation. A characteristic cherry red spot is commonly seen at the macula on examination of the optic fundus. Death occurs before the age of 4 years. An adult form has also been described.

At autopsy there is gross enlargement of the liver and spleen in patients with and without central nervous system involvement. In the infantile form, neurons throughout the brain and gastrointestinal tract are ballooned in a similar way to those in Tay–Sachs disease but the accumulated lipid is sphingomyelin. Lipid also accumulates in glial cells and there is demyelination of the white matter and gliosis with the presence of foamy storage cells (Niemann–Pick cells) in the white matter.[14] The foamy cells are derived from monocytes and are up to 90 μm in diameter with a mulberry-like form and vacuolated cytoplasm. These cells are seen in the red pulp of the spleen and in the sinusoids of the liver, and in the lungs, thymus and most organs. Sea-blue histiocytes are seen in type B Niemann–Pick disease.[14,125]

Sphingomyelin in neurons, in spleen, liver and muscle, and in endothelial cells can be identified in frozen sections or cryostat sections by the ferric haematoxylin method[132] or by the Sudan black B

method which shows positive staining and red birefringence due to the mixture of sphingomyelin and cholesterol crystals in the cells. Acid phosphatase activity is associated with the stored substances, and electron microscopy[133] shows the neuronal inclusions as loosely-packed lamellae in membrane-bound vacuoles 1–2 μm in diameter. Diagnosis can be made prenatally by detecting the enzyme defect in amniotic fluid cells and postnatally in white blood cells and fibroblasts.[134]

In *type C* Niemann–Pick disease, there is hepatosplenomegaly, and soon after birth the onset of dementia, ataxia and fits. A juvenile or adult form may also be seen. Sphingomyelin accumulates in the spleen and other organs but there is no accumulation in the brain and the enzyme defect is unknown. Neuronal ballooning is seen in the basal ganglia and brainstem and spinal cord and in the gastrointestinal tract;[135] the identity of the storage substance in the neurons is unknown—it is not sphingomyelin.

Gaucher's disease

There are three main types of this disease—adult, infantile and juvenile. An autosomal recessive inheritance pattern is seen, with a deficiency of *glucocerebroside β-glucosidase*.[125] In the infantile type of Gaucher's disease, the acute *neuronopathic* type (type 2), severe regression of motor function occurs around 6 months of age, with strabismus and spasticity. Death usually occurs before 2 years of age. In type 3, the onset of the disease is later, the course more protracted, and epilepsy is common.

Type 1 Gaucher's disease (the adult or non-neuronopathic form) involves organs other than the brain, especially the spleen, liver and bone marrow. It is more common than *type 2* (the infantile or neuronopathic form) and *type 3* (the juvenile subacute neuronopathic form).

The basic pathological feature of Gaucher's disease is the accumulation of glucocerebroside within cells that are probably macrophages. Such cells (*Gaucher cells*) occur in almost all organs and may be up to 100 μm in diameter and contain one or more nuclei. There is coarse fibrillary material in the cytoplasm which stains positively with PAS due to the presence of cerebroside; it is also acid phosphatase positive. Electron microscopy[136] reveals the presence of tubular arrangements due to the accumulation of cerebroside in the cytoplasm.

In the adult (type 1) form of the disease there is hepatosplenomegaly, and Gaucher cells accumulate in bone, predisposing to fractures and destruction of vertebrae. In the severe infantile form (type 2), glucocerebroside and ganglioside accumulate in the spleen and liver but not in the brain, although Gaucher cells containing cerebroside are present in the cortex and perivascular regions of the brain.[137] There is loss of neurons and gliosis in the cerebral cortex, basal ganglia and brainstem but no evidence of lipid storage within the neurons. In this form of the disease, the neuronal destruction is more pronounced than the lipid storage.

Diagnosis of Gaucher's disease may be made by bone marrow and liver biopsy showing the presence of PAS-positive lipid and high levels of acid phosphatase activity within the cells. Prenatal diagnosis can be made by detecting the enzyme defect in amniotic fluid cells, and postnatal diagnosis is confirmed by demonstrating the enzyme defect in leucocytes and cultured fibroblasts.

Neuronal ceroid lipofuscinosis (Batten's disease, Kufs' disease)

The term neuronal ceroid lipofuscinosis is applied to this heterogeneous group of diseases which exhibit a common pathology, i.e. the accumulation of ceroid or lipofuscin-like material within neurons.[14,138] Most forms of the disease show an autosomal recessive pattern of inheritance but occasionally dominant forms occur.[139] No consistent abnormality in the chemical analysis of the brain has been found and, as yet, no enzyme defect has been identified.

There are several different forms of the disease and their clinical features vary from family to family. In the rapidly progressive *infantile* form (Batten's disease), there is psychomotor retardation with ataxia starting at 8 months and progressing to death within 3–10 years. Microcephaly is common. In the *late infantile*, *juvenile* and *adult* forms there is less rapid progression of neuro-

logical signs, often with impaired vision, progressive dementia, ataxia and epilepsy.[14]

Pathological changes in the brain are most severe in the infantile form, with gross atrophy of the cerebrum and cerebellum. Neuronal cytoplasm is filled with finely granular brown PAS-positive lipfuscin, although the cell bodies are not ballooned. As neurons are lost, there is gliosis and loss of cerebral white matter. The basal ganglia, brainstem and spinal cord are relatively well preserved. Lipofuscin granules in macrophages in other organs, and in the neurons of the brain and gut wall, can be stained with Sudan black B and PAS and for acid phosphatase. The granules also exhibit autofluorescence and are stained by Luxol–fast-blue in most types except the infantile form of the disease. Electron microscopy shows curvilinear bodies in neurons, astrocytes and oligodendrocytes in the late infantile form,[140] finger print and curvilinear bodies in the juvenile form[141] but no clear ultrastructural uniformity in the deposits of the adult (Kufs') form.[142]

The diagnosis of ceroid lipofuscinosis can be made on rectal biopsy by showing the presence of lipofuscin material in the neurons or by the presence, in some forms of the disease, of vacuolated lymphocytes.

Metachromatic leucodystrophy (sulphatide lipidosis)

In most cases of this disorder there is an autosomal recessive inheritance pattern, but some cases are dominant. *Infantile, juvenile* and *adult* forms are described,[143] with gait disturbances, psychomotor retardation, and educational and behavioural disorders. Adult cases present with psychoses and dementia.[144] CT scan may show decreased attenuation in the cerebral white matter of severely affected individuals. There is slowing of peripheral nerve conduction velocities due to segmental demyelination in all forms of the disease.

There is a deficiency of *arylsulphatase A*[125,144] or possibly a defect in an activator of this enzyme.[145] *Cerebroside sulphate* (*sulphatide*) accumulates in the white matter of the brain and in the peripheral nerves and kidneys.[14]

At post mortem, the brain shows a dull chalky discoloration of the cerebral white matter with a clear demarcation from the cortex. Microscopically, there is loss of myelin, and clusters of macrophages in the white matter containing PAS-positive, metachromatic lipid. Various stains can be used to demonstrate the metachromasia: the abnormal accumulations of cerebroside sulphate show brown metachromasia when stained with acidified cresyl fast violet[146] or with toluidine blue;[14] they stain orange with acriflavine.[40,147] Macrophages and Schwann cells in peripheral nerves contain metachromatic lipid[148] and the presence of lipid is accompanied by segmental demyelination.[149] The lipid has a distinctive electron microscope appearance of stacked discs (Fig. 12.25), known as *Tuffstein inclusions* from their resemblance to the volcanic rocks that are known by this German name.[150]

Diagnosis of the disease may be suspected from the presence of birefringent metachromatic lipid in renal tubular cells discharged into the urine or from the detection of arylsulphatase A deficiency in urine, leucocytes or cultured fibroblasts.[14,125] Sural nerve biopsy is also diagnostic,[40,149] showing segmental demyelination and characteristic metachromatic lipid deposits.

Mucosulphatidosis is a variant of metachromatic leucodystrophy[151] and is characterised by an absence of arylsulphatases A and B and the accumulation of sulphatide mucopolysaccharides. Gangliosides are also found in neurons in this disease.

Krabbe's leucodystrophy (globoid cell leucodystrophy)

This is an autosomal recessive disorder which presents mostly in infancy, at about the age of 4 months, with violent tonic spasms as a reaction to noise or lights and with opisthotonos and myoclonus.[8,14] There is retinal involvement with optic atrophy and blindness; the patients become decerebrate and usually die before the age of 2 years. There is a defect in the activity of the lysosomal enzyme *galactocerebroside β-galactosidase* in the grey and white matter of the brain and in the liver and spleen.[125,152] Deficiency of this enzyme in the serum, leucocytes, fibroblasts and amniotic cells can be used as a diagnostic test.[153]

Pathologically, the brain may be shrunken and there is demyelination of the white matter but subcortical fibres are preserved (Fig. 12.26). Microscopically, there is no storage of lipid in the cortex but the white matter shows gross loss of myelin with gliosis and the presence of *globoid cells*.[14,40] Early in the disease, the globoid cells are mononuclear but often become multinucleate and up to 50 μm in diameter (Fig. 12.26). They accumulate around blood vessels and, as myelin is lost from the white matter and the oligodendrocytes die, globoid cells increase in number, although they subsequently decrease in longstanding cases. Globoid cells are derived from macrophages and their cytoplasm is filled by PAS-positive, weakly sudanophilic *galactocerebroside*. Intense acid phosphatase activity is seen in the cytoplasm. There is often very little evidence of myelin breakdown products within the white matter of longstanding cases as the myelin loss is a combination of myelin breakdown (demyelination) and inhibition of myelin-

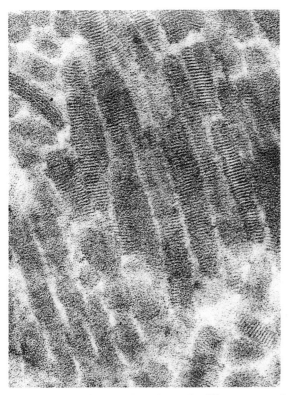

Fig. 12.25 Metachromatic leucodystrophy. Ultrastructure of the lipid deposits showing a lamellar pattern with a 5–6 nm periodicity in the form of stacked discs.
Electron micrograph × 160 000

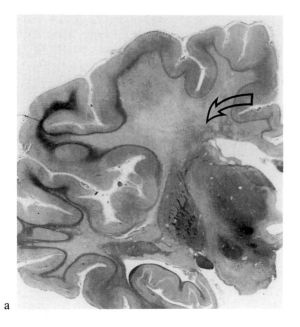

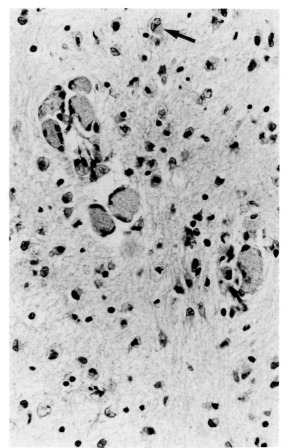

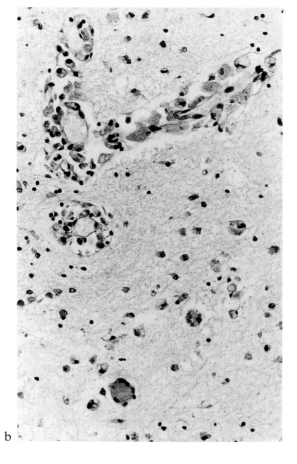

Fig. 12.26a–c Krabbe's globoid cell leucodystrophy.
(**a**) Histological section stained for myelin showing
demyelination in the cerebral white matter (arrow) but with
preservation of a dark line of myelin in the subcortical
regions. (**b**) Cerebral white matter showing the perivascular
accumulation of mononuclear globoid cells (top) and a
multinucleate globoid cell (bottom). (**c**) Multinuclear globoid
cells in the white matter. Mononuclear macrophages and
reactive astrocytes (arrow—top) in the gliotic white matter.
(**b**, **c**) Haematoxylin-eosin (**b**) ×240; (**c**) ×300

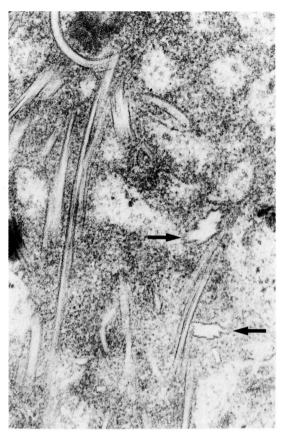

Fig. 12.27 Krabbe's globoid cell leucodystrophy. Ultrastructure of the lipid inclusions showing straight and curved tubular profiles. Irregular crystalloid profiles (arrows).
Electron micrograph × 74 350
Reproduced by permission of the author, editor and publishers from: Suzuki K. In: Johannessen JV, ed. Electron microscopy in human medicine. New York: McGraw-Hill, 1980; 6: 3 (Fig. 1.29).

ation (dysmyelination). There is little neuronal loss except in the dentate nuclei of the cerebellum. Electron microscopy of the lipid inclusions shows straight or curved tubular profiles which have an irregular crystalloid profile on cross-section (Fig. 12.27).[154,155]

Globoid cells accumulate in other organs but are not seen in peripheral nerves despite the segmental demyelination and accumulation of lipid within endoneurial macrophages.[14]

Although high concentrations of galacto-cerebroside, a component of myelin, accumulate within globoid cells, this does not appear to be the main cause of the demyelination and loss of oligo-dendrocytes. Other lipids accumulate, most especially *psychosine* (galactosylsphingosine) and *lactosylceramide*, due to the enzyme defect. It is thought that the presence of psychosine in large amounts is toxic to oligodendrocytes: the loss of these cells results in demyelination and prevents myelination.[156]

Fabry's disease (angiokeratoma corporis diffusum)

This disorder has an X-linked recessive inheritance pattern and is due to a deficiency of α-galactosidase A.[125] It presents in infancy or childhood but is not associated with mental retardation.[157] Angiokeratomas occur on the skin. Severe crises occur, with pains in the hands, feet and abdomen. Lipid composed of birefringent droplets of *trihexosyl ceramide* accumulates in cerebral vessel walls. A similar accumulation in perineurial and endothelial cells in peripheral nerves is associated with peripheral neuropathy and axonal degeneration, mainly involving large myelinated fibres.[158] Extensive lipid deposits occur in the kidneys and renal failure may supervene.

Faber's lipogranulomatosis

Characterised by painful swelling of joints, subcutaneous nodules, hoarse cry, respiratory problems, feeding difficulties and psychomotor retardation in the early months of life,[159] this disease is due to a defect in lysosomal *ceramidase*.[125] Free *ceramide* accumulates in neurons as strongly PAS-positive, weakly sudanophilic birefringent droplets.[14] The basal ganglia, brainstem and anterior horn cells of the spinal cord are affected by the neuronal storage more than the cerebral cortex and neurons of the gastrointestinal tract. Lamellated 'zebra bodies' are found by electron microscopy in neurons and endothelial cells.[14]

Mucopolysaccharidoses (MPS)

There are seven types of mucopolysaccharidosis, classified according to the inherited enzyme defect.[14] All types are characterised by storage of glycosaminoglycans (mucopolysaccharides) within lysosomes in most tissues and organs, and by the presence of glycosaminoglycans (GAG) in the urine. Prenatal diagnosis may be made by the analysis of GAG in amniotic fluid or by the detection of enzyme defects in cultured amniotic cells from the age of 14 weeks gestation.[14] One type, Hurler's disease, has an X-linked recessive inheritance pattern; all other mucopolysaccharidoses have autosomal recessive inheritance.

Mental retardation in childhood is seen in Hurler's disease (MPSI-H), Hunter's disease (MPSII) and Sanfilippo's disease (MPSIII). Other types of MPS show no mental retardation, but bone changes are present and nerve compression may occur.[124]

Hurler's disease presents at around 6 months of age and is the most severe form of mucopolysaccharidosis affecting the nervous system. There is mental retardation, a large head, coarse features, skeletal deformities, large tongue, thickened gums, hepatosplenomegaly, cardiac abnormalities and corneal opacities. Death usually occurs in the first decade of life. The disorder is a defect in the degradation of dermatan sulphate and heparan sulphate, due to a deficiency of *α-L-iduronidase*.[160]

Hunter's disease resembles Hurler's disease but is less severe and there are no corneal opacities. As in Hurler's disease, there is a defect in the degradation of dermatan sulphate and heparan sulphate, both of which are excreted in the urine. There is a deficiency of *idurono-2-sulphate-sulphatase*.[161]

Sanfilippo's disease is characterised by progressive mental retardation which may not become apparent until the first or second year. Deficiencies in at least four enzymes have been identified[162] and there is defective heparan sulphate degradation.

There is accumulation of glycosaminoglycans (GAG) in many organs in MPS but, as these substances are water-soluble, they are extracted during preparation of tissue for pathological examination, leaving ballooned cells. Macroscopically, affected brains may show vacuolation around blood vessels in the white matter. Microscopically, there is ballooning of neurons so that they resemble those in Tay–Sachs disease. GAG does not accumulate within the brain but there is an increase in gangliosides G_{M2} and G_{M3}. *Ganglioside storage* in the neurons can be detected throughout the brain, spinal cord and ganglia of the gut by PAS, Sudan black and Luxol–fast-blue stains on frozen sections. Electron microscopically, neurons contain membranous cytoplasmic bodies (see p. 342) and zebra bodies.[163]

Diagnosis can be made by estimating GAG in the urine, demonstrating enzyme defects in leucocytes and fibroblasts, and by the specific granulation of leucocytes in the peripheral blood.[14]

Mucolipidoses

These diseases resemble the mucopolysaccharidoses and the lipidoses. For example, Austin sulphatidosis presents with a disease similar to metachromatic leucodystrophy but with the physical features of a mucopolysaccharidosis and the presence of GAG in the urine. There are several different lysosomal enzyme disorders in this group of diseases.[124]

Other lysosomal disorders affecting the nervous system

Fucosidosis, due to a deficiency of α-fucosidase,[164] presents with psychomotor retardation, progressing to decerebrate rigidity. There is storage of fucose-containing glycolipid with cardiomegaly and skin thickening. *Mannosidosis* resembles Hurler's syndrome and is due to a deficiency in α-mannosidase.[165] *Type II glycogenosis*, due to a deficiency in the lysosomal enzyme, acid α-1,4 glucosidase (acid maltase), presents with a wide clinical spectrum of disease. In its severe infantile form (*Pompe's disease*) there is accumulation of glycogen in cardiac and skeletal muscle and in anterior horn cells, cranial nerve nuclei and parts of the basal ganglia and in neurons in the gastrointestinal tract.[166]

LEUCODYSTROPHIES

In this group of diseases, the cerebral white matter is selectively damaged and shows demyelination with loss of myelin sheaths but relative preservation of axons. Widespread gliosis occurs throughout the affected white matter. Many of these diseases were grouped originally under the heading of *Schilder's cerebral sclerosis*, but as metabolic disorders and enzyme defects responsible for the white matter damage have become apparent, separate disease categories have been created.

Metachromatic leucodystrophy (sulphatide lipidosis), due to a deficiency of arylsulphatase activity, and *Krabbe's globoid cell leucodystrophy*, associated with reduced levels of galacto-cerebroside β-galactosidase, have been described in the section on lysosomal enzyme deficiency diseases (see p. 344, 345).

Adrenoleucodystrophy

Peroxisomal disorders, in which there is dysfunction of one or more aspects of peroxisomal metabolism, may result in central nervous system disease.[167] Examples include X-linked recessive adrenoleucodystrophy (ALD), infantile Refsum's disease, Zellweger's syndrome and neonatal ALD.

Adrenoleucodystrophy (ALD) can be subdivided into five major clinical types,[168] namely, classical X-linked juvenile ALD, X-linked adult ALD, adrenomyeloneuropathic variant, female ALD and neonatal ALD. A fetal form has also been described.[168] Patients present clinically with visual and motor deterioration and Addison's disease; death may supervene within 5 years. CT scan shows decreased density in the cerebral white matter. At post mortem, the white matter in the hemispheres shows grey discoloration (Fig. 12.28), particularly in the occipital and parietal regions. Subcortical arcuate fibres are preserved.

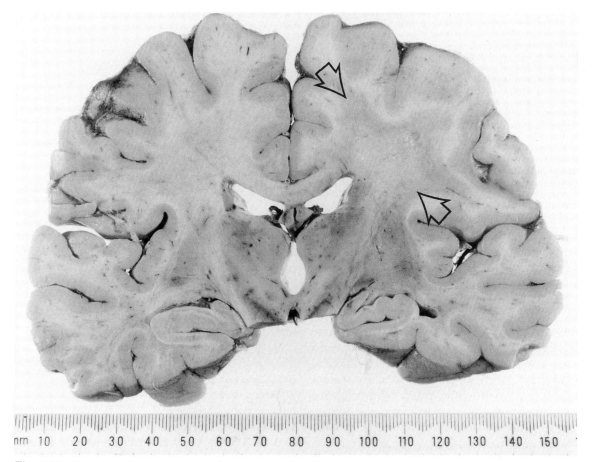

Fig. 12.28 Adrenoleucodystrophy: 45-year-old man. Coronal section of the brain through the frontoparietal region showing grey discoloration of the demyelinated white matter in the right hemisphere (arrows) but with preservation of the subcortical fibres.

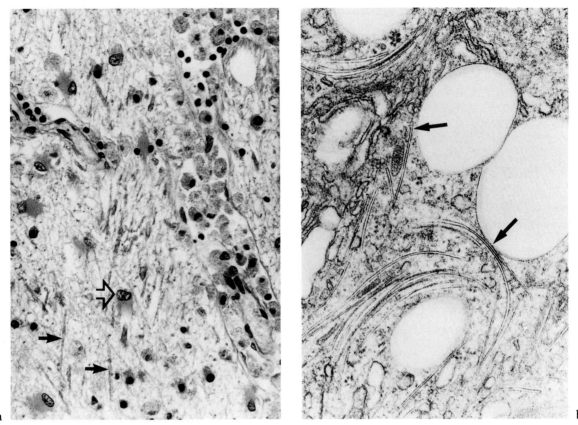

a   b

Fig. 12.29a, b Adrenoleucodystrophy. (**a**) Cerebral white matter showing numerous perivascular foamy macrophages (top and right), reactive astrocytes (open arrow) and preserved axons (solid arrows). (**b**) Trilamellar inclusions (arrow) in the cytoplasm of a macrophage in the brain.
(**a**) Haematoxylin-eosin × 300; (**b**) Electron micrograph × 36 000
Reproduced by permission of Dr K. Suzuki, University of North Carolina, USA

Microscopy of the brain reveals loss of myelin and relative preservation of axons in the cerebral white matter, but the areas of demyelination are not as sharply defined as in multiple sclerosis (see p. 231). Foamy macrophages abound and there is reactive astrocytosis with processes of astrocytes orientated along axonal tracts (Fig. 12.29). Some loss of axons does occur in the white matter and there is atrophy and secondary degeneration of the corticospinal tracts in the brainstem and spinal cord. Neurons in the cortex are well preserved but there may be loss of neurons from the hippocampus, dentate nucleus and the lateral and medial geniculate bodies.[169] Electron microscopy of macrophages in the white matter of the brain reveals characteristic trilamellar inclusions in the cytoplasm (Fig. 12.29).

There is extensive loss of cells from the adrenal cortex, although the zona glomerulosa may be relatively spared; the adrenal medulla is usually unaffected. Adrenocortical cells, particularly those in the zona fasciculata and zona reticularis, become ballooned due to the accumulation of lamellar lipid.[168]

In the *adrenomyeloneuropathic* form of the disease, there is extensive loss of axons from long ascending and descending tracts of the spinal cord. Axonal degeneration is present in the peripheral nerves, with lamellar inclusions in Schwann cells surrounding intact axons.[168]

Patients with X-linked ALD and those with the adrenomyeloneuropathic form of the disease have a defect in the degradation of very long chain fatty acids, probably due to a deficiency in the enzymes of the peroxisomal β-oxidation system. It is possible that the accumulation of the fatty acids plays a rôle in the pathogenesis of the disease.[168] Prenatal diagnosis and the identification of female carriers of the disease are possible through the detection of abnormal amounts of very long chain fatty acids in amniotic cells and skin fibroblasts.[170]

Alexander's disease

This distinctive leucodystrophy presents sporadically in infancy or childhood with progressive dementia, epilepsy and paralysis. There is decreased attenuation of the white matter on CT scan, and extensive demyelination throughout the white matter with little or no preservation of the subcortical arcuate fibres. The histology is characteristic, with large numbers of Rosenthal fibres arranged around blood vessels and on the surface of the brain in the glia limitans (Fig. 12.30). The Rosenthal fibres (see p. 54) are brightly eosinophilic and stain strongly with Luxol fast blue.[171] The metabolic defect is, as yet, unknown.

Cavitating sudanophil leucodystrophy

This probably represents a heterogeneous group of diseases. Patients may present clinically in infancy or in adult life with neurodevelopmental retardation or dementia. On CT scan, the white matter shows decreased attenuation. At autopsy, there is extensive loss of myelin, with oedema of the cerebral white matter (Fig. 12.31). Cavitation may be seen. The cerebellum is also involved.[172] Microscopically, there is loss of myelin but relative preservation of the axons. Foamy macrophages containing sudanophil lipid are seen at the periphery of the lesions but such cells may be uncommon in the central, more cystic, areas of the white matter. An increase in oligodendrocytes may be seen. In some cases a metabolic disorder such as pyruvate carboxylase deficiency has been identified,[173] but in many cases the biochemical defect is unknown.

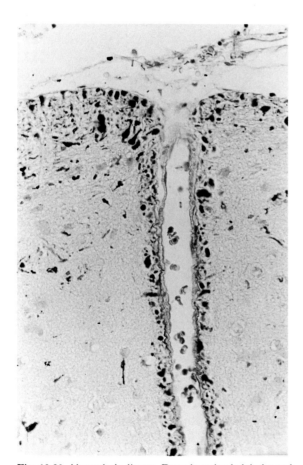

Fig. 12.30 Alexander's disease. Densely stained globular and elongated Rosenthal fibres are seen at the surface of the cerebral cortex (top) and in the glia limitans surrounding a blood vessel (centre).
Klüver–Barrera × 300

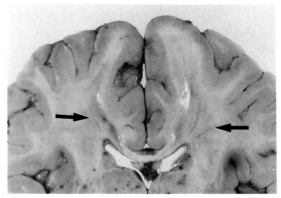

Fig. 12.31 Cavitating sudanophil leucodystrophy. The cerebral hemispheres of a 4-year-old child showing shrinkage and softening of the white matter in the centrum semiovale of both hemispheres (arrows).

Pelizaeus–Merzbacher disease

This is a group of rare diseases which differ clinically and in their mode of inheritance but have a similar pathological appearance in the brain, with patchy demyelination and sparing of perivascular islands of myelin. There are six types;[174] type 5 is X-linked recessive, and type 4 is dominant in inheritance pattern. The disease presents with developmental retardation or dementia in infancy, with death in about 5 years. The brain is atrophic at post mortem and shows a tigroid pattern of demyelination,[175] with small islands of myelin preserved around the blood vessels. There is extensive gliosis but little sign of myelin breakdown products within the affected areas. Axons are relatively well preserved.

Type 6 is *Cockayne's syndrome*,[176] with multiple abnormalities including dwarfism, cataracts, segmental demyelinating peripheral neuropathy and intracranial calcification. There is mental retardation and progressive neurological and retinal degeneration. Skin fibroblasts and amniotic cells are hypersensitive to ultraviolet light[177] and this test forms the basis of prenatal and postnatal diagnosis.

NEUROAXONAL DYSTROPHIES

This group of apparently related disorders is characterised by the formation of dystrophic axon swellings or spheroids similar to those seen following trauma to axons (see p. 131). These appearances suggest that axoplasmic transport is disturbed.

In *infantile* neuroaxonal dystrophy, there is arrest of development at about one year of age, progressive motor disability, dementia and blindness. Half the cases are familial and the metabolic defect is unknown. Widespread axonal swellings 20–60 μm in diameter are seen histologically and are detectable as hyaline, eosinophilic spheroids or, by silver techniques, as strongly argyrophilic bodies. The grey matter areas are most severely affected, particularly the nuclei of the tegmentum of the brainstem and those of the spinal cord. Spheroids are inconspicuous in the cerebral cortex. Cerebellar atrophy with loss of Purkinje

cells is usually present. Electron microscopy suggests that there is also synaptic degeneration.

There are several types of neuroaxonal dystrophy,[178] including the juvenile and adult types of *Hallervorden–Spatz disease*.[179] Hallervorden–Spatz disease may be considered as a localised form of neuroaxonal dystrophy with progressive rigidity, often accompanied by choreoathetotic movement, as a presenting manifestation in the second decade. Progressive dementia and epilepsy are also features. Pathologically, this familial condition is characterised by a rust-coloured pigmentation of the globus pallidus and of the reticular zone of the substantia nigra. Intracellular pigment which stains strongly with the Perls technique for iron is present in the basal ganglia where there is encrustation of blood vessels. Other parts of the brain may also be affected. Axonal spheroids are seen, particularly in the basal ganglia.[179]

OTHER METABOLIC DISEASES

A number of other disorders due to enzyme defects affect the nervous system.

Leigh's disease (infantile subacute necrotising encephalopathy)

First described by Leigh[180] in 1951, this disease is an autosomal recessive disorder with clinical onset usually before the age of 2 years. Adolescent and adult cases have also been described.[179] Patients suffer psychomotor arrest, feeding difficulties, ataxia, loss of vision, external ophthalmoplegia and hypotonia. Pathologically,[181] there is symmetrical damage to the grey matter, particularly in the basal ganglia and diencephalon but also affecting the spinal cord and cerebellum. Microscopic lesions are similar to those seen in Wernicke's encephalopathy (see p. 286) but with a different distribution. Vascular and endothelial proliferation is observed with degeneration of axons, dendrites and myelin sheaths. The degenerative lesions produce areas of low attenuation in the basal ganglia on CT scans. Patients with this disorder have an inhibitor of the mitochondrial enzyme thiamine pyrophosphate-adenosine tri-phosphate phosphoryl transferase in the urine, CSF and blood. This enzyme converts thiamine pyrophosphate to thiamine triphosphate. The inhibitor can also be detected in fibroblasts. It is uncertain whether the inhibitor is the cause of the cerebral lesions: another enzyme defect may be present.[179] 'Ragged-red' fibres containing excessive mitochondria have been reported in muscle biopsies in Leigh's disease.[179]

Menkes' kinky hair disease

This X-linked recessive disorder is characterised by mental and growth retardation and by erect, undulating hair. There is hypocupraemia due to an impaired absorption of copper.[182] Pathologically, the brain is atrophic and shows patchy areas of necrosis and neuronal loss in the cortex. Heterotopia of neurons in the cerebellum and widespread gliosis are also present. Dendritic abnormalities in the Purkinje cells of the cerebellum have also been described.[183]

Disorders of amino acid metabolism

Pathological changes in this group of disorders are rather non-specific.[184] *Phenylketonuria* is a heterogeneous group of disorders characterised by hyperphenylalaninaemia;[13] there is microcephaly with gliosis and spongiosis of the white matter, probably due to delayed myelination. Delay in postnatal neuronal development also occurs.

In *maple syrup disease*[185] children fail to thrive; there is profound acidosis and a characteristic smell to the urine like that of maple syrup. Metabolically, there is a defect in branched chain amino acid metabolism, and pathologically there may be spongiform change in the cerebral white matter. Crystalline proteins may be detected in the cytoplasm of glial cells in alcohol-fixed material.

Urea cycle abnormalities[13]

Brain damage is variable in these (see p. 302). Neurons in the grey matter may be affected rather more than the white matter.

HYPOTHYROIDISM AND IODINE DEFICIENCY

The most important endocrine disorder to affect the central nervous system in children is hypothyroidism;[13] it is accompanied by dwarfism and mental defect (hypothyroid cretinism). A far more common disorder worldwide is *endemic cretinism* due to iodine deficiency. In some severely iodine deficient areas in India, Indonesia and China, daily iodine intake falls below $20\,\mu g$ in contrast to a normal intake of $80-150\,\mu g$.[186] In its fully developed form, endemic cretinism is characterised by mental deficiency, deaf-mutism and spastic diplegia. It can be prevented by iodine supplements during pregnancy. The few neuropathological studies of endemic cretinism show a reduced brain weight and retarded maturation of cerebral and cerebellar cortices. The critical time for the effect of iodine deficiency upon the brain is 14–18 weeks of gestation.[186]

PHACOMATOSES

Gathered under this heading is a group of disorders characterised by malformations and tumours involving mainly the nervous system and other ectodermal structures such as skin and the eyes. Many of them have a genetic basis.[8]

Neurofibromatosis

Two separate disorders are included here, namely, von Recklinghausen's neurofibromatosis (peripheral neurofibromatosis) and bilateral acoustic neurofibromatosis (central neurofibromatosis). They differ in their incidence, in the distribution of abnormalities, and in the chromosomal location of the genetic defect.

Von Recklinghausen's (peripheral) neurofibromatosis

The disorder is characterised by café au lait spots on the skin, which arise early in childhood. Patients develop skin neurofibromas (see p. 469) in increasing numbers through childhood and adult life. Bluish hamartomas of the iris (Lisch nodules) also occur. The estimated prevalence of von Recklinghausen's peripheral neuro-fibromatosis is 1:3000.[187] There is a great variation in the severity of the disease, from minor skin abnormalities to severe disfigurement.[8,188] Among the complications are mental retardation in as many as 45% of patients, epilepsy in 10% and kyphoscoliosis with spinal root compression in 12–40% of patients. Intracranial tumours, including cerebral gliomas, occur in 12–20% of cases, and optic nerve gliomas are seen in 15%.[188] Sarcomatous change occurs in the plexiform neurofibromas arising in peripheral nerves in 11–30% of cases.

There is an autosomal dominant pattern of inheritance with a high penetrance and variable expressivity; there is also a high mutation rate.[189,190] The gene responsible for von Reckling-hausen's peripheral neurofibromatosis has been located on the long arm of chromosome 17 near the centromere and linked to the locus encoding for nerve growth factor.[189,190] There is no hetero-geneity, which suggests that the mutation is at a single gene locus. It is unlikely, however, that mutation of the nerve growth factor gene is the fundamental defect responsible for the von Recklinghausen neurofibromatosis pheno-type.[189,190]

Bilateral acoustic (central) neurofibromatosis

This disease has a prevalence of 0·1 per 100 000,[188] and is very much less common than the peripheral disorder. Patients present with multiple intra-cranial and intraspinal tumours which are mainly schwannomas and meningiomas. Bilateral acoustic schwannomas (neuromas) are common but skin lesions are uncommon. In those patients with multiple intracranial tumours the prognosis is poor,[8] but the prognosis is better when bilateral acoustic schwannomas are the sole manifestation of the disease.

Analysis of tissue from acoustic schwannomas and meningiomas in this condition has shown a gene deletion on chromosome 22,[191] associated with an abnormality of glial growth factor activity.[192] A disorder of nerve growth factor has been detected in both the peripheral and central varieties of neurofibromatosis.[193]

Tuberous sclerosis

Occurring with a frequency in the United Kingdom of 1:15 000,[194] tuberous sclerosis shows considerable variability in its presentation. Most prominent is the combination of neurological and dermatological features.[195] *White macules* of hypo-pigmentation occur on the skin in infancy. Other skin lesions, including *adenoma sebaceum* (fibro-angiomatous nodules), occur on the skin of the face, and dense plaques of collagen (*shagreen patches*) are seen on the trunk and buttocks in adolescence and adult life. *Subungual angio-fibromas* are also found. *Angiomyolipomas* of the kidneys occur and may reach a considerable size. Pits in the enamel of the teeth may also be seen.[8] Patients may present clinically with mental retard-ation and epilepsy.

The pathological changes in the central nervous system consist of gliotic tubers forming irregular superficial thickenings of portions of the gyri (Fig. 12.32), frequently with calcification (Fig. 12.33) deep within the tuber. Para-ventricular nodules are also seen.[14] Histologically, the tubers consist of areas of dense gliosis with large reactive astrocytes staining positively for glial fibrillary acidic protein. Characteristic of the lesions, however, are huge, plump cells, often with numerous short processes which contain vimentin intermediate filaments (Fig. 12.33) but not usually glial fibrillary acidic protein.[40] These cells could represent an immature stage of astrocyte develop-ment.

Tumours of the thalamus, showing the typical histology of a subependymal astrocytoma, occur in 5% of patients with tuberous sclerosis (see p. 436 and Fig. 16.7). Rhabdomyomas of the heart also occur in this disease, and may be a cause of sudden death.

Autosomal dominant inheritance is seen in this condition but 70–90% of cases are new mutations. The tuberous sclerosis gene is linked to an oncogene on the long arm of chromosome 9.[196,197]

Ataxia telangiectasia

This condition presents in infancy or childhood with progressive cerebellar ataxia and involuntary movements. Telangiectases of the skin and conjunctiva appear following the onset of ataxia. Pathological examination of the brain reveals atrophy of the cerebellar cortex with loss of Purkinje cells and granule cells.[198] Atrophy of the posterior columns of the spinal cord is also seen and there may be multiple tiny angiomas in the brain. Angiomatous lesions are also seen in other organs.

Ataxia telangiectasia is inherited as an autosomal recessive disorder.[198] The patients have a reduced level of IgA in the serum and other fluids and hypoplasia of the thymus. Malignant lymphoma is a common complication.[199]

Von Hippel–Lindau disease

This is an autosomal dominant disorder[200] in which there is angiomatosis of the retina and haemangioblastomas of the cerebellum and spinal cord (see p. 476). Cysts occur in the pancreas and kidneys and there is an increased incidence of phaeochromocytoma and renal carcinoma.[14] The renal carcinomas are often multifocal and frequently cause death of the patient at an early age.[201]

The von Hippel–Lindau gene is linked to a locus encoding the human homologue of the RAFI oncogene which maps to chromosome 3p25. The

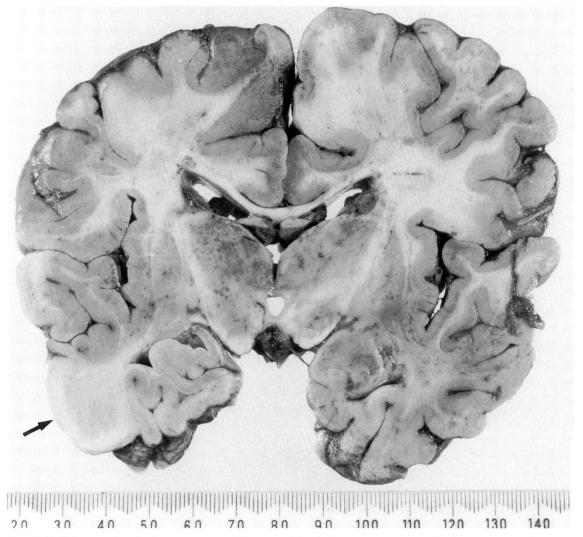

Fig. 12.32 Tubcrous sclerosis. A coronal section of the cerebral hemispheres showing tubers. The largest is in the left temporal lobe (arrow) but other gyri show similar changes.

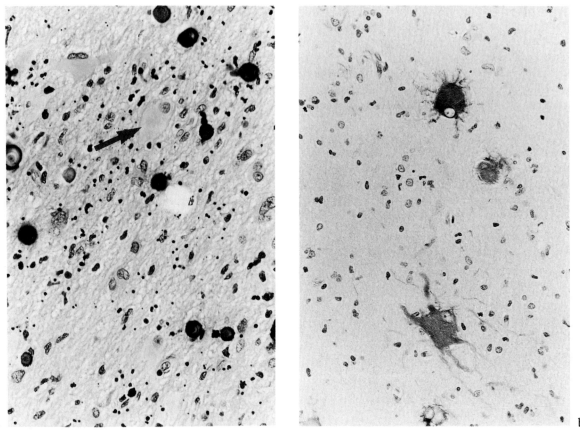

a   b

Fig. 12.33a, b Tuberous sclerosis—histology of a tuber. (**a**) Large, plump cells (arrow) are seen embedded in gliotic tissue and surrounded by densely staining calcospherites. (**b**) The plump cells contain vimentin intermediate filaments and show many short processes.
(**a**) Haematoxylin-eosin × 300; (**b**) Immunoperoxidase for vimentin × 240

defect causing von Hippel–Lindau disease appears to be on the short arm of chromosome 3 and may be related to loss of tumour suppressor factors.[201]

The Sturge–Weber–Dimitri syndrome (encephalofacial angiomatosis)

Strawberry naevus formation in the skin of the territory supplied by the 5th cranial nerve is associated with excessive vascularity and angiomatosis with numerous tortuous small veins in the meninges of the underlying cerebral hemisphere (see page 481). Calcification of the meningeal angiomatosis may be detectable on CT scan.[202] A variable degree of destruction of the brain associated with the meningeal angiomatosis occurs. Clinically, patients may present with epilepsy, mental retardation and hemiplegia.[14] There appears to be no genetic basis for the disease.[8]

REFERENCES

Development of the CNS

1. Hamilton WJ, Mossman HW. Hamilton, Boyd and Mossman's Human embryology. 4th ed. Cambridge: Heffer, 1972.
2. O'Rahilly R, Muller F. J Neuropathol Exp Neurol 1986; 45: 588.
3. Potter EL, Craig JM. Pathology of the fetus and the infant. 3rd ed. London: Lloyd-Luke, 1976.

Aetiology of brain damage in fetus and childhood

4. Creasey MR, Alberman ED. J Med Genet 1976; 13: 9.

5. Leck I. Br Med Bull 1974; 30: 158.
6. Taylor DJ, Howie PW, Davidson J et al. Lancet 1985; 1: 713.
7. Freytag E, Lindenberg R. Johns Hopkins Med J 1967; 121: 379.
8. Bundey S. Genetics and neurology. Edinburgh: Churchill Livingstone, 1985.
9. Baraitser M. The genetics of neurological disorders. Oxford: Oxford University Press, 1985.
10. Warkany J, Lemine L, Cohen MM. Mental retardation and congenital malformations of the central nervous system. Chicago: Year Book, 1981.
11. Edwards JH, Norman RM, Roberts JM. Arch Dis Child 1961; 36: 481.
12. Smith DW. Recognizable patterns of human malformation: genetic, embryonic and clinical aspects. 3rd ed. Philadelphia: Saunders, 1982.
13. Clayton BE. In: Weller RO, Swash M, McLellan DL, Scholtz CL, eds. Clinical neuropathology. Berlin: Springer, 1983: 203.
14. Lake BD. In: Adams JH, Corsellis JAN, Duchen LW, eds. Greenfield's Neuropathology. London: Arnold, 1984: 491.
15. Nicolaides KH, Rodeck CH, Gosden CM. Lancet 1986; 1: 283.
16. Modell B. Lancet 1985; 1: 737.
17. Julien C, Bazin A, Guyot B et al. Lancet 1986; 2: 863.
18. Crome L, Stern J. Pathology of mental retardation. 2nd ed. Edinburgh: Churchill Livingstone, 1972.
19. Larroche J-C. In: Adams JH, Corsellis JAN, Duchen LW, eds. Greenfield's Neuropathology. London: Arnold, 1984: 385.
20. Polani PE, Hamerton JL, Giannelli F, Carter CO. Cytogenetics 1965; 4: 193.
21. Leading article. Lancet 1985; 1: 855.
22. Wisniewski KE, Dalton AJ, Crapper N et al. Neurology 1985; 35: 957.
23. Takashima S, Becker LE. J Neurol Neurosurg Psychiatry 1985; 48: 61.
24. Kang J, Lemaire H-G, Unterbeck A et al. Nature 1987; 325: 733.
25. Robakis NK, Wisniewski HM, Jenkins EC et al. Lancet 1987; 1: 384.
26. Cowen D, Geller LM. J Neuropathol Exp Neurol 1960; 19: 488.
27. Miller RW. Pediatrics 1968; 41: 257.
28. Hicks SP. Physiol Rev 1958; 38: 337.
29. Swan C. J Obst. Gynae 1949; 56: 341.
30. Johnson RT. Viral infections of the nervous system. New York: Raven Press, 1982.
31. Diezel P. Virchows Arch Pathol Anat 1954; 325: 109.
32. Sabin AB, Feldman HA. J Pediatr 1948; 35: 296.
33. Wolf A, Cowen D. J Neuropathol Exp Neurol 1959; 18: 191.
34. Pratt O. Br Med J 1982; 38: 48.

Post-mortem examination

35. Mueller RF, Sybert VP, Johnson J et al. N Engl J Med 1983; 10: 586.
36. Bone J, Bone A, Lazar P. Teratology 1975; 12: 11.
37. Leading article. Lancet 1984; 1: 431.
38. Patrick AD. Br Med Bull 1983; 39: 378.
39. Williams PL, Warwick R. Gray's Anatomy. 36th ed. Edinburgh: Churchill Livingstone, 1980.
40. Weller RO. Colour atlas of neuropathology. Oxford: Miller & Oxford University Press, 1984.
41. Weller RO. A general approach to neuropathological problems. In: Berry CL, ed. Current topics in pathology. Berlin: Springer, 1988; 76: 61.

Patterns of damage

42. Brock DJH, Barron L, van Heyningen V. Lancet 1985; 1: 5.
43. Nakado KK. Dev Med Child Neurol 1973; 15: 383.
44. Nevin NC, Johnston WP, Merrett JD. Dev Med Child Neurol 1981; 23: 155.
45. Menzies RG, Parkin JM, Hey EN. Lancet 1985; 2: 993.
46. Leading article. Lancet 1986; 2: 549.
47. Volpe JJ, Adams RD. Acta Neuropathol 1972; 20: 175.
48. Larroche J-C. Biol Neonate 1986; 50: 61.
49. Cocker J, George SW, Yates PO. Dev Med Child Neurol 1965; 7: 235.
50. Friede RL. Developmental neuropathology. Vienna: Springer, 1975.
51. Larroche J-C. In: Adams JH, Corsellis JAN, Duchen LW, eds. Greenfield's Neuropathology. London: Arnold, 1984: 451.
52. Halsey JH, Allen N, Chamberlin HR. J Neurol Sci 1971; 12: 187.
53. Muir CS. Arch Dis Child 1959; 34: 231.
54. Weller RO, Shulman K. J Neurosurg 1972; 36: 255.
55. Weller RO, Wisniewski H, Shulman K, Terry RD. J Neuropathol Exp Neurol 1971; 30: 613.
56. Weller RO, Wisniewski H. Brain 1969; 92: 819.
57. Weller RO, Williams BN. Arch Dis Child 1975; 50: 763.
58. Margolis G, Kilham L. Lab Invest 1969; 21: 189.
59. Torvik A, Bhatia R, Murthy VS. Acta Neurochir (Wien) 1978; 41: 137.
60. Gardner E, O'Rahilly R, Prolo D. Arch Neurol 1975; 32: 393.
61. Benda CE. J Neuropathol Exp Neurol 1954; 13: 14.
62. D'Agostino AN, Kernohan JN, Brown JR. J Neuropathol Exp Neurol 1963; 22: 450.
63. Raimondi AJ, Soare P. Am J Dis Child 1974; 127: 664.
64. Walton JN. Brain's Diseases of the nervous system. Oxford: Oxford University Press, 1985.
65. Gardener WJ. The dysraphic states. Amsterdam: Excerpta Medica, 1973.
66. Ellis RS. J Comp Neurol 1920; 32: 1.
67. Rorke LB, Fogelson MH, Riggs H. Dev Med Child Neurol 1968; 10: 644.
68. Oppenheimer DR. J Neurol Neurosurg Psychiatr 1955; 18: 199.
69. Altman J. J Comp Neurol 1969; 136: 269.
70. Leviton A, Gilles FH. Ann Neurol 1984; 16: 1.
71. Trounce JQ, Fagan D, Levene MI. Arch Dis Child 1986; 61: 1203.
72. Hambleton G, Wigglesworth JS. Arch Dis Child 1976; 51: 651.
73. Thornburn RJ, Lipscomb AP, Stewart AL et al. Early Hum Dev 1982; 7: 221.
74. Leading article. Lancet 1984; 2: 847.
75. Trounce JQ, Rutter N, Levine MI. Arch Dis Child 1986; 61: 1196.
76. de Vries LS, Dubowitz LMS, Dubowitz V et al. Lancet 1985; 2: 137.
77. Papile LA, Burstein J, Burstein R, Koffler H. J Pediatr 1978; 92: 529.

78. Shankaran S, Slovis TL, Bedard MP, Poland RL. J Pediatr 1982; 100: 469.
79. Leech RW, Kohnen P. Am J Path 1974; 77: 465.
80. Wigglesworth JS, Pape KE. J Perinat Med 1980; 8: 119.
81. Leading article. Lancet 1985; 2: 1280.
82. Flodmark O, Scotti G, Harwood-Nash DC. J Comput Assist Tomogr 1981; 5: 663.
83. Allan WC, Dransfield DA, Tito AM. Pediatrics 1984; 73: 158.
84. McCullough DC, Balzer-Martin A. J Neurosurg 1982; 57: 378.
85. Larroche J-C. J Perinat Med 1982; 10 (suppl 2): 29.
86. Banker BQ, Larroche J-C. Arch Neurol 1962; 7: 386.
87. Lacey DJ, Terplan K. Dev Med Child Neurol 1982; 24: 332.
88. Laurence KM, Cavanagh JB. Brain 1968; 91: 261.
89. Friede RL. Acta Neuropathol 1973; 23: 245.
90. Barmarda MA, Moossy J, Shuman FM. Ann Neurol 1979; 6: 495.
91. Friede R. J Neuropathol Exp Neurol 1972; 31: 548.
92. Shulman ST, Madden JD, Shanklin DR, Esterly JR. Arch Dis Child 1971; 46: 291.
93. Chapman GP, Weller RO, Normand ICS. Br Med J 1978; 2: 398.
94. Kaplan HA, Ford DH. The brain vascular system. Amsterdam: Elsevier, 1966.
95. Jellinger K, Kucsko L, Seitelberger F. Beitr Pathol Anat 1966; 133: 41.
96. Karch SB, Urich H. J Neurol Sci 1972; 15: 89.
97. Long DM, Seljeskog EL, Chou SN, French LA. J Neurosurg 1974; 40: 304.
98. Siqueira EB, Murray KJ. Neurochirurgia 1972; 15: 106.
99. Silverman BK, Breck T, Craig J, Nadas AS. Am J Dis Child 1955; 89: 539.
100. Scott JM. Br Med J 1968; 2: 827.
101. Stern L. Pediatrics 1972; 49: 916.
102. van Bogaert L. Acta Neurol Belg 1949; 49: 961.
103. Dekaban A, O'Rourke J, Corman T. Neurology 1958; 8: 387.
104. Ornoy A, Segal S, Nishini M et al. Am J Obstet Gynecol 1973; 116: 949.
105. Cooper LZ, Krugman S. Arch Ophthalmol 1967; 77: 434.
106. Monif GRG, Sever JL. Neurology 1966; 16: 111.
107. Naeye RL, Blanc W. JAMA 1965; 194: 1277.
108. McCracken GH, Shinefield HR, Cobb R et al. Am J Dis Child 1969; 117: 522.
109. Haymaker W, Girdany BR, Stephens J et al. J Neuropathol Exp Neurol 1954; 13: 362.
110. Anzil AP, Blinzinger K, Dozic S. Virchows Arch Pathol Anat 1970; 351: 233.
111. Frenkel JK. Curr Top Pathol 1971; 54: 28.
112. Binford CH, Connor DH. Pathology of tropical and extraordinary diseases. Washington DC: AFIP, 1976.
113. Overall JC. J Pediatr 1970; 76: 499.
114. Fitzhardinge PM, Kazemi M, Ramsay M, Stern L. Dev Med Child Neurol 1974; 16: 3.
115. Berman PH, Banker BQ. Pediatrics 1966; 38: 6.
116. Barber M, Okubajedo OA. Br Med J 1965; 2: 735.

Brain trauma in infancy

117. Lindenberg R, Freytag L. Arch Pathol 1969; 87: 298.
118. Vowles G, Scholtz CL. J Clin Pathol 1987; 40: 185.

Sudden infant death syndrome

119. Leading article. Lancet 1984; 2: 558.
120. Arneil GC, Brooke H, Gibson AAM et al. Lancet 1985; 1: 740.
121. Valdes-Dapena M. Am J Pathol 1982; 106: 118.
122. Takashima S, Armstrong D, Becker LE, Huber J. Pediatrics 1978; 62: 155.

Inborn errors of metabolism

123. Raine DN. J Clin Pathol 1974; 27 (suppl 8): 156.
124. Whiteman PD. In: Weller RO, Swash M, McLellan DL, Scholtz CL, eds. Clinical neuropathology. Berlin: Springer, 1983: 215.
125. Glew RH, Basu A, Prence EM, Remaley AT. Lab Invest 1985; 53: 250.
126. Rapin I, Suzuki K, Suzuki K, Valsamin MP. Arch Neurol 1976; 33: 120.
127. Purpura DP, Suzuki K. Brain Res 1976; 116: 1.
128. Terry RD, Weiss M. J Neuropathol Exp Neurol 1963; 22: 18.
129. Crocker AC. J Neurochem 1961; 7: 69.
130. Schneider PB, Kennedy DP. J Lipid Res 1967; 8: 202.
131. Elleder M, Jirasek A. Eur J Pediatr 1983; 140: 90.
132. Elleder M, Lojda Z. Histochemie 1973; 36: 149.
133. Wallace BJ, Schneck L, Kaplan H, Volk BW. Arch Pathol 1965; 80: 466.
134. Patrick AD, Young E, Kleijer WT, Niermeijer MF. Lancet 1977; 2: 144.
135. Hagberg B, Haltia M, Sourander P et al. Neuropädiatrie 1978; 9: 59.
136. Fredrickson DS, Sloan HR. In: Stanbury JB, Wyngaarden JB, Fredrickson DS, eds. The metabolic basis of inherited disease. New York: McGraw-Hill, 1972: 730.
137. Banker BQ, Miller JQ, Crocker AC. In: Aronson SM, Volk BW, eds. Cerebral sphingolipidoses. New York: Academic Press, 1962: 73.
138. Zeman W, Dyken P. Pediatrics 1969; 44: 570.
139. Boehme D, Cottrell J, Leonberg S, Zeman W. Brain 1971; 94: 745.
140. Duffy PE, Kornfeld M, Suzuki K. J Neuropathol Exp Neurol 1968; 27: 351.
141. Schwendermann G, Colmant HJ, Elze K-L et al. Neuropädiatrie 1978; 9: 28.
142. Goebel HH, Braak H, Seidel D et al. Clin Neuropathol 1982; 1: 151.
143. MacFaul R, Cavanagh N, Lake BD et al. Arch Dis Child 1982; 57: 168.
144. Austin JH, McAfee D, Armstrong D et al. Biochem J 1964; 93: 15c.
145. Hahn AF, Gordon BA, Gilbert JJ, Hinton GG. Acta Neuropathol (Berl) 1981; 55: 281.
146. von Hirsch T, Peiffer J. Arch Psychiatr Nervenkr 1955; 194: 88.
147. Hollander H. J Histochem Cytochem 1963; 11: 118.
148. Olsson Y, Sourander P. Acta Paediatr Scand 1969; 58: 15.
149. Weller RO, Swash M, McLellan DL, Scholtz CL. Clinical neuropathology. Berlin: Springer, 1983: 261.
150. Bischoff A, Ulrich J. Acta Neuropathol (Berl) 1967; 8: 292.
151. Austin JH. Arch Neurol 1973; 28: 258.
152. Suzuki K, Suzuki Y. Proc Natl Acad Sci USA 1970; 66: 302.

153. Suzuki Y, Suzuki K. Science 1971; 171: 73.
154. Suzuki K. In: Johannessen JV, ed. Electron microscopy in human medicine. New York: McGraw-Hill, 1980; 6: 3.
155. Schochet SS, McCormick WF, Powell GF. Acta Neuropathol (Berl) 1976; 36: 153.
156. Suzuki K, Suzuki Y. In: Fredrickson DS, Goldstein JL, Brown MS, eds. The metabolic basis of inherited disease. New York: McGraw-Hill, 1983: 857.
157. Desnick RJ, Sweeley CC. In: Fredrickson DS, Goldstein JL, Brown MS, eds. The metabolic basis of inherited disease. New York: McGraw-Hill, 1983: 906.
158. Vital A, Vital C, Maleville J. Clin Neuropathol 1984; 3: 168.
159. Moser HW, Chen WW. In: Fredrickson DS, Goldstein JL, Brown MS, eds. The metabolic basis of inherited disease. New York: McGraw-Hill, 1983: 820.
160. Bach G, Friedman R, Weissmann B, Neufeld EF. Proc Natl Acad Sci USA 1972; 69: 2048.
161. Bach G, Eisenberg F Jr, Cantz M, Neufeld EF. Proc Natl Acad Sci USA 1973; 70: 2134.
162. Whiteman P, Young E. Clin Chim Acta 1977; 76: 139.
163. Murphy JV, Hodach AE, Gilbert EF et al. Arch Pathol Lab Med 1983; 107: 495.
164. Durand P, Borrone C, Della Cella G. J Pediatr 1969; 75: 655.
165. Beaudet AL. In: Fredrickson DS, Goldstein JL, Brown MS, eds. The metabolic basis of inherited disease. New York: McGraw-Hill, 1983: 788.
166. Matsuishi T, Terasawa K, Yoshida I et al. Neuropediatrics 1982; 13: 173.
167. Sakai T, Antoku Y, Goto I. Exp Neurol 1986; 94: 149.
168. Powers JM. Clin Neuropathol 1985; 4: 181.
169. Schaumburg HH, Powers JM, Raine CS et al. Arch Neurol 1975; 32: 577.
170. Moser HW, Moser AB, Singh I, O'Neill BP. Ann Neurol 1984; 16: 628.
171. Herndon RM, Rubinstein LJ, Freeman JM, Mathieson G. J Neuropathol Exp Neurol 1970; 29: 524.
172. Anzil AP, Gessaga E. Eur Neurol 1972; 7: 79.
173. Saudubray JM, Marsac C, Charpentier C et al. Acta Paediatr Scand 1976; 65: 717.
174. Seitelberger F. In: Vinken PJ, Bruyn GW, eds. Handbook of clinical neurology. Amsterdam: North Holland 1970; 10: 150.
175. Pamphlett R, Silberstein P. Acta Neuropathol (Berl) 1986; 69: 343.
176. Soffer D, Grotsky HW, Rapin I, Suzuki K. Ann Neurol 1979; 6: 340.
177. Lehmann AR, Francis AJ, Giannelli G. Lancet 1985; 1: 486.

Neuroaxonal dystrophies

178. Seitelberger F. Acta Neuropathol [Suppl] (Berl) 1971; 5: 17.
179. Duchen LW, Jacobs JM. In: Adams JH, Corsellis JAN, Duchen LW, eds. Greenfield's Neuropathology. London: Arnold, 1984: 573.

Other metabolic diseases

180. Leigh D. J Neurol Neurosurg Psychiatr 1951; 14: 216.
181. Montpetit VJA, Anderman F, Carpenter S. Brain 1971; 94: 1.
182. Danks DM, Campbell PE, Stevens BJ et al. Pediatrics 1972; 50: 188.
183. Troost D, van Rossum A, Straks W et al. Brain Dev 1982; 4: 115.
184. Martin JJ, Schlote W. J Neurol Sci 1972; 15: 49.
185. Dancis J, Hutzler BS, Snyderman SE, Cox RP. J Pediatr 1972; 81: 312.

Hypothyroidism and iodine deficiency

186. Hetzel BS, Chavadej J, Potter BJ. Neuropathol Appl Neurobiol 1988; 14: 19.

Phacomatoses

187. Crowe FW, Schull WJ, Neel JV. A clinical, pathological and genetic study of multiple neurofibromatosis. Springfield: Thomas, 1956.
188. Leading article. Lancet 1987; 1: 663.
189. Seizinger BR, Rouleau GA, Ozelius LJ et al. Cell 1987; 49: 589.
190. Barker D, Wright E, Nguyen K et al. Science 1987; 236: 1100.
191. Seizinger BR, Martuza RL, Gusella JF. Nature 1986; 322: 644.
192. Rubenstein AE. Conn Med 1987; 51: 261.
193. Kanter WR, Eldridge R, Fabricant R et al. Neurology 1980; 30: 851.
194. Hunt A, Lindenbaum RH. J Med Genet 1984; 21: 272.
195. Gomez MR. Tuberous sclerosis. New York: Raven Press, 1982.
196. Fryer AE, Chalmers A, Connor JM et al. Lancet 1987; 1: 659.
197. Harper PS. J Med Genet 1987; 24: 513.
198. Oppenheimer DR. In: Adams JH, Corsellis JAN, Duchen LW, eds. Greenfield's Neuropathology. London: Arnold, 1984: 699.
199. Bridges BA, Harnden DG, eds. Ataxia telangiectasia. A cellular and molecular link between cancer, neuropathology and immune deficiency. Chichester: Wiley, 1982.
200. Hudson SM, Harper PS, Hourihan MD et al. Brain 1986; 109: 1297.
201. Seizinger BR, Rouleau GA, Ozelius LJ et al. Nature 1988; 332: 268.
202. Alonson A, Taboada D, Ceres L et al. Pediatr Radiol 1979; 8: 39.

Ageing and dementias

AGEING

The brain undergoes striking morphological and biochemical changes during ageing. The brain weight is reduced, macroscopical, histological and ultrastructural abnormalities develop, and this morphological process is complemented by neurochemical changes.

Gross changes, brain weight and volume

The average weight of the brain in a healthy, 20-year-old male is 1350–1400 g; in a female it is approximately 100 g less at any given age than in the male. There is a gradual loss of cerebral substance during ageing, and the mean loss is 100 g.[1,2]

The cerebral volume is substantially reduced from the age of 20 onwards: 3·5% and 2·0% of brain volume is lost every ten years in men and women respectively,[3] and this loss starts earlier in women than in men.[4] The ratio of brain volume to intracranial volume, however, remains little changed until the age of 60, but falls by 20% between the seventh and tenth decades.[5] The decrease is not evenly distributed between grey and white matter. Quantitative assessment using an image analyser system has revealed that, although the brain is composed of roughly equal amounts of grey and white matter, the latter is lost more rapidly in adult life.[6] This decrease in brain weight and volume is a physiological phenomenon occurring in intellectually intact people and it is not accompanied by clinical or histological evidence of dementia. Although there is a gradual decrease in the weight and volume of the brain, the term atrophy should be used only if the brain weight is 1000 g or less. It has to be remembered that brain weight can be influenced by the nature of the terminal illness, the amount of CSF in the ventricular system and by fixation in 10% formol saline.

The ageing brain shows changes which, although inconsistent, may be obvious to the naked eye. The leptomeninges tend to show fibrous thickening, particularly in the parasagittal areas over the convexity of the cerebral hemispheres; this fibrosis is most noticeable over the age of 60 years. *Cortical atrophy* may or may not be present; its severity can be better appreciated after the arachnoid membrane has been stripped away, revealing the pattern of narrowed gyri and widened sulci (Fig. 13.1). The major cerebral arteries may show *atherosclerosis* of varying

severity, but in many cases they appear to be normal. Coronal or horizontal sectioning of the brain usually confirms the impression of atrophy obtained on external examination. The ventricular system is often dilated;[7] the angles of the lateral ventricles become rounded, the hippocampi do not fill the temporal horns, and even the cerebral aqueduct may be distended. It is important at this stage to exclude any internal or external obstruction of the CSF pathway which can cause ventricular dilatation (hydrocephalus). The wide range of variations in the thickness of the normal cerebral cortex makes macroscopical assessment of the width of the cortical ribbon difficult and unreliable.

The CT scans of ageing brains show widening of the sulci and ventricular dilatation; quantitative

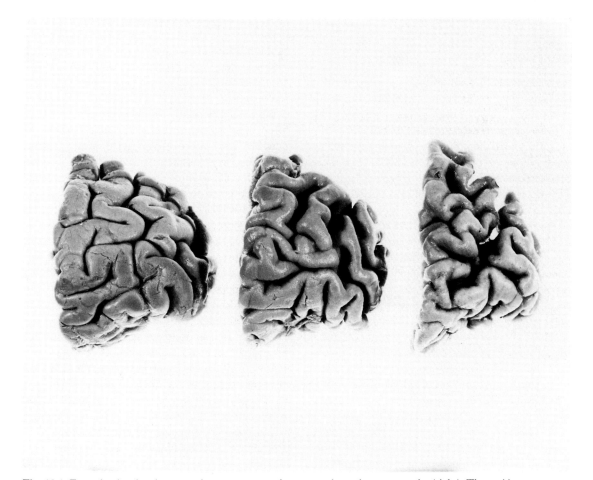

Fig. 13.1 Frontal poles showing normal appearance, moderate atrophy and severe atrophy (right). The gyri become increasingly narrower and the intervening sulci wider.

techniques are now available which give an accurate assessment of these radiological findings.[8] Despite improvements in methodology, however, there is often a discrepancy between neuroradiological and neuropathological examinations: brains which appear atrophied on CT scan may prove to be of normal weight and morphology after death.

Histological changes

Ageing brains, even those which appear normal on gross examination, may reveal a variety of changes affecting nerve cells, glial cells and blood vessels. Some of the abnormalities are intracellular (e.g. neurofibrillary tangles and granulovacuoles in nerve cells), whilst others disrupt the normal organisation of tissues (e.g. neuritic plaques). These changes are described below.

Neuronal loss

Loss of nerve cells from grey matter is difficult to assess, except in extreme cases in which depopulation of the cerebral cortex is obvious. The early observation of a neuronal fall-out of 15–35% in several selected areas of the cerebral cortex[9] was later disputed. However, it is now accepted that neuronal loss does occur during ageing,[2] although there are individual, regional and species differences.

It has been calculated that there is neuronal loss of 1% per annum from the neocortex and medial hippocampus in non-demented individuals between the age of 65 and 95.[10] Nerve cells decrease by about 3.6% per decade between the ages of 15 and 96 years in the Sommer (h1 or CA1) sector of the hippocampus.[11] This is an area of selective neuronal vulnerability (see p. 120) which is usually severely affected in Alzheimer's disease. Other neuronal populations, including Purkinje cells of the cerebellum and the large motor neurons of the lumbar and sacral spinal cord,[2] show cell loss with advancing age. There are, however, two areas which have attracted considerable attention recently: these are the noradrenergic locus ceruleus in the brainstem and the cholinergic nucleus basalis of Meynert in the basal forebrain. During ageing, cell loss occurs in both these areas

and this is relevant to dementia of the Alzheimer type.[12,13]

Neuritic (senile) plaques

These are roughly spherical structures whose diameter ranges from 5 μm to 200 μm. In haematoxylin and eosin preparations, neuritic plaques are hardly discernible but, being argyrophilic, they can be easily demonstrated by silver impregnation techniques. Their size and configuration vary, depending on the stage of development of the plaque and the plane of section. A typical plaque shows a central dense core surrounded by a clear halo which, in turn, is encircled by a ring of filamentous and granular material. This outer rim, like the central core, is argyrophilic (Fig. 13.2). Other plaques appear to lack a central core or a clear halo, or they may consist of a featureless mass of fragmented tissue. Some plaques are discrete; others have a tendency to coalesce. The central core is composed of amyloid fibrils which stain positively with Congo red (see Fig. 13.13, p. 373), whilst the outer rim contains abnormal distended nerve cell processes, filled with mitochondria and dense bodies: these neurites are intermingled with glial processes, occasional microglial cells and surviving normal cortical constituents.[14,15] An astrocyte response around the plaque is occasionally seen (Fig. 13.3).

Neuritic plaques are observed most frequently in the cerebral cortex, where they tend to cluster in the floor of the sulci, but they also occur in the deep grey matter, including the corpus striatum, of the diencephalon and occasionally in the brainstem. The hippocampus, parahippocampal gyrus and amygdaloid nucleus are preferential sites for both neuritic plaques and neurofibrillary tangles in the brains of intellecutally intact individuals. A topographical analysis of different brain areas of non-demented persons aged between 6 and 84 years revealed that plaques develop most often, and in the largest number, in the amygdala, while the hippocampus is most severely affected by tangle formation.[16] Although neuritic plaques increase in frequency with advancing age, unlike neurofibrillary tangles they do not occur in all individuals, even in those who survive into the tenth decade.[1,17]

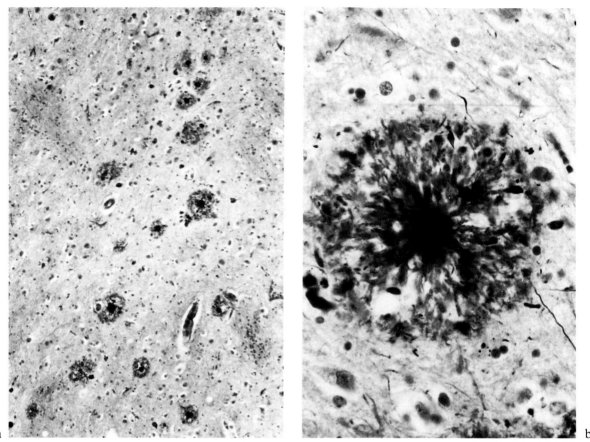

Fig. 13.2a, b Senile (neuritic) plaques. (**a**) A cluster of plaques in the amygdaloid nucleus. (**b**) The densely stained amyloid core of the plaque is surrounded by a crown of abnormal neurites.
Glees and Marsland silver impregnation (**a**) × 120; (**b**) × 500

Three stages in the development of neuritic plaques can be distinguished by electron microscopy; these correspond to the various forms seen in silver-stained sections. In the first stage, the *primitive plaque* is composed of a small collection of abnormal nerve cell processes or neurites, some of which appear to be presynaptic terminals; occasional fibrillary astrocytic processes and microglial cells are found, but amyloid is either absent or only a few fibrils are present. The second stage is the *mature (classical) plaque*, which displays all the typical constituents. The last stage features the *burnt-out plaque* composed mainly of amyloid (amyloid plaque).[18] Recently a fourth type of plaque has been described. This does not contain amyloid or neurites and is recognised by

more intense staining and altered texture of the neuropil. These plaques occur in the lateral entorhinal area of the parahippocampal gyrus and are often associated with microglial cells. Such changes may represent the earliest stages of plaque formation.[19]

Alzheimer's neurofibrillary degeneration

Neurofibrillary tangles are basophilic and are just discernible in sections stained with haematoxylin and eosin. They are more easily demonstrated by silver stains and by Congo red; with the latter stain they are birefringent with polarised light (Fig. 13.4). The tangles are intraneuronal and their configuration is determined by the site and

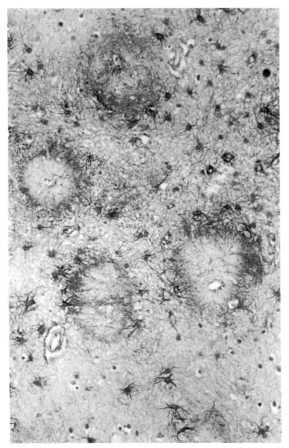

Fig. 13.3 The contour of plaques is outlined by astrocyte processes whose perikarya are present in the vicinity of plaques.
Holzer's stain for astrocytes × 150

type of neuron affected (Fig. 13.5). In the smaller pyramidal neurons of the cortex, the tangles tend to assume a flame-shaped or triangular configuration which extends from the base of the cell towards the apical dendrite. In the hippocampus and in the larger pyramidal nerve cells of the cortex more complex forms develop. A globose configuration occurs in the nerve cells of the basal forebrain and brainstem.[20]

Electron microscopy has shown that neurofibrillary tangles are composed of masses of paired helical filaments (PHF) (Fig. 13.6). Characteristic constrictions appear at regular intervals of 65–80 nm along the PHF as a result of two filaments being wound around each other in a double

helix (Fig. 13.7).[14,15] A recent ultrastructural study has revealed that the protofilaments of paired helical filaments differ from normal neurofilaments; in the protofilaments of the PHF[21] the globular components are larger and the longitudinal bars between them longer. Although straight filaments have also been identified in neurofibrillary tangles, they are rare in Alzheimer's disease and in other pathological conditions in which neurofibrillary degeneration occurs.[2]

Despite intense research in recent years, the chemical composition of neurofibrillary tangles and their relationship to normal components of the cytoskeleton remain largely unresolved. Antiserum against normal human neurotubules was found by immunocytochemistry to label neurofibrillary tangles specifically in isolated neurons and in tissue sections: this suggested that neurofibrillary tangles originated from neurotubules.[22] However, monoclonal antibodies produced against the proteins of neurofilaments were convincingly shown to bind to neurofibrillary tangles, indicating that they and normal neurofilaments share antigenic determinants (Fig. 13.8).[23] It has been realised only recently that neurofibrillary tangles are heterogeneous in their content of neurofilamentous material: they may contain antigens which cross-react with normal neurofilaments, whilst other antigens present may be unique to tangles and consequently are not shared with normal neurofilaments.[24] Paired helical filaments derive, at least in part, from components of the normal neuronal cytoskeleton. They contain not only sequences from neurofilaments and microtubule-associated proteins, but also antigenic determinants which are unique to them.[25] Recently, the microtubule-associated protein tau, which promotes the assembly of microtubules from tubulin, was found to be present in tangles. The abnormal phosphorylation of the tau protein could play an important rôle in tangle formation.[26]

Neurofibrillary tangles occur in ageing and in various cerebral diseases. They are uncommon in non-demented individuals and initially restricted to the hippocampus, but their incidence increases with advancing age and by the ninth decade no individual is spared. The frontal and temporal cortex is usually more affected than the posterior

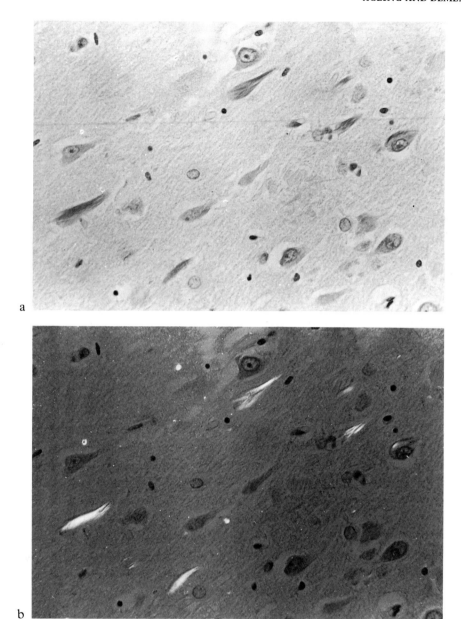

Fig. 13.4a, b Neurofibrillary tangles stained with Congo red (**a**) become birefringent under polarised light (**b**).
× 300

half of the brain, and tangles are more often found in the superficial and middle cortical layers than in the deeper cortex. The hippocampus, parahippocampal gyrus and the corticomedial portion of the amygdaloid nucleus are usually severely involved, whereas the Purkinje cells and large motor neurons appear to be resistant to this degenerative process.[1,2] Pigmented nuclei of the brainstem, the substantia nigra and locus ceruleus contain nerve cells with neurofibrillary degeneration.[20] Neurofibrillary tangles are, of course, encountered in Alzheimer's disease and in adults with Down's

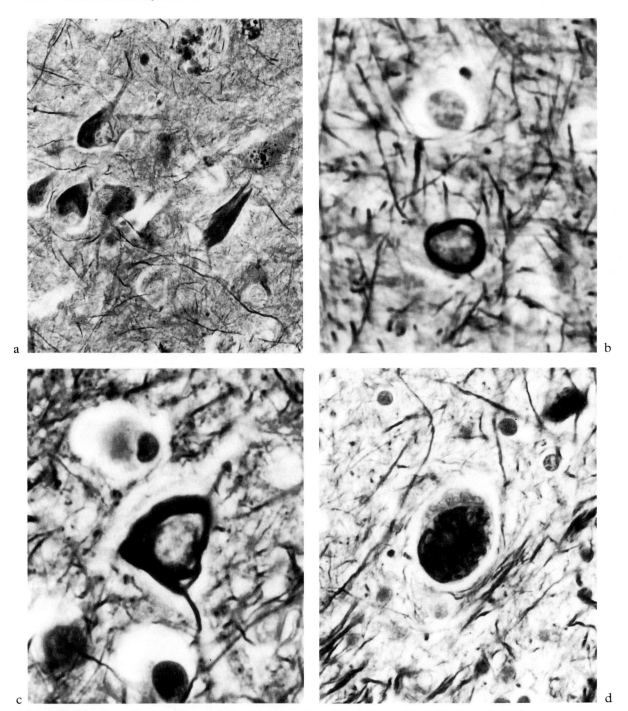

Fig. 13.5a–d The configuration of neurofibrillary tangles varies considerably according to the type and site of neurons affected. (**a**) Hippocampus, (**b**, **c**) neocortex, (**d**) nucleus basalis of Meynert.
a–d Glees and Marsland silver impregnation (**a**) × 500; (**b**) × 640; (**c**) × 960; (**d**) × 640

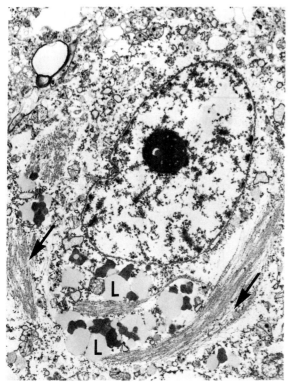

Fig. 13.6 Electron micrograph shows a neuron containing neurofibrillary tangles (arrow). Lipofuscin granules (L) are also present.
Electron micrograph ×7250

syndrome, and they feature in the amyotrophic lateral sclerosis-parkinsonism-dementia complex of Guam, in sporadic motor neuron disease, in subacute sclerosing panencephalitis and following cerebral trauma. In all these disorders, the neurofibrillary tangles display the characteristic configuration of paired helical filaments. There are only two conditions, sporadic motor neuron disease and progressive supranuclear palsy, in which they are composed of straight filaments.[2]

Granulovacuolar degeneration

Granulovacuoles are restricted chiefly to the hippocampus, where they occur in the cytoplasm of pyramidal neurons. A single cell may contain one or more of these inclusions, in which the 3–5 µm diameter vacuole contains a single argyrophilic dot (Fig. 13.9). Electron microscopy shows a dense granular core, embedded in a translucent matrix which, in turn, appears to be separated from the rest of the cytoplasm. Immunocytochemical techniques have shown that granulovacuoles contain abnormal phosphorylated proteins which are also present in neurofibrillary tangles.[27] Granulovacuoles are rare below the age of 65, but their frequency increases

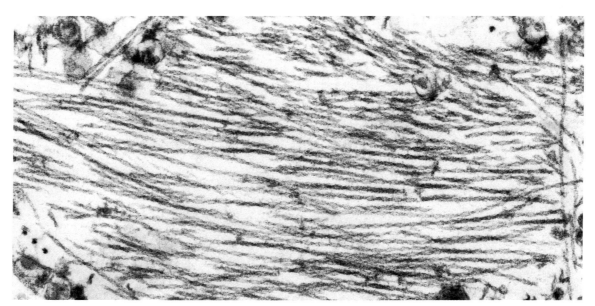

Fig. 13.7 A high-power electron micrograph reveals the typical configuration of filaments wound around each other in double helix.
Electron micrograph ×150 000

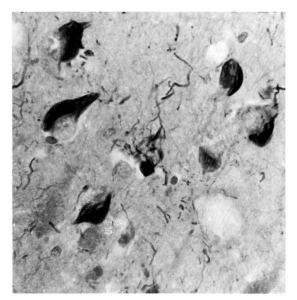

Fig. 13.8 Monoclonal anti-neurofilament antibody binds to neurofibrillary tangles in the hippocampus. Indirect immunoperoxidase × 400

with advancing age and by the ninth decade 75% of all brains have some. However, in normal individuals only 9% of cells are affected in the Sommer sector, whereas in demented cases this proportion rises to over 20%.[28] They have been observed in various diseases, including Down's syndrome and the amyotrophic lateral sclerosis-parkinsonism-dementia complex of Guam, but their occurrence is related to ageing, rather than to a specific disease process. In all these conditions, the hippocampal pyramidal neurons are preferentially vulnerable, with the notable exception of progressive supranuclear palsy in which granulo-vacuolar degeneration develops in cell groups of the brainstem.[1]

Hirano bodies

Hirano bodies, like granulovacuoles, are largely confined to the hippocampus. With haematoxylin and eosin they appear as intensely eosinophilic cylindrical or ovoid structures measuring up to 30 μm in length and 8–10 μm in diameter (Fig. 13.10). Ultrastructurally, they are composed of parallel filaments which alternate with thicker sheet-like material,[29] but Hirano bodies show no

immunostaining with antibodies against neuro-filaments.[30] However, they contain cytoskeletal proteins including actin, α-actinin, vinculin and tropomyosin, indicating that Hirano bodies are derived from abnormal organisation of neuronal cytoskeleton.[31] Their precise localisation is disputed, since they are also found in the neuron-free stratum lacunosum and, even in the pyramidal layer, they often appear to indent rather than to occupy the perikaryon. Although Hirano bodies have been occasionally observed in glial cells,[32] their intraneuronal localisation is now widely accepted. They are present in intellectually normal old people, becoming more frequent with increasing age, but they are particularly abundant in demented patients. Hirano bodies have been

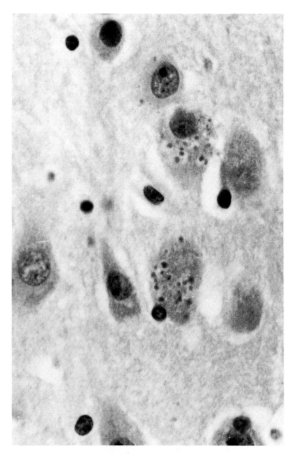

Fig. 13.9 Granulovacuolar degeneration in the pyramidal cells of the hippocampus. Haematoxylin-eosin × 560

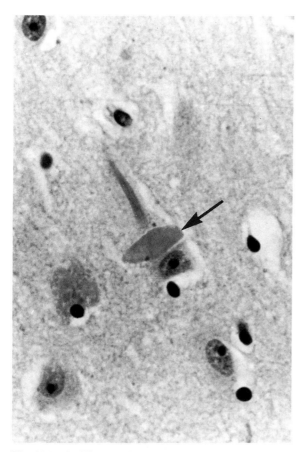

Fig. 13.10 An Hirano body (arrow), closely applied to a hippocampal pyramidal neuron which also contains a neurofibrillary tangle.
Haematoxylin-eosin × 480

abnormalities led to the loss of basilar dendrites and branches of the apical dendrites of the pyramidal neurons. With the devastation of the dendritic tree, the neuron disappears and gliosis ensues.[34] A quantitative ultrastructural study has revealed a statistically significant age-related decrease of synapses in the frontal, but not in the temporal region of human brain at post mortem.[35] Age-related loss of synapses may result from the inability of the presynaptic components to maintain the structural integrity of the synapse in senescence, due to a deficiency of axonal transport.[36,37]

The amount of myelin also decreases with age in the striate cortex of man; this myelin loss is most probably caused by changes in the cortical projection cells and their processes.[38] Axonal abnormalities have indeed been recognised in the ageing brain, with dilated neuronal processes containing a mixture of damaged organelles.[1]

These findings have been confirmed in well-fixed brains of experimental animals. There is a progressive loss of dendritic spines from the pyramidal neurons in the visual cortex of rats with increasing age.[39] However, a considerable degree of plasticity has been demonstrated in the dendritic trees of surviving neurons in the parahippocampal gyrus in man. Dendritic trees were more extensive in non-demented senescent individuals (average age of 79·6 years) than in a group of younger adults (average age of 51·2 years).[40]

Vascular changes

Quantitative changes. Very little is known about quantitative changes which occur in the cerebral microvasculature during ageing. In the human hippocampus, the diameter of both capillaries and arterioles increases, whereas the density of capillaries decreases and that of arterioles increases.[41] In the neocortex, capillary density, diameter and volume show higher values for senescent brains, whereas capillary surface area diminishes.[42] In old rats, aged 124 weeks, the vascularity of the cerebral cortex is severely reduced.[43] The changes in capillaries observed in man and experimental animals suggest that there is a reduced exchange potential between the vascular bed and brain parenchyma during ageing.

observed in a variety of disorders including Alzheimer's disease, Pick's disease and kuru, in different neuronal types and both in man and in experimental animals.[33]

Changes in nerve cell processes

Neuronal loss and the formation of abnormal intraneuronal structures are not the only mechanisms by which neuronal function can be impaired. Damage to dendrites and axons with consequent loss of synaptic activity could play a crucial part in deteriorating mental function. Qualitative changes in dendritic arborisations were observed in Golgi-impregnated sections of human frontal and temporal cortex: thus loss of spines and dendritic

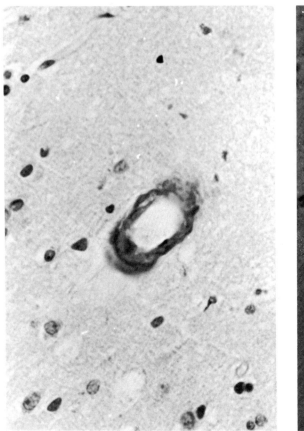
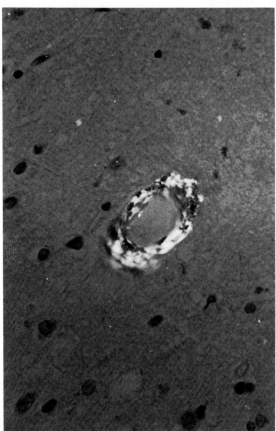

a   b

Fig. 13.11a, b Congophilic angiopathy. An intracerebral blood vessel stained with Congo red (**a**) shows birefringence under polarised light (**b**).
× 250

Amyloid angiopathy. Amyloid is often deposited in cerebral blood vessels: and they thus become 'congophilic' when stained with Congo red. The leptomeningeal vessels, the pial and cortical arterioles, and sometimes the intracortical capillaries are affected (Fig. 13.11). The cortex of the parietal and occipital lobes is more commonly involved than that of the frontotemporal region, and whilst the cerebellar cortex and the deep grey matter of the cerebral hemispheres are occasionally affected, the vascular tree of the brainstem seems to be spared.[2]

Amyloid fibrils accumulate outside the internal elastic lamina, in the media and adventitia and, in some cases, extend in the form of radial spikes into the brain parenchyma. In haematoxylin and eosin preparations the wall of these thickened vessels is brightly and uniformly eosinophilic, whilst positive staining with Congo red renders them birefringent in polarised light. This congophilic or amyloid angiopathy is relatively common in the brains of senescent and demented individuals,[44] but is only very rarely associated with primary, secondary or familial amyloidosis.[45] Ultrastructurally the intravascular deposits show the characteristic features of amyloid fibrils, which tend to accumulate first in the basal lamina and in the pericytes.[45]

The nature and origin of this vascular amyloid and its relationship to the amyloid found in the core of neuritic plaques remain controversial. Immunoglobulins have been demonstrated in both vascular[46] and plaque[47] amyloid, suggesting a common derivation from permeable blood vessels.

Indeed, biochemical analysis indicates a common origin of the amyloid in the plaque core and in congophilic angiopathy.[48] Yet other results show that the amyloid in the core of neuritic plaques has similarities with APUD amyloid and may result from neurosecretion.[49] It is therefore likely that vascular and plaque amyloids are produced by different mechanisms and that even core amyloid may not be homogeneous and could originate from various sources. Moreover, there is now convincing evidence that the fibrillar protein of senile cerebral amyloid differs from that of systemic amyloid of AA type.[50] The pathology, biochemistry and molecular biology of amyloid deposition in the brain have been comprehensively reviewed.[51,52]

Other structural changes. Structural abnormalities associated with ageing are difficult to evaluate, since degenerative disorders, most often atherosclerosis, are liable to occur with increasing frequency in older individuals. With scanning electron microscopy a variety of structural abnormalities have been observed, including thickening of the vessel wall, swelling and proliferation of endothelial cells and pericytes, and loss of the neural plexus from the abluminal surface.[53]

Glial changes

In spite of the important rôle that glial cells play in maintaining normal neuronal activity (see p. 20), little is known about glial changes during ageing. Increase of astrocytic fibrillary processes occurs at the surface of the brain beneath both the pia and the ependyma, and more diffusely around the blood vessels both in grey and in white matter. The number of fibrillary astrocytes increases in both ageing animals and ageing man, and the altered glial–neuronal ratio could disturb the delicate and complex trophic interaction which exists between these two cell types.[54] In rats, the amount of glial fibrillary acidic protein increases with advancing age, reflecting astrocyte hypertrophy which is more likely to be the consequence, rather than the cause, of neuronal degeneration and loss.[55] Moreover, tissue culture studies show that glial cells change their functional characteristics with age;

their response to intrinsic substances, e.g. hormones and nucleotides, becomes altered.[56]

DEMENTIAS

Dementia can be clinically defined as 'an acquired global impairment of intellect, memory, and personality, but without impairment of consciousness'.[57]

The incidence of dementia is difficult to assess, but in industrial countries approximately 0·3% of the population suffer from dementia.[58] It is not until the sixth and seventh decades of life that dementia becomes prevalent, and 4–5% of those over 65 will become severely demented, whilst a further 10% show clinical signs of mild to moderate dementia.[59]

Over 50 diseases have been identified which can result in dementia.[60] Dementias can be arbitrarily divided into two major groups. *Primary dementias* are usually degenerative disorders of the brain, affecting primarily the nerve cells. *Secondary dementias* develop as a consequence of another pathological disorder, either in the brain or another part of the body. Primary dementias, by definition, are associated with profound structural alterations of the brain, whereas some secondary forms can occur without any detectable morphological abnormalities. The term *organic dementia* applies to all those diseases in which the presence of morphological abnormalities can be established. The dementing disease can involve preferentially the cerebral cortex (e.g. Pick's disease), the basal ganglia (e.g. Huntington's disease) or the white matter (e.g. Binswanger's disease).

The prevalence of various causes of dementia has been studied, both under and over the age of 65 years. In a clinical study of a group of 84 demented patients under 65, the most frequent diagnosis (48 cases) was cerebral atrophy of unknown aetiology, followed by space-occupying lesions (8), vascular disease (8), alcoholism (6), normal pressure communicating hydrocephalus (5), Creutzfeldt–Jakob disease (3), Huntington's disease (3), and one case each with trauma, subarachnoid haemorrhage and limbic encephalitis.[61] Since no neuropathological examination was carried out, it can only be assumed that most of the patients with cerebral atrophy suffered from Alzheimer's disease. In a series of histologically verified cases of dementia over 65, half of the patients suffered from Alzheimer's disease and 15% from vascular disease; in about 10% these two degenerative processes were combined. In 15% the abnormalities were not severe enough to provide grounds for a definitive diagnosis and in a further 6% no adequate morphological changes were found to explain the dementia. Pick's disease and cerebral neoplasia accounted for the remaining 4%.[62] These studies have shown that the single most frequent cause of dementia is Alzheimer's disease.

ALZHEIMER'S DISEASE

The first thorough clinical and pathological examination of a case of presenile dementia was reported by Alzheimer in 1907.[63] He observed both argentophilic plaques and neurofibrillary tangles in silver-stained sections of a generally atrophied brain. Presenile dementia (Alzheimer's disease affecting individuals younger than 65 years) was for a long time distinguished from senile dementia and regarded by many as a separate entity. It has now been recognised that presenile and senile dementia of the Alzheimer type are the same nosological entity; it will be referred to, irrespective of the age of onset, as Alzheimer's disease. The only differences between the presenile and senile forms are the more frequent occurrence of parietal lobe symptoms clinically and the greater incidence of atrophy with extensive formation of neuritic plaques and neurofibrillary tangles pathologically in the younger onset group.[2]

Alzheimer's disease is the most frequent cause of dementia, affecting 5% of those in their sixties and increasing to 15% in the eighties and nineties.[64] In the presenile group the disease most often starts between the ages of 50 and 60, but it can occur in young adults and occasionally in children.[2] Women are twice as often affected as men, and after the late seventies the relative number of women suffering from Alzheimer's disease becomes even higher. The average duration of the disease is approximately 5 years, but extremes of a few months and over 20 years have been recorded.[2,65]

The disease evolves through three stages: from a usually insidious onset an early forgetful stage develops, followed by a confusional stage which deteriorates into the final demented phase.[57,65] On admission to hospital the patients may already be disorientated and confused. Deterioration of intellect and personality is rapid, and focal signs develop, mainly localised in the parietal lobes with dysphasia, apraxia, agnosia and acalculia. Extrapyramidal and pyramidal signs are not uncommon, the speech becomes increasingly incomprehensible and in the deepening apathetic dementia the bedridden patient becomes incontinent and usually dies of bronchopneumonia.

Electrophysiological (EEG) and neuroradiological examinations of the brain may show abnormalities which are difficult to distinguish from ageing changes. The EEG is unlikely to be normal in demented patients; diffuse slowing, particularly of the dominant alpha activity, is more severe than that seen in normal ageing. CT scans may reveal cerebral atrophy with widening of the sulci and dilatation of the ventricles, features which are indicative of degenerative disease, but by no means diagnostic of dementia of the Alzheimer type. The improved resolution of brain structures afforded by magnetic resonance imaging (MRI),[66] and the use of positron emission tomography (PET), are expected to increase the accuracy of diagnosis of Alzheimer's disease in life.[67] PET allows the assessment of metabolic activity of various substances in the brain, including glucose.

Morphological changes

General post-mortem examination reveals little abnormality outside the nervous system, apart from the terminal respiratory illness. The brain is often smaller than normal and may weigh less than 1000 g. The atrophy tends to be generalised and symmetrical, although the frontal and temporal lobes may be more severely affected than the rest. The leptomeninges are usually thickened, but rarely more than in normal ageing. The major cerebral arteries often appear normal or may show mild to moderate atherosclerosis. However, it

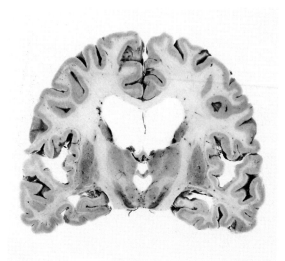

Fig. 13.12 Coronal slice of an Alzheimer brain shows dilated lateral ventricles with rounding of the ventricular angles, distended third ventricle, gaping Sylvian fissures and ample space between the hippocampus and the wall of the temporal horn of the lateral ventricles.

should be borne in mind that combined cases of Alzheimer's disease and vascular dementia exist, and histological examination may reveal striking abnormalities of the small cerebral vessels. Cortical atrophy is chiefly the result of a decrease of cortical length, rather than of width, suggesting that neuronal loss occurs in columns.[68]

The extent of the atrophy is fully appreciated on coronal slices: the widened sulci, the gaping Sylvian fissures and the dilated ventricles all become apparent. The angles of the lateral ventricles often become rounded and the hippocampus, instead of filling the temporal horn, is separated by a sizeable space from the ventricular wall (Fig. 13.12). The mean ventricular volume estimated in a series of Alzheimer patients was twice as large as in age-matched controls. Cerebral atrophy, however, varies considerably, and neither the changes in the cortical pattern, nor the

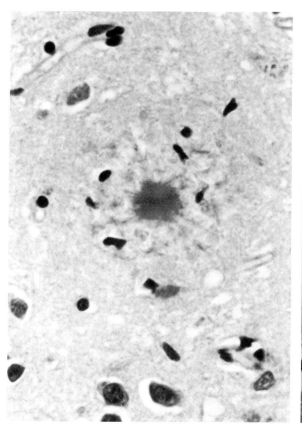
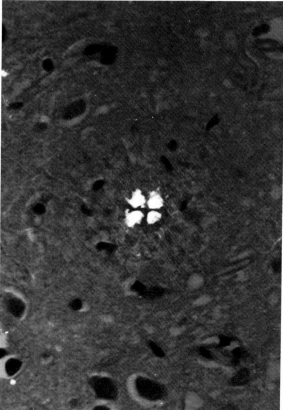

a   b

Fig. 13.13a, b Alzheimer's disease. A neuritic plaque stained with Congo red (**a**) shows birefringence under polarised light (**b**). × 480

ventricular dilatation are reliable diagnostic indicators of Alzheimer's disease. A smaller than average brain and large ventricles may be found in intellectually intact individuals, whereas macroscopically normal brains may be associated with clinically severe dementia and the histology characteristic of Alzheimer's disease.

Histologically, neuritic plaques (senile plaques), neurofibrillary tangles, granulovacuoles and Hirano bodies are all present; the latter two changes are usually restricted to the hippocampus. *Neuritic plaques* (p. 362) are numerous throughout the cortex and groups of these spherical structures disrupt the normal cytoarchitecture of the cortical ribbon. Although no laminae are spared, the plaques are rare in the first cortical layer but abundant in the depths of sulci. The temporal and the parahippocampal gyri usually contain more plaques than any other region. Mostly they are well-defined (Fig. 13.13), but occasionally they coalesce to form irregular configurations. Of the subcortical grey matter, the hypothalamus and the tegmental portion of the midbrain and pons are often affected; in the medulla and cerebellum plaques are rare. A recent quantitative assessment has revealed that plaques occur more frequently in the basal ganglia than was previously considered.[69]

The second most striking histological feature is the presence of *neurofibrillary tangles* (p. 363), distributed throughout the cortex. As with plaques, neurofibrillary degeneration is particularly common in the medial part of the temporal lobe, including the hippocampus, the amygdaloid nucleus and the parahippocampal gyrus (Figs 13.14 and 13.15). Within the hippocampus the Sommer sector is usually most severely affected.[70] Neurofibrillary degeneration also develops in the hypothalamus, thalamus and brainstem and in the anterior olfactory nucleus,[71] but is relatively rare in the basal ganglia.

The application of molecular biology has given new insight into the old problems of plaque and tangle formation. The amyloid core of plaques contains a polypeptide of a relative molecular mass of about 4000, and termed A4; it is possibly derived from a membrane glycoprotein precursor. The gene which codes for the precursor of A4 is located on human chromosome 21. This is of particular interest, since trisomy of this chromo-

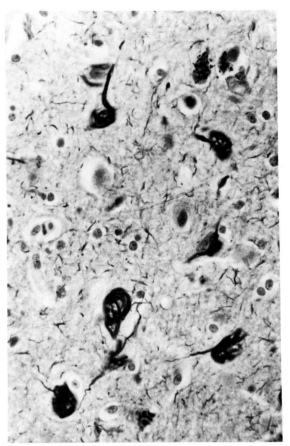

Fig. 13.14 Alzheimer's disease. Neurofibrillary tangles in the neurons of the parahippocampal gyrus.
Glees and Marsland silver impregnation × 300

some results in Down's syndrome, in which plaques are seen at an early age. The gene responsible for a rare familial form of Alzheimer's disease was found also on chromosome 21, indicating that the two genes may be one and the same. Since Alzheimer and adult Down's syndrome brains show morphological similarities, these findings were thought to indicate that the common form of Alzheimer's disease may be linked to chromosome 21. More precise gene mapping has, however, ruled out this possibility and indicated that the gene encoding for the amyloid precursor is not responsible for Alzheimer's disease, either in its familial or sporadic form, or for Down's syndrome.[72,73] More recently a protease inhibitor domain was found in the amyloid precursor, suggesting that abnormal proteolysis of the amyloid precursor may be

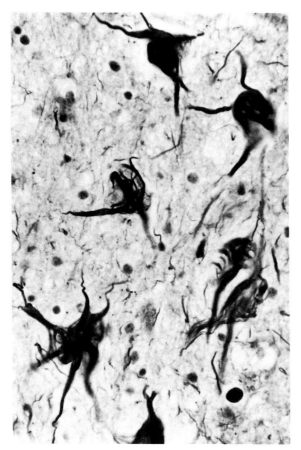

Fig. 13.15 Alzheimer's disease. Severe neurofibrillary change.
Glees and Marsland silver impregnation × 400

instrumental in the formation of neuritic plaques.[74]

The presence of A4 in neurofibrillary tangles is likely to be contamination. But they do contain ubiquitin, which suggests that tangles contain abnormal proteins which the neurons try to remove by the ubiquitin pathway. Indeed, the aberrant phosphorylation of a protein with a relative molecular mass of 60 000 is closely related to tangle formation in neurons, but is not associated with plaque formation or secondary gliosis.[75]

The nucleus basalis of Meynert, a collection of large neurons in the substantia innominata located just beneath the globus pallidus at the level of the infundibulum, has recently attracted considerable attention. Its nerve cells, which give rise to the ascending cholinergic system, are not only sub-

stantially reduced in number, but they also contain neurofibrillary tangles.[76]

Granulovacuolar degeneration (p. 367) and *Hirano bodies* (p. 368) are usually restricted to the hippocampus. Both are found more frequently in Alzheimer's disease than in age-matched controls.

These histological features are, of course, also present in the ageing brains of intellectually intact individuals. It is the quantity and distribution of the abnormalities, particularly of plaques and neurofibrillary tangles, which distinguish Alzheimer's disease from normal ageing. There have been attempts to establish a relationship between the severity of dementia and the frequency of histological abnormalities. Clinical dementia score and biochemically measured cholinergic deficiency appear to correlate well with the number of neuritic plaques,[77] whereas other results suggest a better correlation between dementia and neurofibrillary tangles.[78] The loss of neurons in relatively small and well-defined subcortical nuclei is well documented: there is a substantial decrease of nerve cells in the nucleus basalis of Meynert[79,80] and in the locus ceruleus.[81,82] The depopulation of the cortex is, however, more difficult to assess. Image analysing systems have revealed a significant loss of larger neurons: this depletion amounts to 40% in the mid-frontal region and 46% in the superior temporal gyrus.[83] Neuronal loss, however, is not generalised, but appears to be mainly confined to the frontal and temporal lobes; the parietal and occipital regions are less affected.[84] The loss of the large cortical neurons is age dependent: the volume of these cells is reduced in demented patients under 80 years of age, but appears to be normal for age in older subjects.[85] The cell processes of surviving neurons exhibit abnormalities: the terminal segments of dendrites of pyramidal cells in layer 2 of the parahippocampal gyrus are fewer and shorter than in normal adult brains.[40] Since the major constituents of neuritic plaques are processes of nerve cells, it is hardly surprising that Golgi analysis demonstrates a variety of morphological abnormalities of axons and dendrites which contribute to the plaques.[86] A striking decrease of synapses also occurs, and this loss is likely to contribute to the development of the disease.[87] The number of fibrillary astrocytes is significantly increased when compared to age-matched controls, although there is no correlation between this astrocytosis and the number of neuritic plaques or neurofibrillary tangles. Increased perivascular astrocytes and fibrillary gliosis may be related to a defect in the blood-brain barrier.[54] Amyloid angiopathy occurs in over 80% of Alzheimer's brains[88] and amyloid is deposited in the centre of senile plaques (see pp. 370 and 374). It has been suggested that extracellular deposits of amyloid may be formed in the following way. Coated vesicles in the cytoplasm of amyloid-related cells may fuse with the cell membrane, forming coated pits which then may empty their secretory material into the extracellular space where amyloid filaments become polymerised.[89]

With recent extensive studies, using both quantitative morphometry and neurochemistry, it has become clear that Alzheimer's disease is not a uniformly diffuse disorder, morphologically or neurochemically. Patients who die after the age of 80 years have a relatively pure cholinergic deficit restricted to the temporal lobe and hippocampus together with localised somatostatin deficiency in the temporal lobe, whereas younger patients suffer from a more severe and widespread cholinergic deficit coupled with reduction of other neurotransmitter systems (see below). Morphological abnormalities also tend to be more severe and more extensive in younger patients. The pathological and neurochemical heterogeneity supports the view that early and late onset cases may represent two distinct forms of the disease.[90]

Atypical cases of Alzheimer's disease exist both in familial and sporadic forms.[2] Whilst combined cases of Alzheimer's disease and vascular dementia are common, the simultaneous occurrence of Alzheimer's and Pick's diseases is rare.[91] Although some cases of Alzheimer's disease show no tangle formation, it appears to be the same disease with or without tangles, although the presence of neurofibrillary tangles is associated with dementia of greater severity.[92]

Aetiological and pathogenetic considerations

The cause of Alzheimer's disease is not known. Although recent investigations have revealed pro-found biochemical abnormalities, involving nucleic acids, proteins, neurotransmitters and neuropeptides, their relevance to the morphological changes and their rôle in the pathogenesis of the disorder remain to be determined. Toxic compounds, vascular abnormalities, viral infections and genetic predisposing factors have all been implicated, but the evidence is equivocal and the conclusions are controversial.[93,94]

Changes in neurotransmitters and neuropeptides

Among abnormalities of neurotransmitters, *cholinergic deficit* has been consistently demonstrated: choline acetyltransferase, the synthesising enzyme of acetylcholine, is significantly reduced both in cortical and subcortical structures,[95–97] and accordingly the amount of cortical acetylcholine is decreased.[98] Acetylcholine synthesis in, and release from, biopsy material are also reduced. Since the cholinergic innervation of the cerebral cortex mostly originates from the nucleus basalis of Meynert, its involvement may play a crucial rôle in Alzheimer's disease. Cellular loss and the formation of neurofibrillary tangles in the nucleus basalis are thought to be responsible for the widespread and severe ascending cholinergic deficit.[98] Decreased choline acetyltransferase activity without a decrease in postsynaptic muscarinic or nicotinic receptors suggests the degeneration of presynaptic cholinergic neurons, whilst the postsynaptic nerve cells remain intact. These findings have led to the formulation of the cholinergic hypothesis, which assumes that damage to the cholinergic system is the underlying mechanism of Alzheimer's disease.

This rather simple concept of Alzheimer's disease has been recently challenged. There is now good evidence to suggest that postsynaptic cholinergic receptors, both nicotinic[99] and a subclass of muscarinic receptors,[100] are reduced. Furthermore, neurotransmitter abnormalities in Alzheimer's disease are complex: a deficit of both the noradrenergic and serotoninergic systems has been demonstrated.[101] These biochemical findings correlate with the previously observed loss of noradrenergic cells from the locus ceruleus and of serotoninergic cells from the raphe nuclei.[102] Of the neuropeptides, only somatostatin appears to be

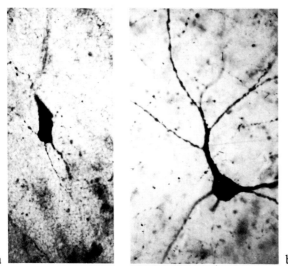

a   b

Fig. 13.16a, b Neuropeptide Y staining of a neuron in the temporal cortex of an Alzheimer brain (**a**) shows an abnormal perikaryon and striking loss of processes compared to a control (**b**).
Immunoperoxidase (peroxidase-antiperoxidase) × 755
Immunocytochemical preparation lent for reproduction by Dr Yvonne S. Allen, Department of Neuropathology, Institute of Psychiatry, London, UK.

consistently reduced in Alzheimer's disease,[103] and immunohistochemical studies have shown that some of the neurofibrillary tangle-bearing neurons[104] and neuritic plaques[105] contain somatostatin. Immunoreactivity of corticotrophin-releasing factor, a hypothalamic peptide which is thought to act as a neurotransmitter in the central nervous system, is reduced in Alzheimer's disease, while there is a reciprocal increase in receptor binding.[106] Immunostaining for neuropeptide Y has revealed striking neuronal abnormalities in the cerebral cortex (Fig. 13.16).[107] Several cortical areas contain reduced concentrations of γ-aminobutyric acid (GABA),[108] and there is also evidence to suggest a loss of cortical glutamate-containing nerve terminals.[109] Evidence is therefore accumulating to show that Alzheimer's disease is associated with the disturbance of several neurotransmitter systems and the cerebral cortex may be primarily affected. Neither the complex clinical symptomatology nor the extensive neuropathology can be satisfactorily explained by the loss of subcortical neurons from the basal forebrain and by the deficit of a single neurotransmitter.

Abnormal nucleic acid and protein metabolism

Alzheimer's disease is associated with profound biochemical changes. In the surviving neurons of the hippocampus, temporal neocortex, locus ceruleus, nucleus basalis of Meynert and dorsal tegmental nucleus, the nucleolar volume and cytoplasmic RNA content are reduced by approximately 30%.[110] Significantly lower levels of RNA in the cortex are related to decreased inhibition of ribonuclease, resulting in an enhanced degradation of RNA.[111] The generalised disturbance of RNA metabolism is, however, unrelated to the severity of the pathology in a given area, since it occurs in regions of both severe and mild neuronal loss and tangle formation.[112] The amount of euchromatin in the neurons is also decreased, suggesting that a smaller proportion of genetic material is available for transcription.[113] These changes will result in impaired RNA metabolism and protein synthesis with inevitable disturbance of neuronal activity. Whether this profound metabolic derangement is a manifestation of Alzheimer's disease or a predisposing factor remains to be seen.

Toxic substances

Data from both human pathology and experimental work suggest that aluminium might be involved in the pathogenesis of Alzheimer's disease. A high concentration of aluminium has been found in the brain of patients with Alzheimer's disease, particularly in areas rich in neurofibrillary tangles. X-ray spectrometry subsequently localised aluminium in the nuclear chromatin of tangle-bearing neurons, supporting the hypothesis that aluminium may interfere with DNA metabolism and thus lead to the synthesis of abnormal proteins of neurofibrillary tangles.[114] Furthermore, aluminium silicates have been demonstrated in the centre of plaque cores, indicating that they may initiate the formation of neuritic plaques.[115] Increased amounts of aluminium are present in four principal sites in the grey matter of Alzheimer's brains: (1) DNA-containing structures of the nucleus, (2) the protein moieties of neurofibrillary tangles, (3) the amyloid cores of plaques, and (4) cerebral ferritin.[116] Other results have, however, shown that increased aluminium levels are associated with advanced age rather than with dementia, and patients suffering from Alzheimer's disease have normal concentrations of aluminium in their serum, CSF and hair.[117] Aluminium has also been implicated in the development of dialysis dementia in which high levels of this metal have been reported both in the serum and in the brain.[118] Dialysis dementia, however, differs from Alzheimer's disease both pathologically and clinically; furthermore, in dialysis dementia the aluminium accumulates in the cytoplasm and not in the nucleus.[119] Aluminium salts injected into rabbits produce neurofibrillary changes, offering an animal model for Alzheimer's disease;[120] however, there are structural differences between the filamentous accumulations of the human disease and those of the experimental condition.[121] Thus, the rôle of aluminium in the pathogenesis of Alzheimer's disease remains controversial.

Increased amounts of silicon were found in association with neuritic plaques, but the presence of this material may only reflect an enhanced avidity of the damaged neural tissue for this element.[122]

Since zinc forms a part of most metallo-enzymes involved in the metabolism of DNA, an interesting hypothesis has envisaged zinc deficiency or the decreased ability to insert zinc into enzymes as a posssible mechanism which triggers off a catastrophic sequence of metabolic events culminating in deranged protein synthesis and finally cell death.[123]

Vascular abnormalities

Increased permeability of cerebral blood vessels could play an important rôle in the pathogenesis of at least one of the structural hallmarks of the disease: i.e. the cores of neuritic plaques. The cores are composed of amyloid fibrils which may originate from the blood and, when deposited in the parenchyma, could initiate a tissue response, leading to plaque formation. Recent immunocytochemical studies indicate that the blood-brain barrier is compromised both in Alzheimer's disease and in non-demented aged controls.[124] Increased levels of brain-specific antibodies have been reported in ageing animals and in patients

with Alzheimer's disease: the breakdown of the blood-brain barrier would facilitate the entry of these antibodies and the consequent auto-immune reaction could play an important rôle in neuronal degeneration.[125] Alternatively, auto-immune injury to the blood-brain barrier by antivascular antibodies could play a precipitating rôle in the pathogenesis of the disease by allowing the entry of injurious substances into the brain.[126] However, the auto-immune mechanism of degenerative changes has not yet been convincingly demonstrated. Neither has it been established whether increased vascular permeability is a primary abnormality responsible for the development of the disease or merely a secondary phenomenon resulting from more fundamental abnormalities of the nervous tissue.

Viruses

Infectious agents, particularly viruses, have been implicated in Alzheimer's disease. The aetiological rôle of viruses has gained support from experiments which claimed that the disease had been transmitted to primates from two cases of familial Alzheimer's disease.[127] Although these results were not confirmed, they focused attention upon a viral aetiology. Aqueous extracts of Alzheimer brains have induced the formation of paired helical filaments in the cultured cells of human fetal neocortex, but these findings have not been reproduced. However, a factor responsible for the assembly of paired helical filaments has been subsequently demonstrated in the CSF of patients with Alzheimer's disease.[128] Scrapie, a transmissible spongiform encephalopathy in sheep, which is now classed with the slow diseases caused by unconventional agents (and not with those caused by conventional viruses), can be transmitted to mice, in which amyloid plaques then develop.[129] Because of similarities between scrapie-associated fibrils, which are thought to be the unconventional infectious agent in scrapie, and amyloid in Alzheimer's disease, it has been postulated that amyloid in Alzheimer's disease is similarly infectious; this hypothesis has gained no support.[130]

It has been suggested that herpes viruses, lying dormant in the trigeminal ganglia and usually travelling centrifugally to cause herpes labialis, may proceed centripetally to induce Alzheimer's changes: this entry and pathway would also explain the preferential involvement of limbic structures.[131] However, even by the application of in situ hybridisation and immunocytochemistry, no viral genomes and antigens could be detected in Alzheimer brain.[132]

Genetic factors

Although the majority of Alzheimer cases are sporadic, familial cases are well documented, and the genetics of the disease have been recently reviewed.[133] The high incidence of Alzheimer's disease in certain families has generated interest in the genetic background of the disorder, but the results of genetic studies are controversial. An excess of Down's syndrome, lymphomas and acute immune disorders has been found in the families of patients suffering from Alzheimer's disease,[134] but these findings have not been confirmed by others.[135] Clinical, histological and genetic study of a family with 51 cases of Alzheimer's disease did not reveal an increased incidence of Down's syndrome or of haematological malignancy.[136] This and other studies indicate an autosomal dominant inheritance, although polygenic involvement cannot be excluded. A clinical study of Alzheimer's patients has confirmed a genetic factor manifested by an increased incidence of dementia and mental retardation in the patients' families and has found a higher frequency of previous thyroid disease and of severe head injury in the patients themselves.[137]

Studies involving monozygotic twins are rare, although an instance of genetically proven identical twins concordant for Alzheimer's disease has been reported.[138] Chromosome abnormalities, particularly hypodiploidy, are known to be associated with ageing.[139] A significant increase in aneuploidy was reported in demented patients, but no difference was found between Alzheimer's disease and multi-infarct dementia. Structurally altered chromosomes, however, were more frequent in Alzheimer's disease than in other types of dementia.[140] It is recognised that nearly all individuals with Down's syndrome who survive beyond 40 years will eventually develop Alzheimer changes.

PICK'S DISEASE

Whilst Alzheimer's disease is a common dementing disorder with diffuse atrophy of the brain, Pick's disease is rare and the pathology is more circumscribed. It develops most often in the sixth decade of life, but both younger and older age groups may be affected. The duration of the illness varies greatly, between 12 months and 10 years; cases starting later in life have a more protracted course. Although the striking female preponderance of Alzheimer's disease does not occur, in Pick's disease women tend to be slightly more often affected than men. Familial cases are known to occur and the examination of a large family has revealed 25 clinically diagnosed cases, 14 of which were confirmed by autopsy, in six generations. The disease is most likely to be transmitted by a dominant gene.[141]

Clinically, the disease usually starts with changes of character and behaviour, suggestive of frontal lobe damage. Impairment of intellect and memory later develops and the patient may become dysphasic, or even mute, dyslexic and dyspraxic. Later stages are marked by advanced dementia with general disintegration of intellect and personality.[57] The electroencephalogram may be normal or may show mild abnormalities; CT scanning may be valuable in the diagnosis by revealing localised atrophy consistent with Pick's disease.

The post mortem usually reveals little outside the nervous system, apart from terminal bronchopneumonia. The most striking feature is severe and circumscribed atrophy of the cerebral hemispheres. The brain may weigh 1000 g or even less. The frontotemporal regions are affected, whilst the parietal and occipital lobes are usually spared. The disease may involve mainly the frontal lobes (25%), or mainly the temporal lobes (17%), but most commonly the entire frontotemporal region bears the brunt of the disease. The atrophy of the two hemispheres is symmetrical in a third of cases, whilst the left hemisphere is more severely damaged in nearly 50% of the patients.[142] Atrophy in the frontal lobes may preferentially involve the inferior aspect, including the medial orbital gyri, or, more rarely, the convexity of the lobe. In the temporal lobes the pole is always affected, with the

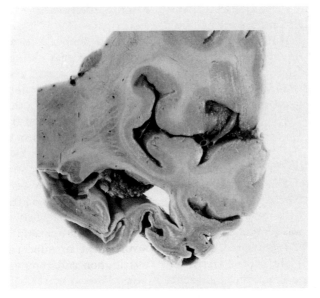

Fig. 13.17 Severe temporal lobe atrophy in Pick's disease: the superior temporal gyrus is well preserved while all the other gyri of the temporal lobe have been devastated.

atrophy extending posteriorly towards the temporal gyri, relatively sparing the posterior two-thirds of the superior temporal gyrus (Fig. 13.17). The severity of cortical atrophy varies, and in extreme cases several gyri are so devastated as to assume a 'walnut' or 'knife-blade' appearance. Occasionally the deep grey matter is involved and the atrophy also spreads to the white matter, which is grey and rubbery.

Histology and ultrastructure. Microscopically, the disease is characterised by neuronal loss, neuronal inclusions and gliosis. The neuronal loss is substantial and, although the pattern is variable, the outer layers tend to be more severely depopulated. In extreme cases the cortex may assume a spongy appearance (Fig. 13.18). Some of the surviving nerve cells become swollen and pear-shaped and their nuclei assume an eccentric position. With the disintegration of the Nissl substance, the cytoplasm becomes homogeneous and

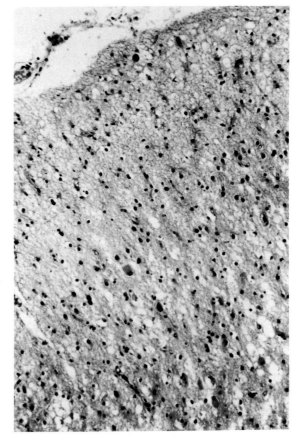

Fig. 13.18 Pick's disease. Histology of the cortex reveals dramatic neuronal loss and spongy appearance. Two large, swollen cells are just discernible (lower centre). Haematoxylin-eosin × 80

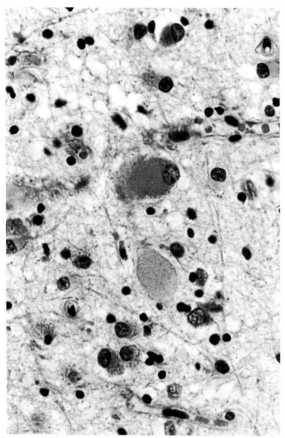

Fig. 13.19 Large, swollen Pick's cells: the abundant cytoplasm is uniformly eosinophilic and the nucleus oval or round.
Haematoxylin-eosin × 300

Neurofibrillary tangles and Pick bodies are both associated with identical phosphorylated neurofilament epitopes.[145] Antibodies to neurofibrillary tangles also react with Pick bodies, suggesting that Alzheimer's and Pick's diseases may share a common molecular pathogenesis which manifests itself in the reorganisation of the filamentous neuronal cytoskeleton.[146]

Astroglial proliferation occurs in atrophied cortical and subcortical areas, in extreme cases justifying the alternative name of 'lobar sclerosis', previously much in use.

The distribution of abnormalities varies and a recent study distinguishes between classical and generalised variants of the disease on the basis of involvement of subcortical structures and the distribution and composition of neuronal inclusions.[147]

eosinophilic (Fig. 13.19). These cells are particularly conspicuous in sections stained with phosphotungstic acid haematoxylin: their pallor contrasts with the darkly stained background. These Pick cells may contain argyrophilic inclusions, the so-called Pick bodies, and are present most frequently in the neocortex: small neurons are affected more often than larger ones. In the hippocampus, area h1 (Sommer sector) is most severely affected.[143] Similar cells also occur in the basal ganglia and in the brainstem. Ultrastructurally, Pick bodies are composed of straight filaments, tubular profiles and paired helical filaments.[144] The use of monoclonal anti-neurofilament antibodies has shown that Pick bodies share antigenic determinants with both neurofilaments and neurofibrillary tangles (Fig. 13.20).

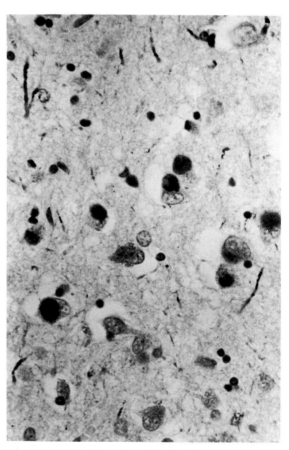

Fig. 13.20 Pick bodies stain positively with a monoclonal anti-neurofilament antibody.
Indirect immunoperoxidase × 320

The cause of Pick's disease is unknown. The rôle of genetic factors, despite the reported familial cases, has not been established. The depletion of neurons in the nucleus basalis of Meynert may indicate a cholinergic deficit,[148] and the reduction in γ-aminobutyric acid (GABA) and substance P in the substantia nigra and the globus pallidus corresponds to the loss of small neurons from the striatum. Dopamine concentrations are markedly reduced in the striatum, in contrast to Huntington's disease.[149] However, biochemical assessments, rare as they are, have not provided clues to the pathogenesis of this dementing disease.

HUNTINGTON'S DISEASE

Huntington's disease is an autosomal dominant degenerative disorder in which dementia and choreiform movements are clinically the most important features. The disease most frequently starts between the ages of 25 and 45 years, although the so-called juvenile form affects children and adolescents. This juvenile type differs from the adult form not only in its clinical manifestations, with akinesia and extrapyramidal rigidity dominating over choreiform movements, but also in the mode of inheritance. Most patients who develop signs and symptoms before the age of 10 years inherit the disease from the father, whereas in the adult form the transmission from either parent is equally likely.[150] The duration of the illness varies considerably, lasting, on average, 15 years.

The prevalence for populations of Northern European origin is 4–7 cases per 100 000, whereas in Japan and amongst blacks in the USA it is much lower.[151] In Britain as many as 3000 people are affected and a further 20 000 carry the risk of developing the disease.[152] The disorder is transmitted by a single dominant gene with a penetrance approaching 100%: each child of an affected parent will have a 50% chance of being affected. Recombinant DNA techniques have localised a genetic marker, a series of DNA sequence polymorphisms, to the terminal band of the short arm of chromosome 4; this may eventually provide a predictive test for those families which are heterozygous for the marker.[153]

Clinically, the disease is relentlessly progressive, but cases with an early onset tend to run a more severe course. There are variations in the sequence of presenting signs and symptoms; in the typical case involuntary movements may precede dementia, but psychiatric disturbances may also appear first. Of the neurological presenting signs, choreiform movements are the most common, but unsteadiness of gait with a tendency to fall or general clumsiness also occurs. Irritability, emotional disturbances and paranoia may precede the appearance of dementia. After the initial stage, both neurological and psychiatric features worsen, occasionally complicated by psychotic episodes.[57] Electroencephalography does not show a definitive pattern, neither is CT scanning diagnostic in itself, although atrophy of the caudate nuclei and cortex together with the pattern of ventricular dilatation may be of confirmatory value.

At autopsy the thoracic and abdominal organs usually appear normal, apart from terminal respiratory infection. The brain occasionally looks

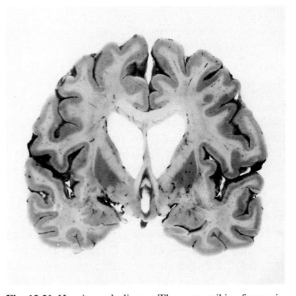

Fig. 13.21 Huntington's disease. The most striking feature is the severe atrophy of the caudate nucleus, rendering the normally convex contour of the lateral aspect of the lateral ventricle flattened. The atrophy of the putamen is less obvious.

normal, but in most cases it is small. Cortical atrophy, manifested by widened sulci and narrowed gyri, is obvious, particularly in the frontoparietal region. The most dramatic feature of the disease is revealed on coronal slices: the corpus striatum, which includes both the caudate nucleus and the putamen, is greatly atrophied. The head of the caudate nucleus which normally bulges into the lateral ventricle may shrink to a narrow, brownish band of tissue and the putamen is also much reduced in size (Fig. 13.21). The substantial loss of the striatum renders the lateral aspects of the greatly dilated lateral ventricles flattened or even concave with rounding of the angle. The internal capsule may appear prominent between the two atrophied parts of the striatum;

with involvement of the white matter, the corpus callosum is thinner than usual. The globus pallidus is also involved, but to a milder degree than the putamen. The brainstem may appear slightly atrophied against the normal-looking cerebellum. Based on naked-eye and histological appearances, a grading system has been established, ranging in severity from grade 0 to 4 and correlating closely with the degree of clinical disability.[154] In a few clinically diagnosed cases, no neuropathological changes were seen (grade 0), indicating that clinical abnormalities may precede morphological damage, whilst in another small group, the alterations could only be recognised by histological examination (grade 1). The earliest changes were seen in the medial paraventricular

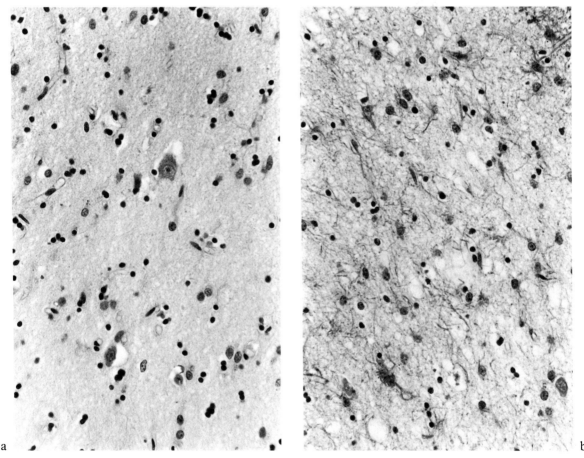

a   b

Fig. 13.22a, b Histology of Huntington's disease. (**a**) There is a considerable loss of neurons in the putamen, but occasional large nerve cells have survived. (**b**) Increase of astrocytes in the putamen.
(**a**) Haematoxylin-eosin × 150; (**b**) Mallory's phosphotungstic acid haematoxylin × 150

portion and tail of the caudate nucleus, and in the dorsal part of the putamen.

Histology and ultrastructure. Microscopical examination shows regionally selective neuronal loss accompanied by glial changes (Fig. 13.22). The most obvious change is the preferential loss of small neurons in the striatum with relative preservation of larger cells. The normal ratio of small to large neurons (160 to 1) is reduced to 40 to 1.[155] However, a recent quantitative analysis reports loss not only of small neurons but also of large cells.[156] Golgi impregnations reveal striking dendritic abnormalities of medium-sized spiny neurons in the striatum, suggesting that a specific population of nerve cells is selectively involved in the pathogenesis of Huntington's disease.[157] The glial changes include frank fibrillary gliosis, whereas the astrocytosis is more apparent than real: astrocytic nuclei appear to be more numerous since they are crowded in a reduced volume of tissue, but in fact there is a 25% loss of astrocytes from the striatum. In decreasing order of severity these changes occur in the caudate nucleus, putamen, and external and internal segments of the globus pallidus. Neuronal loss has been described in the thalamus and hypothalamus, and the Purkinje cells of the cerebellum are sometimes depleted, particularly in the juvenile form of the disease. There is evidence of cortical degeneration in the cerebral hemispheres, with neuronal loss in the third, fourth and fifth layers and accompanying astrocytosis.

Ultrastructural changes include accumulation of lipofuscin, increased Golgi activity, mitochondrial irregularities and degeneration of presynaptic terminals. An increased incidence of nuclear membrane indentations has been observed in the nucleus accumbens, caudate nucleus and frontal cortex, but the significance of this finding remains to be determined; the possibility that it indicates a phase of hyperactive protein synthesis prior to cell death has been considered.[158]

Biochemical abnormalities. γ-aminobutyric acid (GABA), an inhibitory neurotransmitter, and glutamic acid decarboxylase, the enzyme which converts glutamic acid into GABA, are reduced in the corpus striatum and in the substantia nigra.

The number of GABA receptors is reduced in the striatum, but is normal or increased in the globus pallidus and substantia nigra.[159] Reflecting a more generalised abnormality of glutamic acid metabolism, glutamine synthetase has also been found to be reduced in affected brains at post mortem.[160] Dopamine and serotonin measurements have yielded normal results; indeed, striatal dopamine may be even increased, whereas choline acetyltransferase is significantly decreased in the striatum, reflecting the loss of cholinergic interneurons. Increased concentrations of neurotensin, somatostatin and thyrotrophin-releasing hormone have been measured by radio-immunoassay in the caudate nucleus[161] and somatostatin is also increased in the nucleus accumbens.[162] Immunocytochemistry has demonstrated decreased staining for substance P in the internal segment of the globus pallidus and in the substantia nigra, whereas the reaction for met-enkephalin has been similar in both Huntington's and normal brains.[163] The significance of these neurochemical abnormalities is disputed. They may represent selective neuronal degeneration and death in the striatum, but how they relate to the pathology of Huntington's disease remains to be established. The pathogenetic mechanisms and neurotransmitter abnormalities of Huntington's disease have been recently reviewed.[164]

Kainic acid, a rigid cyclic analogue of glutamate, is a potent neurotoxin and, injected into the striatum of experimental animals, produces histological and biochemical abnormalities similar to those of Huntington's disease. This observation raises the possibility of a toxic aetiology; an endogenous kainate-like substance, by overstimulating the corticostriatal system, may cause neuronal death.[165] Since astrocytes influence neuronal activity and play an important rôle in glutamate metabolism, a disturbance of neuronal-glial relationship may be an additional factor in the pathogenesis of the disease.[166]

CREUTZFELDT–JAKOB DISEASE

Creutzfeldt–Jakob disease is a rare dementing disorder of unknown pathogenesis, relentlessly progressive course and fatal outcome. Epidemiological surveys show a worldwide occurrence, and the average annual mortality rate of 0·26 per million in the United States does not vary very substantially from that in other parts of the world, apart from small pockets of higher incidence amongst Libyan Jews and in Slovakia.[167] In England and Wales the annual incidence is 0·3 per million,[168] whilst in France a positive correlation has been demonstrated between frequency of the disease and population density; the annual mortality rate of 0·42 per million in the whole of the country increases to 1·21 in the city of Paris.[169] Approximately 15% of all cases are familial, with incidence as high as 45% in Chile[170] and as low as 6% in Japan[171] and in England and Wales.[172] The pattern of inheritance suggests an autosomal dominant mode.

Although both sexes are usually considered to be equally affected, the most comprehensive epidemiological survey in England and Wales reports a female preponderance of 1·68 to 1.[168] The disease most often starts in middle life and the duration can vary from 3 weeks to 8 years, with the majority of patients dying within 6 months.[172]

Clinically, three variants can be distinguished: subacute, intermediate and amyotrophic. The commonest is the subacute form in which the prodromal symptoms of altered personality, malaise, sleep disturbance and emotional lability are followed by dementia, myoclonus, ataxia, dysphasia, akinetic mutism and cortical blindness. Initial focal cortical disturbance progresses to diffuse deterioration of cortical function and the patients die, demented and usually cachectic, of terminal respiratory infections. In the rare amyotrophic variant, neurogenic muscle atrophy accompanies dementia, whilst in the intermediate form the terminal stage of the disease is preceded by a prolonged period of focal or diffuse neurological signs.[172] Electroencephalography is of considerable diagnostic value and shows characteristic alterations in two-thirds of the patients. CT scan may reveal cerebral atrophy but, since no abnormalities are seen in most cases, its main use is to exclude other diseases.

The autopsy reveals terminal respiratory infection and otherwise normal viscera in the usually cachectic body. The brain may appear normal or may show focal or diffuse atrophy; in

severe cases it may weigh as little as 1000 g. Various subclassifications to encompass all the variants of a clinically and pathologically diverse disease have now been abandoned and replaced by a simple system based on the distribution of morphological abnormalities. To the originally defined four variants of cortical, corticospinal, corticostriatal and corticostriatospinal,[173] the corticostriatocerebellar form was later added.[174] The disease thus characteristically affects the grey matter (neocortex, striatum, thalamus, cerebellar cortex and dentate nucleus), but occasionally the white matter may also be involved, with severe spongiosis, loss of myelin and astrocytic proliferation.[175]

Histology and ultrastructure. Histologically, the disease is characterised by the triad of neuronal

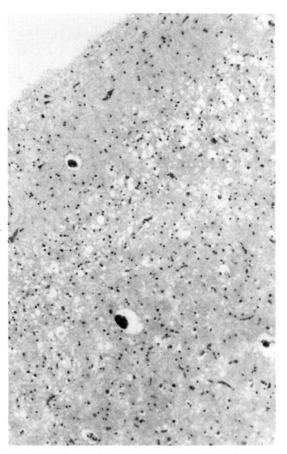

Fig. 13.23 Neuronal loss and vacuolation of the cortex in Creutzfeldt–Jakob disease. Haematoxylin-eosin × 50

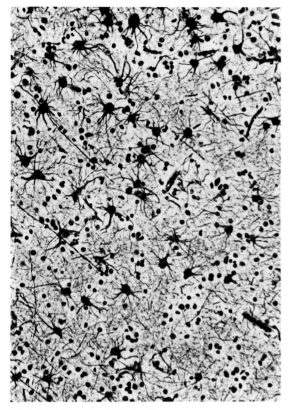

Fig. 13.24 Astrocytosis in the deep cortex.
Hortega's silver carbonate technique × 240

loss, sponginess and astrocytic response (Figs 13.23, 24). The spongy appearance of the grey matter may be caused by fine vacuolation, often referred to as spongiform change, or by a more severe microcystic cavitation, resulting in status spongiosus. The severity of these changes can vary considerably from case to case: the spongy appearance may remain localised or may diffusely involve the entire neocortex and deep grey matter. There is, however, no apparent correlation between the severity of cortical changes and the duration of the disease.[176] When cortical atrophy is severe and extensive, status spongiosus develops and the 'cystic' cortex may collapse to form irregular clefts. This spongy state, however, is non-specific and may occur in elderly individuals, in Alzheimer's disease and other conditions in which there is extensive neuronal loss. Neuronal loss is variable, but tends to be severe in advanced cases and is accompanied by striking astrocytic hypertrophy and hyperplasia. Golgi impregnation may

reveal severe loss of dendritic spines together with focal spherical distensions of dendrites and axons, changes which could partly be responsible for the neurological signs in the absence of severe neuronal loss.[177] Decrease of nerve cells also occurs in the nucleus basalis of Meynert and may be responsible for the cortical cholinergic deficit.[178]

In the corticostriatal variant the caudate nucleus and putamen show similar changes, in the cerebellar form small amyloid plaques may also be observed, whilst in the cases with involvement of the spinal cord the motor pathways are affected. Electron microscopy shows vacuoles in the cell body and processes of neurons and astrocytes (Fig. 13.25). Swollen cell processes in the neuropil tend to rupture to form larger vacuoles.[177] Virus-like particles[179] and spiroplasma-like inclusions[180] have been reported in biopsy material, but the significance of these structures in the pathogenesis of the disease remains unknown.

Spongiform encephalopathies and the transmissibility of Creutzfeldt–Jakob disease

Creutzfeldt–Jakob disease and kuru in man, and two veterinary diseases, scrapie in sheep and mink encephalopathy (scrapie in mink), are classified together on the basis of common morphological features and their transmissibility. Bovine spongiform encephalopathy may also fall into this category. The previously popular term 'slow virus diseases' has now lost favour, since it is far from established that these disorders, despite their infectious nature, are caused by viruses. Indeed, no viruses or viral antibodies have been convincingly demonstrated, and no inflammatory response has been elicited in the affected brains; these features are most unusual in conventional viral infections. Moreover, the agent does not appear to contain nucleic acids. The history of research on these diseases is one of the most exciting in modern medicine and has been recently reviewed.[181] Recognition of the clinical and morphological similarities between Creutzfeldt–Jakob disease and kuru on the one hand and scrapie on the other gave the impetus which led to the successful transmission of the two human diseases to primates.[182] Kuru, now a

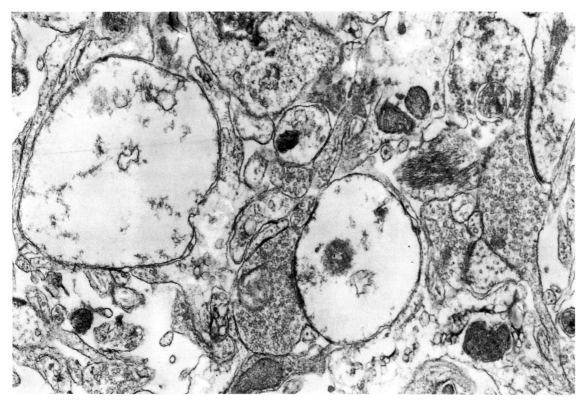

Fig. 13.25 Electron micrograph of the cortex in Creutzfeldt–Jakob disease shows dilated cell processes, one of which (right) can be identified as neuronal, since it forms a synapse.
Electron micrograph × 27 000
Material lent for reproduction by Dr I. Janota, Department of Neuropathology, Institute of Psychiatry, London, UK.

disease of only historical interest, occurred amongst natives of the Fore tribe in Papua New Guinea and was transmitted by cannibalism. The cerebellum, particularly the phylogenetically older parts of the vermis and flocculonodular lobe, showed atrophy. Microscopically, there was loss of Purkinje and granule cells, astrocytosis and fibrillary gliosis throughout the cerebellar cortex and a microglial response in the molecular layer (Fig. 13.26). Amyloid plaques were also abundant. The brainstem showed neuronal loss and degeneration accompanied by fibrillary gliosis; degeneration of the corticospinal and spinocerebellar tracts was also observed. The cerebral hemispheres were affected, with changes similar to those of Creutzfeldt–Jakob disease.[176]

The neuropathology of transmitted kuru and Creutzfeldt–Jakob disease in experimental animals is strikingly similar to that of those diseases in man.[183] The transmission experiments have not

only established the infectious nature of spongiform encephalopathies but also provided a model for the study of their pathogenesis.[184] Creutzfeldt–Jakob disease can be transmitted to a variety of laboratory animals, including guinea pigs, hamsters, mice, rats, cats, goats, ferrets and primates. Moreover, iatrogenic transmission via corneal transplants and stereotactic electrodes has occurred in man.[167,181] Contaminated growth hormone has also been incriminated in the transmission of the disease: 3 neuropathologically confirmed cases have been reported, 2 from the USA[185,186] and 1 from England,[187] after treatment with human growth hormone (see p. 221). All 3 patients died under 25 years of age. Despite extensive experimental and epidemiological studies, the causative agent of Creutzfeldt–Jakob disease remains elusive. It has been suggested that fibrils, first seen in the brains of scrapie-infected mice, are specific for spongiform encephalo-

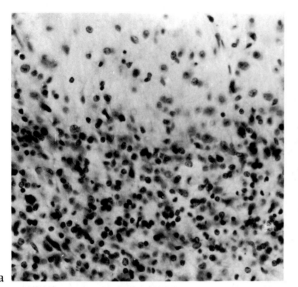 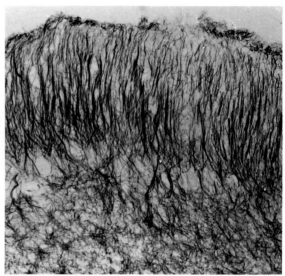

a   b

Fig. 13.26a, b The cerebellum in human kuru. (**a**) Loss of Purkinje and granule cells is accompanied by astrocytic proliferation and microglial response. (**b**) Extensive fibrillary gliosis in the cerebellar cortex.
(**a**) Cresyl violet × 300; (**b**) Holzer × 160
Light micrographs kindly provided by Dr Elisabeth Beck, Department of Neuropathology, Institute of Psychiatry, London, UK.

pathies and represent the aetiological agents.[188] The term 'prion' has been introduced to describe the pathogen, and purified preparations of prions were found to contain a single major protein designated PrP$_{27-30}$.[189] Biochemical analysis suggests that some of these proteins are glycoproteins or sialoglycoproteins which derive from, or reside in, the cell membranes.[190] The molecular biology and biochemistry of prions has been extensively studied[191] but the evidence presently available does not definitely resolve the aetiological rôle of prions.

Precautionary measures for handling Creutzfeldt–Jakob material

The nature of Creutzfeldt–Jakob disease, as a relentlessly progressive, transmissible dementia, and the elusiveness of its aetiological agent, have created considerable uncertainty and confusion as to the safety of carrying out autopsies and handling pathological specimens. The iatrogenic transmission of a few cases and the reported higher incidence of the disease in health professionals, which is more apparent than real, have generated an atmosphere of fear. Clear guidelines for clinical, surgical and pathological practices have now been

established[192] and the pathologist can safely, and should, fulfil his professional duties.

The brain and other parts of the nervous system are the most likely tissues to transmit the disease, even after prolonged formalin fixation, whilst liver, lung, lymph nodes, kidney and CSF carry a lower risk of infection. The causative agent resists standard methods of disinfection and sterilisation by heat, formaldehyde, 70% alcohol, ultraviolet and ionising irradiation, but autoclaving at 121°C for one hour and the use of a 1% dilution of hypochlorite containing 10 000 ppm chlorine are satisfactory disinfectants for instruments and exposed surfaces. Contaminated skin should be disinfected by 1 N sodium hydroxide for 5–10 minutes followed by copious washing with water.[193]

DEMENTIA ASSOCIATED WITH VASCULAR DISEASE

Cerebral vascular disease is the second commonest cause of dementia both in the presenile and in the senile groups. In patients over 65, vascular disease is responsible for 15%, whilst Alzheimer's disease combined with cerebral softening (infarction), the so-called mixed dementia, constitutes a further

10%. The emphasis on the pathogenesis of dementia associated with vascular pathology has shifted from atherosclerosis to hypertension. Although atherosclerotic degeneration may be a contributing factor, the primary underlying cause is usually hypertension, severe and sustained enough to lead to extensive vascular damage and to infarctions of various sizes. These multiple infarctions can produce a condition in which dementia is the predominant clinical manifestation (*multi-infarct dementia*).[194] In addition to dementia, the disease is characterised by focal neurological signs and symptoms and stepwise clinical deterioration. These features, together with a usually sudden onset and the presence of brainstem signs, distinguish multi-infarct dementia from pure Alzheimer's disease. In combined cases of Alzheimer's disease and multi-infarct dementia these distinguishing features become blurred and the final diagnosis depends on the outcome of histological examination. Cerebral infarcts can be present in intellectually intact individuals; quantitative measurements have shown that the volume of brain tissue destroyed when dementia results is of the order of 100 ml. This leaves open the question of distribution, since the location of infarcts is also a crucial factor in the pathogenesis

of dementia. Whilst hypertension is the most frequent underlying cause, other vascular diseases, including collagen vascular disorders, Takayashu disease and moya-moya disease, may produce dementia, as do multiple thromboembolic infarcts (see pp. 102–104 and 99–100).

The pathological examination of the brain shows the familiar picture of infarcts of various sizes (Figs 13.27 and 13.28), and other lesions associated with hypertensive vascular disease (see p. 97).

In other cases of dementia associated with hypertension, the white matter bears the brunt of damage, whilst the cerebral cortex is relatively well preserved. The distribution of lesions in these cases warrants their separation from multi-infarct dementia: the name *Binswanger's disease* has been given to the condition, after its original observer, although he did not appreciate the pathogenetic rôle of hypertension. The patients develop dementia, focal neurological signs and psychiatric disturbances at around the age of 50. Post-mortem examination of the brain reveals a relatively well-preserved cortex and only occasional small scars and cavities in the basal ganglia, thalamus and brainstem, whereas the deep white matter is usually reduced in amount (Fig. 13.29), contains

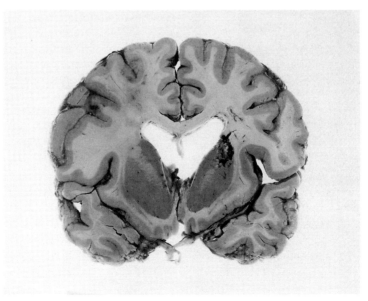

Fig. 13.27 Cerebral vascular disease. Infarcts of various sizes and ages are present in the cortex, white matter and basal ganglia.

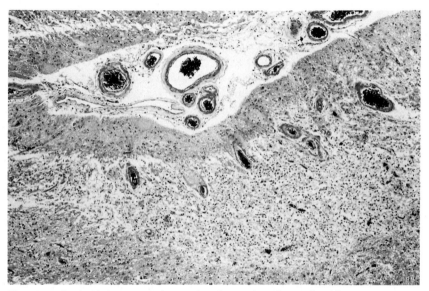

Fig. 13.28 Cortical infarct results in complete devastation of normal architecture. Haematoxylin-eosin × 50

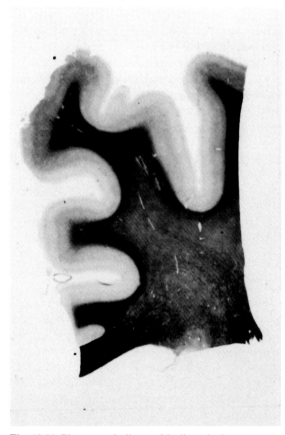

Fig. 13.29 Binswanger's disease. Myelin stain demonstrates pallor as a result of damaged white matter. Klüver–Barrera

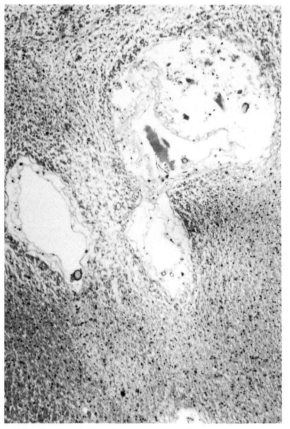

Fig. 13.30 Small cavities in the white matter in Binswanger's disease. Haematoxylin-eosin × 50

cavities of various sizes (Fig. 13.30), and appears to be softened and greyish. The ventricular system is dilated in most cases. Microscopically, there is extensive, patchy loss of myelin and axons, fibrillary gliosis and abnormal small blood vessels with thickened fibrous walls, but without occlusion.[195] The clinical and pathological features of Binswanger's disease and the underlying aetiological factors have been recently reviewed.[196]

A different type of white matter damage has been observed in association with Alzheimer's disease. Symmetrical, incomplete infarctions of the deep white matter are histologically characterised by a partial loss of myelin, axons and oligodendroglial cells, mild astrocytosis, sparsely distributed macrophages and hyaline fibrosis of the arterioles of small vessels. These changes, which do not result in cavitating infarction and are not accompanied by hypertensive vascular degeneration, are thought to be caused by hypoperfusion.[197] The term *leuco-araiosis* has been recently introduced to describe white matter changes which are seen as reduced densities on CT scan in elderly or demented individuals. Similar neuroradiological appearances may be associated with different pathological and pathophysiological processes.[198]

The recognition of multi-infarct dementia and Binswanger's disease is not only of theoretical importance in clarifying nosological entities but also of practical value. These conditions can now often be diagnosed in life by the use of CT scan, and the underlying disease, most often hypertension, can be treated.[194–199]

Congophilic angiopathy is often seen in Alzheimer's disease (see p. 370), but on rare occasions it is a separate entity. The severe vascular involvement leads to occlusion and haemorrhage, and although amyloid-containing plaques are common in the hippocampus and cerebellum, the typical Alzheimer changes are absent.[200]

OTHER DEMENTIAS

Dementia pugilistica

Dementia is a recognised sequel of boxing and the neuropathological changes have been described in retired boxers (page 141).[201] Naked-eye alterations include abnormalities of the septum pellucidum, scarring (chiefly in the cerebellum) and degeneration of the substantia nigra. The cavity of the septum pellucidum often enlarges and its width may reach three or more times that in the normal brain; the laminae of the septum become grossly fenestrated. In the cerebellum, well-defined cortical scarring is seen on the inferior surface of the lateral lobes, and usually the tonsillar regions are most severely affected. Histologically, there is a considerable loss of Purkinje cells which appears to extend well beyond the areas of scarring. Depigmentation of the substantia nigra is common and light microscopy reveals neurofibrillary tangles in the surviving nerve cells, whereas Lewy bodies (pp. 44, 412) are absent: the overall appearances are closer to those of postencephalitic parkinsonism than to Parkinson's disease (paralysis agitans). The most striking histological feature is, however, the presence of neurofibrillary tangles in the absence of neuritic plaques. Neurofibrillary tangles are distributed throughout the cerebral cortex and brainstem, but the medial temporal grey matter is particularly severely affected. These findings indicate that repeated blows to the head may cause wide-ranging changes in the brain, leading to dementia. Indeed, the possible aetiological rôle of head injury has been shown in an epidemiological study in which a significantly increased incidence of head injury with a loss of consciousness has been found in patients suffering from Alzheimer's disease.[202]

Dementia associated with Parkinson's disease

That a proportion of patients suffering from Parkinson's disease develops dementia (see p. 413) is common knowledge, but it has been only recently realised that Lewy bodies (see p. 412) may be widely distributed in the cerebral cortex (Fig. 13.31). The term Lewy body disease has been suggested to describe those cases in which the occurrence of these neuronal inclusions is a prominent feature.[203,204] Based on the distribution of Lewy bodies, three groups can be distinguished: diffuse, transitional and brainstem types of Lewy

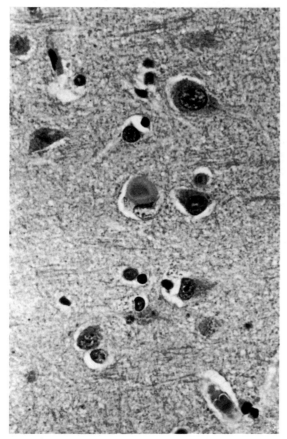

Fig. 13.31 A cortical Lewy body (centre) in a demented patient.
Haematoxylin-eosin × 320

body disease. Cases with the characteristic brainstem pathology (*brainstem type* Lewy body disease) form the largest group: there is no evidence of cortical Lewy bodies. Neuritic plaques and neurofibrillary tangles are in accordance with age, and dementia does not develop. In the *diffuse type*, Lewy bodies are present not only in the brainstem but also in the cortex, neuritic plaques and neurofibrillary tangles are common and progressive dementia develops in addition to the neurological deficit of paralysis agitans. In the *transitional group*, the severity of the cortical changes is between that of the previous two groups. Dementia develops only in those patients whose brains are more severely involved by Lewy bodies or senile changes. Patients who exhibit the cortical changes of diffuse and transitional Lewy body disease may become demented.

An increased incidence of abnormal, pigment-filled axons of pyramidal cells in the third layer of the cortex has also been reported in Parkinson's disease.[205]

The cause of dementia in Parkinson's disease is likely to be multifactorial. The dopaminergic system is not restricted to the basal ganglia, but via the mesocortical and mesolimbic projections it extends to the cortex and hippocampus. Pathology in the locus ceruleus results in damage to the ascending noradrenergic projections to the cortex. Thus cortical dopamine and noradrenaline deficits may play an important rôle in the dementia. Moreover, neuronal loss in the nucleus basalis of Meynert, and Lewy body formation in some of the surviving neurons, may also contribute to the dementia observed in Parkinson's disease.[206]

Dementia associated with AIDS

In acquired immune deficiency syndrome (AIDS, see p. 214) the involvement of the nervous system reaches 80%.[207] In addition to the usual opportunistic infections and neoplasms, practically all parts of the nervous system are affected, including the brain, spinal cord, peripheral nerves, neuromuscular junctions and muscles.[208,209]

A progressive AIDS encephalopathy, often referred to as AIDS-dementia complex, develops in half of the patients. This disease is not merely another complication of AIDS, but a paramount manifestation of HIV infection of the brain. Its onset is usually insidious, but chronic deterioration of cognitive, behavioural and motor functions leads to progressive dementia. CT scans of the brain may show cortical atrophy and ventricular dilatation without any evidence of focal lesions, although white matter changes are better seen on nuclear magnetic imaging. The pathology varies in character and severity. White matter abnormalities range from diffuse pallor to extensive loss of myelin and axons. Scattered microglial nodules and collections of foamy macrophages may be seen throughout the brain. In one-third of cases, multinucleate giant cells, which are pathognomonic of HIV infection,[209a] are accompanied by macrophages, microglial cells and lymphocytes in the deep grey matter, white matter and cortex. This multifocal inflammatory process is the new entity of HIV encephalitis.[209b] There is no clear relationship between the severity of dementia and the degree of neuropathological changes.[210,211] Using in situ hybridisation and immunohistochemistry, HIV infection has been detected in macrophages, giant cells and endothelial cells in affected brains.[212]

Down's syndrome

The aetiology and pathology of Down's syndrome have been described on page 313. The cell biological aspects of the disease, including neurotransmitter abnormalities, have been recently reviewed.[213,214] Patients with Down's syndrome who survive into adulthood develop dementia, and their brains show changes which are indistinguishable from those in Alzheimer's disease.[215] The appearance of neuritic plaques precedes the formation of neurofibrillary tangles and granulovacuoles, and they are most numerous in the frontal lobes and in the hippocampus. Neurofibrillary tangles, although present in the neocortex, are most frequently encountered in the hippocampus, whereas granulovacuolar degeneration is usually restricted to the hippocampus. Within the hippocampus, the distribution of both neurofibrillary tangles and granulovacuoles is similar to that in Alzheimer's disease, suggesting that a common pathogenetic mechanism may underlie these regional predilections.[216] Neuronal loss also occurs; in particular the number of aspinous stellate cells is reduced.[217] Ultrastructurally, synaptic abnormalities, including reduced synaptic parameters, are common, and these may be responsible for the inefficiency of synaptic transmission.[218]

Hydrocephalus and dementia

Longstanding communicating hydrocephalus is frequently associated with the clinical triad of dementia, gait disturbance and urinary incontinence.[219] CSF pressure usually is normal at lumbar puncture, but continuous monitoring may record episodes of increased pressure, particularly during sleep. Thus the term 'intermittently raised pressure hydrocephalus' is more appropriate than the previously used 'normal pressure hydrocephalus'. The underlying cause could be an old subarachnoid haemorrhage, head injury or meningitis, all conditions which have led to fibrous adhesions in the basal cistern; yet in other cases no pathological abnormalities are found. In patients with intermittent hydrocephalus, impaired CSF absorption results in ventricular dilatation and a newly adjusted level of CSF production and absorption.[220] CT scan shows severe dilatation of the ventricles, whilst the sulci are normal or hardly discernible; this latter feature is in contrast with the dilated sulci to be seen in cerebral atrophy. It is of paramount importance to distinguish this form of hydrocephalus, which is likely to be amenable to treatment, from primary degenerative brain disease such as Alzheimer's disease and multi-infarct dementia.

REFERENCES

Ageing
1. Tomlinson BE. In: Smith WT, Cavanagh JB, eds. Recent advances in neuropathology. Edinburgh: Churchill Livingstone, 1979; 1: 129.
2. Tomlinson BE, Corsellis JAN. In: Adams JH, Corsellis JAN, Duchen LW, eds. Greenfield's Neuropathology. 4th ed. London: Arnold, 1984: 951.
3. Corsellis JAN. In: Terry RD, Gershon S, eds. Neurobiology of aging. Aging; vol. 3. New York: Raven Press, 1976: 205.
4. Hubbard BM, Anderson JM. Lancet 1983; 1: 1447.
5. Davis PJM, Wright EA. Neuropathol Appl Neurobiol 1977; 3: 341.
6. Miller AKH, Alston RL, Corsellis JAN. Neuropathol Appl Neurobiol 1980; 6: 119.
7. Hubbard BM, Anderson JM. J Neurol Neurosurg Psychiatry 1981; 44: 631.
8. Bird JM, Prog Neurobiol 1982; 19: 91.
9. Brody H. J Comp Neurol 1955; 102: 511.
10. Anderson JM, Hubbard BM, Coghill GR, Slidders W. J Neurol Sci 1983; 58: 233.
11. Miller AKH, Alston RL, Mountjoy CQ, Corsellis JAN. Neuropathol Appl Neurobiol 1984; 10: 123.
12. Tomlinson BE, Irving D, Blessed G. J Neurol Sci 1981; 49: 419.
13. Arendt T, Bigl V, Arendt A, Tennstedt A. Acta Neuropathol (Berl) 1983; 61: 101.
14. Kidd M. Brain 1964; 87: 307.
15. Terry RD, Gonatas NK, Weiss M. Am J Pathol 1964; 44: 269.

16. Mann DMA, Tucker CM, Yates PO. Neuropathol Appl Neurobiol 1987; 13: 123.
17. Tomlinson BE, Blessed G, Roth M. J Neurol Sci 1968; 7: 331.
18. Terry RD, Wisniewski HM. In: Gaitz CM, ed. Aging and the brain. New York: Plenum Press, 1972: 89.
19. Probst A, Brunnschweiler H, Lautenschlager C, Ulrich J. Acta Neuropathol (Berl) 1987; 74: 133.
20. Ishii T. Acta Neuropathol (Berl) 1966; 6: 181.
21. Wisniewski HM, Wen GY. Acta Neuropathol (Berl) 1985; 66: 173.
22. Grundke-Iqbal I, Johnson AB, Wisniewski HM, Terry RD, Iqbal K. Lancet 1979; 1: 578.
23. Anderton BH, Breinburg D, Downes MJ et al. Nature 1982; 298: 84.
24. Rasool CG, Abraham C, Anderton BH, Haugh M, Kahn J, Selkoe DJ. Brain Res 1984; 310: 249.
25. Perry G, Rizzuto N, Autilio-Gambetti L, Gambetti P. Proc Natl Acad Sci USA 1985; 82: 3916.
26. Joachim CL, Morris JH, Selkoe DJ, Kosik KS. J Neuropathol Exp Neurol 1987; 46: 611.
27. Dickson DW, Ksiezak-Reding H, Davies P, Yen S-H. Acta Neuropathol (Berl) 1987; 73: 254.
28. Tomlinson BE, Kitchener D. J Pathol 1972; 106: 165.
29. Hirano A, Dembitzer HM, Kurland LT, Zimmerman HM. J Neuropathol Exp Neurol 1968; 26: 167.
30. Gambetti P, Shecket G, Ghetti B, Hirano A, Dahl D. J Neuropathol Exp Neurol 1983; 42: 69.
31. Galloway PG, Perry G, Gambetti P. J Neuropathol Exp Neurol 1987; 46: 185.
32. Gibson PH. Acta Neuropathol (Berl) 1978; 42: 165.
33. Gibson PH, Tomlinson BE. J Neurol Sci 1977; 33: 199.
34. Scheibel AB. In: Katzman R, Terry RD, Bick KL, eds. Alzheimer's disease, senile dementia, and related disorders. Aging, vol 7. New York: Raven Press, 1978: 353.
35. Gibson PH. Acta Neuropathol (Berl) 1983; 62: 127.
36. Bondareff W. Mech Ageing Dev 1979; 9: 163.
37. Jones DG. In: Fedoroff S, Hertz L, eds. Advances in cellular neurobiology. New York: Academic Press, 1983; 4: 163.
38. Lintl P, Braak H. Acta Neuropathol (Berl) 1983; 61: 178.
39. Williams RS, Ferrante RJ, Caviness VS Jr. J Neuropathol Exp Neurol 1978; 37: 13.
40. Buell SJ, Coleman PD. Science 1979; 206: 854.
41. Bell MA, Ball MJ. Acta Neuropathol (Berl) 1981; 53: 299.
42. Hunziker O, Abdel'Al S, Schulz U. J Gerontol 1979; 34: 345.
43. Wilkinson JH, Hopewell JW, Rheinhold HS. Neuropathol Appl Neurobiol 1981; 7: 451.
44. Mountjoy CQ, Tomlinson BE, Gibson PH. J Neurol Sci 1982; 57: 89.
45. Mandybur TI. Neurology (Minneap) 1975; 25: 120.
46. Torack RM, Lynch RG. Acta Neuropathol (Berl) 1981; 53: 189.
47. Ishii T, Haga S. Acta Neuropathol (Berl) 1976; 36: 243.
48. Masters CL, Simms G, Weinman NA, Multhaup G, McDonald BL, Beyreuther K. Proc Natl Acad Sci USA 1985; 82: 4245.
49. Powers JM, Skeen JT. J Neuropathol Exp Neurol 1980; 39: 385.
50. Powers JM, Sullivan L, Rosenthal CJ. Acta Neuropathol (Berl) 1982; 58: 275.
51. Vinters HV. Stroke 1987; 18: 311.
52. Landon M, Kidd M, Allsop D. Rev Neurosci 1987; 1: 101.
53. Scheibel AB. In: Wertheimer J, ed. Senile dementia: outlook for the future. New York: Alan Liss, 1984: 137.
54. Mancardi GL, Liwnicz BH, Mandybur TI. Acta Neuropathol (Berl) 1983; 61: 76.
55. Bjørklund H, Eriksdotter-Nilsson M, Dahl D, Rose G, Hoffer B, Olson L. Exp Brain Res 1985; 58: 163.
56. Vernadakis A, Parker K, Arnold EB, Norenberg M. In: Giacobini E, Filogamo G, Giacobini G, Vernadakis A, eds. The aging brain: cellular and molecular mechanisms of aging in the nervous system. New York: Raven Press, 1982: 57.

Dementias

57. Lishman WA. Organic psychiatry. 2nd ed. Oxford: Blackwell, 1987.
58. Mölsä PK, Marttila RJ, Rinne UK. Acta Neurol Scand 1982; 65: 541.
59. Terry RD, Katzman R. Ann Neurol 1983; 14: 497.
60. Haase GR. In: Wells CE, ed. Dementia. 2nd ed. Philadelphia: Davis, 1977: 27.
61. Marsden CD, Harrison MJG. Br Med J 1972; 2: 249.
62. Tomlinson BE, Blessed G, Roth M. J Neurol Sci 1970; 11: 205.
63. Alzheimer A. Allg Z Psychiatrie 1907; 64: 146.
64. Tomlinson BE, In: Wells CE, ed. Dementia. 2nd ed. Philadelphia: Davis 1977: 113.
65. Schneck MK, Reisberg B, Ferris SH. Am J Psychiatry 1982; 139: 165.
66. Besson JAO, Corrigan FM, Foreman EI, Ashcroft GW, Eastwood LM, Smith FW. Lancet 1983; 2: 789.
67. Benson DF, Kuhl DE, Hawkins RA, Phelps ME, Cummings JL, Tsai SAY. Arch Neurol 1983; 40: 711.
68. Duyckaerts C, Hauw JJ, Piette F et al. Acta Neuropathol (Berl) 1985; 66: 72.
69. Rudelli RD, Ambler MW, Wisniewski HM. Acta Neuropathol (Berl) 1984; 64: 273.
70. Ball MJ. Acta Neuropathol (Berl) 1978; 42: 73.
71. Esiri MM, Wilcock GK. J Neurol Neurosurg Psychiatry 1984; 47: 56.
72. Anderton BH. Nature 1987; 325: 658.
73. Anderton BH. Nature 1987; 329: 106.
74. Carrell RW. Nature 1988; 331: 478.
75. Saitoh T, Hansen LA, Dobkins KR, Terry RD. J Neuropathol Exp Neurol 1988; 47: 1.
76. Whitehouse PJ, Price DL, Struble RG, Clark AW, Coyle JT, DeLong MR. Science 1982; 215: 1237.
77. Perry EK, Tomlinson BE, Blessed G, Bergmann K, Gibson PH, Perry RH. Br Med J 1978; 2: 1457.
78. Wilcock GK, Esiri MM, Bowen DM, Smith CCT. J Neurol Sci 1982; 57: 407.
79. Whitehouse PJ, Price DL, Clark AW, Coyle JT, DeLong MR. Ann Neurol 1981; 10: 122.
80. Rinne JO, Paljärvi L, Rinne UK. J Neurol Sci 1987; 79: 67.
81. Marcyniuk B, Mann DMA, Yates PO. J Neurol Sci 1986; 76: 335.
82. Tomlinson BE, Irving D, Blessed G. J Neurol Sci 1981; 49: 419.
83. Terry RD, Peck A, DeTeresa R, Schechter R, Horoupian DS. Ann Neurol 1981; 10: 184.
84. Mountjoy CQ, Roth M, Evans NJR, Evans HM. Neurobiol Aging 1983; 4: 1.

85. Hubbard BM, Anderson JM. Neuropathol Appl Neurobiol 1985; 11: 369.
86. Probst A, Basler B, Bron B, Ulrich J. Brain Res 1983; 268: 249.
87. Davies CA, Mann DMA, Sumpter PQ, Yates PO. J Neurol Sci 1987; 78: 151.
88. Esiri MM, Wilcock GK. J Neurol Neurosurg Psychiatry 1986; 49: 1221.
89. Roher A, Gray EG, Paula-Barbosa M. Proc R Soc Lond [Biol] 1988; 232: 367.
90. Rossor MN, Iversen LL, Reynolds GP, Mountjoy CQ, Roth M. Br Med J 1984; 288: 961.
91. Smith DA, Lantos PL. J Neurol Neurosurg Psychiatry 1983; 46: 675.
92. Terry RD, Hansen LA, DeTeresa R, Davies P, Tobias H, Katzman R. J Neuropathol Exp Neurol 1987; 46: 262.
93. Masters CL. Pathology 1984; 16: 233.
94. Mann DMA. Mech Ageing Dev 1985; 31: 213.
95. Bowen DM, Smith CB, White P, Davison AN. Brain 1976; 99: 459.
96. Davies P, Maloney AJF. Lancet 1976; 2: 1403.
97. Perry EK, Gibson PH, Blessed G, Perry RH, Tomlinson BE. J Neurol Sci 1977; 34: 247.
98. Coyle JT, Price DL, DeLong MR. Science 1983; 219: 1184.
99. Whitehouse PJ, Martino AM, Antuono PG, Lowenstein PR, Coyle JT, Price DL, Kellar KJ. Brain Res 1986; 371: 146.
100. Perry EK. Br Med Bull 1986; 42: 63.
101. Rossor MN. Lancet 1982; 2: 1200.
102. Mann DMA, Yates PO, Marcyniuk B. Clin Neuropathol 1984; 3: 199.
103. Ferrier IN, Cross AJ, Johnson JA et al. J Neurol Sci 1983; 62: 159.
104. Roberts GW, Crow TJ, Polak JM. Nature 1985; 314: 92.
105. Morrison JH, Rogers J, Scherr S, Benoit R, Bloom FE. Nature 1985; 314: 90.
106. De Souza EB, Whitehouse PJ, Kuhar MJ, Price DL, Vale WW. Nature 1986; 319: 593.
107. Chan-Palay V, Lang W, Allen YS, Haesler U, Polak JM. J Comp Neurol 1985; 238: 390.
108. Rossor M, Iversen LL. Br Med Bull 1986; 42: 70.
109. Cross AJ, Slater P, Candy JM, Perry EK, Perry RH. J Neurol Neurosurg Psychiatry 1987; 50: 367.
110. Mann DMA. Neuropathol Appl Neurobiol 1982; 8: 161.
111. Sajdel-Sulkowska EM, Marotta CA. Science 1984; 225: 947.
112. Doebler JA, Markesbery WA, Anthony A, Rhoads RE. J Neuropathol Exp Neurol 1987; 46: 28.
113. Crapper-McLachlan DR, Lewis PN, Lukiw WJ, Sima A, Bergeron C, DeBoni U. Ann Neurol 1984; 15: 329.
114. Crapper DR, Krishnan SS, Quittkat S. Brain 1976; 99: 67.
115. Candy JM, Oakley AE, Klinowski J et al. Lancet 1986; 1: 354.
116. Crapper JM, McLachlan DR. Neurobiol Aging 1986; 7: 525.
117. Shore D, Wyatt RJ. J Nerv Ment Dis 1983; 171: 553.
118. Alfrey AC, LeGendre GR, Kaehny WD. New Engl J Med 1976; 294: 184.
119. Crapper DR, Quittkat S, Krishnan SS, Dalton AJ, DeBoni U. Acta Neuropathol (Berl) 1980; 50: 19.
120. Wisniewski HM, Sturman JA, Shek JW. Ann Neurol 1980; 8: 479.
121. Wisniewski HM, Shek JW, Gruca S, Sturman JA. Acta Neuropathol (Berl) 1984; 63: 190.
122. Rees S, Cragg B. Acta Neuropathol (Berl) 1983; 59: 31.
123. Burnet FM. Lancet 1981; 1: 186.
124. Alafuzoff I, Adolfsson R, Grundke-Iqbal I, Winblad B. Acta Neuropathol (Berl) 1987; 73: 160.
125. Nandy K. In: Hoyer S ed. The aging brain: physiological and pathophysiological aspects. Berlin: Springer, 1982: 123.
126. Fillit HM, Kemeny E, Luine V, et al. J Gerontol 1987; 42: 180.
127. Goudsmit J. Am J Psychiatry 1982; 139: 1380.
128. DeBoni U, Crapper-McLachlan DR. Life Sci 1980; 27: 1.
129. Wisniewski HM, Merz GS, Carp RI. Acta Neurol Scand [Suppl] 1984; 99: 91.
130. Somerville RA. Lancet 1985; 1: 504.
131. Ball MJ. Can J Neurol Sci 1982; 9: 303.
132. Pogo BGT, Casals J, Elizan TS. Brain 1987; 110: 907.
133. Kay DWK. Br Med Bull 1986; 42: 19.
134. Heston LL, Mastri AR, Anderson VE, White J. Arch Gen Psychiatry 1981; 38: 1085.
135. Whalley LJ, Carothers AD, Collyer S, De Mey R, Frackiewicz A. Br J Psychiatry 1982; 140: 249.
136. Nee LE, Polinsky RJ, Eldridge R, Weingartner H, Smallberg S, Ebert M. Arch Neurol 1983; 40: 203.
137. Heyman A, Wilkinson WE, Stafford JA, Helms MJ, Sigmon AH, Weinberg T. Ann Neurol 1984; 15: 335.
138. Kilpatrick C, Burns R, Blumbergs PC. J Neurol Neurosurg Psychiatry 1983; 46: 421.
139. Martin JM. Psychol Med 1982; 12: 231.
140. Nordensson I, Beckman G, Adolfsson R, Bucht G, Winblad B. Age Ageing 1983; 12: 285.
141. Groen JJ, Endtz LJ. Brain 1982; 105: 443.
142. van Mansvelt J. Pick's disease. A syndrome of lobar cerebral atrophy, its clinicoanatomical and histopathological types. Enschede: van der Loeff, 1954.
143. Ball MJ. J Neuropathol Exp Neurol 1979; 38: 614.
144. Takauchi S, Hosomi M, Marasigan S, Sato M, Hayashi S, Miyoshi K. Acta Neuropathol (Berl) 1984; 64: 344.
145. Ulrich J, Haugh M, Anderton BH, Probst A, Lautenschlager C, His B. Acta Neuropathol (Berl) 1987; 73: 240.
146. Rassool CG, Selkoe DJ. N Engl J Med 1985; 312: 700.
147. Munoz-Garcia D, Ludwin SK. Acta Neuropathol (Berl) 1984; 16: 467.
148. Uhl GR, Hilt DC, Hedreen JC, Whitehouse PJ, Price DL. Neurology 1983; 33: 1470.
149. Kanazawa I, Kwak S, Sasaki H, Muramoto O, Mizutani T, Hori A, Nukina N. J Neurol Sci 1988; 83: 63.
150. Went LN, Vegter-Van der Vlis M, Bruyn GW. Lancet 1984; 1: 1100.
151. Schoenberg BS. In: Chase TN, Wexler NS, Barbeau A, eds. Huntington's disease. New York: Raven Press, 1979; 1.
152. Harper PS. Br Med J 1983; 287: 1567.
153. Gusella JF, Tanzi RE, Bader PI et al. Nature 1985; 318: 75.
154. Vonsattel JP, Myers RH, Stevens TJ, Ferrante RJ, Bird ED, Richardson EP Jr. J Neuropathol Exp Neurol 1985; 44: 559.
155. Lange H, Thörner G, Hopf A, Schröder KF. J Neurol Sci 1976; 28: 401.
156. Oyanagi K, Ikuta F. Clin Neuropathol 1987; 6: 71.
157. Graveland GA, Williams RS, Di Figlia M. Science 1985; 227: 770.

158. Roos RAC, Bots GTAM. J Neurol Sci 1983; 61: 37.
159. Marsden CD. Lancet 1982; 2: 1141.
160. Carter CJ. Lancet 1981; 1: 782.
161. Nemeroff CB, Youngblood WW, Manberg PJ, Prange AJ Jr, Kizer JS. Science 1983; 221: 972.
162. Beal MF, Bird ED, Langlais PJ, Martin JB. Neurology 1984; 34: 663.
163. Grafe MR, Forno LS, Eng LF. J Neuropathol Exp Neurol 1985; 44: 47.
164. Martin JB, Gusella JF. N Engl J Med 1986; 315: 1267.
165. Perry TL, Yong VW, Hansen S, Foulks JG, Kish SJ. J Neurol Sci 1985; 67: 351.
166. Vacca LL, Nelson SR. In: Fedoroff S, ed. Advances in cellular neurobiology. Orlando: Academic Press 1984; 5: 221.
167. Masters CL, Harris JO, Gajdusek C, Gibbs CJ Jr, Bernoulli C, Asher DM. Ann Neurol 1979; 5: 177.
168. Will RG, Matthews WB, Smith PG, Hudson C. J Neurol Neurosurg Psychiatry 1986; 49: 749.
169. Brown P, Cathala F, Raubertas RF, Gajdusek DC, Castaigne P. Neurology 1987; 37: 895.
170. Galvez S, Cartier L, Monari M, Araya G. J Neurol Sci 1983; 59: 139.
171. Yamamoto T, Nagashima K, Tsubaki T, Oikawa K, Akai J. J Neurol Sci 1985; 67: 119.
172. Will RG, Matthews WB. J Neurol Neurosurg Psychiatry 1984; 47: 134.
173. Siedler H, Malamud N. J Neuropathol Exp Neurol 1963; 22: 381.
174. Brownell B, Oppenheimer DR. J Neurol Neurosurg Psychiatry 1965; 28: 350.
175. Macchi G, Abbamondi AL, Di Trapani G, Sbriccoli A. J Neurol Sci 1984; 63: 197.
176. Beck E, Daniel PM. In: Prusiner SB, Hadlow WJ, eds. Slow transmissible diseases of the nervous system. New York: Academic Press 1979: 253.
177. Landis DMD, William RS, Masters CL. Neurology (NY) 1981; 31: 538.
178. Arendt T, Bigl V, Arendt A. Acta Neuropathol (Berl) 1984; 65: 85.
179. Horta-Barbosa L, Fuccillo DA, Sever JL, Baringer JR, Birnbaum G. Lancet 1970; 1: 964.
180. Bastian FO. Arch Pathol Lab Med 1979; 103: 665.
181. Manuelidis EE. J Neuropathol Exp Neurol 1985; 44: 1.
182. Gajdusek DC, Gibb CJ Jr. Nature 1971; 230: 588.
183. Beck E, Daniel PM. In: Prusiner SB, McKinley MP, eds. Prions: novel infectious pathogens causing scrapie and Creutzfeldt-Jakob disease. Orlando: Academic Press 1987: 331.
184. Beck E, Daniel PM, Davey AJ, Gajdusek DC, Gibbs CJ Jr. Brain 1982; 105: 755.
185. Koch TK, Berg BO, De Armond SJ, Gravina RF. N Engl J Med 1985; 313: 731.
186. Gibbs CJ Jr, Joy A, Heffner R et al. N Engl J Med 1985; 313: 734.
187. Powell-Jackson J, Weller RO, Kennedy P, Preece MA, Whitcombe EM, Newsom-Davis J. Lancet 1985; 2: 244.
188. Merz PA, Rohwer RG, Kascsak R et al. Science 1984; 225: 437.
189. Bockman JM, Kingsbury DT, McKinley MP, Bendheim PE, Prusiner SB. N Engl J Med 1985; 312: 73.
190. Manuelidis L, Valley S, Manuelidis EE. Proc Natl Acad Sci USA 1985; 82: 4263.
191. Prusiner SB. N Engl J Med 1987; 317: 1571.
192. Acheson ED, Chandler RL, Corsellis JAN et al. Advisory group on the management of patients with spongiform encephalopathy (Creutzfeldt-Jakob disease (CJD)). HMSO: London, 1981.
193. Brown P, Rohwer RG, Gajdusek DC. N Engl J Med 1984; 310: 727.
194. Hachinski VC, Lassen NA, Marshall J. Lancet 1974; 2: 207.
195. Janota I. Psychol Med 1981; 11: 39.
196. Babikian V, Ropper AH. Stroke 1987; 18: 2.
197. Brun A, Englund E. Ann Neurol 1986; 19: 253.
198. Hachinski VC, Potter P, Merskey H. Arch Neurol 1987; 44: 21.
199. Loizou LA, Kendall BE, Marshall J. J Neurol Neurosurg Psychiatry 1981; 44: 294.
200. Griffiths RA, Mortimer TF, Oppenheimer DR, Spalding JMK. J Neurol Neurosurg Psychiatry 1982; 45: 396.
201. Corsellis JAN, Bruton CJ, Freeman-Browne D. Psychol Med 1973; 3: 270.
202. Mortimer JA, French LR, Hutton JT, Schuman LM. Neurology 1985; 35: 264.
203. Yoshimura M. J Neurol 1983; 229: 17.
204. Kosaka K, Yoshimura M, Ikeda K, Budka H. Clin Neuropathol 1984; 3: 185.
205. Stockhausen P, Braak H. Clin Neuropathol 1984; 3: 206.
206. Candy JM, Perry RH, Perry EK et al. J Neurol Sci 1983; 59: 277.
207. Elder GA, Sever JL. Ann Neurol 1988; 23 (suppl): 34.
208. Fischer P-A, Ehrensberger W. J Neurol 1987; 234: 269.
209. Dalakas MC, Pezeshkpour GH. Ann Neurol 1988; 23 (suppl): 538.
209a. Sharer LR, Cho E-S, Epstein LG. Human Pathol 1985; 16: 760.
209b. Lantos PL, McLaughlin JE, Scholtz CL, et al. Lancet 1989; 1: 309.
210. Navia BA, Cho E-S, Petito CK, Price RW. Ann Neurol 1986; 19: 525.
211. Price RW, Sidtis J, Rosenblum M. Arch Neurol 1988; 23 (suppl): S27.
212. Wiley CA, Schrier RD, Nelson JA, Lampert PW, Oldstone MBA. Proc Natl Acad Sci USA 1986; 83: 7089.
213. McCoy EE, Sneddon JM. In: Fedoroff S, Hertz L, eds. Advances in cellular neurobiology. New York: Academic Press, 1983; 4: 249.
214. Coyle JT, Oster-Granite ML, Gearhart JD. Brain Res Bull 1986; 16: 773.
215. Burger PC, Vogel FS. Am J Pathol 1973; 73: 457.
216. Ball MJ, Nuttall K. Neuropathol Appl Neurobiol 1981; 7: 13.
217. Ross MH, Galaburda AM, Kemper TL. Neurology 1984; 34: 909.
218. Scott BS, Becker LE, Petit TL. Prog Neurobiol 1983; 21: 199.
219. Hakim S, Adams RD. J Neurol Sci 1965; 2: 307.
220. Symon L, Dorsch NWC. J Neurosurg 1975; 42: 258.

Epilepsy

INTRODUCTION

Epilepsy can be defined in terms of excessive, synchronous and prolonged electrical activity of a group of neurons. Although the clinical manifestations of a seizure can vary enormously, all forms of epileptogenic activity have a common feature in the increased stereotypy of neuronal behaviour: nerve cells in a given area act simultaneously and approximately in the same way.[1] The presently accepted classifications of epilepsy are based on clinical symptomatology,[2,3] since the aetiology and pathogenesis in most cases are not known or are poorly understood. It is, however, useful, particularly from the point of view of neuropathology, to distinguish *primary or idiopathic epilepsy* and *secondary or symptomatic epilepsy*. In the former, often referred to as cryptogenic epilepsy, no obvious abnormalities are found, although histological examination may reveal neuronal loss and fibrillary gliosis in excess of normal variations. In secondary epilepsy, obvious pathological conditions such as tumours, trauma, or infections are present in the brain: these are the underlying cause of the seizures.

Epilepsy is a common neurological disorder, although the incidence varies in different parts of the world. In the United Kingdom the prevalence rate is 17 per 1000,[4] whilst in the USA it is 6·7 per 1000.[5] The incidence is particularly high in the extremes of life, during the first decade and in senescence. The prevalence rates for the age group between 10 and 20 years depend upon different definitions and upon the methods of calculation. They range from 3·1 to 7·1 per 1000 in various countries. In an unselected national sample in

Britain, 6·7% of children had a history of seizures or other episodes of loss of consciousness, and in 4·1 per 1000 a clear-cut diagnosis of non-febrile epilepsy was established by the age of 11.[6] It is of interest to note that clinically a possible cause of epilepsy was found in only 27%, whilst for the majority there were no obvious precipitating factors. Incidence and prevalence rates are variable, since epidemiological studies of epilepsy are fraught with complex and difficult methodological problems.[7]

The neuropathological examination of an epileptic patient involves the study of biopsy specimens or of the brain post mortem. The most usual source of material from the living patient is a temporal lobectomy specimen, but cortical biopsies of various sizes and from various sites may also be obtained. The method of neuro-pathological investigation will be determined by the amount of tissue available and by the clinical information, including the results of neuro-radiological examination. With increasing sophistication of neuroimaging techniques, the accuracy of the clinical diagnosis of symptomatic epilepsy has greatly improved and the neuropathologist thus will be able to plan the histological, ultrastructural and immuno-histochemical examinations accordingly. The neuropathology of idiopathic epilepsy, however, presents a more complex problem and requires a somewhat different approach. Similarly, temporal lobe epilepsy—characterised by well-defined clinical signs and symptoms—is associated with a spectrum of pathological changes which will be considered separately.

IDIOPATHIC EPILEPSY (CRYPTOGENIC EPILEPSY)

In this form of epilepsy there is no obvious naked-eye abnormality in the brain, but thorough histo-logical examination may reveal changes which could be responsible for the seizures. The pathology of cryptogenic epilepsy has been recently reviewed and the abnormalities separated into three groups.[8] This classification will be adopted here.

Minor dysgenetic lesions

Minor developmental abnormalities occasionally found in the brain may represent the genetic component of primary generalised epilepsy or may be caused by an external noxious factor which has interfered with normal morphogenesis.[8] Whatever their pathogenesis, these small dysgenetic lesions are occasionally found in cases of cryptogenic epilepsy: they take the form of disturbances of the normal cytoarchitecture of neural tissue in the cerebellum, hippocampus and neocortex.[9]

Consequences of trauma

In approximately 11% of patients with chronic epilepsy, superficial damage and scarring of the cerebral cortex are seen, mainly in the orbital, frontal and temporal areas.[10] The relevance of these lesions to the development of epilepsy is somewhat controversial: although they may occasionally precede the onset of epilepsy, as a result of closed head injury, it is more likely that they have been acquired from falls during epileptic fits.[8]

Neuronal loss and gliosis

The areas most subject to neuronal loss and gliosis are the hippocampus and cerebellum, but the neocortex, thalamus and amygdaloid nucleus may also be involved. These changes are common in chronic cryptogenic epilepsy: the hippocampus is damaged in 50–60% of cases, the cerebellum in 45%, and the thalamus, amygdala and neocortex each in 25%.[10] The acute stages of these lesions are occasionally seen in children who die in or shortly after status epilepticus; more commonly, in longstanding cases, only scar tissue is found. The hippocampal damage presents a consistently characteristic pattern in the simplified topography of Scholz.[11] The h1 area (Sommer sector) and h3 (end-plate) are devastated, whereas the intervening h2 is usually spared. The first stage of the lesion is extensive scarring, known as Ammon horn sclerosis (hippocampal sclerosis): the hippocampus in these cases appears to be atrophic to the naked eye (Fig. 14.1). In the cerebellum the loss of Purkinje cells is accompanied by

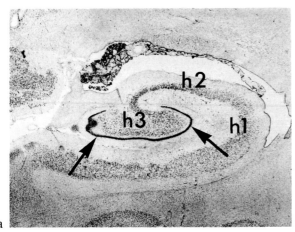
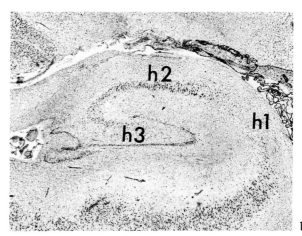

a
b

Fig. 14.1a, b Ammon's horn sclerosis. (**a**) Normal hippocampus (Ammon's horn); h1–h3 areas and the dentate gyrus (arrows). (**b**) Hippocampus with Ammon's horn sclerosis. Sommer sector (h1) and the end plate (h3) are more severely affected than the rest of the hippocampus.
(**a, b**) Cresyl violet × 15
Reproduced by permission of Dr C. J. Bruton, Runwell Hospital, Essex, UK.

proliferation of astrocytes with consequent fibrillary gliosis of the molecular layer (Fig. 14.2). The granule cell layer and even the white matter may become gliosed and in severe cases gross atrophy of several lobules may develop. In the neo-cortex the severity of the damage varies from focal neuronal loss through extensive laminar devas-tation to occasional hemiatrophy. Neuronal loss is patchy and haphazard in the thalamus without preferential involvement of any particular nuclei.

The pathogenesis of these changes is controversial and the question whether neuronal loss and gliosis resulting in scar tissue formation is the cause or the result of epilepsy has not been completely settled. The view that neuronal hypoxia is the primary lesion and not a con-sequence of seizures has gained considerable support and it has been suggested that the initial damage may occur during birth. Deformation of the skull and herniation of the medial part of the temporal lobe through the tentorial opening will interfere with the circulation through the posterior cerebral artery and lead to ischaemia and sclerosis which then becomes the epileptogenic focus.[12] This hypothesis was later expanded to explain the mechanism by which haemorrhage or trauma, occurring in adult life, may cause epilepsy: the common factor in these cases is cerebral oedema with consequent tentorial herniation. This

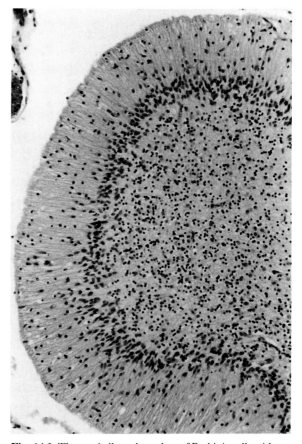

Fig. 14.2 The cerebellum shows loss of Purkinje cells with astrocyte proliferation and fibrillary gliosis in the molecular layer. There is some loss of granule cells.
Haematoxylin-eosin × 80

concept, however attractive it may be, fails to explain the obvious discrepancy between the pattern of damage and the vascular supply: necrotic areas may be far removed from the tentorial opening and lie outside the territory of the compromised blood vessel.

SYMPTOMATIC EPILEPSY

A wide variety of systemic and cerebral diseases can cause epilepsy. The systemic disorders are far too numerous to be considered here, and the metabolic, endocrine and toxic factors have been recently reviewed.[13] Similarly, practically any cerebral disease may be associated with epilepsy, including tumours, malformations (Fig. 14.3), head injuries, infections (both encephalitis and meningitis), vascular diseases and degenerative processes. The incidence of underlying causes varies according to age: metabolic disturbances,

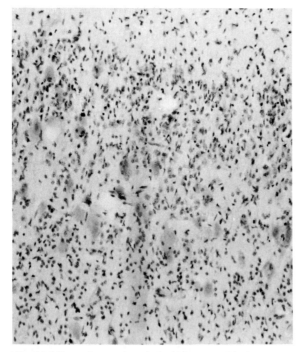

Fig. 14.3 Loss of normal cortical architecture with the presence of many large cells in tuberous sclerosis (see Ch. 12, p. 354).
Klüver–Barrera × 120

birth injuries and cerebral infections are commonest during the neonatal period, tumour and trauma in adults, and cerebrovascular diseases and degenerative disorders in old age.[8]

The single most frequent cause of symptomatic epilepsy is neoplasia, both primary and secondary. Epilepsy is the most common presenting symptom in patients with cerebral gliomas, and by the time the diagnosis is established more than 50% experience seizures.[14] Two factors determine the epileptogenic potential of a given tumour: its site and its type. In general, tumours above the tentorium are more liable to cause seizures than those below, but within the cerebral hemisphere the precise position of the tumour and its nearness to the cortex are most important. The influence of the type of tumour on the incidence of epilepsy is exemplified by the observation that slow growing, relatively benign neoplasms (e.g. oligodendrogliomas) are more frequently associated with fits than fast growing, highly malignant neoplasms (e.g. glioblastomas).

Epilepsy often develops after trauma. The incidence of post-traumatic epilepsy is influenced by the type and severity of the trauma and by the nature of the complications. Open head injury results in a higher incidence of epilepsy than closed wounds: penetrating injuries with torn dura, focal signs and prolonged post-traumatic amnesia particularly carry a high risk. Seizures developing within a few hours of trauma are thought to be caused by focal ischaemic changes, by oedema and by shearing of axons (diffuse axonal injury, p. 130) and capillaries.[8] Epilepsy occurring years after head injury is probably due to scar formation.

Encephalitis, meningitis and cerebral abscess may result in epilepsy. Acute viral encephalitis, particularly herpes simplex with its propensity to destroy the temporal lobes, is a common cause, whilst cerebral malaria, once restricted to tropical countries, is a disease that, because of the expansion of travel, must be considered even in parts of the world that are free of indigenous malaria. Toxoplasmosis and cysticercosis remain important epileptogenic factors, particularly in less developed countries.

In old age, cerebrovascular diseases (e.g. haemorrhages and infarcts) and degenerative disorders (e.g. Alzheimer's disease) carry a risk of seizure. Subdural haematoma and venous thrombosis may lead to epilepsy at any age, but are commonest during the first decade of life and in old age.

TEMPORAL LOBE EPILEPSY

Temporal lobe epilepsy is a focal seizure disorder characterised by a complex and varied clinical symptomatology. Although the association of olfactory and visual hallucinations with the temporal lobe has been known for a century, it is only with the introduction of surgical treatment that the underlying pathology of temporal lobe epilepsy has been established. In an early review of a series of 157 patients, gross or histological abnormalities were found in all specimens obtained by temporal lobectomy performed for epilepsy.[12] Although not all the subsequent reviews reported such a high incidence of structural abnormalities, the range of pathological lesions affecting the temporal lobes and associated with epilepsy has been clarified.[15]

In general, two points deserve consideration in the neuropathological examination of temporal lobectomy specimens. First, since the lesions tend to be situated in deeper, medial structures, in the hippocampus, uncus and amygdaloid nucleus, which are near or at the line of resection, the possibility exists that the afflicted part of the temporal lobe may be sucked away during surgery, lost or even not removed. The neuropathologist may then obtain only fragments of the temporal gyri, which less frequently contain structural abnormalities. Second, not all lesions are obvious macroscopically and many are revealed only after thorough histological examination. It is therefore important that each temporal lobectomy specimen is subjected to a systematic and careful examination: coronal slices of 0·5–0·8 cm thick are cut, numbered consecutively and embedded separately for histology (Fig. 14.4).

A recent review of the neuropathology of temporal lobectomy specimens from 249 cases distinguished eight diagnostic groups histologically.[16] (1) *Ammon's horn sclerosis* was far the commonest abnormality with 107 cases, followed by the (2) *alien tissue lesions*. The latter are usually

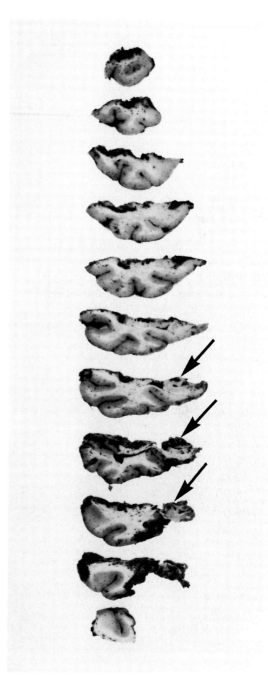

Fig. 14.4 A temporal lobectomy specimen is prepared for systematic histological examination: the coronal slices 0·5–0·8 cm thick are consecutively numbered and embedded separately. The arrows indicate the hippocampus.

localised masses measuring from a few millimetres to a couple of centimetres across. Histologically they can be subdivided into glial (astrocytic,

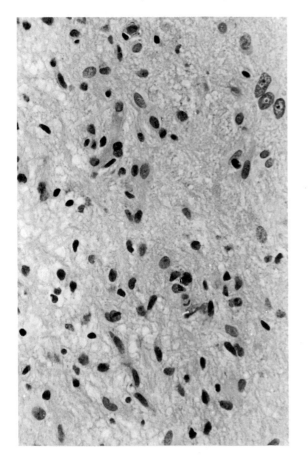

oligodendroglial and mixed), mixed neuronoglial, and vascular lesions. They appear to be long-standing lesions with little or no evidence of invasion or mitotic activity. Their biological behaviour has been disputed and most of them are hamartomas rather than tumours, although occasional cases of frank neoplasms have been noted. This is particularly true of the (3) *glial lesions*; the astrocytic and oligodendroglial masses behave more like neoplasms, although of relatively benign nature: oligodendroglial lesions are the least aggressive. Within the (4) *neuronoglial group* two types of lesions can be distinguished: ganglio-gliomas (Fig. 14.5), which within the temporal lobes appear to behave clinically as malformations rather than true neoplasms, and cortical dysplasias (Fig. 14.6), which are often invisible to the naked eye. The cortical dysplasias[17] are malformations composed of a mixture of abnormal nerve and glial cells scattered throughout the cortex; some of the more bizarre cell forms cannot be positively identified. The presence of large numbers of these

Fig. 14.5 A small tumour of the temporal lobe composed of a mixture of glial and nerve cells (top right). Haematoxylin-eosin × 200

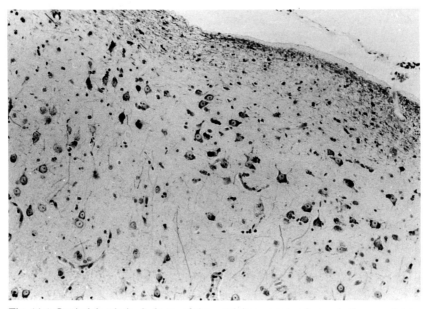

Fig. 14.6 Cortical dysplasia. A cluster of abnormal, large neurons is seen in the superficial cortex. Klüver–Barrera × 120

cells disturbs the cortical architecture, and groups of abnormal cells spread into the underlying white matter. Small tumours of the temporal lobes—the glial or neuronoglial lesions—were considered to form an unusual group of lesions whose neoplastic potential remains to be determined.[18] The (5) *vascular lesions* are clearly angiomatous malformations and all show evidence of previous bleeding.

(6) *Inflammatory processes* included burnt-out leptomeningitis, healed cerebral abscess and quiescent encephalitis. Old (7) *head injuries* left their mark in the form of scarring of cortex and white matter with thickening of the overlying leptomeninges. The (8) *developmental abnormalities* were cystic lesions and cortical malformations (polymicrogyria). A large number of cases had double pathology in which Ammon's horn sclerosis was combined with another lesion. One in ten of the 249 temporal lobectomies was classified as indefinite, since histological appearances were borderline between normal and abnormal. The second largest group of the series (41 cases) showed no abnormalities in the temporal lobes.[16]

From this review a clear clinicopathological problem emerges: one out of four temporal lobes appears to be normal or shows minor non-diagnostic changes even after meticulous histological examination in clinically well-established and carefully investigated cases of temporal lobe epilepsy. However, it is hoped that quantitative assessments of neuronal cell populations in the temporal lobes may improve clinicopathological correlations.[19]

FEBRILE CONVULSIONS AND STATUS EPILEPTICUS

The incidence of febrile convulsions is higher than that of epilepsy: in Great Britain 2·4% of children by the age of 11 and in North America 3·2% of children under the age of 5 have experienced them. Febrile convulsions carry the risk of status epilepticus and permanent cerebral damage. Such damage may include Ammon's horn sclerosis, cerebral hemiatrophy and generalised damage

which preferentially affects those areas which are most vulnerable to hypoxia.[8]

Status epilepticus is a period of seizure activity sustained for at least one hour without regaining consciousness. In most cases it is symptomatic and in both children and adults there is underlying precipitating brain disease; longstanding cryptogenic epilepsy may also be associated with status epilepticus. The neuropathological consequences are revealed only by microscopy, since the naked-eye appearances reveal little damage. The changes are similar to those seen in severe hypoxia and ischaemia. The hippocampus, particularly the Sommer sector and the dentate gyrus, and the uncus are severely affected, whilst the calcarine cortex and parahippocampal gyrus are spared. Other areas of the cortex and the deep grey matter may show necrosis. In the cerebellum, the Purkinje cells display severe degenerative changes and many of them disappear. These neuronal changes are accompanied first by a microglial reaction and then by an astrocytic response leading to fibrillary gliosis. In general, cerebellar pathology in epileptic patients is complex: some changes are not the consequence but the cause of seizures, some lesions are unrelated, and others may result from the toxic action of anti-convulsive drugs.[20]

PATHOGENESIS OF EPILEPTIC BRAIN DAMAGE

Morphological and physiological changes

The relevance of structural changes, particularly those affecting the hippocampus, has been previously discussed (see p. 398). The importance of these alterations has been further elaborated by quantitative measurements: the degree of neuronal loss from the hippocampus is correlated with the frequency of generalised seizures and the overall duration of epilepsy.[21] It is generally accepted that a sequence of major cellular events is involved in the generation, spread and arrest of seizure activity. At a cellular level, various mechanisms have been assessed to be epileptogenic, including loss of inhibitory interneurons, de-afferentation and loss of dendritic spines, overloading of excitatory synapses and the proliferation of fibrous astro-cytes.[13]

Intrinsic membrane excitability, disinhibition (which releases intrinsic burst-generating capacities in a subpopulation of neurons) and excitatory synaptic coupling (which is required to synchronise a population of neurons) are three interacting processes of importance in cortical epileptogenesis.[22]

Since human biopsy and post-mortem material usually shows the end-stage of the pathological process, animal models are necessary for the investigation of the pathogenesis of epilepsy (see Reference 23 for review).

Excitotoxins, compounds which cause neuronal death by excessive depolarisation, have been particularly useful in the study of the evolution, propagation and pathology of epileptic discharge. Of these, kainic acid produces brain damage which is reminiscent of Ammon's horn sclerosis, with a similar pattern of selective vulnerability.[24] Prolonged seizures induced by bicuculline, a γ-aminobutyric acid (GABA) antagonist, in adolescent baboons reproduced the typical pattern of human disease: ischaemic neuronal changes developed in the hippocampus, neocortex, thalamus, amygdala and cerebellum. Damage to Purkinje cells and basket cells in the cerebellum was clearly related to hyperpyrexia and arterial hypotension.[25] More localised damage can be produced by injecting allylglycine, an inhibitor of glutamate decarboxylase, into baboons to produce brief, but recurrent seizures: neuronal loss was detected preferentially in the Sommer sector and the end-folium of the hippocampus in those animals which survived longer than one week.[26] Similarly, systemic administration or local injection into the amygdala of various convulsants, including bicuculline, kainic acid, pilocarpine and picrotoxin, causes limbic seizures: the character-istic pathology, mainly restricted to the hippo-campus, consequently develops.[8] Ultrastructural examination of early hippocampal changes following systemic administration of kainic acid to rats reveals generalised swelling of perineuronal and perivascular astrocytic processes, neuronal hyperchromasia, microvacuolation and swelling of CA1 basal dendrites. Calcium has been demonstrated to accumulate in the swollen mito-

chrondria of the pyramidal neurons in the vulnerable areas CA1 and CA3. This calcium sequestration may lead to impaired metabolic activity and cytotoxic effects in vulnerable neurons which may then develop ischaemic change.[27] Similar abnormalities can also be produced by bicuculline and allylglycine, thus providing evidence for the hypothesis that selective neuronal vulnerability in epilepsy can be explained by high calcium movements associated with burst firing and calcium cytotoxicity.[28] Moreover, calmodulin, the major calcium-binding protein which is present in both pre- and post-synaptic fractions, is thought to play an important rôle in the develop-ment of altered neuronal excitability by regulating calcium movements and thus to be an important factor in the biochemical basis of some forms of epilepsy.[29] In summary, both acutely induced and chronic epilepsies are associated with an increased calcium uptake capability of neurons. This enhanced intracellular calcium may be an important factor which contributes to neuronal degeneration as a consequence of epileptic activity.[30] These studies imply that excessive cellular activity itself may cause neuronal damage, the degree and extent of which are influenced by a variety of systemic factors.

It has been known that subcortical structures, including various thalamic nuclei, the reticular formation and the substantia nigra, may also be important in the propagation and perhaps initiation of generalised seizures in the mammalian brain. The severance of the mamillothalamic tracts prevents seizures in guinea pigs, suggesting that the mamillary bodies with their rostral efferent connections play an important part in controlling the expression and spread of seizures.[31] The cellular phenomena underlying focal epilepsy have been reviewed in terms of cellular and synaptic functions. Interictal discharges result from a com-bination of synaptic events and intrinsic currents; the precise proportion of these varies according to the anatomical and functional state of neurons, and the epileptogenic agents. The transition to seizure is due to increased excitatory activity and decreased inhibitory processes. Although various hypotheses have been suggested to explain increased excitability, there is no single unifying mechanism which could be a common element responsible for the various types of focal epilepsy.[32]

Neurotransmitter abnormalities

Both animal experiments and biochemical studies of human brains suggest that a defect in the GABAergic inhibitory system may be a possible cause of epilepsy. In animals, treatments which interfere with or lower GABA activity result in seizures, including the blockade of GABA receptors by bicuculline or the inhibition of the GABA synthesising enzyme, glutamic acid decarboxylase. In the epileptic foci of human brains the levels of GABA, glutamate and taurine are altered, the amount of glutamic acid decarboxylase is decreased and the number of GABAergic nerve terminals is reduced.[33] These findings are in accordance with the preferential damage to inhibitory interneurons observed in morphological studies.[8] Recent evidence indicates that noradrenaline, serotonin, adenosine 3′,5′-monophosphate and probably dopamine are associated with processes which inhibit or confine seizure activity in the brain, whilst guanosine 3′, 5′-monophosphate is involved in mechanisms which initiate or maintain seizure discharges.[34] In addition, several neuropeptides, particularly opioid-like peptides, adrenocorticotrophic hormone and some hypothalamic releasing factors, have been found to modify neuronal excitability. β-endorphin has a strong anticonvulsant effect, and it is thought that endogenous opioid peptides may limit the spread of seizures or influence postictal (i.e. following a fit or seizure) susceptibility to further seizures.[35] An interesting hypothesis envisages subtle alterations in the anatomical and biochemical relationships between neurons and astrocytes, resulting in excess amounts of glutamic acid in the extracellular space. This, in turn, leads to abnormal functional connectivity between neurons which then become hyperexcitable.[36] For a review of the neurotransmitter and neuropeptide abnormalities see Reference 23.

Metabolic, immunological, viral and genetic factors

In experimentally-induced prolonged seizures, a rapid but reversible decrease of glycogen and glucose in the cortex is accompanied by an increase in lactate. Concentrations of phosphocreatine and adenosine triphosphate (ATP) decline and the ratio of ATP to adenosine diphosphate and to adenosine monophosphate, and the adenylate energy charge are all reduced. Toxic concentrations of lactic acid and free radicals may lead to lipid peroxidation and to breakdown of the cell membrane; thus disturbance of cellular energy metabolism may result in neuronal loss.[37]

It has been suggested that an autoimmune mechanism is involved in the pathogenesis of epilepsy. Antibodies to an antigen released during tissue destruction or to an infective agent may block transmitter receptor sites of inhibitory synapses, in a manner similar to the molecular events of myasthenia gravis (see p. 656).[38] With molecular hybridisation, herpes simplex type 1 DNA sequences were detected in post-mortem and biopsy specimens of temporal lobes from epileptic patients.[39] The presence of herpes virus DNA could provide an epileptic focus, but usually in combination with other factors. Evidence is accumulating to suggest the rôle genetic factors may play in epilepsy. Experimental animal models of epilepsy show that genetic factors can influence the hypersensitivity of neurons. In man, there are apparently over 140 Mendelian traits which increase the risk of seizures. In addition, genetic variation may occur in any of the factors known to be altered in the origin of seizures, including neuronal inhibition, inactivation of excitatory neurotransmitters, feedback control and seizure generation.[40]

REFERENCES

1. Pedley TA, Traub RD. In: Swash M, Kennard C, eds. Scientific basis of clinical neurology. Edinburgh: Churchill Livingstone, 1985; 320.

2. Gastaut H. In: Rose FC, ed. Research progress in epilepsy. London: Pitman, 1983: 8.

3. Dreyfuss FE, Martinez-Lage M, Roger J, Seino M, Wolf

P, Dam M. Epilepsia 1985; 26: 268.
4. Goodridge DMG, Shorvon SD. Br Med J 1983; 287: 641.
5. Hauser WA, Kurland LT. Epilepsia 1975; 16: 1.
6. Ross EM, Peckham CS, West PB, Butler NR. Br Med J 1980; 280: 207.
7. Sander JWAS, Shorvon SD. J Neurol Neurosurg Psychiatry 1987; 50: 829.
8. Meldrum BS, Corsellis JAN. In: Adams JH, Corsellis JAN, Duchen LW, eds. Greenfield's Neuropathology. 4th ed. London: Arnold, 1984; 921.
9. Meencke HJ, Janz D. Epilepsia 1984; 25: 8.
10. Margerison JH, Corsellis JAN. Brain 1966; 89: 499.
11. Scholz W. Die Krampfschädigungen des Gehirns. Berlin: Springer, 1951.
12. Earle KM, Baldwin M, Penfield W. Arch Neurol Psychiatry 1953; 69: 27.
13. Meldrum BS. In: Laidlaw J, Richens A, eds. A textbook of epilepsy. 2nd ed. Edinburgh: Churchill Livingstone, 1982: 456.
14. McKeran RO, Thomas DGT. In: Thomas DGT, Graham DI, eds. Brain tumours. Scientific basis, clinical investigation and current therapy. London: Butterworths, 1980: 194.
15. Corsellis JAN. In: Williams D, ed. Modern trends in neurology. London: Butterworths, 1970; 5: 254.
16. Bruton CJ. The neuropathology of temporal lobe epilepsy. Maudsley Monographs No 31 Oxford, Oxford University Press, 1988.
17. Taylor DC, Falconer MA, Bruton CJ, Corsellis JAN. J Neurol Neurosurg Psychiatry 1971; 34: 369.
18. Cavanagh JB. Brain 1958; 81: 389.
19. Babb TL, Brown WJ, Pretorius J, Davenport C, Lieb JP, Crandall PH. Epilepsia 1984; 25: 729.
20. Gessaga EC, Urich H. Clin Neuropathol 1985; 6: 238.
21. Dam AM. Epilepsia 1980; 21: 617.
22. Prince DA, Connors BW. Ann Neurol 1984; 16 (suppl): S59.
23. Delgado-Escueta AV, Ward AA Jr, Woodbury DM, Porter RJ. Adv Neurol 1986; 44: 3.
24. Ben-Ari Y. Neuroscience 1985; 14: 375.
25. Meldrum BS, Brierley JB. Arch Neurol 1973; 28: 10.
26. Meldrum BS, Horton RW, Brierley JB. Brain 1974; 97: 407.
27. Evans MC, Griffiths T, Meldrum BS. Neuropathol Appl Neurobiol 1984; 10: 285.
28. Meldrum BS, Griffiths T, Evans MC. In: Rose FC, ed. Research progress in epilepsy. London: Pitman, 1983: 78.
29. DeLorenzo RJ. Ann Neurol 1984; 16 (suppl): S104.
30. Heinemann U, Hamon B. Exp Brain Res 1986; 65: 1.
31. Mirski MA, Ferrendelli JA. Science 1984; 226: 72.
32. Dichter MA, Ayala GF. Science 1987; 237: 157.
33. Spero L. Lancet 1982; 2: 1319.
34. Ferrendelli JA. Ann Neurol 1984; 16 (suppl): S98.
35. Bajorek JG, Lee RJ, Lomax P. Ann Neurol 1984; 16 (suppl): S31.
36. van Gelder NM. Neurochem Res 1987; 12: 111.
37. Chapman AG, Meldrum BS, Siesjö BK. J Neurochem 1977; 28: 1025.
38. Ettlinger G, Lowrie MB. Lancet 1976; 1: 1386.
39. Gannicliffe A, Saldanha JA, Itzhaki RF, Sutton RNP. Lancet 1985; 1: 214.
40. Anderson VE, Hauser WA, Rich SS. Adv Neurol 1986; 44: 59.

System disorders

INTRODUCTION

Neurologists use the epithet 'system', in relation to nervous disease, in a partly functional and partly structural sense. The use of the term, and its incorporation into disease classification, is well justified on grounds of physiology, anatomy, history and convenience. Broadly speaking, the nervous pathways which regulate movement can be considered as being of three types. These are the pyramidal system, comprising the cortico-spinal and bulbospinal pathways; the extra-pyramidal system, incorporating numerous sub-cortical neuronal (grey matter) masses and their connections which modulate corticospinal activity; and the cerebellar system, which is involved in motor coordination and comprises deep and cortical cerebellar nerve cells, and the afferent and efferent cerebellar pathways. A large number of diseases affecting the nervous system show striking selectivity for one or other of these three 'systems', and in this chapter many of these will be reviewed. System disorders may be due to identifiable exogenous causes, but the cause of most of the important diseases described here, like motor neuron disease and idiopathic Parkinson's disease, is still unknown. The word 'abiotrophy', coined 90 years ago by Gowers,[1] implied a loss of vitality of nerve cells; in the absence of a defined deficiency, or a toxic or infective cause for the 'neurodegenerative' conditions under scrutiny here, abiotrophy remains a convenient term.

Some system degenerations are sporadic, others are clearly familial and with a recognisable genetic pattern. Such disorders, while affecting pre-dominantly one functional/anatomical system, may also involve other system pathways. In practical pathological terms, abnormalities of cerebral cortex and corticospinal pathways, basal ganglia, thalamus, cerebellum, olives, ascending spinal tracts, dorsal root ganglia and peripheral nerves may occur in varying combinations in some of the diseases outlined in this chapter.

DISORDERS OF PYRAMIDAL PATHWAYS

Motor neuron disease

Motor neuron disease (MND)—in American usage: amyotrophic lateral sclerosis, (ALS)—is fairly frequent, with an annual mortality of up to 2 per 100 000;[2] it has a worldwide distribution, and is generally a sporadic disorder of adult life. It is progressively crippling and eventually fatal, due to loss of upper and lower motor neuron innervation of muscles. The rate of evolution of the disease is generally most rapid in cases with involvement of the tongue and throat muscles, i.e. *progressive bulbar palsy* if of lower motor neuron type, or *pseudobulbar palsy* if spasticity is present indicating involvement of the upper motor neurons; in these cases death may occur within two years of onset. Patients without bulbar disease but with marked limb spasticity and other features of upper motor neuron involvement have an inter-mediate prognosis, while those with the *progressive muscular atrophy* variant, manifested as initially localised or asymmetrical muscle weakness and wasting, evolving slowly into severe paralytic disease of limbs and trunk, may survive for more than ten years.

Clinically, the selective devastation of motor function, with sparing of intellect, sensation and sphincter function, is a striking phenomenon. The name motor neuron disease (MND) recognises this selectivity and the pathological findings in upper and lower motor neurons; it was introduced as a unifying term embracing the historically defined patterns of the disease. Of these, amyotrophic lateral sclerosis (ALS) is a patho-logical as well as a clinical description: Charcot[3] found that in patients with progressive muscular atrophy—'amyotrophy'—degenerative changes ('lateral sclerosis') were present in corticospinal tracts in the cord. However, not all MND patients

show changes in the lateral columns of the spinal cord, and the term MND is thus more com-prehensive than ALS.

Nothing is known of the cause or causes of MND. Although in mice chronic progressive anterior horn cell disease may follow specific viral infection,[4] there is, as yet, no good evidence that this is the case in man. MND due to 'chronic

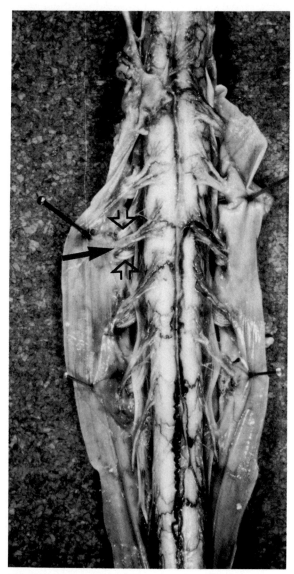

Fig. 15.1 Motor neuron disease. Anterior surface of cervicothoracic spinal cord, showing shrunken anterior nerve roots. Compare the broad, pale posterior root (between the open arrows) and the shrivelled grey anterior root (closed arrow) overlying it.

poliomyelitis' is not proven.[5] Other exogenous causes have been suggested, including lead intoxication, and, recently, cycad nut poisoning (see p. 275). Speculations that nerve cell loss in MND may result from faulty neuronal DNA reparative mechanisms[6] (see p. 423) are also not confirmable by standard methods of investigation.[7] The rare inherited forms of MND, which may be atypical in terms of clinical features and course, have so far failed to provide pathogenetic clues to motor nerve cell loss.

Patients with MND usually die of respiratory insufficiency, and sometimes of pneumonia, consequent on paralysis. Biopsy or autopsy samples of muscle are likely to show the features of denervation (neurogenic) atrophy. Not all muscles are equally affected; lower motor neuron changes indicative of denervation often appear in the legs at a late stage. External ocular muscles are spared. The spinal cord is grossly abnormal, with (Fig. 15.1) shrunken grey anterior roots contrasting strikingly with the normal, thick, white posterior roots. Atrophy of anterior roots is due to loss of large myelinated nerve fibres originating from motor neurons in the anterior horns. Random cross-sections of normal spinal cord of conventional histological thickness contain small and variable numbers of anterior horn cells, and the loss of these in MND may not always be readily appreciated under the microscope. Cell loss in the cord can, however, generally be detected without the use of thick sections and formal quantitation if standard sections from cervical and lumbar regions of the cord are examined; with bulbar involvement neuronal loss is obvious in the hypoglossal nuclei. Affected grey matter areas of the cord may show changes in remaining nerve cells, including neuronophagia (see p. 40) and ballooning (ghost cell change). Gliosis is also evident. Neurofilamentous abnormalities have been demonstrated by electron microscopy in anterior horn cells in both sporadic and familial cases of MND.[8,9]

As already noted, the fibre tracts of the cord show major changes in MND. The chalky appearance of the abnormal lateral columns is visible to the naked eye (Fig. 15.2); they have undergone Wallerian degeneration with lysis of myelin occurring secondary to axonal loss.

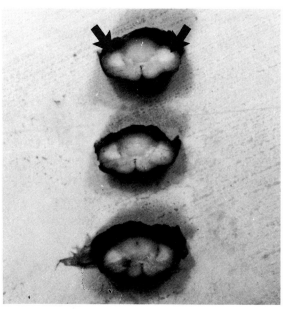

Fig. 15.2 Motor neuron disease. Transverse section of spinal cord showing pale wedge-shaped degenerate lateral corticospinal tracts (arrowed).

Reduced staining for myelin is seen in the anterior as well as the lateral columns of the spinal cord as both are affected (Fig. 15.3). Tract degeneration can often be defined by the Marchi method (see p. 83). Changes in the corticospinal tracts in the spinal cord are absent in about 20% of cases;[10] in others they may extend cranially beyond the cervical region into the brainstem, cerebral peduncles, internal capsule and hemispheric white matter. These changes are the distal manifestation of motor cortex pyramidal cell disease. Precentral gyral atrophy can sometimes be shown, and reduced numbers of giant pyramidal (Betz) neurons are found in histological sections. Notwithstanding the widespread damage to motor nerve cells occurring in MND, certain neuronal groups do not seem to be affected. Sparing of the oculomotor nuclei has been referred to already; there is also sparing of the anteromedial sacral nucleus of Onuf (Onufrowicz), which is the autonomic centre controlling sphincter function, and of the thoracolumbar intermediolateral columns.[11] Minor changes can sometimes be shown in the spinocerebellar tracts and their parent cell bodies in Clarke's column, as well as in

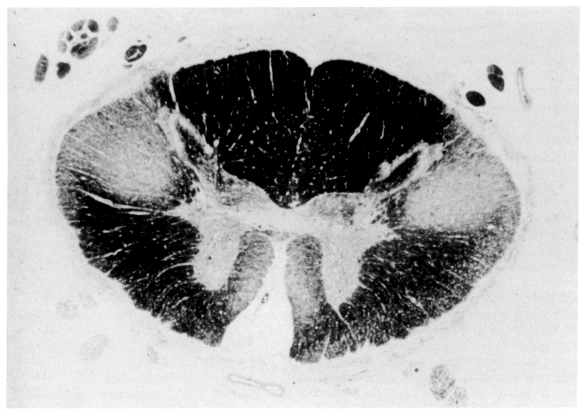

Fig. 15.3 Motor neuron disease. Pallor of myelin staining of anterior and lateral corticospinal tracts is seen. Luxol fast blue × 15

other sensory pathways, but these are of very limited clinical significance.[12] The rare familial cases of MND also show abnormalities of these sensory structures without obvious clinical features of sensory dysfunction. Familial MND is clinically and pathologically distinct from familial spastic paraplegia, which is a complex of genetic disorders with pyramidal tract degeneration but no loss of motor neurons; the legs are affected and there is a prolonged clinical course.[13]

Werdnig–Hoffmann disease

The autosomal recessively inherited infantile spinal muscular atrophy of Werdnig and Hoffmann is one of the most important diseases producing 'floppiness' (muscle weakness and hypotonia) in infancy. It is a rapidly progressive, lethal disorder, often evident at birth. Death results from respiratory insufficiency and

pneumonia consequent on severe and generalised paralysis. As in adult motor neuron disease, eye muscles and sacral and autonomic nuclei in the spinal cord are spared. A major clinical and pathological point of distinction of Werdnig–Hoffmann disease from motor neuron disease is lack of upper motor neuron involvement.

In muscle biopsies, neurogenic patterns of atrophy will again be apparent (see p. 590). At autopsy, atrophy of anterior roots is seen on examination of the spinal cord. Loss of neurons from the anterior horns of the spinal cord, from the facial and hypoglossal nuclei, and from the nuclei ambigui is recognisable under the microscope; some surviving nerve cells in these regions show neuronophagia and chromatolytic change, as in MND. Thalamic neurons may be affected. Long tracts in brainstem and cord characteristically show no alterations of the type seen in motor neuron disease. However, rare atypical cases may show much more extensive changes in the nervous system.[14]

Werdnig–Hoffmann disease is clinically apparent in a third of cases by the time of birth, and in nearly all cases death has occurred by the age of 18 months. The quick, relentless course of infantile spinal muscular atrophy contrasts with the slow, sometimes arrested, progression of weakness in the Kugelberg–Welander form of 'benign' spinal muscular atrophy of childhood, adolescence and early adult life (see p. 609).[15] Between the two extremes of severity are cases of late infantile disease with rapid early progression followed by long survival with severe disability. The classification of the various recessive disorders composing this group is obscure,[16] and pathological data are scanty in late onset cases.

DISORDERS OF EXTRAPYRAMIDAL PATHWAYS

The syndrome of parkinsonism, characterised by tremor, rigidity and inhibition of movement, may result from many causes. However, its commonest form, idiopathic parkinsonism, still has no known cause. It is distinct from genetically determined Parkinson's disease, and studies on identical twins indicate the importance of (as yet undiscovered) exogenous, environmental factors in its pathogenesis.[17] Half a century ago, parkinsonism of known aetiology commonly occurred in patients who had had encephalitis lethargica. Today new cases of postencephalitic parkinsonism are rare, and drugs are the most common identifiable cause. These include the synthetic narcotic agent MPTP (1-methyl-4-phenyl-1,2,3,6-tetrahydropyridine), a pethidine analogue (see p. 284),[18] as well as such therapeutic drugs as phenothiazines (for example chlorpromazine and perphenazine), butyrophenones (for example haloperidol), reserpine, tetrabenazine, methyldopa and procaine. Other recognised causes of parkinsonism include chronic manganese intoxication, carbon monoxide poisoning, boxing, cerebrovascular disease, and local lesions of the substantia nigra. Finally, a number of rare neurological syndromes may show parkinsonian features. In this chapter, the neuropathology of different varieties of parkinsonism will be reviewed.

Idiopathic Parkinson's disease

Until the end of the last century, lack of neurophysiological knowledge and of clinicopathological correlations allowed only guesses at the nature of parkinsonism. James Parkinson himself thought that it originated in a damaged cervical spinal cord and lower brainstem, while preservation of intellectual function suggested to him that the cerebral hemispheres were spared.[19] In contrast, William Gowers noted, ten years before the concept of an extrapyramidal pathway had been formulated, that parkinsonism was a purely motor disorder; he believed it to arise from a disturbance of the cerebral cortex.[20] Blocq and Marinesco, in 1893, were the first to implicate the midbrain and substantia nigra.[21] Their patient, a man of 38 with left-sided parkinsonian signs, was shown at necropsy to have a circumscribed lesion 2·5 cm in diameter replacing the right half of the substantia nigra and adjacent structures. The suggestion that lesions of the substantia nigra might be responsible for idiopathic parkinsonism was made soon afterwards, by Brissaud.[22] In 1919, Trétiakoff examined the brains of 9 patients with parkinsonism and observed a variety of degenerative features and reduction of numbers in the pigmented neurons of the substantia nigra.[23] Besides some non-specific neuronal changes, he found peculiar concentric inclusions in the cytoplasm of these cells. These have become known as Lewy bodies, after the author who first reported them[24] in neurons of the dorsal vagal nucleus and the nucleus of the substantia innominata in idiopathic parkinsonism. With the paper of Foix and Nicolesco, in 1925, knowledge of the morbid anatomy of the disease was practically complete.[25]

In the brain of patients with idiopathic parkinsonism the only naked-eye abnormality is loss of pigmentation of the substantia nigra and of the locus ceruleus (Fig. 15.4). Under the microscope, the substantia nigra shows a decrease in the number of pigmented neurons; shrinkage and vacuolation are often visible in the surviving neurons. Macrophages containing neuromelanin

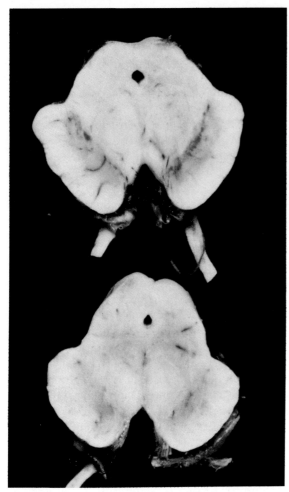

Fig. 15.4 Idiopathic Parkinson's disease. The substantia nigra of the patient's midbrain (lower) is obviously depigmented compared with the age-matched control (upper).

granules, presumably derived from dead nerve cells, are also seen. As well as Lewy bodies, other types of intraneuronal inclusion may be recognisable. These differ from Lewy bodies as they are not concentric; some are ill-defined, while some resemble the corpora amylacea so frequently seen in normal adult brains. Gliosis is present in proportion to the loss of neurons. Similarly affected brainstem structures include the locus ceruleus, reticular formation, and dorsal vagal nucleus. Non-pigmented as well as pigmented neurons are reduced in number in these areas and there are cytoplasmic inclusions in the surviving cells that are well stained by aniline blue; however,

similar inclusions are a common incidental necropsy finding.[26]

Substantia nigra damage is the primary abnormality in parkinsonism; changes in the globus pallidus and putamen are less constant and usually less severe than those in the substantia nigra, and may result from trans-synaptic degeneration.[27] They include patchy atrophy, with disappearance of some neurons and accumulation of lipofuscin in others, reactive gliosis, and loss of myelinated fibres. While the lentiform nuclei are sometimes affected by severe, bilaterally symmetrical degeneration, the lesions are generally minor.

Lewy bodies measure 20 μm or more in diameter. They are usually solitary, but sometimes more than one is present in a cell. They have a hyaline appearance and are concentrically ringed, with a pale halo and a darker core (Fig. 15.5). They may fill the neuronal cell body, compressing the nucleus into a peripheral crescent. In haematoxylin and eosin stained sections they are eosinophilic and they are well shown by trichrome stains such as Lendrum's Martius scarlet blue, which gives a deep red core and a light blue halo.

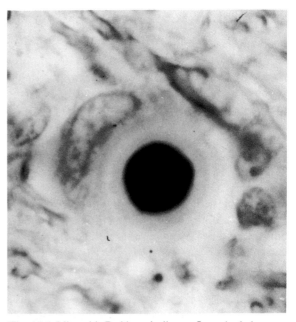

Fig. 15.5 Idiopathic Parkinson's disease. Lewy body in substantia nigra.
Martius scarlet blue × 1000

Those that are free lying are believed to be the remnants of dead neurons. Lewy bodies occur in the brain of up to 5% of old people without apparent neurological disorder,[28] but since parkinsonism is common after 60, in some cases the disease may have been overlooked clinically. Lewy bodies can be found in at least 90% of cases of idiopathic parkinsonism, and only rarely in cases diagnosed as postencephalitic.[29] Thus, there is some reason to believe that they are peculiar to the idiopathic form of parkinsonism. They have been reported as a feature, albeit rare, in cases of olivopontocerebellar atrophy, Shy–Drager syndrome, striatonigral degeneration, Joseph's disease, motor neuron disease, ataxia telangiectasia and Hallervorden–Spatz disease.[30] In many such cases, it is hard to accept that, if correctly identified, they are more than coincidental.

Den Hartog Jager and Bethlem[31] showed that Lewy bodies may be very widely distributed throughout the nervous system. They may be found in neurons of many diencephalic and brainstem nuclei, of lateral and posterior horns of the spinal cord, of ganglia of the sympathetic chain, and of the coeliac ganglion. Thus they are not specifically related to pigmented nerve cells, although it is possible that they are mainly in monoamine-synthesising neurons. Their nature is uncertain and chemical analysis has not contributed any significant data. Histochemical studies have been interpreted as showing the presence of sphingomyelin.[32] Electron microscopy[33,34] appears to show two varieties of intracytoplasmic inclusion in association with parkinsonism: one is the typical concentric Lewy body and is composed of granular and fibrillary material, with more densely packed granules in the core and radiating fibres peripherally in the halo. The other is more clearly marginated, lacks a core, and contains coarse fibrillary material and scattered large dense granules. This latter type closely resembles corpora amylacea. Immunocytochemistry indicates that Lewy bodies contain neurofilaments.[35] How these bodies are formed is quite unknown.

The association of Lewy bodies with dementia (see p. 391), and their occurrence in the cerebral cortex, is of some interest. Abnormalities of the cerebral cortex in idiopathic parkinsonism are generally mild and non-specific, and are in keeping with the fact that intellectual impairment (as distinct from depression) is usually mild or nonexistent. Small numbers of cortical Lewy bodies are found in such cases. Sometimes, cases of severe dementia are associated with the presence of Lewy bodies. Most of these patients have Alzheimer's disease, which can be associated with Lewy bodies in the midbrain in the absence of clinical parkinsonism; the frequency with which Lewy bodies occur in the brain of patients with Alzheimer's disease is similar to that in the general population.[28,36] Rarely, a syndrome of early onset presenile dementia (see p. 391) with subsequent severe extrapyramidal disorder is associated both with the presence of Lewy bodies in the cerebral cortex and with changes of Alzheimer's disease.[37,38]

Progressive supranuclear palsy

Some elderly parkinsonian patients show marked axial rigidity and negligible or absent tremor of the limbs; ophthalmoplegia, dementia, dysphagia and dysarthria are also present and there is a relatively rapid progression of the disease, death occurring within 7 years of the onset of symptoms. The recognition of this characteristic clinical pattern of symptoms and signs led to the description in 1964 of progressive supranuclear palsy (the Steele–Richardson–Olszewski syndrome).[39] Neuropathological findings include evidence of neuronal depletion and neurofibrillary and granulovacuolar degeneration in deep cerebral structures, cerebellum and brainstem; Lewy bodies are absent. The most severely affected areas of the brain are the globus pallidus, subthalamic nucleus (corpus Luysii), red nucleus, substantia nigra, peri-aqueductal grey matter and dentate nucleus. The cerebral cortex is only minimally affected (Fig. 15.6).

Postencephalitic parkinsonism

Cases of postencephalitic parkinsonism may show widespread neurofibrillary degeneration, affecting not only the substantia nigra and locus ceruleus but also the putamen, thalamus and hypothalamus, and sometimes the oculomotor

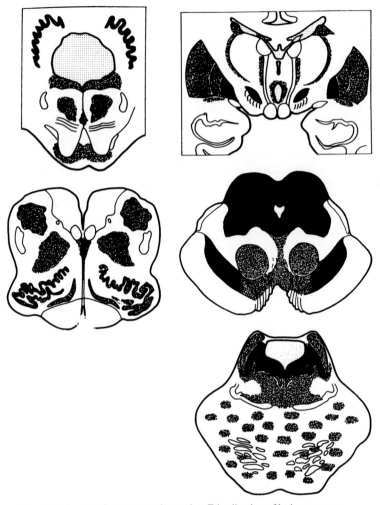

Fig. 15.6 Progressive supranuclear palsy. Distribution of lesions: worst affected areas have the deepest shading.
Reproduced by permission of the authors and editor from: Roy S, Wolman L. J Pathol 1969; 99: 39.

nuclei.[40] In these cases, the pigmented regions of the brainstem may lose all their neuromelanin; very few intact neurons may remain in these regions. Fibrous gliosis in the substantia nigra is marked. This histological picture is diagnostic of postencephalitic parkinsonism. The severe neuro-fibrillary degeneration, gross depigmentation of the substantia nigra and absence of Lewy bodies are often accompanied by small gliotic foci, which are residua of old damage, scattered throughout the brain.

Descriptions from the 1920s of the lesions in recent cases of encephalitis lethargica sometimes noted severe inflammatory changes in deep grey structures and brainstem, and gross damage to the substantia nigra in patients dying more than two weeks after the onset of the disease.

Striatonigral degeneration

The condition known as striatonigral degeneration was first described by Adams, van Bogaert and van der Eecken in 1961,[41] and has been considered in several subsequent publications. Clinically it is indistinguishable from idiopathic Parkinson's disease. Within a range of pathological findings, there is neuronal degeneration in the corpus striatum (notably the putamen) as well as in the substantia nigra. The putamen is usually atrophic, with loss of neurons and myelinated fibres; it is densely gliotic, and contains abnormal pigment. The substantia nigra and locus ceruleus are depigmented and depleted of neurons. In some cases, neuronal loss has been observed in the cerebral cortex, hypothalamic and subthalamic nuclei, and dentate nucleus. In one of the original cases the findings resembled those in olivopontocerebellar atrophy (see p. 418). Lewy bodies are absent, except in the very occasional case. The observation that cases of progressive autonomic failure of Shy–Drager type show lesions resembling those of striatonigral degeneration, together with pontocerebellar atrophy, has led to coinage of the all-inclusive designation *multiple system atrophy*.[42] This term has also been used to encompass a range of rare conditions causing extrapyramidal disorders, with early onset and involving basal ganglia, subthalamic nuclei, red nuclei, dentate nuclei, and superior cerebellar peduncles ('dentatorubropallidoluysian atrophy').[43]

Parkinsonism-dementia complex of Guam

A third parkinsonian disorder in which neurofibrillary change is encountered in the substantia nigra is the endemic disorder affecting the Chamorro population of the Pacific island of Guam (see p. 275). In some cases parkinsonism and dementia are associated with motor neuron disease. Familial occurrence is seen, with onset in middle life and death in a few years.[44] Cycad nut poisoning could be a causal factor. Cortical atrophy and depigmentation of substantia nigra and locus ceruleus are evident macroscopically. Histologically, nerve cell loss and gliosis are seen in many grey structures, cortical and subcortical, and intraneuronal neurofibrillary tangles are numerous.[45]

Other causes of parkinsonism

Toxic causes of parkinsonism

The neuropathology of *drug-induced parkinsonism* is poorly understood, partly because the condition is often reversible. Thus, though a parkinsonian picture is often seen in patients treated with the phenothiazine drugs, very little information about its neuropathology is available. Changes in neurohumoral balance are, of course, not necessarily associated with structural alterations. Nevertheless, patients with phenothiazine-induced oral dyskinesia have been reported to have reduced numbers of cells in the substantia nigra and gliosis of the midbrain,[46] and minor changes of this type could well be related to the Parkinsonian syndrome. Changes seen after *MPTP poisoning* (see p. 284), with resultant gross parkinsonism, are much more marked. Here there is a severe loss of pigmented nigral nerve cells.[18] *Manganese poisoning* (see p. 254) produces a complex neurological disorder in which features of parkinsonism are conspicuous. The very few neuropathological reports describe changes in the caudate and lentiform nuclei; nigral involvement has not been documented.[47] Experimental manganese intoxication in monkeys may cause diffuse cerebral damage but has failed to produce a consistent pattern of lesions in the corpus striatum or substantia nigra.[48] Another toxic cause of parkinsonism is *carbon monoxide poisoning*. Though parkinsonism of this causation is uncommon, its pathology is well documented; hypoxic damage of the globus pallidus is implicated, the substantia nigra being spared in most cases.[49]

Parkinsonism in boxers

In boxers, the punch-drunk syndrome may include extrapyramidal features which resemble Parkinson's disease. The brains of punch-drunk boxers, whether or not there is clinical evidence of parkinsonism, always show loss of cells throughout the substantia nigra. There are no Lewy bodies. Other evidence of neuronal damage is present in the form of neurofibrillary degeneration, mainly in the temporal cortex, without senile plaque formation. The overall neuropathological picture is characteristic (see p. 391).[50]

Parkinsonism associated with arteriosclerosis

Arteriosclerotic parkinsonism has no firm pathological basis. Though occasional patients are reported as having multiple infarcts in the corpus striatum and brainstem and an apparently normal substantia nigra, it is possible in such cases that the changes of idiopathic parkinsonism have been overlooked and that the striatal infarcts are an incidental finding. There is little pathological evidence to support an arteriosclerotic aetiology for parkinsonism, and the case for its existence must be regarded as unproven.

Parkinsonism associated with local lesions of the substantia nigra

Although local lesions affecting the substantia nigra may cause parkinsonism, as in the classic case described by Blocq and Marinesco (see p. 411),[21] by no means all lesions in that situation do so. Small vascular lesions of the substantia nigra may not be associated with parkinsonism.[51] The fact that parkinsonism may be associated with some cerebral tumours that have not invaded the midbrain[52] has been related to midbrain compression; this seems improbable, as brainstem compression is a very common accompaniment of cerebral tumours whereas parkinsonism associated with such tumours is very rare.

Other conditions with parkinsonian features

Parkinsonian features may be seen in Wilson's disease (see p. 302), Creutzfeldt–Jakob disease (see p. 384) and Huntington's disease (see p. 382), as well as in other system disorders such as olivopontocerebellar atrophy (see p. 418) and xeroderma pigmentosum (see p. 422). Batten's disease (neuronal ceroid lipofuscinosis; see p. 344) is a rare disorder in which parkinsonian features (severe rigidity and bradykinesia) sometimes accompany the prominent visual and intellectual symptoms that characterise the metabolic disturbance. Atrophy of cortical and central grey matter occurs, with neuronal loss and lipofuscin deposition in the surviving neurons. The neurons of the substantia nigra are filled with large, protein-containing inclusions.[53]

Other extrapyramidal syndromes

Hallervorden–Spatz disease is described on page 352. Other extrapyramidal syndromes of major clinical importance, notably torsion dystonia and spasmodic torticollis, do not have definable neuropathological changes. In the condition known as palatal myoclonus, in which rapid rhythmic movements of the soft palate interfere with speech, swallowing and breathing, there is striking hypertrophy of the olivary nuclei in the brainstem.[54]

DISORDERS AFFECTING CEREBELLAR FUNCTION

System disorders affecting the cerebellum and its connections (especially Clarke's column and the spinocerebellar tracts in the cord, the inferior olives in the medulla and the vestibular nuclei in the pons) may be secondary to generalised disease or they may be primary, often with a genetic basis. Cerebellar disease with identifiable causal factors (*secondary cerebellar disease*) is associated with some non-neural neoplasms, with chronic mercury poisoning (see p. 251) and chronic alcoholism (see p. 258), and with hypothyroidism[55] and chronic hypoglycaemia.

Primary ataxic diseases involving the cerebellum present complex and controversial problems of classification. One recent classification[56] divides the hereditary ataxias into four groups:

1. congenital disorders of unknown aetiology (a poorly delineated group of syndromes);
2. disorders with known metabolic or other causes (including abetalipoproteinaemia, hexosaminidase deficiency, Hartnup disease, urea-cycle enzyme disorders, ataxia telangiectasia, xeroderma pigmentosum and Cockayne syndrome);
3. early onset ataxic disorders of unknown aetiology, most with recessive inheritance and including, apart from Friedreich's ataxia, syndromes with myoclonus (Ramsay Hunt syndrome), cataracts and mental retardation (Marinesco–Sjögren syndrome), optic atrophy (Behr's syndrome), hypogonadism, deafness, and extrapyramidal features; and
4. late onset ataxic disorders of unknown

aetiology, inherited on an autosomal dominant basis, collectively labelled as olivopontocerebellar atrophies and probably including cases of Machado–Joseph disease (see p. 422).

From the pathological point of view, the primary cerebellar disorders of particular interest include Friedreich's ataxia and olivopontocerebellar atrophy, and these are described in this chapter.

Friedreich's ataxia

First recognised over a century ago,[57] this disorder accounts for at least half of all cases of hereditary ataxia, and has a prevalence in Europe of 1 to 2 per 100 000.[58] It is recessively inherited, with an estimated heterozygote frequency of 1 in 110.[59] The classic clinical syndrome is stereotyped and readily diagnosed. Unsteadiness and dysarthria appear in childhood, and progression of the disease results in many patients being wheelchair-bound before the age of 20 years. It is rare for patients still to be ambulant in middle life. Ataxia, hyporeflexia, extensor plantar responses and proprioceptive sensory loss are characteristic; optic atrophy and deafness occur in some patients. Intellect is generally preserved. Early muscular imbalance causes skeletal deformities (pes cavus and kyphoscoliosis). Cardiac symptoms, recognised by Friedreich, are commonly present. Cardiomyopathy may develop, with angina pectoris, heart failure and emboli as clinical consequences. Patients often die of heart disease. Diabetes with its complications also develops frequently in Friedreich's ataxia. An increased cancer risk is not seen.

Pathology. At autopsy, a reduction in the number and size of Betz cells in the motor cortex is described, and loss of fibres in the optic nerves may

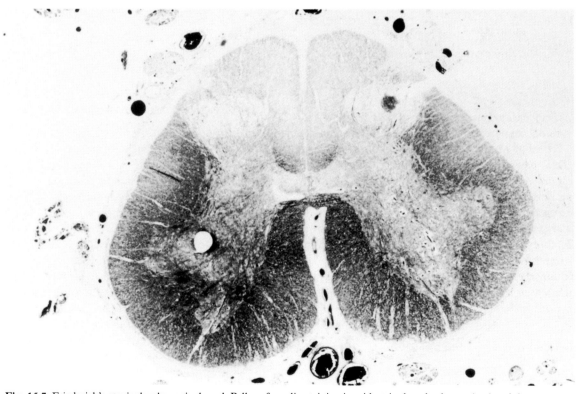

Fig. 15.7 Friedreich's ataxia: lumbar spinal cord. Pallor of myelin staining is evident in dorsal columns (top) and the superficial part of the lateral columns.
Luxol fast blue × 15

be associated with neuronal loss in the lateral geniculate bodies. Otherwise no changes are found in the cerebrum. The important lesions are in the cerebellum, brainstem and spinal cord. In the cerebellum, the cortex is spared but the white matter is gliotic, secondary to degeneration of afferent fibres; the dentate nucleus shows severe neuronal loss with gliosis. Degeneration of the superior cerebellar peduncles extends rostrally into the upper pons, while, in the lower pons and medulla, the vestibular, cochlear, superior olivary and accessory cuneate nuclei all show a degree of cell loss and gliosis. Neuronal changes in the gracile and cuneate nuclei are secondary to degeneration of the posterior columns of the spinal cord. Dorsal root ganglia show marked loss of neurons with the formation of residual nodules of satellite cells; this neuronal loss is the cause of the loss of myelinated fibres in peripheral nerves, in dorsal roots and in the gracile and cuneate tracts of the spinal cord. Loss of neurons in Clarke's column is marked, with resultant severe degeneration of the posterior spinocerebellar tracts (Fig. 15.7). Marked degenerative changes may also sometimes be seen in the corticospinal tracts in the spinal cord, though evidence of 'dying-back' (see p. 540) from damage to Betz cells is generally limited to pallor of myelin staining in corticospinal tracts in the medulla.

The cardiac lesions[60] in Friedreich's ataxia include hypertrophic and congestive cardio-myopathy. Medial hypertrophy and intimal pro-liferation are seen in small coronary arteries, generally without reduction of the lumen; this may be secondary to atrophy and scarring in the myocardium.

Apart from impaired glucose tolerance, Friedreich's ataxia is not associated with any con-sistent metabolic abnormality. However, the patients with this disease are significantly more sensitive to ionising radiation than is general in the population.[7,61,62]

Olivopontocerebellar atrophy

Patients with olivopontocerebellar atrophy (OPCA) show progressive cerebellar ataxia together with other neurological abnormalities in various combinations. These associated abnormalities include corticospinal deficits, bulbar dysfunction, extrapyramidal disorders such as parkinsonism, chorea and dystonia, oculo-motor abnormalities and anterior horn cell and peripheral nerve features. As already noted, the dominantly inherited cerebellar ataxias come into this category. However, many cases of OPCA are sporadic, while recessive inheritance is sometimes encountered. In some recessive cases, a systemic deficiency of glutamate dehydrogenase activity has been reported.[63]

The age of onset and rate of progression in this heterogeneous group of disorders are variable, though typically the diseases present in middle and later life. At autopsy, obvious shrinkage of the pons and middle cerebral peduncles is apparent (Fig. 15.8). Cerebellar cortical atrophy may be present. Atrophy of the inferior olives and loss of olivocerebellar fibres is a major feature. The transverse fibres of the ventral part of the pons show gross myelin pallor, as does the cerebellar white matter. No neuronal loss is seen in the dentate nuclei and the superior cerebellar peduncles are normal. Dorsal column and corticospinal tract degeneration, anterior horn cell loss and neuronal loss in the substantia nigra are among other changes that may be encountered.

Cerebellar cortical degeneration

A minority of patients with progressive ataxic disorders show neuropathological evidence of severe cerebellar cortical degeneration. A heterogeneous group of diseases which selectively involve the cerebellar cortex includes hereditary late onset cerebellar degeneration, ataxia telangiectasia and cerebellar degeneration as a non-metastatic complication of malignant disease.

Hereditary late onset cerebellar degeneration is dominantly transmitted and shows atrophy of the cerebellar hemispheres and vermis with marked loss of Purkinje and granule cells. Changes in the olivary nuclei are seen. A clinical and pathological overlap with olivopontocerebellar atrophy exists.[64]

Ataxia telangiectasia[65,66] has its clinical onset in infancy. With progressive ataxia, immune deficiency predisposing to respiratory infections, and a high incidence of malignant neoplasia, particularly lymphomas, the disorder is generally

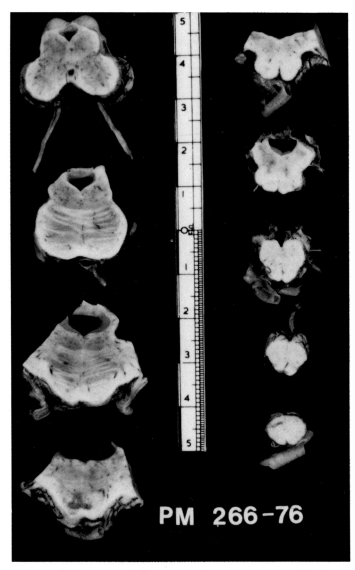

Fig. 15.8 Olivopontocerebellar atrophy. The pons was small and the lower brainstem was pencil-like in the intact brain. Sections of the brainstem shown here confirm pontomedullary atrophy with shrinkage of the cerebellar peduncles.

fatal in the second decade. Telangiectases of the conjunctivae and of the skin of the upper parts of the face and of the ears may be an early feature. Mild cases without susceptibility to infection occur, and with survival into adult life this condition may be misdiagnosed as Friedreich's ataxia. Striking cellular hypersensitivity to ionising radiation is indicative of defective DNA repair,[67] and several patients have died with severe radiation damage to normal tissues after a few fractional doses of X-rays. At autopsy, even in very young children, the cerebellar cortex shows extensive loss of or damage to Purkinje cells (Fig. 15.9). Granule cell loss is apparent. Cerebellar cortical atrophy may be gross. With prolonged survival, changes in the distal neuraxis resembling those of Friedreich's ataxia develop, including nerve cell loss from dorsal root ganglia and marked

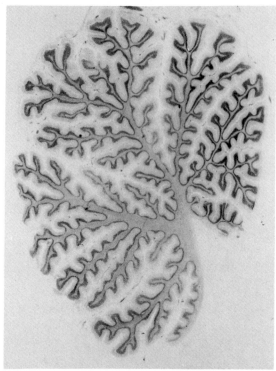

a

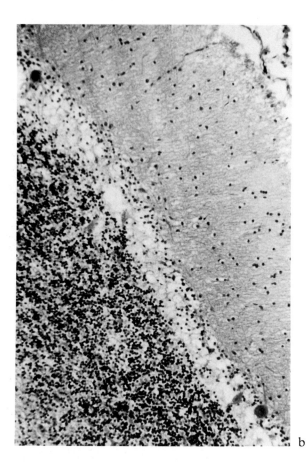

b

Fig. 15.9a, b Ataxia telangiectasia. (**a**) Cerebellar cortex shows mild atrophy at low power, while (**b**) shows that extensive loss of Purkinje cells is evident microscopically. Haematoxylin-eosin (**a**) × 1·6; (**b**) × 105

posterior column degeneration[68] in the spinal cord.

Cerebellar cortical degeneration as a non-metastatic complication of malignant disease (see also p. 494)

It is appropriate to mention here the adult, sporadic, progressive cerebellar syndrome that develops in adults in association with small-cell carcinoma of bronchus, carcinoma of ovary or breast, and sometimes malignant lymphoma. Ataxia and other neurological signs, sometimes associated with encephalomyelitis, may precede the direct clinical presentation of the tumour.

Cerebellar cortical atrophy, Purkinje cell loss and proliferation of the Bergmann glia may be striking features (Fig. 15.10). The cause of this syndrome is unknown; currently an immune pathogenesis is favoured (see p. 494).

Miscellaneous cerebellar disorders of unknown aetiology

It is not appropriate here to review in detail the pathological features of the various metabolic disorders that may cause ataxia. These include *abetalipoproteinaemia* in which there is degeneration of the dorsal columns and spino-cerebellar tracts in the spinal cord,[69] *urea-cycle*

Fig. 15.10a, b Carcinomatous cerebellar cortical degeneration. The patient, aged 40, had an ovarian adenocarcinoma. (**a**) Gross cerebellar cortical atrophy. (**b**) Purkinje cell loss was accompanied by intense Bergmann (left) and stellate astrocytosis in the granule cell layer and white matter (right). Immunoperoxidase for GFAP × 100

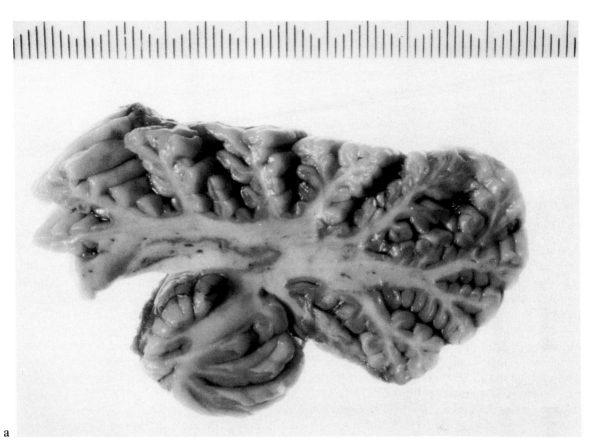

a

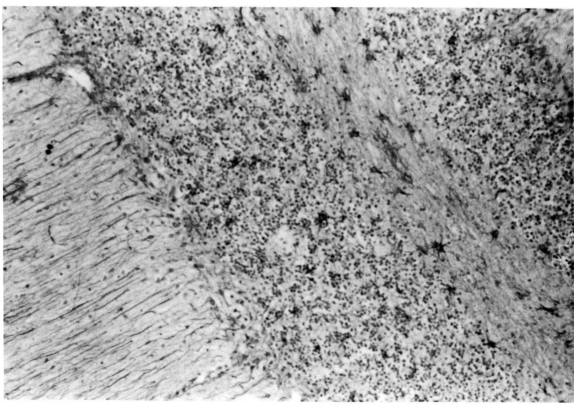

b

enzyme abnormalities in which Alzheimer type II astrocyte change (see p. 302) predominates,[70,71] and *Hartnup disease* in which focal Purkinje cell loss is described.[72] With regard to early onset recessive ataxic syndromes without known cause, the *Ramsay Hunt syndrome* may show, like Friedreich's ataxia, severe neuronal loss in the dentate nuclei.[73] In the *Marinesco–Sjögren syndrome*, two patients who died at the age of 4 showed marked cerebellar atrophy with gross Purkinje cell loss;[74] neuronal loss and gliosis were also present in pontine and inferior olivary nuclei. Pathological data on *Behr's syndrome* are scanty; major lesions that have been described are restricted to the optic nerves and lateral geniculate bodies.[75] In *Machado–Joseph ataxia* (Azorean ataxia, affecting Portuguese families from the Azores) associated clinical features may include pyramidal, extrapyramidal and oculomotor abnormalities and muscle wasting; nerve cell loss in the substantia nigra, dentate nuclei, Clarke's columns and anterior horns has been reported.[76]

OTHER DEGENERATIVE DISORDERS AFFECTING THE NERVOUS SYSTEM

Miscellaneous disorders

A number of neurodegenerative disorders, not readily classifiable into pyramidal, extrapyramidal or cerebellar groups, may be mentioned here.

Ophthalmoplegic syndromes. Paralysis of eye movements is seen in other rare disorders of the central nervous system in addition to the Steele–Richardson–Olszewski syndrome (progressive supranuclear palsy—see p. 413). Some patients diagnosed clinically as 'ocular myopathy' show evidence of neurological system disease, with ataxia, pyramidal signs, peripheral neuropathy, and retinitis pigmentosa. This complex is sometimes referred to as the 'ophthalmoplegia plus syndrome' or Kearns–Sayre syndrome.[77] Loss of cells from oculomotor nuclei may occur in such cases, many of which, however, show evidence of primary disease of eye muscles. In a rare dominantly inherited ophthalmoplegic syndrome with dysarthria, ataxia and rigidity, autopsies showed loss of nerve cells in the sub-stantia nigra, brainstem, cerebellum and cord, as well as in the oculomotor nuclei.[78]

Dysautonomic syndromes. Idiopathic orthostatic hypotension is a system degeneration affecting adults, which is usually but not invariably sporadic.[79] There is loss of normal autonomic reflexes, producing postural hypotension together with other features of autonomic dysfunction, including hypohidrosis, incontinence and impotence. Clinically, cases fall broadly into two types: those (Shy–Drager syndrome) with a complex clinical picture suggestive of olivo-pontocerebellar atrophy[80] and those without associated 'somatic' neurological disease ('pure' progressive autonomic failure). Autopsy in cases of the Shy–Drager type shows features both of striatonigral degeneration and of pontocerebellar atrophy, with loss of nerve cells in the spinal intermediolateral columns (sympathetic) and Onuf's nucleus (parasympathetic).[81] Cases of 'pure' autonomic failure also show inter-mediolateral column cell loss and may have Lewy bodies in the pigmented brainstem nuclei and elsewhere.[82] Such cases may show clinical features of parkinsonism. Occasional reports describe patients with the Shy–Drager syndrome with both olivopontocerebellar lesions and intraneuronal inclusions, and normal numbers of neurons in the intermediolateral columns of the spinal cord.[83] It is possible that there are lesions at the hypothalamic level in cases of idiopathic orthostatic hypotension but no such lesions have yet been identified.

Familial dysautonomia (Riley–Day syndrome)[84] is a rare recessive disorder affecting children and characterised by episodic hypertension, hyper-hydrosis, hyperpyrexia, reduced lacrimation, fits, dysphagia, hyporeflexia and relative insensitivity to pain. Early death occurs from pneumonia or renal failure. Neuropathological studies show loss of neurons in autonomic and spinal sensory ganglia, with secondary changes in the ascending spinal tracts and peripheral nerves.[85,86]

Conditions with increased cellular sensitivity to ultraviolet radiation

Xeroderma pigmentosum. The recessively inherited skin disorder xeroderma pigmentosum

(XP)[87] is of special interest from the neuro-pathological standpoint because its features suggest a possible pathogenetic mechanism in system disorders of the nervous system. Those afflicted by this disease show early cutaneous hypersensitivity to sunlight, and ultimately develop both severe scarring of the skin and basal cell carcinomas, squamous carcinomas and malignant melanomas in exposed areas. Besides skin abnormalities, some patients with XP also develop features of neurological disease. Some of the patients are mentally retarded from infancy; others appear intellectually normal in childhood but subsequently show progressive mental deterioration. Deafness and cerebellar, pyramidal and extrapyramidal signs may be present. Clinical features of peripheral nervous system involvement are sometimes seen. Such patients die of severe neurological disease in their teens or early adult

life. In the few cases of XP in which the nervous system was affected and autopsy was performed, microcephaly has invariably been reported.[88,89] The brain is atrophic, its weight ranging from 700 to 1000 g, suggesting a maldevelopmental as well as a degenerative pathology. Deep cerebral grey structures as well as cortex are atrophic. Olivo-pontocerebellar atrophy and depigmentation of the substantia nigra are seen. The spinal cord is atrophic, with loss of myelinated fibres from the dorsal columns and loss of anterior horn and dorsal root ganglion cells. Peripheral nerves show a gross loss of myelinated fibres of all sizes, in keeping with the spinal cord changes (Fig. 15.11).

In 1968, Cleaver showed that cells from patients with XP were deficient in their capacity to repair ultraviolet (UV) induced damage to DNA.[90] Failure of the excision repair process allowed the DNA strand to be distorted by UV-induced

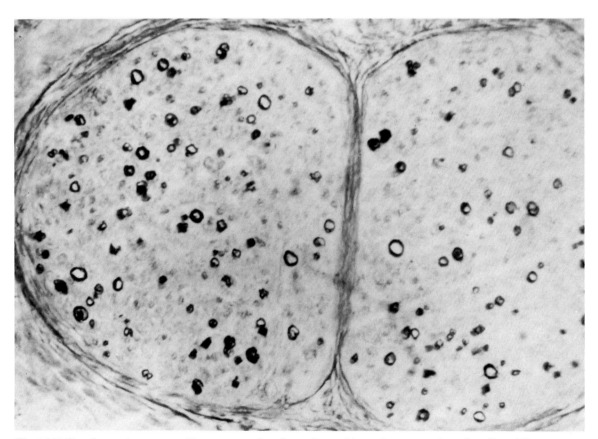

Fig. 15.11 Xeroderma pigmentosum. Transverse section of a sural nerve biopsy shows severe loss of myelinated fibres. Osmium fixation × 100

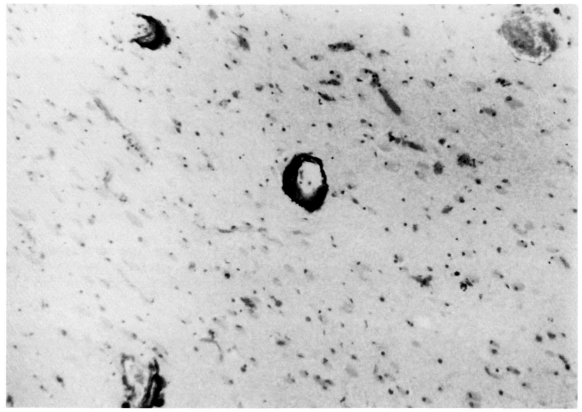

Fig. 15.12 Cockayne's syndrome. Calcified blood vessels (dark circles) are a prominent feature in the basal ganglia. Haematoxylin-eosin × 100

dimers between adjacent pyrimidine bases, providing an explanation for the mutagenic effect of sunlight on XP skin. It was subsequently shown that those XP patients who were most sensitive to the DNA-damaging effect of UV, as measured by inhibition of cell growth, were also those with neurological disease.[91] This observation prompted the hypothesis that neurodegenerative disease might be a consequence of defective DNA repair affecting the viability of large nerve cells.[92] Despite a substantial body of experimental data,[91,92] this hypothesis remains unproven, and indeed much published work contradicts it.[93] Where there is evidence of defective DNA repair in an inherited neurodegenerative disorder, the relation between the two abnormalities may be coincidental, through close chromosomal location, rather than causal.

Cockayne's syndrome. This is another neurodegenerative disorder in which increased cellular sensitivity to ultraviolet radiation has been shown.[94] This syndrome of childhood comprises microcephaly, mental retardation, dwarfism, photosensitive retinitis pigmentosa, deafness, dermatitis, premature ageing and a peculiar bird-like facies. Ataxia with pyramidal signs is seen. Early death occurs. Neuropathological findings include vascular calcification in basal ganglia, cerebral demyelination, and unusual Purkinje cell dendritic morphology (Fig. 15.12)[95,96]

Disorders affecting peripheral nerve function

Charcot–Marie–Tooth disease is discussed on page 573, and Refsum's disease on page 570.

REFERENCES

Introduction

1. Gowers WR. Lancet 1901; 1: 1003.

Disorders of pyramidal pathways

2. Buckley J, Warlow C, Smith P, Hilton-Jones D, Irvine S, Tew JR. J Neurol Neurosurg Psychiatry 1983; 46: 197.
3. Charcot JM. Progr Méd 1874; 2: 325, 341, 453.
4. Gardner MB, Henderson BE, Officer JE et al. J Natl Cancer Inst 1973; 51: 1243.
5. Zilkha KJ. Proc R Soc Med 1962; 55: 1028.
6. Bradley WG, Krasin F. Arch Neurol 1982; 39: 677.
7. Chamberlain S, Lewis PD. J Neurol Neurosurg Psychiatry 1982; 45: 1136.
8. Hirano A, Donnenfeld H, Sasaki S, Nakano I. J Neuropathol Exp Neurol 1984; 43: 461.
9. Hirano A, Nakano I, Kurland LT, Mulder DW, Holley PW, Saccomanno G. J Neuropathol Exp Neurol 1984; 43: 471.
10. Brownell B, Oppenheimer DR, Hughes JT. J Neurol Neurosurg Psychiatry 1970; 33: 338.
11. Mannen T, Iwata M, Toyokura Y, Nagashima K. J Neurol Neurosurg Psychiatry 1977; 40: 464.
12. Jamal GA, Weir AI, Hansen S, Ballantyne JP. J Neurol Neurosurg Psychiatry 1985; 48: 906.
13. Harding AE. J Neurol Neurosurg Psychiatry 1981; 44: 871
14. Steiman GS, Rorke LB, Brown MJ. Ann Neurol 1980; 8: 317.
15. Kugelberg E, Welander L. Arch Neurol Psychiatry 1956; 75: 500.
16. Walton J. Brain's Diseases of the nervous system. 9th ed. Oxford: Oxford University Press, 1985: 384.

Disorders of extrapyramidal pathways

17. Ward CD, Duvoisin RC, Ince SE, Nutt JD, Eldridge R, Calne DB. Neurology 1983; 33: 815.
18. Davis GC, Williams AC, Markey SP et al. Psychiatry Res 1979; 1: 249.
19. Parkinson J. An essay on the shaking palsy. London: Sherwood, Neely and Jones, 1817.
20. Gowers WR. A manual of diseases of the nervous system. London: Churchill, 1888.
21. Blocq P, Marinesco G. C R Soc Biol (Paris) 1893; 5: 105.
22. Brissaud E. Leçons sur les maladies nerveuses. Paris: Masson, 1895.
23. Trétiakoff C. Contribution a l'étude de l'anatomie pathologique du locus niger de Soemmering avec quelques déductions relatives à la pathogénie des troubles du tonus musculaire et de la maladie de Parkinson. Paris: Thesis, 1919.
24. Lewy FH. Dtsch Z Nervenheilkd 1913; 50: 50.
25. Foix C, Nicolesco J. Anatomie cérébrale: les noyaux gris centraux et la région mésencéphalo-sous-optique. Paris: Masson, 1925.
26. Takei Y, Mirra SS. Acta Neuropathol (Berl) 1971; 17: 14.
27. Greenfield JG. Greenfield's Neuropathology. 2nd ed. London: Arnold, 1963: 585.
28. Forno LS. J Neurosurg 1966; 24: 266.
29. Earle KM. J Neuropathol Exp Neurol 1968; 27: 1.
30. Gibb WRG. Neuropathol Appl Neurobiol 1986; 12: 223.
31. Den Hartog Jager WA, Bethlem J. J Neurol Neurosurg Psychiatry 1960; 23: 283.

32. Den Hartog Jager WA. Arch Neurol 1969; 21: 615.
33. Duffy PE, Tennyson VM. J Neuropathol Exp Neurol 1965; 24: 398.
34. Roy S, Wolman L. J Pathol 1969; 99: 39.
35. Goldman JE, Yen SH, Chiu FC, Peress NS. Science 1983; 221: 1082.
36. Woodard JS. J Neuropathol Exp Neurol 1962; 21: 442.
37. Okazaki H, Lipkin LE, Aronson SM. J Neuropathol Exp Neurol 1961; 20: 237.
38. Ikeda K, Yoshimura T, Kato H. Brain Nerve 1975; 27: 733.
39. Steele JC, Richardson JC, Olszewski J. Arch Neurol 1964; 10: 333.
40. Greenfield JG, Bosanquet FD. J Neurol Neurosurg Psychiatry 1953; 16: 213.
41. Adams RD, van Bogaert L, van der Eecken H. Psychiatr Neurol 1961; 142: 219.
42. Takei Y, Mirra SS. Prog Neuropathol 1973; 2: 217.
43. Smith JK. In: Vinken PJ, Bruyn GW, eds. Handbook of clinical neurology, vol 21. Amsterdam: North Holland, 1975; 519.
44. Hirano A, Kurland LT, Krooth RS, Lessell S. Brain 1961; 84: 642.
45. Hirano A, Malamud N, Kurland LT. Brain 1961; 84: 662.
46. Christensen E, Møller JE and Faurbye A. Acta Psychiatr Neurol Scand 1970; 46: 14.
47. Canavan MM, Cobb S, Drinker CK. Arch Neurol Psychiatry 1934; 32: 501.
48. Pentschew A, Ebner FF, Kovatch RM. J Neuropathol Exp Neurol 1963; 22: 488.
49. Schwedenberg TH. J Neuropathol Exp Neurol 1959; 18: 597.
50. Corsellis JAN, Bruton CJ, Freeman-Browne D. Psychol Med 1973; 3: 270.
51. Schwab RS, England AC Jr. In: Vinken PJ, Bruyn GW, eds. Handbook of clinical neurology, vol. 6. Amsterdam: North Holland, 1968; 230.
52. Chorobski J. Arch Neurol 1962; 6: 27.
53. Zeman W, Dyken P. Pediatrics 1969; 44: 570.
54. Koeppen A, Barron KD, Dentiger MP. Neurology 1980; 30: 471.

Disorders affecting cerebellar function

55. Barnard RO, Campbell MJ, McDonald WI. J Neurol Neurosurg Psychiatry 1971; 34: 755.
56. Harding AE. The hereditary ataxias. Edinburgh: Churchill Livingstone, 1984.
57. Friedreich N. Virchows Arch Pathol Anat 1863; 26: 391.
58. Winter RM, Harding AE, Baraitser M, Bravery MB. Clin Genet 1981; 20: 419.
59. Harding AE, Zilkha KJ. J Med Genet 1981; 18: 285.
60. Davies MJ. In: Pomerance A, Davies MJ, eds. The pathology of the heart. Oxford: Blackwell, 1975: 211.
61. Lewis PD, Corr JB, Arlett CF, Harcourt SA. Lancet 1979; 1: 474.
62. Evans HJ, Vijayalaxmi, Pentland B, Newton MS. Ann Hum Genet 1983; 47: 193.
63. Plaitakis A, Berl S, Yahr MD. Ann Neurol 1984; 15: 144.
64. Hoffmann PM, Stuart WH, Earle KM, Brody JA. Neurology 1971; 21: 771.
65. Boder E, Sedgwick RP. Pediatrics 1958; 21: 526.

66. Bridges BA, Harnden DG, eds. Ataxia-telangiectasia. A cellular and molecular link between cancer, neuropathology, and immune deficiency. Chichester: Wiley, 1982.
67. Taylor AMR, Harnden DG, Arlett CF et al. Nature 1975; 258: 427.
68. Strich SJ. J Neurol Neurosurg Psychiatry 1966; 29: 489.
69. Dische MR, Porro RS. Am J Med 1970; 49: 568.
70. Lewis PD, Miller AL. Brain 1970; 93: 413.
71. Bruton CJ, Corsellis JAN, Russell A. Brain 1970; 93: 423.
72. Daute KH, Dietel K, Ebert W. Z Kinderheilkd 1966; 95: 103.
73. Gilbert GJ. In: Vinken PJ, Bruyn GW, eds. Handbook of clinical neurology, vol. 21. Amsterdam: North Holland, 1975: 509.
74. Mahloudji M. In: Vinken PJ, Bruyn GW, eds. Handbook of clinical neurology, vol. 21. Amsterdam: North Holland, 1975: 555.
75. Houroupian DS, Zucker DK, Moshe S, Paterson H de C. Neurology 1979; 29: 323.
76. Sachdev HS, Forno LS, Kane CA. Neurology 1982; 32: 192.

Other degenerative disorders

77. Drachman DA. In: Vinken PJ, Bruyn GW, eds. Handbook of clinical neurology, vol. 22. Amsterdam: North Holland 1975: 203.
78. Woods BT, Schaumburg HH. In: Vinken PJ, Bruyn GW, eds. Handbook of clinical neurology, vol. 22. Amsterdam: North Holland 1975: 157.
79. Lewis P. Brain 1964; 87: 719.
80. Shy GM, Drager GA. Neurology 1960; 2: 511.
81. Sung JH, Mastri AR, Segal E. J Neuropathol Exp Neurol 1979; 38: 353.
82. Johnson RH, Lee G de J, Oppenheimer DR, Spalding JMK. Q J Med 1966; 35: 276.
83. Evans DJ, Lewis PD, Malhotra O, Pallis C. J Neurol Sci 1972; 17: 209.
84. Riley CM, Day RL, Greeley DM, Langford WS. Pediatrics 1949; 3: 468.
85. Fogelson MH, Rorke LB, Kaye R. Arch Neurol 1967; 17: 103.
86. Aguayo AJ, Nair CPV, Bray GM. Arch Neurol 1971; 24: 106.
87. Robbins JH, Kraemer KH, Lutzner ML, Festoff BW, Coon HG. Ann Intern Med 1974; 80: 221.
88. Yano K. Folia Psychiatr Neurol Jpn 1950; 4: 143.
89. Reed WB, Landing B, Sugarman G, Cleaver JE, Melnyk J. JAMA 1969; 207: 2073.
90. Cleaver JE. Nature 1968; 218: 652.
91. Andrews AD, Barrett SF, Robbins JH. Proc Natl Acad Sci USA 1978; 75: 1984.
92. Robbins JH. J Natl Cancer Inst 1978; 61: 645.
93. Brennan S, Lewis PD. J Neurol Neurosurg Psychiatry 1983; 46: 1143.
94. Schmickel RC, Chu EHY, Trosko JE, Chang CC. Pediatrics 1977; 60: 135.
95. Soffer D, Grotsky HW, Rapin I, Suzuki K. Ann Neurol 1979; 6: 340.
96. Leech RW, Brumback RA, Miller RH, Otsuka F, Tarone RE, Robbins JH. J Neuropathol Exp Neurol 1985; 44: 507.

Tumours of the nervous system

INTRODUCTION

Primary tumours which affect the central nervous system arise from cells within the brain and spinal cord, from the meninges and from other intracranial and intraspinal structures. In addition to the primary tumours, carcinomas and other malignant neoplasms may metastasise from various organs throughout the body to involve the nervous system.

Tumours of the peripheral nervous system arise from nerve roots within the confines of the skull and spinal canal, from nerves throughout the body, and from autonomic ganglia.

CLASSIFICATION

There have been many classifications of nervous system tumours[1] and the latest international

Table 16.1 Tumours of the nervous system.

Type of tumour	Principal sites and (age distribution)

1. PRIMARY INTRACRANIAL AND SPINAL TUMOURS

A. *Neuroectodermal tumours*

   1. Astrocytoma

      Pilocytic ⎫

      Fibrillary ⎬   { Cerebrum (young adults)

      Protoplasmic ⎭   { Pons, medulla spinal cord and cerebellum (children)

      Anaplastic astrocytoma   Cerebrum (adults)

   2. Glioblastoma multiforme   Cerebrum (adults)

   3. Oligodendroglioma

      Well-differentiated ⎫

      Anaplastic ⎭   { Cerebrum (usually adults)

   4. Ependymoma

      Well-differentiated   Ventricles and spinal cord (adults and children)

      Ependymoblastoma   Cerebrum and spinal cord (adults and children)

      Anaplastic ependymoma   Lower spinal cord—filum terminale (adults)

      Myxopapillary

   5. Choroid plexus tumours

      Choroid plexus papilloma   Ventricles (all ages)

      Well-differentiated

      Poorly differentiated ('carcinomas')

   6. Primitive neuroectodermal tumours (PNET)

      Medulloblastoma   Cerebellum (children and occasionally adults)

      Cerebral neuroblastoma   Cerebrum (children)

   7. Neuronal tumours

      Gangliocytoma ⎫

      Ganglioglioma ⎬   Cerebrum (children and young adults)

      Ganglioneuroblastoma ⎭

      Paraganglioma-ganglioneuroma   Cauda equina

      Anaplastic gangliocytoma and ganglioglioma   Cerebrum (children and young adults)

B. *Tumours of meninges*

      Meningioma   Cranial and spinal meninges (adults)

      Malignant meningioma (meningeal sarcoma

         including malignant fibrous histiocytoma)   Cranial meninges (adults)

C. *Nerve sheath tumours* (see also Tumours of Peripheral

Nervous System, below)

      Schwannoma (neurilemmoma)   { Spinal and cranial nerve roots (all ages but usually adults)

      Neurofibroma   { von Recklinghausen's disease—Neurofibromas

D. *Primary malignant lymphomas of CNS*

      Cerebral (originally called microgliomas)   (adults)

      Spinal (extradural)   (adults)

E. *Blood vessel tumours and malformations*

      Haemangioblastoma

      Cavernous haemangioma ⎫

      Capillary telangiectasia ⎬   { Cerebellum and spinal cord (adults)

      Arteriovenous malformations ⎬   { Brain, cord and meninges (children and adults)

      Venous malformations ⎭

2. METASTATIC INTRACRANIAL AND SPINAL TUMOURS

   Carcinoma

      Bronchus, lung, breast, kidney, etc.   a. Focal mass anywhere in brain ⎫ mainly

                                       b. Diffuse meningeal involvement ⎬ adults

                                       c. Extradural spinal involvement ⎭

      Malignant melanoma   Focal mass in brain or diffuse meningeal spread (adults)

      Lymphoma   Periventricular, meningeal or extradural involvement (adults)

      Leukaemia   Diffuse meningeal spread (children and adults)

Type of tumour (contd)	Principal sites and (age distribution) (contd)

3. TUMOURS OF THE PERIPHERAL NERVOUS SYSTEM

Schwannoma (neurilemmoma)
Neurofibroma
Malignant schwannoma
Malignant neurofibromas
  Cranial and spinal nerve roots
  Peripheral nerves (adults)
  Skin nerves—neurofibromatosis (mainly adults)

Neuroblastoma
Ganglioneuroma
Ganglioneuroblastoma
  Sympathetic ganglia; thorax, abdomen, adrenal
    (mainly children)

Phaeochromocytoma   Adrenal medulla or sympathetic ganglia (all ages)
Paraganglioma   Eg. carotid body, glomus jugulare
Granular cell tumour   Skin nerves
Nerve sheath myxomas
Tumour-like lesions
  limb nerves

classification was published by the World Health Organization in 1979.[2] Since that time, however, the use of immunocytochemistry has significantly altered concepts regarding nervous system tumours[3] as with tumours elsewhere in the body.[4] The classification in Table 16.1 is based primarily upon the 1979 WHO classification. Some of the very rare subgroups included in other publications[5] have been omitted.

The diversity of histological appearance, especially among astrocytic tumours, has resulted in the creation of many subgroups based upon microscopic appearances. In an effort to simplify the classification of central nervous system tumours, a grading system was introduced by Kernohan and Sayre in 1952.[6] But the attachment of a simple grade to a tumour is often confusing as the appreciation of what the grades actually signify varies widely. In order to avoid confusion, no grading system has been included in this chapter and the classification is based upon the well differentiated, poorly differentiated or anaplastic histological features of the tumours and their biological behaviour.

Although the term *glioma* does not appear in the classification, it is generally used to include a group of neuroectodermal tumours comprising astrocytomas, glioblastoma multiforme, oligodendrogliomas, ependymomas and choroid plexus tumours. Similarly, the terms 'benign' and 'malignant' are avoided as they may be confusing when applied to tumours of the nervous system. Although many meningiomas, schwannomas, haemangioblastomas, colloid cysts, epidermoid and dermoid cysts are well encapsulated and may be excised in their entirety and are thus benign, few of the primary neuroectodermal tumours may be considered benign. Because of the infiltrating nature of even very well differentiated astrocytomas, ependymomas and oligodendrogliomas, these tumours may eventually cause the death of the patient because they are not amenable to complete surgical excision or any other form of treatment. Some choroid plexus papillomas and cerebellar astrocytomas may be completely excised with ultimate cure of the patient; however, the outcome depends very much upon the position and size of the tumour in addition to its degree of differentiation. Metastasis of poorly differentiated neuroectodermal tumours such as anaplastic astrocytomas and glioblastoma multiforme to organs outside the central nervous system is very rare.[5,7] Thus, although these tumours are highly aggressive, and may be referred to as 'malignant gliomas' they do not usually spread from the primary site of origin except by local extension or by cerebrospinal fluid pathways. Care must be taken, therefore, in ascribing the terms benign and malignant to primary neuroectodermal tumours as they do not necessarily have the same meaning as when applied to tumours elsewhere in the body.

INCIDENCE

There were 146 970 deaths from cancer in the United Kingdom (population approximately 55 million) in 1981;[8] 77 940 were male and 69 030 female. Cancer accounted for 22% of all deaths; more than 50% of cancer deaths were due to carcinoma of the lung, breast, stomach and colon. Tumours of the central nervous system are the second most numerous form of cancer in children and account for 3·5% of all deaths in the 1–14 year age group,[9] but CNS tumours are only the sixth most common form in adults. Approximately 2% of all tumours in adults are in the brain and, of these, 35% are neuroectodermal in origin and some 40% are metastatic tumours. The incidences of nervous system tumours recorded in a number of surveys are roughly comparable.[10] Gliomas have an annual incidence of approximately 4 per 100 000 in the adult population, glioblastoma multiforme and anaplastic astrocytoma having the highest incidence with a peak annual incidence of 7·3 per 100 000 in the sixth decade. Glioblastoma is slightly more common in males whereas meningiomas tend to occur more frequently in females.

AGE AND SITE

There is a general pattern to the occurrence of tumours in the nervous system according to age and site (Table 16.1) although exceptions do occur. About 75% of intracranial tumours in children under the age of 16 years arise in the posterior fossa.[11] They are mainly well-differentiated astrocytomas of the pons, medulla and cerebellum, ependymomas of the fourth ventricle,[12] or primitive neuroectodermal tumours (medulloblastoma)[13] arising in the midline of the cerebellum. In young adults, astrocytomas are generally well differentiated and usually occur in the cerebral hemispheres; they may undergo anaplastic change after a few years. Medulloblastoma may also occur in the cerebellar hemispheres of young adults. Oligodendrogliomas arise mainly in the cerebral hemispheres of young or middle-aged adults[14] but can occasionally occur in children. Ependymomas present at all ages and may involve the cerebral ventricles and spinal cord. Glioblastoma multiforme and anaplastic astrocytoma account for approximately 65% of all primary neuroectodermal tumours.[5] They arise almost exclusively in the cerebral hemispheres,

most frequently in the frontal and temporal lobes and least frequently in the occipital lobes. Glioblastomas occasionally occur in the spinal cord. Meningiomas arise from the arachnoid mater and may be found at any site over the brain or spinal cord or, more rarely, in the ventricles; they are more frequent in older women[10] but may occur at any age. Schwannomas (neurilemmoma, neurinoma) affecting the central nervous system most commonly arise from the 8th cranial nerve (acoustic neuroma) or from the dorsal spinal roots;[15] they usually occur in adults. In overall incidence, metastatic tumours are the most common tumours to involve the central nervous system;[15,16] carcinoma of bronchus, carcinoma of breast, leukaemias, adenocarcinoma of lung and kidney and malignant melanoma are the commonest primary sources of metastatic involvement.

CLINICAL FEATURES AND INVESTIGATIONS

Familiarity with the clinical features of intracranial and spinal lesions is usually essential if the pathologist is to reach a logical diagnosis, particularly from a surgical biopsy. With intracranial and spinal tumours, the signs, symptoms and rate of progression of the clinical picture depend upon the nature and site of the tumour.[17–19] Patients may present with symptoms either due to focal destruction of neural tissue, or due to oedema, distortion of intracranial structures and raised intracranial pressure. Clinical localisation of a tumour causing focal neurological signs due to involvement of the motor cortex, brainstem or spinal cord may be relatively straightforward. However, tumours do arise in 'silent areas' of the brain such as the non-dominant temporal lobe, the corpus callosum, the frontal lobes and the thalamus.[18] The first indication of the presence of a tumour in these regions may be signs of raised intracranial pressure with headache, nausea, alteration in level of consciousness, papilloedema and visual failure. In general, tumours present with progressive neurological signs as opposed to the sudden onset of focal neurological signs with a stroke. Epilepsy occurs in one-third of patients with brain tumours and is more frequent with slowly growing tumours than with rapidly growing tumours such as metastatic carcinoma.

Computerised axial tomography (CT scanning)[20] and magnetic resonance imaging (MRI)[21] have largely replaced skull X-rays and isotope scans for the localisation of intracranial tumours. Although calcification within well-differentiated astrocytomas, oligodendrogliomas and craniopharyngiomas may be seen on skull X-ray, as may the bony changes associated with meningiomas and pituitary adenomas, tumours are more easily visualised on CT scan.

With CT images produced in the horizontal plane (Figs 16.33 and 16.75) and reconstructions in the coronal (Fig. 16.36b) and sagittal planes, intracranial tumours can be accurately localised within the skull. Unenhanced CT scans may reveal the presence of a tumour through differences in radiological density of the tissue. In addition, distortion and shift of the brain or dilatation of the ventricles and hydrocephalus may be seen. Enhanced CT scans are produced by the intravenous injection of contrast medium which leaks into areas of the brain in which the blood-brain barrier is defective.[20] Well-differentiated astrocytomas and oligodendrogliomas do not usually enhance, whereas viable tumour tissue in glioblastomas and anaplastic astrocytomas enhances and thus appears as a white region on CT scan contrasted with the non-enhancing areas of surrounding oedema (Fig. 16.9b). Other tumours which regularly enhance are meningiomas (Fig. 16.36), metastatic carcinomas (Fig. 16.75), lymphomas, schwannomas and primitive neuroectodermal tumours such as medulloblastomas (Fig. 16.33). Ring-like enhancement is seen in cerebral abscesses. Infarcts may enhance during the first few days.

Tumours involving the spinal cord may be intrinsic (intramedullary), such as astrocytoma, or they may be extrinsic (extramedullary) intrathecal tumours, e.g. meningiomas or schwannomas. Extradural (epidural) spinal tumours are usually metastatic carcinomas, myeloma or lymphomas; they may extend from vertebral bone or involve only the extradural fat. Myelography[22] is used to localise extradural, intradural and intramedullary spinal tumours; such lesions are more clearly demonstrated by MRI (Fig. 16.2).[21]

PATHOLOGICAL INVESTIGATION OF NERVOUS SYSTEM TUMOURS

The clinical history, the age of the patient and the site of the tumour, together with the results of CT scan investigations, may be a very good guide to the identity of a tumour involving the central nervous system. A definitive diagnosis, however, can only be obtained by histological or cytological examination of a biopsy or autopsy specimen of the tumour.

Tumour biopsies

Tumour biopsies taken at craniotomy, by burrhole needle biopsy or under CT scan guidance, may be fixed in buffered formalin in the operating room. However, the receipt of fresh tumour tissue in the laboratory allows the pathologist to make a rapid diagnosis of the tumour and to plan further investigation of the tissue. These are essential steps if full use is to be made of the immunocytochemical and electron microscopic techniques now available.

Rapid diagnosis of intracranial and spinal tumours may be made with smear or touch preparations or with cryostat sections. Smears[23] are particularly suitable for small pieces of soft tumours such as gliomas. The cytology is well demonstrated when smears are stained in 1% toluidine blue in 1% borax, as are the large blood vessels and capillary endothelial proliferation of glioblastomas.[23,24] Soft meningiomas and metastatic tumours can also be smeared. Cryostat sections are more suitable for firm tumours such as meningiomas, schwannomas, tough gliomas and metastatic tumours. Although the cytology may not be as clear in a cryostat section as in a smear, tissue patterns are more easily appreciated and a variety of histological stains and immunohistochemical techniques can be applied to the sections.[25,26] Touch preparations[26,27] are particularly valuable for the examination of lymphomas and metastatic carcinomas. The technique involves gently dabbing a piece of tissue onto a slide, air drying the preparation and staining by a Giemsa method.

Histological diagnosis of a tumour is often easier on *paraffin sections* than on smears and cryostat sections. Staining with *haematoxylin and eosin* will reveal histological patterns, mitoses, and the presence of necrosis and nuclear pleomorphism, whereas the *haematoxylin van Gieson* technique is valuable for detecting bands of collagen in meningiomas and metastatic tumours as an aid to distinguishing them from gliomas. The Gordon and Sweet *reticulin* technique[28] allows capillary endothelial proliferation in glioblastoma multiforme to be easily detected, the intimate reticulin network of schwannomas to be demonstrated, and the characteristic proliferation of reticulin around blood vessels in lymphomas to be revealed. Mucus in metastatic carcinomas can be stained with *periodic acid-Schiff* (PAS) or *Alcian blue* techniques. *Immunocytochemistry*[29] has proved to be a very valuable tool in the diagnosis of neurological tumours.[3,30,31] Astrocytic tumour cells and reactive astrocytes can be identified by the presence of glial fibrillary acidic protein (GFAP). Tumour cells in malignant melanoma and schwannomas stain for S100 protein, and many metastatic carcinomas contain cytokeratins.[32] Panels of polyclonal[33] or monoclonal[26,34] antibodies can be used to identify tumours when no single antibody is suitable. Such panels of monoclonal antibodies are particularly valuable for the identification of lymphomas.[25]

Electron microscopy still has a rôle in the diagnosis of brain tumours.[35] For example, the detection of cilia[36] may confirm a diagnosis of ependymoma, the presence of desmosomes may be used to identify a meningioma, and dense core vesicles within cells suggest a neuronal tumour.

Some malignant melanomas and metastatic carcinomas may diffusely involve the leptomeninges—'carcinomatous meningitis'. Lymphomas and leukaemias may invade in a similar pattern. Examination of *cytospin* preparations of very fresh cerebrospinal fluid from such cases often reveals the presence of tumour cells, and this procedure may be the major diagnostic test.[24,25]

Autopsy examination

Fixation of the uncut brain and spinal cord at autopsy, together with thorough examination[37,38] of the cranial cavity and spinal column, is essential in the documentation of brain or spinal tumours. In the firm fixed brain or cord, the shape and extent of the macroscopic extension of the tumour may be assessed and suitable blocks may be taken for the histological study of the identity of the tumour and its degree of involvement of the surrounding tissues. Although the histological preservation of autopsy tumour tissue may not be as good as that in biopsy material, the anatomical relationships are much better preserved and the extent of the involvement of the brain is more easily appreciated. Gliomatosis cerebri,[39] with diffuse involvement of the cerebral hemisphere or even larger areas of brain, is often only substantiated at autopsy.

PRIMARY INTRACRANIAL AND INTRASPINAL TUMOURS

NEUROECTODERMAL TUMOURS

Approximately 50% of primary intracranial tumours arise from neuroectoderm.[5] The majority are gliomas, i.e. astrocytomas, glioblastoma multiforme, oligodendrogliomas, ependymomas and choroid plexus papillomas, but neuronal tumours and primitive neuroectodermal tumours such as medulloblastoma and cerebral neuroblastoma are also included in this group.

Astrocytoma

Well-differentiated astrocytomas of the brainstem and cerebellum comprise approximately 45% of primary neuroectodermal tumours in children. In adults, approximately 10% of neuroectodermal tumours are moderately well differentiated astrocytomas and they occur mainly in the cerebral hemispheres under the age of 30. Although initially moderately well differentiated, many cerebral astrocytomas undergo anaplastic change.

Clinical presentation

This depends upon the site at which the tumour arises.[17-19] Astrocytomas in general are slow-growing, so that if they arise in the brainstem there is a gradual onset of spastic quadriparesis as the corticospinal tracts become involved, or cranial nerve palsies as the floor of the fourth ventricle becomes infiltrated by tumour. Hydrocephalus may ensue due to tumour growing into the fourth ventricle and occluding the CSF drainage pathways. Cerebellar astrocytomas may present with ataxia; hydrocephalus may develop due to distortion of the fourth ventricle.

Astrocytomas of the cerebral hemispheres may present with focal neurological signs, epilepsy, or signs of raised intracranial pressure. Rapid progression of clinical signs suggests the development of anaplastic foci. Astrocytomas arise less commonly in the spinal cord than in the brain. They slowly expand the spinal cord, and not only damage the corticospinal tracts, dorsal columns and other long tracts, but may cause muscle weakness and wasting due to focal loss of anterior horn cells. At the lower end of the cord, astrocytomas involve the conus medullaris and cauda equina, inducing incontinence and lower limb weakness.

Astrocytomas may also arise in the optic nerves (see p. 696).

Skull X-rays in patients with astrocytomas may reveal little except foci of calcification. On CT scan,[20] these tumours are seen as low attenuation areas, sometimes containing a large cyst. Well-differentiated astrocytomas do not usually enhance; focal enhancement may indicate anaplastic change within an astrocytoma. An exception to this rule is that well differentiated pilocytic astrocytomas may show enhancement. Spinal cord astrocytomas may be localised by myelography, CT scan or, more satisfactorily, by MRI.

Prognosis and treatment

These depend upon the site of the tumour and its histology.[40] Cerebellar astrocytomas can be totally excised in approximately 70% of cases, resulting in a 25-year survival rate of 90% for well-differentiated pilocytic cerebellar astrocytomas and of 30–40% for tumours with cellular atypia.[41] Brainstem gliomas are usually inoperable due to involvement of vital structures and have a 15–20% 5-year survival rate following irradiation.[11] It is not often that cerebral astrocytomas can be

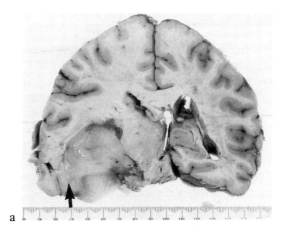

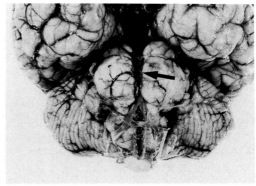

Fig. 16.1a, b Astrocytomas. (**a**) An astrocytoma in the left temporal lobe is seen as a soft gelatinous cream mass replacing the normal brain structures. The border is ill-defined (arrow). (**b**) Astrocytoma causing enlargement of the medulla and pons. The basilar artery passes in a deep groove (arrow) anterior to the expanded pons.

completely excised, so that reduction of the bulk of the tumour together with irradiation is often the treatment of choice. A significant number of astrocytomas eventually undergo anaplastic change (see p. 437). The prognosis of cerebral astrocytomas is more favourable in children, with a 45% survival rate at 5 years and 38% at 10 years.[11]

Macroscopic appearances

Well-differentiated astrocytomas are usually cream in colour. In the centre of the tumour the anatomy of the brain is obliterated but, at the edges, the tumour merges diffusely with the normal brain (Fig. 16.1). Astrocytomas vary in consistency; protoplasmic astrocytomas are soft and gelatinous whereas pilocytic astrocytomas may be firm and rubbery. The pons, medulla or midbrain may be expanded by the tumour (Fig. 16.1). Cerebellar astrocytomas frequently contain either a large single cyst or many smaller cysts.

As with other space-occupying lesions in the brain (see p. 66), the mass effect of tumour in the cerebral hemisphere may cause parahippocampal herniation, with brainstem compression and haemorrhage. Branches of the posterior cerebral artery and companion veins may be compressed, causing infarction of the temporal and occipital lobe on the affected side. Cerebellar tonsillar herniation through the foramen magnum may also occur, particularly with cerebellar tumours.

Astrocytomas of the spinal cord may cause diffuse enlargement (Fig. 16.2): on cross-section the cord is featureless and soft or rubbery. At the lower end of the cord the tumour may expand into

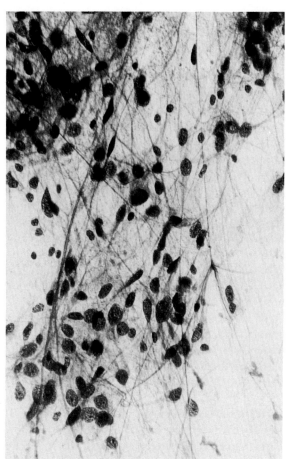

Fig. 16.3 Smear preparation of a well-differentiated astrocytoma. Fine astrocytic processes extend from oval or elongated astrocytoma cell nuclei.
Toluidine blue × 270

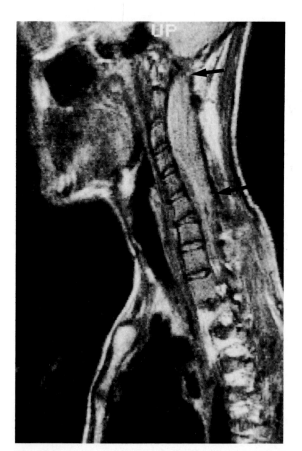

Fig. 16.2 Astrocytoma causing gross expansion of the spinal cord (arrows). Magnetic resonance imaging (MRI).

the subarachnoid space and involve the roots of the cauda equina.

Histology

Well-differentiated astrocytomas are composed of cells with varying numbers of fine fibrillary processes (Fig. 16.3). The nuclei show little variation in shape, size or staining, and very few mitoses.

The presence of fibrillary cell processes and indistinct cell borders in haematoxylin and eosin stained sections may be sufficient evidence to make a diagnosis of an astrocytoma. Other stains, such as haematoxylin van Gieson or Gordon and

Sweet, are often useful for showing the absence of collagen and reticulin fibres within the tumour. Glial fibrillary acidic protein is present in most astrocytoma cells.

In the central regions of an astrocytoma, the normal tissue elements are usually replaced by tumour, but at its infiltrating edge, tumour cells mingle with the neurons and myelinated nerve fibres of normal brain.

There is some variation in the histological pattern of astrocytomas.[2,5] *Protoplasmic astrocytomas* are composed of stellate cells with fine processes containing glial fibrils (Fig. 16.4). Microcystic spaces are common (Fig. 16.5). Such tumours are usually soft and they smear easily to reveal a uniform pattern of fine delicate cells and thin-walled blood vessels.[23,24]

Fibrillary astrocytomas, on the other hand, may be firmer in consistency and the cytoplasmic processes contain abundant glial filaments. In *pilocytic astrocytomas* (Fig. 16.6) the tumour cells are elongated and often polar with long tenuous processes containing glial filaments; they seldom undergo anaplastic change.

Rosenthal fibres[42] are seen in pilocytic astrocytomas but also occur in ependymomas and in longstanding gliosis. They appear as elongated brightly eosinophilic club-like structures with a slightly nodular profile (Fig. 16.6); although they are probably derived from astrocyte processes, the

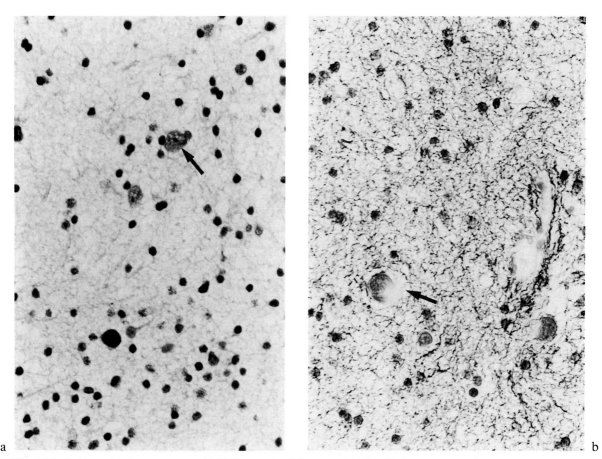

a   b

Fig. 16.4a, b Protoplasmic astrocytoma. (**a**) Well-spaced nuclei separated by fine fibrillary processes. An entrapped neuron (arrow). Occasional large nuclei are seen. (**b**) The fine darkly stained processes within the tumour contain glial fibrils. Some cells (arrow) with large nuclei contain no GFAP in the cytoplasm.
(**a**) Haematoxylin-eosin × 380; (**b**) Immunocytochemistry for GFAP × 380

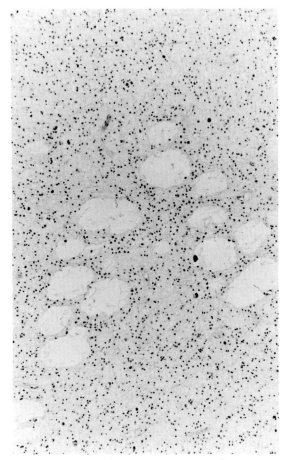

Fig. 16.5 Protoplasmic astrocytoma showing microcystic change.
Haematoxylin-eosin × 75

central mass of the Rosenthal fibre does not contain glial fibrillary acidic protein.[42a] Spherical, granular eosinophilic (protein) droplets are also seen in pilocytic astrocytomas.

Gemistocytic astrocytomas in their pure form are rare; they are composed of large plump astrocytes with abundant paranuclear cytoplasm.[5,43] The cells resemble reactive astrocytes, but nuclear abnormalities and the abundance of the cells in the absence of obvious tissue damage and inflammation are usually sufficient to distinguish tumour from areas of reactive gliosis. In general, reactive astrocytes in smears and in tissue sections have more abundant fine fibrillary processes than do astrocytoma tumour cells.

Two uncommon variants of astrocytoma also occur. *Subependymal giant-celled astrocytomas*

arise in the thalamus in patients with tuberous sclerosis;[2] they are composed of large plump cells with eccentric nuclei (Fig. 16.7). However, their origin is in doubt as many of the cells lack glial fibrillary acidic protein and some express neurofilament proteins.[31,44] These tumours grow slowly and have a relatively good prognosis. *Pleomorphic xanthoastrocytomas* are composed of large cells with foamy cytoplasm containing lipid.[45,46] There is often a reticulin network between the cells but their astrocytic nature is suggested by the presence of glial fibrillary acidic protein. Such tumours usually occur in young people near the meningeal surface of the cerebral hemisphere; they have a good prognosis and should be distinguished from giant cell glioblastomas.[46]

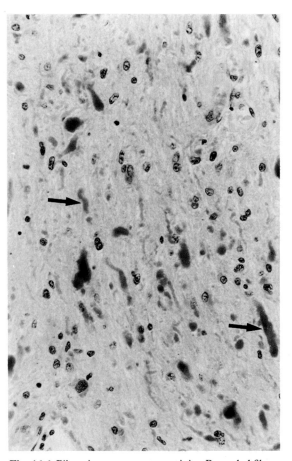

Fig. 16.6 Pilocytic astrocytoma containing Rosenthal fibres (arrows). Nuclei are widely separated by glial processes and show little variation in shape or size.
Haematoxylin-eosin × 240

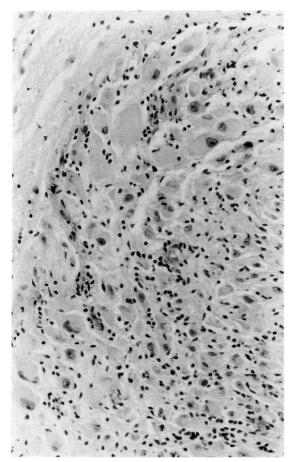

Fig. 16.7 Subependymal giant-celled astrocytoma in the thalamus of a patient with tuberous sclerosis. Large cells with abundant cytoplasm and prominent nucleoli are seen mixed with smaller tumour cells.
Haematoxylin-eosin × 190

Less well differentiated astrocytomas are distinguished histologically by an increase in nuclear pleomorphism and by the presence of a few mitoses. In some cases tumour cells form rosettes, or pseudorosettes around blood vessels, producing the pattern of *astroblastoma*.[5,40] These tumours usually arise in the cerebral hemispheres of young adults or children;[47] focal areas of astroblastoma may be seen in glioblastomas and in anaplastic astrocytomas.[24]

Anaplastic astrocytoma

These tumours arise from previously well differentiated astrocytomas.[5,40] Clinically, the change in the character of the tumour may present with sudden deterioration in a patient with a known astrocytoma or the symptoms may present de novo. Histologically, two elements are present: a well-differentiated astrocytoma and a focus of anaplastic change. The well-differentiated areas of astrocytoma show little hypercellularity or pleomorphism, few mitoses and no capillary endothelial proliferation or necrosis. Anaplastic regions (Fig. 16.8) show an increase in the number of nuclei per unit area, more pleomorphism, more mitoses and higher cell proliferation rates[47a] than the well-differentiated areas; in some cases, capillary endothelial proliferation is seen. Glioblastomas (see next page) can be distinguished from anaplastic astrocytomas as they lack areas of

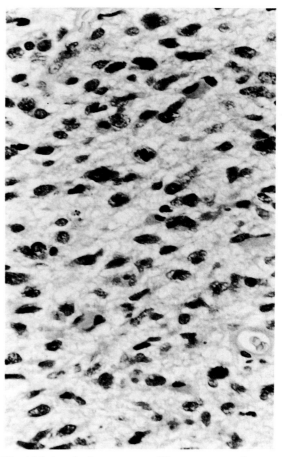

Fig. 16.8 Anaplastic astrocytoma. There are more cells per unit area, greater pleomorphism and more mitoses than in a well-differentiated area of astrocytoma (cf. Fig. 16.4).
Haematoxylin-eosin × 380

well-differentiated tumour and exhibit more pleo-morphism and capillary endothelial proliferation; they also contain larger areas of necrosis, with or without pseudopalisading (see p. 441).[40] The prognosis of anaplastic astrocytomas (50% survival at 2 years) is more favourable than glioblastoma multiforme (less than 10% survival at 2 years).[40] Anaplastic astrocytomas usually occur in the cerebral hemispheres of adults and are rare in the cerebellum and brainstem.

Glioblastoma multiforme

Glioblastomas are the commonest primary neuro-ectodermal tumours. They arise in middle-aged and elderly patients, with a peak annual incidence of 7·3 per 100 000 in the sixth decade.[10] Approximately 73% of glioblastomas arise in the frontal and temporal lobes of the cerebral hemi-spheres, and 20% in the parietal lobes; the occipital lobes are uncommon sites for these tumours.[17] Occasionally glioblastoma is seen in the brainstem or spinal cord.

Clinical presentation

This depends upon the site of the tumour.[17–19] There is usually a short history of a few months with either progressive personality change, focal neurological deficit, or epilepsy. Some patients present initially with raised intracranial pressure due to the mass effect of the tumour or due to hydrocephalus from obstruction of the lateral or third ventricles.

On CT scan,[20] a glioblastoma is visualised as an enhancing mass lesion (Fig. 16.9). There is often a rim of enhancement around a central cystic or necrotic region of the tumour. The enhancement

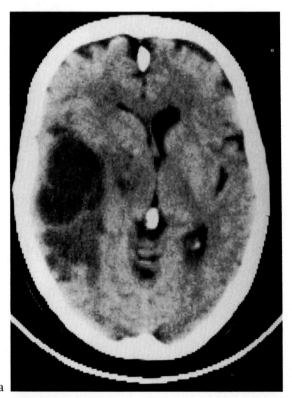

a

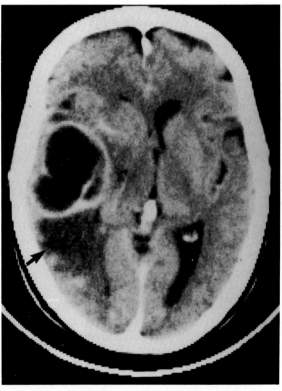

b

Fig. 16.9a, b Glioblastoma multiforme—CT scans. (a) An unenhanced scan showing an area of low density (black) in the left temporal lobe. Pineal (lower centre) and choroid plexus (lower right) are calcified. (b) Same case: enhanced scan showing a white rim of enhanced tumour around a necrotic or cystic centre. An area of oedema (arrow) is seen in the white matter posterior to the tumour.

represents viable tumour in which the blood-brain barrier is defective and thus allows leakage of oedema fluid and contrast medium into the tissue. Peritumoral oedema may be very extensive and is seen on CT scan as a low attenuation area which does not enhance (Fig. 16.9). Considerable distortion of the brain and ventricular system may be seen. The oedema associated with glioblastomas may be dramatically reduced initially by steroids[19] and the bulk of the tumour may be further reduced by evacuation of cyst fluid. Treatment by surgical excision of glioblastomas, particularly those in the frontal lobe, together with radiotherapy, gives the best prognosis, especially in patients under the age of 50 years.[40,48] Despite treatment, however, most patients do not survive longer than one year.

Chemotherapy has, as yet, had little effect on the overall survival of patients with glioblastoma.[49]

Macroscopic appearances

Many patients dying with glioblastoma multiforme have a swollen, heavy brain with flattening of the cerebral gyri, transtentorial herniation and brainstem compression (see p. 67). In the sliced, fixed brain (Fig. 16.10), glioblastoma appears as a more clearly defined tumour than a well-differentiated astrocytoma. However, histologically there is tumour cell invasion of surrounding brain tissue. Usually the tumour is single and irregular in shape, but satellite nodules may be seen. A thin grey rim of viable tissue is

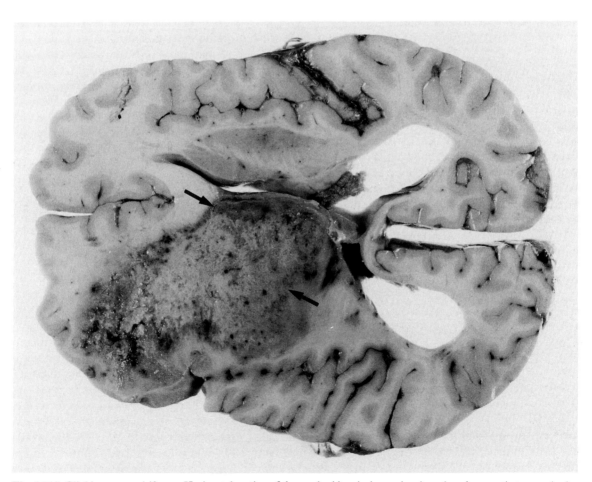

Fig. 16.10 Glioblastoma multiforme. Horizontal section of the cerebral hemispheres showing a largely necrotic tumour in the left frontal lobe and basal ganglia. Thin, viable rim of tumour (arrows).

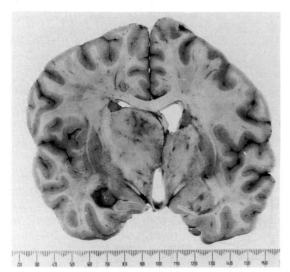

Fig. 16.11 Glioblastoma multiforme of left thalamus obstructing the foramina of Monro and distorting the ventricular system (coronal section).

usually present around the edge of the tumour but the centre is often yellow, necrotic (Fig. 16.10) and haemorrhagic, or contains protein-rich encysted fluid. The tumour may be confined to one hemisphere and surrounded by soft, swollen, oedematous white matter. In some cases, however, glioblastomas spread from one hemisphere to the other through the corpus callosum; occasionally they appear to be multicentric in origin. Centrally placed thalamic glioblastomas may compress the third ventricle and cause hydrocephalus (Fig. 16.11). Glioblastomas only rarely metastasise to lymph nodes or lung[5] but they may spread through the cerebrospinal fluid of the ventricular system and over the surface of the spinal cord. Very diffuse invasion by tumour cells may occur in gliomatosis cerebri (see p. 444)[39] in which the cerebral hemispheres, brainstem and parts of the spinal cord may be involved, but with little macroscopic abnormality in the brain and no localised tumour mass.

Histology

There is considerable histological variation between different glioblastomas and also between different areas of the same tumour. Many glioblastomas show astrocytic features in some regions, but the major feature which distinguishes

these tumours from anaplastic astrocytomas is that no area of well-differentiated astrocytoma is present in glioblastomas. A further distinction is the relatively narrow front of tumour invasion into normal brain in glioblastomas compared with the diffuse border in anaplastic astrocytomas. The presence of anaplastic tumour cells throughout glioblastomas suggests that these tumours arise de novo as glioblastomas rather than as anaplastic foci in previously well differentiated tumours.

When large histological sections of post-mortem specimens of glioblastomas are examined the full range and regional variation of the histology can be appreciated. The presence of the following features can also be sought in biopsy material as an aid to diagnosis.

1. *Necrosis.* Much of the central region of a glioblastoma is necrotic and haemorrhagic. Large dilated blood vessels may be occluded by thrombus and may thus be associated with central infarction of the tumour. Compared with areas of infarction in non-tumorous brain, there are relatively few macrophages associated with the areas of necrosis in glioblastomas but macrophages are distributed widely throughout most tumours and can be identified by immunocytochemistry.[50] A variable degree of lymphocytic cuffing of vessels, both within glioblastomas and in the surrounding brain, is seen. Most of the cells are T-cells,[51] usually suppressor/cytotoxic cells and sometimes helper cells. The presence of such inflammation appears to have little significance for the prognosis of the tumour.[40]

2. *Cellular pleomorphism.* There is considerable variation in nuclear shape and size in most, but not all, glioblastomas. Large giant cells with bizarre hyperchromatic nuclei and abundant cytoplasm (Figs 16.12 and 16.13) may be seen, particularly near the centre of the tumour. Abnormal mitoses may also be observed in these regions. Large, hyperchromatic nuclei are well demonstrated in smears of glioblastomas (Fig. 16.12a) and are a useful diagnostic feature.[23,24] Very little normal mitotic activity may be seen in the pleomorphic cells, and although thymidine labelling suggests that many of the bizarre cells are unable to divide,[52]

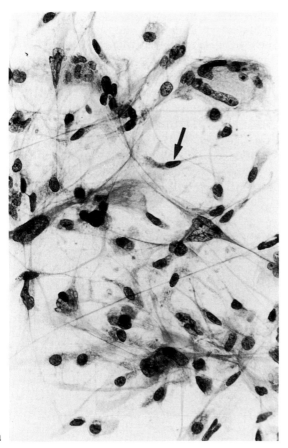 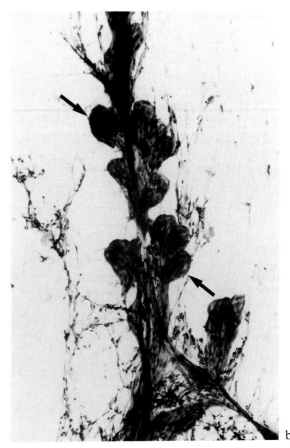

a

b

Fig. 16.12a, b Glioblastoma multiforme—smears. (**a**) Cytology of the smear showing bizarre, multinucleate cells (upper right) and small bipolar cells with rod-shaped nuclei (arrow). (**b**) Low-power view of blood vessel showing club-like projections of capillary endothelial proliferation (arrows). Toluidine blue (**a**) × 350; (**b**) × 100

other studies indicate that they are capable of cell division.[47a]

3. *Pseudopalisading* is uncommon in tumours other than glioblastomas. Serpiginous areas of necrosis are surrounded by cells with rod-shaped nuclei orientated perpendicular to the area of necrosis (Fig. 16.14).[5] Such an arrangement of nuclei in a palisading pattern is readily visible at low power. The term 'pseudopalisading' implies that the cells do not align themselves spontaneously (as in schwannomas) but are induced to do so by the presence of necrosis.

4. *Small rod-shaped anaplastic cells* are characteristic of glioblastoma multiforme. Such cells can be distinguished from the rod-shaped microglial cell by their irregular hyper-chromatic nuclei. In smears (Fig. 16.12a), such cells are often bipolar with fine processes extending from each end.[23] Although they are distributed throughout the tumour (Fig. 16.14), small rod-shaped cells are particularly prominent at the infiltrating edge (Fig. 16.15). Thymidine labelling studies suggest that these cells are an actively proliferating element in glioblastomas.[52] Mitoses are more common in glioblastomas than in well-differentiated astrocytomas, and monoclonal antibodies have been used to demonstrate proliferating cells in a variety of gliomas. Some 12–19% of cells are proliferating in glioblastomas, compared with 0·6 in pilocytic astrocytomas.[47a,53] Immunocytochemistry for glial fibrillary acidic protein has shown that many of the cells in glio-

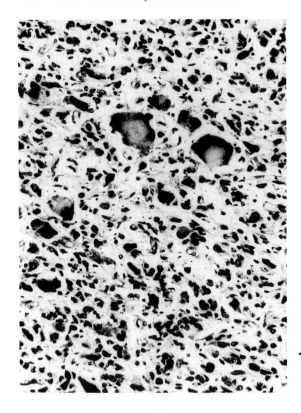

blastomas stain for this astrocytic marker although a proportion of the large bizarre giant cells in the centre of the tumour may have little or no GFAP in their cytoplasm.[30] Typically, the rod-shaped anaplastic cells at the periphery of glioblastomas are negative for GFAP, although the surrounding reactive astrocytes stain strongly for this marker (Fig. 16.15b).

5. *Capillary endothelial proliferation.* This may be seen in some anaplastic astrocytomas and even in some well-differentiated astrocytomas, but it is much more frequently observed in glioblastomas. In smears, thick-walled blood vessels are seen, with short, thick branches ending as a club-like tangle of capillaries (Fig. 16.12b). In paraffin sections (Fig. 16.16) and by electron microscopy, these glomerulus-like structures are seen as individual capillaries

Fig. 16.13 Glioblastoma multiforme—central pleomorphic region showing multinucleate giant cells and many small rod-shaped anaplastic cells. Haematoxylin-eosin ×240

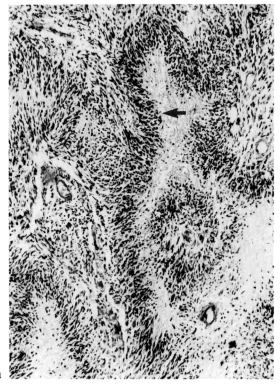

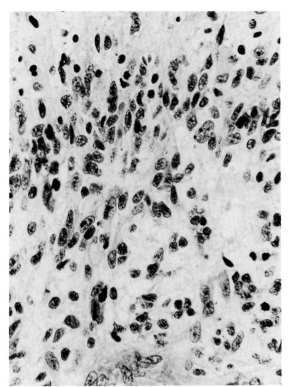

a

b

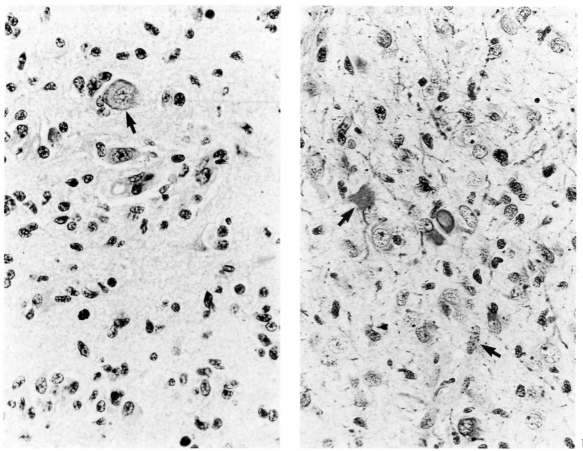

a   b

Fig. 16.15a, b Glioblastoma multiforme—infiltrating edge. (**a**) Anaplastic tumour cells with small nuclei are infiltrating the cortex. Preserved neuron (arrow). (**b**) Similar field to (a). Reactive astrocyte (arrow, middle left) is darkly stained for GFAP whereas anaplastic tumour cells (arrow, bottom right) do not stain.
(**a**) Haematoxylin-eosin × 380; (**b**) Immunocytochemistry for GFAP × 380

bound together by pericytes.[54,55] Such areas of capillary endothelial proliferation are well demonstrated in reticulin stains as they stand out against the reticulin-free background of the rest of the tumour (Fig. 16.16b). Although capillary endothelial proliferation may be seen throughout a glioblastoma, it is often concentrated around areas of necrosis.

Histological variants. In some examples of glioblastoma multiforme, large bizarre giant cells

predominate (*monstrocellular glioblastoma*).[42] The tumour cell nuclei are large, hyperchromatic, often multiple and set within copious eosinophilic cytoplasm. These tumours behave in a similar way to other types of glioblastoma. In some glioblastomas, areas resembling oligodendroglioma may be present interspersed with more overtly astrocytic regions.

Gliosarcomas[56] may cause diagnostic difficulty, especially if only small portions of the tumour are examined histologically. They occur at the same

◀ **Fig. 16.14a, b** Glioblastoma multiforme—pseudopalisading. (**a**) Low-power view showing pale areas of necrosis surrounded by pseudopalisades of densely packed nuclei (arrow). (**b**) Detail of pseudopalisade showing cells with oval or rod-shaped nuclei.
Haematoxylin-eosin (**a**) × 75; (**b**) × 380

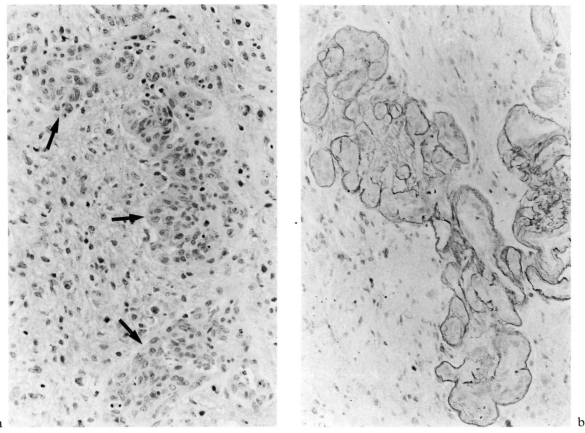

a   b

Fig. 16.16a, b Glioblastoma multiforme—capillary endothelial proliferation. (**a**) Compact areas of endothelial proliferation (arrows) with few capillary lumina. (**b**) Capillary buds are outlined by black-stained reticulin. (**a**) Haematoxylin-eosin × 160; (**b**) Gordon and Sweet × 160

ages and sites as glioblastomas. On CT scan they may be confused with metastatic carcinoma or meningioma. Gliosarcomas may appear to be well circumscribed at surgery and may be removed as spherical, firm, fibrous and partly necrotic nodules resembling metastatic carcinomas. Histologically, there are two main elements (Fig. 16.17): a spindle cell component, with reticulin-rich sheaths of elongated cells, and poorly-differentiated astrocytic tumour cells, forming reticulin-poor islands. In haematoxylin and eosin stained sections, the glial element may be difficult to detect, but the lack of reticulin (Fig. 16.17b) and the presence of GFAP in the glial areas may be diagnostic in a tumour that is otherwise pre-dominantly composed of spindle cells. Myxoid change may be present[57] and in some cases the spindle cell element resembles a malignant fibrous

histiocytoma. Despite the apparently circum-scribed nature of the tumour, neoplastic glial elements infiltrate the normal brain surrounding the tumour, and the prognosis of these tumours is similar to that of glioblastoma.[56]

Gliomatosis cerebri is the diffuse invasion of wide areas of the brain by small spindle-shaped anaplastic glial tumour cells which insinuate themselves between the normal neural elements and are often seen orientated along myelinated fibre tracts.[39] There is comparatively little destruction of the normal brain elements and there may be no localised tumour mass. Clinically, patients may present with behavioural and intellectual disturbances, epilepsy and localised neurological signs. On CT scan, the tumour may not enhance but there may be diffuse swelling of the affected areas of the brain.

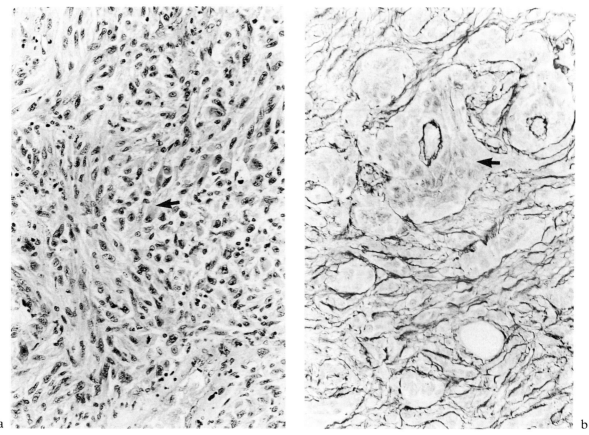

a   b

Fig. 16.17a, b Gliosarcoma. (**a**) The spindle-cell element (left) can be distinguished from the glial element (right) which is composed of plump glial cells with fine processes (arrow). (**b**) The reticulin-rich spindle-cell elements surround the areas of glial tumour (arrow) which is free of reticulin except around the blood vessels.
(**a**) Haematoxylin-eosin × 190; (**b**) Gordon and Sweet × 190

Oligodendroglioma

The majority of oligodendrogliomas arise in the cerebral hemispheres, particularly in the frontal lobes;[58] they are rare in the posterior fossa and spinal cord. These tumours may occur at any age, but only 6% occur in children. Comprising 3–6% of all glial tumours,[59] oligodendrogliomas often grow slowly but aggressive, anaplastic forms do occur and they mimic anaplastic astrocytoma or glioblastoma multiforme in their clinical course.[41] Typically, a slowly growing oligodendroglioma presents with epilepsy or slowly progressive focal neurological signs and eventually with raised intracranial pressure. Patients under 45 years of age have a better prognosis than older patients.[60]

Calcification can be detected in skull X-rays in 28% of oligodendrogliomas.[58] Well-differentiated oligodendrogliomas do not usually enhance on CT scan and there may be little associated oedema; any calcification will be evident on CT scan. More aggressive anaplastic oligodendrogliomas do enhance on CT scan and usually have associated peritumoral oedema.

Macroscopic appearances

Oligodendrogliomas often have a distinctive plum-coloured hue and, although they may appear well circumscribed (Fig. 16.18), the majority show infiltration of the surrounding brain. Nodules of tumour may be present on the surface of the brain but spread of the tumour through the cerebro-spinal fluid is uncommon.[59] If large, oligoden-

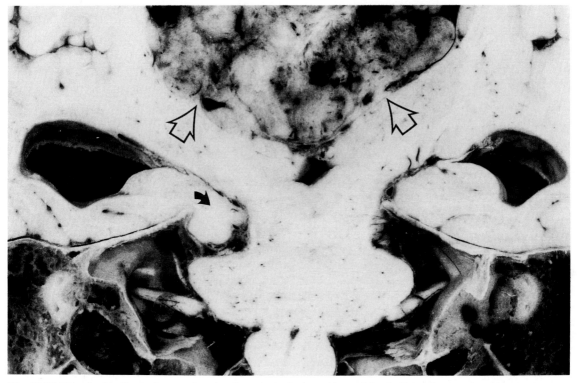

Fig. 16.18 Oligodendroglioma. A coronal section through the brain and base of the skull showing an apparently well-demarcated oligodendroglioma (top, open arrows) arising in the wall of the third ventricle. The left parahippocampal gyrus (solid arrow) has herniated through the opening in the tentorium cerebelli and the midbrain is compressed. Temporal horns of lateral ventricles are both dilated. The 7th and 8th nerves can be seen entering the internal auditory meatus on each side (bottom).
Reproduced by permission of Dr M.S. Kearney, Regional Hospital, Tromsø, Norway.

drogliomas produce brain distortion with transtentorial herniation and brainstem compression (Fig. 16.18). Areas of haemorrhage or necrosis may be seen in the tumour.

Histology

Oligodendrogliomas are composed of cells with small round nuclei which usually vary little in shape and size (Fig. 16.19), although in some tumours there may be moderate nuclear pleomorphism. In many oligodendrogliomas a clear space of swollen cytoplasm around the tumour cell nucleus is seen (Fig. 16.20) giving the cells a box-like appearance. Oligodendroglioma cells have few processes, so that in smear preparations (Fig. 16.19) a uniform sheet of nuclei is seen, with only sparse fine fibrillary processes extending from the cells.

Characteristically, oligodendroglioma cells spread diffusely through white matter and cortex, often accumulating as small nodules on the subpial surface. As they spread through the cortex, the tumour cells are frequently widely spaced although they do accumulate in small groups around cortical neurons (Fig. 16.21). Occasionally, the nuclei are arranged in small palisades, producing a 'rhythmic' arrangement. Capillaries in oligodendrogliomas are typically thin-walled and branching; this pattern is seen particularly well in reticulin stains (Fig. 16.20). Larger blood vessels may show endothelial proliferation, producing a rather thick vessel wall, but the capillary endothelial buds seen in glioblastomas are not usually present in oligodendrogliomas. Calcospherites are often distributed throughout the tumour.

The cellularity of oligodendrogliomas varies. A

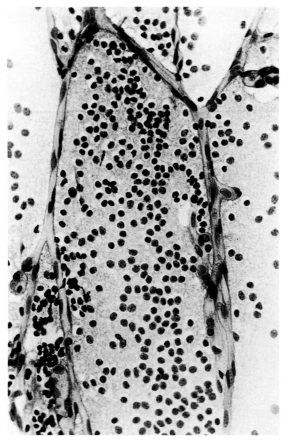

Fig. 16.19 Oligodendroglioma. A smear showing uniform tumour cell nuclei and thin-walled branching tumour vessels. Toluidine blue × 240

minority have a low cellularity and few mitoses. In more than 60% of pure oligodendrogliomas[59] there is a medium cellularity (Fig. 16.20) with a few astrocyte processes between the cells. In some 20% of cases, cellularity is high (Fig. 16.22) and in these tumours there may be many mitoses (more than 10 per high-power field). However, mitoses are found in most oligodendrogliomas and their frequency by itself does not appear to have prognostic significance.[59]

In a series of 208 oligodendrogliomas in which 75% of the cells were oligodendroglial tumour cells, survival of the patient was related to a number of histological features.[59] Patients with tumours of low cellularity, microcysts and no necrosis had a median survival of 91 months, a 5-year survival of 67% and a 10-year survival of

17%. Those patients with tumours showing a combination of medium or high cellularity, areas of necrosis, but no microcysts had a median survival of 18 months and a 5-year survival of only 9%. The correlation of high cellularity, necrosis and poor prognosis has been found in other studies,[14] in which most of the tumours with low cell density were in patients under 40 years of age whereas those with high cell density and necrosis were over 40 years of age.

The frequency of mitoses and nuclear atypia alone does not seem to have a significant effect upon prognosis, but subpial infiltration by tumour cells is associated with a poor prognosis.[59]

Immunocytochemistry has shown that there are GFAP-positive oligodendroglial cells in over 40% of oligodendrogliomas.[31,61] These GFAP-positive tumour cells are distinct from the reactive astrocytes within the tumour and from the astrocytic component of oligoastrocytomas (see below). GFAP has been detected in human fetal oligodendrocytes at 15–16 weeks,[62] but it is not present in oligodendrocytes later in fetal or postnatal life. Markers such as carbonic anhydrase C and myelin basic protein, which can be used to identify oligodendrocytes and myelin in normal adult brain, are usually not detectable by immunocytochemistry in oligodendrogliomas.[30,33]

A number of histological variants occur in oligodendrogliomas; these include the presence of globular cells with paranuclear eosinophilic cytoplasm and tumours which contain mucoid material and even signet-ring cells.[43]

Oligoastrocytomas.   Some 25% of oligodendrogliomas have a prominent astrocytic component, comprising more than 25% of the total cells. Such tumours are mixed gliomas[63] and the astrocytic element may be a prominent neoplastic component of the tumour.

Ependymoma

Ependymomas have a bimodal age distribution with a peak at 5 years and a broad peak in adult life.[64] They arise from the ependymal lining of the lateral, third and fourth ventricles and in the spinal cord and cauda equina. In children, ependymomas comprise 10% of all intracranial tumours: 60%

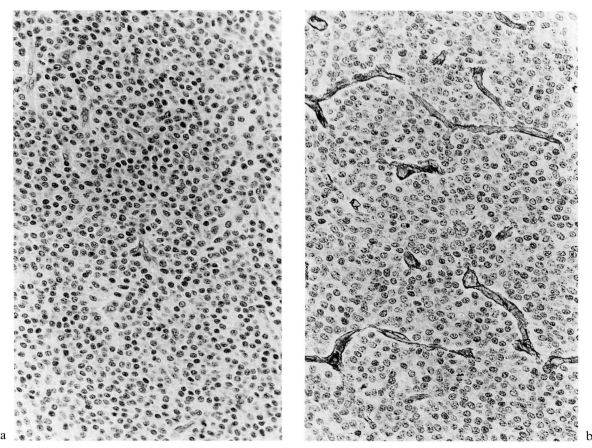

Fig. 16.20a, b Oligodendroglioma of medium cellularity. (**a**) The tumour is composed of uniform cells with round or oval nuclei. A few pale perinuclear halos are seen (top). (**b**) Thin-walled branching blood vessels typical of an oligodendroglioma are outlined by their black-stained reticulin coats.
(**a**) Haematoxylin-eosin × 240; (**b**) Gordon and Sweet × 240

arise below the tentorium cerebelli and 40% above.[11]

Over all ages, approximately 39% of ependymomas arise in the posterior fossa from the floor of the fourth ventricle, 20% in the cerebral ventricles, 14% in the cervicothoracic spinal cord and 28% from the cauda equina.[64,65] The majority of ependymomas in children are intracranial whereas in adults they are equally distributed between the cranial cavity and the spine. Although they may spread through the subarachnoid space, especially caudally, ependymomas only rarely metastasise outside the CNS,[66] usually by local spread into paraspinal tissues.

Clinical presentation

Ependymomas may present with raised intra-cranial pressure due to hydrocephalus as the tumour grows into the ventricular system.[19] Some patients exhibit focal brainstem signs due to invasion of the floor of the fourth ventricle. Spinal ependymomas may involve the nerve roots, particularly of the cauda equina, and cause backache and focal lower motor neuron signs. Long tract signs in the spinal cord result from local invasion by the tumour. In slowly growing ependymomas of the spinal cord the history may extend back several years. Ependymomas also present as intracerebral mass lesions.

On CT scan, ependymomas show moderate to marked enhancement and may exhibit cystic change and calcification.[67] Posterior fossa and spinal ependymomas are particularly well demonstrated by magnetic resonance imaging.

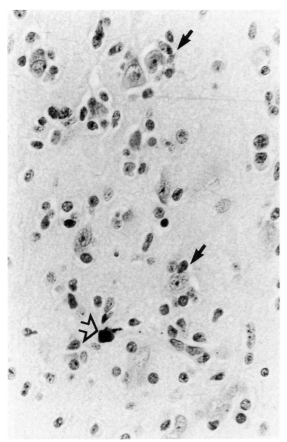

Fig. 16.21 Oligodendroglioma invading cerebral cortex. Groups of tumour cells surround neurons (solid arrows). Calcospherite (open arrow). Haematoxylin-eosin × 385

Treatment of ependymomas has improved in recent years with surgical excision and post-operative irradiation so that, in children, the 5-year survival rate is now 40–50%.[19,68]

Macroscopic appearances

Ependymomas are seen as soft, pale pink or cream-coloured tumours within the ventricular system (Fig. 16.23) or coating the spinal cord and cauda equina. In some 12% of cases, the tumour is widely distributed over the surface of the spinal cord.[19] Some tumours, especially subependymomas, have a very firm consistency, are lobulated, white, and well localised.

Histology

Microscopically, ependymomas show a variety of histological patterns, more than one of which may occur within the same tumour.[65] Short lengths of ciliated, cuboidal epithelium (Fig. 16.24) resembling normal ependyma may be present within the tumour, or ependymal cells may form small circular *rosettes* with a lumen into which cilia project. Far more typical of most ependymomas is the formation of *pseudorosettes*, in which tumour cells extend fine fibrillary processes onto the walls of blood vessels so that, in a haematoxylin and eosin stained section, a broad pink halo is seen around the vessels (Fig. 16.25). In well-differentiated ependymomas there is little variation in nuclear shape and size, and cyto-plasmic processes may be abundant. In smears of

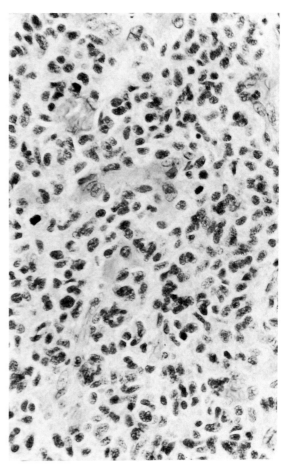

Fig. 16.22 Oligodendroglioma—high cellular density. There is variation in nuclear shape and size and mitoses are present in this field (cf. Fig. 16.20a). Haematoxylin-eosin × 385

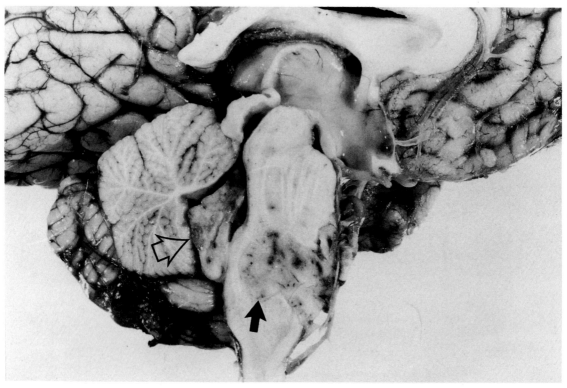

Fig. 16.23 Ependymoma in a 2-year-old child. A sagittal section through the brain showing ependymoma filling the fourth ventricle (open arrow) and invading the medulla (solid arrow); the aqueduct, third ventricle and foramen of Monro are seen towards the top of the picture. The tumour caused hydrocephalus.

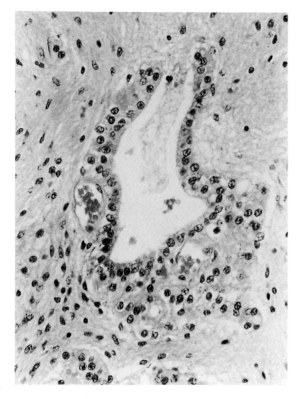

these tumours, the small round or oval nuclei are seen to contain small nucleoli.

Subependymomas are firm, lobulated tumours, often arising in the fourth ventricle as small white nodules but sometimes forming large tumour masses. Histologically, the tumour cell nuclei are gathered in small nests separated by large areas of interweaving glial processes (Fig. 16.26). Rosenthal fibres may be present in subependymomas and in other types of ependymoma.

Many ependymoma cells have cilia although these may not be apparent in haematoxylin and eosin stained sections. The basal bodies of the cilia (blepharoplasts) may be seen as small blue dots with the phosphotungstic acid haematoxylin stain;[5] they are more easily identified by electron microscopy (Fig. 16.27).[35]

Fig. 16.24 Well-differentiated ependymoma showing solid areas of tumour and a lumen surrounded by ciliated, cuboidal epithelium resembling normal ependyma. Haematoxylin-eosin × 240

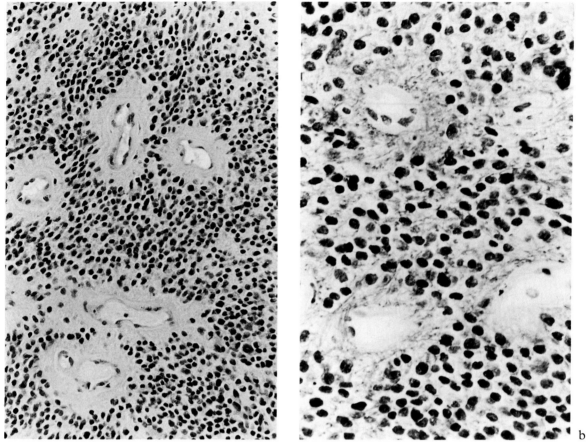

Fig. 16.25a, b Poorly differentiated ependymoma from a 3-year-old child. (**a**) There is a high cellular density and many mitoses. Pseudorosettes have formed as pale halos around the blood vessels. (**b**) Fine ependymoma cell processes in the pseudorosettes contain GFAP (e.g. top left).
(**a**) Haematoxylin-eosin × 190; (**b**) Immunoperoxidase for GFAP × 385

Poorly-differentiated ependymomas are uncommon; they mainly occur in children.[65] There is an increase in cellularity and mitotic activity within the tumour, and few glial processes are present, but the perivascular pseudorosette pattern is usually maintained (Fig. 16.25). *Ependymoblastomas*[69] are poorly-differentiated tumours which occur mainly in children, with a peak incidence at 5 years of age. They resemble medulloblastomas[69] but may still show prominent pseudorosette formation around blood vessels; they have been grouped with the primitive neuroectodermal tumours by Rorke.[13] In some cases the perivascular cells have thick processes directed towards blood vessels. *Anaplastic ependymomas*[70] are rare; occasionally they arise

from well-differentiated ependymomas or subependymomas and they may show bizarre cellular features similar to those seen in anaplastic astrocytomas. Other anaplastic forms are composed of small rod-shaped cells (Fig. 16.28) which spread widely through the cerebrospinal fluid pathways and invade the surface of the brain and the periventricular areas.

One variant of ependymoma has a particularly striking histological appearance. The *myxopapillary ependymoma*[65] occurs at the lower end of the spinal cord and is thought to arise from the filum terminale.[5] Histologically, the tumour cells are arranged in loosely-packed sheets bordered by rows of columnar cells which themselves surround mucoid areas (Fig. 16.29). The mucus stains

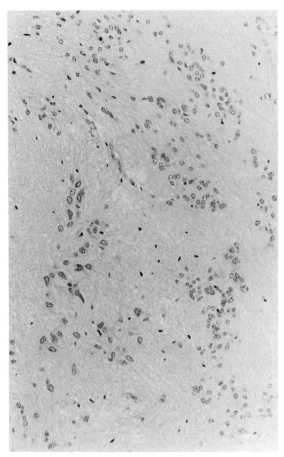

Fig. 16.26 Subependymoma. Nests of small round or oval nuclei are separated by dense interweaving glial processes. Haematoxylin-eosin × 150

positively with PAS and Alcian blue. An extensive connective tissue stroma may be seen in these tumours; this is not a characteristic feature of other types of ependymoma. Myxopapillary ependymomas may, on rare occasions, invade through the tissue surrounding the spinal cord and present as subcutaneous tumours over the spine.

Immunocytochemical techniques have shown that most ependymomas, even the poorly-differentiated tumours, express glial fibrillary acidic protein (GFAP) in the fine cellular processes surrounding blood vessels (Fig. 16.25b). Similarly, the tough glial tissue in sub-ependymomas contains GFAP. Most normal adult ependymal cells do not contain GFAP but it is expressed in fetal ependyma.[71] In some cases, a papillary pattern is seen in ependymomas which may thus be confused with metastatic carcinoma or with choroid plexus papillomas (see below).

Choroid plexus tumours

Choroid plexus papillomas may occur at any age from birth to late middle age; 50% of choroid plexus tumours arise in patients under 20 years of age.[5] They are uncommon and account for less than 1% of all intracranial tumours; most are well-differentiated choroid plexus papillomas but malignant choroid plexus carcinomas also occur.[72] Papillomas arise from the choroid plexuses in the lateral and fourth ventricles, and their main clinical effect is due to hydrocephalus—either from obstruction of cerebrospinal fluid drainage pathways or possibly from overproduction of CSF.

On CT scan, choroid plexus tumours are seen as

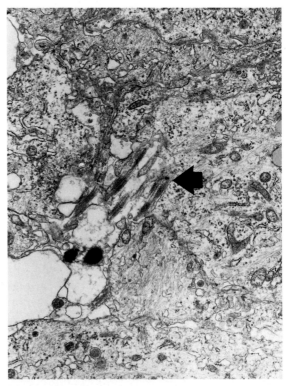

Fig. 16.27 Ependymoma showing obliquely cut basal bodies and cilia (arrow). Electron micrograph × 7000

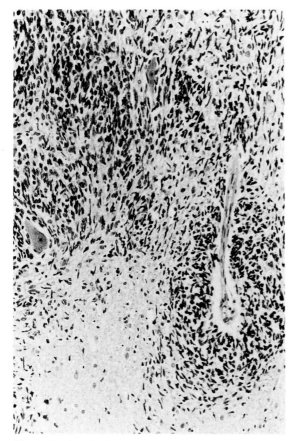

Fig. 16.28 Anaplastic ependymoma invading the medulla. Cells with small rod-shaped nuclei have surrounded neurons (top and left) and a blood vessel (right) as they invade the medulla.
Haematoxylin-eosin × 150

enhancing nodules within a dilated ventricular system. A high mortality (40–65%) or residual neurological damage (25–30%) has been reported with these tumours, regardless of the degree of histological differentiation.[73]

Macroscopically, choroid plexus papillomas are pink, friable, papilliferous tumours attached to the choroid plexus. Choroid plexus carcinomas invade the walls of the ventricles, and seeding may occur throughout the ventricular system. Calcification within the stroma gives a gritty consistency to some choroid plexus tumours.

Histologically,[74] a papillary structure with thin cores of connective tissue coated by epithelium is seen. The epithelium is, in general, more columnar than the low cuboidal epithelium of the normal choroid plexus (Fig. 16.30). In well-differentiated tumours, there is little variation in shape and size of the epithelial cells, and few mitoses are present (Fig. 16.31). In poorly-differentiated choroid plexus carcinomas,[75] however, there is nuclear pleomorphism, irregularity of the papillary structure, moderate numbers of mitoses (Fig. 16.32) and, in some cases, invasion of the ventricular wall by tumour cells. Calcification is frequently seen in choroid plexus papillomas as in the normal adult choroid plexus.[76]

Immunocytochemistry has facilitated the diagnosis of choroid plexus tumours and their distinction from ependymomas and from papillary metastatic adenocarcinomas, particularly those arising in the lung.[33] Choroid plexus tumour

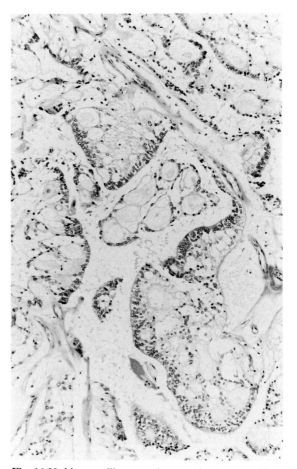

Fig. 16.29 Myxopapillary ependymoma showing mucoid areas and lengths of cuboidal and columnar epithelium.
Haematoxylin-eosin × 75

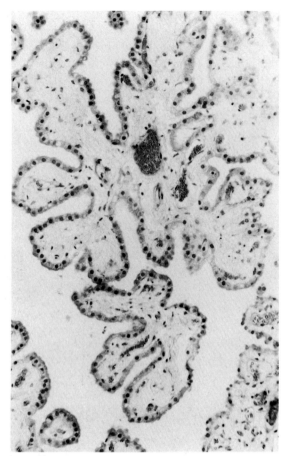

Fig. 16.30 Normal choroid plexus showing a low cuboidal epithelium.
Haematoxylin-eosin × 150

epithelium contains carbonic anhydrase C and S100 protein; in many tumours patches of epithelium stain for glial fibrillary acidic protein and cytokeratins. Metastatic papillary carcinomas stain for cytokeratins but none of the other markers. Ependymomas on the other hand contain S100 protein and glial fibrillary acidic protein but no carbonic anhydrase C. A further point of distinction between choroid plexus tumours and ependymomas is the absence of a collagenous stroma in ependymomas.

Primitive neuroectodermal tumours (medulloblastoma and cerebral neuroblastoma)

Primitive neuroectodermal tumours (PNET)[13,77]

are 'small blue cell' tumours of the nervous system. This group[13] includes neuroblastomas arising from autonomic ganglia in the abdomen (see p. 494), aesthesioneuroblastomas of the nasal mucosa (see p. 495), retinoblastoma (see p. 708), medulloblastoma, cerebral neuroblastoma, pinealoblastoma (see p. 510), ependymoblastoma and polar spongioblastoma.[13] PNET share certain histological characteristics: the cells have a high nuclear–cytoplasmic ratio and fine fibrillary processes. The nuclei themselves are small, oval and hyperchromatic. Mitoses are common. Evidence of glial, ependymal or neuronal differentiation may be detected, either histologically or immunocytochemically, in many primitive neuroectodermal tumours.[13] In some

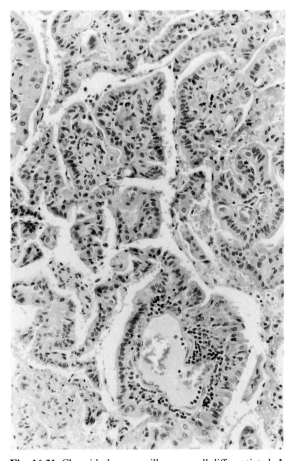

Fig. 16.31 Choroid plexus papilloma—well differentiated. A papillary tumour with a fibrous stroma and an epithelium that is taller than normal choroid plexus.
Haematoxylin-eosin × 150

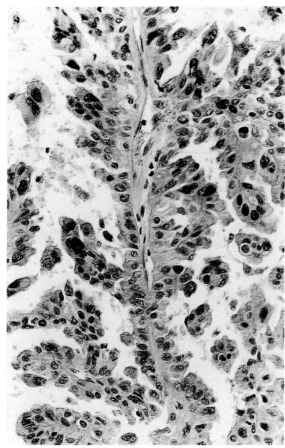

Fig. 16.32 Poorly differentiated choroid plexus tumour (carcinoma) showing minimal stroma, and pleomorphism in the epithelial cells. Mitoses are present in this tumour. Haematoxylin-eosin × 240

cases there is mesenchymal or mesodermal differentiation with recognisable striated muscle fibres.[24,78]

PNET: medulloblastoma

This is the most common primary brain tumour in childhood; 80% of cases occur under the age of 15 years with two peaks of incidence at 3–4 years and 8–9 years.[11] There is a further peak in the early twenties. In children, medulloblastomas arise

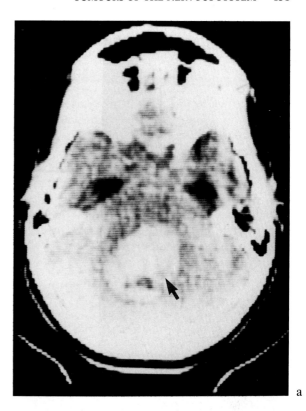

a

Fig. 16.33a, b PNET: medulloblastoma of the cerebellum— CT scans. (**a**) The tumour is seen as an enhancing mass (arrow) in the posterior fossa. (**b**) Obstruction of the fourth ventricle has resulted in hydrocephalus with dilatation of both lateral ventricles.

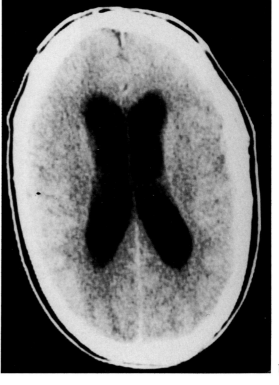

b

almost exclusively in the vermis in the midline of the cerebellum, but in young adults a more lateral site in the cerebellar hemispheres is common.[79] Clinically, patients present with ataxia due to cerebellar damage or with hydrocephalus following blockage of the fourth ventricle by the tumour (Fig. 16.33). Brainstem signs with cranial nerve palsies indicate spread of tumour to the floor of the fourth ventricle. On CT scan (Fig. 16.33), medulloblastomas appear as enhancing nodules in the cerebellum[20] and examination of the lumbar CSF may reveal the presence of tumour cells.[24] Partial surgical removal of medulloblastomas with whole cerebrospinal axis irradiation has significantly increased the survival of patients with this tumour. 40–55% of those irradiated survive for 5 years and 30–40% for 10 years; the overall 5-year survival rate is 38%.[11]

Macroscopic appearances. Medulloblastomas appear as soft white nodules in the cerebellum or as a gelatinous white coating over the surface of the cerebellum and extending into the fourth ventricle. Spread of the tumour may be very extensive over the surface of the cerebral hemispheres and the spinal cord. Secondary invasion of the brain and cord may occur from the sub-arachnoid space. Metastases in other organs, especially bone, have been reported but are rare.[5]

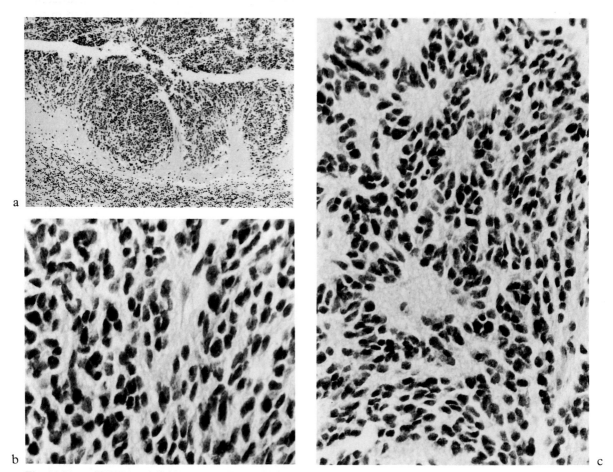

Fig. 16.34a–c PNET: medulloblastoma. (**a**) Low-power view of cerebellar cortex showing invasion of the surface by medulloblastoma (top). (**b**) Detailed cytology showing small hyperchromatic nuclei and the fine fibrillary processes of the tumour cells. (**c**) Rosettes have formed in this part of the tumour; nuclei are arranged in a circle and the fine fibrillary processes project into the centre of the rosettes.
Haematoxylin-eosin (**a**) × 70; (**b**) × 480; (**c**) × 385

Histology. Medulloblastomas are composed of sheets of cells with small oval hyperchromatic nuclei and small amounts of fibrillary cytoplasm (Fig. 16.34). Occasionally the cells are arranged in rosettes in which the fibrillary processes are directed towards the centre of the rosette with the nuclei at the periphery. Larger areas of fibrillary processes are seen in many medulloblastomas. Thymidine labelling has shown that some 14% of cells are proliferating;[80] numerous mitoses are seen.[80] There is individual cell necrosis together with small and large areas of necrosis within the tumour. Numerous macrophages may be present and can be identified by the immunoperoxidase technique for α_1-antichymotrypsin or by anti-macrophage monoclonal antibodies.[50] In smear preparations, medulloblastomas appear as monomorphic sheets of cells with small, slightly elongated hyperchromatic nuclei which can be distinguished from the smaller round nuclei of the internal granule cells of the cerebellum.[23]

The pattern of invasion of the cerebellum may be helpful in the biopsy diagnosis of medulloblastoma. Much of the spread of medulloblastoma occurs through the subarachnoid space over the surface of the folia. Tumour cells invade the molecular layer of the cerebellum as diffuse sheets of cells or as small nodules (Fig. 16.34). Both morphologically and in their pattern of invasion, medulloblastoma cells bear some resemblance to the external granule cell layer of the infant cerebellum (see p. 326).[24] As the cells invade intact tissue, most of the normal elements are destroyed but some reactive astrocytes may remain. Although many areas of medulloblastoma may be virtually free of fibrous connective tissue, in those regions where the tumour invades the leptomeninges and the subarachnoid space, an intense fibrous reaction may be induced with the formation of an extensive reticulin network. This *desmoplastic* variant of medulloblastoma is often much firmer in consistency than other medulloblastomas.[5]

A monomorphic cellular pattern is seen in the majority of medulloblastomas but in *medullomyoblastoma*, striated muscle cells and epithelial elements may be present.[78] These tumours behave in a similar way to other medulloblastomas. Very rarely, *medulloepitheliomas* occur in very young children. Histologically, the tumour cells are arranged in tubular patterns resembling the 'epithelial' arrangement of the primitive neural tube.[5]

Immunocytochemistry for glial fibrillary acidic protein reveals varying numbers of reactive astrocytes within medulloblastomas, particularly around blood vessels and at the invading edge of the tumour. About 50% of medulloblastomas, however, contain small numbers of tumour cells with GFAP in the cytoplasm.[81] Often these cells are arranged in small clusters. Areas rich in fibrillary cell processes stain for neuron-specific enolase (NSE) and for the neuronal protein PGP 9.5. Focal staining for synaptophysin is also seen. This staining pattern suggests neuronal differentiation within the tumour and can be used in the diagnosis of primary medulloblastomas and their rare metastases. Striated muscle cells within medullomyoblastomas contain myoglobin.[24]

Correlation between immunocytochemical evidence of glial and neuronal differentiation in medulloblastomas and survival of the patient has yet to be firmly established.[81]

PNET: cerebral neuroblastomas

These comprise approximately 3% of brain tumours in children.[82] Although commonest in children, they may also occur in adults of up to 50 years, in whom they may be confused with glioblastoma multiforme.[83] Clinically, neuroblastomas may present as mass lesions in the cerebral hemispheres with raised intracranial pressure and epilepsy or with focal neurological signs. Neuroblastomas enhance on CT scan.[20] Following surgical extirpation and irradiation, patients with cerebral neuroblastoma have a 20–25% 5-year survival.[11]

Macroscopic appearances. Invasion of the ventricular system by tumour is frequently seen, in addition to infiltration of the cerebral hemispheres.

Histology. The majority of the tumours resemble medulloblastoma, with small oval hyperchromatic nuclei and little intervening fibrillary cytoplasm.[83] There is focal glial or neuronal differentiation in about 50% of tumours, and choroid plexus differentiation has also been reported.[84] In some cases there is a biphasic histological pattern with one part of the tumour as PNET and the other as a differentiating astrocytoma.[83] In adults, PNET: neuroblastoma can usually be distinguished from glioblastoma multiforme by histology; the PNET nuclei are larger and less pleomorphic and the tumour itself is more cellular. Although necrosis occurs in both types of tumour, the capillary endothelial proliferation so characteristic of glioblastoma multiforme is not as prominent in PNET.

PNET arising in the cauda equina of adults have been reported.[85] They have a similar histology to PNET elsewhere in the CNS and spread through the spinal subarachnoid space to invade the surface of the spinal cord and nerve roots.

Neuronal tumours

Tumours showing firm histological (as opposed to immunocytochemical) features of neuronal differentiation are uncommon in the central nervous system and account for less than 1% of primary intracranial or spinal tumours.[5] There is a variable degree of cytological differentiation, allowing division of this group of tumours into the subgroups outlined below. Neuronal tumours occur mainly in the cerebral hemispheres of children or young adults, but they may be seen in the brainstem. The well-differentiated forms are slowly growing, often well localised, and cause epilepsy or focal neurological signs. More aggressive tumours such as *ganglioneuroblastoma* may grow to a large size and cause problems due to the mass effect of the tumour with distortion of the brain. Calcification within neuronal tumours may be seen on CT scan; well-differentiated *gangliocytomas* and *gangliogliomas* do not usually enhance whereas the more *anaplastic* tumours show some enhancement.

Macroscopic appearances

Gangliocytomas and gangliogliomas may appear to be well circumscribed although they infiltrate surrounding brain.[5] They are frequently pink in colour and may be associated with a cyst. Those arising in the brainstem cause diffuse swelling of the pons or medulla with extension into the ventricle or subarachnoid space.[86] Ganglioneuroblastomas may reach a large size and contain substantial areas of necrosis and haemorrhage.

Histology

Neuronal tumours reveal a variety of patterns.

Gangliocytomas.[2] These tumours are characterised by the presence of mature neurons, often pyramidal in shape, with well-defined Nissl substance in the cytoplasm and the large vesicular nuclei and prominent nucleoli characteristic of normal neurons. Smaller cells are also present in the tumour, some of which may be glia. Immunocytochemistry for GFAP reveals the slender processes of reactive astrocytes within the tumour. Some of the tumour cells may stain positively for neurofilament protein. Most of the tumours are well differentiated and the prognosis is good if the tumour can be excised; if the tumour recurs it may not be for many years. Anaplastic change in these tumours is uncommon.

Gangliogliomas. These are mixed neuronal and glial tumours; both cell types are probably neoplastic.[2,87] Thus, neuronal cells can be identified and the glial element is similar to that seen in an astrocytoma. Anaplastic change may occur, in which case the tumour resembles an anaplastic astrocytoma in its behaviour and histological appearance, although distinguishable from the latter by the presence of mature neuronal tumour cells.

Ganglioneuroblastomas. These tumours usually occur in the cerebral hemispheres of adolescents or young adults and produce neurological signs due to their mass effect.[5] Histologically, they show varying degrees of neuronal differentiation. They have a distinctive pattern[24] which separates them on morphological criteria from primitive neuroectodermal tumours such as medulloblastoma and cerebral neuroblastoma. Many of the cells have small, round nuclei (Fig. 16.35) lacking the hyperchromasia of PNET, and mitoses are usually few. There is a profuse fibrillary background, part of

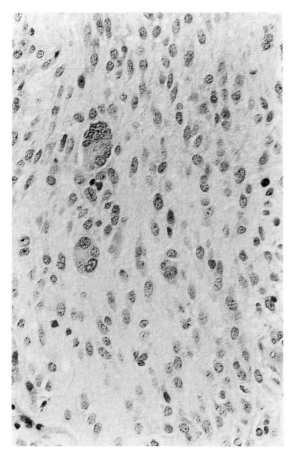

Fig. 16.35 Ganglioneuroblastoma in a 17-year-old girl. The pale oval nuclei are separated by a fine fibrillary background. Multinucleate neuronal cells are seen (centre left). Haematoxylin-eosin × 240

more rapidly and recur following partial surgical removal.

Immunocytochemistry for GFAP usually shows astrocytes distributed throughout neuronal tumours, but there is no staining of tumour cells. Many of the neuronal tumour cells contain neurofilament protein[88] and although this helps to distinguish neuronal tumours from astrocytomas, neurofilament proteins are also present in some PNET.[89] Neuron-specific ($\gamma\gamma$) enolase (NSE) is a useful marker for normal neurons[90] and is present in the cells of neuronal tumours. But this enzyme, together with the α, α-isoenzyme, is also present in reactive and tumour astrocytes.[91] Thus, NSE should be used with caution as a marker for neuronal tumours. Dense core vesicles (see Fig. 16.85, p. 496) may be seen in neuronal tumour cell cytoplasm by electron microscopy.[35]

Paragangliomas. These tumours occasionally arise in the central nervous system.[92] Some present as well-circumscribed tumours in the cauda equina,[93] and although most of the tumour consists of polygonal cells with round, pale nuclei, mature neurons may be seen in some examples (*paraganglioma-ganglioneuroma*).[94]

TUMOURS OF THE MENINGES

Meningiomas

These tumours are rare in children, infrequently seen in adolescents and young adults, and most common in older adults. Comprising some 15% of intracranial tumours in Western Europe and the USA, meningiomas have a much higher incidence in parts of Africa.[5,95] They are commoner in women, with a ratio of 2·5:1 female to male for cranial meningiomas and 9:1 female to male for spinal meningiomas. In a survey in southern Britain, there was a peak annual incidence in the sixth decade of 4 per 100 000.[10] There is an increased incidence of meningiomas in association with von Recklinghausen's disease[96] and there is a correlation between meningiomas and carcinoma of the breast.

Clinical presentation

This depends largely upon the rapidity of growth

which is due to the presence of astrocytes within the tumour. A characteristic feature is the presence of fine, fibrovascular strands of tissue traversing the tumour.[2,24] Ganglion cells similar in appearance to mature neurons may be seen scattered throughout the tumour. Some of these cells have hyperchromatic abnormal nuclei, others are binucleate and some may have large amounts of cytoplasm (Fig. 16.35). Care must be taken not to mistake normal neurons entrapped in a tumour for evidence of ganglioneuroblastoma. Usually, the neoplastic neurons are in disorganised groups or show some cellular atypia. Foci of calcification are frequently seen in ganglioneuroblastomas.

The prognosis of ganglioneuroblastomas is not as good as that of the gangliocytomas as they grow

and the site of origin. Meningiomas arise from the arachnoid mainly over the surface of the brain and spinal cord, although they may occasionally arise

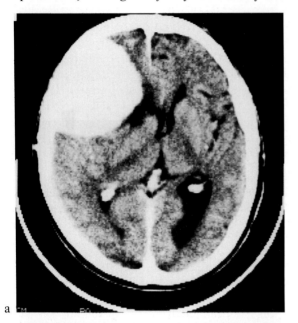

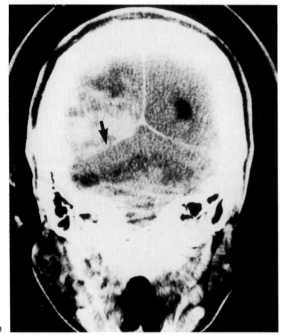

from arachnoid cells in the choroid plexuses and expand into the deeper areas of the brain. At the base of the skull, meningiomas may cause focal neurological deficits by compressing the olfactory bulbs, the optic nerves, or structures in the cerebellopontine angle. Meningiomas may reach a large size (10 cm in diameter) over the superior aspects of the cerebral hemispheres before the patient presents with signs of raised intracranial pressure. These tumours are attached to the falx cerebri.

Spinal meningiomas are common, particularly in older women; they grow as extramedullary, intradural tumours and compress the long tracts of the spinal cord or the nerve roots, giving rise to upper motor neuron deficits, incontinence or nerve root lesions.

A variety of extracranial sites has been described for meningiomas[5,95] including the nose, various viscera, skin, orbit, eye and extraspinal tissue.[97]

In general, meningiomas are slowly growing and they may be localised by skull X-ray due to the presence of an exostosis, particularly on the calvaria. Spinal meningiomas may be suspected when there is erosion of vertebral pedicles; the tumour can be localised by myelography. Meningiomas enhance brightly on CT scan (Fig.

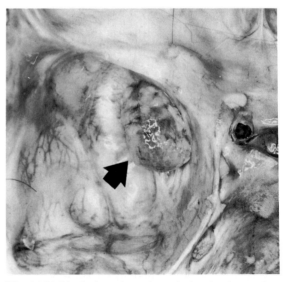

Fig. 16.36a, b Meningioma—CT scans. (**a**) Horizontal cut showing a large enhancing mass displacing the left frontal lobe and apparently attached to the skull. (**b**) Coronal view showing the lambda-shaped falx cerebri and tentorium cerebelli with an irregularly enhancing meningioma attached mainly to the superior surface of the tentorium (arrow).

Fig. 16.37 Meningioma (arrow) attached to the dura at the base of the skull just below the lesser wing of the sphenoid bone. Pituitary fossa and carotid artery are at centre right.

16.36) and are frequently associated with oedema of the underlying brain.

The majority of meningiomas are benign and can often be completely excised. Inadequate excision may lead to recurrence[98] but widespread seeding of the tumour through the cerebrospinal fluid is uncommon. Metastases in the lung and other sites are seen in approximately 0.1% of cases. Such distant spread may be from meningiomas of all histological types[98,99] but occurs mainly in tumours with a high mitotic rate and cellular atypia.[98] Angioblastic and papillary meningiomas are more likely to recur than other types. Local spread of all types of meningioma into the diploe of the skull is associated with the formation of exostoses.

Macroscopic appearances

A typical meningioma is a roughly spherical, lobulated, firm, well-encapsulated tumour with a fibrous cream-coloured or pink cut surface. The tumour is usually adherent to the dura (Fig. 16.37) and in most cases separates easily from the underlying brain (Fig. 16.38). Some meningiomas, however, are adherent to the brain, and there may be substantial underlying cerebral oedema (Fig. 16.39). Occasionally, meningiomas are very soft and sometimes gelatinous in consistency. When the tumour is attached to the falx cerebri, meningioma tissue may be found on both sides of the falx (Fig. 16.38) and invading the superior sagittal sinus; such tumours may be inoperable as excision of the sinus might result in substantial venous infarction of the cerebral hemispheres. Meningiomas similarly penetrate the tentorium cerebelli. In some cases the meningioma forms a flat sheet of tumour on the inner aspect of the dura (*meningioma en plaque*).

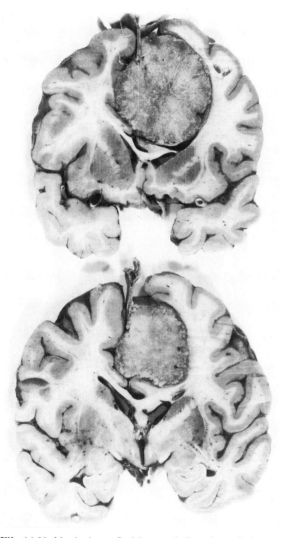

Fib. 16.38 Meningioma. Serial coronal slices through the cerebral hemispheres show a large meningioma attached to the falx cerebri. There is a clear plane of separation between tumour and brain.

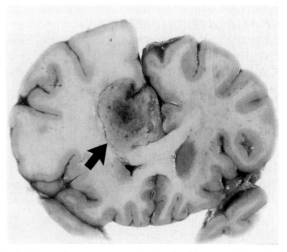

Fig. 16.39 Meningioma attached to the falx cerebri (arrow). The adjacent left cerebral hemisphere shows extensive oedema, particularly of the white matter.

Many spinal meningiomas are gritty due to numerous psammoma bodies (see below) within their substance, but the tumours are usually well circumscribed and separate easily from the underlying nervous tissue.

The uncommon malignant or aggressive meningiomas may be firmly adherent to underlying brain, and these tumours are more likely to recur than other types.

Major complications of meningiomas result from their mass effect—either with compression of underlying brain or, if large, with raised intracranial pressure, transtentorial herniation and brainstem compression or cerebellar tonsillar herniation (see p. 66).

Histology

The histology of meningiomas varies widely, and the resemblance of different patterns to gliomas, schwannomas and metastatic tumours may cause diagnostic difficulties.[95,98] However, in the majority of meningiomas the nuclei vary little in shape and size; they are rather pale and open, with one or two small but prominent nucleoli. The nuclear features are well demonstrated in smears of meningiomas, as is the delicate fibrillary nature of the tumour cytoplasm (Fig. 16.40). The cells tend to form whorls and in most meningiomas there are desmosomes between adjacent cells.[100,101,101a] In the more unusual variants, the diagnosis may be suspected from the clinical history and the site of the tumour.

Meningothelial, fibroblastic, transitional and psammomatous meningiomas are the most common types.[95] In the *meningothelial meningiomas* (Fig. 16.41a) sheets of tumour cells are seen, with or without whorl formation. The nuclei are oval, rather pale and have one or two small nucleoli typical of the arachnoid cells in arachnoid granulations[102] and in other parts of the arachnoid mater.[103] Cell borders may be indistinct by light microscopy (syncytial pattern), and there is no reticulin between the cells. *Fibroblastic meningiomas* (Fig. 16.41b) are characterised by sheets of elongated cells that have typical arachnoid cell nuclei. *Transitional meningiomas* (Fig. 16.41c) have areas of both meningothelial and fibroblastic pattern, together with the typical

meningioma cellular whorls. In *psammomatous meningiomas*, calcified spheres (psammoma bodies) with concentric lamellae are seen (Fig. 16.42); these may be very numerous in spinal meningiomas. Psammoma bodies result from calcification of whorls of collagen fibres produced by meningioma cells.[76] Similar calcification of collagen occurs to form the calcospherites in the stroma of the choroid plexus.[76]

Detailed examination of meningioma nuclei in histological sections reveals several features which may aid diagnosis. In addition to the small nucleoli, nuclei often show prominent grooves and cytoplasmic invaginations (Fig. 16.43). Large hyperchromatic nuclei may be seen in many types

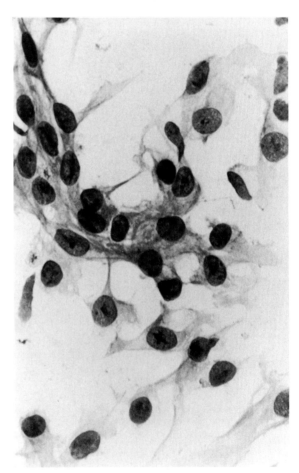

Fig. 16.40 Meningioma—smear. The oval or round nuclei have small but prominent nucleoli. The cytoplasm is delicate and finely fibrillar.
Toluidine blue × 600

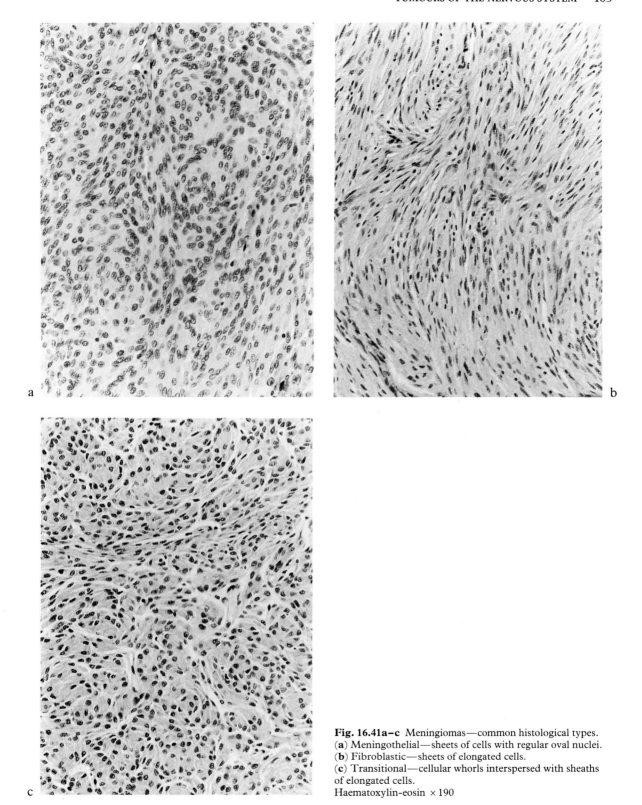

Fig. 16.41a–c Meningiomas—common histological types.
(**a**) Meningothelial—sheets of cells with regular oval nuclei.
(**b**) Fibroblastic—sheets of elongated cells.
(**c**) Transitional—cellular whorls interspersed with sheaths
of elongated cells.
Haematoxylin-eosin × 190

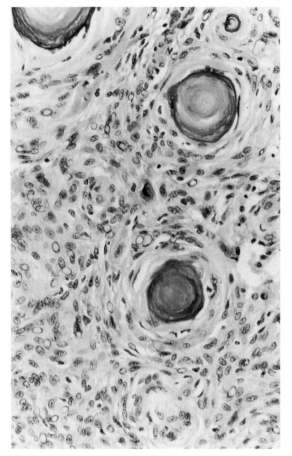

Fig. 16.42 Psammoma bodies in a meningioma. Haematoxylin-eosin × 240

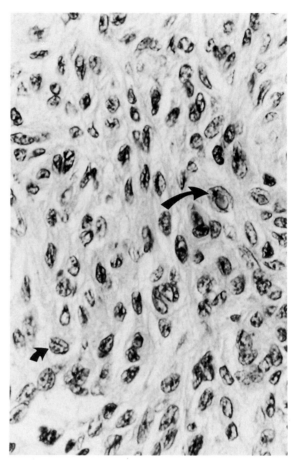

Fig. 16.43 Meningioma—details of nuclear morphology in a meningothelial meningioma. Deep grooves are seen in some nuclei (small arrow) and cytoplasmic invaginations in other nuclei (large arrow). Haematoxylin-eosin × 600

of meningioma (Figs 16.45a and 16.47), and the chromosomal abnormalities (polyploidy) in benign, slowly-growing meningiomas are well recorded.[104]

For distinguishing meningiomas from other intracranial and spinal tumours, particularly in frozen sections, a number of other histological features are useful. Fibrous collagenous bands are seen in meningiomas but they are uncommon in gliomas. Most types of meningiomas can be distinguished from schwannomas by a reticulin stain. There is a rich reticulin network investing each tumour cell in a schwannoma whereas most meningiomas, except for the angioblastic type, contain little or no reticulin between the tumour cells.

Electron microscopy (Fig. 16.44) shows that

meningioma cells have numerous intermediate filaments in the cytoplasm (Fig. 16.44a) and that the cells are closely packed with intervening gap junctions and desmosomes (Fig. 16.44b).[95] The vimentin intermediate filaments and desmosomes can be demonstrated by immunocytochemical staining.[100,101,101a] Hormone receptors for oestrogen, progesterone and androgens are present on the cells of many meningiomas.[105,106]

In addition to the more common histological types of meningioma, a number of histological variants are seen.

Angiomatous meningiomas contain large numbers of blood vessels, but the typical meningioma cells are recognisable in the inter-

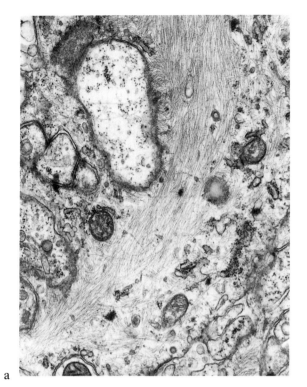

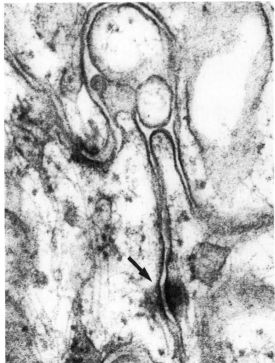

Fig. 16.44a, b Meningioma—electron microscopy.
(**a**) Numerous intermediate filaments are seen within
the cytoplasm. (**b**) Interdigitating cell processes form
desmosomes (arrow).
(**a**) × 18 750; (**b**) × 81 000

vening tumour tissue (Fig. 16.45). Furthermore,
the reticulin is concentrated around the blood
vessels (Fig. 16.45b), which helps to distinguish
angiomatous from angioblastic meningiomas (see
below).

Two forms of *angioblastic meningioma* are
described;[107] the *haemangioblastic variety* resembles haemangioblastomas of the cerebellum
(see p. 476) whereas the *haemangiopericytic
variety* resembles haemangiopericytomas elsewhere in the body. The main importance of
haemangiopericytic meningiomas lies in their
aggressive behaviour;[108] they tend to recur and
may invade the skull and scalp. Histologically,
(Fig. 16.46) the haemangiopericytic meningiomas
contain large numbers of thin-walled blood vessels
and a widely distributed reticulin network which
encloses the cells in small packets. There is little
resemblance between the cells in this tumour and
other types of meningioma as their nuclei are
rather elongated and do not have the characteristic
morphology of arachnoid cell nuclei.

Xanthomatous change and microcystic regions
(Fig. 16.47)[95] may occur in many of the varieties of
meningioma but there are usually areas within the
tumour which retain the typical histological
pattern of meningioma.

Papillary meningiomas (Fig. 16.48)[109] are uncommon and this particular pattern may only be
present in part of the tumour. They tend to recur
and may metastasise.

In malignant or *anaplastic meningiomas*, which
comprise about 1% of meningiomas,[110] there is not
only an increased variability in the nuclear shape,
size and density of staining but also an increased
mitotic rate. These tumours may still retain some
of the whorled pattern of meningiomas but they
tend to invade the underlying brain, recur at the
site of excision and in the operation scar on the
skin; they may also metastasise.

Meningeal sarcomas[95,110] may resemble fibrosarcomas or malignant fibrous histiocytomas.
They are uncommon but they invade the underlying brain, tend to recur when excised, and also
metastasise to distant sites. In those tumours
which resemble fibrosarcomas (Fig. 16.49), sheets
of elongated cells surrounded by reticulin are seen,
and there are many mitoses. In those which
resemble malignant fibrous histiocytomas, a

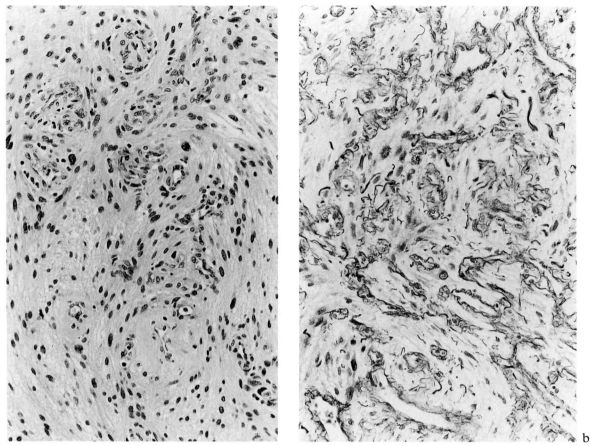

a

b

Fig. 16.45a, b Angiomatous meningioma. (a) Numerous blood vessels are seen embedded in an otherwise typical meningioma. There is some nuclear hyperchromasia. (b) The reticulin is concentrated around the blood vessels and there is little reticulin within the sheets of tumour cells.
(a) Haematoxylin-eosin × 190; (b) Gordon and Sweet × 190

storiform pattern is seen with an intimate reticulin network surrounding the cells.[24] Mitoses may also be common in these tumours.

NERVE SHEATH TUMOURS

Schwannomas and neurofibromas are the commonest tumours of peripheral nerves. Both types of tumour arise from cranial and spinal nerve roots as well as from more peripheral nerves. They are, therefore, discussed here. Other peripheral nerve tumours and tumour-like lesions are dealt with on page 499.

Schwannomas (synonyms: neurilemmoma, neurinoma, acoustic neuroma)

Arising mainly from the vestibular portion of the 8th cranial nerve and from the dorsal spinal (sensory) nerve roots, intracranial and spinal schwannomas occur at any age but are seen mainly in middle-aged adults. Schwannomas account for approximately 8% of intracranial tumours and they are more common in females. Some 80% or more intracranial schwannomas arise from the 8th nerve; a few arise from the trigeminal nerve and others from the vagus. Occasionally, schwannomas arise from meningeal nerves at the base of the cerebral hemispheres.

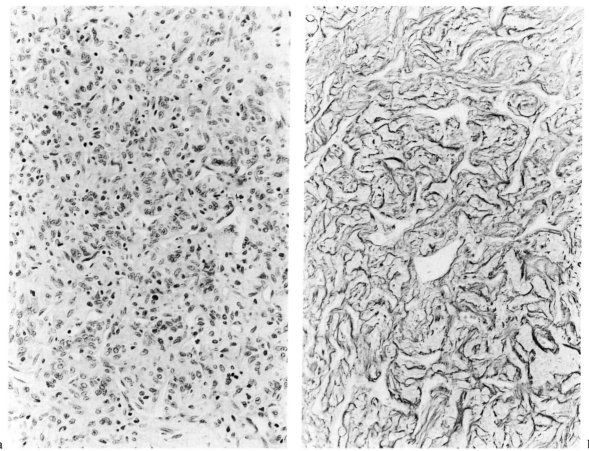

Fig. 16.46a, b Angioblastic meningioma—haemangiopericytic type. (**a**) Tumour cells with elongated nuclei surround numerous thin-walled blood vessels. (**b**) The numerous blood vessels are emphasised by the reticulin network which also extends into the tumour to enclose small packets of cells.
(**a**) Haematoxylin-eosin × 190; (**b**) Gordon and Sweet × 190

Clinical presentation

This depends upon the site of the tumour.[19] Acoustic schwannomas present with deafness and tinnitus on the affected side and, if the tumour reaches a large size (3–4 cm in diameter), its mass effect in the cerebellopontine angle may distort the brainstem and cause hydrocephalus. Schwannomas arising on other nerves may interfere with their function by compression of the nerve. In the spine, the most common sites for a schwannoma are the lumbar region and cauda equina. Bladder function may be affected or back pain may be the main symptom. Compression of the spinal cord may result from schwannomas in the thoracic region, and nerve root compression in the intervertebral foramen may occur if the schwannoma grows through the foramen as a dumb-bell or hour-glass tumour.

Acoustic schwannomas enhance brightly on CT scan.[20] Spinal schwannomas can be localised by myelography,[22] which shows an intradural block or irregularity. The spinal tumours are very well demonstrated by magnetic resonance imaging.[21]

Macroscopic appearances

Schwannomas are smooth, lobulated, encapsulated tumours which may be white and firm or rubbery, or soft with a pink or light brown colour

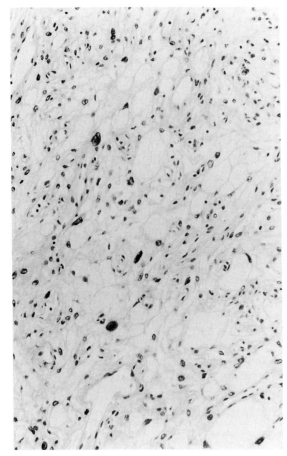

Fig. 16.47 Meningioma—microcystic change. Elongated spindle cells surround the microcystic spaces. Some nuclear hyperchromasia is seen.
Haematoxylin-eosin × 150

(Fig. 16.50). They are usually attached to a nerve or a nerve root. Although large acoustic schwannomas may distort the brainstem and may be adherent to the meninges of the cerebellum, they do not invade brain tissue.

Histology

There are two major patterns recognised in schwannomas (Figs 16.51 and 16.52).[15] In *Antoni type A* areas, there are broad and narrow sheaths of spindle cells with long, narrow nuclei and fine tapering interweaving cytoplasmic processes (Fig. 16.52a). Palisades in which the nuclei are arranged in bands are also typical of schwannomas. *Verocay bodies* are seen when palisading forms a regular

repeating array (Fig. 16.53). *Antoni type B* areas are composed of loosely packed cells with small round nuclei and fine cytoplasmic processes (Fig. 16.52b); these areas are usually intermixed with Antoni type A areas. Mast cells are common in the type B areas but are not present in the type A areas. Typically, schwannomas are attached to the sides of nerves, unlike neurofibromas which infiltrate and expand the nerve itself (see below). Compressed nerve fascicles may be identified in the capsule of a schwannoma.

A variety of secondary changes may occur in schwannomas. *Ancient change* is characterised by scattered hyperchromatic, large, pleomorphic nuclei and is seen especially in longstanding

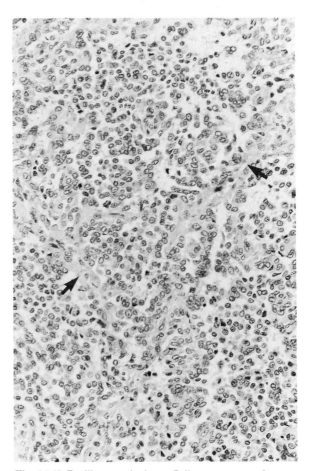

Fig. 16.48 Papillary meningioma. Collagenous cores of papillae (arrows) are coated by meningioma cells. Other tumour cells appear to lie in loosely associated sheets.
Haematoxylin-eosin × 190

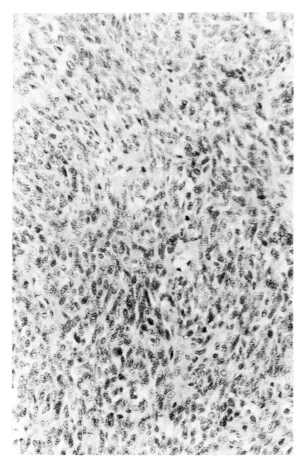

Fig. 16.49 Meningeal sarcoma. Sheets of cells of elongated nuclei resembling a fibrosarcoma.
Haematoxylin-eosin × 190

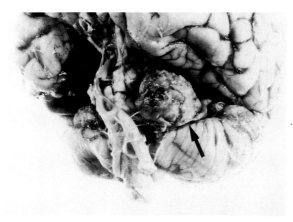

Fig. 16.50 Schwannoma of the 8th cranial nerve (acoustic neuroma) presenting as a lobulated nodule in the left cerebellopontine angle (arrow).

acoustic neuromas.[5] In the absence of a significant number of mitoses, these changes are not associated with malignancy.[111] There may be little recognisable Antoni A or Antoni B tissue in long-standing acoustic schwannomas; large areas of tumour may be replaced by collagenous fibrous tissue and blood vessel walls may be thickened and hyaline. Cysts also occasionally form in acoustic schwannomas. Xanthomatous areas may be present in schwannomas: in some tumours the foamy, fat-filled cells may be predominant, but usually elongated cells with some nuclear palisading are seen even within these tumours. Metaplasia with bone formation has also been described.[15]

Schwannomas are usually difficult to smear, so that cryostat sections are better for rapid diagnosis. They have a rich reticulin network between the cells which distinguishes them from the majority of meningiomas (see p. 464). Schwann cells contain S100 protein and although it is not specific for Schwann cells[30] S100 protein remains a useful immunocytochemical marker for schwannomas. Electron microscopy has shown that the Antoni type A areas are composed predominantly of compacted, elongated cellular processes, each covered by a distinct basement membrane.[112,113]

Malignant schwannomas

Malignant schwannomas are uncommon within the cranium or spine and more commonly occur in peripheral nerves. They differ histologically from benign schwannomas in showing an increase in the number of mitoses, hyperchromasia and pleomorphism of the nuclei, and an increased nuclear–cytoplasmic ratio.[114,115] When they metastasise, it is usually to the lungs.

Neurofibromas and von Recklinghausen's disease

Schwannoma and neurofibroma are often incorrectly used as interchangeable terms. However, although they may be associated in a given case, they are distinct entities which can be distinguished in the majority of cases by their histology. The distinction may have important

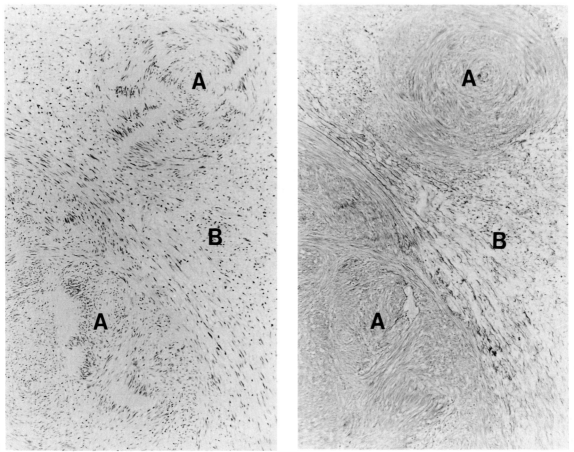

a

b

Fig. 16.51a, b Schwannoma. (**a**) Low-power picture showing Antoni type A and Antoni type B areas. (**b**) Same field as (**a**) showing a rich reticulin network especially in the Antoni type A areas.
(**a**) Haematoxylin-eosin × 75; (**b**) Gordon and Sweet × 75

implications for the patient; schwannomas are frequently solitary and sporadic whereas neurofibromas may be multiple and associated with inherited von Recklinghausen's (peripheral) neurofibromatosis (see p. 353).[15] Histologically, schwannomas are encapsulated tumours of Schwann cells and grow on the sides of nerves. Neurofibromas, in contrast, are of mixed composition, containing Schwann cells, fibroblasts and other cellular elements which infiltrate and expand nerve fascicles and spread into the surrounding tissue;[15,112] they are not usually encapsulated.

Von Recklinghausen's (peripheral) neurofibromatosis is a phacomatosis (see p. 353) inherited as an autosomal dominant trait.[116,117] The disorder is characterised by café au lait spots on the skin and by the presence of cutaneous neurofibromas which may, in some cases, cover large areas of the skin; they often develop during the second decade. In *elephantiasis nervosa*,[15,112] an overgrowth of soft tissue around enlarged nerve trunks may cause the skin to hang in thickened redundant folds. Neurofibromas may involve the peripheral nerve trunks in the limbs and small nerves in the viscera.

Malformations of the base of the skull, and central nervous system malformations such as heterotopias and cortical dysplasias, occur in von Recklinghausen's (peripheral) neurofibromatosis, but the major complications affecting the brain and spinal cord arise from the presence of the tumours themselves.[118,119] There may be multiple

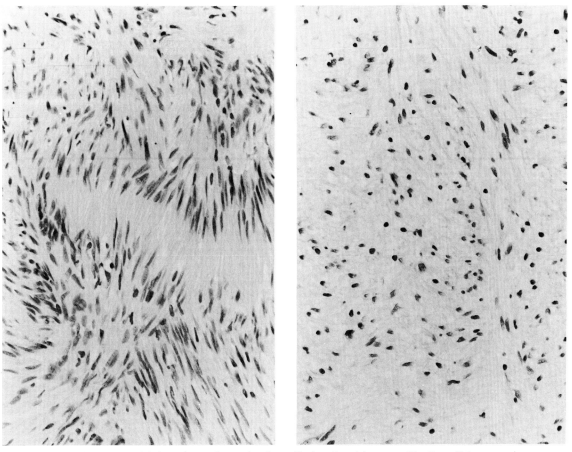

Fig. 16.52a, b Schwannoma. (**a**) Antoni type A area showing palisades of nuclei separated by fine cellular processes. (**b**) Antoni type B area showing loosely packed sheaths of elongated cells cut transversely and longitudinally. Haematoxylin-eosin × 240

schwannomas, and bilateral acoustic schwannomas occur in central neurofibromatosis (see p. 354). Meningiomas, cerebral glioblastomas, astrocytomas of the optic nerves and phaeochromocytomas all have an increased incidence in von Recklinghausen's disease. Neurofibromas may become malignant (see p. 472).

Neurofibromas are not in themselves painful but compression of nerve roots may cause pain. Those arising on spinal nerve roots may grow as dumbbell or hour-glass tumours within intervertebral foramina, compressing roots and spinal cord. Occasionally neurofibromas exhibit aggressive behaviour with erosion and destruction of bone. In peripheral nerves in the limbs, neurofibromas form fusiform or spherical expansions of the nerve, and several nerve trunks may be matted together as a plexiform neurofibroma.[15]

Histology

Neurofibromas in the skin are usually poorly circumscribed and composed of loosely packed infiltrating spindle cells (Fig. 16.54). Nerve fascicles, expanded by tumour, are often seen within these lesions.[15] When neurofibromas involve nerve trunks or roots, there is diffuse enlargement of the nerve fascicles (Fig. 16.54) and axons entering the lesion are widely separated by tumour cells (Fig. 16.55). Prominent bands of collagen may traverse the tumour (Fig. 16.55) and

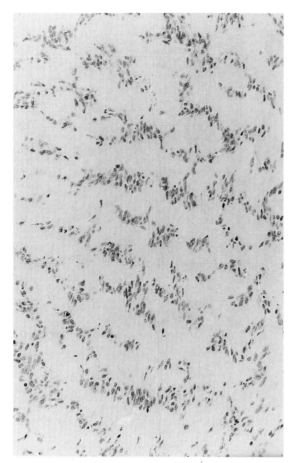

Fig. 16.53 Schwannoma—Verocay bodies. Nuclear palisades are separated by fibrillar cytoplasmic processes. Haematoxylin-eosin × 150

there may be large amounts of interstitial mucoprotein. No recognisable Antoni type A tissue is seen in neurofibromas. If the spinal roots are involved, dorsal root ganglion cells may be entrapped within the neurofibromas and should not be confused with ganglioneuroma (see p. 495). Axons can be demonstrated within neurofibromas by silver stains (e.g. Glees and Marsland)[28] or by immunocytochemistry for neurofilament proteins. The presence of nerve fibres (Fig. 16.55) distinguishes neurofibromas from schwannomas, which displace nerves rather than invade them.

Malignant neurofibromas

Malignant neurofibromas occur in patients with neurofibromatosis[120] in association with the benign neurofibromas. There is an increase in the number of mitoses and in nuclear pleomorphism (Fig. 16.56). A variety of divergent sarcomatous elements may occur within malignant nerve sheath tumours, including embryonal rhabdomyosarcoma and chondrosarcoma.[120]

PRIMARY MALIGNANT LYMPHOMAS

Primary cerebral lymphomas were originally called microgliomas or reticulum cell sarcomas. They present clinically at a similar age to glioblastomas and often in a similar way. Lymphomas also arise as primary tumours in the extradural tissues of the spine and may cause spinal cord compression.

Primary cerebral lymphomas

These uncommon tumours account for approximately 1% of all cerebral tumours and less than 1% of lymphomas from all sites.[121,122] They occur mainly in patients over the age of 40 years but they are also seen in younger patients; most are B-cell lymphomas[25,123,124] but a few are T-cell lymphomas.[25,125] They are potentially treatable.[25] Some primary cerebral lymphomas have no known predisposing factors, whereas in other cases there are well recognised predisposing features: thus there is an increased incidence of primary cerebral lymphomas in immunosuppressed patients, e.g. with acquired immune deficiency syndrome (AIDS) (see p. 214), with Hodgkin's disease, and following renal transplantation.

Clinical presentation

Primary cerebral lymphomas present with focal neurological signs, epilepsy or signs of raised intracranial pressure. There is no clear pattern of presentation and the signs and symptoms depend upon the location of the tumour. The length of history may be a month to two years or more. CT scan[126] reveals one or more brightly enhancing lesions, often in the corpus callosum or in the periventricular regions. Occasionally, primary lymphomas arise in the cerebellum.[25] Once the

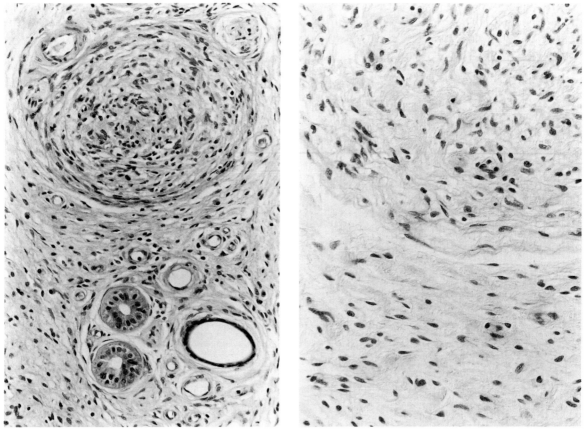

a

b

Fig. 16.54a, b Neurofibroma. (**a**) Low-power showing infiltration and expansion of a nerve fascicle (top) by neurofibroma cells and an extension of the same cells into the surrounding dermis. Preserved sweat gland elements (bottom). (**b**) Details of (a) showing part of a nerve fascicle invaded by neurofibroma cells (top), perineurium (centre) and neurofibroma in the dermis (bottom).
Haematoxylin-eosin (**a**) × 190; (**b**) × 300

diagnosis has been made, the patient should be investigated in order to exclude generalised lymphoma.[27,127] But, primary lymphomas usually present in a different way from metastatic lymphoma and probably they are an entity distinct from nodal lymphoma.

Treatment of primary cerebral lymphomas by irradiation and chemotherapy has resulted in an 8% 5-year survival rate.[128]

Macroscopic appearances

Primary cerebral lymphomas are recognisable in slices of fixed brain as diffuse areas of granular, white, softened tissue either in the white matter or basal ganglia of one hemisphere or in the corpus callosum (Fig. 16.57) and periventricular regions;

they may be multiple. Lymphomas can be distinguished from metastatic carcinomas, which are usually well circumscribed, and from glioblastomas, which usually have a central area of necrosis. Although they are soft, cerebral lymphomas usually do not disintegrate in the fixed brain like infarcts. Occasionally, there is an intense fibrous reaction and the lymphoma has a hard consistency.

Histology

Affected areas of the brain are diffusely invaded by sheets of lymphoid cells which have larger and more open nuclei than reactive lymphocytes (Fig. 16.58). Lymphoma cells characteristically accumulate around blood vessels and a typical

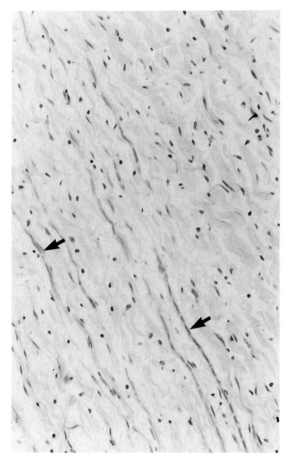

Fig. 16.55 Neurofibroma showing entrapped myelinated nerve fibres (arrows). Broad collagen bands in the tumour (top right).
Haematoxylin-eosin × 150

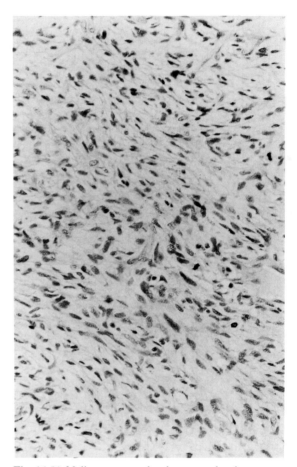

Fig. 16.56 Malignant nerve sheath tumour showing an increased density of cells, nuclear pleomorphism and mitoses (cf. Fig. 16.54b).
Haematoxylin-eosin × 240

concentric reticulin pattern is seen around the vessels in areas of tumour invasion (Fig. 16.59).

Rapid diagnosis of lymphoma can be made on touch preparations (see p. 431) using fresh tumour tissue. As they demonstrate the cytology so clearly (Fig. 16.60), touch preparations are also valuable for characterisation of the tumour.[25,127]

Immunocytochemistry is useful for the identification and categorisation of lymphomas and can be performed on cryostat sections of fresh biopsy material and on paraffin sections; post-mortem material can give misleading results. Using monoclonal antibodies, the lymphoma cells can be first identified by pan-leucocyte markers and then characterised as either B-cell or T-cell by

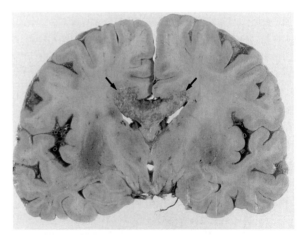

Fig. 16.57 Primary cerebral lymphoma seen here as a granular (soft) region in an expanded corpus callosum (arrows).

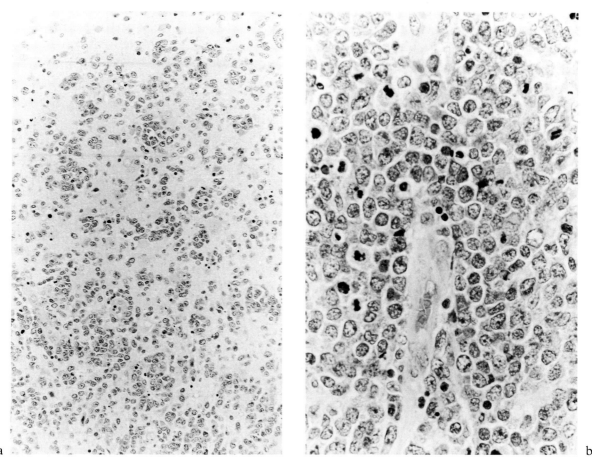

a

b

Fig. 16.58a, b Primary cerebral lymphoma. (**a**) Edge: groups of lymphoma cells are diffusely invading brain tissue. (**b**) The detail of the cytology shows tumour cells resembling centroblasts. There is a blood vessel at the centre of the field. Haematoxylin-eosin (**a**) × 150; (**b**) × 430

appropriate antibodies.[25] Nuclear morphology in the touch preparations is valuable for the rapid diagnosis of lymphomas. The majority of primary cerebral lymphomas that have been fully characterised are B-cell lymphomas showing a diffuse growth pattern; the predominant cell resembles the centroblastic type using the Kiel terminology[127,129] (large non-cleaved lymphomas of the Working Formulation[127]). Occasional T-cell lymphomas have been identified.[25]

Immunocytochemistry on paraffin sections of lymphomas shows a mixture of different cell types within the tumour. GFAP staining (Fig. 16.61) reveals how reactive astrocytes are intimately mixed with the tumour cells. Using monocyte–macrophage markers, large numbers of microglial cells and macrophages are seen distributed throughout the tumour (Fig. 16.62). It is these reactive histiocytic cells which were originally identified in cerebral lymphomas and resulted in the misnomer 'microglioma'. True histiocytic primary lymphomas have not, as yet, been reported in the central nervous system.

Spinal lymphomas

Lymphoma deposits in the epidural tissue of the spinal canal cause spinal cord compression in approximately 3% of cases of lymphoma.[130] In some cases the lymphoma is confined to the epidural space and spinal cord compression may be the presenting lesion;[131] in other cases, the

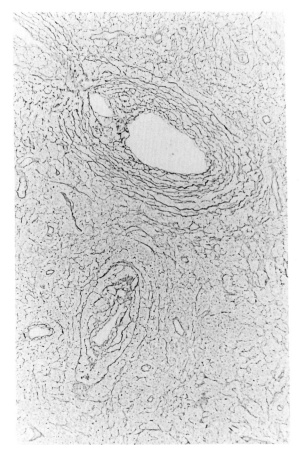

Fig. 16.59 Cerebral lymphoma showing concentric rings of reticulin around blood vessels.
Gordon and Sweet × 60

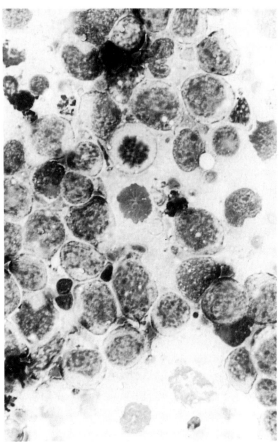

Fig. 16.60 Primary cerebral lymphoma—touch preparation showing lymphoma cells resembling centroblasts in morphology. Mitosis is seen (top centre).
Giemsa × 500

tumour is widely disseminated. Thus, although metastatic carcinoma remains the major cause of malignant epidural disease, lymphoma should always be suspected in cases with an unknown primary tumour. Characterisation of lymphoma from tissue obtained at laminectomy is often essential for the diagnosis.

Immunocytochemical studies of epidural lymphomas have shown that the majority are follicle centre cell lymphomas—diffuse centroblastic/centrocytic by the Kiel terminology.[129] Occasional T-cell lymphomas and lymphoblastic lymphomas are also seen at this site.[130] Following treatment by laminectomy, radiotherapy and chemotherapy, some patients make a good recovery, especially when the disease is localised to the spine.

BLOOD VESSEL TUMOURS AND MALFORMATIONS

Haemangioblastomas

Occurring mainly in adults, haemangioblastomas constitute 1–2% of intracranial tumours and some 7% of tumours in the posterior fossa.[5] Haemangioblastomas usually arise in the cerebellum but also occur on the surface of the upper and lower parts of the spinal cord.[132] Supratentorial haemangioblastomas are rare.

Clinical presentation

Patients with cerebellar haemangioblastomas present with cerebellar ataxia and nystagmus or with raised intracranial pressure, vomiting, headache and alteration in consciousness due to hydrocephalus. Spinal haemangioblastomas may compress the spinal cord or its roots or the lower part of the medulla.[132] In some patients, there is polycythaemia due to the production of erythropoietins by the tumour.[133] A familial incidence of haemangioblastomas has been observed, especially in Lindau's syndrome, in which intracranial haemangioblastomas may be multiple and may be associated with cysts in the pancreas and kidneys and with renal carcinomas. Haemangioblastomas of the retina (von Hippel's disease) may also be associated with intracranial haemangioblastomas.

On CT scan, haemangioblastomas in the cere-

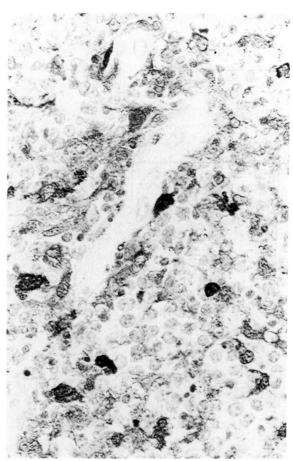

Fig. 16.62 Primary cerebral lymphoma. Darkly stained macrophages are seen, particularly around blood vessels (centre). Unstained tumour cells are also seen. Immunocytochemistry: polyclonal anti-macrophage antibody S22 × 430

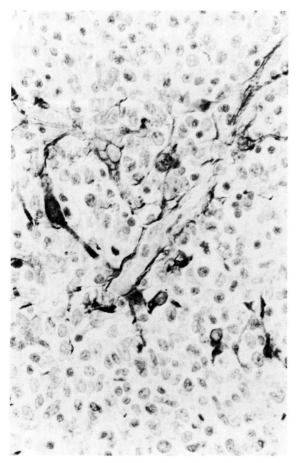

Fig. 16.61 Primary cerebral lymphoma. Darkly stained astrocytes and their processes encompassing a blood vessel (centre) are seen between the unstained tumour cells. Immunocytochemistry for GFAP × 430

bellum are seen as enhancing nodules, often associated with a fluid-filled cyst;[20] they may compress the fourth ventricle. Angiography shows a highly vascular tumour. Following complete surgical excision, the prognosis is usually very good.

Macroscopic appearances

Haemangioblastomas are well-circumscribed light brown or yellow nodules embedded in the cerebellar hemisphere or attached to the surface of the spinal cord. Cysts associated with haemangioblastomas in the cerebellum are filled with proteinaceous straw-coloured fluid (Fig. 16.63).

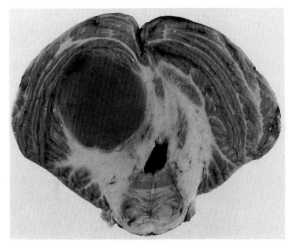

Fig. 16.63 Haemangioblastoma of the cerebellum associated with a large cyst (left) containing proteinaceous fluid.

The smooth gliotic walls of the cyst often show brown discoloration due to the deposition of blood pigment; the haemangioblastoma may be seen as a nodule attached to the wall of the cyst.

Histology

Haemangioblastomas are well demarcated from the surrounding gliotic cerebellum and are composed of small packets of cells with foamy cytoplasm, fairly uniform nuclei and few, if any, mitoses (Fig. 16.64). The packets of cells are surrounded by a fine reticulin network which also defines the large number of thin-walled branching blood vessels within the tumour (Fig. 16.65). Lipid stains (e.g. oil red O) on frozen sections reveal neutral lipid droplets within the cytoplasm

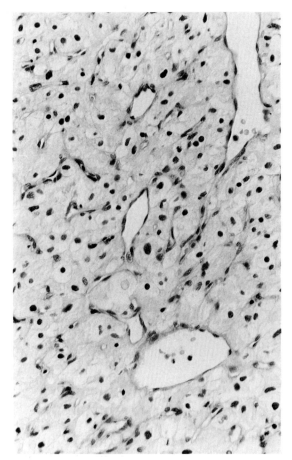

Fig. 16.64 Haemangioblastoma. Thin-walled blood vessels are separated by pale, foamy cells. Haematoxylin-eosin × 240

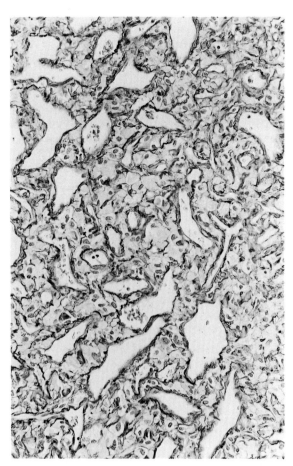

Fig. 16.65 Haemangioblastoma—low-power view showing an extensive reticulin network around blood vessels and around small packets of tumour cells. Gordon and Sweet × 150

of the tumour cells. Electron microscopy shows an abundant extracellular glycoprotein matrix in the tumour.[134]

The origin of the tumour is still unclear; although endothelial markers such as factor-VIII-related antigen are present in the thin-walled blood vessels, the tumour cells are negative for this marker.[55,135] A neuroendocrine origin for these tumours has been suggested.[136]

Cavernous angiomas

These lesions (see also p. 114) are often multiple in the central nervous system and are well shown as enhancing lesions on CT scan,[137] but they may be difficult to demonstrate by angiography. The cerebral hemispheres and pons are most commonly affected but cavernous angiomas also occur in the spinal cord.

Clinically, patients present mainly in the third to fifth decade but also in childhood with intracranial haemorrhage (23–30%), epilepsy (38–53%), headache (28%) or focal neurological signs (12–15%).[138,139] Cavernous angiomas in the spinal cord may present with paraparesis. Occasionally angiomas occur in the epidural tissue and, more commonly, in the vertebral bone. Such lesions rarely cause symptoms but may result in root or even cord compression.[140] Treatment of accessible cerebral and spinal lesions is by local excision.

On CT scan, cavernous angiomas enhance brightly and are well visualised.

Macroscopically, cavernous haemangiomas are well defined, up to 2–3 cm in diameter and reddish-brown in colour. They often have a honeycomb appearance.

Histology reveals a mass of blood vessels which may be thin-walled or have thick collagenous walls and show little differentiation into arteries and veins (Fig. 16.66). The vessels are packed together with little intervening brain tissue; this is one feature which distinguishes them from arteriovenous malformations, in which brain tissue is clearly seen between the vascular elements (see Fig. 16.68).[43] Calcification is frequently present in the vessel walls, and macrophages containing haemosiderin together with reactive astrocytes are observed around the periphery of the tumours.

Capillary telangiectases

Such lesions (see also p. 114) may be found incidentally in the cerebral white matter, pons or medulla at any age. However, lesions in the cerebrum may cause epilepsy; if large, those in the brainstem may cause destruction of neural pathways in the medulla or pons.[43] Occasionally they bleed. Telangiectases are usually not detectable by CT scan or by angiography.

Macroscopically, they appear as red–brown patches in the cerebrum or brainstem or as a series of dilated vessels just visible to the naked eye (Fig. 16.67).

Microscopically, multiple dilated capillaries are seen;[24,43] their walls are composed only of a layer of endothelial cells and a small amount of connective

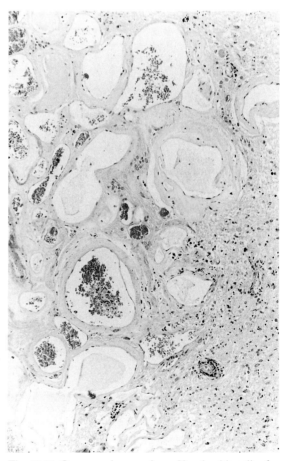

Fig. 16.66 Cavernous haemangioma. Vessels with walls of varying thickness are tightly packed in the angioma. Adjacent brain tissue (lower right) is gliotic. Haematoxylin-eosin × 60

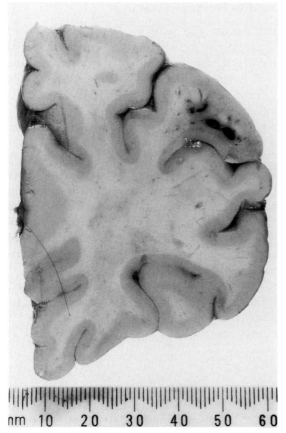

nm 10 20 30 40 50 60

Fig. 16.67 Capillary telangiectasis in the white matter of a frontal lobe gyrus (upper right).

tissue. In some cases, the capillaries are widely separated by normal brain tissue; in others, the vessels are closely packed together. Perfusion studies have shown that the calibre of individual vessels varies widely, with focal varicosities and dilatations.[5] There is usually little or no gliosis or iron deposition around capillary telangiectases.

Vascular malformations

Arteriovenous malformations

Arteriovenous malformations (AVM) (see also p. 113) account for approximately 1% of intracranial tumorous lesions.[5] They are most commonly seen in the distribution of the middle cerebral arteries but also occur in the cerebellum. Although they are probably congenital lesions, AVM commonly present in the second to fourth

decade.[141] Some are situated on the surface of the brain; others are deep within the cerebral hemispheres.[142]

Clinical presentation

AVM present with focal neurological signs, epilepsy or intracerebral or subarachnoid haemorrhage. The majority of cerebellar and posterior fossa AVM[143] present with haemorrhage and a sudden rise in intracranial pressure; patients may die unless the haematoma is evacuated. Intact malformations enhance on CT scan and haematomas are revealed as dense localised lesions. Angiography defines the extent of the malformation, the feeding vessels and the presence of saccular aneurysms, which are commonly found on arteries feeding arteriovenous malformations.[144] Treatment is by evacuation of blood clot and excision of accessible malformations. Neither ligation of feeding vessels nor embolisation usually leads to long-term obliteration of vascular malformations, but stereotactic radiotherapy may be used to treat small lesions. Some arteriovenous malformations regress spontaneously, possibly following thrombosis of component vessels.[145]

Macroscopic appearances

Inspection of surgically removed specimens often reveals a malformation partly destroyed by haemorrhage, but fragments of the lesion may be recovered by careful examination of the blood clot. In intact post-mortem specimens, an arteriovenous malformation appears as a tangled mass of blood vessels (see Fig. 5.28, p. 000); often the lesion is no larger than 2–3 cm in diameter but has large dilated feeding vessels.

Histology

Surface malformations are seen to extend into the underlying cerebral cortex, and frequently much of the malformation lies within brain tissue (Fig. 16.68). Thick-walled and thin-walled dilated blood vessels are seen in the overlying leptomeninges and within the brain itself. An elastic van Gieson stain identifies some arteries with a well-marked internal elastic lamina and smooth muscle

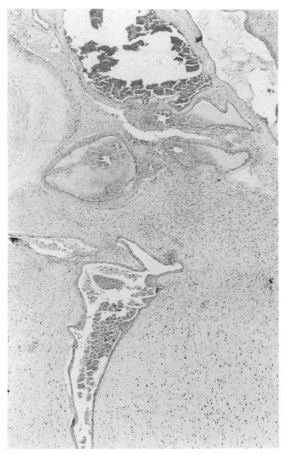

Fig. 16.68 Arteriovenous malformation. Large vessels from the surface (top) extend into the cerebral cortex. They are separated by gliotic brain tissue.
Haematoxylin-eosin ×25

media. Other vessels, however, are dilated and have thin fibrous walls; some may be necrotic and invaded by polymorphonuclear leucocytes. In addition to fresh haemorrhage, there may be evidence of old haemorrhage with macrophages containing haemosiderin surrounding the vascular malformation. The vessels themselves are separated by gliotic brain tissue.[43]

Spinal AVM

Arteriovenous malformations or fistulae involving the spinal cord (see p. 113)[146] usually affect the lower part of the cord. They are characterised by dilated venous varices on the posterior aspect of the cord (see Fig. 5.29, p. 113). Microscopically,

the veins have thick fibrous walls and the intervening spinal cord is necrotic and gliotic.[147] The syndrome, which presents with paraparesis and bladder paresis, is referred to as the subacute, necrotic myelitis of Foix and Alajouanine. Spinal angiography (see Fig. 5.29, p. 113) reveals dilated radicular arteries forming arteriovenous fistulae with the veins of the spinal cord.[147]

Sturge–Weber–Dimitri syndrome

This syndrome (encephalofacial angiomatosis: see p. 356) is a rare condition characterised by a port wine stain (capillary haemangioma) on the face, localised to the region supplied by the trigeminal nerve, and a vascular malformation on the surface of the ipsilateral cerebral hemisphere composed of dilated capillaries and veins. There is atrophy and calcification in the surrounding brain. Other lesions such as glaucoma and choroidal angiomas may be present. Patients present with hemiparesis and epilepsy; some are affected at birth.[148]

Venous malformations[149]

These lesions are composed mainly of dilated venous channels and are less common than arteriovenous malformations but they may be very extensive. Those involving the cerebral veins and the vein of Galen[150] may present at birth with high output cardiac failure or with hydrocephalus due to compression of the midbrain and aqueduct. Angiography in these cases reveals a dilated, tangled mass of veins in the vicinity of the pineal extending into the central regions of the brain and onto the surface of the occipital lobes. At postmortem, the veins collapse but may still be readily identified.

TUMOURS OF MISPLACED TISSUE ELEMENTS

Colloid cysts

Colloid cysts are found in a constant position at the anterior end of the third ventricle at the level of the foramina of Monro (Fig. 16.69).[5] They comprise some 2% of intracranial tumours and they present clinically with the signs and symptoms of hydro-

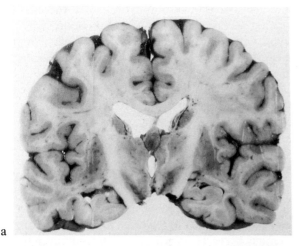

a

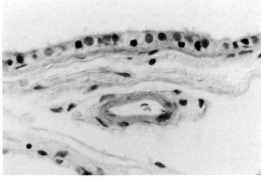

Fig. 16.70 Colloid cyst showing a lining of ciliated cuboidal epithelium (top) lying on a fibrous stroma. Haematoxylin-eosin × 400

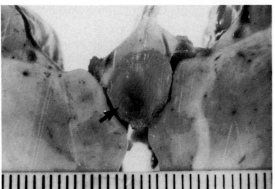

b

Fig. 16.69a, b Colloid cyst of the third ventricle. (a) Coronal section of cerebral hemispheres showing slightly dilated lateral ventricles; a colloid cyst occludes the foramina of Monro. (b) Details of the colloid cyst (arrow) in (a). It is nestling between the thalami on either side and the fornix (top).

cephalus due to obstruction of the ventricular system. On CT scan they enhance brightly. They can be effectively treated by surgical removal.

Macroscopically, they are thin-walled cysts containing grey, soft colloid material (Fig. 16.69). Histologically, the thin wall of the cyst is typically lined by columnar or cuboidal epithelium, often bearing cilia (Fig. 16.70); the cyst contains PAS-positive material.[24] The outer part of the wall is composed of a collagenous stroma.

The origin of colloid cysts is still uncertain; it has been suggested that they arise from the embryonic paraphysis at the anterior end of the third ventricle, from the ependyma, or from the choroid plexus.[5] However, immunocytochemistry has shown that they do not contain the choroid plexus marker carbonic anhydrase C or the glial-ependymal marker, glial fibrillary acidic protein.[33] In addition, the epithelium is mounted on a fibrous stroma which is not seen in ependymomas. Squamous cells have been described in colloid cysts, which suggests that the origin is from an embryonic remnant of the stomatodeum.

Although most colloid cysts[151] are thin-walled and contain colloid, some become inflamed and a thick wall of xantho-granulation tissue forms;[24,152] the epithelium in these cases has usually been destroyed so that a firm diagnosis of colloid cyst may be difficult.

Craniopharyngiomas and suprasellar cysts

Although they are more common in children, with a peak incidence in the second decade, these lesions also occur in adults and make up 3–5% of intracranial tumours.[153] They present as cystic or solid masses at the base of the brain; 94% are above the sella turcica, 18% extend into the sella but extension through the floor of the sella is rare.[153]

Clinical presentation[154]

78% of patients present with headache and 71% with visual disturbances due to compression of the optic chiasma. Raised intracranial pressure—due to distortion of the ventricular system—and hydrocephalus may occur. Abnormal psychological features and aggression, together with a variety of other neurological signs, have been described in patients with craniopharyngiomas.[154] Hypopituitarism is seen in 32% of patients,[154] and raised serum prolactin levels in 16%.[155] Radiographs may reveal calcification within craniopharyngiomas. On CT scan these tumours are seen as enhancing cystic lesions above the pituitary fossa. Radical surgical excision and radiotherapy may be curative but the tumours often recur.[153]

Macroscopic appearances

Craniopharyngiomas and suprasellar cysts appear as yellow or white, often multilocular, cystic structures. The solid areas may have a gritty consistency due to calcification; there may be semisolid keratin or a colloidal fluid in the cystic areas. In some tumours there is an abundance of cholesterol crystals in the fluid, identifiable by polarising microscopy of a wet film.[24] The tumour may be firmly attached to the base of the brain and the meninges and may extend up into the third ventricle or beyond.

Histology

Suprasellar cysts are lined by keratinising squamous epithelium like that of epidermoid cysts elsewhere in the body. There is a surrounding fibrous stroma, and granulation tissue may replace part of the lining of the cyst where the epithelium has been destroyed.

Craniopharyngiomas are composed of distinctive sheets of squamous cells (Fig. 16.71) with well-defined basal layers separating the squamous areas from the connective tissue in the tumour. The squamous areas resemble ameloblastomas of the jaw, which arise from the enamel organ. Calcification and areas of keratin accumulation are frequently seen in these tumours and granulomas may form around accumulated cholesterol crystals. Some craniopharyngiomas invade the surrounding brain tissue as small buds of squamous cells which make complete excision of the tumour very difficult.

Craniopharyngiomas and suprasellar cysts are considered to be basically the same tumour, possibly with a more mature squamous epithelium in the cystic lesions.[153] They are thought to arise from the hypophysial recess (Rathke's pouch) in

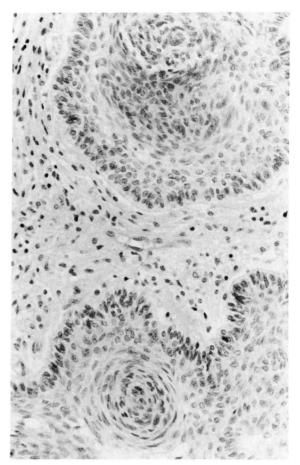

Fig. 16.71 Craniopharyngioma infiltrating brain. Islands of squamous epithelium (top and bottom) are separated by gliotic brain tissue (centre). Haematoxylin-eosin × 240

the roof of the stomatodeum, the structure from which the anterior pituitary is derived. In addition to the local mass effect, rupture of these tumours with the release of keratin or cholesterol crystals into the basal meninges may cause severe sterile fibrosing meningitis.

Epidermoid cysts

Accounting for less than 1% of intracranial and spinal tumours, epidermoid cysts may arise at a number of intracranial sites and at all ages. Most commonly they occur in the cerebellopontine angle,[156] or in the bones of the base of the skull. In the spine, they may be intramedullary. When they

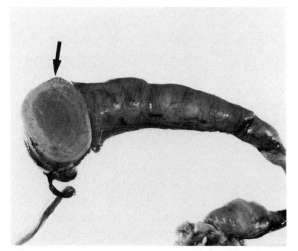

Fig. 16.72 Epidermoid cyst of the filum terminale. An elongated epidermoid cyst with a smooth surface is attached to the filamentous filum terminale (lower left). Transverse section (arrow) reveals the pultaceous contents of the cyst.

involve the cauda equina and filum terminale (Fig. 16.72) there is usually spina bifida.[157]

The clinical picture depends upon the site of the cyst. There may be raised intracranial pressure due to disturbance of cerebrospinal fluid flow caused by brainstem and fourth ventricle distortion from an epidermoid cyst in the cerebellopontine angle. Sterile meningitis may result from the release of cyst contents into the cerebrospinal fluid. Intramedullary cysts may expand within the cord to compress the corticospinal tracts or dorsal columns, producing paraparesis and sensory loss. Back pain and disturbances of bladder function may be present when the cyst is in the region of the cauda equina.

Intracranial or spinal cysts are revealed on CT scan[20] or by MRI[158] as enhancing ring-like structures with contents of low density. Myelography may be useful in localising spinal epidermoid cysts.[22]

Macroscopically, epidermoid cysts have a fibrous wall and pultaceous keratin within their lumen (Fig. 16.72). The lining of the cyst often has a pearly white appearance[156] due to the keratinised epithelium forming its wall. There may be many cholesterol crystals in the cyst contents (cholesteatoma). Microscopically, the cyst is lined by keratinising squamous epithelium which is separated from adjacent brain, cord or meninges by a fibrous stroma. In some cysts, the epithelial lining is destroyed and replaced by granulomatous inflammatory tissue.

Dermoid cysts

These are much less common than epidermoid cysts.[43] They occur in the posterior fossa, in the ventricles, at the base of the brain, in the lumbosacral spine and within the spinal cord (intramedullary dermoid) or filum terminale. They present in a similar way to epidermoid cysts. Microscopically, skin appendages such as hair and sebaceous glands can be detected within the wall of the cyst.

Teratomas

Teratomas mainly occur in the pineal region (see p. 509) but may also be seen in the suprasellar region and in the posterior fossa.[5]

Lipomas

As there is no adipose tissue within the confines of the dura in the skull or spine, lipomas are developmental abnormalities. They are probably present from birth and are usually located in the midsagittal plane above the corpus callosum, or in relation to the cerebellum or in the fourth ventricle. Spinal lipomas may be embedded in the cord; if they are in the cauda equina they may be associated with spina bifida.[43,159]

Clinically, it is mainly the spinal lipomas that cause neurological problems. Cord compression may occur with lipomas in the thoracic region. Most of the lipomas are in the region of the cauda equina,[159] where they cause tethering of the lower end of the spinal cord and nerve roots of the cauda equina: pain, bladder symptoms and weakness of the legs result. Lipomas may be localised by CT scan,[20] MRI[158] or myelography.

Macroscopically, intracranial lipomas are usually well-defined masses of adipose tissue.[5] When they involve the cauda equina, the fatty tissue is frequently intermixed with the nerve roots and is difficult to excise without damaging them.

Microscopically, lipomas are similar to those elsewhere in the body, with large, lipid-filled cells and scanty intervening fibrous stroma. Nerve roots and small blood vessels may be seen embedded within lipomas of the cauda equina.

Other cysts

A variety of cystic lesions may present in intracranial[160] or spinal[161] sites. Spinal *enterogenous cysts* containing elements of gut may be associated with defects in the vertebral bodies.[161] *Arachnoid cysts* may be related to the lateral fissures of the brain[162] or to the surface of the spinal cord; the arachnoid over the surface of these cysts may be fibrotic and thickened. *Mucoceles* arising from nasal sinuses may involve the orbit or the brain; they are lined by mucus-secreting columnar respiratory epithelium.[43]

PITUITARY TUMOURS

This is not the place for a full account of pituitary tumours, which are described in the volume of *Systemic Pathology* that deals with the endocrine system. Some mention of them is required here as their local intracranial extension may affect neural structures.

Clinical presentation

Pituitary adenomas may present at any time of life, either with hypopituitarism or with hormonal effects due to excessive secretion of prolactin, growth hormone, or adrenocorticotrophic hormone.[153] 25–30% of tumours, however, are clinically hormonally inactive,[153,163] and may pre-

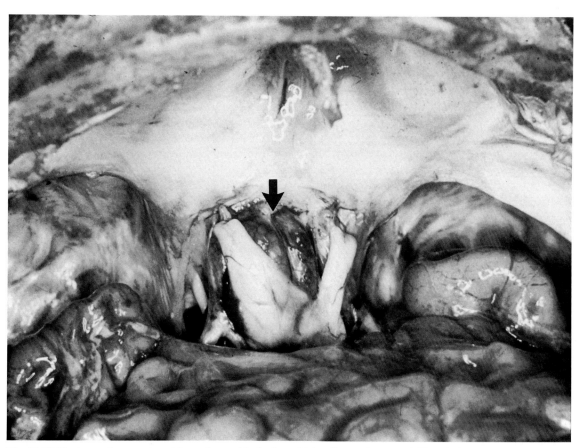

Fig. 16.73 Pituitary adenoma viewed from above with the frontal lobes (bottom) retracted. The pituitary adenoma (arrow) is seen bulging from the sella turcica. The optic nerves and chiasma are stretched over the tumour. Both optic nerves have been detached from the optic canal.
Reproduced by permission of Dr P. J. Gallagher, Pathology, University of Southampton, UK.

sent with bitemporal hemianopia or with visual field loss due to upward extension of the adenoma and compression of the optic chiasma or optic nerves (Fig. 16.73). The hormone-producing tumours may also cause visual disturbance or they may remain as microadenomas confined within the pituitary gland itself.[153] Very occasionally, there is involvement of the third cranial nerve due to lateral extension of a pituitary adenoma; this complication does not necessarily mean that the tumour is malignant.

Skull radiography often reveals enlargement of the pituitary fossa. On CT scan, pituitary adenomas enhance brightly and this technique may even locate microadenomas within the pituitary in cases in which there is no enlargement of the pituitary fossa.

Although prolactinomas may be treated medically with bromocriptine, many tumours require surgical excision, especially those with suprasellar extension causing visual failure. Many of the hormonally active tumours are excised surgically, either by trans-sphenoidal hypophysectomy or by a frontal approach.

Macroscopic appearances

Pituitary adenomas are usually well circumscribed, and those with suprasellar extension are seen bulging from the pituitary fossa with the optic chiasma stretched over the superior surface (Fig. 16.73). When very large, the tumours may expand upwards to block the third ventricle and cause hydrocephalus.

Histology

Pituitary adenomas may appear as diffuse sheets of cells with some variation in nuclear size, or as a sinusoidal pattern in which the cells are arranged around blood vessels.[24] Adenomas can be distinguished from normal pituitary by staining with PAS-orange G; normal pituitary shows a heterogeneous population of equal numbers of acidophil, PAS-positive and chromophobe cells whereas pituitary adenomas have a uniform staining pattern of chromophobe, acidophil or PAS-positive cells.[153] Touch preparations or smears can be used to rapidly identify pituitary adenomas during a surgical operation.[23] Immunocytochemistry for pituitary hormones has shown that approximately 50% of adenomas secrete prolactin, 8% growth hormone, 2% follicle stimulating hormone and luteinising hormone, 6% adrenocorticotrophic hormone, and 34% no hormone at all.[163] Electron microscopy may be useful for confirming a diagnosis of pituitary adenoma by showing secretory granules of characteristic size and density.[153] A proportion of adenomas are oncocytomas: there are very few granules in the cells of these tumours, but they contain large numbers of mitochondria.[153]

PINEAL TUMOURS

Pineal tumours are considered in the next chapter (pp. 507–514).

TUMOURS OF BONE

Tumours arising in the skull and spine may affect the central nervous system by local extension or by compression.

Chordomas

Chordomas are uncommon tumours which arise from the sacrum and from the clivus at the base of the skull.[164] Spinal chordomas may cause compression of the cauda equina or present as a pelvic or retrosacral mass. In the skull, chordomas may compress the brainstem or cause cranial nerve palsies. Radiographs of the skull show destruction of bone at the site of the chordoma.[22] Treatment is by local excision; complete removal may not be possible and recurrence then ensues.

Macroscopically, chordomas are seen as grey, gelatinous tumours which are locally invasive. Histologically, they are characterised by sheets of physaliphorous ('bubbly') cells (Fig. 16.74) containing PAS-positive material.[164] Fragments of bone may be present within the tumour. The physaliphorous nature of the cells is well seen in smear preparations.[24] Immunocytochemistry has

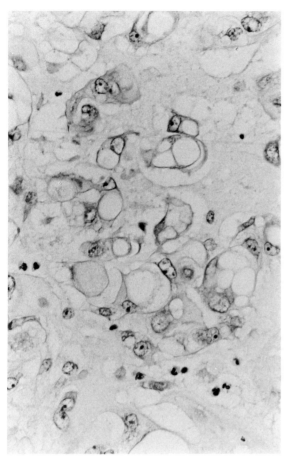

Fig. 16.74 Chordoma showing the typical 'bubbly' physaliphorous cells.
Haematoxylin-eosin × 385

shown that chordomas stain for cytokeratins, epithelial membrane antigen, S100 protein and vimentin;[165,166] these findings distinguish them from chondromas, chondrosarcomas, liposarcomas and carcinomas.

Chordomas are thought to arise from remnants of the notochord.[167]

Chondromas

Also arising in the base of the skull as well as in the vault, chondromas[168] have similar histological appearances to cartilaginous tumours elsewhere in the body. They should not be confused with chordomas. Chondrosarcomas are very uncommon, occurring in the base of the skull.

Ivory osteomas

Ivory osteomas of the nasal sinuses are uncommon. They may present as hard, craggy, chalky masses which slowly extend into the orbit and into the base of the skull.[168] There may be an associated mucocele of the related nasal sinuses.

Other tumours

Chemodectomas of the glomus jugulare may extend from the middle ear cavity into the posterior fossa. They present in a similar way to other cerebellopontine angle tumours.[169] Histologically, they are characterised by thin-walled vessels and clear cells packed into small groups by reticulin.

Osteosarcomas of the skull are uncommon[170] but may arise in the vault, especially in association with Paget's disease. The tumour adheres to the dura and infiltrates the underlying brain, causing focal neurological signs, or symptoms of raised intracranial pressure due to the mass effect of the tumour.

Fibrous dysplasia[170] may affect the base of the skull causing damage to cranial nerves and distortion of the bone.

Haemangiomas of bone[170] are uncommon. They occur in the spine where they compress the spinal cord.

METASTATIC INTRACRANIAL AND SPINAL TUMOURS

Carcinomas and melanomas are the main tumours which give rise to intracranial and spinal metastases.[5,43] Direct spread of nasopharyngeal carcinoma through the base of the skull may cause cranial nerve palsies or directly invade the base of the brain. Haematogenous spread of carcinomas and melanomas is much more common than direct spread. Metastases may involve the central nervous system as deposits in the brain, in the cranial and spinal meninges, or in the bones of the skull and vertebral column. It is not possible to give exact figures for the incidence of metastases involving the central nervous system, but it is estimated that 20–40% of all intracranial tumours are metastatic[5] and that 24% of patients dying from carcinoma have metastases in the brain. This gives an annual incidence for brain metastases of 8·5 per 100 000.[16] With the increasing use of CT scanning, a more exact figure for the incidence of brain metastases may become available. In Britain, carcinomas of bronchus, breast, lung and kidney, malignant melanoma and leukaemias account for most metastatic cancer of the nervous system. However, almost any malignant tumour may metastasise to involve the nervous system. In regions where choriocarcinoma is common, cerebral metastases are found in 20–30% of cases.[171]

Intracranial metastases

These mainly occur as discrete, often spherical lesions in the brain, but carcinomas and malignant melanomas may also cause meningeal carcinomatosis ('carcinomatous meningitis') with diffuse spread through the cerebrospinal fluid involving the surface of the brain and spinal cord and the leptomeninges.[5] Deposits of carcinoma in the dura are uncommon but they may spread to involve underlying brain or spinal cord.

Clinical presentation. Intracranial metastases give rise to a wide variety of symptoms depending upon the site and multiplicity of the lesions.[18,19] There may be focal neurological signs with motor or sensory deficit. Epilepsy may be seen, or the patient may present due to the mass effect of the tumour and surrounding oedema with headache, papilloedema, vomiting and alteration in consciousness due to raised intracranial pressure. Cerebral metastases enhance brightly on CT scan and are usually multiple (Fig. 16.75). Extensive areas of low density oedema may be seen around the metastases, although in some cases there may be remarkably little oedema and little distortion of the brain from the presence of metastases.

Carcinomatous meningitis may cause cranial nerve palsies or obstruct the cerebrospinal fluid pathways, resulting in hydrocephalus. In such cases, diagnosis may be made by identifying carcinoma or melanoma cells in cytospin preparations of cerebrospinal fluid.[24,25] The malignant cells are larger than the accompanying inflammatory cells and have irregular nuclei;

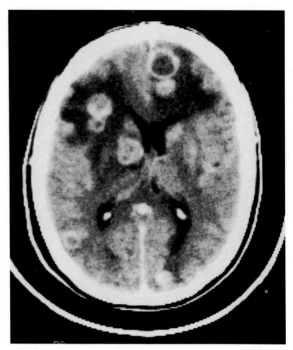

Fig. 16.75 Metastatic carcinoma—CT scan. Ring-like and solid enhancing lesions (white) are seen distributed throughout both cerebral hemispheres. The metastases in the frontal lobe are surrounded by oedema (dark areas).

metastatic carcinoma cells may also contain globules of mucus in the cytoplasm which can be stained with PAS or mucicarmine as an aid to diagnosis.

Macroscopic appearances

Cerebral metastases are often distributed randomly throughout the cerebral hemispheres and cerebellum (Fig. 16.76). They may range in size from 1 mm to several centimetres in diameter; the smaller metastases are spherical in shape and well demarcated from the surrounding brain. Larger metastases may be irregular in shape due to distortion by the contours of the brain. Metastases can usually be distinguished from glioblastoma multiforme by their multiplicity, spherical shape and sharp margins of demarcation from surrounding brain. Melanomas are usually brown and frequently haemorrhagic; carcinomas may be chalky white in colour and granular in consistency with central areas of necrosis. Metastatic

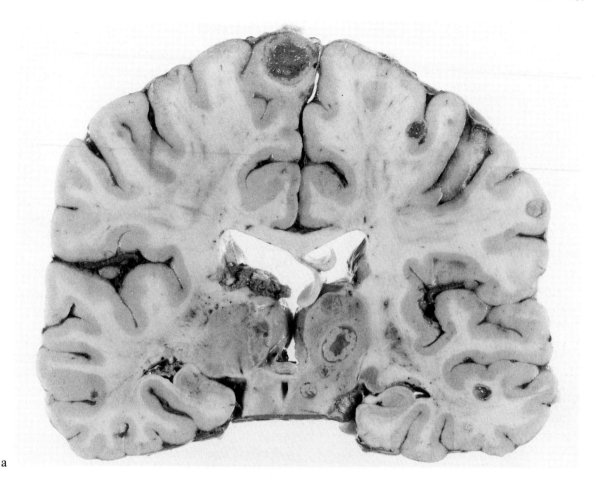

a

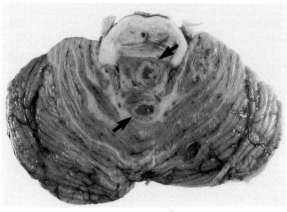

b

Fig. 16.76a, b Metastatic carcinoma. (**a**) Multiple mucus-secreting adenocarcinoma metastases are seen distributed throughout both cerebral hemispheres. (**b**) Metastases in the pons and cerebellum (arrows) have caused compression and occlusion of the fourth ventricle. Other metastases are seen in the right cerebellar hemisphere.

adenocarcinomas, especially from colon and stomach, often have a mucoid consistency (Fig. 16.76). Soft, necrotic metastases should be distinguished from multiple cerebral abscesses which are filled with liquid pus and, in their more chronic stage, surrounded by a firm, fibrous capsule (see p. 169) which is not present around metastases.

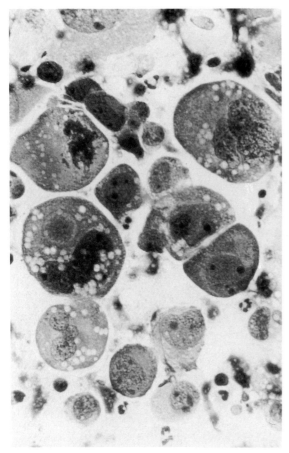

Fig. 16.77 Metastatic adenocarcinoma—smear. Individual cells show large hyperchromatic pleomorphic nuclei and multiple vacuoles in the cytoplasm.
Toluidine blue × 430

Histology

With surgical specimens, smears, touch preparations and cryostat sections can be used for rapid diagnosis.[23,24,38] Groups of rounded carcinoma cells can be identified in smears (Fig. 16.77) as they remain separate from the fibrillary and often gliotic surrounding brain tissue. The morphology of the cells is often well depicted in touch preparations, and the histological form of the tumour can be appreciated in cryostat sections.

Histological sections of metastases confirm the sharp demarcation between the tumour and the surrounding brain tissue in the majority of cases (Fig. 16.78). Small groups of carcinoma cells may bud into the surrounding brain but only

lymphomas and, more rarely, malignant melanomas and small cell carcinomas of the lung diffusely invade the surrounding brain. Frequently there is little tissue reaction around metastatic carcinomas; in some cases, however, there may be extensive oedema and reactive astrocytosis.

Sections stained for mucus by PAS and Alcian blue are often useful as a guide to the site of the primary tumour. Immunocytochemistry may also be valuable. Metastatic carcinoma cells do not stain for the glial marker GFAP, in contrast to reactive astrocytes which may be included within the tumour. Carcinomas, however, may contain cytokeratins[32] and human milk factor globulin which can be identified by immunocytochemistry as an aid to diagnosis. Prostatic carcinoma cells usually contain prostatic acid phosphatase which can be localised by immunocytochemistry. With the rare exception of non-pigmented tumours, malignant melanomas may be readily recognised by the presence of melanin; the cells are also positive for S100 protein on immunocytochemical staining.

In *carcinomatous meningitis*,[172] the surface of the cerebral hemispheres, cerebellum, brainstem and spinal cord may be coated by a thin layer of white tumour tissue, or brown tissue in the case of malignant melanoma (Fig. 16.79).

Primary malignant melanoma[173] of the meninges is rare and probably arises from melanocytes in the arachnoid mater.

Histologically, malignant cells are diffusely distributed throughout the subarachnoid space and invade the surface of the brain and perivascular spaces. Adenocarcinomas are the tumours that metastasise most commonly in this way (Fig. 16.80). Tumour cells can be identified in the CSF.[24,36] Cranial and spinal nerve roots may also be heavily invaded by tumour cells in carcinomatous meningitis (Fig. 16.81).

Lymphomas and leukaemias

High-grade non-Hodgkin's lymphomas and leukaemias, particularly lymphoblastic, may involve the central nervous system either as primary CNS lymphomas (see p. 472) or, more commonly, as lymphomatous meningitis with

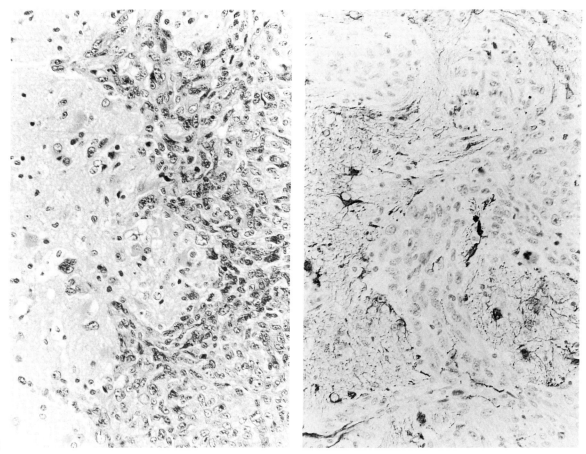

a   b

Fig. 16.78a, b Metastatic carcinoma—edge. (**a**) Carcinoma (right) is sharply demarcated from the gliotic brain (left).
(**b**) Darkly stained, reactive astrocytes in the gliotic brain are sharply contrasted with the unstained metastatic carcinoma cells.
Some astrocyte processes are included in the tumour tissue.
(**a**) Haematoxylin-eosin × 190; (**b**) Immunocytochemistry for GFAP × 190

widespread lymphoma in other parts of the body.[174] The dura may be invaded or there may be diffuse involvement of the leptomeninges by lymphoma and by leukaemia. Neoplastic cells may fill the subarachnoid space and invade the surface of the brain and cranial and spinal nerve roots. Up to 30% of patients with non-Hodgkin's lymphoma have CNS involvement, especially in the late stages of the disease.[175] Some 5% of patients with leukaemia have CNS involvement at presentation of the disease[176] and 95% will have CNS involvement if specific and effective treatment is not applied to the cerebrospinal fluid.[177] Leptomeningeal involvement by lymphoma and leukaemia may present with cranial nerve palsies,

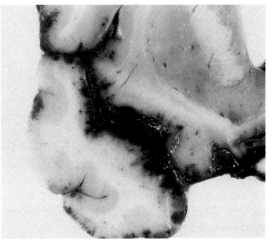

Fig. 16.79 Metastatic malignant melanoma. Darkly stained melanoma deposits are seen in the meninges and invading the surface of the temporal and frontal lobes.

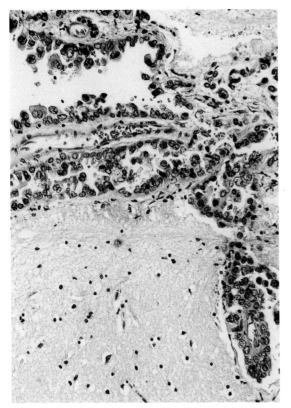

Fig. 16.80 Carcinomatous meningitis. Rows of metastatic adenocarcinoma cells are seen lining the pia mater and covering the vessels in the subarachnoid space (top). Carcinoma cells are also seen around blood vessels within the brain (bottom right).
Haematoxylin-eosin × 150

meningism and raised intracranial pressure. Neoplastic cells are recovered from the CSF in a high proportion of cases (Fig. 16.82).[178]

In some cases of lymphoma, there is direct involvement of the substance of the brain itself, particularly in the periventricular regions.

Neoplastic angioendotheliosis is a rare condition most commonly presenting with a rapidly progressive neurological illness characterised by dementia and multiple small infarcts within the brain. Histology reveals the occlusion of small blood vessels in the brain and elsewhere in the body by neoplastic cells in the absence of significant extravascular tumour. Skin nodules with a similar occlusive vascular pathology are also seen.

Immunocytochemistry suggests that the tumour cells are of B-lymphocyte origin.[179]

Spinal metastases

Although lymphomas (see p. 475) metastasise to involve the spinal meninges and extradural tissue, they are not as common as carcinomas in this site. Virtually any carcinoma may metastasise to the spine but carcinomas of the bronchus, breast, lung and prostate are those that do so most commonly. Intramedullary spinal cord metastases are very rare;[180] roughly half are from the lung. They present with signs of long tract destruction and local anterior horn cell loss due to the focal nature of the lesion.

Extramedullary intradural metastatic deposits may be focal or may be diffusely spread throughout the subarachnoid space as meningeal carcinomatosis. Nerve roots may also show focal deposits of metastatic tumour (Fig. 16.81). Extradural metastases are probably the commonest

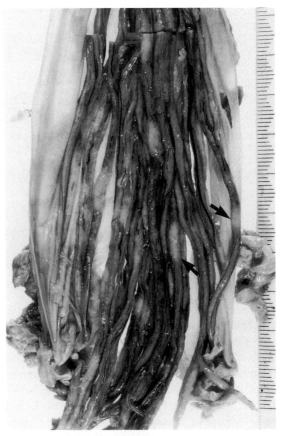

Fig. 16.81 Metastatic carcinoma in the cauda equina. Pale tumour deposits (arrows) are seen expanding nerve roots.

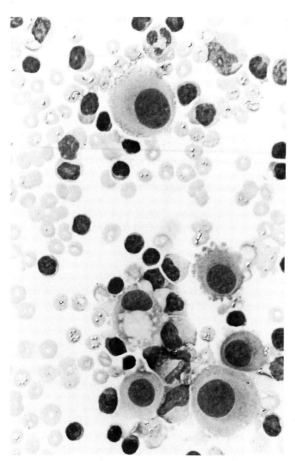

Fig. 16.82 Lymphoma cells in a cytospin preparation of CSF. The smaller normal lymphocytes and erythrocytes can be used for size comparison.
Giemsa × 575

myelography can be used to define the level of spinal cord compression. Intramedullary, intradural and extramedullary tumours can also be distinguished by myelography.[22] CT scan[20] or magnetic resonance imaging[158] is used to define the extent of tumour involvement.

NON-METASTATIC NEUROLOGICAL MANIFESTATIONS OF MALIGNANT DISEASE

There are several well recognised neurological syndromes which are associated with tumours but are not due to the direct metastatic spread of those tumours to the brain or spinal cord.[181]

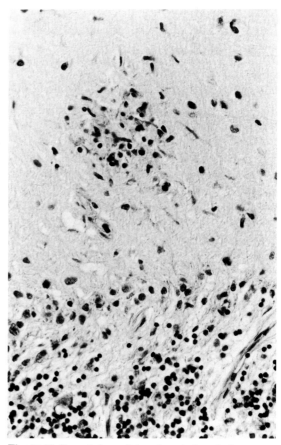

Fig. 16.83 Encephalomyelitis and cortical cerebellar degeneration in a patient with lymphoma. There is necrosis with microglial accumulation in the molecular layer of the cerebellum (top) and loss of Purkinje cells. The granule cell layer is seen at the bottom of the field.
Haematoxylin-eosin × 300

form of spinal involvement. The extradural layer of fat may be infiltrated by metastatic carcinoma or there may be deposits of tumour in the vertebral bodies, laminae and pedicles, later expanding into the extradural space.

Spinal cord compression may result from extradural deposits of lymphoma, including Hodgkin's lymphoma, either in the bone or in extradural fat. Bone destruction by myeloma is also a cause of spinal cord compression.

Clinically, extradural metastases produce spinal cord compression either from the mass in the extradural space or from collapse of an affected vertebra. Patients may present with sudden onset of paraparesis, bladder malfunction or back pain. X-rays of the spine reveal erosion of bone, and

Encephalomyelitis may occur with perivascular cuffing by lymphocytes, damage to neurons and proliferation of microglial cells (Fig. 16.83). There is diffuse and focal damage within the brain, often affecting the grey matter. The distribution of the changes varies: the limbic system, bulbar region (pons and medulla), cerebellum, spinal cord and dorsal root ganglia are the main sites. All areas may be affected or one area may be predominantly involved. It is suggested that the disorder is due to an auto-immune phenomenon; no virus has been isolated. This form of encephalomyelitis is associated mainly with carcinoma of the bronchus (77%);[181] in the majority of cases the tumour is an oat cell carcinoma; most other cases are associated with small anaplastic primary tumours. A small proportion of tumours causing this syndrome are from other sites, especially carcinoma of the ovary, stomach and larynx and occasionally Hodgkin's disease.

Cerebellar cortical degeneration is also seen as a non-metastatic complication of malignant disease.[182,183] Cerebellar atrophy may be widespread with severe or total loss of Purkinje cells (Fig. 16.83) and in some cases an inflammatory reaction in the dentate nucleus. The syndrome is usually associated with bronchial and ovarian carcinomas or with lymphoma.[182,183] It appears to be due to an auto-immune response with anti-Purkinje cell antibodies in the serum of half the patients.[184]

Peripheral neuropathies (see p. 565) with axonal degeneration, segmental demyelination or a Guillain–Barré-type chronic relapsing neuropathy have been described.[181] *Muscle disease* associated with malignant tumours includes polymyositis, an acute necrotising myopathy, disorders of neuromuscular transmission (the Eaton–Lambert syndrome) and selective type 2B fibre atrophy (see pp. 627, 632).[181]

A range of *unclassifiable disorders*, some with a doubtful association with tumours, has been described.[181] They include necrotising myelopathy, central pontine myelinolysis and motor neuron disease. Peripheral neuropathies with paraproteinaemias are also well recorded.[185]

Opportunistic viral and mycotic infections occur in the brain in patients who are immunosuppressed either due to a lymphoma or due to chemotherapy. Such virus infections include progressive multifocal leucoencephalopathy, cytomegalovirus and herpes simplex (see p. 217–221); the main fungi involved are aspergillus, candida and cryptococcus (see p. 173–176). Toxoplasma infection may also occur (see p. 184).

TUMOURS OF THE PERIPHERAL NERVOUS SYSTEM

Schwannomas and neurofibromas

Two of the commonest tumours involving peripheral nerves are schwannomas and neurofibromas. As they may affect the central nervous system, they are discussed earlier in this chapter (p. 469). Other tumours of the peripheral nervous system are discussed below and include those derived from peripheral neuronal elements.

Neuroblastoma

Neuroblastomas occur mainly in the first three years of life and can be present at birth. They account for 7–10% of cases of malignant disease in children;[186,187] 86% occur under the age of 2 years and they are rare in adults.[188] 76% arise in the abdomen from the adrenals, from sympathetic ganglia and in the retroperitoneal tissue;[189] they may also arise from sympathetic ganglia in the thorax.

Clinical presentation

Neuroblastomas present as a mass at the primary site of origin or following metastatic spread—either locally to abdominal viscera or to lymph nodes, liver and bone. Although metastases to the skull and dura may occur, the brain is virtually never the site of blood-borne metastases. Despite treatment by chemotherapy there is only a 30% 2-year survival rate;[190] the prognosis is poor in children over one year of age. Intermediate products of catecholamine metabolism are secreted by neuroblastomas, and increased levels may be detected in the urine.[191] They include dopa, dopamine, 5-hydroxyindoleacetic acid, homovanillic acid and especially vanillylmandelic acid (VMA). Raised levels of VMA in the urine are

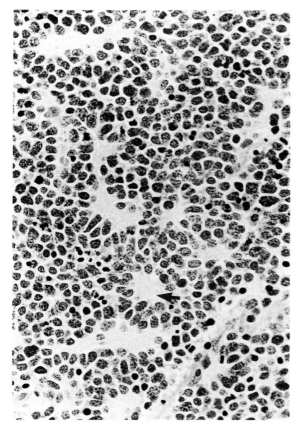

Fig. 16.84 Neuroblastoma arising in the abdomen. Sheets of cells with hyperchromatic nuclei are seen. Rosettes with pale fibrillary centres (arrow) are also present. Haematoxylin-eosin × 385

found in 75% of cases of neuroblastoma and this test has been used to screen populations of young children for the tumour.[187]

Macroscopic appearances

Neuroblastomas appear as soft, friable, grey tumours infiltrating surrounding structures. There may be areas of necrosis and haemorrhage.

Histology

There are sheets of small uniform cells with darkly staining nuclei and little cytoplasm (Fig. 16.84). Some larger cells may also be present. Neuroblastomas have been included among the primitive neuroectodermal tumours (PNET) (see p. 454).[13] Rosettes occur in 10–15% of cases; they

are recognised by a peripheral ring of nuclei with fine fibrillary processes in the centre of the ring (Fig. 16.84).[5] In some cases, the processes are argyrophilic, suggesting neuronal differentiation. Occasionally, mature neurons are seen and may represent maturation of tumour cells. The prognosis of neuroblastomas is more favourable when there is neuronal maturation.

Electron microscopy[113] reveals the presence of specialised intercellular junctions and, in the cytoplasm, dense core vesicles 100 nm in diameter resembling catecholamine granules (Fig. 16.85). Dense core vesicles are more numerous in those tumours showing neuronal differentiation. Choline acetyltransferase has also been detected in neuroblastoma.[192]

Olfactory neuroblastomas (aesthesioneuroblastomas)[5] are uncommon; they exhibit a relatively slow growth rate and respond best to a combination of surgery and radiotherapy. They may spread to the nasal sinuses, palate, orbit and brain.[193] Metastasis may occur to the lymph nodes in the neck and to the lungs. Histologically, olfactory neuroblastomas consist of small cells with fibrillary cytoplasm; the cells are often gathered in groups or Zellballen similar in arrangement to paragangliomas.[193a] These tumours have been categorised as PNET.[13] Immunocytochemistry has shown that many of the tumour cells contain small amounts of low molecular weight cytokeratin and that cells at the periphery of the cell groups are positive for S100 protein.[193a] Electron microscopy reveals the presence of dense core vesicles, synapses and axons.[194] These tumours behave in a less aggressive manner than neuroblastomas elsewhere in the body.[5]

Ganglioneuroma

Peripheral ganglioneuromas occur mainly in adults but are also found in children.[195] Most commonly they arise in the posterior mediastinum or in the retroperitoneal regions of the abdomen in association with the gut or from paraspinal autonomic ganglia.[189] They present clinically due to the mass effect of the tumour.

Macroscopically, ganglioneuromas are well-circumscribed, firm white fibrous tumours. The

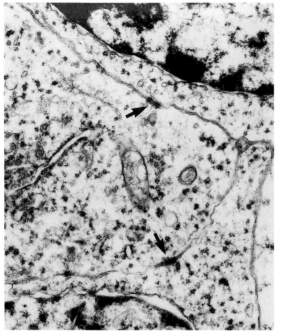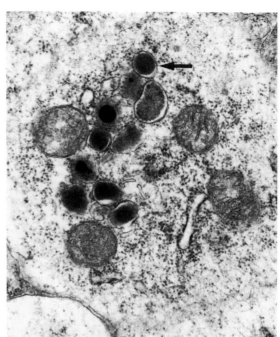

a

b

Fig. 16.85a, b Neuroblastoma (same case as Figure 16.84). (**a**) Intercellular junctions (arrows) have formed between the closely applied tumour cells. (**b**) Dense core vesicles (arrow) in the cytoplasm.
Electron micrographs (**a**) × 18 000; (**b**) × 27 000

presence of necrotic areas within the tumour suggests malignancy.

Microscopically,[5] thoracic and abdominal ganglioneuromas consist of a mixture of neurons, capsule cells and connective tissue elements; in this way they differ from ganglioneuromas of the central nervous system, which are composed of neurons and supporting astroglia but no satellite cells. The fibrillary structure of abdominal and thoracic ganglioneuromas may be reminiscent of neurofibromas, but groups of mature ganglion cells are seen (Fig. 16.86); these cells often lack Nissl granules and they may be binucleate or even multinucleate. Schwann cells abound and there may be a rich reticulin network. Many axons are seen within the tumour but few are myelinated. Mitoses are not usually observed within these tumours.

Electron microscopy[196] reveals the presence of 100 nm dense core vesicles, resembling catecholamine granules, in the neurons; larger granules may also be observed.[112] Unmyelinated axons and a few myelinated axons are seen together with Schwann cells. Satellite cells surround the ganglion cells but synapses are uncommon.

Ganglioneuromas are essentially benign tumours and are treated by local excision. They may be multiple in the gut or at other sites.

Ganglioneuroblastoma

Peripheral ganglioneuroblastomas are rare tumours which are biologically intermediate between benign ganglioneuromas and malignant aggressive neuroblastomas.[5] They usually occur in children under 6 years of age in retroperitoneal and thoracic sites similar to the distribution of ganglioneuromas. Macroscopically, they may resemble ganglioneuromas but foci of calcification, necrosis, local invasion and metastasis may be evident.

Histologically, there are two patterns of ganglioneuroblastoma.[5] In the *imperfect type*, all stages of differentiation are seen, from cells resembling neuroblasts to pleomorphic and immature neurons with delicate axons. They may be considered as differentiating neuroblastomas, and similar

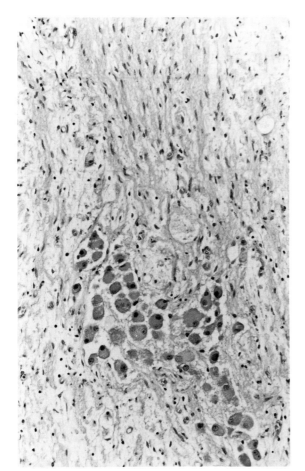

Fig. 16.86 Ganglioneuroma showing a group of ganglion cells and parallel arrays of nerve fibres. Haematoxylin-eosin × 150

the better the prognosis.[197,198] A detailed classification based on the stromal content of the tumour and maturation or differentiation of the cellular elements allows length of survival to be correlated with the tumour histology.[199]

Phaeochromocytoma

Phaeochromocytomas arise from chromaffin cells of the adrenal medulla or sympathetic ganglia. They occur at all ages, but most present in the third to sixth decade. A typical triad of symptoms is seen with sweating attacks, tachycardia and headaches; these symptoms are associated with hypertension.[200] The diagnosis is established by the detection of excessive catecholamine secretion through the measurement of catecholamines or

patterns may be seen in central nervous system ganglioneuroblastomas (see p. 458).

The other histological type is the *immature ganglioneuroblastoma*, in which there are areas resembling ganglioneuroma and others resembling a highly cellular neuroblastoma. These tumours usually lack the pleomorphic neurons seen in the imperfect type. Electron microscopically, ganglion cells containing dense core neurosecretory granules are seen, together with non-myelinated axons and Schwann cells.

The behaviour of ganglioneuroblastomas is unpredictable; they may be locally invasive and the immature types may metastasise in a similar way to neuroblastomas. In general, the greater the number of mature ganglion cells that are present,

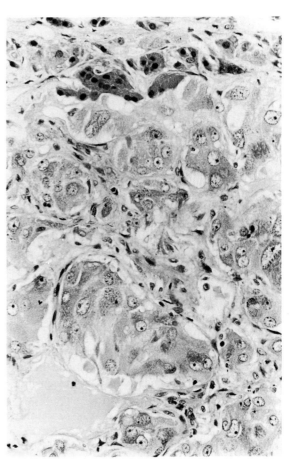

Fig. 16.87 Phaeochromocytoma. Large cells with copious darkly staining cytoplasm are gathered in small packets. Haematoxylin-eosin × 240

their metabolites, vanillylmandelic acid and total metanephrins, in the urine.[200] Radio-iodinated meta-iodobenzylguanidine (MIGB) can be used to localise phaeochromocytomas.[201] It has a high affinity for the adrenal and for phaeochromocytomas; it appears to follow the uptake and release pathways of noradrenaline. In addition to imaging, therapeutic doses of radio-iodinated MIBG can be used to treat malignant phaeochromocytomas and neuroblastoma.[201]

Macroscopically, phaeochromocytomas are usually well-circumscribed nodules, 1–10 cm in diameter, attached to the adrenals; they are bilateral in 10% of cases.[112] The cut surface is plum-coloured and histologically there is an alveolar pattern of polygonal or spheroidal cells (Fig. 16.87). In haematoxylin and eosin stained sections the large amounts of cytoplasm exhibit a dusky blue appearance and it is from this feature that the name of the tumour is derived. Chromated tissue shows brown granules in the cells (chromaffin reaction). On electron microscopy the cells contain osmiophilic granules 100–300 nm in diameter.[112,202] They are highly vascular tumours. A small proportion of phaeochromocytomas metastasise.

Paraganglioma

The extra-adrenal paraganglion system[203] consists of small macroscopic bodies and microscopic cell groups associated with the autonomic nervous system. They tend to be distributed in the para-axial regions of the trunk but they are also found in the peripheral portions of the autonomic nervous system. These organs all act as chemoreceptors and store catecholamine granules as dense core vesicles. Major components of the paraganglion system are found in the glomus jugulare, carotid bodies, around the aortic arch, and distributed along the abdominal aorta. The adrenal medulla is a major paraganglion in which phaeochromocytomas arise (see above).

Paragangliomas may be non-functioning tumours or they may secrete catecholamines.

Histologically, the tumour cells are gathered in cell nests by a reticulin stroma in a pattern similar to that seen in the normal paraganglion. The tumour cells are usually ovoid or polyhedral, with

more pleomorphism than the normal cells. The tumours are highly vascularised by vessels that often are thin-walled.

Para-aortic paragangliomas (paragangliomas of the organ of Zuckerkandl) and abdominal paragangliomas undergo malignant change slightly more frequently than paragangliomas in other sites. An incidence of 38% metastatic spread has been reported[204] with metastases usually in the regional lymph nodes or in bone.

Granular cell tumours

Also known as *granular cell myoblastomas*, these tumours arise as small nodules in the dermis or

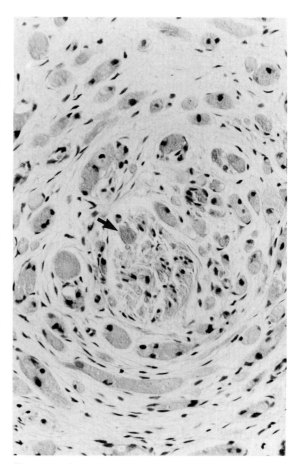

Fig. 16.88 Granular cell tumour of peripheral nerve. Large bulbous cells with granular cytoplasm are arranged concentrically around a nerve fascicle (centre). A tumour cell is seen within the nerve bundle (arrow). Haematoxylin-eosin × 240

may form much larger tumours in deeper tissue. They usually do not recur if completely excised. Microscopically, the tumour cells have a distinctive appearance with a small round nucleus and copious cytoplasm which contains granules which are usually slightly basophilic.[15,24,115] In the smaller tumours, the granular cells may be seen actually within small nerve bundles (Fig. 16.88). On electron microscopy[113] the granular cells contain polymorphic lysosomal granules and some angulate bodies. Ultrastructural features and positive immunocytochemical staining for S100 protein suggest that the tumour cells are derived from Schwann cells.

Nerve sheath myxomas

Dermal nerve sheath myxomas (neurothecoma) are benign cutaneous tumours growing mainly on the face, arms and shoulders.[205] They are treated by excision and rarely recur. Histologically, the tumours consist of nests of large stellate or spindle cells. The abundant matrix of mucous substance is mainly chondroitin sulphate which stains with Alcian blue and is sensitive to hyaluronidase.[206] Ultrastructural aspects of the tumour cells and their positivity for S100 protein[207] suggest that the tumours are derived from Schwann cells.

Tumour-like lesions of peripheral nerves

There are a number of swellings or tumour-like lesions that occur on peripheral nerves and appear, in general, to be a result of trauma.

Amputation neuromas[15,112,208] may develop as painful swellings at the distal ends of amputated limbs. They also occur if small nerve branches are damaged. Pain from the amputation neuroma[101] may be referred to the amputated limb (phantom limb). Histologically, amputation neuromas consist of disorientated bundles of axons and Schwann cells often divided into compartments by perineurial cells.[24,209]

Morton's neuroma (plantar neuroma)[209] involves the plantar interdigital nerves, which undergo local degeneration and scarring to form a painful mass. A small swelling on the nerve is seen with nerve fibre loss, fibrosis of the endoneurium and perineurium and the accumulation of mucosubstances. Morton's neuromas are thought to be due to trauma.[209]

A *pseudocyst* or *ganglion* of peripheral nerve (*nerve sheath myxoma*) contains mucinous material which stains with Alcian blue.[15,112] The cyst may have a thick fibrous wall, is attached to the nerve and may reach a size several times the diameter of the nerve trunk. There may be an increase in mucopolysaccharide within the nerve bundles themselves, with separation of the nerve fibres due to an increase in endoneurial mucosubstance. The usual sites of these cysts, on the common peroneal nerve and the ulnar nerve, suggest a traumatic origin.

Localised hypertrophic neuropathy has been described especially at sites of trauma,[210] usually on the radial nerve and its deep terminal branch (posterior interosseous nerve), and the lateral terminal branch of the deep peroneal nerve. Histologically, the nerve is enlarged, there is loss of myelinated axons and there is formation of cellular whorls.[211] The cellular whorls are probably formed from perineurial cells[212] as they do not contain S100 protein.[213] These lesions are probably due to nerve compression[214] with an exaggeration of the compartmentalisation of the nerve fascicles which occurs following damage to axons and perineurium.[215] Such a picture should not be confused with hypertrophic polyneuropathy, which is due to recurrent segmental demyelination (see p. 573).[112,210]

REFERENCES

Introduction

1. Graham DI. In: Thomas DGT, Graham DI, eds. Brain tumours: scientific basis, clinical investigations and current therapy. London: Butterworths, 1980: 268.
2. Zulch KJ, ed. Histological typing of tumours of the central nervous system. Geneva: World Health Organization, 1979.
3. McComb RD, Bigner DD. Clin Neuropathol 1984; 3: 93.
4. Gould VE. Hum Pathol 1986; 17: 212.
5. Russell DS, Rubinstein LJ. Pathology of tumours of the nervous system. 5th ed. revised by Rubinstein LJ. London: Arnold, 1989.
6. Kernohan JW, Sayre GP. Atlas of tumour pathology.

Washington DC: Armed Forces Institute of Pathology, 1952; section X, fascicle 35.

7. Friedman JH, Liu HM, Sprenivelli E, Calabresi P. J Neurol Neurosurg Psychiatry 1987; 50: 237.

8. Mortality statistics: cause, England and Wales 1981. London: HMSO, 1983.

9. Jones RD. Food Chem Toxicol 1986; 24: 99.

10. Barker DJP, Weller RO, Garfield JS. J Neurol Neurosurg Psychiatry 1976; 39: 290.

11. Bloom HJG. In: Bleehan NM, ed. Tumours of the brain. Berlin: Springer, 1986: 121.

12. Albright AL, Price RA, Guthkelch AN. Cancer 1983; 52: 2313.

13. Rorke LB. J Neuropathol Exp Neurol 1983; 42: 1.

14. Ludwig CL, Smith MT, Godfrey AD, Armbrustmacker VW. Ann Neurol 1986; 19: 15.

15. Harkin JC, Reed RJ. Tumors of the peripheral nervous system. 2nd series. Fascicle 3. Washington DC: Armed Forces Institute of Pathology, 1969; suppl 1983.

16. Greig NH. Cancer Treat Rev 1984; 11: 157.

Clinical features and investigations

17. McKeran RO, Thomas DGT. In: Thomas DGT, Graham DI, eds. Brain tumours: scientific basis, clinical investigations and current therapy. London: Butterworths, 1980: 194.

18. Weller RO, Swash M, McLellan DL, Scholtz CL, eds. Clinical neuropathology. Berlin: Springer, 1983: 105.

19. Walton JN. Brain's Diseases of the nervous system. Oxford: Oxford University Press, 1985.

20. Gonzalez CF, Grossman CB, Marsden JC, eds. Head and spine imaging. New York: Wiley, 1985.

21. Bydder GM. In: Bleehan NM, ed. Tumours of the brain. Berlin: Springer, 1986: 51.

22. Burrows EH, Leeds NE. Neuroradiology. Edinburgh: Churchill Livingstone, 1981.

Pathological investigation

23. Adams JH, Graham DI, Doyle D. Brain biopsy. The smear technique for neurosurgical biopsies. London: Chapman & Hall, 1981.

24. Weller RO. Colour atlas of neuropathology. Oxford: Miller and Oxford University Press, 1984.

25. Grant JW, Gallagher PJ, Jones DB. Arch Pathol Lab Med 1986; 110: 897.

26. Coakham HB, Garson JA, Allan PM et al. J Clin Pathol 1985; 38: 165.

27. Wright DH. Diagn Histopathol 1982; 5: 73.

28. Bancroft D, Stevens A, eds. Theory and practice of histological techniques. Edinburgh: Churchill Livingstone, 1982.

29. Sternberger LA. Immunocytochemistry. New York: Wiley, 1979.

30. Bonin JM, Rubinstein LJ. J Neurosurg 1984; 60: 1121.

31. Rubinstein LJ. Neuropathol Appl Neurobiol 1986; 12: 523.

32. Makin CA, Bobrow LG, Bodmer WF. J Clin Pathol 1984; 37: 975.

33. Weller RO, Steart PV, Moore IE. In: Walker MD, Thomas DGT, eds. Biology of brain tumour. Dordrecht: Nighoff & Junk, 1986: 115.

34. Bullard DE, Bigner DD. J Neurosurg 1985; 63: 2.

35. Moss TH. Tumours of the nervous system; an ultrastructural atlas. London: Springer, 1986.

36. Rosenthal DL. Cytology of the central nervous system. Basel: Karger, 1984.

37. Adams JH, Murray MF. Atlas of post mortem techniques in neuropathology. Cambridge: Cambridge University Press, 1982.

38. Weller RO. A general approach to neuropathological problems. In: Berry CL, ed. Current topics in pathology. Berlin: Springer, 1988: 61.

39. Artigas J, Cervós-Navarro J, Iglesias JR, Ebhart G. Clin Neuropathol 1985; 4: 135.

Primary tumours

40. Burger PC, Vogel FS, Green SB, Strike T. Cancer 1985; 56: 1106.

41. Gjerris F, Klinken L. J Neurosurg 1978; 49: 179.

42. Smith DA, Lantos PL. Acta Neuropathol 1985; 66: 155.

42a. Lowe J, Morrell K, Lennox G. et al. Neuropathol Appl Neurobiol 1989; 15: 45.

43. Rubinstein LJ. Tumors of the nervous system. 2nd series. Fascicle 6. Washington DC: Armed Forces Institute of Pathology, 1972; supplement 1982.

44. Nakamura Y, Becker LE. Acta Neuropathol 1983; 60: 271.

45. Kepes JJ, Rubinstein LJ, Eng LF. Cancer 1979; 44: 1839.

46. Grant JW, Gallagher PJ. Am J Surg Pathol 1986; 10: 336.

47. Husain AN, Leestma JE. J Neurosurg 1986; 64: 657.

47a. Raghavan R, Steart PV, Weller RO. Neuropathol Appl Neurobiol 1990 (in press)

48. EORTC Brain Tumour Group. J Neurosurg 1981; 55: 27.

49. Walker MD, Alexander E, Hunt WE et al. J Neurosurg 1978; 439: 333.

50. Weller RO. In: Bleehen NM, ed. Tumours of the brain. Berlin: Springer, 1986: 19.

51. von Hanwehr RI, Hofman FM, Taylor CR, Apuzzo MLJ. J Neurosurg 1984; 60: 1138.

52. Hoshino T, Townsend JJ, Muraoka I, Wilson CB. Brain 1980; 103: 967.

53. Burger PC, Shibata T, Kleihues P. Am J Surg Pathol 1986; 10: 611.

54. Weller RO, Foy M, Cox S. Neuropathol Appl Neurobiol 1977; 3: 307.

55. Weller RO, Davis BE, Wilson POG, Mitchell J. In: Cervós-Navarro J, Fritschka E, eds. Cerebral microcirculation and metabolism. New York: Raven Press, 1981: 41.

56. Morantz RA, Feigin I, Ransohoff J. J Neurosurg 1976; 45: 398.

57. Kishikawa M, Tsuda N, Fujii H et al. Acta Neuropathol 1986; 70: 44.

58. Mørk SJ, Lindegaard K-F, Halvorsen TB et al. J Neurosurg 1985; 63: 881.

59. Mørk SJ, Halvorsen TB, Lindegaard K-F, Eide GE. J Neuropathol Exp Neurol 1986; 45: 65.

60. Wilkinson IMS, Anderson JR, Holmes AE. J Neurol Neurosurgry Psychiatry 1987; 50: 304.

61. Herpers MJHM, Budka H. Acta Neuropathol (Berl) 1984; 64: 265.

62. Choi BH, Kim RC. Science 1984; 223: 407.

63. Hart MN, Petito CK, Earl KM. Cancer 1974; 33: 134.

64. Mørk S, Loken C. Cancer 1977; 40: 907.

65. Ilgren EB, Stiller CA, Hughes JT et al. Clin Neuropathol 1984; 3: 113.
66. Patterson RH, Campbell WG, Parsons H. J Neurosurg 1961; 18: 145.
67. Centano RS, Lee AA, Winter J, Barba D. J Neurosurg 1986; 64: 209.
68. Read G. Clin Radiol 1984; 35: 163.
69. Mørk SJ, Rubinstein LJ. Cancer 1985; 55: 1536.
70. Mørk SJ, Risberg G, Krogness K. Neuropathol Appl Neurobiol 1980; 6: 307.
71. Roessmann U, Velasco ME, Sindley SD, Gambetti P. Brain Res 1980; 200: 13.
72. Lewis P. Brain 1967; 90: 177.
73. Coffin CM, Wick MR, Braun JT, Dehner LP. Am J Surg Pathol 1986; 10: 394.
74. Nakashima N, Goto K, Tsukidate K et al. Virchows Arch [Pathol Anat] 1983; 400: 201.
75. Nakashima N Goto K, Takeuchi J. Virchows Arch [Pathol Anat] 1982; 395: 303.
76. Alcolado JC, Moore IE, Weller RO. Neuropathol Appl Neurobiol 1986; 12: 235.
77. Hart MN, Earle KM. Cancer 1973; 32: 890.
78. Smith TW, Davidson RI. Cancer 1984; 54: 323.
79. Pobereskin L, Treip C. J Neurol Neurosurg Psychiatry 1986; 49: 39.
80. Hoshino T, Kobayashi S, Townsend JJ. Cancer 1985; 55: 1711.
81. Packer RJ, Sutton LN, Rorke LB et al. J Neurosurg 1984; 61: 296.
82. Gaffney CC, Sloane JP, Bradley NJ, Bloom HJG. J Neurooncol 1985; 3: 23.
83. Grant JW, Steart PV, Gallagher PJ. Clin Neuropathol 1988; 5: 228.
84. Janzer RC, Kleihues P. Clin Neuropathol 1985; 4: 93.
85. Kepes JJ, Belton K, Roessmann U, Ketercherside WJ. Clin Neuropathol 1985; 4: 1.
86. Southall DP, Lewis GM, Buchanan R, Weller RO. Dev Med Child Neurol 1987; 29: 789.
87. Rubinstein LJ, Herman MM. J Neurol Sci 1972; 16: 27.
88. Trojanowski JQ, Lee V. Acta Neuropathol (Berl) 1983; 59: 155.
89. Roessmann U, Velasco ME, Gambetti P et al. J Neuropathol Exp Neurol 1983; 42: 131.
90. Royds JA, Taylor CB, Timperley WR. Neuropathol Appl Neurobiol 1985; 11: 1.
91. Vinores SA, Rubinstein LJ. Neuropathol Appl Neurobiol 1985; 11: 349.
92. Llena JF. Paraganglioma in the cerebrospinal axis. Progr Neuropathol 1983; 5: 261.
93. Anderson JR, Gullan RW. J Neurol Neurosurg Psychiatry 1987; 50: 100.
94. Lerman RI, Kaplan ES, Daman L. J Neurosurg 1972; 56: 280.
95. Kepes JJ. Meningiomas: biology, pathology and differential diagnosis. New York: Masson, 1982.
96. Battersby RDE, Ironside JW, Maltby EL. J Neurol Neurosurg Psychiatry 1986; 49: 362.
97. Ibrahim AW, Satti MB, Ibrahim EM. J Neurosurg 1986; 64: 328.
98. Kepes JJ. J Neuropathol Exp Neurol 1986; 45: 95.
99. Miller CD, Ojemann RG, Proppe KG et al. J Neurosurg 1985; 62: 763.
100. Moll R, Cowin P, Kaprell H-P, Franke WW. Lab Invest 1986; 54: 4.
101. Parrish EP, Garrod DR, Mattey DK et al. Proc Natl Acad Sci USA 1986; 83: 2657.
101a. Vilela MJ, Parrish EP, Wright DH, Garrod DR. J Pathol 1987; 153: 365.
102. Upton M, Weller RO. J Neurosurg 1985; 63: 867.
103. Alcolado R, Weller RO, Parrish EP, Garrod D. Neuropathol Appl Neurobiol 1988; 14: 1.
104. Sandberg AA. The chromosomes in human cancer and leukaemia. Amsterdam: Elsevier, 1980: 535.
105. Cahill DW, Bashirelahi N, Solomon LW et al. J Neurosurg 1985; 60: 985.
106. Poisson M. Clin Neuropharmacol 1984; 7: 320.
107. Pitkethly DR, Hardman JM, Kempe LG, Earl KM. J Neurosurg 1970; 32: 529.
108. Skullerud K, Loken AC. Acta Neuropathol (Berl) 1974; 29: 337.
109. Ludwin SK, Rubinstein LJ, Russell DS. Cancer 1975; 36: 1363
110. Jaaskeläinen J, Haltia M, Servo A. Surg Neurol 1986; 25: 233.
111. Pesce CM, Sanguineti G, Reale A. Clin Neuropathol 1984; 3: 153.
112. Weller RO, Cervós-Navarro J. Pathology of peripheral nerves. London: Butterworths, 1977.
113. Henderson DW, Papadimitriou JM, Coleman M. Ultrastructural appearances of tumours. Edinburgh: Churchill Livingstone, 1986.
114. Chen KTK, La Torraca R, Fablich D et al. Cancer 1980; 45: 1585.
115. Enzinger FM, Weiss SW. Soft tissue tumors. St Louis: Mosby, 1983.
116. Bundey S. Genetics and neurology. Edinburgh: Churchill Livingstone, 1985.
117. Riccardi VM. N Engl J Med 1981; 305: 1617.
118. Blatt J, Jaffe R, Dentsch M, Adkins JC. Cancer 1986; 57: 1225.
119. Hope DG, Mulvihill JJ. Adv Neurol 1981; 29: 33.
120. Ducatman BS, Scheithauer BW, Piepgras DG et al. Cancer 1986; 57: 2006.
121. Henry JM, Heffner RR, Dillard SH et al. Cancer 1974; 34: 1293.
122. Jellinger K, Scowik F, Sluga E. Clin Neurol Neurosurg 1979; 81: 173.
123. Letendre L, Banks PM, Reese DF et al. Cancer 1982; 49: 939.
124. Allegranza A, Mariani C, Giardini R et al. Histopathology 1984; 8: 781.
125. Marsh WL, Stevenson DR, Long HV. Cancer 1983; 51: 1125.
126. Enzman DR, Krikorian J, Norman D et al. Radiology 1979; 130: 165.
127. Wright DH, Isaacson PG. Biopsy pathology of the lymphoreticular system. London: Chapman & Hall, 1983.
128. Merchut MP, Haberland C, Naheedy MH, Rubino FA. Neurology 1985; 35: 552.
129. Lennert K, Stein M, Kaiserling E. Br J Cancer 1975; 31 (suppl 2): 29.
130. Grant JW, Kaesch D, Jones DB. Histopathology 1986; 10: 1191.
131. Haddad P, Thaell JF, Kiely JM et al. Cancer 1976; 38: 1862.
132. Sanford RA, Smith RA. J Neurosurg 1986; 64: 317.
133. Jeffreys RV, Napier JAF, Reynolds SG. J Neurol Neurosurg Psychiatry 1982; 45: 264.
134. Spence AM, Rubinstein LJ. Cancer 1975; 35: 326.

135. Epstein JI, White CL, Mendelsohn G. Am J Clin Pathol 1983; 81: 285.
136. Ismail SM, Jasani B, Cole G. J Clin Pathol 1985; 38: 417.
137. Pozzati E, Padorani R, Morroni B et al. J Neurosurg 1980; 53: 826.
138. Globini S, Morello G. Acta Neurochir (Wien) 1978; 40: 61.
139. Tagle P, Huete I, Mendez J, del Villar S. J Neurosurg 1986; 64: 720.
140. Lavi E, Jamieson D, Granat M. J Neurol Neurosurg Psychiatry 1986; 49: 709.
141. Graf CJ, Peret GE, Torner JC. J Neurosurg 1983; 58: 331.
142. Guidetti B, Delitala A. J Neurosurg 1980; 53: 149.
143. Drake CG, Friedman AH, Peerless SJ. J Neurosurg 1986; 64: 1.
144. Weller RO. In: Adams JH, Corsellis JAN, Duchen LW, eds. Greenfield's Neuropathology. 4th ed. London: Arnold, 1984: 208.
145. Wakai S, Chen C-H, Wuk Y, Chiu C-W. Arch Neurol 1983; 40: 377.
146. Logue V. J Neurol Neurosurg Psychiatry 1979; 42: 1.
147. Hughes JT. In: Adams JH, Corsellis JAN, Duchen LW, eds. Greenfield's Neuropathology. 4th ed. London: Arnold, 1984: 779.
148. Alonso A, Taboada D, Ceres L et al. Pediatr Radiol 1979; 8: 39.
149. Biller J, Toffol GJ, Shea JF et al. Arch Neurol 1985; 42: 367.
150. Lagos JC. In: Vinken PJ, Bruyn GN, eds. Handbook of clinical neurology. Amsterdam: North Holland, 1977; 31: 137.
151. Yagishita S, Itoh Y, Shiozawa T, Tanaka T. Acta Neuropathol (Berl) 1984; 65: 41.
152. Matsushima T, Fukui M, Kitamura K et al. Surg Neurol 1985; 24: 457.
153. Kovacs K, Horvath E. Tumors of the pituitary gland. 2nd series. Fascicle 21. Washington DC: Armed Forces Institute of Pathology, 1986.
154. Petito CK, De Girolami U, Earle KM. Cancer 1976; 37: 1944.
155. Thomsett MJ, Conte FA, Kaplan SL, Grumbach MM. J Pediatr 1980; 97: 728.
156. Tytus JS, Pennybacker J. J Neurol Neurosurg Psychiatry 1956; 19: 241.
157. Saunders RL. J Neurosurg 1969; 86: 83.
158. DiChiro G, Doppman JL, Dwyer AJ et al. Radiology 1985; 156: 689.
159. Leading article. Lancet 1986; 2: 549.
160. Walls TJ, Purohit DP, Aji WS et al. J Neurol Neurosurg Psychiatry 1986; 49: 438.
161. Agnoli AL, Laun A, Schönmayr R. J Neurosurg 1984; 61: 834.
162. Harsh GR, Edwards MSB, Wilson CB. J Neurosurg 1986; 64: 835.
163. Martinez AJ, Lee A, Moosy J, Maroon JC. Ann Neurol 1980; 7: 24.
164. Volpe R, Mazabrand A. Am J Surg Pathol 1983; 7: 161.
165. Coindre J-M, Rivel J, Trojani M et al. J Pathol 1986; 150: 61.
166. Miettinen M, Lehto VP, Dahl D, Virtanem I. Am J Pathol 1983; 112: 160.
167. Ho L-K. Clin Neuropathol 1985; 4: 77.
168. Bingas B. In: Vinken PJ, Bruyn GW, eds. Handbook of clinical neurology. Amsterdam: North Holland, 1974; 17: 136.
169. Schermer KL, Pontius EE, Dziabis MD, McQuinston RJ. Cancer 1966; 19: 1273.
170. Dahlin DC. Bone tumors. 3rd ed. Springfield: Thomas, 1978.

Metastatic tumours

171. Wolf AL, Adcock LL, Hachiya JT, Klassen A. Cancer 1986; 57: 1432.
172. Gonzalez-Vitale JC, Garcia-Bunuel R. Cancer 1976; 37: 2906.
173. Bamborschke S, Ebhardt G, Szelies-Stock B et al. Clin Neuropathol 1985; 4: 47.
174. Mackintosh FR, Colby TV, Podolsky WJ et al. Cancer 1982; 49: 586.
175. Johnson GJ, Oken MM, Anderson JR et al. Lancet 1984; 2: 685.
176. Price RA. In: Mastrangelo R, Poplack DG, Riccardi R, eds. CNS leukaemia: prevention and treatment. Boston: Martinus Nighoff, 1983: 1.
177. Leading article. Lancet 1985; 1: 1196.
178. Riceruti G, Savoldi F, Piccolo G et al. Arch Neurol 1986; 43: 466.
179. Theaker JM, Gatter KC, Esiri MM, Easterbrook P. Histopathology 1986; 10: 1261.
180. Schwechheimer K, Lemminger JM. Clin Neuropathol 1985; 4: 28.
181. Henson RA, Urich H. Cancer and the nervous system. Oxford: Blackwell, 1982.
182. Kearsley JH, Johnson P, Halmagyi M. Arch Neurol 1985; 42: 1208.
183. Ang LC, Zochodne DW, Ebers GC et al. Acta Neuropathol (Berl) 1986; 69: 171.
184. Jaeckle KA, Graus F, Houghton A et al. Ann Neurol 1985; 18: 592.
185. Thomas PK, Landon DN, King RHM. In: Adams JH, Corsellis JAN, Duchen LW, eds. Greenfield's Neuropathology. London: Arnold, 1984: 807.

Tumours of the peripheral nervous system

186. Young JL, Miller RW. J Pediatr 1975; 86: 254.
187. Sawada T, Hirayama M, Nakata T et al. Lancet 1984; 2: 271.
188. Allan SG, Cornbleet MA, Carmichael J et al. Cancer 1986; 57: 2419.
189. Stowens D. Arch Pathol 1957; 63: 451.
190. Breslow N, McCann B. Cancer Res 1971; 31: 2098.
191. Gitlow SE, Bertani LM, Rausen A et al. Cancer 1970; 25: 1377.
192. Prasad KN, Mandal B, Kumar S. J Pediatr 1973; 82: 677.
193. Hamilton AE, Rubinstein LJ, Poole GJ. J Neurosurg 1973; 38: 548.
193a. Taxy JB, Bharani NK, Mills SE, et al. Am J Surg Pathol 1986; 10: 687.
194. Schochet SS, Peters B, O'Neal J, McCormick WF. Acta Neuropathol (Berl) 1975; 31: 181.
195. Wilson, LMK, Draper GJ. Br Med J 1974; 2: 301.
196. Yokoyama M, Okada K, Tokue A, Takayasu H. Virchows Arch A 1973; 361: 195.

197. Gitlow SE, Dziedzic LB, Strauss L et al. Cancer 1973; 32: 898.
198. Hughes M, Marsden HB, Palmer MK. Cancer 1974; 34: 1706.
199. Shimada H, Chatten J, Newton WA et al. JNCI 1984; 73: 405.
200. Bravo EL, Gifford RW. N Eng J Med 1984; 311: 1298.
201. McEwan AJ, Wyeth P, Ackery D. Appl Radiat Isot 1986; 37: 765.
202. Cervós-Navarro J, Bayer JM, Käser H. Virchows Arch [Pathol Anat] 1973; 361: 51.
203. Glenner GG, Grimley PM. Tumors of the extra-adrenal paraganglion system (including chemoreceptors). 2nd series. Fascicle 9. Washington DC: Armed Forces Institute of Pathology, 1974.
204. Olson JR, Abell MR. Cancer 1969; 23: 1358.
205. Gallagher RL, Helwig EB. Am J Clin Pathol 1980; 74: 759.
206. Fletcher CDM, Chan JK-C, McKee PH. Histopathology 1986; 10: 135.
207. Angervall L, Kindblom L-G, Haglid K. Cancer 1984; 53: 1752.
208. Mathew GJ, Osterholm JL. Surg Clin North Am 1972; 51: 1313.
209. Asbury AK, Johnson PC. Pathology of peripheral nerve. Philadelphia: Saunders, 1978.
210. Weller RO. Lancet 1974; 2: 592.
211. Lallemand RC, Weller RO. J Neurol Neurosurg Psychiatry 1973; 36: 991.
212. Johnson PC, Kline DG. J Neuropathol Exp Neurol 1986; 45: 352.
213. Hirose T, Sano T, Hizawa K. Acta Neuropathol (Berl) 1986; 69: 103.
214. Ochoa J, Neary D. Lancet 1975; 2: 632.
215. Ahmed AH, Weller RO. Neuropathol Appl Neurobiol 1979; 5: 469.

Pineal gland

NORMAL ANATOMY

The pineal (pineal body, epiphysis cerebri) is present in the embryo by the seventh week of development as an evagination of the roof of the third ventricle. It is a small truncated conical glandular body, slightly flattened in the vertical plane, which in the developed brain lies behind the third ventricle. Above it is the splenium of the corpus callosum and the origin of the great vein of Galen, while below it and on either side are the superior corpora quadrigemina. The normal adult pineal is 5–9 mm long and 3–6 mm in diameter. Its weight varies with age. Pineal weights of 30–150 mg have been reported up to the age of about 30 years. In the following two decades the range is 30–90 mg, while from the sixth decade onwards, a range of 50–900 mg is described.[1]

The pineal is covered by pia mater which is continuous with vascular connective tissue septa, penetrating the gland and dividing it into lobules. The pineal arterial supply comes from the medial posterior choroidal branches of the posterior cerebral artery. Small veins drain into the great vein of Galen or the internal cerebral veins. The pineal capillary endothelium is flat and fenestrated in a way comparable to that in other endocrine organs.

Pineal blood vessels are accompanied by un-myelinated post-ganglionic sympathetic nerve fibres which originate from the superior cervical ganglia.[2] The slender pineal stalk also contains nerve fibres of cerebral origin;[3,4] these include some recurrent fibres and appear to be unimportant in the control of pineal function.

Concentric calcified bodies, *corpora arenacea*

(also known as acervuli and psammoma bodies), are found in the pineal parenchyma. They are present in children and their number increases with age; they are the structural basis of the radiological phenomenon of pineal calcification, which is of great diagnostic value in the detection of cerebral midline displacement. Pineal calcific concretions are believed to be of two types, those of connective tissue origin and those derived from parenchymal cells. The latter are composed of a carbonate-containing hydroxyapatite; they are formed in cytoplasmic vacuoles and extruded into the extracellular space.[5]

The pineal parenchyma (Fig. 17.1) consists largely of pinealocytes. These are polygonal cells which stain positively for the 'neuroendocrine' marker, neuron-specific enolase. There is a minority population (about 5%) of glial cells, astrocytic in morphology and staining for glial fibrillary acidic protein.[6] Pinealocytes form sheets or cords arranged into lobules; they have large vesicular nuclei with prominent nucleoli, and a weakly basophilic cytoplasm containing organelles suggestive of active secretory function.[7] Cell processes containing parallel microtubules end in terminal expansions close to capillaries. These expansions contain dense core vesicles, mitochondria and endoplasmic reticulum. Ultrastructurally, the glial cells are typical fibrillary astrocytes with bundles of 5–6 nm microfilaments. Glial processes form a limiting lamina at the periphery of the gland and constitute the boundaries of lobules. Many glial end-feet are apposed to capillaries. Terminal varicosities of post-ganglionic sympathetic fibres are found in perivascular spaces. Some sympathetic terminals may be found between parenchymal cells, but do not appear to synapse with them.

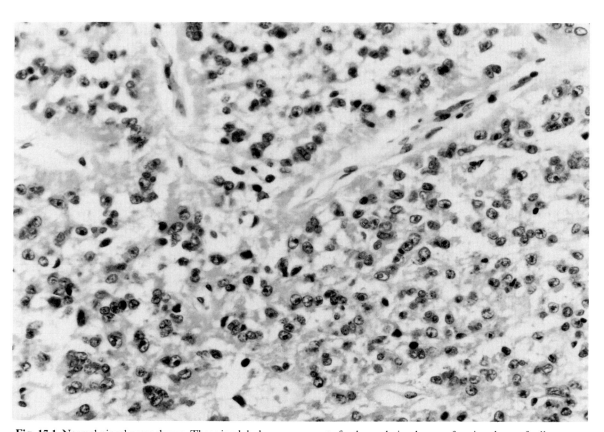

Fig. 17.1 Normal pineal parenchyma. There is a lobular arrangement of polygonal pinealocytes, forming sheets of cells. Haematoxylin-eosin × 900

PHYSIOLOGY

The scientific investigation of pineal physiology has been under way since the beginning of this century. Following early descriptions of embryology, gross and microscopic anatomy, vasculature and nerves, the similarity of the mammalian pineal to the third eye or photosensory epiphyseal organ of other vertebrates was noted. Ablation experiments and administration of pineal extracts were carried out on the supposition that the gland had an endocrine function, notably with respect to the control of the onset of puberty. The early suggestion[8] that the endocrine activity of the pineal gland was influenced by light via the nervous system was developed through the melatonin studies of Wurtman and Axelrod and their colleagues[9,10] into the concept of 'neuroendocrine transduction'. In the following decades experimental studies in animals strengthened the idea that the pineal is a light-influenced regulator of endocrine function. It is now generally held that the gland receives environmental information through the brain and relays this information systemically by humoral action. A number of monoamine and peptide transmitter substances are known to be present in the pineal. Amongst these the indoleamine *melatonin* (N-acetyl-5-methoxytryptamine) is the humoral agent most clearly related to the endocrine function of the gland. Melatonin was identified in 1958[11] as the agent present in pineal extracts which is capable of producing perinuclear aggregation of melanin in amphibian and reptile dermal melanophores, thus causing skin blanching.[12] Melatonin is the product of O-methylation of N-acetylserotonin in pinealocytes under the influence of the enzyme hydroxyindole-O-methyltransferase. The substrate for this reaction is derived from serotonin (present in higher concentration in the pineal than in any other organ), which is itself produced from tryptophane by hydroxylation and decarboxylation.[13] Melatonin biosynthesis is regulated by the influence of noradrenaline, released from sympathetic nerve terminals, on cell membrane β-adrenergic receptors.[14] Melatonin levels in the pineal show cyclical changes in relation to daylight and darkness in a number of mammalian species, peaking during the dark phase.[15] Melatonin synthesis is thus stimulated by lack of external light. Plasma levels of this hormone correlate well with pineal levels, and available evidence indicates that the pineal is probably the only source of circulating melatonin. Melatonin in the circulation is metabolised rapidly; its half-life in rats is about 20 minutes.[16] Cyclical changes in melatonin levels in man have been detected; human urinary excretion of melatonin is also rhythmic, being maximal during the night under normal conditions and during the dark period within a week of artificial phase reversal.

The neural pathway enabling light (or its lack) to regulate melatonin output is believed to involve the retina, suprachiasmatic nuclei (in the ventromedial region of the hypothalamus), the lateral regions of the hypothalamus, the intermediolateral columns of the spinal cord and the superior cervical ganglia.[17]

Melatonin is thought to be a mediator of the seasonal reproductive changes that occur in some species of mammals and that are related to the changing length of day. It has been shown to have a gonadal inhibitory effect. The rôle of melatonin and the pineal in the control of puberty is unclear, despite many clinical observations that pineal neoplasms can produce precocious or delayed puberty. The mechanisms whereby the dark-activated pineal influences reproductive activity are also quite unknown. It has been suggested that melatonin may increase the susceptibility of the hypothalamus to the inhibitory feedback effects of steroid sex hormones on luteinising hormone (LH) and follicle stimulating hormone (FSH) secretion, and that it may act as a temporal coordinating influence in the hypothalamic-pituitary-gonadal axis. It is not known if melatonin acts directly on the CNS, despite observations of sedative and hypnotic effects.

PATHOLOGY

DEVELOPMENTAL DISORDERS

Aplasia or hypoplasia of the pineal occurs rarely. The association of pineal agenesis with retinal dysplasia and other congenital abnormalities has been reported, with the suggestion that pineal maldevelopment was the consequence of the ocular lesion.[18] *Hyperplasia* of the pineal has been described in a family with hirsutism, sexual and mental precocity, adrenal cortical hyperplasia and diabetes mellitus,[19] and in two siblings with acanthosis nigricans, dental dysplasia, genital enlargement and diabetes.[20] It may also occur in Albright's syndrome (polyostotic fibrous dysplasia).[21]

PINEAL CYSTS

Small cysts are often found in the pineal at autopsy.[7,22] They have a glial wall in which Rosenthal fibres, derived from the proliferation of normal benign astrocytes, are sometimes prominent. Clinical manifestations rarely accompany large cysts of this type. Benign cysts of epithelial origin, dermoid and epidermoid, are very uncommon and most are of small size.[23,24] Larger cysts of this type are likely to be part of a mature teratoma of the pineal (see p. 509).

PINEAL NEOPLASMS

Tumours of the pineal will be considered under four categories: (1) germ cell tumours, (2) pinealocytic tumours, (3) miscellaneous primary tumours, and (4) secondary tumours.

General observations

Pineal tumours are rare, and account at most for 1% of all intracranial tumours[25] (though up to 4% in paediatric neurosurgical practice[26]). The overwhelming majority (at least 80%) are of germ cell type. These tumours are far more frequent in males than females (in a ratio of between 6 to 1 and 18 to 1); thus, as a group, pineal tumours occur predominantly in males. Most patients with pineal tumours present clinically below the age of 16, with an average duration of symptoms of about one year. The symptoms and signs of a pineal tumour are related to the pattern of growth. Thus, blockage of the upper end of the aqueduct, which lies very close to the pineal, produces features of hydrocephalus and raised intracranial pressure. Antero-inferior expansion may damage the superior colliculi and the pretectal region of the midbrain to produce characteristic oculomotor disorders which are of value, clinically, for localising the tumour. Downward growth of a tumour, which compresses the cerebellum from above without blocking the aqueduct, causes loss of balance. Extension of the tumour anteriorly into the third ventricle, with involvement of the thalamus, hypothalamus and optic chiasma, may be responsible for mental changes, endocrine abnormalities (including sexual precocity) and visual field defects. Finally, since the pineal is surrounded by cerebrospinal fluid and many of its tumours are highly malignant, multifocal neurological signs, including signs of spinal cord and root damage, may occur as a result of tumour metastasis through the subarachnoid space.

In CT scans, pineal tumours show a slight increase in density with intense enhancement by contrast medium.[27]

Germ cell tumours

The majority of pineal tumours are neoplasms of germ cell type, which are histologically identical to tumours found in the testis and elsewhere. Testicular germ cell tumours have been divided into four classes: seminoma, embryonal carcinoma, choriocarcinoma, and teratoma (mature and immature).[28] Mixed tumours may also occur. As a group, germ cell tumours of the pineal contain representatives of each of these categories.

Germinoma

The pineal counterpart of the testicular seminoma is the germinoma (seminoma-like tumour, atypical teratoma); it is the most frequent (about 60%) of all pineal tumours.[29] Histologically, it is composed of two distinct cell types. Large round or polygonal tumour cells with large nuclei, sometimes in mitosis, showing coarse chromatin and prominent nucleoli, are mingled with small mature lymphocytes (Fig. 17.2). Scanty connective tissue trabeculae are present in these very cellular tumours. The lymphocytes probably represent a host response to the tumour cells. With transplantation of human pineal germinoma to rat brain, the large tumour cells proliferate but the

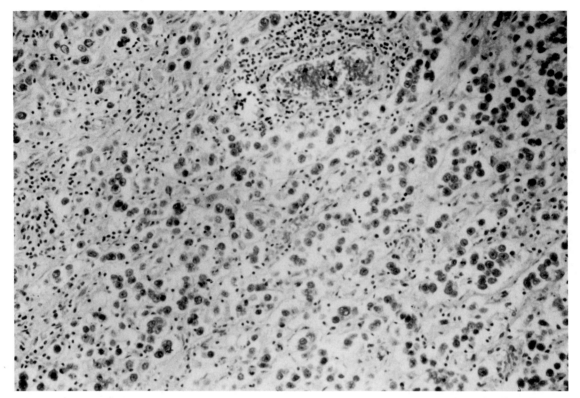

Fig. 17.2 Germinoma. The tumour is composed of diffusely arranged, large, polygonal cells interspersed with small lymphocytes.
Haematoxylin-eosin × 250

lymphocytes disappear.[30] The lymphocytes within the tumour are reported to be T-cells,[31] and both lymphocytes and large tumour cells can sometimes be identified in CSF.[32] A giant-cell granulomatous reaction is seen in some pineal germinomas, as in some testicular seminomas. Pineal germinomas nearly always occur in males and are most common late in the second decade; they are highly malignant tumours. Macroscopically soft, cellular and friable, they destroy the pineal gland, infiltrate adjacent structures, and cause the clinical problems noted above. Germinomas may metastasise widely within the CSF and may spread systemically, usually after craniotomy and shunting.[33,34]

Histologically identical tumours not only develop in the testis as seminomas, but also occur as dysgerminomas in the ovary, and may occasionally be found, apparently as primary tumours, in the mediastinum. Intracranial germinomas are not confined to the pineal. *Supra-sellar germinomas* occur above the pituitary in females as well as males, and primary intracerebral germinomas have been reported.[35] No satisfactory explanation has been offered for the axial scattering of this tumour, or for the simultaneous multifocal occurrence of germ cell tumours in brain, mediastinum and testis.[29,36]

Pineal germinomas may contain heterologous elements other than lymphocytes. Glandular structures, squamous epithelial foci, mesenchyme, muscle, cartilage and trophoblast may be seen in some germinomas, implying that at least part of the tumour is a teratoma (Fig. 17.3).

Embryonal carcinoma, choriocarcinoma and teratoma of the pineal

Both *embryonal carcinoma* and *choriocarcinoma* may be histologically uniform; sometimes, the histological elements of each may be found in the same tumour or they may be mixed, as germi-

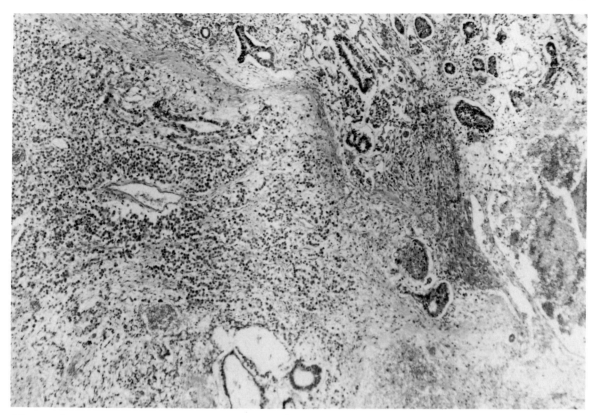

Fig. 17.3 Teratomatous elements in germinoma. Typical germinoma is present to the left of this field. There are neoplastic glandular structures at the top, right.
Haematoxylin-eosin × 60

nomas may be, with mature teratomatous components. These tumours, again like germinomas, typically occur in males in the second decade. Embryonal carcinoma has the most primitive morphology, being composed of sheets or bands of undifferentiated polygonal cells. Foci of trophoblastic or yolk sac differentiation are sometimes seen, as are teratoid elements. Yolk sac differentiation in embryonal carcinoma may be extensive, producing a histological appearance resembling that of the testicular endodermal sinus tumour. α-fetoprotein can be detected in serum, CSF and by immunocytochemistry in tissue sections.[37] Choriocarcinoma is a haemorrhagic tumour which responds to radiotherapy and methotrexate; it shows a histological picture of malignant trophoblastic tissue. High levels of chorionic gonadotrophin in the urine and CSF may be a diagnostic feature.[38] This tumour is reported to occur in the lateral ventricles as well as in the pineal.[38]

Well-differentiated pineal *teratomas* resemble ovarian dermoid cysts (benign teratomas) in showing a wide range of tissue components, including squamous epithelium, hair, glands, cartilage and neural tissue. They are slow-growing, circumscribed tumours, spherical or lobulated, with a variegated and often cystic cut surface. They are sometimes totally cured by surgery. However, as already noted, the histological features of mature teratoma are often found in mixed germ cell tumours with areas of germinoma or embryonal carcinoma.

Pinealocytic tumours

As well as tumours of germ cell type, the pineal may give rise to neoplasms that are morphologically related to the main parenchymatous cell, the pinealocyte. These rare neoplasms can be divided into the more mature pinealocytoma (pineocytoma) and the more primitive pinealoblastoma (pineoblastoma).

Pinealocytoma

This tumour is generally circumscribed and slowly growing; it presents mainly in adolescence and adult life. Males and females are equally affected. Pinealocytomas are composed of small cells with darkly staining nuclei, arranged in lobules separated by slender connective tissue septa (Fig. 17.4). Mitoses are not seen. An arrangement of cells in ribbons interspersed with acellular areas showing weakly eosinophilic, fibrillated material may be a striking feature in the tumour. Eosinophilic polar cytoplasmic processes, often orientated towards blood vessels, have also

been described. Argyrophilia of such processes can be demonstrated. Electron microscopy shows features like those of normal pineal parenchyma, with intracytoplasmic dense core vesicles and numerous slender cytoplasmic processes; many of the processes are closely related to capillary basement membranes (Fig. 17.5).

Pinealocytomas may be amenable to surgical removal, and do not usually metastasise via the cerebrospinal fluid, though some histologically typical cases follow an aggressive course and seed widely throughout the neuraxis. Survival for as long as 13 years has been reported, though most patients die within 6 years.[39,40]

Pinealoblastoma

In contrast to the pinealocytoma, the pinealoblastoma behaves in a uniformly aggressive manner, comparable to that of medulloblastoma

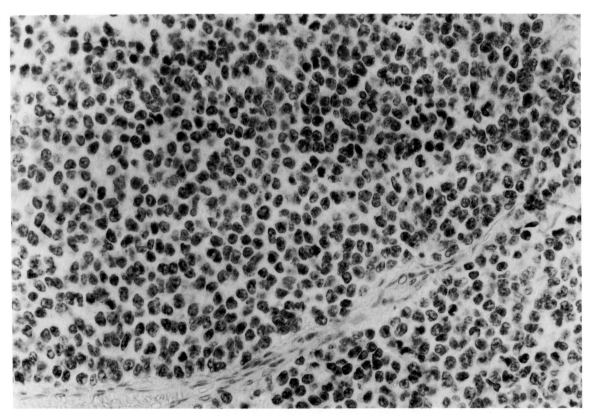

Fig. 17.4 Pinealocytoma. Sheets of cells resembling normal pinealocytes are arranged in lobules. Haematoxylin-eosin × 900

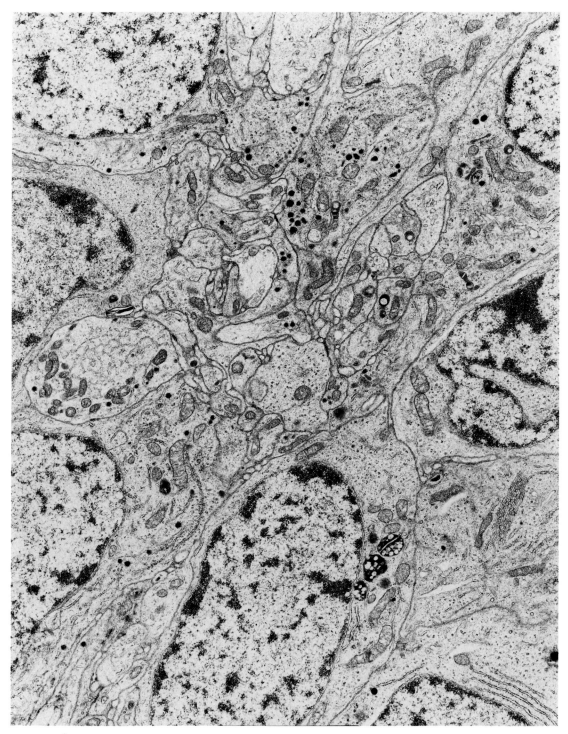

Fig. 17.5a Pinealocytoma. Electron micrograph of a solid area of the tumour showing clumps of tumour cells separated by numerous fine interlacing processes. Small dense core vesicles can be seen in many cells and processes. (See Fig. 17.5b.) × 6825

Reproduced by permission of Dr T. H. Moss, Department of Neuropathology, Frenchay Hospital, Bristol, UK.

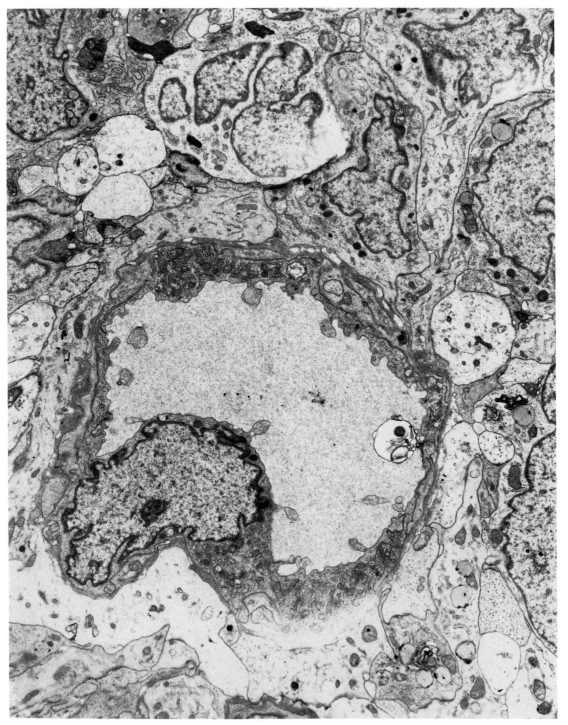

Fig. 17.5b Pinealocytoma. The tumour cells and their processes are closely related to the capillary basement membrane, as in normal pineal tissue. (See Fig. 17.5a.)
×4560
Reproduced by permission of Dr T. H. Moss, Department of Neuropathology, Frenchay Hospital, Bristol, UK.

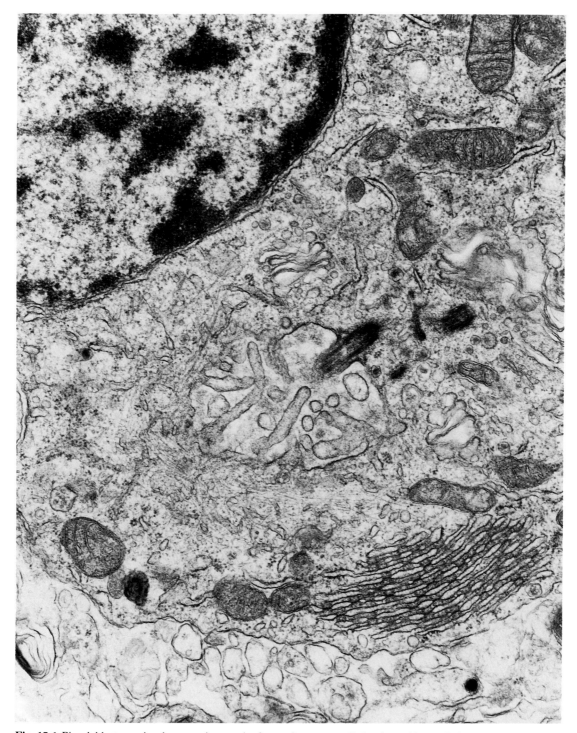

Fig. 17.6 Pinealoblastoma. An electron micrograph of part of a tumour cell showing evidence of photoreceptor differentiation. Cilia are seen projecting into an intracytoplasmic lumen; a well-formed annulate lamella is present at the bottom, right.

× 22 780

Reproduced by permission of Dr T. H. Moss, Department of Neuropathology, Frenchay Hospital, Bristol, UK.

(see p. 455). It resembles this tumour morphologically, being composed of closely packed small primitive cells with a high nucleus–cytoplasmic ratio; these cells may form rosettes of neuroblastic type. Mitoses and pyknoses are evident. Lobulation may be seen. Retinoblastomatous differentiation may also occur, with the formation of the rosettes characteristic of retinoblastoma occurring in the eye; cilia with the $9+0$ configuration, characteristic of photoreceptor cells as well as some endocrine cells, are also seen (Fig. 17.6). As with neuroblastoma, pinealoblastoma may show evidence of histological differentiation; a mosaic pattern, with larger pinealocytic cells interspersed with smaller pinealoblastic cells, may be seen. Nevertheless, all such tumours are highly aggressive, with local invasion and a tendency to metastasise through the CSF. They occur mainly in young children and, although radiosensitive, they are generally fatal within two years. Pinealoblastoma may be familial.[41] It has been reported in association with retinoblastoma ('trilateral retinoblastoma' or 'ectopic intracranial retinoblastoma').[42]

Miscellaneous primary tumours

The glial cells of the normal pineal can potentially give rise to a variety of *gliomas*. Clinically, these would present in a way indistinguishable from the other pineal neoplasms. *Glioblastoma*[43] and more highly differentiated astrocytic tumours such as *astroblastoma* have been reported. It should be noted that the precise site of origin of an infiltrative astrocytic tumour in the region of the pineal, the third ventricle and the tectum of the midbrain might be impossible to ascertain at autopsy.[29]

Glial and neuronal elements may be combined in pineal tumours of neuroectodermal type. Pineal *ganglioglioma* and *ganglioneuroma* have been des-

cribed. Neoplastic ganglion cells interspersed with fibrillary astrocytic tissue may be incorporated in a tumour showing areas of pinealocytoma.[29]

Meningiomas sometimes originate from the pineal.[44] They may be large enough to occlude the great vein of Galen.[45] Various histological types, including angioblastic meningioma, have been described.[46] *Chemodectoma* has been reported to arise from the pineal.[47] Its cells, which morphologically are the same as those of a pinealocytoma, are arranged in lobules separated by sinusoids, with an overall pattern resembling both normal pineal and chemodectomas elsewhere in the body. Other primary tumours reported as arising in the pineal include *cavernous haemangioma*[48] and *craniopharyngioma*.[49]

A *tuberculoma* may mimic a pineal neoplasm.[50]

Secondary tumours

Adult patients presenting with hydrocephalus and features of a tectal plate lesion are occasionally found to have metastatic carcinoma in the pineal. In different series, 1–4% of cases with metastases in the brain show pineal involvement.[51,52] Even at the lower figure, the pineal would appear to be affected disproportionately often, taking into account its size and weight. However, this apparently high incidence of secondary deposits can probably be accounted for by its rich blood supply, with a minimum flow per gram of tissue greater than that of most endocrine organs.[53]

Pineal weights are increased in middle-aged and elderly patients who have died of cancer, and it has been claimed that the heaviest glands are found in those with either carcinoma of breast or melanoma.[54] Histological findings suggest that this phenomenon is not due to occult metastasis.[55]

As well as a variety of carcinomas, myeloma may be deposited in the pineal.[56]

REFERENCES

1. Rodin AE, Overall J. Cancer 1967; 20: 1203.
2. Kappers JA. Z Zellforsch 1960; 52: 163.
3. Rønnekliev OK, Møller M. Exp Brain Res 1979; 37: 551.
4. Dafney N. Life Sci 1980; 26: 737.
5. Welsh MG. Pineal Res Rev 1985; 3: 41.
6. Higley HR, McNulty JA, Rowden G. Brain Res 1984; 304: 117.
7. Erlich SS, Apuzzo MLJ. J Neurosurg 1985; 63: 321.
8. Bargmann W. In: Mollendorf W, ed. Handbuch der mikroskopischen Anatomie des Menschen, vol 6. Berlin: Springer, 1943: 309.
9. Wurtman RJ, Axelrod J, Chu EW. Science 1963; 141: 277.
10. Wurtman RJ, Axelrod J, Phillips LS. Science 1963; 142: 1071.

11. Lerner AB, Case JD, Takahashi Y et al. J Am Chem Soc 1958; 80: 2587.
12. McCord CP, Allen FP. J Exp Zool 1917; 23: 207.
13. Axelrod J, Weissbach H. Science 1960; 131: 1312.
14. Axelrod J. Science 1974; 184: 1341.
15. Ozaki Y, Lynch H, Wurtman RJ. Endocrinology 1976; 98: 1418.
16. Pang SF. Pineal Res Rev 1985; 3: 115.
17. Moore RY. In: Ganong WF, Martini L, eds. Frontiers in neuroendocrinology, vol 5. New York: Raven Press, 1978: 185.
18. Mori W, Okeda R. Acta Pathol Jpn 1973; 23: 359.
19. Rabson SM, Mendenhall EN. Am J Clin Pathol 1956; 26: 283.
20. West RJ, Borin HZ, Turner WML, Lloyd JK. Arch Dis Childh 1972; 47: 153.
21. McMahon H. Pathol Annu 1971; 6: 81 [p. 135].
22. Smith RA, Estridge NM. In: Vinken PJ, Bruyn GW, eds. Handbook of clinical neurology, vol 17. Tumours of the brain and skull, part II. Amsterdam: North Holland, 1974: 648.
23. Sambasivan M, Nayar A. J Neurol Neurosurg Psychiatry 1974; 37: 1333.
24. McDonnell DE. Surg Neurol 1977; 7: 387.
25. Russell DS, Rubinstein LJ. Pathology of tumours of the nervous system. 5th ed. revised by Rubinstein LJ. London: Arnold, 1989: 380.
26. Zülch, KJ. In: Voth D, Gutjahr P, Langmaid C, eds. Tumours of the central nervous system in infancy and childhood. Berlin: Springer, 1982: 3.
27. Jooma R, Kendall BE. J Neurosurg 1983; 58: 654.
28. Mostofi FK, Price EB. Tumors of the male genital system. Washington DC: Armed Forces Institute of Pathology, 1973: 16.
29. Rubinstein LJ. Tumors of the central nervous system. Washington DC: Armed Forces Institute of Pathology, 1972: 269.
30. Miyakawi H, Ishii S. Arch Pathol 1960; 70: 508.
31. Neuwalt EA, Smith RG. Ann Neurol 1979; 6: 133.
32. Gindhart TD, Tsukuhara YC. Acta Cytol (Baltimore) 1979; 23: 341.
33. Rubery ED, Wheeler TK. J Neurosurg 1980; 53: 562.
34. Howman-Giles R, Besser M, Johnson IH, da Silva M. J Neurosurg 1984; 60: 835.
35. Tanaka R, Ueki K. Surg Neurol 1979; 12: 239.
36. Dayan AD, Marshall AHE, Miller AA, Pick FJ, Rankin NE. J Pathol Bacteriol 1966; 92: 1.
37. Arita N, Bitoh S, Ushio Y et al. J Neurosurg 1980; 53: 244.
38. Kawakami Y, Yamada D, Tabuchi K, Ohmoto T, Nishimoto A. J Neurosurg 1980; 53: 369.
39. Herrick MK, Rubinstein LJ. Brain 1979; 102: 289.
40. Borit A, Blackwood W, Mair WGP. Cancer 1980; 45: 1408.
41. Lesnick JE, Chayt KJ, Bruce DA et al. J Neurosurg 1985; 62: 930.
42. Bader JL, Meadows AT, Zimmerman LE et al. Cancer Genet Cytogenet 1982; 5: 203.
43. Kalynaram UP. Arch Neurol 1979; 36: 717.
44. Sachs E, Avman N, Fisher RG. J Neurosurg 1962; 19: 325.
45. Sakaki S, Shiraishi T, Takeda S, Matsuoko K, Sadamoto K. J Neurosurg 1984; 61: 1136.
46. Olson JR, Abell MR. J Neurol Neurosurg Psychiatry 1969; 32: 445.
47. Smith WT, Hughes B, Ermocilla R. J Pathol Bacteriol 1966; 92: 69.
48. Vaquero J, Carrillo R, Cabezudo J, Leunda G, Villoria F, Bravo G. J Neurosurg 1980; 53: 833.
49. Solarski A, Panke ES, Panke TW. Arch Pathol 1978; 102: 490.
50. Whittle IR, Allsop JL, Besser M. J Neurosurg 1983; 59: 875.
51. Ortega P, Malamut N, Shimkin MG. Arch Pathol 1951; 52: 518.
52. Halpert B, Erickson EE, Fields WS. Arch Pathol 1960; 69: 93.
53. Goldman H, Wurtman RJ. Nature 1964; 203: 87.
54. Tapp E. Prog Brain Res 1979; 52: 481.
55. Tapp E, Blumfield M. Br J Cancer 1970; 24: 67.
56. Holness RO, Sangalang VE. Surg Neurol 1976; 5: 97.

PART 2

Peripheral Nervous System

J. B. Cavanagh

Normal peripheral nerve

INTRODUCTION

The principal function of peripheral nerves is to act as lines of communication bringing information from sensory transducers in the skin, muscle and other organs to the central nervous system (CNS) and to convey motor commands from the CNS to somatic muscle and to other effector organs controlled by the autonomic nervous system. To perform these tasks, peripheral nerves must be able to convey signals rapidly over considerable distances, to supply terminal axonal regions with material necessary for cell-to-cell transmission and at the same time to maintain their own integrity, by rapid transport of materials both from the perikaryon (cell body) as well as in the reverse direction. Unlike the central nervous system, peripheral nerves must also be able to regenerate and repair any damage that may be inflicted by minor trauma due to their exposed situation. In this last property they differ strikingly from the CNS fibres, in which repair mechanisms have been discarded during the course of evolution in favour of the development of synaptic complexity and the organisation of integrative circuitry.

To achieve these specialised ends, peripheral nerves are enclosed by the *perineurial sheath* from the site where they leave the pia-arachnoid meningeal sheath to the point where they are surrounded by the special cells encasing their terminals (Fig. 18.1). This sheath encloses a unique compartment, the *endoneurium*, which must provide the optimal milieu for the conduction of the nerve impulse and, at the same time, possess the mechanical properties necessary for protecting the delicate nerve fibres from trivial injury. In addition, the endoneurium provides the lubrication needed for the longitudinal slippage of nerve fibres required during body and limb movements. The milieu of the endoneurium is protected from the general body tissues by a selectively permeable *blood-nerve barrier* and by the absence of lymphatics. The endoneurium is, however, in continuity with the extracellular space of the CNS proximally, as shown by injection studies, and with the extracellular space of muscles at the nerve terminals. Thus substances, including viruses and toxins, which find their way to muscles, are able to pass fairly freely into the endoneurial space and thus gain access to uptake mechanisms at the axon surface. Peripheral nerves, therefore, in addition to being subject to the pathological processes that affect the CNS, are subject to other factors, not shared by the CNS,

which play significant rôles in the genesis of disease.

PERINEURIUM, EPINEURIUM AND ENDONEURIUM

The *perineurium* (Fig. 18.1) consists of one to many sheets (usually not more than 8) of flattened cells surrounding the endoneurial space in which the nerve fibres lie. This sheath is continuous proximally with the pia-arachnoid sheath;[1,2] both are probably derived, together with Schwann cells, largely from the neural crest. Perineurial cells are surrounded by basement membrane and bound together by tight junctions so that, as with the blood-nerve barrier, all materials must pass through the cells by means of numerous caveoli and pinocytotic vesicles. External to the peri-

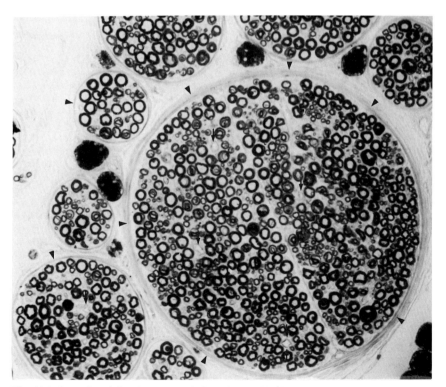

Fig. 18.1 A small peripheral nerve consisting of several fascicles, each surrounded by a perineurial sheath (arrow heads) within which the endoneurium contains myelinated fibres of various sizes. Septa divide the large fascicle, and blood vessels (small arrows) are faintly visible. Outside the perineurium, the epineurial tissue contains a few large (black) fat cells. Specimen from a normal cat.
Osmium-fixed, iron haematoxylin × 100

neurium is the *epineurium*, composed of connective tissue, normal diameter (70–85 nm) collagen fibres and lymphatics. Internal to the perineurium lies the endoneurial space, which is thus a closed compartment, for the perineurium is impermeable to substances applied to its outer surface and both its barrier and its transport functions are energy-dependent.

The *endoneurium* is essentially a specialised extracellular space containing, as well as the nerve fibres and the vascular bed, small diameter (50–60 nm) collagen fibres and a matrix of neutral and acidic glycoproteins that stain with the PAS reaction, with Alcian blue and with colloidal iron.[3] This material is viscous and impedes the move-

ment of substances injected into the endoneurial space, but this resistance to flow can be overcome by adding hyaluronidase to the injected material. The source of the matrix material is unknown but may be the perineurial cells, the fibroblasts of the endoneurium or the Schwann cells themselves. It not only provides lubrication for the longitudinal sliding of nerve fibres within nerve bundles during limb and body movements, but also controls the ionic environment of the nerve fibres. Mast cells are seen in the endoneurial space, and their number increases in any form of injury. Their rôle is unknown.

The *vascular bed* of peripheral nerves is supplied with blood from arteries in the local region, and the

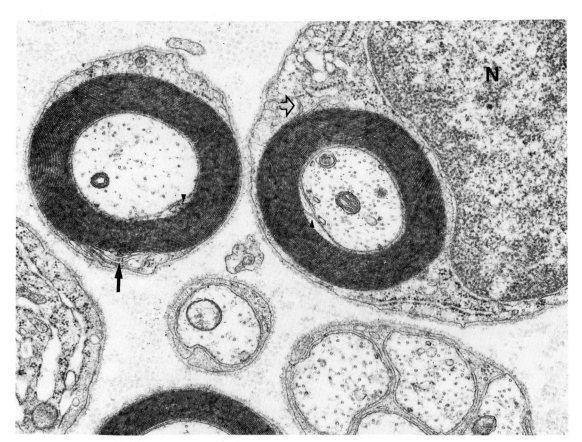

Fig. 18.2 Electron micrograph of two myelinated axons. Right, a Schwann cell nucleus (N) with little surrounding cytoplasm containing a few short strands of rough endoplasmic reticulum. Note an inner mesaxon (arrowhead) in each fibre and an outer mesaxon also visible (open arrowhead): in one sheath there are desmosome-like junctions visible (arrow). Note also abundance of microtubules, often lying close to mitochondria, both in these small myelinated axons and in nearby unmyelinated axons (bottom).
× 30 000
Reproduced by permission of Dr D. N. Landon, Institute of Neurology, London, UK.

presence of many collaterals prevents local ischaemia unless a major artery is blocked or many small vessels become obstructed by disease. Like that of the CNS, the capillary bed of peripheral nerves is a closed system, the endothelial cells being welded together by tight junctions; there are no fenestrations. The blood-nerve barrier has, with minor differences, the properties of the blood-brain barrier (see p. 30),[4] except in sensory ganglia where there are tight junctions but there are also occasional fenestrations through the endothelial cells.[5] As a result, substances in the plasma can easily enter the extracellular space of sensory ganglia, passing readily between satellite cells to reach the surface of nerve cells. Because of this it must be supposed that primary sensory cells have their own protective mechanisms against harmful substances from the plasma. Indeed, sensory neurons are unusually exposed to damage by toxic and other damaging agents.

SCHWANN CELLS AND MYELIN

Development

Axons everywhere outside the CNS are ensheathed by Schwann cells. These cells are probably derived from the neural crest whence they migrate along the developing nerve paths, and come eventually to ensheath all the bundles of immature axons. With increasing functional activity, maturing axons enlarge and, when about 0.5 µm or so in diameter, become segregated from their smaller fellows and enveloped by a chain of Schwann cells that initially lie at regular intervals of about 200 µm along their length. At this point, the Schwann cells begin to spin out a spiral of plasma membrane that after ten or more turns becomes the compacted myelin sheath around the axon. Each Schwann cell forms a separate segment or internode of myelin and, as the compaction process of the loosely wound membrane proceeds, the contained cytoplasm is extruded and at the same time the two external faces of the plasma membrane come into close contact. The final result is a compacted sheath which has a regular periodicity of membrane profiles, when seen in section, with the major dense line representing the two inner surfaces coming together with exclusion

of the cytoplasm, while the minor dense line is the remnant of the external surfaces of the membranes (Fig. 18.2).

The internodes of any one axon do not all begin to myelinate at the same time. Myelination proceeds in a proximo-distal direction, and once begun it continues slowly for many years until all body growth has ceased. Moreover, different axons do not all begin to myelinate at the same time. In consequence, the earliest internodes to myelinate will be elongated by the process of growth of the part in which they lie, and myelinating internodes coming later into the system will show a correspondingly smaller amount of longitudinal growth. In this way, in the adult nerve, a range of internodal lengths is produced (Fig. 18.3) from about 250 µm up to 1000 µm or more in those parts of the body, such as the limbs, that have grown the most.[6] Proximally lying nerves, such as cranial nerves, show the least amount of internodal growth. By the same token the distribution of fibre sizes seen in transverse section of any peripheral nerve is a historical record of the ages of onset of myelination in the different fibres. Myelination thus begins first in the group I sensory fibres that run from the annulospiral formation of muscle spindles and many Golgi tendon organs, and in α-motor fibres going to somatic muscle. Muscles with spindles will thereby tend to have nerves with a bimodal fibre size distribution, while those without will tend to have a unimodal fibre diameter distribution.[7]

The adult Schwann cell

In the peripheral and autonomic nervous systems, the chief function of Schwann cells is the formation and maintenance of myelin; one Schwann cell forms one distinct internode of myelin. This special membrane formation provides the electrical resistance that enables the increase in velocity of impulse conduction from about 1–2 metres/second in unmyelinated fibres to 50–60 metres/second or more in the largest diameter myelinated fibres. While one major function of the Schwann cell is to maintain the myelin sheath for the life of the individual, a second and equally important function is to aid in some, as yet, undefined way the ionic functions

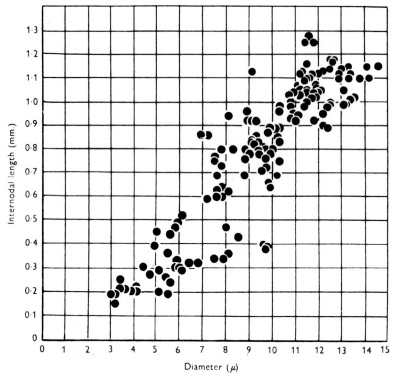

Fig. 18.3 Graph of internodal lengths versus fibre diameter in the ulnar nerve of a 67-year-old woman. Note the general linear relationship, but there are several fibres with abnormally short internodes that are likely to have been produced in adult life, when growth has ceased, as the result of minor nerve injury and remyelination.
Reproduced by permission of the author and editor from: Vizoso A. J Anat 1950; 84: 342.

concerned in the propagation of the action potential at the nodes of Ranvier. Both functions, if disturbed by disease, lead to profound slowing or cessation of conduction of the nerve impulse even though the axon itself may remain in contact with the peripheral organ.

The nucleus of the resting Schwann cell is long and relatively thin with rather square-cut ends (see Fig. 19.1a). The cytoplasm seen by electron microscopy contains moderate amounts of rough-surfaced endoplasmic reticulum, polyribosomes, an inconspicuous Golgi apparatus and many longitudinally running microtubules. Occasionally π-granules are seen in the region of the nucleus. These stain metachromatically with basic dyes and ultrastructurally consist of partly compacted membrane lamellae of doubtful origin.

Myelin formation and general structure have

been described above. In the adult peripheral nerve, myelin has a spiral structure with a repeat distance of the lamellae in aldehyde-fixed nerves of about 13·5 nm, but from X-ray diffraction and other studies on unfixed nerve a more accurate figure of about 18·0 nm is obtained. The difference is likely to be due to shrinkage during tissue preparation. In electron micrographs of transverse sections of myelinated fibres a mesaxon is invariably seen running from the surface plasma membrane and is continuous with the first turn of the myelin. There is not infrequently a zonula adherens in the double membrane, and tight junctions have also been found in this region which may hinder the entry of small molecules into the space between the two myelin membranes. At the inner or adaxonal region of the myelin spiral there is a bleb of Schwann cell cytoplasm which may also have tight junctions between the two investing membranes. Very occasionally, and especially in the spinal roots, there are clusters of fine filaments (7–8 nm) in the adaxonal region of Schwann cell cytoplasm[8] which have similarities with Hirano bodies and stain for actin.[9]

Schmidt–Lantermann clefts or incisures are apparent splits that extend through the compact internodal myelin. They increase in numbers as the myelin becomes thicker with growth, and represent a systematic loosening of the compact myelin to allow the cytoplasm to extend through the compacted lamellae to the adaxonal region of the cell. The opening, or splitting, is in the major dense (cytoplasmic) line; microtubules and an occasional mitochondrion can be identified within the cytoplasmic space so formed.[10] Tight junctions have been seen between the membranes here as in other regions where the myelin opens out. It should be noted that myelin compaction appears to be unstable adjacent to these clefts, and artefactual swelling and disorganisation of the lamellae are often seen here in suboptimally prepared specimens.

Nodes of Ranvier

At regular intervals along a myelinated fibre, individual Schwann cells make contact with one another and with the axon in a highly organised manner at the nodes of Ranvier.[11] These regions (Fig. 18.4) are concerned specifically with the ionic and metabolic events involved in saltatory propagation of the action potential along nerve fibres. They are, in fact, the only points where the axon is directly exposed to the extracellular space and through which it is possible for substances in the endoneurial space to enter the axon, as shown experimentally by the local introduction of horse-radish peroxidase (molecular weight 48 000). At each node of Ranvier (Fig. 18.5) the adjacent Schwann cell forms numerous microvilli (about 75 nm diameter) that make contact with the surface of the axon plasma membrane so that in larger axons little more than about 10% of the surface may be uncovered. Between the microvillous processes there is an acidic glycoprotein covering ('gap substance') which has the capacity to bind cations and may thus act as a cationic 'sink' to limit

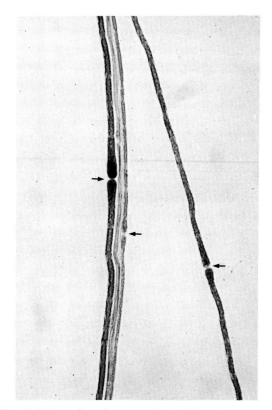

Fig. 18.4 Nerve fibres from cat stained with osmium tetroxide and teased in araldite. Note that the fibres vary in size. Nodes of Ranvier (arrows), where two internodes of myelin make contact; the proximal paranode is very slightly bigger than the distal paranode.
× 370
Reproduced by permission of Professor T. W. Boulding, University of North Carolina, Chapel Hill, NC, USA.

the flow of ions away from the nodal region.[12] This material is specifically stainable by the copper ferrocyanide method. Immediately beneath the axolemma there is another electron dense layer that stains selectively with the ferricyanide-osmium method.[13] This layer is very similar in appearance and staining property to the sub-axolemmal density present at the initial segment of the axon.[14] It has been suggested that such a structure may be in some way related to the concentration of sodium channels known to occur at these sites.

The juxtanodal region lying immediately on either side of the nodal region is the site of attachment of the loops of myelin that form the lower and upper limits of adjacent internodes. Here, the

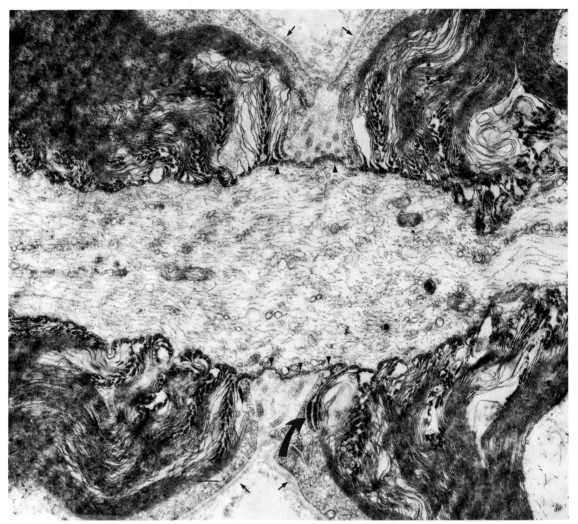

Fig. 18.5 Electron micrograph of a longitudinal section of a node of Ranvier. Externally there is fluffy basement membrane (small arrows): Schwann cell processes, surrounded by amorphous gap-substance material, are seen reaching to make contact with the axon membrane between the two myelinated internodes. The nodal axon membrane has a characteristic dense undercoat (arrowheads). Note that the loops of Schwann cell cytoplasm, seen as dark 'commas', are reflected away from the surface of the axon in a herring-bone pattern. Each contains one or two microtubules not visible at this magnification. Desmosomal junctions sealing the myelin membranes are present (curved arrow).
× 5000
Reproduced by permission of Dr D. N. Landon, Institute of Neurology, London, UK.

compact myelin opens at the major dense (cyto-plasmic) line and there is a tongue of cytoplasm containing several microtubules and an occasional mitochondrion. It is in fact the main spiral passage from the outer Schwann cell cytoplasm to the inner adaxonal regions of the cell. It is also the point where the internode will grow in length during development by the addition of further

membrane. The spiral of the myelin loops is closely applied to the axon and indents it to some extent, and indeed large diameter axons are significantly constricted thereby in the juxtanodal regions. While the two membranes are thus closely applied, there is no good evidence that they are in fact attached to one another, though there appear to be particles in the axonal membrane that further restrict the space between the two membranes.[15] Lanthanum ions can enter the axonal-Schwann cell space with difficulty[16] so that it is probable that here too there is restriction of ionic flow between the two cells.

In the paranodal regions lying beyond the juxta-nodal region there is usually some expansion of the axons, especially visible in large diameter fibres; at the same time there is folding or fluting of the myelin. Within the troughs formed by the fluted myelin, the Schwann cell cytoplasm contains many small mitochondria crowded together that may well provide energy for the functions of the microvilli that spread out into the nodal region from this part of the cytoplasm. It is probable that this region of the Schwann cell actively controls the concentration of Na^+ ions, perhaps by providing energy for the ionic pumping process at the axon membrane, which itself is poorly provided with mitochondria. Within the axon of the paranodal region it is not unusual, especially in the spinal root regions, to see intrusions of Schwann cell cytoplasm pushing into the axoplasm; it is suspected that such formations may be a way of removing effete or abnormal material from the axon. Such intrusions are said to be increased in number in experimental pathological conditions, such as acrylamide intoxication (see p. 272).[17]

Schwann cells are surrounded throughout their length by a sleeve of basement membrane and outside this there is a layer of small diameter collagen which in silver preparations for reticulin

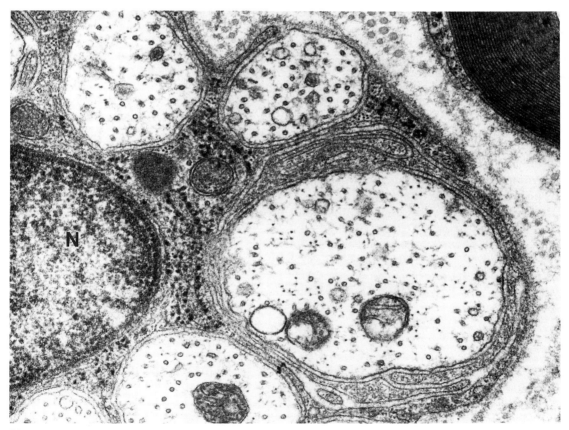

Fig. 18.6 Part of a Remak cell (nucleus, N) with a few strands of rough endoplasmic reticulum, and electron dense processes surrounding several unmyelinated axons. Basement membrane lies outside. Note conspicuous microtubules in axons, related particularly to mitochondria and smooth endoplasmic reticulum: there are very few filaments.
Electron micrograph × 53 000
Reproduced by permission of Dr D. N. Landon, Institute of Neurology, London, UK.

is seen to form a distinct sheath (Plenk–Laidlaw sheath). This is part of the collagenous matrix of the endoneurium[18] and the tropocollagen needed for its formation is probably secreted by the Schwann cells. The Plenk–Laidlaw sheath is minimal or absent in the spinal roots, which may account for the greater delicacy of the latter and the greater difficulty experienced in teasing out single nerve fibres from them than from more peripheral nerve.

REMAK CELLS

Of the same lineage as Schwann cells, Remak cells surround bundles of unmyelinated axons to serve a similar rôle in segregating the axons from endoneurium (Fig. 18.6). As many as 10 or more small axons may be thus buried in the cytoplasm of the cell, each with a small mesaxon attaching it to the exterior.[19] Remak cells form a continuous sheath for the unmyelinated fibres, but show no special modifications at any site.

NEURONAL SATELLITE CELLS

All neurons of sensory ganglia are surrounded by satellite cells that are analogous to Schwann cells and Remak cells. They are flattened cells which overlie the surface of the neurons (Fig. 18.7) and cover them completely, with their edges interdigitating. They maintain a constant numerical relationship with the surface area of the neuron; the surface area they cover remains more or less the same regardless of neuronal size.[20] Satellite cells have no special structural features other than occasionally showing villus-like processes in the space adjacent to the neuronal plasma membrane. They are occasionally found in mitosis, presumably as part of the normal process of growth, and they react to axonal section by a burst of mitoses—in response, perhaps, to the slight increase in neuron size following that event. When the sensory nerve cell dies for any reason, the satellite cells proliferate and there is left behind a ball of cells known as a residual nodule (*nodule résiduelle* of Nageotte).

NEURONS

Apart from the special sense organs, there are three types of neuron that are the source of axons in peripheral nerves: the sensory cells of spinal and cranial nerve ganglia, the motor nerve cells of the spinal cord and of the cranial nerve nuclei in the brainstem, and the cells of the autonomic nervous system. The second set of neurons has very different origins and environment from the other two, but all have the same basic internal organisation and show the same responses to injury.

Sensory ganglion cells

Primary sensory cells are gathered in the dorsal root and cranial nerve ganglia and are referred to as sensory ganglion cells. Their axons carry information from sensory transducers in the skin, muscles and other body organs to the CNS. In common with Schwann cells, melanoblasts, cells of the adrenal medulla, and certain derivatives of the branchial arches, sensory ganglion cells are derived from the neural crest tissue. They and the autonomic ganglion cells are the only neurons unprotected by vascular barriers. They are, however, surrounded everywhere by satellite cells, described briefly above, that may well have protective and nutritional functions.[20] Unlike the neurons of the CNS and the autonomic nervous system, sensory ganglion cells receive no somatic synaptic contacts; all their synaptic relationships are in their terminal regions within the CNS.

The cell body, or perikaryon, of sensory cells is round or oval and varies greatly in size, ranging from rather less than 20 μm to more than 60 μm in diameter (Fig. 18.7b). Two principal morphological forms can be distinguished—a large palely staining cell (large light cell, or type A), and a small darkly staining cell (small dark cell, or type B).[21] The former has well demarcated blocks of Nissl material scattered throughout the cytoplasm; about 5% of these cells contain abundant neurofilaments, sufficiently distinctive to warrant distinguishing them as A2 cells. The type B cells have less well ordered Nissl material and are more electron dense with fewer neurofilaments in the cytoplasm. The smaller cells and a few of the larger cells stain positively for peptides such as substance

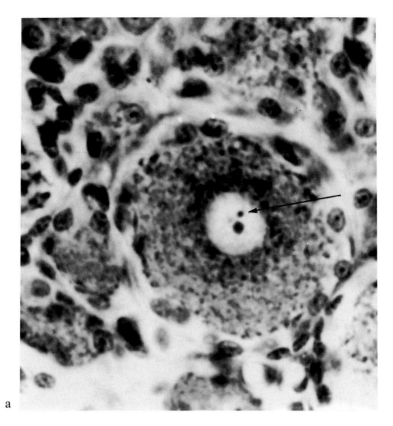

a

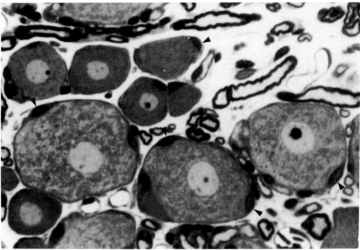

b

Fig. 18.7a, b (**a**) Paraffin section of cat spinal ganglion fixed by perfusion of formol-acetic acid, showing a large neuron with conspicuous flakes of Nissl material. Note the large nucleus; a female sex body (arrow) lies next to the nucleolus. (**b**) Resin section of rat spinal ganglion fixed by perfusion with glutaraldehyde. Note the greater clarity of detail, the large light neurons with flakes of Nissl material and the small dark neurons, the satellite nuclei (arrow heads), and the conspicuous nucleoli.
(**a**) Cresyl fast violet × 750. (**b**) Toluidine blue × 930

P, metenkephalin, etc. The larger cells usually stain for acetylcholinesterase. In contrast, satellite cells stain positively for pseudocholinesterase. Small dark cells almost exclusively serve autonomic functions and less discriminative senses, while large light cells are mainly concerned with more discriminatory somatic sensations from muscle, skin and other tissues.

The nucleus and the nucleolus of sensory cells are large and there is a well-correlated linear size relationship between these and the cell. Cell size, indeed, appears to depend upon the projection field of the peripheral fibre[22] and is likely to be, therefore, a reflection of the amount of synthetic activity in the cell necessary for providing maintenance materials for the axon and its terminal regions.

Ultrastructurally, there is an abundance of rough endoplasmic reticulum (RER) and polyribosomes in the perikaryon, but there are few if any single ribosomes in the normal cell. The Golgi apparatus is abundant, while the smooth endoplasmic reticulum (SER) forms a relatively sparse network between the blocks of Nissl substance.[23] Mitochondria are small and numerous everywhere in the cell, while dense bodies are not uncommon.

Large molecular weight materials, such as horseradish peroxidase (MW 48 000), can be shown to reach the surface of the sensory neuron readily from the bloodstream, through fenestrations in the capillary endothelial cells; indeed, such tracers may pass into the nerve cell. With age, there is an increasing amount of lipofuscin in these cells and granules of this material may be found in the extracellular space and within macrophages nearby. The normal large light cell has a conspicuous axon hillock region which lies just above the point of emergence of the axon. It is an area of the cell devoid of Nissl substance within which neurofilaments and microtubules pass towards the entrance of the axon. In this region there is also a fine network of SER, continuous with the network within the axon. The latter can only be well seen ultrastructurally in thick (1·0 μm) sections stained with uranyl acetate.[24] Thin sections show this organelle poorly.

Initial segment of axon. All sensory ganglion cells other than those in the ganglia of the vestibulocochlear nerves are unipolar. The axon emerges at one point of the cell and, after making a few twists and turns surrounded by Schwann and satellite cells, it escapes into the adjacent tissue where it bifurcates. There is usually no myelin before the bifurcation, though one or more internodes may be found. In the ganglia of the vestibulocochlear nerves the body of the bipolar nerve cells is covered with a multilamellar sheath of satellite cells resembling myelin.

There does not appear to be any initial segment specialisation as there is in motor and many other CNS neurons (see p. 12). The axons of the sensory neuron run both proximally into the CNS as well as distally into the peripheral nerves. While there has been much discussion in the past as to whether the proximally directed axons have the properties of a dendrite or not, there seems little point in pursuing this since there are very few differences in the structure of the two branches, except at their terminals. At the peripheral terminals, there are the special relationships with the cells that form the transducers which initiate the sensory input. At the end of the proximal axon there are the typical synaptic endings on other neurons in the spinal cord and in the lower medulla (gracile and cuneate nuclei).

Motor nerve cells

All motor nerve cells of the peripheral nervous system lie within the CNS and are, therefore, protected by the blood-brain barrier. Whether they lie in the cranial nerve motor nuclei or in the grey matter of the spinal cord, the cells have the same general characteristics. They are usually large, and angular in outline; in the spinal cord they lie in clusters in the grey matter, organised in such a way that those supplying the limbs tend to lie in the lateral parts of the cord, while those running to the proximal muscles lie in the medial columns of the grey matter.

Motor neurons have large pale-staining nuclei and prominent nucleoli which emphasise their synthetic activity. To this end they also show an abundance of rough endoplasmic reticulum (RER) and polyribosomes that often form well stacked and organised clumps of Nissl substance, which are strongly stained in paraffin or celloidin sections by aniline dyes, such as cresyl fast violet. An abundant Golgi apparatus surrounds the nucleus and usually runs for some distance into the dendrite of the cell, accompanied by some RER. Microtubules and 10 nm neurofilaments run in all directions within the cell, and many small mitochondria are scattered apparently at random. Smooth endoplasmic reticulum (SER) is not conspicuous in thin sections (see p. 530) and dense bodies are few except in older individuals. Acid-fast lipofuscin granules, staining for lipid with Sudan black B and giving a positive PAS reaction, are frequent as the subject becomes older.

In general, motor nerve cells have large, long and much branched dendrites which in the spinal cord may stretch for several segments. They usually contain some Golgi membranes and small clumps of RER, particularly in areas close to the cell body, but more conspicuous throughout the rest of the dendrite are many microtubules, mitochondria and irregular clusters of varicose SER tubuli and vacuoles. While neurofilaments are numerous in large anterior horn cells they are usually quite absent from the dendrites. The large dendrites of the anterior horn cells reflect the large synaptic input into the final common path to the effector organ.

As in sensory cells, cell size is a reflection of the size of the projection field or of the motor unit,[22] and nucleolar, nuclear and cell sizes are linearly correlated, all three being a reflection of the synthetic commitment of these cells.

Specialised regions

Synapses make contact with dendrites and with the soma of the neurons and there is an accompanying thickening of the plasmalemma as with other neurons. At the initial segment of the emerging axon, proximal to the first segment of myelin, there is a conspicuous coating of the inner surface of the plasmalemma which is very similar to the coating underlying the axon membrane of the nodes of Ranvier, and it gives the same staining reactions with ferricyanide-osmium technique.[14] In addition, this region of the axon shows a curious clustering of the microtubules, so that they appear to be bound together for a short distance before they pass into the shaft of the axon,[25] and in this region, too, there are many small groups of polyribosomes.[26] While the membrane of this specialised axonal region is clearly important in the initial generation of the action potentials, the meaning of the other intra-axonal features is obscure.

The axon hillock of large motor nerve cells is a conspicuous region near the point of exit of the axon. Nissl bodies are absent here. There are, however, still many polyribosomes and the SER is continuous with that which runs into the axon. Microtubules and neurofilaments course through this zone on their way into the axon, and mitochondria and dense bodies are often conspicuous.

THE AXON

All axons, whether sensory or motor, myelinated or unmyelinated, have essentially the same general structure although marked quantitative differences develop as they increase in size. The cytoskeleton of the axon consists of three elements: microtubules, 10 nm filaments and a branching network of smooth endoplasmic reticulum (SER). The microtubules are similar to microtubules found in any other cell type and consist of polymerised dimers (molecular weight about 100 000) of tubulin protein forming an apparently hollow tube, 20–26 nm in diameter. The wall consists of a ring of 11–13 globular units with a central core, occasionally showing as an electron dense dot. On the surface, wispy arms of slightly electron dense material are visible; they associate with adjacent organelles and may represent actin filaments. Microtubules appear randomly scattered through the cross-section of the axon, but they often lie beside mitochondria (Figs 18.2 and 18.6), small tubules of SER or vesicles of the size of synaptic vesicles. Microtubular proteins are synthesised in the cell body, but their assembly into microtubules may occur anywhere along the axon though no organising centre is ever seen in the normal nerve cell, in contrast to other cell types. There is, however, substantial evidence that they move along the axon at 1–3 mm/day. Their length is indeterminate but may not be much more than a millimetre or so.[27]

Neurofilaments (10 nm diameter) are considerably more numerous than microtubules, especially in the larger diameter axons, and they too are synthesised and assembled in the perikaryon and move down along the axon at 1–3 mm/day. In the normal axon they appear to be randomly scattered throughout. Both microtubule numbers and neurofilament numbers are related to axon diameter,[28] but in slightly different ways. Microtubules are proportionately more numerous in small diameter axons, whereas neurofilaments are greatly in excess in the larger fibres. Axon circularity may be related to the numbers of neurofilaments, for small diameter fibres are significantly less circular than larger diameter fibres.[29] Circularity is of importance both to the electrical properties of the axon[30] and for minimising the surface area of its membrane and thus reducing the level of membrane maintenance. Whether neurofilaments are continuous or in segments of indeterminate length is unknown, but probably the latter is true so that breakage and reassembly may take place within the axon. They must be able to slip through the axon constrictions at each node of Ranvier, which in larger diameter fibres may be reduced to as much as one-quarter of the internodal diameter.[31] Filaments are normally degraded by Ca^{++} activated proteases in the terminal regions of the axon.

Smooth endoplasmic reticulum (SER)

The third major structural component of the axon is the network of SER that runs a continuous course from the perikaryon to the terminal regions.[32] This component seems to be responsible for the rapid transport of large molecular weight proteins and presumably also for much of the local metabolism required for axonal maintenance. The SER accumulates as many small vesicles both proximal to a nerve crush and above other forms of transport block, such as cold or colchicine. The SER network is poorly visible in thin sections and is best appreciated in 1 μm sections photographed by scanning-transmission electron microscopy (STEM) or high voltage transmission electron microscopy (TEM) and viewed by stereoscopy. Since many large molecular weight materials are transported in membrane-bound packets along the length of the axon, the SER seems to be the best structure to effect such transport.[33]

Other intra-axonal organelles are mitochondria, multivesicular bodies and dense bodies. The mitochondria are often unusually long (3–5 μm) and can often be found lying in close contact with microtubules along which they are conveyed, probably by an actin-myosin interaction. Multivesicular bodies are not infrequently seen lying near the axon membrane at nodes of Ranvier. Their rôle is uncertain, but when stained for calcium, using the pyroantimonate method, each vesicle within them contains an electron dense granule that X-ray diffraction indicates may contain calcium. This organelle may well be a calcium trap. Both multivesicular and dense bodies accumulate in distal paranodal regions in the 4 mm or so proximal to a nerve crush and are thus probably moving towards the perikaryon. Intrusions of adaxonal Schwann cell membrane are occasionally seen pushing into the axon, especially at the proximal paranodal regions.

Axoplasmic transport

The normal processes of intracellular movement are accentuated in neurons by the need to convey large amounts of materials along axons and dendrites, from the perikaryon to the periphery and back. Indeed, the total dependence of the axon for health and survival upon cell transport processes is underscored by the frequency with which large and longer axons are earliest affected in any metabolic disease associated with neuropathy. In essence, it is now established that most organelles, large molecular weight substances and other intermediates are conveyed by rapid transport processes at rates of up to 400 mm/day.[34] This rate is constantly found in all types of axon in both the central and peripheral nervous systems, in all species that have been examined; it seems to vary very little with age or with direction of flow. The transport process is dependent upon oxidative energy mechanisms and can be halted by O_2 lack, by iodoacetate and by other inhibitors of adenosine triphosphate (ATP) generation. It is also halted by cold and by agents that depolymerise microtubules, such as colchicine. Moreover, transported materials accumulate proximal to, and to a lesser degree distal to, a ligature around a nerve; measurement of the accumulation rate is a convenient measure of the transport rate. In general, organelle transport is mediated through microtubules, probably by the intervention of an actin-myosin system. Since most, if not all, major substances are transported in membrane-bound forms,[33] this is a major route of intra-axonal movement. It is, furthermore, important to realise that, apart from materials specifically required for the functions of the terminal axonal regions, most (95%) materials made in the cell's body and passed into the axon are used up along their route, presumably in axon maintenance processes, and never reach the terminal regions.[35] This observation further emphasises the logistical problems faced by long, large diameter axons in the face of adverse environmental or metabolic circumstances.[36] Retrograde transport appears to be carried out by the same general mechanism and at the same rate as anterograde transport. The materials conveyed, however, will be distinctly different in each case. Control signals, possibly in a chemical form and determining the rate of supply of the various components, must be envisaged as constantly passing upwards towards the cell body giving information about the metabolic state of the periphery. This will change from hour to hour and from day to day. What these signals are is unknown but they must be carried by rapid transport processes.[37] There is a growing awareness that in some neuropathies there may be an important defect in anterograde or retrograde fast transport mechanisms,[38] although whether this plays a primary rôle in the condition is not clear.

Slow axonal transport is concerned with the steady distal movement of the cytoskeletal elements of the axon. Neurofilaments, microtubules, actin, etc. move at the rate of 1–3 mm/day and this appears to be the same whatever the nerve, the region or the species. It is a one-way process, unlike rapid transport, as befits the limited and rather inflexible rôle of the cytoskeletal elements. These move down the axon in performance of their rôles in transport, stability and structure, and then are ultimately broken down in the terminal and preterminal regions of the axon. Neurofilaments are broken down by Ca^{++} activated proteases, enzymes sensitive to sulphydryl-reacting agents[39] relying upon the release of Ca^{++} ions sequestered in the smooth-surfaced endoplasmic reticulum (SER) of the terminal regions. Microtubules, in contrast, are readily depolymerised in the presence of mild local increases in Ca^{++} ion concentration.

REFERENCES

1. Shanthaverappa TR, Bourne GH. J Anat 1962; 96: 527. 96: 527.
2. Shanthaverappa TR, Bourne GH. J Cell Biol 1962; 14: 343.
3. Abood LG, Abdul-Haj SK. J Neurochem 1956; 1: 119.
4. Bradbury M. The concept of the blood-brain barrier. London: Wiley, 1979.
5. Jacobs JM, MacFarlane RM, Cavanagh JB. J Neurol Sci 1976; 29: 95.
6. Vizoso A. J Anat 1950; 84: 342.
7. Fernand VSV, Young JZ. Proc R Soc Lond [Biol] 1951; 139: 38.
8. Jacobs JM, Cavanagh JB. J Neurocytol 1972; 1: 161.
9. Goldman JE. J Neuropath Exp Neurol 1983; 42: 146.
10. Hall SM, Williams PL. J Cell Sci 1971; 8: 541.
11. Berthold C-H, Rydmark M. J Neurocytol 1983; 12: 475.
12. Langley OK, Landon DN. J Histochem Cytochem 1968; 15: 722.
13. Jones HB, Cavanagh JB. J Neurocytol 1983; 12: 459.
14. Waxman SG, Quick DC. J Neurol Neurosurg Psychiatry 1977; 40: 379.
15. Wiley CA, Ellisman MH. J Cell Biol 1980; 84: 261.
16. Hirano A, Dembitzer HM. J Ultrastruct Res 1969; 28: 141.
17. Spencer PS, Thomas PK. J Neurocytol 1974; 3: 763.
18. Thomas PK. J Anat 1963; 97: 35.
19. Ochoa J. J Anat 1971; 108: 231.
20. Pannese E. Adv Anat Embryol Cell Biol 1981; 65.
21. Jacobs JM, Carmichael N, Cavanagh JB. Neuropathol Appl Neurobiol 1975; 1: 1.
22. Donaldson HH, Nagasaka G. J Comp Neurol 1918; 29: 529.
23. Rambourg A, Clermont Y, Beaudet TA. J Neurocytol 1983; 12: 47.
24. Droz B, Rambourg A, Koenig HL. Brain Res 1975; 93: 1.
25. Palay SL, Sotelo C, Peters A, Orkand PM. J Cell Biol 1968; 38: 193.
26. Kosaka T. J Neurocytol 1980; 9: 861.
27. Bray D, Bunge MB. J Neurocytol 1981; 10: 589.
28. Friede RL, Samorajski T. Anat Rec 1970; 167: 379.
29. Hoffman PN, Griffin JW, Price DL. J Cell Biol 1984; 99: 705.
30. Arbuthnott ER, Ballard KJ, Boyd IA, Kalu KU. J Physiol 1980; 308: 99.
31. Rydmark M. Neurosci Lett 1981; 24: 247.
32. Droz B, Rambourg A. In: DG Weiss, ed. Axoplasmic transport. Berlin: Springer, 1982: 384.
33. Tytell M, Black MM, Garner JA, Lasek RJ. Science 1981; 214: 179.

34. Ochs S. J Physiol 1972; 227: 627.
35. Muñoz-Martinez EJ. In: DG Weiss, ed. Axoplasmic transport. Berlin: Springer, 1982: 267.
36. Cavanagh JB. Lancet 1984; 1: 1284.
37. Cragg BG. Brain Res 1970; 23: 1.
38. Jakobson J, Sidenius P, Braendgaard H. J Neurol Neurosurg Psychiatry 1986; 49: 986.
39. Pant HC, Gainer H. J Neurobiol 1980; 11: 1.

Reactions of neurons and Schwann cells to injury

THE AXON

WALLERIAN DEGENERATION (*Axonal degeneration*)

Probably no pathological change in nervous tissue has been studied more intensively than the consequences of axon interruption. Augustus Waller[1] described it first in the glossopharyngeal nerve of the frog, in 1850; he drew attention to the different responses between the distal and proximal parts of the severed nerve. What we now clearly understand is that separation of a large portion of the cytoplasm (the distal portion of the axon) from its sources of essential materials in the cell body leads to its inevitable decline and disintegration. All energy-demanding vital activities, especially those of ion exclusion and pumping, begin to fail, and the isolated piece of cytoplasm can no longer maintain itself in a hostile environment. The sequence of events that we thus see below the point of section reflects the heavy responsibilities of the perikaryon towards the axon, and stresses the indivisibility of this cellular unit. Any pathological process that affects one part of the cell must inevitably also involve the remainder.

For many hours after nerve transection, there is little decline in the axon's ability to carry the nerve impulses; their transmission does not cease for up to 71–78 hours.[2] Conduction velocity decrease is small during the first 48 hours, but there is a steady decline in the size of the action potential as the number of surviving fibres gradually becomes less. Fragmentation of the severed fibres becomes visible with the light microscope 26–28 hours after section, but the delay depends greatly upon the type of axon: small fibres tend to break down faster than large fibres, and terminal and preterminal fibres disintegrate particularly rapidly. Sensory fibres are said to break down slightly faster than motor fibres, and a proximo–distal gradient of response of the Schwann cells to events in the axon is known to develop,[3,4] although axon changes are said to take place simultaneously along its whole length.[5] Schlaepfer,[6] in a careful study of the early events after axon section, concluded that loss of energy to maintain Ca^{++} ion exclusion from the axon is a vital first step in the process. Normally there is a CA^{++} ion concentration difference by a factor of 4800 on the two sides of the axon membrane (0·3 μmol inside to 1600 μmol outside) and by 16 hours after section, Ca^{++} ions begin to leak into the axon in significant amounts. The earliest ultrastructural changes are disintegration of the neurofilaments and microtubules: this stems directly from the catastrophic entry of calcium ions which then activate proteases and initiate depolymerisation of microtubules.

From this moment on, there is a stereotyped sequence of events in the nerve fibre beginning with break-up of the axon and myelin into ovoids of various sizes (digestion chambers of Cajal). During the ensuing days there is an incursion of blood-borne macrophages into the nerve (Fig. 19.1); axonal and myelin debris are broken down to simpler proteins and the cholesterol and other lipids are esterified by these cells. Lipid droplets of cholesterol esters stain more readily and brightly with oil red O and Sudan III than does the original myelin. Schwann cells probably play little rôle in the actual breakdown of the axon

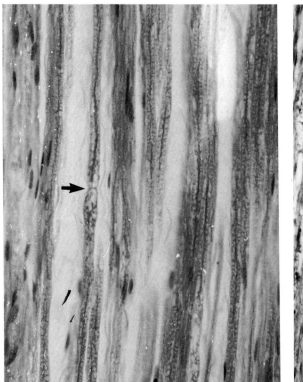
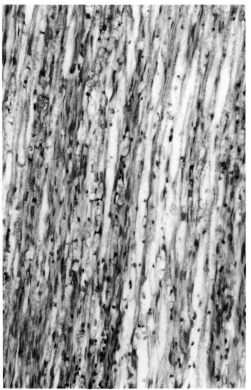

a   b

Fig. 19.1a, b (**a**) Normal nerve. Note the slender Schwann cell nuclei and the straight haematoxyphil axons surrounded by (eosinophilic) reticulated myelin sheaths; the reticulation is the result of the tissue processing. A node of Ranvier is arrowed. (**b**) Wallerian degeneration in a nerve cut one week previously. Note the increase in nuclei, the chains of vacuoles as axons and myelin disintegrate, and the many macrophages with short round or oval nuclei.
Haematoxylin-eosin (**a**) × 370; (**b**) × 240

and myelin debris but, over the first 24 hours, their nuclei and nucleoli enlarge, preceding the first cell divisions that appear at about 36 hours. From then onwards the nuclear population increases linearly over the subsequent 10 to 14 days or so.[7,8] After two weeks, the rate of cell increase falls and as the macrophage population returns to the blood-stream the total cell population declines. However, the Schwann cells continue to multiply until they form continuous columns, each within a sleeve of basement membrane, and each cell about 25–50 μm in length. These continuous chains of cells (*bands of Büngner*) act both as guides for regenerating axons, leading them to their end organs, and as a source of cells for future myelination of these newly grown axons. Should

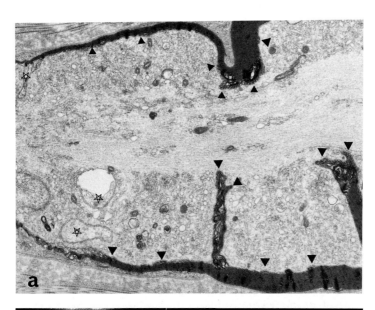

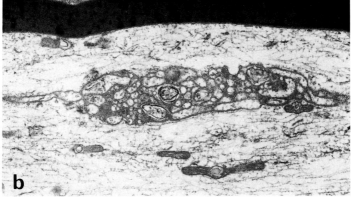

Fig. 19.2a, b (a) Paranodal region proximal to a ligature applied 3 days previously. Node of Ranvier to the left. Note axonal expansion into the paranodal myelin (myelin loops marked by triangles), the expansions containing large amounts of smooth endoplasmic reticular vesicles and occasional mitochondria. Schwann cell intrusions into the axon at asterisks. The central axonal region contains filaments, tubules and mitochondria. (**b**) Schwann cell intrusions into the axon in a proximal paranodal region, proximal to and 3 days after nerve ligature. Note the double membranes, from Schwann cell and from axon, around each of the intrusions which contain dense bodies and other debris.
Electron micrographs × 9900

no regenerating axons grow into the cell columns, either because their cell bodies have been destroyed or because they were lost at the point of interruption, the bands of Büngner may persist for many months, finally undergoing atrophy. On entry of a neurite into the cell column, myelination by Schwann cells begins even before an effective end organ is reached.

In the process of degradation of axon and myelin sheath materials by macrophages, phospholipids are broken down to triglycerides, cholesterol is esterified, and proteins are hydrolysed by proteases; final removal of the breakdown products is relatively rapid in peripheral nerve by comparison with the CNS. By two months there may be little residual evidence of degeneration in small nerves, other than an increase in cell population made up of Schwann cells and endoneurial fibroblasts; most of the macrophages have migrated away by this time. In the CNS, in contrast, myelin may remain trapped among astroglial processes for many months or, in man, for many years.

Retrograde axonal changes

Proximal to the level of a nerve section or crush, another set of stereotyped changes occurs, but they are limited largely to 4 mm above the point of injury. Within this narrow zone, which may involve 6 to 8 internodes of myelin, degeneration occurs back to the next node of Ranvier or perhaps the one beyond that, though rarely further. The axon lying proximal to these nodes of Ranvier becomes distended with mitochondria and large numbers of smooth endoplasmic reticulum (SER) vesicles derived from the SER network within the axon (Fig. 19.2). These organelles tend to lie peripherally in the axon, with the microtubules and filaments lying in the core of the axon.[9] The myelin overlying such swollen paranodal regions is stretched by this distension process, the paranodal myelin loops become attenuated, and, in larger fibres, axoplasm may expand into spaces between clusters of myelin loops. The same events also occur in the distal paranodal regions of each node within this narrow zone, but in them the accumulated material is largely made up of dense bodies, mitochondria and large multivesicular bodies. In both juxtanodal regions, abundant pro-

trusions of Schwann cell adaxonal cytoplasm may be seen apparently taking part in disposing of intra-axonal materials, for these protrusions often contain electron dense debris resembling dense bodies. The material in distal paranodal regions is probably moving back towards the cell body while that in the proximal paranodal regions would normally be passing in an anterograde direction.

Beyond 4 mm proximal to the point of nerve transection, little abnormality is to be seen, but measurements of axonal diameter will show that after a nerve crush there is a transitory reduction of axon calibre that may last for several weeks. This reduction is a reflection of reactive changes in synthesis and of slow transport of neurofilaments into the axon in response to nerve injury.[10]

Recognition of Wallerian degeneration in a nerve

From a practical standpoint, in conditions where the question of recent nerve fibre degeneration arises, this is best looked for in longitudinal sections of nerve (Fig. 19.3). Haematoxylin and eosin stained sections will readily show increase in nuclear populations, increase in nuclear and nucleolar size of Schwann cells, and the presence of increased numbers of macrophages. Important also is the increased number of mast cells, recognisable by their characteristic basophilic cytoplasm; their number always increases whenever there is any kind of abnormality in peripheral nerves. Vacuoles running in chains, accompanied by darkly staining nuclei, are characteristic of isolated degenerating fibres. Normally, in well-stained haematoxylin and eosin preparations of nerve, axons are pale blue, and the presence of eosinophilic rounded masses should suggest that axons have recently undergone degeneration. This should be confirmed by staining for axons with the Glees and Marsland or similar silver stains; these show swollen and fragmented material, readily visible under low magnification of the microscope. Later in the process of Wallerian degeneration there is only the nuclear increase to show where degeneration has occurred. Frozen sections from the cryostat, 25–50 μm thick and stained with Sudan black B, are valuable for detecting fine lipid

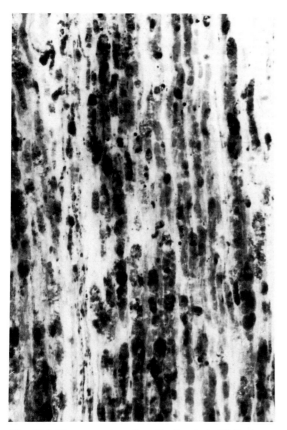

Fig. 19.3 Fragmentation of myelin sheaths in Wallerian degeneration. Granules of sudanophilic lipid form chains; small fibres seem to become broken into small fragments earlier than large fibres. Case of polyarteritis nodosa. Sudan black B × 390

granules that may remain later in the process. Examination of semi-thin (1 μm) resin sections tends to underestimate the amount of degeneration because of the smallness of the sample, but if fixation has been good the increase in resolution that these sections give may be valuable; such semi-thin sections of transverse sections of the nerve are essential for quantitative work on fibre sizes. Finally, a clear separation of Wallerian degeneration from segmental myelin loss can only be obtained by teasing small bundles of nerve in glycerine or in Araldite® after staining respectively with Sudan black B or with osmic acid. This should always be carried out in any newly observed condition affecting peripheral nerves.

RESPONSES OF THE PERIKARYON TO AXONAL DAMAGE (AXON REACTION)

'Chromatolysis' simply means loss of stainable material from the cell, but behind this term lies a series of changes that are of importance in preparing the nerve cell for the process of axon regeneration. Unfortunately, the term is also often loosely used for analogous changes which occur in the neuron but are due to causes other than axon damage. For that reason, it should be reserved for a general description of an affected neuron; when specifically discussing the perikaryal response to axon section, the more precise term *'axon reaction'* should be used.

The classical change of chromatolysis involves swelling of the cell body, displacement of the nucleus to one side, usually away from the axon hillock, and dispersal of the Nissl bodies into a dust-like basophilia. This dispersal is more marked at the centre of the cell than at the periphery, where Nissl granules often persist (Fig. 19.4). Folding of the nuclear membrane and

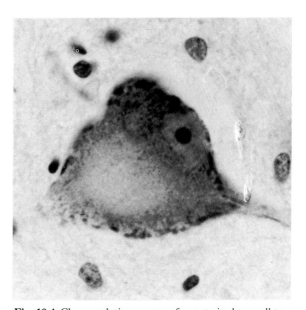

Fig. 19.4 Chromatolytic response of an anterior horn cell to loss of its axon (axon reaction). Note clearing of Nissl material from the central region of the cell, the eccentric nucleus, enlarged nucleolus, and persistence of peripheral Nissl material. Dendrite to the right and axon hillock to the left. Case of acute intermittent porphyria. Cresyl fast violet × 825

the appearance of a basophilic nuclear 'cap' are also frequent findings.[11] In addition, there is often a short burst of proliferation of the microglial cells near the motor nerve cell body or of the perineuronal satellite cells in sensory ganglia.

Biochemical studies have shown that there is no loss of RNA from a chromatolytic neuron though cell water is increased, as are protein and lipid.[12] There is also evidence of increased energy utilisation and a decrease of transmitter synthesis in the early weeks of the axon reaction. The stimulus for these events in the cell is unknown. But an identical reaction of the perikaryon occurs following local injection of botulinum toxin into muscle,[13] when release of acetylcholine from motor nerve terminals is prevented, although no loss of axon substance occurs. It has been suggested that the need for the neurite to increase membrane surface area may be the essential stimulus for the axon reaction; this response ultimately leads to regeneration of damaged axons, and restoration of the neuron's effectiveness. Or, in the case of botulinum toxin, restoration of function by production of terminal sprouts that eventually induce new myoneural junctions.

In essence, therefore, the axon reaction is the visible sign of a change in the neuron's functional state from the fully differentiated condition, concerned with synthesis of transmitter and the maintenance of the large volume and surface area of the axon, to a simpler, less specialised, metabolic state concerned primarily with the regrowth of axoplasm and the re-establishment of contact with an effector organ. Not all the features of this reaction are understood and there are several features of the process that need further study. For example, cutting the distal axon of a sensory ganglion cell produces a typical axon reaction, whereas cutting the proximal axon in the dorsal root close to the spinal cord produces no apparent cell response, although the volume of axoplasm lost is often very little different in the two cases. Another unresolved problem is why severance of the axon a long way distal from the perikaryon should cause little obvious change in the neuron cell body, but if the cut is made at the spinal root level just distal to the neuron, the typical response takes place. Moreover, if a second distal cut is made a few days later only a short

distance proximal to the first distal lesion, once more a marked chromatolytic response occurs.

Other states of 'chromatolysis' have been reported in recent years, particularly in experimental conditions in animals, that superficially resemble the axon reaction, but without any preceding axon degeneration. Thus, in methyl mercury intoxication (see p. 251) in the rat, focal clearing of Nissl material from the cytoplasm of spinal ganglion cells is seen a few days *before* the onset of axon degeneration.[14] In acrylamide intoxication (see p. 271) in the rat 'chromatolytic' changes also occur in sensory ganglion cells before any axon dysfunction or degeneration can be found. In this case it may be a response on the part of the perikaryon to accumulation of neurofilaments and other changes in the nerve terminals that precede axon degeneration.[15] In trimethyltin intoxication (see p. 257) 'chromatolytic' clearing of Nissl material occurs, especially in hippocampal neurons, associated with accumulation of large numbers of dense bodies but without axonal degeneration.[16] The 'chromatolysis' of pontine and other nuclei that is a classical post-mortem feature of pellagra in man (see p. 292) is also unassociated with axonal degeneration and probably indicates a severe metabolic disturbance of RNA metabolism in the perkaryon.

REGENERATION AND REPAIR PROCESSES

An outstanding characteristic of peripheral nerves is their capacity for regeneration after injury. The property is essential for survival, due to the daily minor injuries to which the peripheral nervous system is exposed and which must be repaired. The frequent occurrence of numerous short myelin internodes in the nerves of the elderly, indicating that remyelination has taken place at some time during adult life,[17] is strong evidence for past regeneration (see Fig. 18.3, p. 522).

Within a few hours of interruption of axons, signs of sprouting can be seen in the preserved proximal nerve stump.[18] After nerve crush, where the Schwann cell basement membrane and the Plenk–Laidlaw sheath of individual axons are not severed, newly sprouted axons find their way into appropriate channels that will guide them back to their end organs. After complete transection of the nerve, the gap between the severed ends will form a significant barrier both to penetration of neurites into the distal nerve trunk and to the connections with appropriate bands of Büngner. Unless the two cut ends of the nerve are carefully sutured, many neurites will wander aimlessly into adjacent connective tissue. With time, this mixture of neurites and connective tissue will come to form a significant and often painful swelling, an *amputation neuroma*. In the late repair of damaged peripheral nerve tissue, clean excision of this mass before suturing of the cut ends is essential to obtain the greatest chance of a satisfactory reinnervation of the distal stump.

Factors that control successful regeneration of neurites are not fully understood, but the axon reaction in the perikaryon described above is vital to 'switching on' of the metabolism of nerve cells to synthesise new axoplasm and, at the same time, for 'switching off' production of materials no longer needed.

The growing tip of the regenerating neurite consists of an active membrane in constant movement, mitochondria to provide energy, small vesicles, cytoplasm and microfilaments, probably actin. As the fibre grows, 10 nm neurofilaments push into the advancing tip together with microtubules.[19] The tip grows at the rate of 1 mm/day, about the same rate as the movement of cytoskeletal structures, though, over long distances, this growth rate may decline substantially. That the cytoskeleton is necessary for the forward growth of the advancing tip is shown by the finding that inhibition of the growth of microtubules by vincristine and the impairment of normal functions of neurofilaments by 2,5-hexanedione both significantly slow regeneration of neurites after nerve crush.[20] The blood-nerve barrier that was broken down while nerve degeneration was in progress is, with time, restored as the nerve fibres grow along the distal stump. With this restoration, myelination of the new axon takes place and nerve conduction properties are restored.[21]

Collateral sprouting

When partial denervation occurs with loss of a

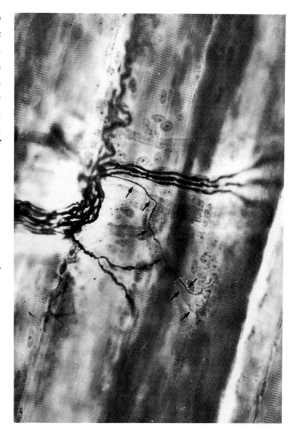

Fig. 19.5 Collateral sprout in a partially denervated muscle of a cat given tri-*ortho*-cresyl phosphate. The sprout (arrows) runs to enter a denervated muscle end-plate. Glees and Marsland × 300

proportion of nerve fibres innervating muscles, surviving axons within a day or so produce fine sprouts from nodes of Ranvier that lie near the terminal and preterminal regions, i.e. near the partially denervated muscle fibres (Fig. 19.5). Such collateral sprouts are best seen with methylene blue stained preparations or with well-stained silver preparations. They migrate towards denervated muscle end-plates, re-innervate them and, with time, may become myelinated. They function sufficiently well to prevent denervation atrophy of muscle fibres. When partial denervation is the consequence of nerve cell loss, such as in motor neuron disease, surviving neurons come to bear a greater burden of terminal fibres and effector organs than would normally be the case. The *terminal innervation ratio*, i.e. the ratio of neurite terminals to motor end-plates, which normally is about 1·1, can thereby become substantially greater, with neurite terminals innervating many end-plates. Chronic neuronal atrophies, such as amyotrophic lateral sclerosis (motor neuron disease) and poliomyelitis, commonly show this phenomenon. The polyphasic spike potentials noted electromyographically in such conditions are in large part explicable on the basis of the spatial growth and spread of the terminal innervation, with asynchronous contractions of the muscle fibres innervated in this way. While the effects of such change upon the motor nerve cell have not been studied experimentally, they have been examined in sensory root ganglion cells by Terni,[22] who found a significant increase in size of the spinal ganglion cells with parallel enlargement of the nuclei and nucleoli; these changes (compensatory neuronal hypertrophy) reflect increased synthetic activity of the perikaryon in response to an increased work load.

Ultraterminal sprouting

After partial denervation of a muscle, and in addition to collateral sprouting, surviving nerves begin to sprout from terminals lying within motor end-plates and grow out to innervate empty end-plates on adjacent muscle fibres. How functionally satisfactory such a union becomes cannot be stated, but it is yet another response on the part of terminal neurites to muscle denervation. What initiates these growth reactions is unknown. There is evidence that denervated muscle fibres send some kind of signal to nerve endings, demanding innervation; if this request is not satisfied, muscle fibres will ultimately undergo atrophy. Such a response is typically seen with local botulinum intoxication of muscle. Even though, in this case, there is no nerve fibre degeneration, nerve terminals produce a remarkable dense sprouting response within a few hours of the institution of blockade of acetylcholine release. Within a few days, large numbers of small new neuromuscular junctions are formed on the surfaces of adjacent muscle fibres. On the basis of this concept of mutual support between nerve and muscle, it is suggested that active terminal sprouting is in response to muscle signals of a chemical nature initiated by loss of end-plate function.

THE 'DYING BACK' PHENOMENON

In many diseases of the nervous system in which peripheral nerves, long spinal tracts or other tract systems are specifically affected, it had been observed, both clinically and pathologically, that the longest axons, and often too those of greatest diameter, tend to be affected earliest in the degenerative process. This pattern of selective degeneration dominates the clinical picture, so that in motor neuron disease (see p. 408), for instance, in which there is a system degeneration of both lower and upper motor neurons, the hands and the feet show weakness and other evidence of denervation long before more proximal regions are affected. It is also a characteristic clinical feature of Friedreich's ataxia that the more discriminative aspects of sensation are affected earliest in the limbs and a large measure of the ataxia is the result of loss of primary sensory afferent fibres running from muscle spindles, these being amongst the largest diameter sensory axons. In many deficiency diseases and toxic neuropathies the same selectivity of long and large diameter axons is noted. It can be shown in experimental animals, by sampling nerves at suitable moments, that long axons show degeneration in their more distal parts in the earliest stages of the disorder. A condition which characteristically shows this pattern of change is the neuropathy due to organophosphorus intoxication (see p. 269). In tri-*ortho*-phosphate poisoning in cats, if the dose is not too large, there may be extensive degeneration of nerve terminals and preterminals and of axons in intramuscular nerve bundles in distal muscles, but examination of the nerve emerging from the muscle may show little or no sign of axon degeneration. With a low dose, degeneration may not progress much further back towards the cell body than this, and on recovery affected axons thus have very little distance to travel to re-innervate muscle end-plates; recovery is consequently relatively rapid. The same relatively short retrograde degeneration may be found in the neuropathy of acute intermittent porphyria when the attack is relatively mild; but when the attack is severe, and life-threatening, axon degeneration may occur as far back as the spinal roots. This degree of severity is the state usually described in cases coming to post-mortem; milder cases, with only clinical weakness to indicate denervation, survive.

From the clinical progress of such conditions it has been envisaged that affected long and often large diameter axons are withering from the distal regions in a proximal direction. The name 'dying back' was coined by Greenfield to describe this phenomenon, by analogy with the withering of branches of a tree affected by fungal disease impairing the transport mechanisms in xylem and phloem. The analogy is a good one, for in such conditions as thiamine deficiency and arsenical intoxication there is good evidence that energy supplies to the axon from the perikaryon are impaired. In these conditions, large diameter and long axons, especially from spinal sensory neurons, are at greatest risk—first, from their greater work load and therefore their greater demand for energy and, secondly, because if all parts of the axons are equally affected by the primary problem, supplies from the perikaryon will reach more proximal regions and the shortest axons first. This simple concept of the underlying mechanism of selective vulnerability of long axons has been borne out by the steadily increasing knowledge of the transport and supply problems that neurons with long axons are prone to; it also helps our understanding of the clinical signs and symptoms of disease. It has, furthermore, been demonstrated in several experimental neuropathies that axoplasmic transport processes may be significantly slowed before or at the onset of the distal degenerative changes. Whether this phenomenon is the cause or the result of the disturbed axonal maintenance that leads to the degeneration is undecided.[23]

REACTIONS OF THE SCHWANN CELL TO INJURY

SEGMENTAL DEMYELINATION

In normal circumstances each Schwann cell will continue to maintain, during the life of the individual, that segment of myelin sheath it made during infancy. Schwann cells may be transiently damaged so that they are unable to maintain the stability of their segment of myelin. Such damage may result from local causes, such as pressure from a tourniquet or local ischaemia due to a transient vascular event, or from general disease, such as diphtheria or lead intoxication. As a result the segment will degenerate and be removed from around the axon. Since Schwann cells are quite separate one from another, any segmental demyelination that occurs will tend to be randomly scattered among the axons in the damaged region.

The only satisfactory way to identify segmental (primary) demyelination, and to separate it clearly

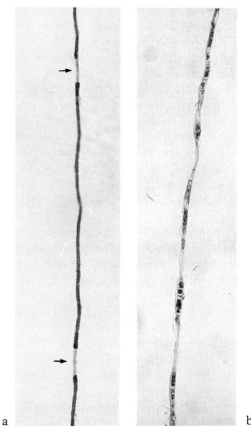

a   b

Fig. 19.6a, b (a) Segmental myelin degeneration (segmental demyelination) (arrows) at the distal ends of an internode. Such a change is found in diphtheria, lead neuropathy, ischaemia and other local processes damaging peripheral nerve. (b) By comparison, a teased single fibre showing only Wallerian degeneration with fragmentation of myelin all along its length.
(a) Osmic acid: nerve fibres teased in Araldite® ×55;
(b) Osmic acid ×55

from secondary demyelination due to axon degeneration, is by teasing nerve fibres apart after staining them with Sudan black B or osmic acid (Fig. 19.6). Alternatively, electron microscopy can be used though the sample examined is disappointingly small, and quantitative methods cannot be satisfactorily employed to gauge the severity of the changes.

In some conditions, such as diphtheria intoxication, whole internodes of myelin may undergo degeneration, though the Schwann cell itself usually survives. In most instances only a short length of internode adjacent to nodes of Ranvier breaks down, so that perhaps only 100 μm or so of myelin internode is affected; this is a small part of the whole internode, which may be as long as 500–1000 μm or more. Whatever the length of myelin segment that breaks down, the effect on nerve function is the same, since it is the associated loss of function at the affected nodes of Ranvier that is important, not the demyelination as such. It is true that severe slowing of conduction, down to 2-5 metres per second (m/s) (normal 40-50 m/s in large fibres), will occur over the zone of myelin loss. But damage to the nodal apparatus, if this cannot be jumped by the action potential, is liable to block conduction completely in that fibre.[24]

In all conditions in which segmental myelin loss occurs, Schwann cells are rarely, if ever, completely destroyed; only their ability to maintain the myelin sheath is impaired by disease. This is an important characteristic of the Schwann cell, since it will, thus, be always available to repair the loss of myelin once the causal process has ceased. Even when the whole myelin internode is destroyed, the surviving Schwann cell immediately divides to make sufficient cells to fill the gap in the cell chain caused by the internodal loss. Since internodes in the limbs have been stretched by the process of growth from the basic length of 250–300 μm at the time of myelin initiation to 800 –1000 μm or more in the adult, three to four myelin-forming cells are needed to replace a whole myelin internode. In contrast, when only part of an internode has degenerated, and the gap is more than about 15 μm long, a new cell is needed to fill the gap by forming a short, intercalated internode. If the damage has produced a gap less than 15 μm long, the existing Schwann cell is able to extend the myelin loops into the damaged paranodal region.[25]

Cold injury

People exposed to intense and prolonged cold and wet, such as immersion in arctic sea-water, develop a condition known as 'immersion foot'. In this, both sensory and motor peripheral nerve disturbances occur, in addition to ischaemic vascular changes. Examination of the peripheral nerves from such cases shows extensive Wallerian degeneration;[26] it is uncertain how much of this is of vascular origin and how much directly due to cold. Since cold alone is now known to have a depolymerising action upon microtubules and is thus capable of blocking rapid axoplasmic transport in axons, there is no doubt that cold alone would impair nutrition, especially of longer axons. Experimental studies have shown that cold alone has indeed a profound effect upon conduction of the action potential and upon the integrity of peripheral nerve axons. Small fibres are more susceptible to loss of conduction while larger fibres degenerate.[27] It is of interest that axonal microtubules reappear within an hour of warming the nerve from 2°C to 25°C, so that their repolymerisation must occur within axons, as the response is too rapid for the regenerated microtubules to have been produced in the cell body.

Tourniquet paralysis

The transient paralysis that may follow application of a tourniquet to a limb was at one time thought to be due entirely to ischaemic vascular effects.[28] More recent experimental studies have shown, however, that the upper and lower edges of the tourniquet may exert sufficient local pressure upon the nerve to cause paranodal myelin from one internode to herniate beneath the paranodal myelin of the adjacent internode. The resulting intussusception leads to local disruption of the myelin and, more importantly, of the nodal region itself. The paranodal myelin disturbances are readily repaired, however, usually with an intercalated segment of myelin and with reconstruction of the nodal regions on either side of this.[29]

Chronic nerve entrapment syndrome

In many situations in the body, nerves need to run beneath ligaments and aponeuroses; with the action of the limbs they thus become exposed to repetitive flexion and extension as well as stretching. The resulting syndrome is particularly often seen in the wrist (*carpal tunnel syndrome*), but may also be found at the elbow, and at several other sites. These include the points where the lateral cutaneous nerve of the thigh passes through the inguinal ligament and where the posterior branch of this nerve pierces the fascia lata: in both instances troublesome sensory disturbances (meralgia paraesthetica) occur in the skin of the thigh. Such general conditions as myxoedema, hormonal disturbances and increasing age may play a rôle in precipitating the lesion, which is more common in women than men. The damage to the nerve is expressed partly as segmental demyelination and partly as axonal degeneration, depending upon the severity of the lesion and its duration. There may, indeed, be some element of vascular insufficiency in its development.[30]

REFERENCES

1. Waller A, Proc R Soc Lond 1862; 12: 89.
2. Gutman E, Holubar J. J Neurol Neurosurg Psychiatry 1950; 13: 89.
3. Lubinska L. Brain Res 1977; 130: 47.
4. Joseph BS. Brain Res 1973; 59: 1.
5. Donat JR, Wisniewski HM. Brain Res 1973; 53: 41.
6. Schlaepfer WW. Brain Res 1974; 78: 71.
7. Abercrombie M, Johnson MJ. J Anat 1968; 41: 37.
8. Cavanagh JB. Br J Radiol 1968; 41: 275.
9. Martinez AJ, Friede RL. Brain Res 1970; 19: 183.
10. Hoffmann PN, Griffin JW, Price DL. J Cell Biol 1984; 99: 705.
11. Lieberman AR. Int Rev Neurobiol 1971; 14: 49.
12. Brattgard S-M, Edstrom J-E, Hyden H. J Neurochem 1957; 1: 316.
13. Watson WE. J Physiol (Lond) 1969; 202: 611.
14. Carmichael N, Cavanagh JB, Rodda RA. Acta Neuropathol 1975; 32: 115.
15. Cavanagh JB. Neuropathol Appl Neurobiol 1982; 8: 315.
16. Brown AW, Cavanagh JB, Verschoyle RD, Gysbers MF, Jones HB, Aldridge WN. Neuropathol Appl Neurobiol 1984; 10: 267.
17. Visozo AD. J Anat 1950; 84: 342.
18. Cajal SR. Degeneration and regeneration of the nervous system. Trans R May, 1928.
19. Lasek RJ, Hoffman PN. In: Goldman RD, Pollard T, Rosenbaum J, eds. Cell Motil 1976: 1021.
20. Shiraishi S, LeQuesne PM, Gajree T, Cavanagh JB. J Neurol Sci 1986; 71: 165.
21. Mellick RS, Cavanagh JB. Brain 1968; 91: 141.
22. Terni T. Arch Ital Anat Embriol 1920; 17: 507.
23. Jakobsen J, Sidenius P, Braendgaard H. J Neurol Neurosurg Psychiatry 1986; 49: 986.
24. Rasminsky M, Sears TA. J Physiol 1972; 227: 323.
25. Cavanagh JB, Jacobs JM. Br J Exp Pathol 1964; 45: 309.
26. Blackwood W. Br J Surg 1944; 31: 329.
27. Roderiguez-Echandia EL, Piezzi PS. J Cell Biol 1968; 39: 491.
28. Denny Brown D, Brenner C. Arch Neurol Psychiatry 1944; 51: 1.
29. Ochoa J, Danta G, Fowler TJ, Gilliatt RW. Nature 1971; 233: 265.
30. Thomas PK, Fullerton PM. J Neurol Neurosurg Psychiatry 1963; 26: 520.

Pathology of peripheral nerve diseases

INTRODUCTION

There are numerous pathological processes which affect peripheral nerves, and they are discussed in this chapter. However, the reactions of peripheral nerves to damage or insult are relatively limited, as illustrated in Chapter 19. The most common finding in peripheral neuropathies is axonal damage, expressed as axonal degeneration and regeneration. Segmental demyelination may occur to a minor degree in many neuropathies but is the predominant feature in only a few neuropathies (see p. 541). If recurrent and repeated segmental demyelination occurs, hypertrophic changes may result with the formation of onion-bulb whorls (see p. 572). Hereditary disorders are also seen in which there is a defect in myelin formation as part of a primary defect of Schwann cell metabolism.

The clinical presentation of peripheral nerve disease[1] must depend upon the anatomical site of the pathological lesion, the kind of nerve damage and its speed of progression. There may be a symmetrical polyneuropathy affecting peripheral nerves and particularly in the limbs, or there may be a mononeuropathy affecting one particular nerve, or several nerves (mononeuritis multiplex). Sensory signs such as loss of sensation, paraesthesiae, and pain may predominate, and are often distal and symmetrical in the hands and the feet. While most neuropathies are mixed motor and sensory neuropathies, pure motor neuropathies do occur and such cases usually present with loss of power and muscle bulk in the distal parts of the limbs. Electrophysiological investigations such as nerve conduction studies and electromyography may be valuable in defining the distribution of the neuropathy and perhaps also the type of pathological process involved. For example, a gross reduction in nerve conduction velocity is seen in segmental demyelinating neuropathies.

Pathological investigation of a peripheral neuropathy may be by nerve biopsy or at autopsy.[2] Careful and accurate clinical descriptions of the distribution of the neuropathy, the length of the patient's history, the family history, and the speed of progression of the neuropathy will be helpful in deciding which nerve to biopsy or which specimens to take at autopsy to provide a full topographical analysis of the condition of the peripheral nervous system.

Biopsies of peripheral nerves are usually taken from a superficial skin nerve and the sural nerve is the most popular. The biopsy can either be full-thickness or fascicular. Peripheral nerves are very fragile and the surgeon should be encouraged to treat the nerve extremely gently; otherwise crush artefact may make histological interpretation of the biopsy very difficult.[3] A variety of histological techniques can be employed to detect pathological changes in a peripheral nerve biopsy, and in all these techniques it is essential that exact transverse as well as longitudinal sections are cut. Paraffin sections stained with haematoxylin and eosin, elastic–van Gieson, and a myelin technique such as Klüver–Barrera, are particularly valuable for detecting overall loss of myelinated fibres and the presence of arteritic lesions. Cryostat sections of nerve may be used for lipid histochemistry and cryostat or paraffin sections for immunohistochemistry. Cytological abnormalities, damage to individual myelinated fibres, the presence of regenerating clusters, and the pathology of non-myelinated nerve fibres are most adequately demonstrated in transverse sections of epoxy resin embedded nerve, either in sections 1 μm thick stained with toluidine blue or in electron microscope preparations. Teased fibres should be used to detect segmental demyelination and remyelination in addition to axonal degeneration and regeneration.

A post-mortem examination on a patient who has died with a peripheral neuropathy should be planned according to the clinical distribution of the neuropathy, and in a similar way to that outlined for toxic neuropathies (see p. 245) with the general aim of defining the topography of the degenerative changes. The brain should be removed and fixed, and the spinal cord removed together with as many dorsal root ganglia as possible. The Gasserian (Vth cranial nerve) ganglion should always be examined. Specimens should be taken from proximal and distal locations along the nerves affected by the neuropathy in order to gauge the severity of any 'dying back' change. Tissue should be taken from the muscles affected by the neuropathy so that the degree of neurogenic atrophy can be assessed and the degree of involvement of intramuscular motor and sensory nerves can be estimated.

VASCULAR AND IMMUNE DISEASES

INTRODUCTION

While these two disease agencies seem at first sight essentially different, changes in peripheral nerves associated with abnormal immune reactions often occur from vascular insufficiency because the primary immunological reaction may lie in the walls of neural blood vessels. It is, thus, frequently difficult to determine what is primary immunological disease and what is secondary to the many small vascular lesions that occur. The peripheral nerves may be involved in a generalised vascular disease without the primary immune responses being directed specifically towards nerve fibres. This group of diseases, therefore, has a wide spectrum, ranging from purely vascular occlusions due to inflammatory changes in vessel walls to those conditions where an apparently pure immune response is directed specifically towards some component of the nerve fibre, such as the myelin sheath. Where the vascular element predominates, peripheral nerve lesions are likely to be chiefly Wallerian degeneration with varying degrees of primary myelin (segmental) degeneration. But where an abnormal immune response is directed mainly against myelin or its components, segmental demyelination is usually the major component, with lesser amounts of axonal degeneration. These generalisations may not, however, be applicable in every instance, for immunologically determined peripheral neuropathies are still not well understood; only recently have immunocytochemical techniques become available for their study.

regenerating myelinated fibres, although the total nerve fibre population is reduced.

Ageing in the peripheral nervous system

Little is known about the effects of age upon the peripheral nervous system in man; most studies have been concerned with growth and maturation up to middle age. Corbin and Gardner[9] found a reduction in the numbers of nerve fibres in dorsal roots, but the methods available to them have since been replaced by new and more informative and sophisticated techniques. Although it is generally believed that loss of nerve fibres regularly occurs with increasing age, the evidence for this is scanty.

DISEASES WHOLLY OR PREDOMINANTLY VASCULAR IN NATURE

Ischaemic neuropathy

In a healthy individual it is difficult to cause damage to peripheral nerves by obstruction of blood vessels due to the considerable network of collaterals.[4] In a patient with *arteriosclerosis* or with other kinds of chronic vascular disease, such as *thromboangiitis obliterans (Buerger's disease)*,[5] chronic ischaemia, from obstruction of large numbers of small as well as large vessels, plays an important part in the production of the peripheral nerve signs and symptoms. Paraesthesiae, patchy loss of sensation, muscular weakness and wasting, and loss of tendon reflexes are found in a high proportion of cases in direct relation to the severity of the vascular insufficiency.[6] Examination of nerve biopsy material[7] and of nerves from amputations for peripheral vascular disease[8] has shown an abundance of short intercalated myelin internodes in the surviving nerve fibres as well as marked loss of large diameter axons. Abundant Wallerian degeneration will be seen as well as evidence of segmental demyelination in such material: both indicate progression of the disease. In addition, signs of active nerve fibre regeneration are detectable through the preponderance of small diameter axons in histograms of nerve fibre diameter and by the presence of clusters of small

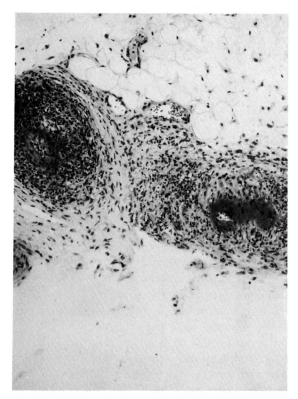

Fig. 20.1 Medium-sized artery lying in the epineurium of a peripheral nerve from a case of polyarteritis nodosa. Note loss of structure in the top vessel due to fibrinoid necrosis and the marked infiltration of the walls of both vessels by chronic inflammatory cells. The vessel at the bottom is occluded. The adjacent nerve showed patchy Wallerian degeneration.
Haematoxylin-eosin × 115

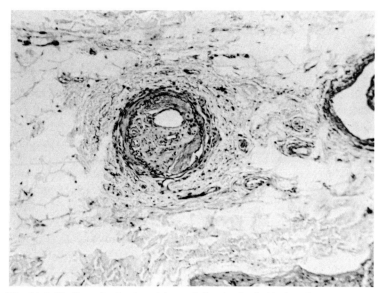

Fig. 20.2 Medium-sized epineurial vessel showing healed lesion of polyarteritis nodosa with a central recanalised thrombus, and patchy loss of elastic lamella and of media. There is an increase in surrounding fibrous tissue. Haematoxylin-eosin × 110

VASCULAR IMMUNE DISEASE

Polyarteritis nodosa, Wegener's granulomatosis and rheumatoid necrotising arteritis

These are three conditions in which major changes of an inflammatory nature take place in the walls of medium-sized and small arteries in various parts of the body; peripheral nerves are frequently involved. Thus, peripheral neuropathy occurs in about 50% of cases of polyarteritis nodosa,[10] in up to 70% of cases of rheumatoid arthritis with arteritis,[11] and in about 15% of cases of Wegener's granulomatosis.[12]

While it is not understood exactly how the altered immune state initiates the vessel lesions, the changes have a close structural similarity with those seen in the Arthus phenomenon, in which antigen-antibody immune complexes are deposited within the vessel wall. The characteristic histological change is fibrinoid degeneration of the vessel wall with destruction of the muscularis and, particularly, of the elastica (Fig. 20.1). Varying amounts of inflammatory infiltration of the wall and of the surrounding connective tissues are also seen. In *polyarteritis*

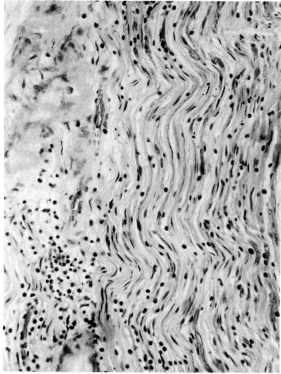

Fig. 20.3 Longitudinal section of peripheral nerve from a case of polyarteritis nodosa showing inflammatory infiltration within the endoneurium and around a small vein (bottom left), general increase in cell population and evidence of Wallerian degeneration in the nerve fibres. Haematoxylin-eosin × 190

nodosa there may be considerable variation from case to case in the size of the vessels involved (Fig. 20.2), and the clinical neuropathy presents typically as a mononeuritis multiplex (see p. 545). Only very rarely are the signs symmetrical in distribution, indicating a much more diffuse vascular process.

Changes in the nerves are typically those of Wallerian degeneration (Fig. 20.3) with varying amounts of regenerative activity. Segmental demyelination may also be found, but this is less obvious. In transverse sections of larger nerves patchy myelin loss may be seen from one fascicle to another (Fig. 20.4), emphasising the variable distribution of the vascular lesions. Severe chromatolysis may be seen in anterior horn cells (Fig. 20.5) due to damage to motor axons.

The major pathological features of *Wegener's granulomatosis* are lung lesions, nephritis and arteritis. But since the latter two features are also common to polyarteritis nodosa and the under-lying pathology is somewhat similar, distinction between the two diseases is usually made on clinical criteria. Some believe Wegener's granulomatosis to be merely a variant of polyarteritis nodosa.

The *neuropathy complicating rheumatoid arthritis* may take several distinct clinical forms. Vascular lesions are responsible for the mono-neuritis multiplex and there is nerve entrapment in the inflamed connective tissues around the affected joints and beneath ligaments and aponeuroses. All nerve lesions are associated with arteritic changes càpable of producing ischaemia of varying degrees of intensity.[13] The more local forms of neuropathy are usually mild and improve with time. However, distal sensory and motor polyneuropathy, associated with rheumatoid nodules and wide-spread vasculitis, carries a poor prognosis.[14] As with the other conditions in this group of diseases, Wallerian degeneration of nerve fibres is the principal form of nerve damage found. Segmental

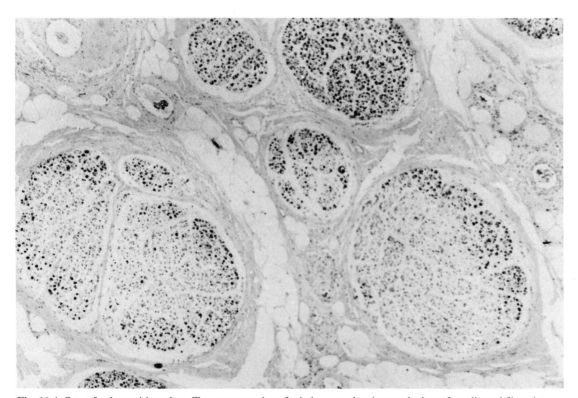

Fig. 20.4 Case of polyarteritis nodosa. Transverse section of sciatic nerve showing patchy loss of myelinated fibres in several larger fascicles.
Iron haematoxylin × 95

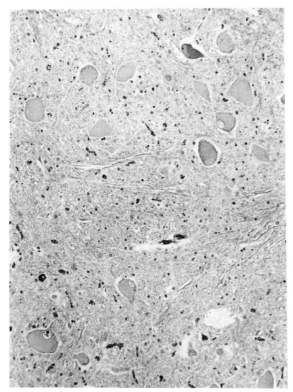

Fig. 20.5 Spinal cord from a case of polyarteritis nodosa showing severe chromatolysis of all visible anterior horn cells. A typical 'axon reaction' to extensive axon damage. Haematoxylin-eosin × 280

demyelination may also be seen, but always in relatively small amounts: it is perhaps due to less severe ischaemia or to mild local compression of swollen nerves beneath ligaments.

Giant cell (or temporal) arteritis

This condition is considerably more indolent than other forms of arteritis, and typically shows foreign-body type giant cells within the inflammatory lesions (Fig. 20.6). There is a striking and unexplained tendency to affect temporal arteries and other extracranial vessels, so that cranial nerves frequently become implicated in the lesions. Rarely, cases with more widespread distribution have been reported.[15]

Systemic lupus erythematosus and scleroderma (systemic sclerosis)

Among other neuropathies with an immune-

vascular basis is that associated with systemic lupus erythematosus (SLE). This may take the form of a symmetrical distal neuropathy or of a mononeuritis multiplex; the former perhaps reflects the widespread nature of the vascular changes. Neuropathy has been noted also in *scleroderma*, considered by some to be a varient of SLE. It is interesting that the Spanish toxic oil syndrome (due to ingestion of contaminated rape seed oil) has many clinical similarities with scleroderma, and peripheral neuropathy was a common feature as the condition advanced to a more chronic stage.[16]

AMYLOID NEUROPATHY

Deposition of amyloid within nerves occurs in several different circumstances.

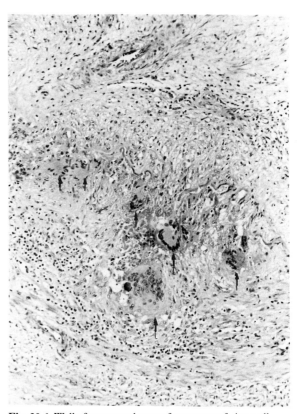

Fig. 20.6 Wall of a temporal artery from a case of giant cell arteritis (post-mortem specimen). Note the badly damaged elastica running across the centre of the field and giant cells (arrows) on its endothelial side. Both the endothelium and much of the media are replaced by granulation tissue. Haematoxylin-eosin × 110

In *secondary amyloidosis*, accumulation of amyloid material in many tissues, particularly in liver, spleen and kidneys, occurs as a complication of chronic inflammatory processes, including chronic rheumatoid arthritis and chronic infections. This type of amyloidosis is now less common. It rarely, if ever, involves peripheral nerves.

Primary amyloidosis, without any recognisable precipitating cause, may affect many different tissues, but has a definite predilection for the cardiovascular, neuromuscular and gastrointestinal systems; it generally spares the organs conspicuously involved in secondary amyloidosis. The deposits of amyloid tend to be focal and nodular, but may eventually become diffuse. This is conspicuous in the heart which may become diffusely enlarged. In peripheral nerves and in the autonomic system,[17] amyloid occurs as small deposits within the walls of vessels (Fig. 20.7) and also more diffusely within the extracellular spaces of the endoneurium, the perineurium and the epineurium. In all these sites it expands the tissue spaces and compresses the neighbouring structures. Sensory and autonomic ganglia are particularly prone to involvement.[18]

Amyloid is seen with the light microscope as a hyaline, eosinophilic, rather structureless material. It stains positively with the periodic acid-Schiff reaction, indicating the presence of a carbohydrate moiety. In polarised light it shows a greenish birefringence after staining with Congo red. This very characteristic phenomenon, termed 'dichroism', is due to the arrangement of the amyloid protein filaments. Ultrastructurally, all types of amyloid consist of 10 nm straight and unbranched filaments arranged in bundles, sheaves or fan shapes.

The origin of the deposited material is not known. Chemically it lacks the characteristics of collagen or of elastin, while antigenically it has features that identify it with κ-immunoglobulin light chains. However, there appear to be other protein constituents within it, derived from the plasma; these are of uncertain rôle and may be non-specifically bound to the principal deposited proteins.[19]

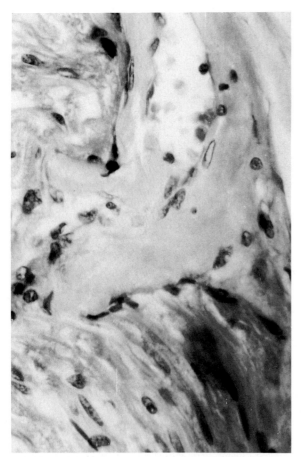

Fig. 20.7 Endoneurial vessel thickened and hyalinised by amyloid.
Haematoxylin-eosin × 335

Amyloid deposits in other conditions

In addition to sporadic primary amyloidosis, referred to above, neuropathy is occasionally associated with the deposition of abnormal proteins formed by the cells of *myelomatosis*.[20] A similar neuropathy is associated with *Waldenström's macroglobulinaemia* and with *cryoglobulinaemia*[21] (see p. 554). This type of neuropathy should be distinguished from the condition that occasionally results from infiltration of the peripheral nerves by myeloma cells.

Four forms of *inherited amyloid neuropathy* have been recognised in various parts of the world; each is distinguished by somewhat differing clinical features.[22]

Pathogenesis of neuropathy in amyloidosis

In all forms of amyloidosis, both sporadic and inherited, the mechanism of production of the neuropathy is complex. The rôle of nerve compression at constriction sites, e.g. the carpal tunnel, is clearly important when nerves are swollen by the deposited proteins. Some degree of ischaemia in other parts of the nerve must also play a rôle in leading to axonal degeneration, as must impairment of the nerve cells in spinal and autonomic ganglia. In addition, disturbance of Schwann cell nutrition may contribute towards any segmental demyelination that may occur. The frequent occurrence of residual nodules (of Nageotte) (see p. 565) in these ganglia reflects the ganglion cell loss which accompanies amyloid deposition. Such neuronal loss may be an important component of the nerve lesions.

Histologically, Wallerian degeneration is the principal change in the affected peripheral nerves. It is almost certainly due to the effects of the amyloid deposition.

GUILLAIN–BARRÉ SYNDROME

This disease has now become the commonest paralytic condition in developed countries since the occurrence of poliomyelitis was reduced by immunisation programmes. It was originally described as 'acute ascending paralysis', a term that aptly draws attention to the acuteness of onset and the rapid advance of the flaccid paresis that characterises the illness. Usually developing over the course of 2–4 weeks, the condition may occasionally progress within as little as 2–4 days to

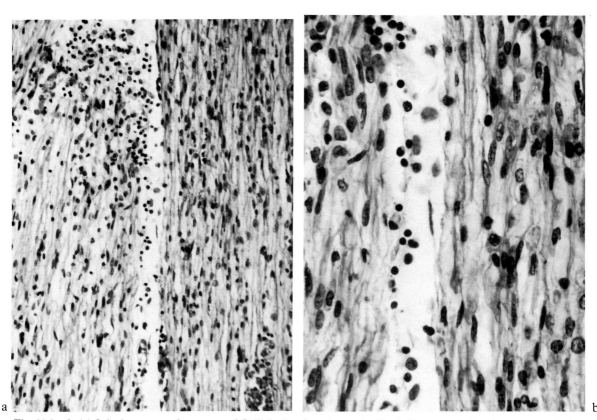

a   b

Fig. 20.8a, b (a) Spinal nerve root from a case of Guillain–Barré syndrome showing inflammatory infiltration, more marked in the left bundle, which also shows oedema and separation of nerve fibres. There is extensive myelin loss from both nerve bundles. (b) Higher magnification of a to show round cells in endoneurial space, activation of Schwann cell nuclei and infiltration of the nerve by macrophages. Haematoxylin-eosin (a) × 155; (b) × 385

complete flaccid quadriplegia, bulbar paralysis and respiratory difficulties. Despite this occasionally dramatic onset, more than 75% of cases recover completely without sequelae, though serious and persistent paresis follows in 15–20% of cases. About 5% of patients die during the course of the illness.

Clinical features. There is profound motor paresis with little sensory disturbance other than subjective dysaesthesiae, especially distally in the limbs. If objective sensory signs, such as loss of vibration and joint position sensations, are present, there is likely to be severe inflammatory involvement of the sensory roots.[22] Extension to the cranial nerves occasionally occurs. The autonomic nervous system is commonly affected, as evidenced by the frequent occurrence of tachycardia. The principal objective sign that characterises the illness is the presence of a marked increase in the protein content of the CSF that follows the onset of the paralytic illness, without a concomitant rise in inflammatory cells. This striking and diagnostically important sign is probably the result of increased permeability of the vascular barrier in the spinal roots to protein.

Pathological features. The earliest changes found

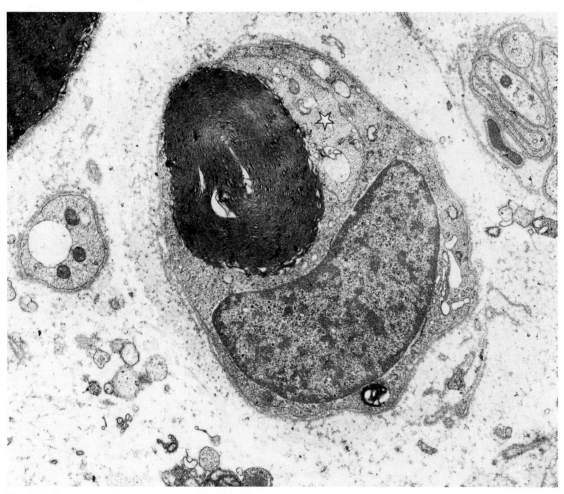

Fig. 20.9 Sural nerve biopsy from a case of Guillain–Barré syndrome showing a Schwann cell containing an axon (asterisk) with a coiled mass of myelin lying to one side, and no longer covering the axon.
× 14 875

in patients dying in the acute phase of the illness are pronounced oedematous swelling of the endoneurial spaces, especially in the spinal roots and in the spinal ganglia, and an accompanying steady increase with time in inflammatory cell infiltration.[23] The inflammatory cells enter the endoneurial spaces from the blood vessels, not only in the spinal roots but in a patchy manner throughout the peripheral nervous system (PNS). They are macrophages and lymphocytes, with a small admixture of plasma cells (Fig. 20.8). Macrophages are aggressive and actively insinuate themselves into the myelin sheaths, between the lamellae and between the myelin and the axon; the myelin is stripped from the axon and destroyed. The Schwann cells themselves remain viable and may take part in the myelin degradation once it has begun (Fig. 20.9); axons bare of myelin are often surrounded by a ring of Schwann cells (Fig. 20.10). Schwann cell proliferation continues side by side with phagocytic removal of myelin debris; this cell replication is necessary to fill the gaps left by disintegrating internodes (see p. 542).

Both the inflammatory infiltration and the myelin destruction are essentially focal throughout the PNS, seen principally in spinal ganglia and roots, and scattered without apparent pattern in the remainder of the peripheral nerves. For this

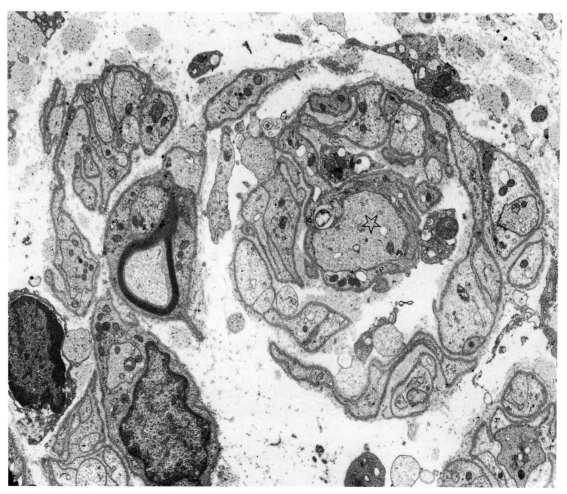

Fig. 20.10 From the same nerve as Figure 20.9, showing a naked axon (asterisk) surrounded by a concentric array of Schwann cell processes. The naked axon is too large to be a normally unmyelinated axon.
× 7395

reason a sural nerve biopsy, for instance, may show no inflammatory changes although they may be abundant elsewhere along the nerve; there may be secondary axonal degeneration visible due to involvement of the nerve elsewhere on its course.

Axons are thus essentially unaffected in the primary disease process, which is selectively directed towards myelin. Spinal ganglia are often more intensively involved than many other regions, and many sensory ganglion cells may die in the acute inflammatory phase of the illness. Transient swelling of peripheral nerves during the acute phase of the illness, together with some degree of associated ischaemia, will cause degeneration of some axons passing through such areas.

Underlying causative mechanisms. A majority of patients with Guillain–Barré syndrome have suffered some kind of infective illness during the 2–3 weeks before the onset of the neurological symptoms. No one specific type of infection can be identified and there is a clear parallel here with post-infectious encephalomyelitis (see p. 207), though the two diseases rarely, if ever, overlap. Three analogous conditions strongly suggest the importance of preceding infection in producing an abnormal cell-mediated immunological reaction directed against peripheral nerve myelin.

1. Following the widespread use as a prophylactic agent against human influenza in the USA of a vaccine prepared from swine influenza virus (Hsw1 N1), cases of an illness indistinguishable from Guillain–Barré syndrome began to occur in a proportion of those vaccinated. Neurological signs began within 4 weeks of vaccination, and the condition ran an identical course to Guillain–Barré syndrome with almost exactly the same fatality rate (5·2%) as in cases of the disease among un-vaccinated people (4·7%).[24] When the vaccination programme was stopped, the occurrence of new cases ceased within a few weeks.

2. Dogs used for the hunting of raccoons (coon hounds) may develop a condition similar to Guillain–Barré syndrome within 2–3 weeks following a bite from a raccoon. The pathological changes are also essentially the same.[25] The agent responsible has never been recovered from these animals.

3. It is possible, by the injection of peripheral nerve myelin or extracts of myelin, particularly P_2 protein, combined with Freund's adjuvant, to produce *experimental allergic neuritis* (EAN) in animals; this disease of peripheral nerves closely resembles Guillain–Barré syndrome in many features.[26] In addition to the delayed hypersensitivity reaction (cellular responses) induced in EAN, circulating antibodies directly toxic to myelin in cell cultures are also produced. The immunological response in Guillain–Barré syndrome, however, is a cellular immune response rather than a humoral antibody-mediated process. Although potentially damaging antibodies may gain entrance to peripheral nerve, either through the normal fenestrations of the capillary bed in spinal and other ganglia, or into nerves once the blood-nerve barrier has been lowered by the inflammatory and degenerative changes, they do not appear to play a major rôle in the destruction of myelin. All the events relate only to the cell-mediated immune responses.

PARAPROTEINAEMIC NEUROPATHY (benign monoclonal gammopathy)

A group of patients can be identified in whom peripheral neuropathy is associated with the presence of abnormal proteins in the plasma.[27] While a proportion of these cases may have associated Waldenström's macroglobulinaemia, cryoglobulinaemia, or myelomatosis (see p. 550), others have none of these conditions, yet the plasma contains raised levels of γ-globulin for reasons as yet unknown. To this condition the name benign monoclonal gammopathy has been given.

Clinical features. Benign monoclonal gammopathy usually affects males between the ages of 50 and 70 years. The history is of a slow onset of diminished sensory and motor function, especially in the limbs, with accompanying loss of reflexes.[28] Electrophysiologically there is marked slowing of the conduction velocity, suggesting the presence of *segmental demyelination* in the nerves. In severe examples almost complete denervation may be found.

In many of these cases, there is a moderate increase of IgM in the serum, up to 2–3 times the normal level (0·4–3·0 g/l), with a discernible monoclonal band on electrophoresis. The IgM has κ light chains. CSF globulin levels also may be mildly raised, perhaps due to an increase in capillary permeability.

Pathological features. Nerve biopsy material typically shows segmental demyelination, sometimes of severe degree, with abundant evidence of remyelination and the occasional finding of hypertrophic changes with 'onion skin' formation, indicating chronicity of the demyelinating process (see p. 573). Ultrastructurally, the characteristic feature of the changes, in addition to the demyelination, is widening of the interperiod line of the myelin sheath to give a repeat distance of 37 nm instead of the normal 23 nm. This is usually seen in the outer lamellae of the remyelinating sheaths. In addition, there may be varying amounts of axonal loss, but it is a striking feature that cellular infiltration, beyond that expected for the demyelination process, is mild or even absent.[28,29]

Direct immunocytochemistry reveals the deposition of IgM in the remaining myelin sheaths, but there is no staining for complement. It has been found that the IgM has specificity for myelin-associated glycoprotein (MAG), a protein of molecular weight 100 000, of which one-third is composed of carbohydrate, but whose function in the economy of the myelin sheath is unknown. If the destruction of the myelin sheath is the direct result of the reaction between the circulating antibody and a component within the myelin sheath, then this is the first time that attack by circulating antibodies has been shown to result in pathological changes in a defined structure within the nervous system.[30]

DIABETIC NEUROPATHY

One of the commonest kinds of peripheral neuropathy, with persistent and painful consequences, is that found in patients with diabetes mellitus; this condition is now regarded as essentially a vascular pathological process. Three principal varieties of neuropathy are seen; mixtures of the different types are not uncommon. The first, symmetrical neuropathy, has a more or less symmetrical distribution of sensory signs and symptoms, frequently accompanied by evidence of damage to the autonomic nervous system. The second form, a group of mononeuropathies, is a variety of mononeuritis multiplex in which any region of the peripheral nervous system might become involved, including the cranial nerves. The third, diabetic amyotrophy, is the least common, and has been the subject of much clinical controversy as to its nature and underlying mechanism; evidence suggests that it is a special example of mononeuritis.

Symmetrical neuropathy

This condition is usually of insidious onset and occurs in either the milder forms of diabetes mellitus seen in adult life or the more severe forms in younger patients. The symptoms of distal paraesthesiae and numbness are mild at first, but later are accompanied by loss of reflexes and of vibration sense in the lower limbs, although motor weakness is uncommon. In more severe cases, glove and stocking anaesthesia, ataxia and episodes of spontaneous severe burning or lancinating pains, as well as the occurrence of Argyll Robertson pupil (loss of the pupillary reflex to light but not to accommodation) may suggest tabes dorsalis (diabetic pseudotabes). The presence of trophic changes in the lower limbs, especially the feet, with deep penetrating ulcers and joint disturbances of neuropathic type, might further suggest the presence of tabes.

Autonomic disturbances are common in diabetic neuropathy but rarely occur on their own. There may be loss of control of sweating and body temperature, loss of circulatory and pupillary reflexes, and hypersensitivity of the peripheral vessels to temperature changes. These signs and symptoms are not only very distressing, but contribute to the development of chronic foot ulceration and to joint disturbances.

Electrophysiological studies reveal mild to moderate slowing of the conduction velocity with normal latencies and reduction of the size of the action potentials. Sensory-evoked responses are depressed.

Mononeuropathies

In the more *chronic mononeuropathies* of insidious onset, more than half the cases have involvement of nerves in the upper limb, either radial or ulnar, and usually in the dominant arm, suggesting the operation of a work factor. There is evidence of entrapment either at the wrist or at the elbow. The majority of the patients are women and many already show some evidence of the symmetrical type of neuropathy (see above).

By contrast, *acute mononeuropathy* is usually restricted to the lower limbs or to cranial nerves, and males and females are more equally affected. It presents as dull aching pains with evidence of weakness and wasting in one group of muscles, and muscle fasciculation, but little accompanying sensory change. Recovery is often slow and incomplete.

There is little doubt that, in both forms of mononeuritis, ischaemia plays a major part. Where entrapment is largely responsible, ischaemia ensues from pressure within the constriction beneath the ligament. In the mononeuritis affecting the lower limbs and cranial nerves, it is generally presumed that obstruction to larger vessels is responsible for the ischaemic changes in the nerves.[31]

Diabetic amyotrophy

Amyotrophy complicating diabetes mellitus forms a small percentage of cases of diabetic neuropathy.[32] The syndrome of deep muscle pain, weakness and areflexia, mainly restricted to the thighs and the pelvic regions, is one that has caused considerable clinical speculation as to its origins. There is very little sensory change and it was originally suggested that the condition arose from lesions in the spinal cord. However, there is little post-mortem evidence for this[33] and the best suggestion is that it is vascular in origin.[32]

Pathological features

Examination of the peripheral nerves in the symmetrical form of diabetic neuropathy reveals changes in almost every element of their structure,[34] and there has long been controversy whether the primary lesion is in the vascular bed,

in the Schwann cells or in the nerve cells themselves.[35] Variable degrees of axon degeneration are constantly present and are more severe in the distal parts of the limbs, but teased fibre studies have shown that there may also be evidence of marked segmental demyelination accompanied by re-myelination.[36] Significantly, this may also be present in the spinal roots.[37] Schwann cell hypertrophy and the formation of 'onion-bulb' whorls are indications of the continuing activity of the demyelination process.

The underlying mechanism that leads to these changes in such a complex and longstanding condition as diabetes is not fully known. It has been suggested that the neurons themselves are primarily damaged,[38] but the evidence for this is not good. The fibre loss is multifocal within the peripheral nerves and there is no suggestion of a systematic axonal loss.[39] There is an accumulation of the intermediates in the sorbitol pathway in nerve and spinal cord, due to general metabolic disturbances. This has led to suggestions that the relative preponderance of segmental demyelination in the symmetrical form of the neuropathy may be due in some way to this disturbance.[40] The most persuasive suggestion is that there is a reduction in the number of small blood vessels in the peripheral nerves and thus a decrease in the appropriate nourishment to the nerve fibres.[41] This idea has much to commend it, and would bring the pathological problem into line with the pathogenesis of diabetic retinopathy and nephropathy as being a disease of small vessel integrity.

INFLAMMATORY NEUROPATHIES

LEPROSY

In terms of the number of cases of leprosy and the chronicity of the disease, this must be one of the world's most common disorders and certainly the most common peripheral neuropathy. An estimated total of 15 million cases has been made by Dastur and Porwal;[42] the majority of those infected live in tropical or subtropical areas of the world. Indigenous cases in Europe are very few, but with increasing ease of travel, patients with leprosy are now more often seen in low incidence areas.

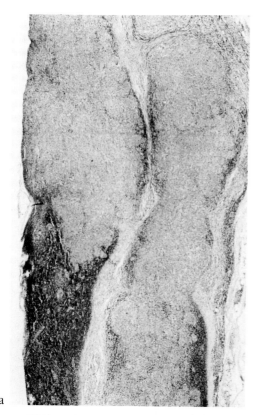

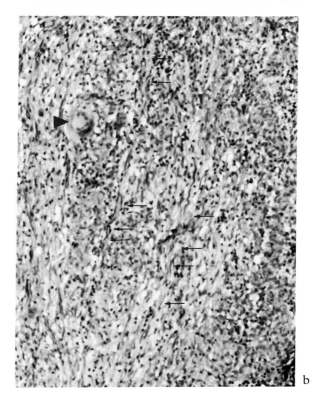

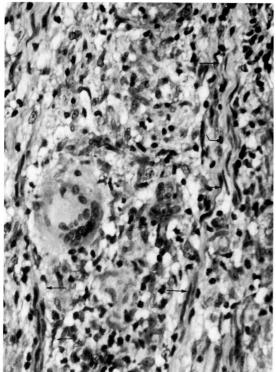

Fig. 20.11a–c Tuberculoid leprosy. Cutaneous nerve showing intense inflammatory infiltration causing gross disorganisation of the nerve structure. (**a**) The dark zones are areas of lymphocytic infiltration both inside and outside the perineurium. The lighter areas are filled with epithelioid cells. The original nerve can only be recognised by the general form of the tissue. (**b**) In the pale zone of (a) there are sheets of epithelioid cells with many lymphocytes and occasional giant cells (arrowhead). Nerve bundles (small arrows) can just be made out at this magnification. (**c**) Higher magnification of (b) to show a giant cell, epithelioid cells, small dark lymphocytes and slender nerve bundles (small arrows).
Haematoxylin-eosin (**a**) × 125; (**b**) ×115; (**c**) ×290
Photomicrographs provided by Dr D. S. Ridley, Hospital for Tropical Diseases, London, UK.

Three principal forms of the disease occur, constituting part of a continuous spectrum of clinical conditions related to the responsiveness of the host to the bacillus,[43] namely tuberculoid, lepromatous and dimorphic forms.

Tuberculoid leprosy

Clinical features. This is usually a localised condition involving both skin and the underlying nerves, though very occasionally nerve alone is affected. The skin lesion, which is usually single, is round, oval or serpiginous in form and sharply outlined, with a scaly centre and slightly raised borders. There is usually a sharply localised patch of sensory loss, often with palpable thickening of the underlying nerve. The lesion is commonly located on the face, outer surfaces of the arms or legs or the buttocks. The lepromin test, analogous to the tuberculin test, is positive and the prognosis of this form of leprosy is good.

Pathological features. The skin lesion on biopsy shows intense granulomatous cellular infiltration of the dermis and the epidermis. The inflammatory cells consist of epithelioid macrophages and histiocytes, giant cells of Langhans and foreign-body type, and lymphocytes. Small areas of caseous necrosis may be present. Bacilli are exceedingly difficult to find in the lesions.

In the greatly swollen underlying nerves, a similar severe granulomatous infiltration is present. The nerve may be severely disorganised by the presence of large numbers of epithelioid cells with many giant cells and large areas of lymphocytic infiltration (Fig. 20.11). The cellular infiltration thus causes gross disorganisation of the nerve architecture and frequently it is difficult to detect the nerve fibres. Small bundles of nerve fibres may be seen and many show signs of Wallerian degeneration. In small nerve bundles the loss of fibres may seem to be complete, but in larger trunks fibre loss is partial and dependent upon the amount of inflammatory activity present. Again, bacilli are exceedingly sparse.

Lepromatous leprosy

Clinical features. This form of leprosy lies at the opposite end of the clinical spectrum to tuber-culoid leprosy. Proliferation of lepra bacilli takes place in the tissues unchecked by any inflammatory activity. Skin lesions are macular, papular, nodular or plaque-like in form and are often numerous, while in other areas, such as the face, the skin may be diffusely infiltrated. There is also often involvement of the eyes, the nose or the throat, and lepra bacilli are numerous in the secretions.

Neurologically, large areas of sensory loss may be found; these are often more or less symmetrical in distribution. But there are important areas of predilection, which are related to the cooler parts of the skin surface. Thus the ears, the brows, the malar regions of the face, the external surfaces of the arms and legs, and the hands and feet are frequently the sites of sensory loss, whereas the perineum, neck, back and abdomen are rarely affected.[44] Sensory loss is almost always associated with palpable enlargement of the underlying nerve trunks; varying degrees of motor weakness are present, especially in the distal parts of the limbs.

Pathological features. By contrast with the tuberculoid form of the disease, there is remarkably little inflammatory cell infiltration in lepromatous lesions, other than an abundance of actively phagocytic macrophages. These cells contain large numbers of acid-fast lepra bacilli and many more bacilli lie free in the tissues (Fig. 20.12). Foam cells (lepra cells) filled with bacilli are numerous and characteristic, and infiltration of lymph nodes by macrophages is striking. In the same way, peripheral nerves also show infiltration by foamy macrophages and here too there are enormous numbers of bacilli. There is extensive loss of axons and of myelin sheaths as well as considerable fibrosis of the endoneurium (Fig. 20.12b). Whether the axon and myelin loss is secondary to fibrotic changes in the blood vessels, or due to the large numbers of bacilli in the Schwann cells impairing their capacity to maintain the myelin sheath, is still debatable.[45] Bacilli are everywhere in large numbers and may be seen in small clumps even in axons.[46] Surviving myelinated axons may show evidence of remyelination, and there are often signs of axonal regeneration.

Ultrastructurally, bacilli are present in Schwann cells of unmyelinated as well as

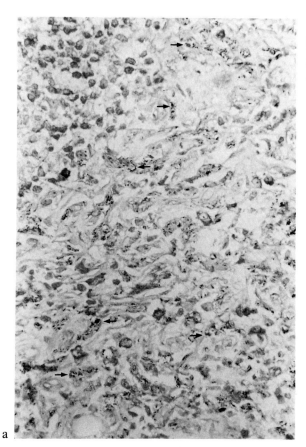

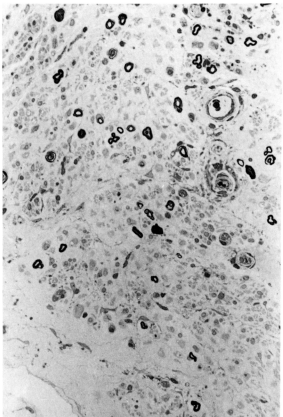

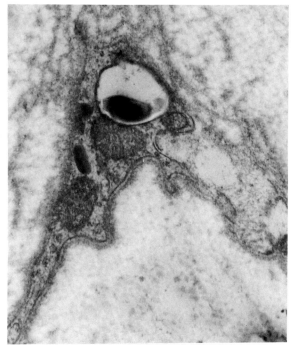

Fig. 20.12a–c Lepromatous leprosy. (**a**) Ziehl-Nielsen stain for acid-fast bacilli. These appear as dark clusters (some of which are arrowed) mostly lying within macrophages and foam cells (lepra cells). (**b**) Cutaneous nerve showing severe reduction of myelinated nerve fibres; the space between the fibres is filled with histiocytic macrophages and surviving Schwann cells. (**c**) A lepra bacillus within a denervated Schwann cell of a band of Büngner; the Schwann cell is identified by its basement membrane.
(**a**) × 450; (**b**) Toluidine blue; 1 μm section × 280;
(**c**) × 28 500
(**a, b**) *Photomicrographs provided by Prof. P. K. Thomas, Royal Free Hospital School of Medicine, London, UK.*
(**c**) *Electron micrograph provided by Dr R. O. Barnard, Maida Vale Hospital (National Hospitals for Nervous Diseases), London, UK.*

myelinated fibres (Fig. 20.12c). But a large proportion of the bacilli, both in Schwann cells and in macrophages, are dead.

It is probable that in lepromatous leprosy the bacilli are dispersed by the bloodstream, but they proliferate and induce damage only in superficial cooler regions of the body. They never damage the CNS or muscle although bacilli may be found in both sites. The lepromin test is negative in lepromatous leprosy and the prognosis is always poor, despite treatment.

Dimorphous leprosy

Clinical features. The wide degree of variation of skin and nerve involvement between the two extremes of the clinical spectrum of leprosy, the tuberculoid and lepromatous forms, depends greatly upon the amount of resistance by the host to the presence of the bacilli. At the same time, the rôle of temperature is important in the localisation of the lesions.

Skin lesions may thus be either numerous or few; thickening of nerves and areas of patchy sensory loss also vary very widely in extent. The importance of coolness is shown by the predilection for the ears, the malar regions of the face and the outer aspects of the limbs.

Pathological features. All degrees of severity of cellular infiltration in the skin and nerves are found, according to whether the patient's response to the infection leans towards the tuberculoid or the lepromatous form of the disease. Since the disease state may be unstable, the clinical condition may vacillate between one extreme and the other, but the essential character of leprosy will be maintained. The numbers of bacilli present depend upon the degree of host resistance. The outcome depends upon the development of host resistance as well as upon treatment.

Immunological basis of the tissue changes

There is still some debate regarding the initial route of infection but entry through minor injury involving the skin is thought to be most likely. As with other mycobacteria, *Mycobacterium leprae* has the capacity to excite cell-mediated immune responses, and indeed the tuberculoid form, as the name indicates, has many similarities with the lesions of tuberculosis. It is the intensity of the cell-mediated tissue response that controls the infection; at the same time, it is this response that causes the destruction of the skin and nerve tissue. The positive lepromin reaction, closely analogous to the tuberculin test, is an indication of the delayed hypersensitivity response generated by the bacilli.

In lepromatous leprosy, in contrast, there is evidence that the cell-mediated responses are markedly reduced, but not entirely lacking. Thus, in some typical lepromatous cases it may not be possible to sensitise the skin to dinitrochlorobenzene as occurs in normal people and in patients with tuberculoid leprosy. In such insensitive patients, however, keyhole-limpet haemocyanin, another agent inducing cell-mediated immune responses, may be quite capable of causing sensitisation. Moreover, patients can still successfully combat virus and other infections, and the life span in lepromatous leprosy may not be substantially shortened by the depressed immune state.[47] It is probable that infiltration of the paracortical areas of lymph nodes by very large numbers of actively phagocytic macrophages, often containing bacilli, may displace the normal lymphocyte population and thereby profoundly depress delayed hypersensitivity responses. The position of any patient within the spectrum of clinical leprosy is thus probably a reflection of the degree of immunological depression.

THE NEUROPATHY OF ACUTE INTERMITTENT PORPHYRIA

There are four main types of *acute hepatic porphyria. Acute intermittent porphyria* (AIP) is the commonest form in Europe and America; the *variegate (mixed) form* is more prevalent in South Africa. Neither the rare *hereditary coproporphyria* nor the *symptomatic (acquired) forms of hepatic porphyria* caused by drugs or other chemicals are associated with neurological disturbances. A proportion of cases of AIP and of variegate porphyria (42% of 143 cases of AIP in Waldenström's series)[48] shows a closely similar type of sensory and motor peripheral neuropathy, with many clinical features that sharply distinguish it from the more common forms of peripheral neuropathy.

Clinical features. Acute intermittent porphyria is hereditary and transmitted by an autosomal dominant gene. Only about 1 in 3 of the carriers eventually expresses the trait. It presents at almost any age, though most commonly in the third or fourth decade. The acute attack begins with complaints of 'nagging' or 'colicky' abdominal pain of variable localisation. Vomiting and constipation are characteristic and sometimes severe, and these symptoms not infrequently lead to exploratory laparotomy.

Many patients never show more than these symptoms. Neurological complications occur in less than half of such attacks, presenting only as persistent weakness in the limbs following the acute episode. A few cases, however, show severe degrees of motor weakness that may rapidly advance over a few days to almost total limb paraparesis or even quadriparesis. More usually the neuropathy is of slower onset, gradually becoming worse over the course of two to three weeks; rarely, if ever, does the neuropathy begin contemporaneously with the onset of the abdominal crisis.

The distribution of the motor weakness and sensory changes is unusual for peripheral neuropathy. Muscle weakness commonly involves chiefly the antigravity muscles, and thus is proximal in distribution, though peripheral weakness also occurs and wasting in hand muscles is not uncommon. Sensory disturbances, too, are less frequently purely distal and more often are found in 'bathing trunk', 'long john' or 'sleeve' and 'garter' areas. Dysaesthesiae, numbness and loss of temperature and light touch senses are common. Weakness of sphincters is not infrequent, especially during the acute period of the neurological illness. Progress of all these changes and their spread to involve other areas may be relatively rapid over the course of a few days or may take a week or two to reach a climax, gradually regressing thereafter.[49] In the fully developed neuropathy, cranial nerves may also be involved, especially the facial and vagus nerves, spreading perhaps to the oculomotor nerves. Evidence of autonomic disturbances is frequent; persistent

tachycardia continues as long as recovery progresses.[50] Transient, fluctuating hypertension is also seen and is related to involvement of carotid sinus nerves.[51] Skin photosensitivity, which is often present in other forms of porphyria, due to fully formed porphyrins accumulating in the dermis, does not occur in acute intermittent porphyria but may be seen in variegate porphyria.

Mental disturbances are frequent, and may dominate the clinical picture. They consist of insomnia, confusion, hallucinations, dreams (often of a nightmarish nature), depression and emotional disturbances. Sometimes occurring in the early phases of the attack and always preceding the neurological changes, the psychiatric symptoms may be sufficiently serious to lead to admission to a mental institution.

Laboratory findings. It is characteristic that the urine, at some time during the course of the acute attack, shows dark red ('port wine') discoloration on exposure to air or light, due to the presence of porphobilinogen (PBG). The urine should, thus, never be thrown hastily away in the presence of such symptoms. Excess urinary porphobilinogen and its precursor, δ-aminolaevulinic acid, are essential for the diagnosis. There may be also an increased pyruvate tolerance following a loading dose of glucose. The significance of this last finding is not clear; it occurs in a number of peripheral neuropathies, not necessarily related to vitamin B_1 deficiency. Interestingly, 5-hydroxyindoleacetic acid may also be increased in the urine, presumably indirectly related to lowered activity of liver tryptophan pyrrolase, a haem-containing enzyme.

Electrophysiological studies reveal evidence of muscle denervation, even when there is little more than mild weakness; the conduction velocity is only mildly slowed, indicating axonal degeneration rather than segmental demyelination.

Precipitation of the attacks. A large proportion of patients with acute intermittent porphyria endure acute attacks, accompanied by excessive amounts of δ-aminolevulinic acid and porphobilinogen in the urine, without evident neurological involvement other than persisting leg weakness after the attack. However, certain agents, particularly drugs, when taken by patients with this condition have precipitated attacks that are followed by neuropathy. Sulphonal, which is 2,2-bis(ethylsulphonyl)propane, formerly prescribed as a hypnotic, was the first drug reported to be regularly followed by an attack with dark red urine and neuropathy.[52] More recently, barbiturates have been principally responsible, and sulphonamides the next most common culprits. A full list of such agents is given by de Matteis.[53] How these drugs induce the attacks is not known. The variegate form of porphyria is extremely sensitive to induction in this way; attacks of the hereditary forms can also be precipitated.

Pathological features. Since the earlier post-mortem studies,[54,55] it has been plain that the essential pathological change is a *denervation* process involving only peripheral sensory and motor neurons; central neurons do not show degenerative changes. Peripheral nerves show widespread Wallerian degeneration (Fig. 20.13) with greatest emphasis on more distal regions. Muscles of hands and feet in severe cases may be almost completely denervated, while the nerves to more proximal muscles are less severely affected. If there has been a previous acute attack in the not-too-distant past, many new regenerating and myelinating fibres may be seen intermingled with active degeneration; this is well demonstrated in preparations silver-stained to show axons. Such appearances should not be mistaken for segmental demyelination for, in fact, there is little or no selective myelin damage in this condition. There is also axonal degeneration in dorsal columns, especially in the cervical region, but in no other spinal tract. Occasional reports of focal demyelination in the CNS have all been in patients previously maintained on a respirator and this is

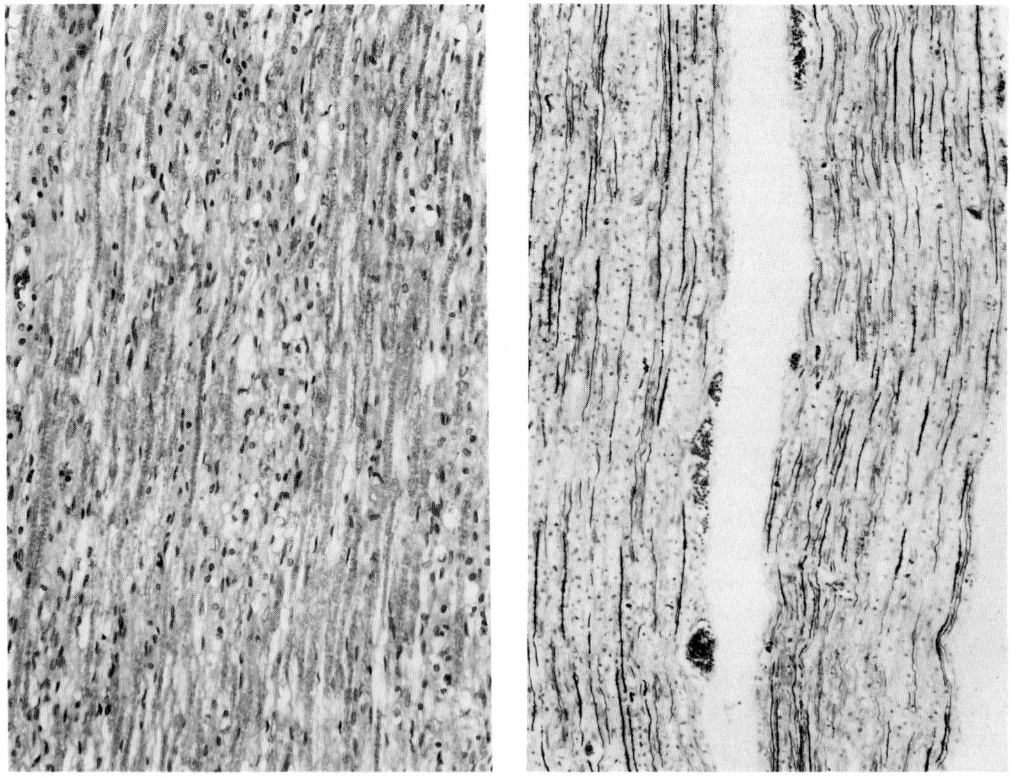

a b

Fig. 20.13a, b Denervation in acute intermittent porphyria. (**a**) Nerve root showing active Wallerian degeneration of nerve fibres with an increase in macrophages in the form of foam cells, but with many surviving myelinated fibres. (**b**) Nerve stained for axons to show axonal loss and large numbers of reactive cells lying between the surviving fibres.
(**a**) Haematoxylin-eosin × 150; (**b**) Glees and Marsland × 95

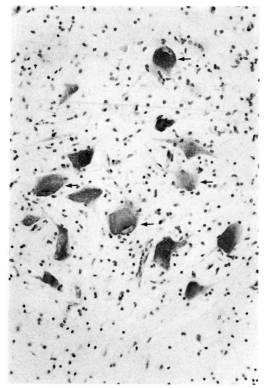

Fig. 20.14 Chromatolysis of anterior horn cells (arrows) from a case of acute intermittent porphyria with severe denervation.
Cresyl fast violet × 150

likely to have been responsible. Anterior horn cells and dorsal root ganglion cells show chromatolysis (Fig. 20.14), often to a striking degree; the severity is related to the extent to which the degenerative 'dying back' process (see p. 540) has occurred. When this has progressed back to the spinal roots, the neuronal changes will be most severe.[56]

Metabolic basis of the attack and the neuropathy. The genetic disturbance in acute intermittent porphyria (AIP) is associated with an instability of the mechanism controlling the synthesis of haem. This important substance is required not only for the formation of haemoglobin, but perhaps more importantly in the formation of haemproteins, especially cytochromes. Haemproteins are synthesised in all cells and nowhere more actively than in the liver and the brain. The activity of this pathway is tightly controlled by a feedback mechanism in which the end product, haem, regulates the primary and

rate-limiting enzyme, δ-aminolaevulinic acid (δ-ALA) synthetase. This is an amino decarboxylating enzyme requiring pyridoxal phosphate as a co-factor, conjugating glycine and succinyl-coenzyme A to form δ-ALA. Repression and derepression of the operon responsible for the formation of δ-ALA synthetase appears to be controlled by the levels of haem in the cell.[57] How instability of the control of this pathway comes about in the genetic defect is unknown, but it leads to uncontrolled synthesis of the enzyme with resultant excessive urinary excretion of δ-ALA and of porphobilinogen (a product of the next step in the pathway).[58] Of considerable therapeutic interest is the capacity of administered haem to inhibit the uncontrolled formation of δ-ALA synthetase and to stop the clinical attacks. Administration of glucose has the same effect though the reason for this response is not clear. Stopping the attacks in the early stage prevents the development of the much more life-threatening neurological changes.

Whether the early abdominal symptoms of the acute attack are related to plasma levels of intermediates of haem synthesis is not known, but it is certain that the latter have never been shown to be capable of producing neuropathic changes in experimental animals. It is of interest, however, that reduction in haemproteins in the liver is associated with parallel reduction in tryptophan pyrrolase and a resulting increase in circulating tryptophan. Injection of this amino acid is known to cause abdominal symptoms and psychiatric changes and, thus, could be responsible for many of the symptoms found with the acute episodes,[59] including the psychiatric features.

There is some doubt as to how the neurological changes are produced and it seems unlikely that the primary metabolic changes in haem metabolism are directly responsible. The neurological disorder does not constantly accompany acute attacks; it never occurs at the same time as, but always follows, the acute illness; and there is no known mechanism by which excess δ-ALA, porphobilinogen or tryptophan is able to produce neurotoxic changes. This suggests that another mechanism must be involved. What seems to be important is that, during the acute attacks, patients are significantly depleted in pyridoxal phosphate (PPO_4). One consequence is a serious inability to metabolise tryptophan to nicotinamide (as estimated by the tryptophan load test), because this metabolic route is dependent upon PPO_4.[60,61] There is also a significant reduction of pyridoxal phosphate in the plasma.[62] Such findings only occur during the acute phase of the illness, not during remission. It has been suggested that since δ-ALA synthetase is a PPO_4-requiring enzyme, and becomes many times more active during the acute attack than normally, an intense over-utilisation of PPO_4 occurs in the tissues, with resulting depletion of those cells with the greatest demand.[63] This suggestion is of relevance to the development of the neuropathy, since the pattern of denervation found at post mortem[56] is exactly similar to that found in experimental animals given large doses of the anti-PPO_4 drug, isoniazid (p. 280). It is difficult to believe that such a coincidence is not significant, and it is considered likely that the neuropathic changes are secondary to consumptive tissue depletion of PPO_4.[64]

URAEMIC NEUROPATHY

Patients with longstanding chronic renal disease may develop a distal symmetrical sensory and motor neuropathy.[65] During the early stages of the development of dialysis for renal failure many patients so treated showed signs of neuropathy. The neuropathy develops regardless of the type of renal lesion and will stabilise, if not improve, with intensive dialysis treatment. This has become a strong positive criterion for renal transplantation.

Clinical features. The earliest signs are muscle cramps and dysaesthesiae in the distal regions of the lower limbs. Unpleasant sensations, numbness, and loss of sensation, particularly of more discriminative modalities, are associated with variable degrees of muscular weakness and wasting, and loss of reflexes. All these features are regularly and characteristically concentrated in the distal parts of the lower limbs and in the upper limbs to a lesser degree. Cranial nerves are not involved nor is the autonomic system. Occasionally, the paresis is severe and rapid in

onset, but in general the progress of the condition varies greatly from case to case.

Electrophysiological studies show relatively mild slowing of conduction velocity, but occasionally there is a fairly close correlation between conduction velocity and the uraemic state.[66] Electromyography shows denervation in distal muscles.

Pathological features. Histologically, the peripheral nerves show only Wallerian (axonal) degeneration with perhaps evidence of re-innervation. The distribution is always very distal in the limbs. Abundant degeneration is thus found below the knee, while the sciatic nerve and spinal roots are usually normal. Changes in upper limb nerves are similarly distal. In the spinal cord, anterior horn cells may be chromatolytic, according to the severity of the denervation. Neurons in spinal ganglia are similarly chromatolytic and the upper regions of the gracile tracts may also show degeneration of axons with accompanying gliosis. No other tracts are affected.

While most of the degenerative change is axonal in nature, segmental demyelination has been reported[67] and even 'onion bulb' formation (see p. 573) has been found in sural nerve biopsies.[68] The significance of these changes is uncertain, but atrophy of axons (see below) appears to be the primary pathological feature and the Schwann cell changes secondary.

Electron microscopy shows no specific features in the Wallerian degeneration, but measurement of the size of axons and myelin sheaths not only demonstrates that larger diameter fibres are selectively lost from distal peripheral nerves, but that there is evidence for a significant *axonal atrophy* in surviving fibres when axon diameter is correlated with myelin thickness.[69] Whether such selective axonal atrophy is specific for uraemic neuropathy, or whether other 'dying back' types of neuropathy (p. 540) with similarly distributed degenerative changes show it has yet to be determined.

Metabolic basis of the neuropathy. The biochemical basis of this disorder is unknown. However, the pattern of the clinical disturbances and the distribution of the degenerative changes are closely similar to those found in the chronic energy deprivation syndromes (see p. 286) that are associated with peripheral neuropathy, such as vitamin B$_1$ deficiency. There is little to relate the neuropathy to the particular type of renal lesion, but there does appear to be some relationship to the uraemic state. Certainly renal transplantation has a dramatically beneficial effect upon the neuropathy, most of the cases either recovering completely or being greatly improved.[70] It has been suggested that myoinositol levels in the plasma, which are strikingly increased, may be causally related to the neuropathy,[71] but exactly how is unclear. Perhaps of more interest, in view of the similarity of the denervation pattern to the energy deficient neuropathies, is the appearance of a dialysable factor in the plasma of these patients which is capable of inhibiting the enzyme transketolase.[72] This factor is lost on dialysis. Transketolase is thiamine-dependent but its specific rôle in the metabolism of peripheral nerves is unknown.

CARCINOMATOUS NEUROPATHIES

Apart from infiltration, compression and local destruction of peripheral nerves by metastatic deposits, particularly at their emergence from the cranium and the spinal canal, there are several kinds of neuropathy that are the indirect result of malignant growths. The pathogenesis of these so-called remote effects of malignant disease is still unknown.[73-75] Non-metastatic complications of malignancy that affect the central nervous system are considered on page 493.

Electrophysiological studies have shown some disturbance in peripheral nerve function in almost half of cases of advanced malignant disease.[76] However, this frequency of effects on peripheral nerves has not been confirmed by pathological examination. Clinically identified cases of neuropathy are substantially less numerous;[77] the condition presents in about 5% of cases of lung cancer, about 3% of stomach cancer and slightly more than 1% of breast, colon and other major types of cancer.

Three principal types of neuropathy are encountered: sensory neuropathy, demyelinating neuropathy, and sensorimotor neuropathy. Other kinds of pathological process in peripheral nerves, such as vasculitis, may also occasionally complicate malignant disease.

Carcinomatous sensory neuropathy

Clinical features. This type of neuropathy is relatively uncommon. It is comparatively slow in onset and development and may precede the first direct manifestations of the associated malignant growth. At the outset there may be asymmetrical disturbance and loss of sensation in distal regions of the limbs, but this spreads to produce a severe and extensive sensory disability. Since large diameter fibres are selectively destroyed, there is often severe loss of proprioceptive sensation with inability to determine the position of the limbs in space. Control of movements may thereby be severely impaired and this may even produce a pseudoathetosis. Sensory conduction velocity is significantly slowed and sensory action potentials are severely reduced.[78]

Pathological features. Examination of peripheral nerves shows extensive loss of nerve fibres and active Wallerian degeneration in many of the remainder, but few signs of regeneration. In the spinal cord there is marked degeneration of the cuneate and gracile tracts, sometimes resulting in almost complete myelin loss from the dorsal columns (Fig. 20.15). In spinal ganglia loss of ganglion cells is characteristic; their original position is marked by clumps of satellite cells, termed residual nodules of Nageotte (Fig. 20.16). Varying amounts of focal perivascular chronic inflammatory cell infiltration are also not uncommon, but whether this is part of the primary process or secondary to the degenerative changes is uncertain. Such changes in spinal ganglia are not associated with any encephalomyelitis and this distinguishes the sensory neuropathy from the sensorimotor neuropathy described below.

Demyelinating carcinomatous neuropathy

Clinical features. This condition may be difficult to distinguish from Guillain–Barré syndrome (see p. 551). Both motor and sensory functions are

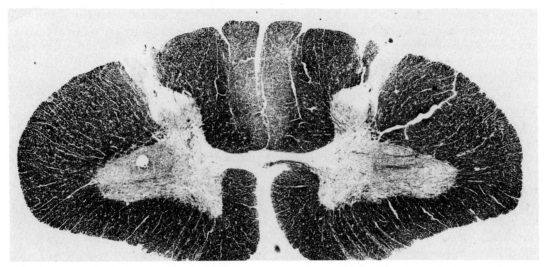

Fig. 20.15 Cervical spinal cord from a case of carcinomatous sensory neuropathy. Note the myelin loss from the gracile tracts from loss of axons, but in this instance very little loss from the cuneate tracts. Loyez × 12·5

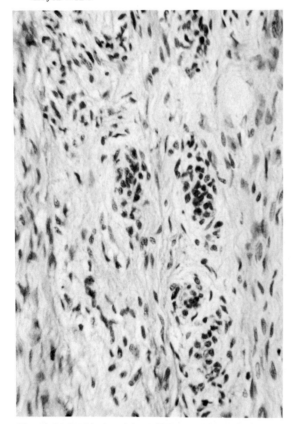

Fig. 20.16 Residual nodules (of Nageotte) in a spinal ganglion from a case of carcinomatous sensory neuropathy. Very few ganglion cells were left in this ganglion; only the satellite cell clusters remained to show their positions. Haematoxylin-eosin × 110

disturbed and the progress of the illness may be acute with severe subsequent paresis. Relapsing and remitting forms may be encountered. Conduction velocity is consistently, and often severely, slowed.

Pathological features. The significant lesion found in teased nerve preparations is segmental demyelination, often paranodal in distribution, and accompanied by focal inflammatory infiltration of the nerve. The changes are, thus, very similar to those found in Guillain–Barré syndrome, and the conditions can often only be distinguished by the discovery of the primary tumour. In addition, there may be loss of axons with detectable Wallerian degeneration. Whether the axonal degeneration is due to secondary involvement of the axons in the inflammatory changes or to other causes may be difficult to determine.

Sensorimotor carcinomatous neuropathy

This type of pathological process is less easy to identify clinically but the variety of signs and symptoms encountered in a patient with malignant disease may be a guide.

Pathological features. Chromatolysis and loss of anterior horn cells in the spinal cord are accompanied by inflammatory perivascular infiltration. Comparable changes are present in the CNS generally and in the spinal ganglia. The nature and extent of these changes indicate a disease of the nervous system which is generalised although expressed principally as a peripheral neuropathy.[79] In the peripheral nerves, widespread loss of nerve fibres and Wallerian degeneration will be seen. In the CNS, perivascular inflammatory infiltrates may be found in the cerebrum, particularly in the limbic regions, and in the brainstem, cerebellum and spinal cord.

Underlying pathogenetic mechanisms (see also p. 493).

These remain speculative. There is a high possibility that a virus infection is responsible for the encephalomyelitic forms in which inflammatory cell infiltration is abundant, particularly in view of the changes that occur in the immune state in malignant disease. No virus, however, has yet been convincingly demonstrated.[80]

The second possibility is an abnormal immune response to antigens in nervous tissue. Although circulating antibodies that bind to Purkinje cells have been found in cases of cerebellar cortical degeneration associated with cancer (see p. 494),[81] there is little evidence that such a phenomenon occurs in the peripheral nervous system except for the unconfirmed finding of circulating antibodies binding to spinal ganglion neurons in a few cases.[82] Unfortunately, there is considerable doubt as to whether these were primary or secondary to the progressive neuronal destruction.

The third possibility, particularly in the sensory form of carcinomatous neuropathy, is that the malignant tumour may interfere with the metabolism of peripheral nerves in some, as yet, undefined way.

IONISING RADIATION NEUROPATHY

Ionising radiations have little immediate effect upon normal peripheral nerve function with doses of less than 30 000 rads (300 Gy).[83]

On the other hand, there have been many reports of neuropathic lesions involving the brachial and lumbar plexuses, following therapeutic exposures.[84,85]

Pathological features. It is difficult to determine the causes of changes that appear in peripheral nerves following irradiation. Factors that may be responsible include local spread of the tumour itself, fibrosis accompanying the tumour or caused by radiation, vascular obliteration by radiation, or direct damage to the peripheral nerves by radiation. This is especially so because of the marked variability of radiotherapeutic regimens and doses. All the above features will be found on histological examination of the irradiated tissues. Wallerian degeneration is marked in involved nerves.

Experimental studies have shown delayed radiation damage in peripheral nerves after doses ranging from 2000 to 5000 rads (20–50 Gy). Lumbosacral roots seem to be most susceptible. The changes may be delayed for several months after the course of radiation. In the peripheral nervous system of irradiated rats there is the additional problem of the normal ageing processes found in this species that could enhance the changes.[86] Ventral roots seem to be more susceptible than dorsal roots, and some hypertrophic Schwann cell changes follow in about one-quarter of the animals.[87]

Mechanisms of damage. Just as in the case of delayed radiation effects in the CNS (see p. 147), the mechanisms of radiation damage to peripheral nerve cells are not fully understood. Injury to vascular cells and to Schwann cells by X-rays plays a rôle in producing the changes. Doses of 2000 rads or more cause extensive damage to DNA in the majority of cells exposed, but peripheral nerve tissue, being in normal circumstances non-proliferative, tolerates the damage, which therefore is not expressed. However, with increasing age and steady accumulation of minor degrees of nerve damage, the defect in proliferative activity that results from radiation-induced DNA damage begins to have an effect upon the repair capacity of the Schwann cells and upon the responsiveness of the vascular bed.[88-90] Evidence of radiation damage can be seen as chromosome breaks, chromosome 'bridges' and other abnormalities in dividing cells, as well as multinucleate and polyploid forms and cell death. Just how much these radiation-induced basic cell defects contribute to the individual tissue changes in any particular case is always difficult to decide.

HEREDITARY NEUROPATHIES

INTRODUCTION

Hereditary diseases of the peripheral nervous system are rare, although the literature contains many individual reported cases. In general, these diseases can be separated into disturbances of lipid metabolism (which include metachromatic leucodystrophy, Krabbe's disease and Fabry's disease), various forms of hereditary amyloid disease and a large group of heterogeneous sensory and/or motor neuropathies. This last group includes the hypertrophic neuropathies of Déjérine and Sottas in children and young adults, two varieties of Charcot–Marie–Tooth disease, as well as other sensory and motor neuropathies with less conspicuously striking features. Some of these diseases may form links with well-defined hereditary conditions such as Friedreich's ataxia and other systematised degenerations of the CNS. These *abiotrophies*, to use Gowers' term, often vary somewhat from one affected family to another in the details of their clinical state and in the precise anatomical pathways involved. Such expression of genetic diversity is undoubtedly one important reason for the differing views of these conditions that have prevailed among clinicians for many years and may in part account for the confusion that has surrounded them. The underlying mechanisms of these sensory and motor neuropathies are still unknown in the great majority of cases.

DEFECTS IN LIPID METABOLISM

Fabry's disease (angiokeratoma corporis diffusum)

This is a hereditary X-linked recessive disorder of homozygous males in whom there is a defect in the activity of α-galactosidase A in the tissues. The enzyme defect leads to the accumulation of glycosphingolipids in lysosomes in many tissues. Particularly affected are the vascular endothelium leading to angiokeratosis of skin and mucous membranes, the kidneys (which may in time become severely damaged), the sensory neurons in spinal and autonomic ganglia, and the cornea and lens tissues, which often develop opacities. The extensive involvement of vascular tissues may lead eventually to cardiovascular problems and to cerebrovascular disease, both of which are causes of disability or death.

Clinical features. Pain is the principal complaint in a large proportion of patients with this disease and particularly affects the lower limbs. The pain is burning and persistent, often lasting several days, although acute episodes of excruciating pain may also occur, occasionally simulating renal or intestinal colic.

Pathological features. In peripheral nerves accumulations of lipid are present in endothelial cells of capillaries as well as in perineurial cells, but not apparently in Schwann cells.[91] Degeneration of myelinated nerve fibres is found, especially those of small diameter, i.e. those serving pain sensations and the autonomic system.[92] Lipid accumulation occurs in the neurons of the dorsal root and autonomic ganglia and many affected neurons are lost from these sites. Neurons of the CNS are also affected, particularly in the intermediate cell columns of the thoracolumbar regions of the cord, in the peri-aqueductal regions of the brainstem and in other nuclei of the brainstem concerned with autonomic functions.[93]

Ultrastructurally, lipid accumulations are membrane bound within secondary lysosomes and have a lamellar structure with an irregular periodicity varying from 4–5 nm to 9 nm or more. The accumulated material is birefringent under polarised light and stains with lipid stains as well as by the PAS method.

The metabolic basis of the changes. Defective activity of the α-galactosidase leads to storage of glycosphingolipids in many cells, but it is uncertain why there is such localised accumulation in some neurons but not in others. The cells at risk are those of the autonomic nervous system, both motor and sensory, while somatic motor and sensory neurons as well as the majority of the cells of the CNS are apparently unaffected. There is also unexplained accumulation in neurons of the hippocampus, the substantia nigra and brainstem centres, some of which are known to be related to autonomic functions. The major neuron regions of the cerebrum and the cerebellum are not, however, involved.

Evidence of the metabolic defect is found in reduced degree in heterozygotes. They show at most only minor signs of the disease.

Metachromatic leucodystrophy

The condition is characterised by accumulation of galactosyl sulphatide (cerebroside sulphate) in the white matter of the CNS (see p. 344) and in peripheral nerves. It is due to a deficiency of arylsulphatase, an enzyme necessary for hydrolysis of sulphatides. Various genetically distinct forms of the condition are known; they are inherited as autosomal recessive traits. Peripheral neuropathy is a minor component of the condition.

Clinical features.   Congenital cases are rare, the most frequent age of appearance of the disease being in late infancy or between the ages of 3 and 16 years (juvenile form). Adult cases are also rare but when they occur they tend to progress more slowly than the younger forms.

In the younger cases the onset is indicated by failure of development, weakness, hypotonia and unsteady gait. With time, spasticity develops and there is increasing loss of control of limb movements as well as mental retardation which becomes severe. The effects on the CNS are described further on page 344. The peripheral neuropathy is a relatively minor association and is related to the myelin loss consequent upon faulty metabolism of essential myelin lipids.

Pathological features.   In peripheral nerves segmental demyelination occurs extensively, and myelin debris can be found lying between nerve fibres in the endoneurium as well as within Schwann cells. The lipid material is metachromatic and stains brown with cresyl violet, a reaction best shown by polarised light. It also stains with Sudan black B, with Alcian blue and with the PAS method; these latter stains are abolished by previous extraction with lipid solvents, such as alcohol and chloroform. In the younger cases, the myelin breakdown is more intense and widespread than it is in the cases of later onset. However, the older cases show more complete nerve fibre degeneration, more 'onion bulb' formation and a greater amount of endoneurial fibrosis; these features reflect the slower progress and greater chronicity of the disease.

As judged from the ultrastructural characteristics, the metachromatic inclusion material is complex, probably being made up of both lipid and protein. The lamellar inclusions are bound by unit membranes within secondary lysosomes, and show a periodic banding with a repeat pattern of 5–6 nm. Protein material probably lies between the osmium-binding lipid, and stains readily with phosphotungstate to give a pseudohelical pattern to the structures.[94]

Globoid cell leucodystrophy (Krabbe's disease)

This condition affects infants and young children, and is rarely encountered in adults. It is due to a defect in galactocerebroside metabolism involving galactocerebroside-β-galactosidase and it is transmitted as an autosomal recessive trait. All tissues are affected, but the white matter of the CNS is particularly involved (see p. 345) leading to progressive flaccid paresis with severe mental and psychomotor deterioration. Peripheral nerves are incidentally affected and because of the overwhelming nature of the central disturbances their involvement has often in the past been overlooked. However, marked slowing of the conduction velocity and increased distal latencies have indicated segmental demyelination in nerves.[95,96]

Pathological features.   Teased portions of nerves show variable amounts of myelin loss in many nerve fibres, and loss of axons with Wallerian degeneration may occasionally be severe. Foamy macrophages are numerous both in the endoneurium and around blood vessels, but the big clusters of globoid cells formed from macrophages that characterise the CNS changes are not found in nerves. Ultrastructurally, the straight or curved tubular inclusions seen in macrophages are similar to those already noted in the CNS (see p. 347); these are sometimes found also within Schwann cells.

Refsum's disease

The principal clinical features of this hereditary condition are retinitis pigmentosa, peripheral neuropathy and ataxia. These changes result from a defect in the degradation of a 20-carbon branch-chain fatty acid of exogenous origin (phytanic acid) that in consequence accumulates in blood and many other tissues. The connection between the tissue accumulation and the cellular pathological changes is obscure. The defect is inherited as an autosomal recessive trait.

Clinical features. The onset of the clinical condition is in children or young adults and begins insidiously with distal weakness and wasting of the lower limbs. This gradually becomes more severe and extensive, and on electrophysiological examination a profound slowing of conduction velocity is found in peripheral nerves. Sensory loss of glove and stocking distribution is frequent, and subjective sensory disturbances are noted as well as loss of reflexes. The frequent occurrence of hearing loss and of anosmia suggests that involvement of peripheral nerves is widespread.

Pathological features. In most cases, the peripheral nerves are enlarged but not greatly so. The enlargement extends to the spinal roots and spinal ganglia. On cross-section, the nerves are watery and mucoid in appearance. Histologically, a characteristic 'onion bulb' pattern is seen in which the Schwann cells are neatly arranged around an axon that may or may not have lost its myelin sheath. In the later stages, axons may also be lost from the 'onion bulb' formations. There is an abundance of endoneurial collagen between and among the 'onion bulb' formations; Schwann cell and other nuclei are more numerous than is normal. Many of the remaining axons are demyelinated and the myelin around the rest is thinner than usual, suggesting remyelination. Chromatolysis is seen in the anterior horn cells and in spinal ganglion cells. The dorsal columns show varying degrees of axon and myelin loss[97] due to destruction of spinal ganglion cells; residual nodules may be numerous in the spinal ganglia.[98] There are very few other changes in the CNS.

Ultrastructurally, peripheral nerves show evidence of segmental demyelination and of remyelination in the form of inappropriately thin myelin sheaths. Within Schwann cells, lipid inclusions are numerous, and crystalline bodies are also described, often lying close to the nucleus.[99]

Metabolic basis of the lesions. The phytanic acid that accumulates in the tissues is derived from intestinal absorption and normally it is rapidly degraded by β-oxidative steps after an initial α-hydroxylation. The α-hydroxylase required for the latter is absent in cases of Refsum's disease, so that the phytanic acid cannot be removed and thus accumulates in the tissues. It is suggested that during development and myelination this may become incorporated into myelin sheath membranes and lead to their instability. Other possibilities exist, however, and one is that the occurrence of low levels of linoleate in the tissues, which may be an indirect effect of excess phytanic acid, may be detrimental to cell membrane metabolism.[100]

The neuropathy associated with Tangier disease (high density lipoprotein deficiency)

This rare autosomal recessive condition is characterised by hyperplastic orange-coloured tonsils, corneal opacities, relapsing neuropathy and storage of cholesterol esters in the tissues. There is a profound reduction of high density lipoproteins in the plasma.[101]

Clinical features. Most, but not all, reported cases show evidence of a peripheral nerve disorder, and this may be the presenting complaint. The severity of the neurological condition varies considerably from case to case and milder cases show patchy loss of pain and temperature sensation that is more marked in the feet and the legs than in the hands, although all parts of the body, including the face, may, in more severe instances, be affected. The more discriminating aspects of sensation, such as light touch and vibration sense, are usually spared.[102]

On the motor side, there may be slowly progressive weakness and wasting of the hand and foot muscles, but transient weakness of ocular and facial muscles has also been noted, as well as various local muscle palsies. The condition is essentially a mononeuritis multiplex rather than a systemic neuropathy. Loss of reflexes is frequent and signs of disturbance to the autonomic nervous system, as demonstrated by episodes of excessive sweating, are seen.

Pathological features. The cellular changes consist of infiltration of the tissues by lipid-laden macrophages, especially in the reticuloendothelial tissues of the liver, spleen, lymph nodes and bone marrow. The orange colour of the tonsils and their enlargement reflect their infiltration by these lipid-filled cells. The liver and spleen may be enlarged and there may be thrombocytopenia and other evidence of bone marrow damage. Yellowish infiltration is seen in the mucosa of the intestine and in the skin.[103]

In peripheral nerves, lipid-laden macrophages infiltrate the endoneurium and there is an increase in endoneurial collagen. Some sural nerve biopsies may not show severe involvement; in other cases there may be extensive axonal loss. On the whole, the infiltration and nerve fibre loss take place principally in the more peripheral terminal regions of the nerves. The Schwann cells contain lipid vacuoles and myelin figures, but segmental demyelination is not a feature of this condition.[104]

It should be noted that a somewhat similar neuropathy has occasionally been encountered in *biliary cirrhosis with hypercholesterolaemic xanthomatosis*, which is a much milder and more chronic disorder of cholesterol metabolism.[105] Neuropathy is not recognised in other forms of xanthomatosis.

In abetalipoproteinaemia, in which there is a peripheral neuropathy associated with an hereditary deficiency of *low density lipoproteins*, the neurological changes are recognised to be secondary to a tissue deficiency of vitamin E (α-tocopherol) which is normally transported by this class of lipoproteins. The condition is therefore considered in the section concerned with vitamin deficiencies (see p. 297).

HEREDITARY SENSORY NEUROPATHIES (HSN)

Hereditary radicular sensory neuropathy of Denny Brown (HSN I)

Clinical features. Denny Brown[106] described the first case of this autosomal dominant condition in which there was a steadily progressive distal loss of sensation from the limbs. Young adults are particularly affected, with loss of pain and temperature sensation from the feet and to a lesser degree from the hands. There is a parallel loss of sweating in the limbs as well as of other autonomic functions. In consequence, and as the result of unnoticed minor trauma in the anaesthetic limbs, chronic ulcers in the feet begin to appear and become infected. The infection spreads more deeply to involve underlying tissues, bones and joints. Neuropathic (Charcot) joints also may develop.

Pathological features. There is loss of the longer axons of smaller diameter from sensory nerves. Accompanying this there is loss of cells from the spinal root ganglia. Larger diameter axons and their cell bodies are also lost,[107] and degeneration of dorsal columns as well as loss of neurons from the dorsal ganglia characterise the condition. Motor nerve cells in the spinal cord and their nerve fibres appear to be unaffected.

Congenital sensory neuropathy (HSN II)

In marked contrast to Denny Brown's hereditary radicular sensory neuropathy, congenital sensory neuropathy is an autosomal recessive condition presenting in young children with progressive loss of sensation distally in the limbs without any major disturbance of motor or autonomic functions. The sensory loss affects the limbs distally and symmetrically, spreading incompletely to involve the trunk; it does not involve the face. Severe secondary ulceration of the feet and hands and Charcot's type of neuropathic joints are likely to occur.[108]

Pathological features. Biopsy studies, particularly of the sural nerve, have shown severe loss of sensory nerve fibres, especially distally in the limbs, the loss becoming less apparent in more proximal samples of the nerve. This suggests that there is a degeneration of the longer fibres, but unmyelinated fibres are also reduced in numbers. A small proportion of surviving myelinated fibres show also segmental loss of myelin, suggesting that

there may be axonal atrophy preceding ultimate axonal degeneration.[109]

Dysautonomia (Riley–Day syndrome) (HSN III)

Also inherited as an autosomal recessive trait, this rare condition chiefly, but not entirely, affects Ashkenazi Jewish infants and young children. It is separable from other sensory neuropathies by the striking disturbances of autonomic functions. Fluctuations in blood pressure, poor temperature control, reduced tear flow and abnormalities of sweating combined with insensitivity to pain are

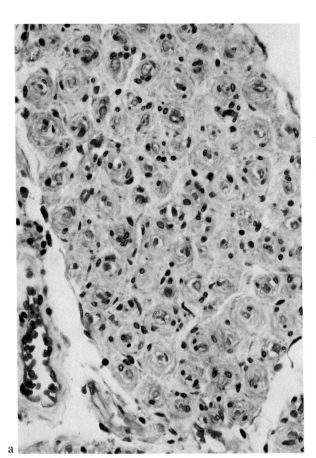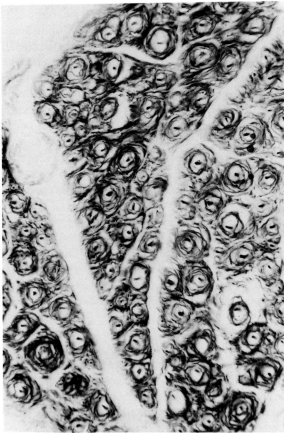

Fig. 20.17a, b Charcot–Marie–Tooth Disease (HMSN I). Onion-bulb formation around axons in lumbar spinal nerve root. In **b**, axons can still be seen in the majority of the concentric formations, and this stain also picks out the reticulin lying between the concentrically arranged Schwann cells.
(**a**) Van Gieson ×250; (**b**) Glees and Marsland ×250
Photomicrographs provided by Prof. P. L. Lantos, Institute of Psychiatry, London, UK.

characteristic of the condition. Reduced reflexes and poor coordination of the limbs also occur.

HEREDITARY MOTOR AND SENSORY NEUROPATHIES (HMSN)

Charcot–Marie–Tooth disease (HMSN I and II)

Recent studies have shown that there are in fact two forms of Charcot–Marie–Tooth disease (HMSN I and HMSN II), which lead to slow distal loss of motor functions with muscular wasting. Both are hereditary and both may be transmitted either as dominant or as recessive traits. They may also present as sporadic cases.

Charcot–Marie–Tooth disease I (peroneal muscular atrophy—HMSN I)

Clinical features.   This first form of the disease is the commoner and accounts for about 85% of cases. The mean age of onset is in the first decade, and the condition progresses very slowly over many years with distal weakness and wasting of the lower limbs; the weakness later spreads to the hands and arms. Pes cavus is a common early sign and scoliosis is frequently found. With time, reflexes are lost and there is mild sensory impairment, with later development of ataxia, probably the result of sensory deprivation. Peripheral nerves may become thickened and palpable.

Electrophysiological findings are important for identifying this condition. There is pronounced slowing of nerve conduction velocity, while sensory action potentials are either grossly diminished or completely lost.

Pathological features.   Nerve biopsies cut in transverse section show characteristic 'onion bulb' formations with extensive loss of myelin sheaths but persisting axons. In the more advanced cases, many of the axons are also lost from within the 'onion bulb' formations. This curious cellular arrangement is due to concentric proliferation of the Schwann cells around the nerve fibre as the result of repeated segmental demyelination and remyelination.

Post-mortem studies show that the 'onion bulb'

arrangement of Schwann cells is present throughout the peripheral nervous system, even including the spinal roots (Fig. 20.17). In addition, there is abundant mucoid (glycoprotein) material and collagen in the endoneurial spaces between the 'onion bulb' formations. Anterior horn cells may show severe chromatolysis (Fig. 20.18). Examination of teased nerve fibres and morphometric measurements of different nerves at post mortem[110] confirm the presence of segmental demyelination and remyelination. These features certainly account for the striking slowing of conduction found clinically; the probability of a primary defect in the Schwann cell's capacity to maintain myelin is suggested by a study which has shown that Schwann cell transplants from such

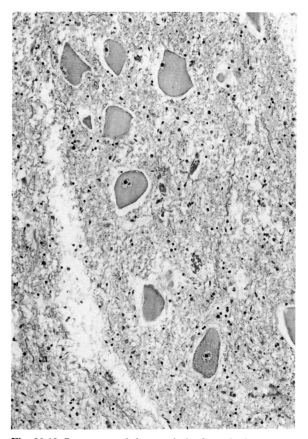

Fig. 20.18 Severe general chromatolysis of anterior horn cells in a case of Charcot–Marie–Tooth disease (HMSN I). Haematoxylin-eosin × 145
Photomicrograph provided by Prof. P. L. Lantos, Institute of Psychiatry, London, UK.

individuals into immune-suppressed mice are markedly less efficient at myelinating regenerating axons than similar transplants from control subjects.[111] The pronounced reduction in axon calibre that is also present implies that there is also a neuronal defect. Since myelin thickness and stability are both dependent upon axon calibre, substantial reduction in size of the axon would be expected to destabilise the myelin.

The locus for the genetic defect has been found in 5–10% of families to lie on chromosome 1 close to the Duffy locus; the chromosome locus of the majority is obscure.[112]

Charcot–Marie–Tooth disease II (HMSN II)

Pathological features.   As noted above, this condition is less common than HMSN I and has been

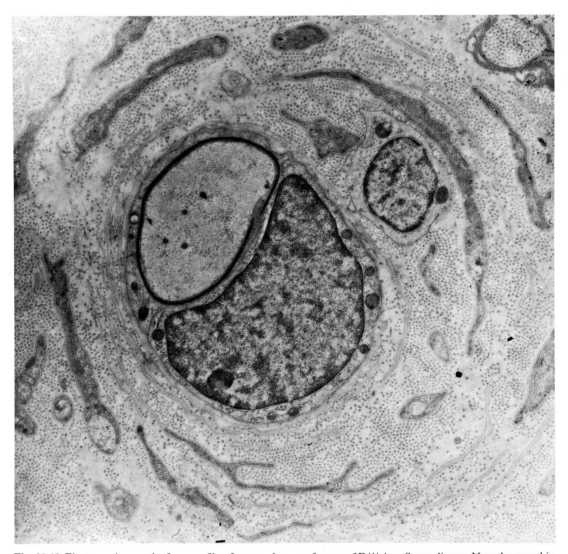

Fig. 20.19 Electron micrograph of a nerve fibre from sural nerve of a case of Déjérine–Sottas disease. Note the very thin, recently reformed myelin sheath around the axon within a Schwann cell, and the concentrically arranged Schwann cell processes, each with a basement membrane and separated by collagen fibres.
× 7000
Electron micrograph provided by Prof. R. O. Weller, University of Southampton, Southampton, UK.

studied less, but biopsy material has shown that 'onion bulb' formation, so characteristic of HMSN I, is much less in evidence, nerves are not significantly enlarged and segmental demyelination is less frequently seen. There is, however, evidence of fibre loss from both sensory and mixed motor nerves that fits the clinical picture of distal sensory deprivation and distal motor weakness with muscle wasting. There is still debate as to whether this is merely a milder form of the more common Charcot–Marie–Tooth disease or whether it is a separate pathological entity, however clearly the two conditions may be separated clinically.[110,113] The fact that the condition does not appear to be linked to the Duffy locus is a priori evidence for regarding it as a separate entity; however, the genetic linkage is not found in all the families with the common form of this condition.

Déjérine–Sottas hypertrophic neuropathy (HMSN III)

This condition differs in two features from Charcot–Marie–Tooth disease, namely a strong hereditary recessive trait and the clinical onset of the disease in infancy or in early childhood. In other ways the two conditions are very similar.

Clinical features. The onset of muscle weakness may be in young children or in the first few months of life so that the developmental milestones are delayed and the child becomes confined to a wheel chair from an early age. The muscle weakness is always distal in the limbs and later there is muscle atrophy. Sensory loss is also distal in distribution and affects all modalities; truncal ataxia and abnormal limb movements, both resulting from sensory deprivation, may develop later. Peripheral nerves become enlarged and are readily palpable and perhaps visible through the skin. Nerve conduction velocities are greatly slowed and the tendon reflexes are lost.

Pathological features. Peripheral nerves are visibly and palpably enlarged due to striking development of 'onion bulb' thickening of the nerve fibres from Schwann cell hyperplasia.[114,115] In the early stages many of these formations have centrally placed axons that either are naked (demyelinated) or have a thin myelin sheath (Fig. 20.19); later an increasing number become empty as denervation becomes complete. Teased preparations of nerves, whether from biopsy or from post-mortem material, show long lengths of segmental demyelination and shorter segments of recent remyelination; each individual nerve fibre shows considerable numbers of Schwann cell nuclei clustered around it.

It is not clear whether the Schwann cell's apparent incapacity in this disease to maintain the myelin sheath is a primary defect or whether, as suggested for Charcot–Marie–Tooth disease, this is secondary to a basic slow neuronal atrophy. The analogy with Refsum's disease (see p. 570) is also apparent, but a clearly defined analogous defect in lipid metabolism has not been shown.

TUMOURS

The tumours and tumour-like conditions of the nerves are considered in Chapter 16 (pages 466 to 472 and 494 to 499).

REFERENCES

Introduction

1. Walton JN. Brain's Diseases of the nervous system. 9th ed. Oxford: Oxford University Press, 1985.
2. Weller RO. A general approach to neuropathological problems. In: Berry CL, ed. Current topics in pathology. Berlin: Springer, 1988: 61.
3. Weller RO. A colour atlas of neuropathology. Oxford: H. Miller & Oxford University Press, 1984: 148.

Vascular and immune diseases

4. Blunt MJ, Stratton K. J Anat 1956; 90: 508.
5. Erbsloh F, Katzmeier F. Arch Psychiatr Nervenkr 1950; 183: 703.
6. Eames RA, Lange LS. J Neurol Neurosurg Psychiatry 1967; 30: 215.
7. Chopra JS, Hurwitz LJ. J Neurol Neurosurg Psychiatry 1967; 30: 207.

8. Garven HSD, Gairns FW, Smith G. Scott Med J 1962; 7: 570.
9. Corbin KB, Gardner ED. Anat Rec 1937; 68: 63.
10. Conn DL, Dyck PJ. In: Dyck PJ, Thomas PK, Lambert EH, eds. Peripheral neuropathy. Philadelphia: Saunders, 1975: 1149.
11. Scott DGI, Bacon PA, Tribe CR. Medicine (Baltimore) 1981; 60: 288.
12. Fauci AC, Wolff JR. Medicine (Baltimore) 1973; 52: 535.
13. Weller RO, Bruckner FE, Chamberlain MA. J Neurol Neurosurg Psychiatry 1970; 33: 582.
14. Pallis CA, Scott JT. Br Med J 1965; 1: 1141.
15. Warrell DA, Godfrey S, Olsen EGJ. Lancet 1968; 1: 1010.
16. Ricoy JR, Cabello A, Roderiguez J, Tellez I. Brain 1983; 106: 817.
17. French JM, Hall G, Parish DJ, Smith WT. Am J Med 1965; 39: 277.
18. de Nevasquez S, Treble HA. Brain 1938; 61: 116.
19. Glenner GC, Ignaczak TF, Page DL. In: Stanbury JB, Wyngaarden JB, Fredrickson DS, eds. Metabolic basis of inherited disease. New York: McGraw-Hill, 1978: 1308.
20. Victor M, Banker BQ, Adams RD. J Neurol Neurosurg Psychiatry 1958; 21: 73.
21. Ritzman SE, Thurm RH, Truax WE, Levin WC. Arch Intern Med 1960; 105: 939.
22. Asbury AK, Arnason BGW, Adams RD. Medicine (Baltimore) 1969; 48: 173.

Guillain–Barré syndrome

23. Haymaker W, Kernohan JW. Medicine (Baltimore) 1949; 28: 59.
24. Langmuir AD. J R Soc Med 1979; 72: 660.
25. Cummings JF, Haas DC. Am J Pathol 1972; 66: 189.
26. Liebowitz S, Hughes RAC. Immunology of the nervous system. London: Arnold, 1983.

Paraproteinaemic neuropathy

27. Kelly JJ, Kyle RA, O'Brien PC, Dyck PJ. Neurology 1981; 31: 1480.
28. Smith IS, Kahn SN, Lacey BW, King RM, Eames RA, Whybrew DJ, Thomas PK. Brain 1983; 106: 169.
29. Meier C, Vandervelde M, Steck A, Zarbriggen A. J Neurol Sci 1983; 63: 353.
30. Gregson NA, Liebowitz S. Neuropathol Appl Neurobiol 1985; 11: 329.

Diabetic neuropathy

31. Raff MC, Asbury AK. N Engl J Med 1968; 279: 17.
32. Garland H, Taverner D. Br Med J 1953; 1: 1405.
33. Matthews WB. Proc R Soc Med 1958; 51: 859.
34. Woltman HW, Mulder RM. Arch Intern Med 1929; 44: 576.
35. Dolman CL. Neurology 1963; 13: 135.
36. Thomas PK, Lascelles RG. Brain 1966; 35: 489.
37. Ohnishi A, Harada M, Tateishi J, Ogata J, Kawanami S. Ann Neurol 1983; 13: 541.
38. Greenbaum D, Richardson PC, Salmon MV, Urich H. Brain 1964; 87: 201.
39. Sugimura K, Dyck PJ. J Neurol Sci 1982; 53: 501.
40. Gabby KH, Merola LO, Field RA. Science 1966; 151: 209.

41. Dyck PJ, Yasuda H, Karnes J. In: Recent advances in neuropathology, vol III. Cavanagh JB, ed. Edinburgh: Churchill Livingstone, 1986.

Inflammatory neuropathies

42. Dastur DK, Porwal GL. Clin Exp Neurol 1979; 16: 277.
43. Sabin TD, Swift TR. In: Dyck PJ, Thomas PK, Lambert EH, eds. Peripheral neuropathy, vol. II. Philadelphia: Saunders, 1975: 1166.
44. Sabin TD, Hackett ER, Brand PW. Int J Lepr 1974; 42: 33.
45. Dastur DK, Ramamohan Y, Shah JS. Int J Lepr 1973; 41: 47.
46. Astbury AK, Johnson PC. Pathology of peripheral nerve. Philadelphia: Saunders 1978: 186.
47. Turk JL, Waters MFR. Lancet 1969; 2: 243.

Neuropathy of acute intermittent porphyria

48. Waldenström J. Acta Med Scand 1937; 82 (Suppl): 1.
49. Ridley A. Brain 1969; 83: 307.
50. Ridley A, Hierons R, Cavanagh JB. Lancet 1968; 2: 708.
51. Kezdi P. Arch Intern Med 1954; 94: 122.
52. Harley V. Br Med J 1890; 2: 1896.
53. de Matteis F. Pharmacol Rev 1967; 19: 523.
54. Mason JR, Courville C, Ziskind E. Medicine 1933; 12: 355.
55. Hierons R. Brain 1957; 870: 176.
56. Cavanagh JB, Mellick RS. J Neurol Neurosurg Psychiatry 1965; 28: 320.
57. Meyer UH, Schmid R. Res Publ Assoc Res Nerv Ment Dis 1974; 53: 211.
58. Granick S. Ann NY Acad Sci 1965; 123: 188.
59. Litman DA, Correia MA. Science 1983; 222: 1031.
60. Price JM, Brown RR, Peters HA. Neurology 1959; 9: 456.
61. Elder TD, Mengel CE. Am J Med 1966; 41: 369.
62. Hamfelt A, Wetterberg L. Ann NY Acad Sci 1969; 166: 361.
63. Cavanagh JB, Ridley A. Lancet 1967; 2: 1023.
64. Cavanagh JB. Lancet 1984; 1: 1284.

Uraemic neuropathy

65. Asbury AK, Victor M, Adams RD. Arch Neurol 1963; 8: 413.
66. Jebsen RH, Tenckhoff H, Honet JC. N Engl J Med 1967; 277: 327.
67. Dayan AD, Gardner-Thorpe C, Down PF. Gleadle RI. Neurology 1970; 20: 649.
68. Appenzeller O, Kornfeld M, MacGee J. Arch Neurol 1971; 24: 499.
69. Dyck PJ, Johnson WJ, Lambert EH, O'Brien PC. Mayo Clin Proc 1971; 46: 400.
70. Nielsen VK, Acta Med Scand 1974; 195: 163.
71. Clements RS, DeJesus PV, Winegrad AI. Lancet 1973; 1: 1137.
72. Sterzel RB, Semar M, Lonergan ET, Treser G, Lange K. J Clin Invest 1971; 50: 2295.

Carcinomatous neuropathies

73. Brain WR, Henson RA. Lancet 1959; 2: 971.
74. Croft PB, Urich H, Wilkinson M. Brain 1967; 90: 31.

75. Horwich MS, Cho L, Porro K, Posner JB. Ann Neurol 1977; 2: 7.
76. Teravainen H, Larsen A. Ann Neurol 1977; 2: 495.
77. Croft PB, Wilkinson MIP. Brain 1965; 88: 427.
78. McLeod JG. In: Dyck PJ, Thomas PK, Lambert EH, eds. Peripheral neuropathy. Philadelphia: Saunders, 1975: 64.
79. Henson RA, Urich H. Cancer and the nervous system. Oxford: Blackwell Scientific Publications, 1982.
80. Walton JN, Tomlinson BE, Pearce GW. J Neurol Sci 1968; 6: 435.
81. Jaeckle KA, Graus F, Houghton A et al. Ann Neurol 1985; 18: 592.
82. Wilkinson PC, Zaromski J. Brain 1965; 88: 529.

Ionising radiation neuropathy

83. Gaffey CT. In: Haley TJ, Snider RS, eds. Responses of the nervous system to ionizing radiation. New York: Academic Press, 1962.
84. Mumenthaler J. Eur Neurol 1969; 2: 257.
85. Greenfield MM, Stark FM. Am J Roentgenol 1978; 60: 617.
86. ven der Kogel AJ, Barendson GW. Br J Radiol 1974; 47: 393.
87. van der Kogel AJ. Acta Neuropathol (Berl) 1977; 39: 139.
88. Cavanagh JB. Br J Radiol 1968; 41: 275.
89. Hopewell JW. Neuropathol Appl Neurobiol 1979; 5: 329.
90. Love S. Brain 1983; 106: 39.

Hereditary neuropathies

91. Kocen RS, Thomas PK. Arch Neurol 1970; 22: 81.
92. Ohnishi A, Dyck PJ. Arch Neurol 1974; 31: 120.
93. Sung JH. J Neuropathol Exp Neurol 1979; 38: 87.
94. Gregoire A, Perier O, Dustin P. J Neuropathol Exp Neurol 1966; 25: 617.
95. Hogan GR, Gutmann L, Chou SM. Neurology 1969; 19: 1094.
96. Dunn HG, Lake BD, Dolman DL, Wilson J. Brain 1969; 92: 329.
97. Cammermeyer J, Haymaker W, Refsum S. Am J Pathol 1954; 30: 643.
98. Gordon N, Hudson REB, Brain 1959; 82: 41.
99. Fardeau M, Engel K. J Neuropathol Exp Neurol 1969; 28: 278.
100. Steinberg D. In: Stanbury JB, Wyngaarden JB, Fredrickson DL, Goldstein JL, Brown MS, eds. The metabolic basis of inherited disease. 5th ed. New York: McGraw Hill, 1983; 35.
101. Fredrickson DS, Gotto AM, Levy RI. In: Stanbury JB, Wyngaarden JB, Fredrickson DS, eds. Metabolic basis of inherited disease. New York: McGraw Hill, 1972: 493.
102. Haas LF, Austad WI, Bergin JD. Brain 1974; 97: 351.
103. Ferrans VJ, Fredrickson DS. Am J Pathol 1975; 78: 101.
104. Kocen RG, King RHM, Thomas PK, Haas LF. Acta Neuropathol (Berl) 1973; 26: 317.
105. Thomas PK, Walker JG. Brain 1965; 88: 1079.
106. Denny Brown D. J Neurol Neurosurg 1951; 14: 237.
107. Dyck PJ, Lambert EH, Nichols PC. In: Cobb WA, ed. Handbook of EEG and clinical neurophysiology, vol. 9. Amsterdam: Elsevier, 1971: 83.
108. Johnson RH, Spalding JMK. J Neurol Neurosurg Psychiatry 1964; 27: 125.
109. Ohta M, Elletson RD, Lambert EH, Dyck PJ. Arch Neurol 1973; 29: 23.
110. Dyck PJ. In: Dyck PJ, Thomas PK, Lambert EH, Bunge R, eds. Peripheral neuropathy. 2nd ed. Philadelphia: Saunders, 1984.
111. Aguayo A, Perkins S, Bray G, Duncan I. J Neuropathol Exp Neurol 1978; 37: 582.
112. Guiloff RJ, Thomas PK, Contereas M, Armitage S, Schwarz G, Sedgwick EM. J Neurol Neurosurg Psychiatry 1982; 45: 669.
113. Vogel P, Gabriel M, Goebel HH, Dyck PJ, Ann Neurol 1985; 17: 455.
114. Dyck PJ, Gomez MR. Mayo Clin Proc 1968; 43: 280.
115. Weller RO. J Neurol Neurosurg Psychiatry 1967; 30: 11.

PART 3

Muscle

D. G. F. Harriman

Normal muscle

INTRODUCTION

Skeletal muscle is often referred to as the largest organ in the human body. It is dependent for its function on neural control. This provides for a convenient broad classification of muscle disorders into those which are due to failure of neural control and those which are primary diseases of muscle. The first are the *neurogenic diseases* of muscle and the second are the *myopathies*. Both are further subdivided according to pathogenesis.

Muscle is subject to the same general principles of pathology as the rest of the body, and the study of these principles is vital for an understanding of muscle diseases.

Interest in muscle disease grew slowly during the nineteenth century owing to the difficulty in handling and fixing a vigorously contractile tissue. Better results were obtained with autopsy muscle but in general this had the disadvantage that muscle could be examined only at a late stage of disease. Histological study of muscle was considered to be limited in scope and no real progress was made until cryostat sectioning, histochemical examination and electron microscopy became available. Myopathology now flourishes in collaboration with clinical disciplines and is ever more dependent upon help from biochemists.

ANATOMY

The arrangement of muscle fibres in muscles, both large and small, is subject to variation. In some long muscles, fascicles run in sequence from origin to tendinous insertion whereas in others they run obliquely, transversely or towards the core of the muscle. As individual motor end-plates lie on the midpoint of each muscle fibre, they form a distinct transverse band (the innervation zone) only when the fascicular pattern is simple, as in the vastus medialis muscle, or when the fibres are short, as in the peroneus brevis. Knowledge of the disposition of muscle fibres is of practical importance to the surgeon when he takes specimens for histology; such specimens should be orientated along the length of the muscle fascicles.

Muscle fibres are grouped into fascicles of varying size, each containing up to several hundred fibres. The fascicle is enclosed by a thin capsule of fibrous tissue, the perimysium, and groups of fascicles lie in abundant fibrofatty tissue, the epimysium, which contains the larger arteries, veins and lymphatic vessels. Capillaries encircle individual muscle fibres. Normally, adipose tissue is confined to the epimysium but it does extend into muscle fascicles in obese individuals. An increase in intramuscular adipose tissue is seen in many chronic myopathies, and when accompanied by excessive fibrosis it gives rise to pseudo-hypertrophy, as in Duchenne dystrophy.

HISTOLOGY

Each skeletal muscle fibre is a syncytium formed by the fusion of fetal myoblasts to produce a cylinder whose length is often many thousand times greater than its diameter. Muscle fibre nuclei are usually situated at the periphery of the fibre in a subsarcolemmal position, but they become internalised as fibres approach their insertions into fibrous tissue or tendon. It is rare for muscle fibres to terminate within the muscle belly; thus, the small round profiles of tapering muscle fibres are rarely seen in the centre of a muscle.

Each muscle fibre is enclosed by a delicate fibrous membrane, the endomysium. It contains the capillaries that encircle the muscle fibres; five or six capillaries surround each type 1 fibre whose metabolism is oxidative, but fewer surround type 2 fibres whose metabolism is anaerobic and glycolytic. The nuclei of endomysial cells are less conspicuous than the subsarcolemmal nuclei but are distinguished by their slightly larger size and their tendency to lie transversely across longitudinally sectioned muscle fibres.

There is some variation in the diameter of the muscle fibres, particularly between individual muscles. Fibre measurements should always be made in transverse cryostat sections of muscle and the shortest diameter of the muscle fibre should be calculated; this avoids distortion of the fibre measurement due to obliquity of the section. No detailed tables are yet available comparing all the individual muscles in all somatotypes. However, normal muscle fibres vary between 40 and 80 μm in adult males and between 30 and 70 μm in adult females.[1] At birth, the mean muscle fibre diameter is 15 μm, increasing to 16 μm by one year and to 40 μm by 10 years of age; it is not until the age of 14–15 years that adult fibre sizes are attained.[1]

Fibre types

In man, muscles vary only slightly in colour but in other species, e.g. chicken, there are distinct red and white muscles. The white muscles are composed mainly of the fast-twitch type 2 fibres whereas red muscles are composed of slow-twitch type 1 fibres. Myoglobin is responsible for the red colour of the type 1 fibres. The muscles of diving amphibians may be almost black because of the high concentration of myoglobin needed to provide extra oxygen-binding capacity. All muscles in man are composed of a mixture of fibre types. The slow-twitch fibres are type 1 and the fast-twitch fibres are type 2. Fibre types can be identified by different histochemical reactions. Type 2 fibres stain strongly for phosphorylase, for glycogen with the PAS technique, and for α-glycerophosphate dehydrogenase. Other dehydrogenases are more abundant in type 1 fibres.[1-4]

In diseased muscle, most of the histochemical techniques listed above are unreliable for fibre typing. The most reliable technique is the myosin adenosine triphosphatase (myosin ATPase). By a series of pre-incubation steps, demonstrating the alkali-stable and acid-stable myosin ATPases, type 1 and type 2 fibres can be reliably demonstrated (Fig. 21.1).[1-4] Staining for the alkali-stable

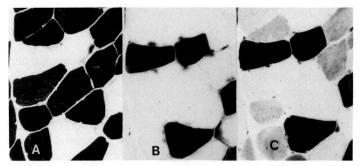

Fig. 21.1a–c Muscle fibre types. Serial sections stained for myosin adenosine triphosphatase (myosin ATPase) at various levels of pH. (**a**) pH 9·4: type 1 fibres light, type 2 fibres dark. (**b**) pH 4·35: type 1 fibres dark, type 2 fibres light. (**c**) pH 4·63: type 1 fibres dark, type 2A fibres light, type 2B fibres intermediate level of staining.   (**a–c**) × 160

ATPase at pH 9·4 reveals a pattern with the type 2 fibres darkly stained and the type 1 fibres pale. The acid-stable ATPase requires pre-incubation at pH 4·35 and stains the type 1 fibres darkly whereas the type 2 fibres are virtually unstained. Pre-incubation at an intermediate pH of 4·63 produces an intermediate picture, presumably due to reaction with reduced concentrations of the two forms of ATPase. At pH 4·63, two forms of type 2 fibre can be distinguished, namely 2A and 2B. 2A fibres are virtually colourless and 2B are intermediate, whereas type 1 fibres stain darkly. Strict control of the pH at every stage is essential. Another fibre type is seen in some diseases and is present in normal infants and children but is not normally seen in adults. This is the undifferentiated or regenerating type 2C fibre which stains darkly or at an intermediate level at all three levels of pH.

The proportions of each fibre type vary in man, not only in different muscles but also in different parts of the same muscle. Type 1 fibres may form up to 80% of fibres in the large tonic back muscles whereas type 2 fibres predominate in the phasic limb muscles such as the gastrocnemius. There is, however, no constant relationship to muscle function. The greatest variation in fibre type proportions is shown by type 2B fibres, which can be either very numerous or totally absent. It was thought originally that absence of type 2B fibres in one biopsy was representative of the musculature in general, but it is now well known that a second biopsy a few millimetres away could contain such fibres.

The admixture of fibre types in normal human muscle produces an apparently random pattern (Fig. 21.2). When first described, it was likened to a chequerboard (chessboard) and it was thought that grouping of even two or three fibres of the

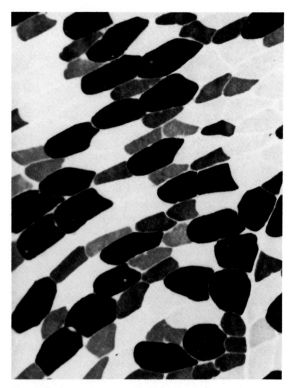

Fig. 21.2 Muscles vary in their distribution of fibre types but this section shows the typical mosaic (chequerboard) pattern in a female of 21 years.
Cryostat section, myosin ATPase at pH 4·63   × 160

same type must be abnormal and a sign of denervation (see p. 591).

Innervation of muscle

The innervation of muscle consists of motor nerve fibres which terminate on motor end-plates on muscle fibres, and nerves which supply muscle spindles, tendon organs, and a variety of free-ending sensory fibres.

The innervation of muscle spindles is complicated (Fig. 21.3) and pathological changes are only routinely observed in myotonic dystrophy.[5]

Axons from motor neurons do not branch until they reach the muscle, after which a series of branchings occurs at the division of intramuscular nerve trunks. From the smallest nerve bundles, single subterminal myelinated axons fan out to the

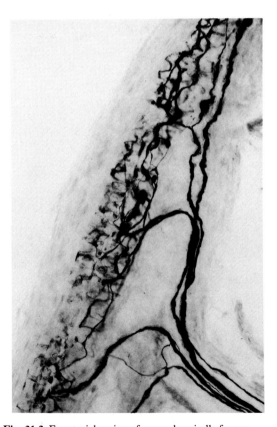

Fig. 21.3 Equatorial region of a muscle spindle from a normal infant. Annulospiral endings are seen. Motor endings are plentiful towards the poles.
De Castro silver, dissection × 300

motor end-plate zone. Each subterminal fibre forms one end-plate (Fig. 21.4a) but one in ten may supply two end-plates by distal division of the subterminal fibres. The number of subterminal nerve and muscle fibres comprising the motor unit varies with the size and function of the muscle; thus only 8 to 10 fibres form a motor unit in extra-ocular muscles whereas up to 1000 fibres or more form a motor unit in the largest limb muscles. Each motor unit within the muscle is formed from the same type of fibre. Thus the admixture of fibre types in normal muscle indicates an intimate inter-mingling of motor units.

Ultrastructure

Transmission electron microscopy has shown that the normal human muscle has a smooth plasma membrane (sarcolemma) covering most of its surface and closely surrounded by a basement membrane. However, in the motor end-plate region, the plasma membrane is thrown into complicated folds and it is here that the innervating axon is in close proximity to the fibre (Fig. 21.4b).

Within the muscle fibre, the narrow dense black Z lines are separated by the lightly staining I bands and the more densely fibrillar A bands (Fig. 21.5). A sarcomere is the distance between two Z lines. During contraction, the actin filaments in the I band interleave with the myosin filaments of the A band. Mitochondria are regularly spaced between the myofibrils. Coarse, darkly stained, granular glycogen is also seen within the muscle. Mitochondria are more numerous in type 1 fibres, whose Z bands tend to be wider than those of type 2 fibres. In type 2 fibres, the muscle end-plates have more numerous, narrower and longer synaptic folds than type 1 fibres. A T-tube system, intimately involved in the spread of depolarisation from the motor end-plate, penetrates the fibre from its external surface. Within the muscle fibre (Fig. 21.5b), the T-tubes are in apposition to lateral sacs of the sarcoplasmic reticulum. Following spread of the wave of depolarisation along the T-tube, calcium ions are released during the initiation of muscle contraction.

A detailed account of mammalian muscle ultra-structure is given by Landon.[2]

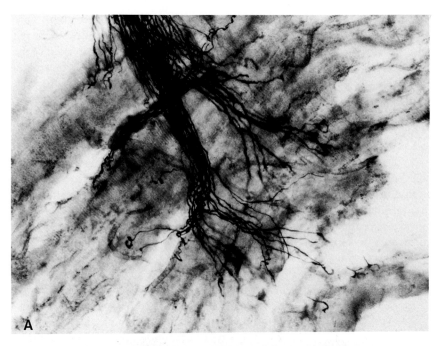

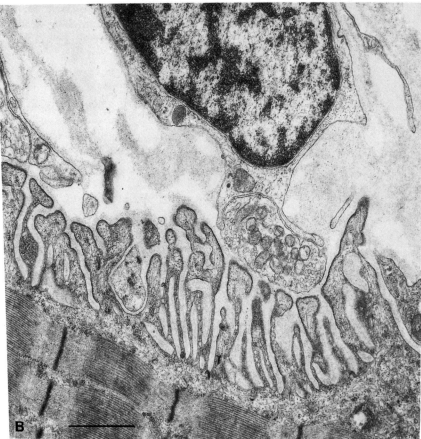

Fig. 21.4a, b (**a**) Normal motor innervation in a child at post mortem. Subterminal fibres do not branch. (**b**) Part of a normal motor end-plate. Note Schwann cell cytoplasm (top), axonic expansion with mitochondria and synaptic vesicles (centre) and secondary synaptic folds (bottom). (**a**) De Castro silver, dissection × 145; (**b**) Electron micrograph; bar = 1 μm

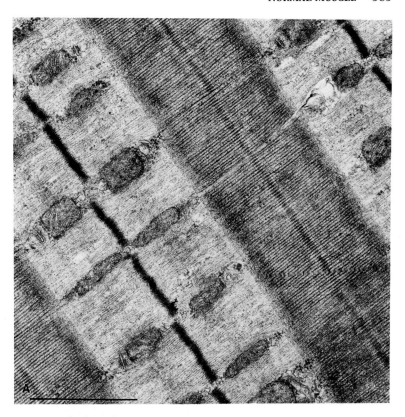

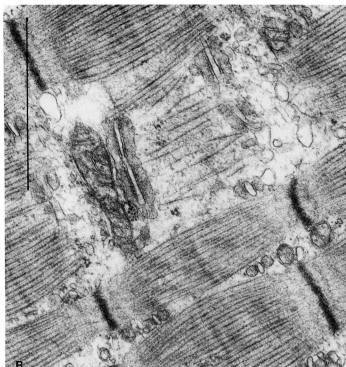

Fig. 21.5a, b Electron micrographs of skeletal muscle. (**a**) Type 1 fibre. (**b**) Type 2 fibre: sarcoplasmic reticulum and normal triads (T tube and lateral sacs) (left). Bar = 1 μm

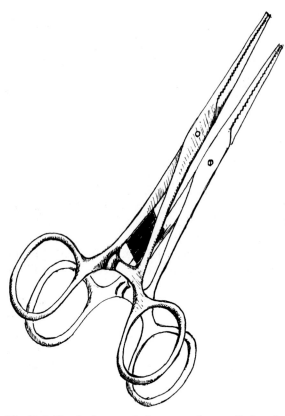

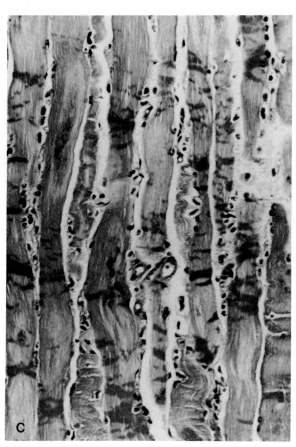

Fig. 21.6 Muscle clamp made from artery forceps. Each end of the muscle strip can be manipulated separately. The smallest available forceps ('mosquito' forceps) are used for electron microscope preparations.

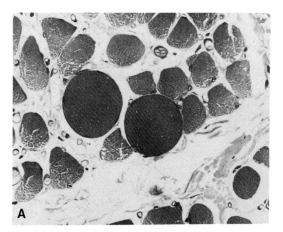

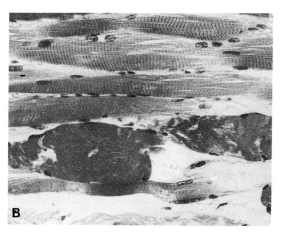

Fig. 21.7a–c (**a**) Swollen hyaline fibres in Duchenne dystrophy in transverse section. (**b**) Hyaline fibres in longitudinal section. (**c**) Extreme contraction artefact following immediate fixation in formalin.
Paraffin section, haematoxylin-eosin (**a, b**) ×280; (**c**) ×200

TECHNIQUES FOR THE EXAMINATION OF SKELETAL MUSCLE

Details of the preparation of skeletal muscle biopsies and of their histochemical staining are found elsewhere.[1,3,5] As a general principle, muscle biopsies must be carefully planned, with full clinical information available. The biopsy should be performed by an experienced surgeon, so that the correct amount of muscle is taken with as little trauma as possible. It is important to plan the techniques that will be used for evaluation of the biopsy before the operation commences.

Routinely, three specimens of muscle are taken. The first is a thin strip for electron microscopy; the muscle is clamped in the jaws of the pair of rigidly fixed mosquito forceps (Fig. 21.6) so that the fibres do not contract when the biopsy is placed in cold glutaraldehyde.

The second specimen, which is for histochemical study, should be about 5 mm in diameter and 10–20 mm in length. It should be left in a damp environment or on ice for 15 minutes until it will no longer contract. There are various techniques for freezing the tissue, either in liquid nitrogen[1,3] or in propane chilled by liquid nitrogen.[5] Exact transverse sections of the muscle are cut and stained with haematoxylin and eosin, and with the enzyme stains necessary for determining muscle fibre types and the presence of abnormal organelles.[1,3] The remains of the block used for histochemistry may be stored in a liquid nitrogen refrigerator and recut if necessary.

The third specimen is fixed in formalin and embedded in paraffin wax; exact transverse and longitudinal sections of formalin-fixed muscle are often valuable for detecting vasculitis and for study of longitudinal sections.

Artefact may occur in pathological and in normal muscle (Fig. 21.7), either from crushing or from excessive contracture of the muscle fibres during preparation.

In metabolic myopathies in which the patient exhibits an enzyme defect, fresh muscle biopsy tissue should be frozen in liquid nitrogen for biochemical assays.

If the innervation of the muscle is to be stained, the technique of motor-point muscle biopsy should be used.[6]

REFERENCES

1. Dubowitz V. Muscle biopsy: a practical approach. 2nd ed. London: Baillière Tindall, 1985.
2. Landon D. Skeletal muscle—normal morphology, development and innervation. In: Mastaglia FL, Walton J, eds. Skeletal muscle pathology. Edinburgh: Churchill Livingstone, 1982: 1.
3. Weller RO. Muscle biopsy and the diagnosis of muscle disease. In: Anthony P, MacSween RNM, eds. Recent advances in histopathology, 12. Edinburgh: Churchill Livingstone, 1984: 259.
4. Weller RO. Colour atlas of neuropathology. Oxford: Miller & Oxford University Press, 1984.
5. Anderson JR. Atlas of skeletal muscle pathology. Lancaster: MTP Press, 1985.
6. Harriman DGF. Preanesthetic investigation of malignant hyperthermia: microscopy. Int Anesthesiol Clin 1979; 17: 102.

General pathological reactions of muscle fibres

HYPERTROPHY

Hypertrophy of a muscle fibre indicates an increase in its calibre above the normal range for age and sex in response to increased muscular activity or hormonal stimulation, or to compensate for muscular weakness. The enlargement of the fibre comes about through the formation of additional myofibrils, and, in pronounced hypertrophy, nuclei become internalised and fibre splitting may occur. Hypertrophy occurs in some myopathies, especially in Duchenne and other dystrophies.[1]

When whole muscles are increased in size they also are referred to as hypertrophied and this is the result of hypertrophy of the fibre population. There is, as yet, no evidence that muscle fibre hyperplasia occurs.

ATROPHY

There are many ways by which fibres can be made to become smaller, and it must be decided whether fibres are small by nature or have really undergone atrophy. Some fibres are small because they are fragments split off from parent fibres. Immature or undifferentiated small fibres are seen in some congenital myopathies.[2,3] Here, the term *hypotrophy* is sometimes used. *True atrophy* develops following *denervation*, and it is also seen in individual fibres or small groups of fibres in *myopathies*. *Selective type 2B fibre atrophy* occurs in muscle wasting due to malnutrition, systemic disease and chronic infections and is the commonest of the remote effects of neoplasm.[1,4,5] When atrophy occurs, peripheral myofibrils disappear from the fibre. Local muscle atrophy occurs in limbs immobilised by joint disease or fracture.

Atrophy of large groups of muscle fibres is usually due to *neurogenic disorders*, e.g. peripheral neuropathy or motor neuron disease (amyotrophic lateral sclerosis). Causes of small group atrophy are less well defined. Fibres that lose peripheral myofibrils may retain their central ones intact for a considerable time; they remain striated. When striations are eventually lost, fibre shrinkage becomes more obvious; in transverse section atrophic fibres stain more heavily, especially with non-specific esterase, and an angular excavated shape is adopted (Fig. 22.1). By electron micro-

scopy, folding of the basement membrane is seen and the sarcolemma may be scalloped. Basement membrane redundancy alone is not totally reliable evidence of atrophy; it also depends upon the state of contraction of the muscle fibre at the moment of fixation. Severely atrophic fibres eventually show loss of structure and striations; little remains, apart from scattered organelles, fibrils and fragments of Z bands (Fig. 22.2).[1] In the longitudinal plane, nuclei congregate in rows but most retain their subsarcolemmal position. If the cause of the atrophy is removed, the muscle may recover its mass and power but only if the fibres are still striated and innervated.

In some disorders *type-specific atrophy* occurs. In wasting due to severe infections or other

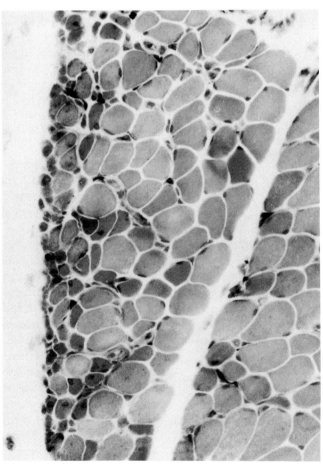

Fig. 22.1 Perifascicular atrophy (left) in chronic dermatomyositis. Cryostat section, non-specific esterase × 290

Out

 Due

 truncated

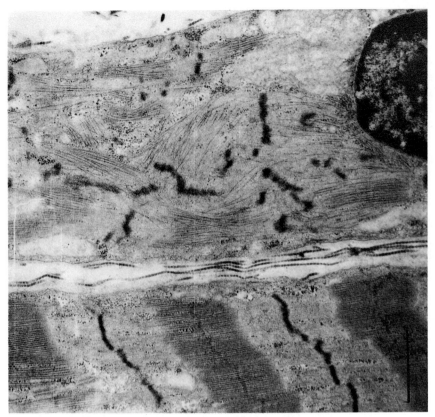

Fig. 22.2 Myofibril disintegration in a fibre (top). Collagen fibres separate this fibre from a normal fibre at the bottom of the picture.
Electron micrograph; bar = 1 μm

systemic disease, type 2B fibres are selectively atrophied[1,4,5] long before the type 1 and type 2A fibres are affected. The reduction in fibre size can be as much as 50%. Type 2B fibre atrophy may be caused by immobilisation but there are other mechanisms which can produce it. Cryptic or overt cancer can be a cause of type 2B fibre atrophy even in patients who are still active and mobile, and it develops as a reaction to many other systemic diseases, whether or not the patients are immobilised in bed.

Neurogenic atrophy

The muscular atrophy that follows denervation differs from the type-specific atrophy described above. When an anterior horn cell or a motor axon in a peripheral nerve degenerates, the function of the whole motor unit which it supplies is abolished. No histological changes can be discerned in the very early stages (1–2 days) either in nerve terminals, muscle end-plates or muscle fibres. Then, the subterminal nerve fibres fragment, but as this is a short-lived phenomenon it is only rarely detected in biopsy material. A reaction occurs in neighbouring healthy subterminal nerve fibres, resulting in the development of *nerve sprouts* from nodes of Ranvier. The nerve sprouts are attracted to the recently denervated motor end-plates and reinnervate them. Sprouts that are supernumerary are unable to form extra end-plates on the muscle fibres and degenerate. The result is that muscle fibres of one motor unit are reinnervated by the nerve supply of a neighbouring motor unit. From this it will be appreciated that the early stages of progressive forms of neurogenic disease (e.g. motor neuron disease) can remain clinically silent so long as

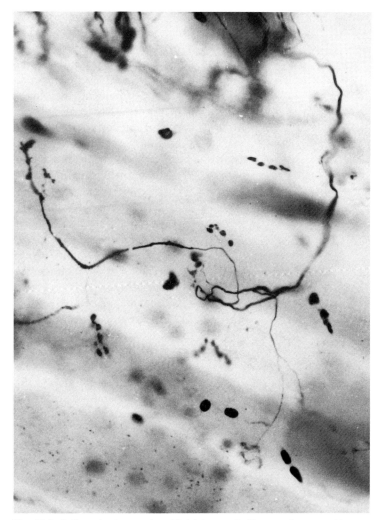

Fig. 22.3 Collateral reinnervation. Multiple muscle fibres are innervated by branches from a single axon.
Methylene blue × 360

collateral reinnervation (Fig. 22.3) is effective.[6] The muscle innervation in these patients changes from that of single subterminal fibres to a pattern of subterminal fibres with collateral branches, each of which will have reinnervated an end-plate. One subterminal fibre now innervates up to 17 or 18 muscle fibres through its collateral branches. Collateral reinnervation is the most sensitive indicator of neurogenic disease;[4] it persists indefinitely or until the nerve supply is ultimately lost due to degeneration of the motor neuron or the axon. It is the first abnormality to appear in de-nervation, but can still be found when neurogenic atrophy is firmly established.

Regeneration of the nerve supply with collateral sprouting is responsible for *fibre type grouping*, another useful sign of denervation which occurs mainly in very slowly progressive neuropathies. When one motor unit is reinnervated by the nerves from a neighbouring motor unit whose muscle fibres are of another type, the re-innervating axons convert the muscle fibres to their own fibre type. If cross-innervation happens over a large enough area, large groups of uniform

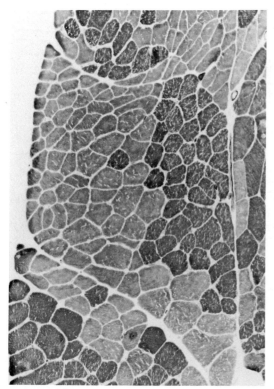

Fig. 22.4 Fibre type grouping due to reinnervation. Large blocks of type 1 (pale) and type 2 (dark) fibres are seen in the biopsy.
Cryostat section, myosin ATPase at pH 9·4   × 70

type result (Fig. 22.4). Groups of about one hundred fibres all of the same type are considered to be diagnostic of neurogenic disease, but if there are several groups in a given area they may be smaller. Formerly, quite small groups (10–15 fibres) were thought to be diagnostic of neurogenic disease but experience has shown that this is probably not correct. Groups of type 1 and type 2 fibres should be detected in order to confirm a diagnosis of neurogenic muscle disease, otherwise fibre type predominance[1] may be mistaken for type grouping.

Large group atrophy (Fig. 22.5d) has long been accepted as evidence of neurogenic muscle disease. Three or four weeks after the muscle fibres are denervated they undergo atrophy, eventually to neonatal size. Striations persist, sometimes for years. Within the atrophied fibres, most nuclei retain their normal peripheral position, but a few may become internal or even central within the

fibre. As time passes, different degrees of atrophy can be distinguished and the atrophic groups become very large, reflecting the progressive involvement of more motor units. Unaffected fibres remain normal in diameter and therefore appear prominent; they may even undergo compensatory hypertrophy. The end stage of neurogenic atrophy is similar to that seen in myopathies; the few intact fibres that remain are scattered within large areas of fat and fibrous tissue. Little sarcoplasm may remain in the chronically denervated fibres and they remain merely as clumps of darkly staining nuclei, often resembling multinucleate giant cells.[1]

Small group atrophy and *single fibre atrophy* both occur most often in neurogenic disease (Fig. 22.5), especially in predominantly distal peripheral neuropathies; however, neither is specific for neurogenic disease. Small groups of atrophied fibres are not uncommon in myopathies but are usually accompanied by other abnormalities, such as necrosis and regeneration, which are recognisable as myopathic. A small biopsy may show small group atrophy only; this presents difficulty in diagnosis and it is in such cases that staining of the innervation is valuable. It has been claimed that scattered atrophic fibres that stain darkly by non-specific esterase are always denervated, but this has not been borne out in my experience. The ultrastructural features of atrophic fibres are not helpful in deciding the cause of the atrophy. When the atrophy is gross, no specific features remain; when moderate, it is nearly always complicated by signs of regeneration.

NECROSIS, PHAGOCYTOSIS, REGENERATION

In skeletal muscle necrosis, phagocytosis and regeneration may involve only short lengths or segments of the fibre, leaving the remainder of the very long fibre unaffected. Segmental necrosis and phagocytosis occur in many actively progressing myopathies and are occasionally seen in neuropathies.[1] The pathogenesis of the muscle necrosis is not known in many myopathies, including polymyositis, but it is thought that a number of different insults may cause focal damage to the

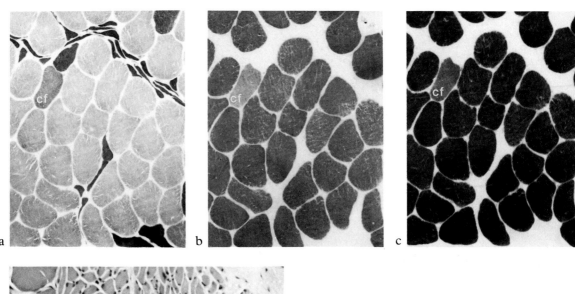

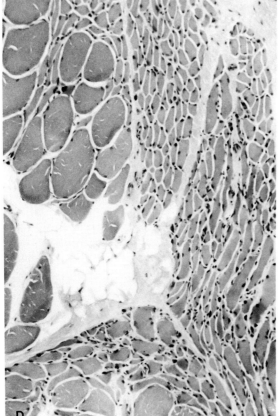

Fig. 22.5a–d Neurogenic atrophy. (**a–c**) Serial sections of muscle stained for myosin ATPase at various levels of pH showing small group atrophy of type 2 fibres. (**a**) pH 9·4: the atrophic group of type 2 fibres is darkly stained. (**b**) pH 4·35: the atrophic type 2 fibres are unstained. (**c**) pH 4·63: the atrophic type 2 fibres are unstained. Solitary fibre (cf) shows moderate to dark staining throughout the range; it is a type 2C fibre. (**d**) Large group atrophy.
(**a, b, c**) Myosin ATPase × 110; (**d**) Haematoxylin-eosin × 125

sarcolemma and local flooding of the fibre with calcium. Necrosis occurs in two forms, *pan-necrosis* and *segmental necrosis*. Both may cause a rise, sometimes massive, in the plasma creatine

kinase (CK) level by increasing the permeability of the cell membrane to this soluble enzyme. *Rhabdomyolysis* occurs and, if sufficiently extensive, will liberate myoglobin and sarcoplasm into the blood

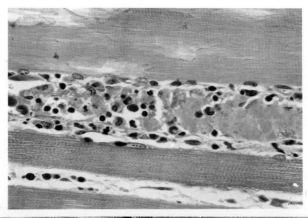

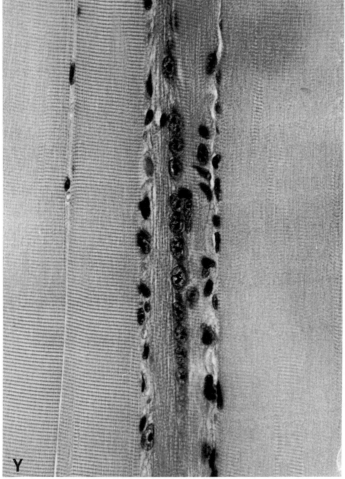

Fig. 22.6a–c Muscle fibre destruction and regeneration. (**a**) Segmental necrosis (centre). A few elongated regenerating myoblasts have appeared in the necrotic portion of the fibre. (**b**) A regenerating fibre showing large internal nuclei with prominent nucleoli. (**c**) A regenerating fibre. The nucleus has a large nucleolus (top left) and the sarcoplasm contains many clusters of regenerating muscle filaments.
(**a**) Paraffin section, haematoxylin-eosin × 280; (**b**) paraffin section, haematoxylin-eosin × 450; (**c**) electron micrograph: bar = 4 μm

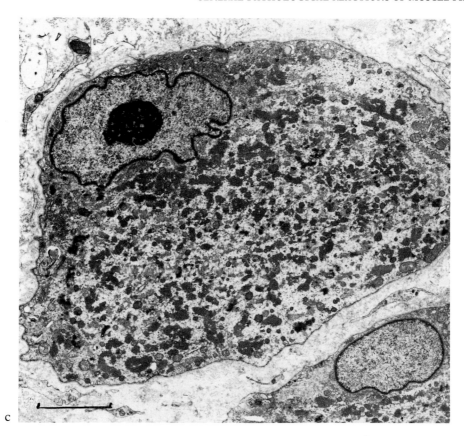

c

and subsequently into the urine, causing myo-globinuria and sometimes renal failure.[7]

Segmental necrosis

In segmental necrosis, granular, hyaline or coagulative change develops in the affected part of the muscle fibre. During the first few hours, before any cellular reaction develops, it may be difficult to distinguish a necrotic segment from contraction artefact. The sarcolemma in the affected segment disintegrates but the basal lamina and endomysium are unaffected and may act as a guide for the future reconstitution of the segment. It takes several days for macrophages to enter and invade the whole necrotic segment (Fig. 22.6). During this time, large and spindle-shaped regenerating myoblasts form a layer on the inner aspect of the basal lamina. They are derived from satellite cells, which are resting myoblasts lying so close to the surface of mature muscle fibres that they cannot be detected by light microscopy.[8] Satellite cells indent the sarcolemma and are covered by the basal lamina. The regenerating myoblasts develop myofibrils, fuse together in the longitudinal and transverse planes to form multi-nucleate cells and eventually restore the continuity of the muscle fibre segment as the macrophages leave. During regeneration the mononuclear and fused multinuclear myoblasts develop large nucleoli, and their cytoplasm, full of ribosomes, becomes basophilic. Basophilia may persist for two to three months, and affected fibres show heavy mitochondrial staining. Thereafter the only evidence of previous regeneration may be the presence of internal nuclei. While fusion is still incomplete in the regenerated segment, the fibre may appear to fork, giving a false impression of fibre splitting.

Segmental necrosis and regeneration often occur in scattered single fibres and less frequently in small groups of fibres. However, large groups of necrotic or regenerating fibres are seen in Duchenne dystrophy (see p. 614). Even the largest groups of regenerating fibres are easily distinguished from neurogenic group atrophy as the regenerating fibres are basophilic whereas the denervated fibres have eosinophilic cytoplasm.

Pan-necrosis

This differs from segmental necrosis by involving all the muscle fibres within a given area; it also affects the basal laminae and endomysium. Histologically, it is similar to infarction. Ischaemia,[9] toxins (including those of anaerobic gas-forming organisms), and blunt trauma may all cause pan-necrosis of large areas of muscle. Unlike segmental necrosis, total regeneration of such an area is not possible unless it is very small. The necrotic tissue soon loses its normal staining qualities and stains a uniform pink with haematoxylin and eosin. Within 24 hours inflammatory cells invade the affected area; they spread inwards from the periphery and may take many days or weeks to reach the central area. Phagocytosis and regeneration of muscle fibres occur at the edge of the lesion but not in the centre of large areas of necrosis. The end result, after weeks or months, is a fibrous scar and possibly the deposition of adipose tissue. This is bounded by a zone of regenerated muscle in which ring fibres and internal nuclei are often seen (Fig. 22.7).

Regeneration following muscle cell necrosis was

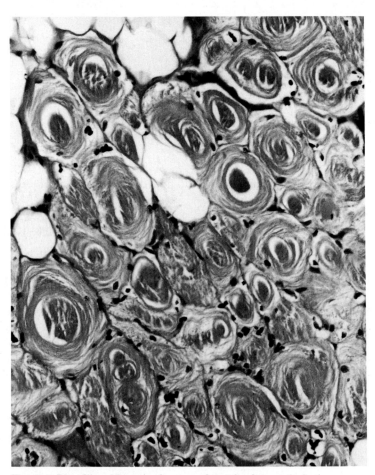

Fig. 22.7 Ring fibres. Necrosis of an area of muscle often results in the formation of ring fibres at its edge during the healing phase.
Transverse section. Paraffin section, haematoxylin-eosin × 290

thought to be impaired by the destruction of the basal lamina and therefore by the loss of its guiding framework. But recent experimental work shows that this is unlikely, as regeneration occurs within areas of muscle necrosis in which the basement membrane has been destroyed; the basal lamina itself reforms as the muscle regenerates following necrosis.[10]

FIBRE SPLITTING

This phenomenon is relatively common and non-specific. It occurs with increasing age, with muscle hypertrophy and in many slowly progressive myopathies, especially dystrophies, and in neuropathies. It is particularly noticeable in muscles subject to severe stretching as with the abdominal muscles in pregnancy and obesity (Fig. 22.8). Splitting is easily recognised when a cleft forms part way across a fibre; if it traverses the fibre completely it is then difficult to distinguish a split from the space between two normally apposed fibres. Two splits across the same fibre are obvious even when complete, and the same applies to the splitting off of small fibre fragments. The narrowness of some splits may help in their recognition except when they contain endomysial connective tissue. The phenomenon is more easily recognised in transverse sections, but does occur over some length of the fibre. The unusual occurrence of a capillary apparently lying in the middle of a transversely cut muscle fibre is due to its presence at the tip of a fibre split.

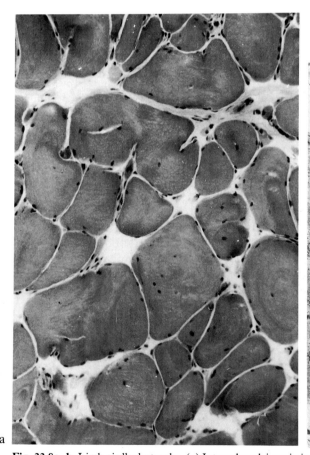
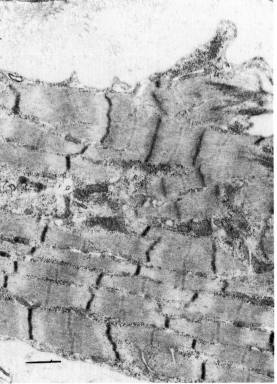

a   b

Fig. 22.8a, b Limb girdle dystrophy. (**a**) Internal nuclei, variation in fibre size, obvious fibre splitting and fragment formation are seen. (**b**) Electron micrograph showing an atrophic fibre which appears to be shedding a fragment (top). (**a**) Cryostat section, haematoxylin-eosin × 145; (**b**) Electron micrograph: bar = 1 μm

There may be several different mechanisms at work in the pathogenesis of splitting.[4,11] The effects of abnormal tension on the muscle fibre in the longitudinal plane and the extrusion of unwanted, diseased parts of the parent fibre have been proposed. Sometimes the fusion of regenerating myoblasts resembles splitting, as when four or five of these cells become apposed inside a sarcolemmal tube.

NUCLEI: INTERNAL AND CENTRAL

In normal muscle most nuclei lie peripherally in the fibre, apposed to the internal aspect of the sarcolemma: only a few lie between the myofibrils. Such internal nuclei are found in no more than 3% of fibres under normal circumstances (Fig. 22.9). By 'internal' is meant any site within the fibre other than subsarcolemmal, whereas the much rarer abnormally placed 'central' nuclei are

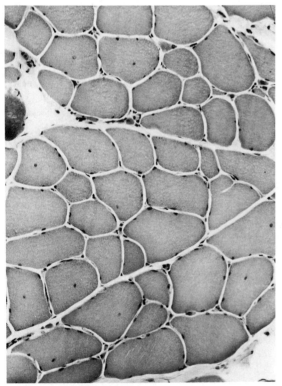

Fig. 22.9 Limb girdle dystrophy showing internal nuclei at an early stage of the disease.
Cryostat section, haematoxylin-eosin × 145

confined to the central axis of the fibre (Fig. 23.26 —p. 641). Myoblasts and myotubes contain central nuclei, and this nuclear position is thought to persist in certain congenital myopathies, notably centronuclear myopathy.[2,3] Some writers use the terms 'internal' and 'central' synonymously.

When counting the number of fibres with internal nuclei it is necessary to exclude those at or near their tendinous insertions, where nuclei are normally internal, often in clusters. Fibres may also be inserted into fascia, thus explaining internal nuclei close to that structure, or even into the perimysium. Fibres so placed should be ignored when establishing the percentage of fibres with internal nuclei. In general, significant increases in internal nuclei involve fibres distributed diffusely throughout the histological section.

Internal nuclei are a feature of many myopathies, but are especially numerous in long-established myotonic syndromes[1] and in some patients with malignant hyperthermia myopathy; in both these diseases up to 30% of fibres may be affected. They may also be seen in chronic denervation, but less often, and a small proportion may be central. Central nuclei are common in the denervated muscle of small mammals.

RING FIBRES

In transverse sections of muscle, ring fibres show a typical striated ring of one or more myofibrils at the edge of the fibre, spiralling around a core of longitudinally orientated myofibrils (Fig. 22.10). Ring fibres are commonly found near muscle insertions and only rarely elsewhere in normal muscle. They occur in small numbers in many myopathies and are often prominent in myotonic dystrophy;[1] they are sometimes seen in larger numbers as a late result of focal regeneration, especially following trauma.

CYTOPLASMIC BODIES

Cytoplasmic bodies are found, usually in very small numbers, in almost any disorder as well as in normal muscle. A myopathy has been recorded in

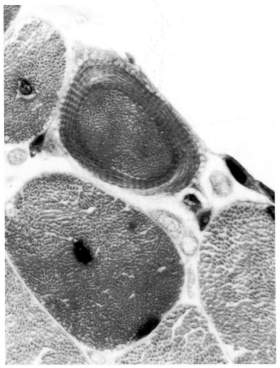

Fig. 22.10 A ring fibre (top) close to the palmaris longus tendon.
Paraffin section, haematoxylin-eosin × 720

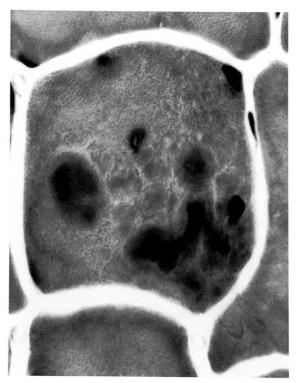

Fig. 22.11 Cytoplasmic bodies. Several darkly stained cytoplasmic bodies are seen in a single muscle fibre; the light halos can just be distinguished.
Cryostat section, modified Gomori[1] × 920

two patients in whom the bodies were numerous.[12] By electron microscopy, cytoplasmic bodies consist essentially of actin-like filaments which form a dense central mass; less tightly packed filaments radiate from its edge.[1] A fibre in transverse section can accommodate one or several bodies (Fig. 22.11). By light microscopy, protoplasmic stains demonstrate a round or irregular central dark mass enclosed by a light halo. By the modified Gomori method,[1] the central mass should be red and the halo should be relatively clear.

CORES, 'MOTH-EATEN' FIBRES AND TARGETS

Cores

Cores[1,13] are best seen in type 1 fibres in frozen sections stained for oxidative enzymes. Against the dark background of mitochondria and inter-myofibrillar substance the core forms a sharply defined area of pallor which is not an empty space but contains unstained myofibrils (Fig. 22.12a).

In some longer established cores, the central area appears to have coagulated or disintegrated and is then shown by other stains and is visible in paraffin sections. The cores with intact myofibrils are called 'structured cores' and are short in longitudinal section. The second type of core is unstructured and long. Cores are best shown by fibre dissection (Fig. 22.12b). In addition to central core disease, cores may be found in denervation, malignant hyperthermia and, in small numbers, in some other myopathies. Core-like lesions can be produced experimentally by tenotomy; they consist of foci of myofibrillar lysis and not of intact or distorted myofibrils. Such cores (pseudocores) develop only if the motor nerve supply is intact, if permanent shortening of muscle fibres has occurred, and if fibrous healing of tenotomy is underway. They are usually present

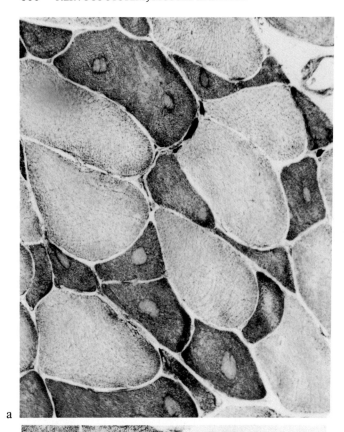

a

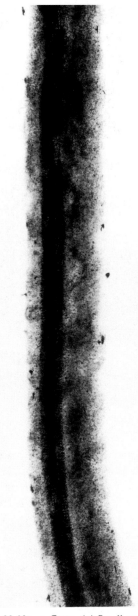

b

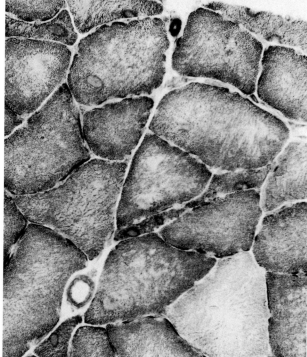

c

Fig. 22.12a–c Cores. (**a**) Small cores in type 1 fibres in malignant hyperthermia myopathy. No type 1 fibre predominance is seen. (**b**) A long core (dark) in central core disease. (**c**) Central core disease. There is type 1 fibre predominance; few cores are seen but there is prominent 'moth-eaten' change.
(**a**) Cryostat section; NADH-tetrazolium reductase × 290;   (**b**) de Castro silver; dissection of single fibre × 290;   (**c**) Cryostat section; NADH-tetrazolium reductase × 230

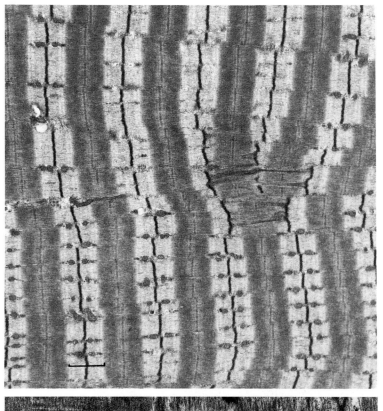

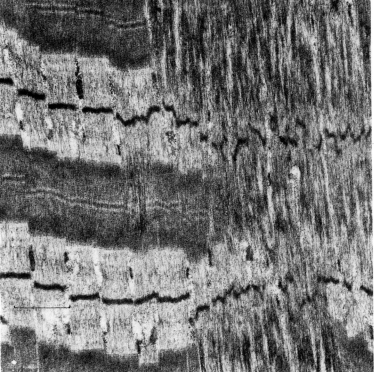

Fig. 22.13a, b 'Moth-eaten' fibre.
(**a**) An electron micrograph showing part of the 'moth-eaten' area with few mitochondria and minimal Z-line streaming. (**b**) Electron micrograph of an unstructured core (right).
a, b Electron micrographs: bar = 1 μm

in type 1 fibres only, but they may occur also in type 2 fibres.[14]

'Moth-eaten' fibres

These may be seen alone but also may accompany cores in type 1 fibres (Fig. 22.12c). Only oxidative enzyme stains such as NADH-tetrazolium reductase will show them.[1,5] Areas of pallor occur as in cores, but instead of being sharply defined and punched out, the edges are irregular and diffuse. The moth-eaten appearance is due to partial or complete loss of mitochondria and the absence of staining of intermyofibrillar sarcoplasm and myofibrils. As in structured cores, the myofibrils within the 'moth-eaten' areas are intact. It is possible to detect transitional forms between the two abnormalities: thus 'moth-eaten' change may be an early stage of the core. When detected in a single frozen section, 'moth-eaten' change can resemble staining artefact, so confirmation in a serial section should be sought. Their apparent presence in type 2 fibres is pathognomonic of artefact. 'Moth-eaten' change is common in some myopathies[1,5,15] and following denervation, but artefact cannot always be excluded.

Ultrastructure of 'moth-eaten' and core fibres. It is not easy to identify 'moth-eaten' fibres in electron micrographs if absence of mitochondria is the only criterion. Fortunately, one or two very small foci of Z-line streaming[1] direct one to the affected area (Fig. 22.13a). Structured cores present less difficulty and show loss of mitochondria within the sharply outlined edge of the lesion; there is also a greater degree of Z-line streaming than is visible in 'moth-eaten' foci. Ultrastructural studies confirm the impression that 'moth-eaten' fibres and cores

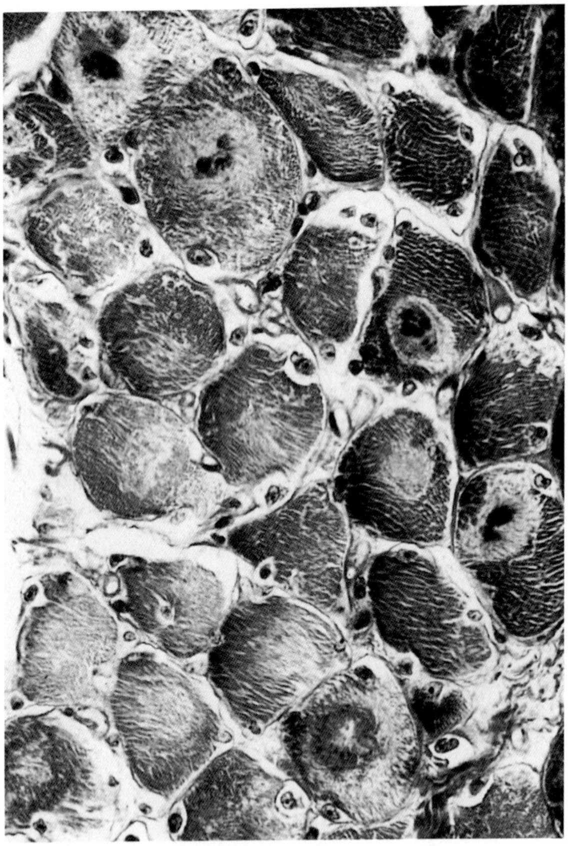

Fig. 22.14 Target fibres. In this section, the three zones in the targets are well demonstrated (particularly in the fibres on the right).
Paraffin section, phosphotungstic acid haematoxylin × 260

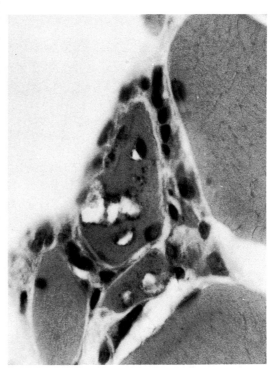

Fig. 22.15 Rimmed vacuoles. These are so called because the filamentous and granular contents project above the level of the section.
Cryostat section; modified Gomori × 720

are related. The unstructured core seems to be a further development of the structured core, as disintegration of central myofibrils and Z lines occurs or there is gross, closely packed streaming (Fig. 22.13b).

Target fibres

These are a variant of cores seen occasionally in slowly progressive denervations and in motor neuron disease (amyotrophic lateral sclerosis). They are best visualised in paraffin sections or in cryostat sections stained by the NADH-tetrazolium reductase technique. The affected fibre is only moderately atrophic or is normal in size. Within it, the three zones of a target are formed by a central granular mass, an intermediate pale ring and an outer zone formed by normal peripheral myofibrils. As with cores, the central part is composed of varying amounts of Z-line streaming and granular material, with pallor in the intermediate zone (Fig. 22.14). Targets are invariably short in their longitudinal extent. In frozen sections the three ring structure is not usually seen.

VACUOLES

Vacuoles are spaces of variable size and content within a muscle fibre. In longitudinal section they are ovoid. Most are bounded by a single or double membrane, presumably derived from local organelles, but some are unbounded. The contents consist of fragments of membrane, lipid and unidentifiable granular material; some vacuoles may be empty. Those with visible contents are likely to be derived from lysosomes, which can be confirmed by the staining of hydrolytic enzymes such as acid phosphatase; they are thus autophagic vacuoles. In *rimmed vacuoles*, filamentous material (stained red with the modified Gomori technique[1]) collects at the edge of the vacuole and projects up away from the section (Fig. 22.15). They were first identified in oculopharyngeal dystrophy but have since been seen in several other conditions.[1] Vacuoles in otherwise normal fibres suggest one of the forms of periodic paralysis (see p. 652). However, non-specific vacuolation occurs in inflammatory myopathies, in ischaemia, in systemic lupus erythematosus and in some toxic myopathies such as that caused by chloroquine.

REFERENCES

1. Dubowitz V. Muscle biopsy: a practical approach. 2nd ed. London: Baillière Tindall, 1985.
2. van Wijngaarden GK, Fleury P, Bethlem J, Meijer AEFH. Neurology (Baltimore) 1969; 19: 901.
3. Collins JE, Collins A, Radford MR, Weller RO. Clin Neuropathol 1983; 2: 79.
4. Swash M, Schwartz M. Neuromuscular diseases. Berlin: Springer, 1981.
5. Weller RO. In: Anthony PP, MacSween NM, eds. Recent advances in histopathology. London: Churchill Livingstone, 1984; 12: 259.
6. Walton JN. Brain's Diseases of the nervous system. 9th ed. Oxford: Oxford University Press, 1985.
7. Di Bona FJ, Morens DM. J Paediatr 1977; 91: 943.
8. Landon D. Skeletal muscle—normal morphology, development and innervation. In: Mastaglia FL, Walton JN, eds. Skeletal muscle pathology. Edinburgh: Churchill Livingstone, 1982: 1.
9. Harriman DGF. J Clin Pathol 1977; 30 (Suppl 11): 94.
10. Caldwell CJ, Weller RO. Neuropathol Appl Neurobiol 1987; 13: 492.
11. Carpenter S, Karpati G. Pathology of skeletal muscle. New York: Churchill Livingstone, 1984: 125.
12. Wolburg H, Schlote W, Langohr HD, Pfeiffer J, Reiher KH, Heckl RW. Clin Neuropathol 1982; 1/2: 55.
13. Dubowitz V, Roy J. Brain 1970; 93: 133.
14. Baker JH. Muscle Nerve. 1985; 8: 115.
15. Weller RO. Colour atlas of neuropathology. Miller & Oxford University Press, 1984.

Pathology of muscle diseases

INTRODUCTION

Clinical features

In general, disorders of muscle, whether neurogenic or myopathic, cause weakness and muscle wasting. Clinicopathological correlation is very important for the diagnosis of muscle disease, from biopsy or at autopsy; full clinical details should be provided. Detailed discussions between clinician and pathologist are very useful.

In addition to weakness and muscle wasting, pain at rest or on exercise is not infrequently seen in both categories of muscle disease. Pain is obviously a primary manifestation in the inflammatory myopathies; pain on exercise immediately suggests that a glycogenosis should be considered. In the more advanced stages of many of the disorders pain may be secondary to contractures or to compression of nerves or muscle.

There is a form of *chronic myalgia*, often cripplingly severe, in which biopsy reveals normal muscle, and which may persist for years defying diagnosis. Many of the patients obtain relief from rest, and most physicians have discarded any idea that the condition is a functional disorder. Viral studies have so far been negative. But, in view of the difficulty, originally, of isolating viruses in the acute viral myositides, and the remarkably few occasions on which inflammatory reactions are found on biopsy, it is possible that chronic myalgia will also prove to be of viral origin.

As a general rule the myopathies produce symmetrical proximal weakness and wasting, whereas the weakness and wasting in neurogenic muscle diseases tend to be distal in the limbs initially and neither quite symmetrical nor totally asymmetrical. There are many exceptions: Duchenne dystrophy (p. 611), the most severe of the inherited myopathies, clearly affects the proximal lower limb muscles at an early stage but causes enlargement of the calves at the same time, giving the dystrophy its original name—pseudo-hypertrophic muscular dystrophy. In the neurogenic disorder spinal muscular atrophy (SMA) type 1, better known as Werdnig–Hoffmann disease (see p. 606), the proximal muscles are more severely affected. The degree of paresis in this disease is not easily assessed because of gross hypotonia, but the distal tendon reflexes are preserved longer than the proximal reflexes. In another denervating disorder, adult motor neuron disease (see p. 609), there is an increase in deep tendon reflexes in the presence of weak muscles, at least in the early phases of the disease. The reason for this is the association of degeneration of the upper motor neuron with that of the lower motor neuron. The same association can be seen on occasion in SMA type 3 (see p. 609). With these exceptions, neuropathies and myopathies manifesting weakness generally show diminution and eventual loss of deep reflexes.

In longstanding muscle disease with extensive fibrosis within the muscle, there is a danger that patients develop contractures and deformities of great severity. These were seen in large numbers in the nineteenth century, but with better clinical management they are much less common now, apart from those few disorders which actually present with contractures. In the presence of contractures, the site of biopsy should be carefully chosen; two small biopsies close to and distant from a contracture will be more helpful than a single larger biopsy. Some congenital myopathies present not with contractures but with associated malformations such as scoliosis or congenital dislocation of the hip. Contractures are encountered in the newborn in arthrogryposis (see p. 638),[1] a syndrome comprising several different congenital disorders.

A clinical feature in adults which is almost always due to denervation is true *migratory fasciculation*. The exception is *benign fasciculation*, which is rare and without known cause. Both must be distinguished from the even rarer, almost continuous, undulating or rippling movements of *myokymia* in which both muscle and motor end-plates are normal.

Investigations

Electromyography

Electromyography (EMG) is very useful, especially in the hands of an experienced practitioner.[2,3] It is complementary to muscle biopsy in mapping out the distribution of muscle disease, though biopsy can be more effective in showing abnormalities confined to one or two areas of the muscle. Fibrillation or fasciculation potentials on EMG or large amplitude volitional motor unit potentials are diagnostic of the various forms of denervation but occasionally none may be present in these conditions. Myotonic discharges are easily detected by EMG; the fatigue of myasthenia gravis may be less convincing electrically. Short-duration action potentials of reduced amplitude suggest a myopathy. Slowing of nerve conduction velocities may help to distinguish demyelinating peripheral neuropathies from those with mainly axonal degeneration (see p. 573). There is no doubt that EMG reduces considerably the number of patients who would otherwise require muscle biopsy. The presence of EMG needle tracks in biopsy material is undesirable (see p. 659) and can be avoided by an agreement between electromyographer and pathologist to confine their respective investigations to muscles on opposite sides.

Creatine kinase

The serum level of creatine kinase (CK), formerly known as creatine phosphokinase, is the most sensitive indicator of activity of neuromuscular disease available. Its only limitations are that, firstly, muscular exercise in the healthy individual causes the serum CK to rise so that a day of rest should precede the estimation. Secondly, different laboratory techniques result in different normal levels. Laboratory reports should always indicate their normal range. The enzyme is present in the muscle fibre cytosol and leaks into the circulation in the presence of fibre necrosis and regeneration. It is thought that increased membrane permeability short of necrosis may produce seepage to an equal degree. The serum levels vary considerably, e.g. from many thousands of international units (iu) per litre in early or pre-clinical Duchenne dystrophy to levels of 100–200 iu/l in many chronic myopathies (normal = 60 iu). As fibre destruction is reduced and regeneration is no longer seen, CK levels become normal, as is therefore often the case in the last stages of disease. Neurogenic disorders mostly do not cause a rise in CK level in the serum, but occasionally may do so even in the chronic forms. A biopsy taken at this stage will show regeneration in the undenervated parts of the muscle.

In the inflammatory myopathies the levels of serum CK may be high or low; thus CK levels help to assess the extent and activity of these focal disorders.

NEUROGENIC MUSCLE DISEASE

Any disorder affecting any part of the lower motor neuron may cause neurogenic disease of muscle, whether it is the cell body in the anterior horn, the axon in the spinal root or the peripheral nerve and branches as far distal as, and including, the neuromuscular junction, which is damaged. Many patients do not require a muscle biopsy when EMG can show unequivocally the presence of neurogenic muscle disease. The cause of the neurogenic disease must be sought by other means, clinical and radiological. A nerve biopsy can be helpful in appropriate cases (see p. 545). When neurogenic disease is known to be present in an adult, a muscle biopsy is not performed unless the clinical findings are uncharacteristic or a rare but demonstrable cause such as polyarteritis is suspected. The most frequent neurogenic disorders to require histological study of muscle are the spinal muscular atrophies and, occasionally, motor neuron disease; hereditary motor and sensory neuropathies require nerve biopsy principally, but a small muscle biopsy through the same incision helps to indicate the degree of motor nerve involvement.

Spinal muscular atrophies (SMA)

Type 1: infantile spinal muscular atrophy (Werdnig–Hoffmann disease)

The classification of the spinal muscular atrophies into four types, depending on clinical features, and especially age at onset, has done much to eliminate earlier confusion; only a few patients do not fit easily into the proposed categories. All SMA are due to disease of anterior horn cells of unknown cause; the affected neurons show ballooning and chromatolysis more often than degeneration and shrinkage.[4] Type 1 spinal muscular atrophy (SMA 1, Werdnig–Hoffmann disease) is the most lethal type of SMA and probably begins in utero; a biopsy taken as early as one week of age can show established signs of denervation. It is usually not helpful to biopsy at such an early age, as group atrophy may not be apparent in the biopsy until later. Clinically, the infant is severely hypotonic, has no head control and lies in the frog-leg position. The degree of hypotonia can be such as to mask underlying paresis or paralysis. Fasciculation of the tongue is diagnostic. Some infants appear not be be affected at birth, but signs always develop by the age of six months. Progressive deterioration with respiratory muscle involvement and death by the age of 18 months is characteristic, although some die later. A necropsy should be obtained to help in genetic counselling. Inheritance is usually autosomal recessive, but an autosomal dominant pattern has been reported in a small number of families.

Histology. Histological diagnosis on muscle biopsy depends on the discovery of large groups of atrophic fibres interspersed with obviously hypertrophied fibres occurring singly or in groups (Fig. 23.1). The small fibres are nearly all round in transverse section, in contrast to the angularity or irregularity of fibres in group atrophy at a later age. They are not distinctly smaller than normal neonatal fibres.

Histochemically, both type 1 and type 2 fibres

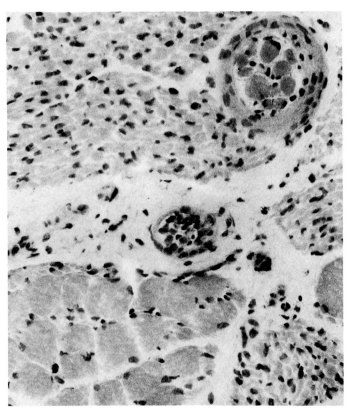

Fig. 23.1 Type 1 spinal muscular atrophy (Werdnig–Hoffmann disease). Neurogenic atrophy showing large group atrophy with hypertrophy of unaffected fibres. Note normal spindle.
Frozen section, haematoxylin-eosin × 290

are represented among the small fibres, whereas the hypertrophied fibres may be all type 1, predominantly type 2 or of both types. The hypertrophied fibres are easily distinguished from Wohlfart type B fibres which are large type 1 fibres that persist from antenatal muscle for some months after birth. The Wohlfart type B fibres do not occur in groups and are few in number, less than one per muscle fascicle. They may be more numerous in the premature infant.

Type 2: intermediate spinal muscular atrophy

Type 2 spinal muscular atrophy (SMA 2) also affects babies but is much less severe than SMA 1. No signs are observed for the first six months of life but thereafter motor development is delayed.

Sitting and standing are achieved as a rule but a characteristic feature is the inability to walk unaided at any stage. The disease may affect the respiratory muscles, resulting in early death, but the majority survive for over 10 years, even into adulthood. Limb involvement is usually asymmetrical and the CK is only slightly raised, but may increase in later years. The inheritance pattern is uncertain but is often autosomal recessive.

Histology. Although less severe than in SMA 1, large group atrophy in a muscle biopsy often provides a diagnosis. However, in some cases there is only small group atrophy, diffusely distributed and simulating the early stages of some slowly progressive myopathies. A focal myopathic pattern

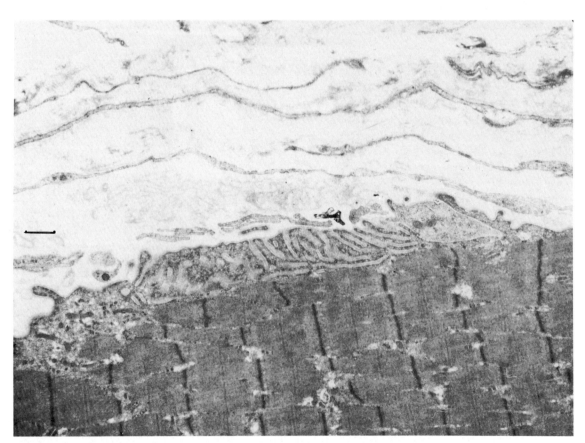

Fig. 23.2 Type 3 spinal muscular atrophy (Kugelberg–Welander syndrome). Denervated muscle end-plate. The convoluted sole-plate on the muscle fibre surface is preserved, but little or nothing remains of the axonic expansions. Later the junction will be covered by collagen.
Bar = 1 μm

with fibre necrosis and regeneration may be misleading if seen in small biopsies, especially needle biopsies, and may lead to an incorrect diagnosis. A motor point biopsy is useful in such cases as collateral reinnervation can be clearly demonstrated. Definite fibre type grouping is not often present.

Type 3: juvenile spinal muscular atrophy (Kugelberg–Welander syndrome)

The time of onset of type 3 spinal muscular atrophy (SMA 3) varies widely, but is always after the age of two years. SMA 3 is commonly described as juvenile onset SMA, and more popularly as Kugelberg–Welander syndrome, following the definitive descriptions by the Swedish workers of a slowly progressive muscle disease with neurogenic features on histology. They described the proximal muscle involvement, sometimes with pseudohypertrophy and often asymmetrical. Their cases were familial with an autosomal dominant inheritance pattern. Since then autosomal recessive patterns have been reported, and apparently sporadic cases. Hypertrophy of the calves has been noted as an early sign. It is not surprising that such patients were formerly diagnosed as suffering from muscular dystrophy even when a biopsy was made, for in the earlier stages the classical features of denervation may be absent. The diagnosis depends upon the demonstration of fibre type grouping and collateral reinnervation. The pseudomyopathic pattern of SMA 2 is not common in SMA 3 but end-plate ultrastructure may show denervation (Fig. 23.2). The CK level in the serum may be moderately raised.

Type 4: adult onset spinal muscular atrophy

This type of SMA (SMA 4) begins after 30 years and develops slowly, usually permitting a normal life span. Histologically, it is like SMA 3 but if the patient is first seen in old age, the muscle will have progressed to end-stage disease, with only a few fibres surviving along with nuclear clumps (see p. 589) (Fig. 23.3) in an abundance of fat and fibrous tissue. It is not possible to decide whether such advanced degeneration and loss of muscle bulk is neuropathic or myopathic. Three necropsies in this group[5] showed no loss of Betz cells from the motor cortex, no pyramidal tract degeneration and only a decrease in numbers of anterior horn cells in the spinal cord.

There are other syndromes of spinal muscular atrophy, such as a distal form[6] and a form with facioscapulohumeral distribution, but they are rare. Sometimes the same syndrome may have a myopathic or neuropathic basis, such as the scapuloperoneal syndrome. Whether some of the conditions mentioned are distinct entities or merely clinical variants of SMA remains to be seen. At the present time it is suggested that at least the four main types of SMA described above are closely related.

Motor neuron disease

Like spinal muscular atrophy, this disorder is characterised by degeneration of anterior horn

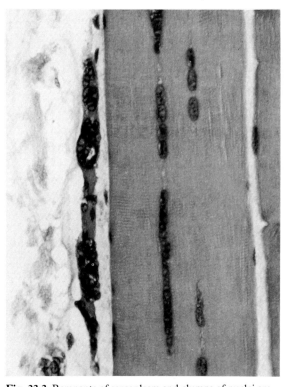

Fig. 23.3 Remnants of sarcoplasm and clumps of nuclei are seen on the left of a normal muscle fibre. This is from longstanding denervated muscle in Type 4 spinal muscular atrophy.
Paraffin section, haematoxylin-eosin × 430

cells, but is more widespread. In addition to neurons in the spinal cord, bulbar motor neurons are often affected, except for those supplying the extraocular muscles. Betz cells of the motor cortex are commonly involved and there is corticospinal tract degeneration. At post mortem some other long tracts, including the posterior columns, may show axonal loss but without symptoms during life.

Clinically, the disease affects adults, mostly in middle age, but patients as young as 19 years have been affected. There are three forms. The most frequent is *amyotrophic lateral sclerosis*, a term descriptive of both the firmness of the lateral columns of the spinal cord, produced by lateral corticospinal tract degeneration and consequent gliosis, and the accompanying atrophy of muscle. The names of the other two forms are self-explanatory: *bulbar palsy* and *progressive muscular atrophy*. The classical mode of onset is with wasting and weakness of the small muscles of the hands spreading up the arms painlessly and then affecting the legs later. Deep tendon reflexes are exaggerated and bulbar muscles are affected causing a very troublesome dysphagia.

The tongue atrophies and fasciculates, and the limbs also show fasciculation. But there are many patients in whom the pattern of limb involvement is asymmetrical, even markedly so, affecting one arm and one leg; others suffer increasing pain. Mononeuritis multiplex may be simulated.

Muscle biopsy is required only when the presentation is not typical. Provided a moderately affected muscle is selected for biopsy, large group atrophy is usually seen. Fibre type grouping is uncommon. If large group atrophy is unusually extensive few motor nerve fibres will be found. Target fibres may be present and oxidative enzyme stains may show 'moth-eaten' change in the fibres of normal size.

Motor neuron disease is common throughout the world, but there are small areas in the Far East, on the Pacific island of Guam, in New Guinea and in the Kii peninsula of Japan where the disease appears to differ from that elsewhere.[7,8] In Guam it is responsible for a high proportion of the deaths in the Indian Chamorro population, and the proportion of familial cases is much higher than in the West. The disease appears to be associated with regular ingestion of food derived from the nuts of the cycad trees (see p. 275).

Peripheral neuropathies

Peripheral neuropathies are considered in Chapters 18–21. It can be added here that it is often useful to take a muscle biopsy at the same time as a nerve biopsy. Intramuscular nerves may confirm the findings in the nerve biopsy, or even provide a diagnosis when the latter has not done so, as in hypertrophic neuropathy, polyneuritis or the rare infantile neuroaxonal dystrophy. Most often the muscle will show whether the neuropathy being investigated is purely sensory (rare) or has a motor component which has not been detected clinically. The extremely slowly progressive hereditary motor and sensory neuropathies are the most likely of all neuromyopathies to show unequivocal fibre type grouping.

Poliomyelitis—chronic syndrome

In the acute phase of poliomyelitis there may be a severe degree of paralysis (see p. 205); later, as the inflammation in the anterior horns of the spinal cord recedes, there is some recovery, limited by the number of anterior horn cells destroyed. The degree of permanent paralysis depends also on the amount of collateral reinnervation possible; much occurs, as shown by the enlargement of motor units on electromyography.

Many patients disabled by poliomyelitis have a normal life span and show no change in their clinical condition after recovery from the acute phase. Very rarely, after a period of 30 or 40 years, occasionally more, there is a focal increase in weakness in one arm, or leg or shoulder,[9] often diagnosed as a coincidental dystrophy or amyotrophic lateral sclerosis. This condition was predicted by Charcot over 100 years ago. If a muscle is biopsied, the usual features of longstanding denervation alone may be shown, but examination of the muscle fibres unaffected by denervation shows abnormalities (Fig. 23.4): these include variation in fibre size, splitting, internal nuclei, necrosis and regeneration similar to that seen in myopathies. But innervation studies show

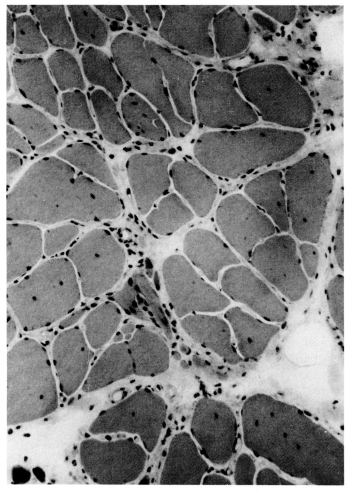

Fig. 23.4 Man, aged 43 years. Poliomyelitis at age of 2, leaving severe disability. Recent progressive weakness of his 'good' arm. Biopsy shows pseudomyopathy.
Frozen section, haematoxylin-eosin × 180

that collateral innervation is present to a degree in the myopathic areas. Myopathic changes in the muscle may lead to an incorrect diagnosis, as such changes do occur, but rarely, in other neuro-pathies, e.g. the Kugelberg–Welander syndrome (p. 609). The pathogenesis is not clear, but it has been suggested that anterior horn cells, long overloaded by enlarged motor units, may be responsible for the development of the 'myopathic' changes. Under some circumstances, denervation is associated with muscle fibre hypertrophy as well as atrophy.[10]

THE MYOPATHIES

PRIMARY MYOPATHIES

Duchenne muscular dystrophy

This is the best known and the most lethal of the inherited myopathies. With an X-linked recessive inheritance pattern, it affects young boys; their sisters may be carriers. The mutation rate is high, 30%, which may cause diagnostic difficulty. It is often necessary to seek the carriers by means of the family history, electromyography and repeated creatine kinase (CK) estimations. Muscle biopsy is a last resort and is often unhelpful in the detection of carriers although a few may have minor clinical signs of myopathy.

Duchenne muscular dystrophy may occur in girls, who show a translocation on the short arm of the X-chromosome with a break point at the locus Xp21.[11] The affected Xp21 gene in male Duchenne dystrophy is large, with about 2000 kilo-base pairs which may account for the high (30%) mutation rate. Dystrophin is the sarcolemma-associated protein product of the Xp21 gene[11] and is absent or at very low levels in muscle in Duchenne dystrophy.[11a] Estimation of dystrophin levels in muscle by electrophoresis or of Xp21 disorders by DNA analysis can now be used to confirm the diagnosis of Duchenne dystrophy.[11]

When affected boys present, at the age of 3 or 4 years, some awkwardness in gait may have been noticed, or difficulty in climbing stairs or even toe walking (because of shortening of the calf muscles). Muscle enlargement is almost always seen, not only of the calves but of other muscles such as the quadriceps, deltoid and scapular muscles. One of the first cases recorded by Duchenne de Boulogne in the mid-nineteenth century had the appearance of an infant Hercules.[11b] That is now known to be rare, but the enlargement of several proximal muscles is not. If the enlarged muscle is weak, the increase in size is due to replacement of degenerated muscle by adipose and fibrous tissue, and the muscle is therefore *pseudohypertrophic*. If the power of the muscle is normal it is *hypertrophic*. On general examination many of the patients show some intellectual impairment. At the onset of clinical signs the CK is 10 000 iu/l or more (normal = 60 iu/l) and this continues in the first few years, gradually falling to near normal levels as the disorder progresses. The heart is involved, at first slightly; anaesthetists consider it good practice always to monitor the electrocardiogram during operations. At post mortem the heart shows disseminated focal fibrosis in the presence of normal coronary arteries.[12] The surviving myocardium shows no changes comparable to those present in the skeletal musculature.

Histopathology. A moderately affected muscle should be chosen for biopsy, usually some part of the quadriceps, e.g. the vastus medialis at the motor point. It is striking how advanced the myopathy can be in a boy who can still run. The incision reveals obviously abnormal muscle, not quite the fish flesh appearance of an advanced dystrophy but a pinkish–white muscle of increased firmness still able to contract on stimulation. Transverse section of the muscle will show fascicles separated by broad fibrous bands composed partly of perimysium and partly of epimysium (Fig. 23.5a).

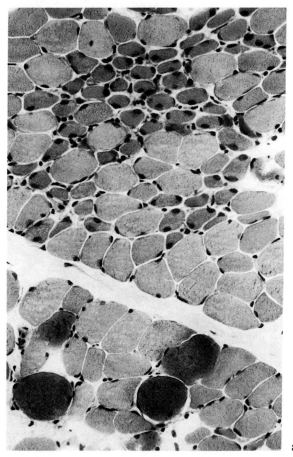

a

Fig. 23.5a–d Duchenne dystrophy. Boy, aged 4 years. (**a**) Cluster of darkly stained regenerating fibres (top), endomysial and perimysial fibrosis, and a few hyaline fibres (bottom). (**b**) Electron micrograph of small regenerating fibres. (**c**) Regenerating fibres contain polyribosomes and prominent clusters of developing myofibrils cut in transverse section. (**d**) Normal motor end plate.
(**a**) Haematoxylin-eosin × 190; (**b–d**) Electron micrographs: (**b**) Bar = 10 μm, (**c**) Bar = 1 μm, (**d**) Bar = 0·5 μm

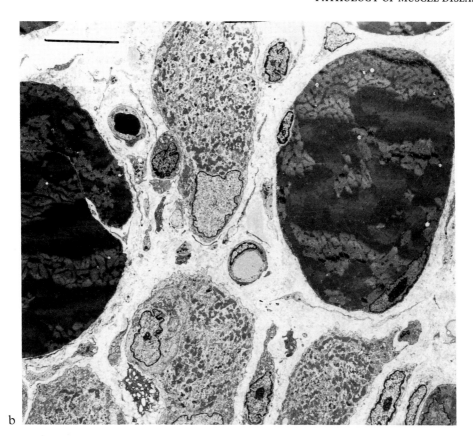

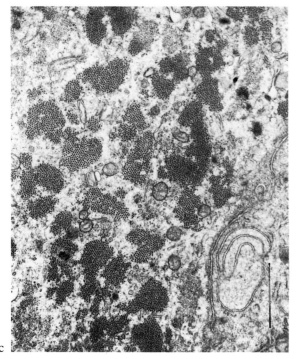

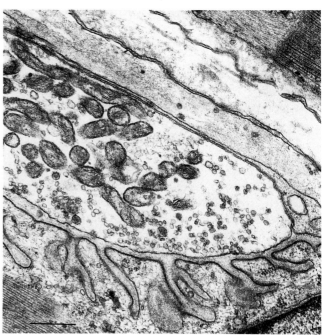

At this stage there is little or no increase in endomysial fibrous tissue, but there is if the biopsy is taken at a later age, at 6 or 7 years. In haematoxylin and eosin preparations an unusually large number of fibres of normal size stain darkly; their nuclei are dark and shrunken, suggesting artefact despite the usual technical precautions (Fig. 23.5a). The dark fibres are greater in number than in similarly treated biopsies of other muscular disorders. If they are followed in longitudinal section, the hyaline appearance gives way to a short pale segment suggestive of contraction artefact, followed again by a hyaline segment. Rarely, if the pale zone is seen in transverse section, there is infiltration by an occasional histiocyte, an undoubted vital reaction indicating that fibre contraction or hypercontraction must have occurred well before the biopsy commenced. It is generally thought, however, that fibres free of inflammatory cells are artefactually contracted (the fibres are unduly susceptible to excessive contraction). Whatever their pathogenesis may be, the presence of hyaline fibres in large numbers is helpful in the diagnosis of Duchenne dystrophy. They have been noted in small numbers in other myopathies, and are relatively frequent in normal and abnormal neonatal muscle.

Other equally striking changes occur in the earlier phases of Duchenne dystrophy. There is variation in fibre size, eventually covering a wide range but with relatively few internal nuclei and little or no fibre splitting. Groups of small regenerating fibres form islands with a delicate fibrous stroma (Fig. 23.5a). When sectioned longitudinally these fibres can appear shrunken and darkly stained. Lymphocytes and macrophages are difficult to detect in most biopsies, but in others there is obvious perivascular or interstitial infiltration by both types of cell as a reaction to muscle fibre necrosis. Rarely, the inflammatory cell infiltrates are large enough to simulate polymyositis; however, muscle fibre hypertrophy, so common in Duchenne dystrophy, is rarely seen in polymyositis and may indicate the correct diagnosis.

Ultrastructure. There are no specific findings. The small basophilic fibres have the features of regenerating muscle fibres (Fig. 23.5b and c). The

end-plates are normal (Fig. 23.5d). Hyper-contracted fibres are again seen in resin sections as structureless and dark or pale. Despite their variation in size, many fibres are normal in structure. Some are enclosed by a duplicated basal lamina. Delta-like defects in the sarcolemmal membrane have been thought to be the prime defect in the disease,[13] but similar defects can be found in other myopathies.

Malignant hyperthermia and Duchenne dystrophy

Some interest has been shown recently in the possible association of Duchenne dystrophy with malignant hyperthermia (MH) (see p. 649) as several patients with Duchenne dystrophy have shown a rise in temperature during surgery. The diagnosis of MH has been confirmed only once so far by in vitro testing.[14] The association seems to be rare, and is perhaps coincidental. The development of MH in any myopathy and indeed in any surgical procedure lasting more than ten minutes can be detected early by monitoring core body temperature.

Becker muscular dystrophy

Becker dystrophy is allied to Duchenne dystrophy; both show X-linked recessive inheritance and affect young boys, who develop proximal muscle weakness and calf pseudohypertrophy. But there are differences. In families in which affected children conform to the Becker type,[15] the onset is several years later than Duchenne dystrophy, even as late as the second decade, and the course is relatively benign. Some patients attain the age of 50. The CK levels vary between very high (similar to Duchenne dystrophy), and only ten times the normal value. Dystrophin (see p. 612) has an abnormal molecular weight in Becker dystrophy.[11a]

Histopathology. Variation of fibre size is similar to that seen in Duchenne dystrophy (Fig. 23.6a), but there is in addition fibre splitting which seems to increase during the course of the disease. Some nuclei are internal. Necrosis and regeneration are less prominent than in Duchenne dystrophy. In some children a fine fibrosis separating individual fibres develops, but not until late in the course of

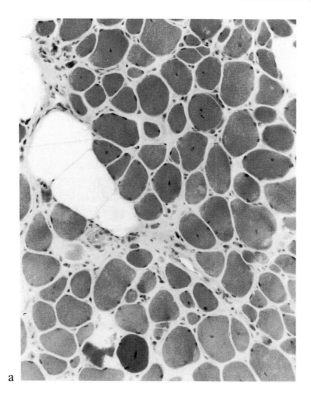

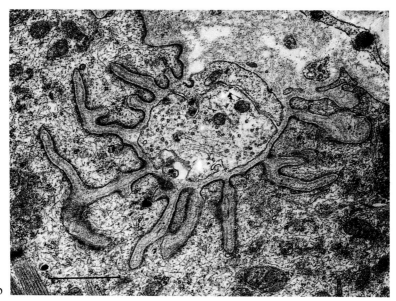

Fig. 23.6a, b (**a**) Becker dystrophy showing variation of fibre size. Internal nuclei, an increase in adipose tissue, fibre splitting and endomysial fibrosis. (**b**) Motor end-plate showing only an insignificant retraction of the axon terminal (centre). (**a**) Frozen section, haematoxylin-eosin × 170; (**b**) Electron micrograph: bar = 1 μm

the disease do extensive fibrosis, adipose tissue, nuclear clumps and isolated atrophic fibres appear, as they may at the end stage of any chronic muscle disorder.

Ultrastructure. Apart from non-specific degenerative changes (Fig. 23.6b), abnormalities in the motor innervation[16] have been reported in 3 patients, in whom there was some dilatation of secondary synaptic clefts (but only in type 1 fibre end-plates), an increase in glycogen, myelin figures and disorganised neurofilaments. These findings have been used to support the neural hypothesis of the cause of muscular dystrophies but are more likely to be a reaction to muscle fibre degeneration, as suggested by light microscopy of the nerve supply. Muscle fibre degeneration which happens to include the end-plate zone gives rise only to distal sprouting of the nerves, not to true collateral innervation.

Limb girdle muscular dystrophy

Several slowly progressive disorders of muscle, such as type 3 spinal muscular atrophy, Becker dystrophy and various metabolic myopathies, may present with weakness and wasting of proximal and limb girdle musculature and sometimes with enlargement of the calves. It has thus been suggested that limb girdle dystrophy is not a specific diagnosis but one only arrived at after exclusion of other possibilities. This suggestion is mistaken: limb girdle muscular dystrophy is as well defined as any other, provided that a diagnosis is not attempted either from clinical features alone or on muscle biopsy alone. In the past it has been overdiagnosed, especially in children, in whom it is rare.

Pelvic girdle weakness or scapuloperoneal weakness and wasting may present first; with scapular muscle weakness, winging of the scapulae becomes prominent and later very marked. The onset of the clinical signs is usually in the second decade, and sometimes in the third decade. Progress of the disease is so slow that the patient may deny any disability despite obvious winging of the scapulae and lordosis. The life span can be normal. Autosomal recessive inheritance with equal involvement of males and females has been suggested but this may not be accurate in what is still a heterogeneous condition.

Histology. The changes are those of almost any slowly progressive chronic myopathy, with variation in fibre calibre, internal nuclei and a moderate amount of fibre splitting. Occasional atrophic fibres are seen, sometimes gathered in small groups; there may be occasional regenerating fibres. Fibrosis occurs late. The muscle fibre abnormalities occur in both main fibre types (Fig. 23.7). As would be expected in a primary muscle disorder, the motor innervation only shows changes distally, with distal and ultraterminal sprouting. Small groups of atrophic fibres or small fragments formed by fibre splitting should not be regarded as evidence of neurogenic muscle disease in this disorder. In some biopsies there is a moderate preponderance of one or other fibre type, but this is not abnormal. A non-specific abnormality is the presence of 'moth-eaten' or partially 'moth-eaten' fibres containing scattered mitochondria. Ring fibres and 'spotted' fibres may also be found.

Ultrastructure. Only non-specific features have been reported.[17]

Childhood muscular dystrophy

This is another dystrophy of slow progression with quite marked variation of muscle fibre size, internal nuclei, fibre splitting, scattered necrosis and regeneration and delayed fibrosis similar to that in limb girdle dystrophy and Becker dystrophy.[18] 'Moth-eaten' and occasional ring fibres may complicate all three. It is unwise, and usually impossible, to distinguish between any of these on biopsy without detailed clinical correlation. Childhood muscular dystrophy is quite rare, but not as rare as limb girdle dystrophy in young children. It occurs in girls predominantly and there is not infrequently a family history of consanguinity. The onset is between the ages of 2 and 14 years of age, with pelvifemoral weakness and on occasion enlargement of the calves and sometimes of proximal muscles. This is due to a high proportion of greatly hypertrophied abnormal muscle fibres rather than to fibrofatty

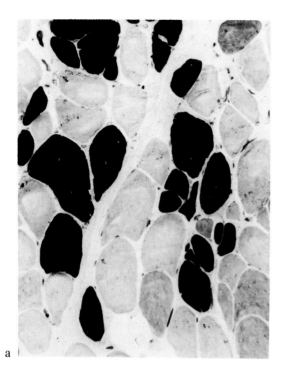

a

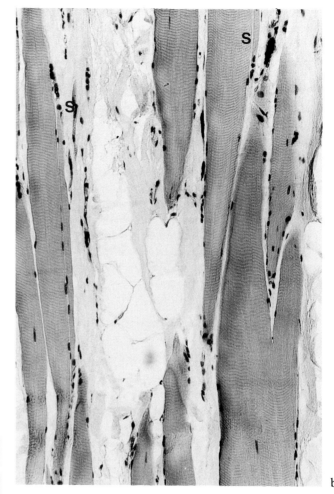

b

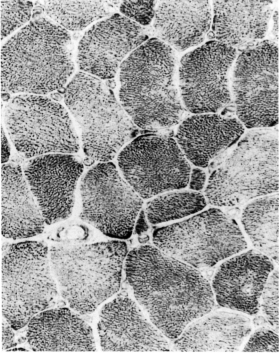

c

Fig. 23.7a–c Limb girdle dystrophy. Man, aged 25 years.
(**a**) Myosin ATPase pH 9·4. Size variation and splitting
affecting both fibre types. (**b**) Fibre splitting is seen in muscle
fibres cut in the longitudinal plane. Very thin fibres could be
long thin extrusions of split fibres. (**c**) Daughter of the above
patient, aged 5 years, showing an early stage of the disorder
with only a few small angular fibres (lower centre).
(**a**) Frozen section, myosin ATPase × 245; (**b**) Paraffin
section, haematoxylin-eosin × 245; (**c**) Frozen section,
NADH-TR × 400

infiltration. Progress of the dystrophy is slow, eventually involving the upper limb girdle and sometimes the face to a limited degree. Life expectancy is little affected but walking becomes impossible by the age of 20.

Investigations. The CK level varies but can be quite high at the onset (5000 iu/l), reflecting the amount of necrosis and regeneration. The electrocardiogram may show minor changes, but less than in Duchenne dystrophy at the same stage. The mode of inheritance, like that in limb girdle dystrophy, is autosomal recessive but often indeterminate. It remains to be seen whether recombinant DNA techniques will in future assign some or even all children in this category to the X-linked Becker disorder (see p. 614) despite the fact that most are girls.

Facioscapulohumeral muscular dystrophy (FSH dystrophy)

The title refers to a dystrophy involving the facial muscles, the shoulder girdle and the upper arm; it is slow or even intermittent in its evolution and benign in its course. FSH dystrophy is quite common, with dominant inheritance and variable expression. There is great variation in the severity of the symptoms and signs, but even the mildest cases are affected to some degree, however slight and difficult the signs are to recognise. The onset is insidious, between 5 and 20 years of age, and is usually first noticed in the face, progressing to the sternomastoid and shoulder girdle muscles. The extraocular muscles are not affected. The deltoid muscles may be spared for a time and so should be avoided for biopsy in the earlier stages. Many patients go on to develop pelvifemoral and anterior tibial weakness in addition.

Histopathology. In children, a biopsy of triceps or biceps may show little change, with mild variation in fibre calibre which is hardly abnormal, and a small number of apparently atrophied triangular or rectangular fibres which stain darkly. As a single finding, such atrophic darkly stained fibres must be considered as non-specific until other evidence—either of denervation or of fibre splitting—is available. In FSH, fibre splitting will

be seen, possibly several years after the onset (Fig. 23.8a), but at no stage will the innervation show collateral reinnervation, and hence this excludes neurogenic disease (Fig. 23.8b). With further progress of the dystrophy, variation in fibre calibre increases and many internal nuclei appear. In some patients, necrosis and regeneration develop and affected muscle segments are ringed by inflammatory cells. Lymphocytes and macrophages may be numerous and infiltrate between neighbouring muscle fibres, as happens rarely in Duchenne dystrophy. This feature may cause confusion with polymyositis.

The appearance, in haematoxylin and eosin

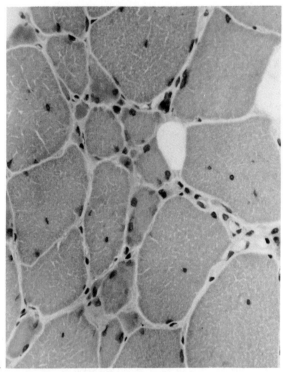

a

Fig. 23.8a–e Facioscapulohumoral dystrophy. (**a**) Shows size variation, splitting and small fragments of muscle fibres. Some smaller fibres with prominent nuclei may be spotted fibres. (**b**) Subterminal nerve fibres show no collateral reinnervation. (**c**) Spotted fibres, mainly smaller than the average. (**d**) Electron micrograph showing abnormal mitochondria; two contain crystalline inclusions (top left and bottom centre). (**e**) Ring fibre (centre), and spotted fibres containing glycogen.
(**a**) Frozen section, haematoxylin-eosin × 315; (**b**) Methylene blue, squash preparation × 125; (**c**) Frozen section, NADH-TR × 255; (**d**) Electron micrograph × 16 500; (**e**) Frozen section, PAS × 395

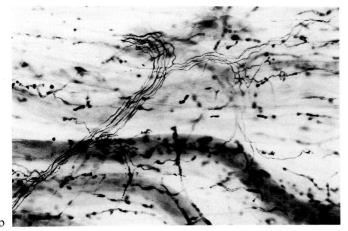

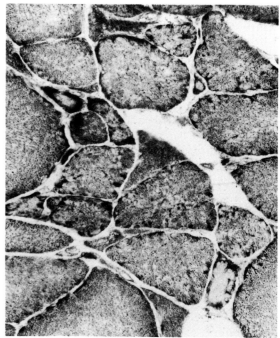

c

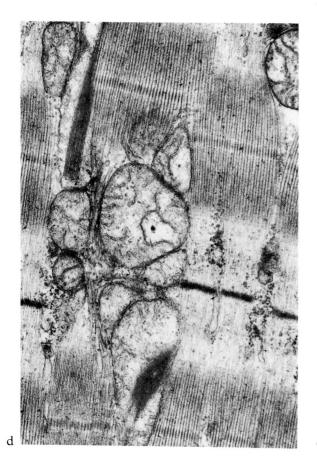

d

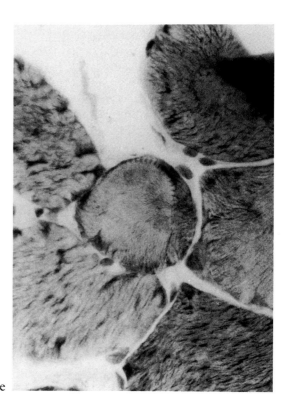

e

stained sections, of indistinct tiny peripheral masses of pale blue material in type 1 muscle fibres has resulted in the term 'spotted' fibres.[19] They are clearly seen with NADH-tetrazolium reductase and PAS stains (Fig. 23.8c). Black reaction product is deposited in affected fibres as small triangular or rounded masses, usually at the periphery and based on the sarcolemma, while the inter-myofibrillar pattern may show small foci of absent staining. Electron microscopy of spotted fibres reveals accumulations of glycogen and sometimes of mitochondria and sarcoplasmic reticulum, probably the result of a minor degree of myofibril loss or atrophy. Spotted fibres were first described as 'lobulated', on account of indentations sometimes produced in the myofibrillar pattern;[19] later they became known as 'cartwheel' fibres.

FSH dystrophy is probably the condition in which spotted fibres appear most regularly and in

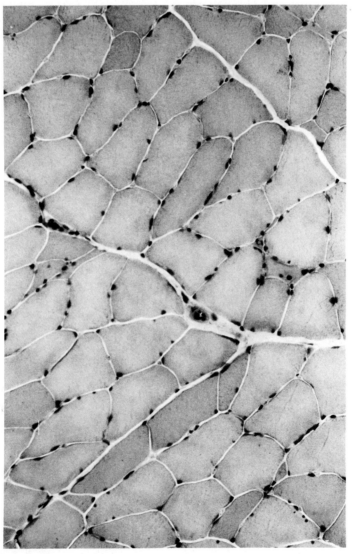

Fig. 23.9 Emery–Dreifuss dystrophy showing a mild myopathic picture with variation in muscle fibre size.
Frozen section, haematoxylin-eosin × 290

the largest numbers. They are an undoubted help in diagnosis, but do occur in other chronic myopathies and in some normal old people. Other findings may include 'moth-eaten' fibres, very occasional ring fibres (Fig. 23.8e), rod bodies and abnormal mitochondria (Fig. 23.8d); all these are also found in other dystrophies.

Emery–Dreifuss humeroperoneal muscular dystrophy

This is an unusual dystrophy, first reported in 1966.[20,21] Its features are an X-linked inheritance, a skeletal muscle myopathy of generally benign course, a cardiomyopathy often more severe than the skeletal myopathy, and the early appearance of contractures. 73 cases in 6 major families have now been reported, with a striking incidence of sudden death due to a cardiac conduction defect. The insertion of a pacemaker is advisable. The contractures may affect many joints but those most often affected are in the neck and the elbows and ankles. The patient characteristically presents with arms semiflexed and ankles plantar-flexed, all virtually immovable. But there is much variation and diagnosis may not be apparent in patients seen apart from the family. The onset of the disorder is between 5 and 15 years and the clinical course is slow. Walking is still possible at 45 years of age. The predominant histological findings are fibre size variation, with smaller type 1 fibres and hypertrophied type 2, some fibre splitting, and 'moth-eaten' and spotted fibres. The relationship of the contractures to the skeletal muscle myopathy is not clear.

No matter how severe the contractures, the myopathy is usually mild (Fig. 23.9).

Distal muscular dystrophy

As dystrophies commonly affect proximal muscles predominantly, it is unusual to encounter a myopathy of undoubted distal distribution. In Sweden, Welander in 1951 described a large group of cases of distal dystrophy with autosomal dominant inheritance. Distal dystrophy elsewhere in the world is rare and genetically distinct from the Welander type. In one patient in whom the histological changes of myopathy were in doubt

staining of the innervation confirmed primary muscle disease.[22]

Ocular myopathies

Normal extraocular muscles. The extraocular muscles are more complicated in function, and therefore in structure, than limb skeletal muscle. Their specialised functions include extremely rapid and coordinated movement, fixed gaze, following gaze, reflex blinking, etc., and necessitate small motor units, numerous spindles, a rich nerve supply and muscle fibres of six types.[23,24] In all extraocular muscles except the levator palpebrae superioris there are multiply innervated muscle fibres, similar to those in amphibians, in addition to limb-type skeletal muscle fibres (Fig. 23.10). There are also species differences, particularly in the outer zone of each extraocular muscle. Here, in man, the zone is broad and consists of fibres of uniform small size

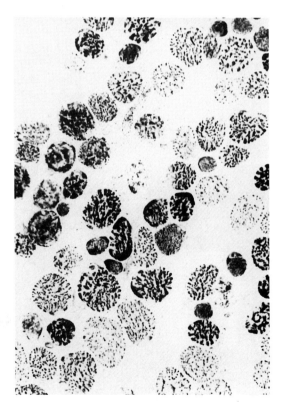

Fig. 23.10 Normal extraocular muscle. Coarse, fine and sparsely granular fibres of varying size are shown by this NADH reaction.
Frozen section, NADH-TR × 450

when compared with the large fibres in the core. Compared to limb skeletal muscle extraocular muscle appears quite peculiar.

Most work on the histopathology of extraocular muscle was done before histochemistry was available. 'Progressive external ophthalmoplegia' was at first thought to be a neuropathy, but histological post-mortem examination threw doubt on this. Very little has been learnt in the past from tiny biopsies of abnormal extraocular muscle, but post-mortem histochemical examination is becoming useful. There is a general tendency to assume that extraocular muscle in man will react to denervation in the same way as skeletal muscle elsewhere in the body, but in fact its peculiar structure and especially the small size of its motor units demand new criteria of collateral re-innervation, type grouping and group atrophy.

Ocular myopathy with progressive external ophthalmoplegia

The patient presents with ptosis and weakness of extraocular muscles, usually after the age of 20. The time of onset is sometimes difficult to determine because the patient may not be aware of his condition for some years, as he can compensate for lack of eye movement by moving his head. Autopsy studies show end stage, probably myopathic, disease; the 3rd, 4th and 6th cranial nerve nuclei are normal, confirming that ocular myopathy is a dystrophy. Biopsy of the deltoid muscle shows virtually no change. Many cases are sporadic, but autosomal dominant inheritance has been described. There are thorough reviews in the older and modern literature, including autopsy studies.[25,26]

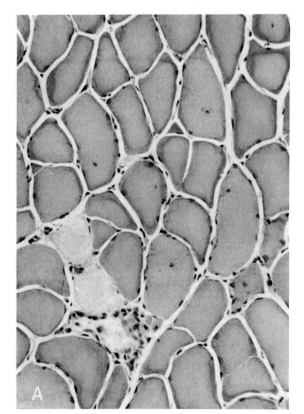
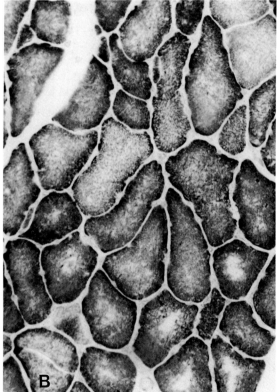

Fig. 23.11a, b Oculopharyngeal dystrophy. Pharyngeal biopsy showing (**a**) fibre necrosis (lower left), and fibre fragments; (**b**) 'moth-eaten' fibres which are almost cores.
Frozen section (**a**) Haematoxylin-eosin × 190; (**b**) NADH-TR × 190

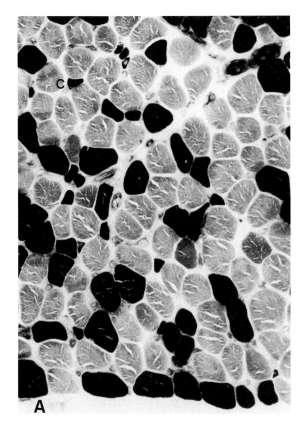
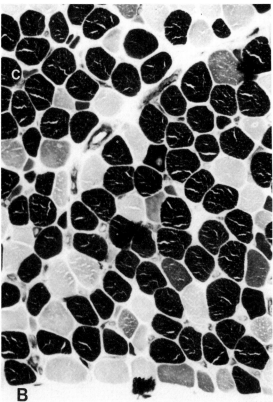
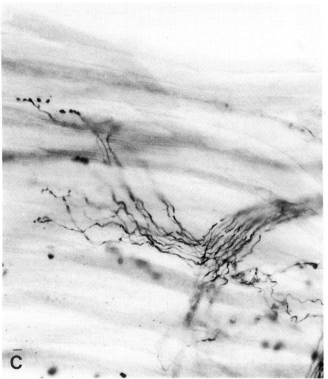

Fig. 23.12a–c Congenital dystrophic myopathy, mild form (**a and b**) Serial myosin ATPases, pH 9·4 and 4·3 respectively. Variation in fibre size affects mainly type 2 fibres (dark in A and pale in B). Some tiny fibres (e.g. indicated by letter C) are dark at both pH and are type 2C. (**c**) The innervation is normal.
(**a, b**) Frozen section, myosin ATPase ×290;
(**c**) Methylene blue, squash preparation ×290

Oculopharyngeal muscular dystrophy

This presents in the same way as ocular myopathy, with extraocular muscle weakness and progressive ptosis, but later in life, mostly after the age of 50. As in ocular myopathy, the precise time of onset is difficult to determine. As its name implies, oculopharyngeal dystrophy is not confined to the eyes but spreads relentlessly in a caudal direction to cause a severe progressive dysphagia, and eventually proximal weakness of upper and lower limbs. Even if the deltoid muscles appear to be of normal power, a biopsy is likely to show mild myopathic features (Fig. 23.11) and a number of autophagic vacuoles ('rimmed vacuoles'). A biopsy of pharyngeal muscle may show advanced myopathic changes but no characteristic vacuoles. Two complete autopsies have been reported.[27]

Mitochondrial ocular myopathy

The mitochondrial myopathies affect many different organs and tissues but the Kearns–Sayre syndrome, in particular, presents with involvement of the extraocular muscles (see p. 652).

Congenital dystrophic myopathy

Some infants who are hypotonic at birth display, on biopsy, a histological picture very like that of a muscular dystrophy. There may be minimal changes at first, or variation of fibre size with occasional necrotic and regenerating segments may be seen. In some cases, variation in fibre size (Fig. 23.12) is accompanied by groups of small undifferentiated fibres (type 2C), with adipose tissue and fibrosis in the muscle. It has been noted by some authors that babies with such an apparently severe myopathy, which is sometimes accompanied by contractures, have a good chance of survival if they can pass their second birthday. Others,[28] who have reported many cases, regard the prognosis as mostly poor. Most affected infants provide no evidence of genetic inheritance of the myopathy, but in some it appears to be autosomal recessive. Early clinical arrest in a few babies suggests that the disorder may be heterogeneous, some cases having an intrauterine cause, such as myositis. It is for this reason that the term 'dystrophic myopathy' is preferred at the present time to 'congenital muscular dystrophy'.

An infantile myopathy with the same histological characteristics is sometimes associated with cerebral malformations such as polymicrogyria or pachygyria, or with hydrocephalus. This is the Fukuyama type of congenital dystrophic myopathy,[29] rare except in Japan, suggesting an environmental factor. Again, in a minority there is evidence of autosomal recessive inheritance.

The myotonic syndromes

Myotonia is an uncommon sign of several disorders of skeletal muscle in which active contraction of a muscle continues after voluntary effort ceases. It can be demonstrated by asking the patient to grip an object and then to relax his grip; this cannot be done until involuntary contraction wears off after a relatively short period. Percussion of any muscle with a patellar hammer produces a dimple which also holds its shape for a time. The disability can be serious for some patients, causing them to stiffen up at awkward moments, drop objects and fall, but in others it causes only minor disability.

Myotonic dystrophy

This is a multi-system disorder of dominant inheritance in which myotonia and muscular atrophy are combined with frontal baldness, cataracts, facial wasting, bilateral ptosis, striking wasting of the sternomastoids, a poor smile and gonadal atrophy. The limb weakness is distal. The dystrophy appears to start with myotonia, wasting and weakness occurring later. The myotonia then tends to disappear. Many patients are mentally mildly subnormal and apathetic so that symptoms may not be noticed early. There is much variation within families.

The onset is in adult life, generally after 20 years of age. The heart is quite often involved and at autopsy shows patchy myocardial fibrosis. The life span may not be reduced.

In recent years neonatal onset has been recognised, producing hypotonia and sometimes severe respiratory difficulty. The babies do not

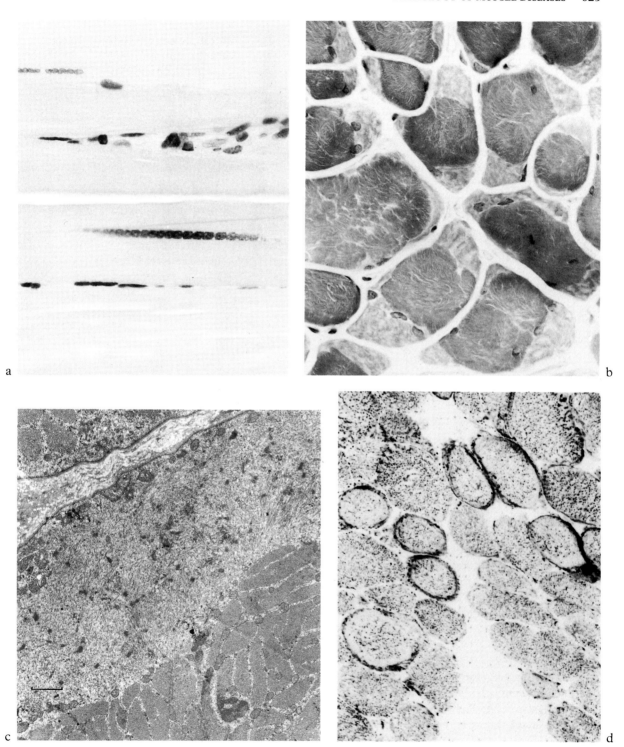

Fig. 23.13a–d Myotonic dystrophy. Girl, aged 9 years. (**a**) Internal nuclei in long closely packed rows. (**b**) Sarcoplasmic masses. (**c**) Electron micrograph showing the fibrillary nature of a sarcoplasmic mass. (**d**) Ring fibres.
(**a, b**) Paraffin section, (**a**) Haematoxylin, Van Gieson, NADH-TR ×325; (**b**) Haematoxylin-eosin ×495; (**c**) Electron micrograph, bar = 1 μm; (**d**) Frozen section, NADH-TR ×260

show myotonia and some years may pass before the characteristic histopathology develops in the muscles. The diagnosis can be made very early, however, if the infant's parents, especially the mother, are examined. The clinical features of myotonic dystrophy, especially the facial expression, can often be recognised at a glance in the adult.

Histopathology. The most obvious feature in the established syndrome is a great increase in the number of fibres with internal nuclei, sometimes with four or five nuclei in the same transverse plane. Muscle fibres vary in size, considerably so in the later stages, and obviously hypertrophied fibres (usually type 2) mingle with others of variable calibre and of both types. In longitudinal section the internal nuclei lie close together and form long chains (Fig. 23.13a). Some very small fibres occur, probably the result of fibre splitting. Other changes that may be seen are sarcoplasmic masses, where fibrillar material collects near the periphery of the fibre and separates the sarcolemma from the myofibrils (Fig. 23.13b and 13c). In some biopsies, ring fibres are quite frequent (Fig. 23.13d). Muscle spindles in distal muscles may be abnormal. The upper limit of the number of intrafusal muscle fibres in human spindles is 15; if more are found there is usually evidence of intrafusal fibre splitting (Fig. 23.14). When this process is advanced, as many as 60 thin fibres may be counted.[30] Other myopathic changes may be noted, but are non-specific.

The pathogenesis of the characteristic, if not specific, trio of long internal nuclear chains, sarcoplasmic masses and the extraordinary intrafusal fibre splitting is not known, but it is tempting to link it to longstanding myotonia.

Myotonia congenita

In this disorder, myotonia is more severe than in myotonic dystrophy and of much longer duration although it abates later in life. There is no sign of a structural myopathy. The onset of myotonia is during the first decade, and in many patients the muscles hypertrophy. A biopsy at this stage will show hypertrophy, of type 2 fibres predominantly, and large motor end-plates. When hypertrophy

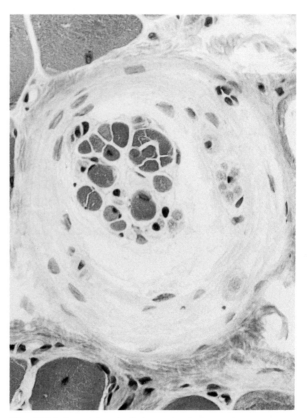

Fig. 23.14 A muscle spindle in myotonic dystrophy at a relatively early stage shows an increase of intrafusal fibres which must be due to longitudinal fibre splitting. Frozen section, haematoxylin-eosin × 405

has been present for a long period, the muscle shows an increase in internal nuclei and some evidence of fibre splitting. Anaesthetists are well acquainted with the myotonic syndromes and of the difficulties that may arise during anaesthesia such as a paradoxical response to relaxants and respiratory impairment. Patients with myotonia congenita can react to anaesthesia in a similar way to patients carrying the malignant hyperthermia (MH) gene (see p. 649). Three patients with myotonia congenita were identified in a group of 1400 individuals tested for susceptibility to MH during anaesthesia. All three had suffered a reaction to anaesthesia, including a rise in temperature, but none had MH.[31] MH has been diagnosed in myotonic dystrophy on grounds such as these, but in none of the cases was that diagnosis confirmed by the in vitro tests.

Inheritance. There are two distinct forms of myotonia congenita. They are similar clinically. The first has been known for over a century as *Thomsen's disease.* Julius Thomsen was a Danish physician who suffered from the disorder and who described it in 1876 in 20 members of four generations of his own family.[31a] It is autosomal dominant, and appears equally in both sexes.

The second variety of myotonia congenita is the *Becker type*, with more widespread myotonia and in later years the development of weakness of the limbs. It is autosomal recessive.

Paramyotonia

Eulenberg[32] described families who suffered from myotonia only on exposure to cold. Myotonia in general can be elicited or made worse by cold, so that symptom alone would not characterise an in-dependent disorder. The affected members also suffered from periodic unexplained weakness. As myotonia may occur in periodic paralysis it is possible that paramyotonia is a form of that disease (see p. 652).

REACTIVE MYOPATHIES

Introduction

Skeletal muscle reacts to adverse stimuli in a number of different ways but the reactions are not stereotyped: a cryptic carcinoma, for example, may induce type 2B fibre atrophy in one patient, and a necrotising myopathy in another. The main causes of reactive myopathy are malnutrition and starvation, malignant tumours, systemic diseases and drugs. The latter may produce specific reactions whether given therapeutically or by

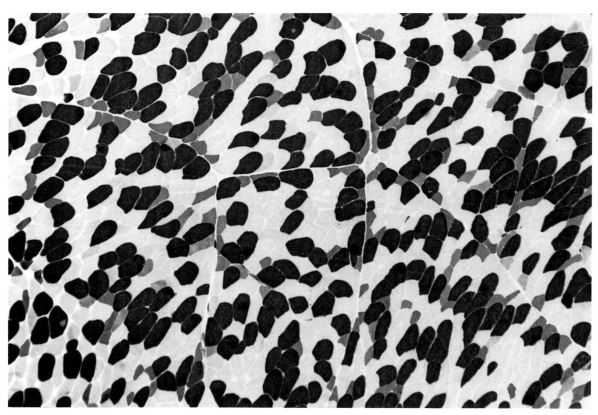

Fig. 23.15 Selective type 2 fibre atrophy. There is moderate atrophy of the relatively few type 2B fibres (intermediate staining) in this preparation.
Frozen section, myosin ATPase, pH 4·63 × 80

overdosage.[33,34] The reactive myopathies cause weakness initially, followed by wasting. Usually their cause is obvious and no biopsy is required, but when the origin of wasting and weakness is obscure, it is important to include reactive myopathy in the differential diagnosis.

Reactive myopathy appears in many histopathological forms. The commonest are type 2B fibre atrophy, cachectic atrophy and necrotising myopathy. Less common are vacuolar myopathy and myotonia.

Type 2B fibre atrophy

At one time this was referred as as type 2 fibre atrophy, but when 2B fibres were defined it was found that the atrophied fibres were of type 2B. This is therefore a selective fibre-type disorder and sets these fibres apart from 2A fibres as an independent form. The atrophy is insidious and progressive, affecting some of the 2B fibres initially (partial type 2B atrophy) but later they all shrink and become misshapen while type 1 and 2A fibres remain unaffected (Fig. 23.15). Common causes are a cryptic malignant neoplasm, focal sepsis, therapeutic drugs, rheumatoid arthritis and polymyalgia rheumatica. It occurs in severe form in chronic alcoholism, but is not found in acute alcoholism, which initially causes accumulation of large amounts of intracellular lipid in type 1 fibres.

Cachectic atrophy

This is familiar as the effect of malnutrition, starvation, chronic infections, malignancy and combinations of these. It may develop in senile dementia despite all attempts to maintain good nutrition, and in some endocrine disorders such as Addison's disease. A rare cause of unexpected cachectic atrophy in children without other signs or symptoms is a slowly growing astrocytoma of the medulla oblongata.

Cachectic atrophy appears to be a more severe form of type 2B fibre atrophy. The loss of fibrillary protein probably starts in 2B fibres, but soon spreads to the other fibre types, which eventually are reduced to one-third or one-quarter of their normal diameter. In paraffin sections, fibre types cannot be distinguished as they can in ATPase-

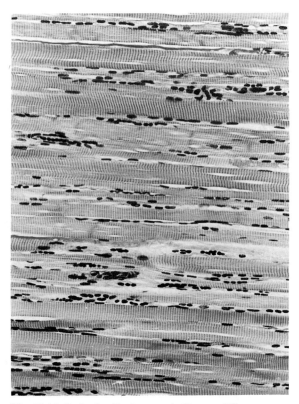

Fig. 23.16 Cachexia affecting muscle fibres to different degrees in a patient with severe rheumatoid arthritis. The biopsy served to exclude myositis and rheumatoid neuropathy.
Paraffin section, haematoxylin-eosin × 405

stained cryostat sections but, nevertheless, fibres of different sizes are seen in these sections in severe cachexia (Fig. 23.16).

Necrotising myopathy

This reaction is quite different from type 2B fibre atrophy. It consists of fibre necrosis and regeneration, mainly in proximal muscles and more pronounced in the lower limbs than in the upper limbs. The degree of involvement may range from as little as one segment of necrosis per low-power field to widespread necrosis and macrophage invasion (Fig. 23.17). Despite this, most of the necrosis is segmental, permitting good regeneration. In some patients there is an inflammatory cell reaction; this can generally be ascribed to the muscle fibre necrosis. When the myopathy is extensive, the patient is very ill and suffers from myoglobinuria.

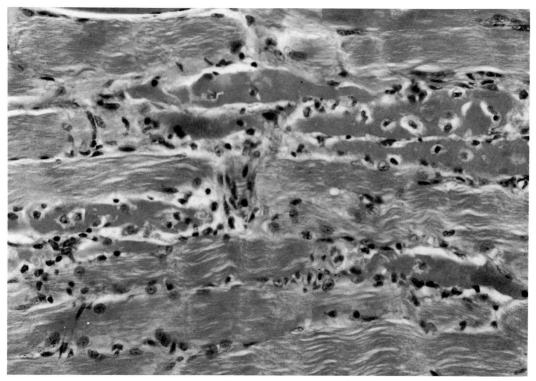

Fig. 23.17 Necrotising myopathy. Many necrotic segments are invaded by macrophages with, as yet, little regeneration.
Paraffin section × 290

The causes of a mild or moderately severe necrotising myopathy will include general factors like systemic disease, carcinoma, chronic infections and drugs, but the most severe are almost always due to drugs, including both therapeutic drugs and drugs of addiction. When extensive rhabdomyolysis occurs, there is always the danger of renal failure (as in the 'crush syndrome'). An autopsy on a patient who has died in unexplained renal failure should always include examination of skeletal muscle.

Vacuolar myopathy and myotonia

Drugs may also cause a *vacuolar myopathy*, e.g. those drugs causing hypokalaemia, and *myotonia*, as with drugs that lower serum cholesterol such as 20,25-diazocholesterol.

Myositis

As myositis is more often a primary inflammatory disorder of muscle (inflammatory myopathy), its histology will be described with polymyositis (see p. 632). It is a reactive phenomenon when it is the presenting manifestation of a cancer. Certain drugs can precipitate a myositis similar to that seen in lupus erythematosus. Examples of such drugs are sulphacetamide and hydralazine. This reaction is apparently more common in patients who are slow acetylators.[35]

INFLAMMATORY MYOPATHIES DUE TO KNOWN INFECTIVE AGENTS

Inflammation is a relatively frequent feature in the pathology of skeletal muscle, but cases in which the cause of the inflammation is known are in a minority. Whitaker[36] discusses the possible rôle of viruses, cell-mediated immunity and genetic influences in the majority of inflammatory myopathies. However, he stresses that viruses cannot be identified on morphological grounds alone (i.e. by electron microscopy of muscle), and high levels of antibody to the suspected virus are often more reliable.

Viral infections

Influenzal myopathy

Many people have experienced muscle aching, starting about a week after the onset of influenza and persisting for another week or two. On the few occasions on which it has been investigated, the level of creatine kinase in the blood has been raised; on biopsy a necrotising myopathy has been found. Influenza virus has been recovered from muscle at least once, but the clinical timing of the myalgia suggests mediation by an immunogenic mechanism.

Other viruses

The following have occasionally been implicated in myopathy: echovirus 9 (myositis), Coxsackievirus B6 (acute myositis) and Coxsackievirus B5 (Bornholm disease). Other viruses that have been blamed for myopathy, including hepatitis B, are a less certain cause of muscle disease.

Bacterial myositis

Suppuration in the skeletal musculature is characterised by the formation of large abscesses. Multiple small abscesses suggestive of pyaemia are apparently no longer seen. In temperate climates, local abscesses in muscle are seen most frequently in two categories of people—the elderly bedridden who develop abscesses which spread from bedsores, and those who use dirty injection needles, especially when immunity is impaired. Abscesses also complicate suppurative arthritis. Streptococci and staphylococci are commonly the infecting organisms.

Gas gangrene still occurs, particularly in some tropical regions but also certainly in temperate climates. The organisms which flourished under the conditions of trench warfare and affected muscle in particular were the anaerobic gas-forming bacilli, particularly *Clostridium welchii*. Being anaerobic and toxin-forming, this organism caused extensive necrosis; bubbles of gas formed

and could be recognised on clinical examination by the peculiar crepitant feel of the tissues. An inflammatory reaction was confined to the edge of the necrotic area, with little pus.

True pyogenic abscesses are not common in temperate climates. They do occur in hot and humid environments where it is not uncommon to encounter a large abscess, often gluteal, and more often in men, but without any obvious source for the infection.

Tuberculous pseudo-abscess. The so-called tuberculous psoas abscess is still encountered. The infection spreads into the muscle as a caseating granulomatous mass originating in an infected vertebral body. It is not a true abscess unless secondarily infected by pyogenic organisms.

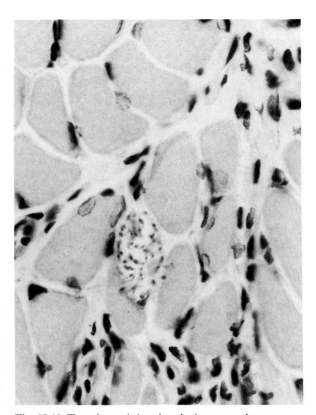

Fig. 23.18 Toxoplasmosis in a dog. An intramuscular cyst containing the tiny crescentic protozoa, with minimal neighbouring inflammation.
Paraffin section, haematoxylin-eosin × 520

Protozoal infections

Toxoplasmosis

Toxoplasma gondii (see p. 184) is a widely distributed pathogenic protozoon. It may infect many organs, and often antibodies are formed in the absence of symptoms. A large proportion of the population has raised antibody levels to toxoplasma and it is often tempting to ascribe various illnesses to the parasite. The serious consequences of eye infection in infants are well known (see p. 682). A multifocal myositis occurs in toxoplasmosis but is rare. The organisms in muscle are not usually well preserved in man; a clearer picture is obtained in dogs (Fig. 23.18). The myositis is characterised by necrosis and regeneration, and infiltration by lymphocytes and plasma cells and, not infrequently, also by eosinophils.[37]

Infection by Sarcocystis *species*

Species of the protozoal parasite *Sarcocystis* are occasionally found encysted in skeletal and cardiac muscle fibres of various domestic and wild animals in many parts of the world. These cysts, ingested by the definitive host, are the source of the characteristic intestinal infection in the latter. Sarcocystis infection was formerly a very frequent finding in laboratory rodents but has become rare since the introduction of modern methods of feeding and housing. The parasite is sometimes

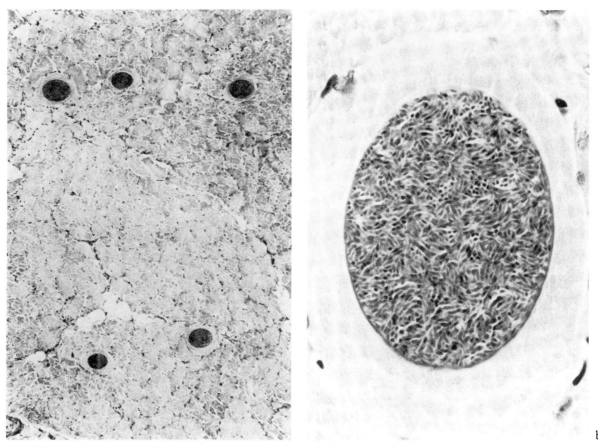

a   b

Fig. 23.19a, b (a) The thick-walled cysts of *Sarcocystis* within muscle fibres. (b) Individual cyst containing trophozoites. Paraffin section, haematoxylin-eosin (a) ×65; (b) ×630
Photomicrographs provided by W. St C. Symmers.

referred to as a sarcosporidium. Sarcocystis cysts have been found incidentally in human muscle, both cardiac and skeletal. The organism in these cases is *Sarcocystis lindemanni*: its intestinal phase is probably passed in non-human primates. When symptomatic infection occurs in man, the affected muscles show localised swelling and there is an accompanying fever.

The histology of the infected muscles in man is unaltered, apart from the presence of the cysts themselves, provided these remain intact; on rupture an inflammatory reaction is induced, often with numerous eosinophils. The cysts measure from 50 to 300 μm in length and lie lengthwise in the fibre (Fig. 23.19). The trophozoites are usually 10–14 μm, but some are shorter and can be mistaken for the trophozoites of *Toxoplasma gondii*.

Metazoal infestations

Cysticercosis

The adult forms of *Taenia solium* (pig tapeworm) and of *T. saginata* (beef tapeworm) live in the intestine of their definitive host, which is man (see p. 186). If man ingests free ova, larvae hatch and are distributed to skeletal and heart muscle as well as to other organs, giving rise to cysticercosis *Taenia solium* is by far the more frequent cause of human cysticercosis. The larvae encyst, and part of the cyst wall is formed of the host's connective tissue. Eventually the cysts calcify. When the parasite dies, soluble antibodies diffuse into the surrounding tissues, in some cases inducing an inflammatory reaction. Eosinophils are present in the cellular infiltrate and may make up its greatest part. Several cases have been reported with gross enlargement of affected muscles. As the muscle strength is not impaired, the enlargement may largely be due to the number of cysts present; each cyst measures about 1 cm across. Jolly and Pallis[38] illustrate such pseudohypertrophy and also the appearance of the muscle exposed at biopsy; the entire surface of the muscle is studded with cysts.

Trichinosis

The adult *Trichinella spiralis* lives in the intestine of many species, including man. The embryos pass through the intestinal mucosa and thence by the bloodstream to the muscles. Human infestation is due to eating undercooked pork. In the muscles, the larvae can be seen curled up in oval cysts that are about 0·5 mm long and lie within muscle fibres. The cyst wall is derived from host tissue and, once completed, renders the parasite harmless. Cysts in the heart and brain, however, may cause complications.

MYOPATHIES DUE TO IMMUNOLOGICAL OR UNKNOWN CAUSE

Polymyositis and dermatomyositis

Both these conditions are characterised by inflammatory changes in muscle.[39] In dermatomyositis there are, in addition, skin rashes and an inflammatory cellular infiltrate in the dermis. Both may occur at any age. The majority of cases of both disorders occur in adults and the elderly. In children, dermatomyositis is more often diagnosed than polymyositis. Clinically, the face may be slightly swollen and have a reddish or violaceous tinge, Raynaud's phenomenon may be seen in both upper and lower limbs, and the paravertebral muscles are often involved. Unlike the dystrophies there is no constant pattern of involvement or even of symmetry. The distribution of the myositis is usually multifocal, so that it is a matter of chance if the site chosen for biopsy is affected. There is a high incidence of 'normal' biopsies in polymyositis, but this can be reduced by taking two small biopsies from different sites rather than a standard biopsy from a single site. Rarely, there is a single diffuse swelling within a muscle, which is tender and painful. The naked eye appearance of muscle exposed at biopsy can help with the diagnosis; if inflammation is present, the muscle assumes a bright red colour and is unduly firm.

Histopathology. The classical features in the muscle consist of a combination of large infiltrates of lymphocytes, plasma cells and histiocytes, occasionally with a few eosinophils, along with segmental necrosis, phagocytosis and vigorous regeneration of muscle fibres. Immunoperoxidase techniques help to distinguish the various types of

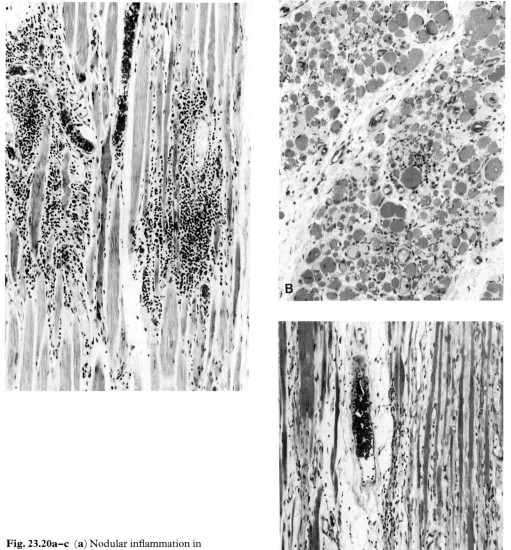

Fig. 23.20a–c (**a**) Nodular inflammation in polymyositis. (**b**) Transverse section of muscle showing a diffuse pattern of inflammation. (**c**) Longitudinal section showing separation of fibres and swelling of perimysium and epimysium. Paraffin section, haematoxylin-eosin (**a**) × 120; (**b**) × 40; (**c**) × 110

mononuclear cells. The fibrous bands between muscle fascicles are usually swollen during the period of cellular infiltration and tend to remain so thereafter: this is likely to account for atrophy of the peripheral muscle fibres in some fascicles (perifascicular atrophy) that is seen especially in dermatomyositis in the chronic phase (Fig. 22.1, p. 589). The cellular infiltrates may be nodular (Fig.

23.20a), taking the form of long oval deposits of lymphocytes in the interstitial tissue, on occasion forming germinal centres. In other cases the infiltration may spread diffusely throughout fascicles (Fig. 23.20b and c). Lymphocytes may encircle blood vessels but a true arteritis is rare except in childhood dermatomyositis, in which evidence of active or healed arteritis is found in about 50% of cases. It has been proposed in consequence that all childhood dermatomyositis is due to arteritis. A similar arteritis has been found in adults also, but this is usually only seen at necropsy when many samples of muscle tissue can be examined. Often the histological picture is incomplete in this focal disorder, showing muscle fibre necrosis and regeneration alone, or even completely normal muscle if the biopsy sample has not included the lesions. Histopathology of the skin taken at the same time as the muscle biopsy shows non-specific lymphocytic infiltration.

Innervation of muscle shows quite marked changes with distal sprouting and enlargement and distortion of end-plates. On occasion there is collateral reinnervation in addition, which is thought to be due to inflammatory destruction of intramuscular nerves and consequent collateral re-innervation. This has been designated *neuro-myositis*.

The heart in polymyositis.[40]   Although electrocardiographic (ECG) evidence of myocardial involvement is not uncommon, pathological evidence is confined to three post-mortem reports. In two of these the myositis appeared to be 'burnt out', with fibrosis of the vessel walls in both skeletal and cardiac muscle; in only one was there active inflammation. It would not be surprising for skeletal and cardiac muscle to be involved at times, for they share similar immunogenic properties.

Investigations.   Electromyography shows features of myopathy, often accompanied by patchy fibrillation potentials and spikes, due no doubt to scattered collateral reinnervation.

Creatine kinase levels may be little above normal in the presence of a fulminant myositis, but more often they are considerably raised. The same is true of the erythrocyte sedimentation rate.

Differential diagnosis.   In children, the most important differential diagnosis is with Duchenne dystrophy, in which a few patients show an excessive unexplained inflammatory reaction. This, in the presence of active necrosis and regeneration, may mimic polymyositis. In the same way, polymyositis in a chronic or non-inflammatory phase may be mistaken for Duchenne dystrophy (see p. 611).

Precipitating factors.   Myositis is one form of reactive myopathy (see p. 627). Polymyositis in young adults rarely heralds a neoplasm but in the fifth and sixth decades the incidence of association with a cryptic malignant tumour rises to 80%.

Sarcoid myopathy

It is well known that sarcoidosis has a predilection for the nervous system (see p. 163), especially the hypothalamus and the peripheral nerves. It is probably present just as often in the skeletal muscles, for the diagnosis of sarcoidosis can be sought and often confirmed by a random muscle biopsy. Overt involvement of muscle is less common and presents as a predominantly proximal myopathy with muscle weakness, tenderness, and sometimes pain. Women are more often affected than men, and in the USA the disease is much more frequent among black patients than among whites.

Histology.   The main changes are in the interstitial tissue of the muscle; there is minimal secondary necrosis, regeneration and atrophy of the muscle cells. The sarcoid infiltration takes two forms. In one, sarcoid granulomas resemble those in other organs; they are composed of epithelioid histiocytes, lymphocytes and Langhans type giant cells. Necrosis is exceptionally rare and is not caseous in type but fibrinoid (Fig. 23.21). The granulomas may be widely spaced and are more likely to be found by open than by needle biopsy. The second form of sarcoid infiltration of muscle consists of lines of single small epithelioid cells between muscle fibres: diagnosis then depends on being aware of the possibility of sarcoidosis.

It should be recalled that sarcoidosis also involves peripheral nerves and thus induces denervation atrophy in muscles, especially the distal limb muscles.

Other forms of granulomatous myositis

In some patients, granulomas, or the linear infiltrates of small epithelioid cells noted in the preceding section, appear to be present only in muscle.[41]   The concept of a granulomatous disorder confined to muscle has been proposed but

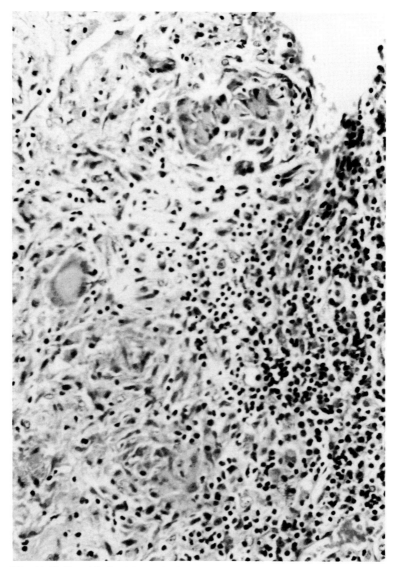

Fig. 23.21 Sarcoidosis of the orbit. Several granulomas are present; there is no necrosis.
Paraffin section, haematoxylin-eosin × 250

is difficult to prove, as it has been shown only once at necropsy.[42] Similar granulomas may be seen in other organs, such as the liver and the lymphoid tissues, which, on investigation, prove not to be associated with sarcoidosis. Most of these are of unknown cause. Thus it is not justifiable to assume that every granulomatous myopathy must be a manifestation of sarcoidosis; other evidence of sarcoidosis must be sought and, in the absence of this evidence, a non-specific diagnosis is necessary.

Arteritis

Wasting, weakness and tenderness of muscle may be attributable to arteritis. The affected muscle may show myositis, generally less florid than in acute polymyositis. Following arteritic thrombosis

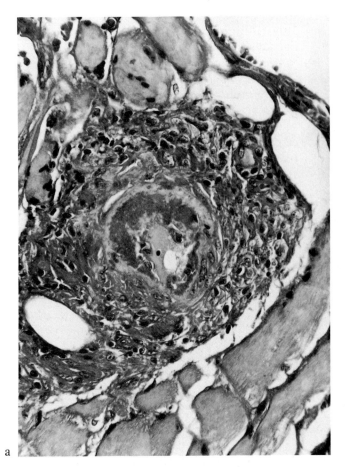

a

Fig. 23.22a, b (**a**) Arteritis. A small intramuscular artery shows medial fibrinoid necrosis and endothelial prominence. There is pronounced cellular infiltration of the adventitia. (**b**) Healed arteritis in chronic polyarteritis showing endothelial and subendothelial hyperplasia.
(**a**) Paraffin section, Martius Scarlet Blue × 360;
(**b**) Haematoxylin-eosin × 200

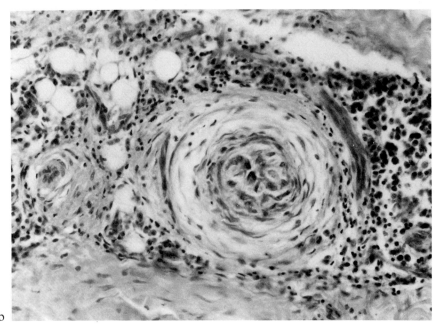

b

there may be an area of infarction, although this is rare. If a major nerve is affected, as in polyarteritis, the biopsy may show neurogenic atrophy alone, in which case the diagnosis will only be suspected because of the clinical picture of mononeuritis multiplex.

The involvement of skeletal muscle in arteritis can be clinically silent and, as in the case of sarcoidosis, clinical suspicion of arteritis is investigated by a random muscle biopsy. The muscle chosen is often proximal, but no one site has a greater success rate than others. Enough muscle must be obtained to provide at least one paraffin block for longitudinal sections as well as those for transverse sections of reasonable size.

Polyarteritis nodosa affects large and medium-sized arteries. Characteristically, the acute phase shows necrosis of a crescent of media which is infiltrated by fibrin (fibrinoid necrosis—Fig. 23.22a), accompanied by cellular infiltration of the media and adventitia. In the larger arteries fibrinoid necrosis can be so severe that there is aneurysmal dilatation of the vessel wall, producing the nodose appearance of the vessel. Not infrequently there is subintimal fibrous hyperplasia with or without thrombosis.

In *giant cell arteritis*, the target tissue is primarily the internal elastic lamina, which fragments and is ingested by histiocytes, often in the form of giant cells, in the midst of an inflammatory cell infiltration. It is most often seen in the cranial arteries, especially the temporal arteries, but is found at times in most organs and tissues, including muscle and nerve.

Not much is known of the ultimate fate of blood vessels affected by arteritis except that recovery is frequent, especially with the appropriate treatment, and that some undergo thrombosis. In cases of longstanding polyarteritis observed at post mortem, fibrotic areas of muscle contain arteries with gross subintimal fibrosis and a small central lumen bordered by proliferating endothelium (Fig. 23.22b). This appearance has been attributed to recanalisation of fibrin thrombi or healing of the arteritis by fibrous scarring.

Inclusion-body myositis

This is a recently described condition[43]

characterised by muscle weakness and severe fatigability occurring predominantly in the elderly but also at any age from the late teens onward. Males predominate. Most patients remain ambulant but are frustrated by the early development of their fatigue. Treatment by steroids or immunosuppressive drugs is ineffective and may cause deterioration. The condition is said to be rare, but the diagnosis may be overlooked in some patients with the symptoms mentioned because no changes were found on examination of only one biopsy. As in other myositides, its distribution is focal and the severity of histopathological changes is extremely variable.

The main features at biopsy are lymphocytic infiltration of the fibrous perimysium. This varies in intensity from large masses to one or two cells. There are numbers of small autophagic vacuoles which stain with a blue granular pattern with haematoxylin and eosin, and red with the modified Gomori technique[43a] (Fig. 23.23).

In some cases there are no lymphocytes in the biopsy. There may be more than one vacuole in an

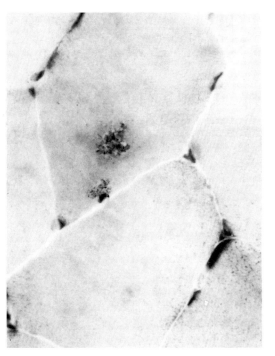

Fig. 23.23 Inclusion body myositis. One muscle fibre (top) contains two small granular autophagic vacuoles. Frozen section, modified Gomori technique.[43a] × 720

affected fibre, each containing several dark granules. Intranuclear inclusions are the most characteristic electron microscopic feature.[43,43a] They consist of closely packed filaments which in a single plane may be seen both in longitudinal and in transverse section.

CONGENITAL MYOPATHIES

Infantile hypotonia

Mild hypotonia at birth is not uncommon in premature infants or in the presence of some degree of perinatal hypoxia. Severe hypotonia, on the other hand, is very serious as it may herald the appearance of a number of congenital myopathies or neuropathies or it may be the first sign of abnormality in the CNS such as a malformation, birth hypoxia (see p. 120) or tumour (secondary hypotonia).

Not uncommonly, equally severe hypotonia is found in the absence of any demonstrable cause, either in the muscles or in the brain. This is *benign congenital hypotonia* (formerly known as amyotonia congenita) which may persist for many months or even years before it disappears. There is delayed motor development. In some cases muscle biopsy shows a moderate degree of type 2B fibre atrophy.

A floppy baby who feels like a rag doll, who lies in the prone, frog-leg, position unable to raise his head, and in whom an experienced clinician finds it difficult or impossible to decide whether paralysis underlies the hypotonia, obviously requires investigation. But severe forms of some congenital myopathies may involve the respiratory muscles and make invasive procedures impracticable.

Arthrogryposis[44]

This term is used to describe an infant born with multiple congenital contractures, giving rise to pronounced curvature of the wrist and ankle joints (the name means curved joints). Muscle biopsies are sometimes difficult to interpret in these cases, but when taken at a suitable distance from deformity the muscle may be normal, or show neurogenic atrophy or congenital dystrophic myopathy. At autopsy there may be several abnormalities of the brain and spinal cord and of the skeletal structures and integuments. Those babies who survive long enough for assessment are mentally subnormal.

Central core, multicore and minicore diseases

Central core disease was recognised and described in 1956[45] before frozen section histochemistry was available, and was the first of a number of congenital muscle disorders that seemed at the time to be invariably mild and of benign prognosis. Later it was found that some of these disorders were progressive, and a few appeared in forms that were fatal in infancy. Hypotonia was often present at birth. The 'cores' were sharply defined circular areas, within muscle fibres (Fig. 23.24a), in which staining was absent or pale. Although most of the cores were centrally placed in the fibre, a proportion were eccentric and up to five cores could be found in the same transverse section of a fibre. With some routine stains the central part of each core stained intensely.

In later reports incorporating histochemistry and ultrastructure, it was found that the whole area of the core was devoid of mitochondria. In some cores, myofibrils were intact throughout except for a few small foci of Z-line streaming, and these were referred to as structured cores; the remaining unstructured cores showed advanced Z-line streaming (Fig. 23.24b) and eventual myofibrillar coagulation in their central zone; it was this inspissated material which had enabled the cores to be recognised in the original studies of paraffin sections of muscle. The structured cores could only be clearly seen in frozen sections, particularly in reactions such as dihydronicotinamide adenine dinucleotide tetrazolium reductase (NADH-TR), which demonstrate mitochondria.

Cores are not confined to central core disease (see p. 599), but in the congenital myopathy they have two distinctive features: they are associated in most cases at least with a marked preponderance of type 1 muscle fibres, and when seen in dissected single muscle fibres they are long, and limited only by the length of dissection (Fig. 23.24c). In some patients, very few cores are present but they show type 1 fibre preponderance.

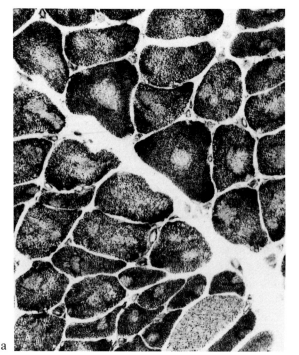

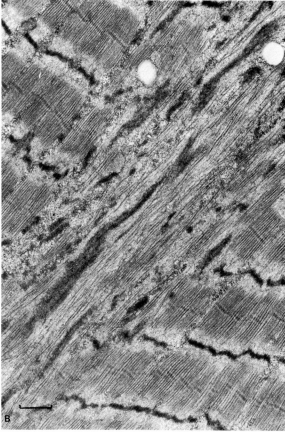

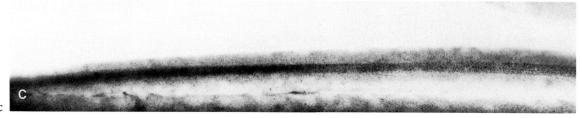

Fig. 23.24a–c Central core disease. (**a**) There is marked predominance of type 1 fibres; many pale circular cores are seen as well as irregularly stained 'moth-eaten' fibres. (**b**) The centre of a core is unstructured but not yet showing coagulation. There is a virtual absence of mitochondria. (**c**) Dissected fibre showing a long core with a dark unstructured centre.
(**a**) Frozen section, NADH-TR × 205; (**b**) Electron micrograph, bar = 1 μm; (**c**) de Castro silver × 170

The number of cores appears to increase with age: in one female patient biopsied at the age of 5 years and again at the age of 16, there was a marked increase in the number of cores. The second biopsy was taken in the investigation of susceptibility to malignant hyperthermia (see p. 649).

As more cases of central core disease were reported, clinical and genetic heterogeneity became evident.[46] In some families there was a dominant pattern of inheritance, in at least one it was recessive, and there was clinical variation. Cases were described in which there were pain on exercise and unusual patterns of muscle weakness such as a facioscapulohumeral distribution.

As noted on page 649, members of families with

central core disease should be offered the in-vitro test for susceptibility to malignant hyperthermia (MH) or at least advised of the need to inform their anaesthetist of the association between central core disease and MH.

Several histological variants of central core disease have been described, among them *multicore disease*[47] and *minicore disease*.[48] Multicores are very much shorter than average cores, and their long axes lie transversely in the muscle fibres. The breadth of a fibre can accommodate two, perhaps three multicores. As in central core disease, there is type 1 fibre predominance, but multicores can also be found in type 2 fibres. The clinical features are variable but weakness is as a rule non-progressive. Minicore disease differs in that the lesions are tiny. They consist of very small foci of Z-line streaming occupying about one-tenth of the width of the muscle fibre. Such tiny lesions may be visible in cryostat and paraffin sections of muscle;[48] in most

cases there is a mixture of minicores and multicores.

Rod-body myopathy (nemaline myopathy)

This congenital myopathy, described several years after central core disease (see above), was also thought at first to be non-progressive. The infants were hypotonic at birth but slowly improved. They often suffered from skeletal deformities such as a high arched palate or congenital dislocation of the hip as well as mild, mainly proximal, weakness and occasionally ptosis. The first report, in 1963,[49] named the condition 'nemaline myopathy' as the authors observed threadlike bodies within muscle fibres; later observations revealed that the bodies were not threads but short rods 2 μm or more in length (Fig. 23.25a). Recently, it has been recognised that severely affected infants may die of the effects of the condition. If a biopsy is not possible during life, it is always worth while taking

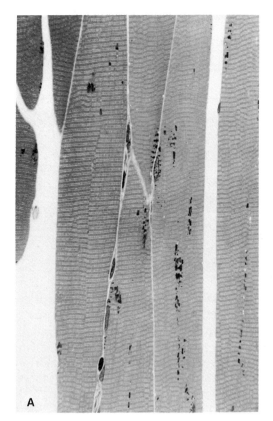

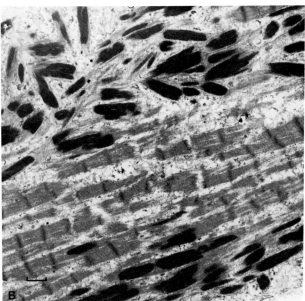

Fig. 23.25a, b (a) Asymptomatic rod-body myopathy in a female aged 16 years. (b) Female, 13 months, with severe rod-body myopathy. Post-mortem specimen. Electron micrograph showing numerous dense rod bodies.
(a) Semi-thin section × 470; (b) Electron micrograph: bar = 1 μm

muscle at post mortem, even 24 hours after death; rods are smaller in infants than in older patients and may be difficult to see in frozen sections, but they resist post-mortem autolysis quite well and can be identified in semi-thin sections and electron micrographs (Fig. 23.25b). At the opposite end of the spectrum, rod-body myopathy has been reported with onset in adult life. With such a variety of clinical presentations, it is not surprising that the mode of inheritance is not always clear. In the majority it is autosomal dominant, but it is often stressed that most patients are female, and that sex-linked inheritance with poor penetrance may eventually be proved.

The rods are usually present in a high proportion of muscle fibres, characteristically in type 1 fibres; there may or may not be type 1 fibre predominance. Rods tend to be in little groups or sheaves under the sarcolemma and are often also scattered within the fibre. They stain well by the modified Gomori method[43a] in frozen sections, where they should be bright red. In paraffin sections they look like poorly defined granules, but can be well shown by the phosphotungstic acid haematoxylin stain. The muscle fibres in general show a mild variation in fibre size, but other features of myopathy are rare. It is now generally accepted that rod bodies are derived from the Z-discs. Rod bodies are of greater volume than the discs, since they are roughly oblong; they are thought to be formed by longitudinal protrusions into the I-band from the Z-discs. Both Z-discs and rod bodies have an identical lattice ultrastructure.

The discovery of rod bodies alone is not necessarily diagnostic of the myopathy. They may be incidental findings in other myopathies and neuropathies, and thus may be seen to develop from fragmenting myofibrils within atrophic or degenerating fibres and still have actin filaments attached to them.

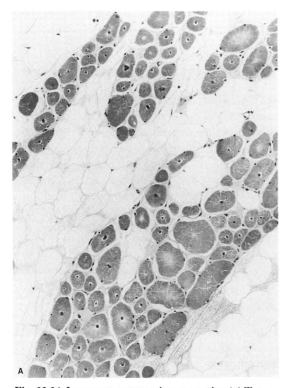
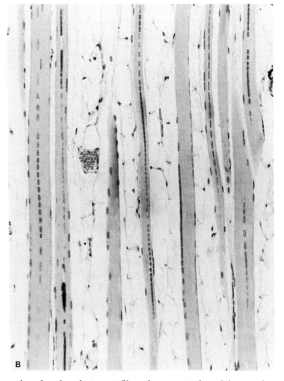

Fig. 23.26 Late onset centronuclear myopathy. (**a**) Transverse section showing that most fibres have central nuclei; some have inconspicuous sarcolemmal nuclei. There is extensive variation in fibre size. (**b**) Longitudinal section. Central nuclei are often closely packed.
Paraffin section, haematoxylin-eosin × 80

The curious finding of numerous rod bodies in leg muscle in a patient with Adie's syndrome (pseudo-Argyll Robertson pupils with absent tendon reflexes) remains unexplained.[50]

Centronuclear myopathy

This myopathy was described in 1966.[51] As in other congenital myopathies, there was weakness from birth and very slow progression in the first case. But there were unusual features. Patients showed extraocular muscle involvement, especially ptosis, and also facial weakness and predominantly distal limb weakness. A more extensive involvement of muscle than in the previously described congenital myopathies was suggested.

The histological findings were unique. Type 1 fibres were smaller than type 2 and frequently contained central (axial) nuclei with a small perinuclear halo. In longitudinal sections, rows of central nuclei could sometimes be found. The appearance recalled fetal myotubes and the name myotubular myopathy was used for the condition. It was suggested that the fibres with central nuclei had undergone arrest of maturation at about the fifth month of gestation. Later, the name centronuclear myopathy was preferred as the comparison with myotubes was not close with regard to nucleus:fibre ratio, fibre diameter and the presence of normally sited sarcolemmal nuclei in addition to the central nuclei.

In later reports it became obvious that there were three different forms of centronuclear myopathy; an early infantile form, sometimes with small type 1 fibres, and childhood and late onset forms (Fig. 23.26).[52] A common problem is posed by the last named: do the centronuclear fibres not develop until middle age, or have they been present since before birth but focal and asymptomatic until affected by ageing? With such a variety of presentations, almost all forms of inheritance have been claimed in centronuclear myopathy.

Congenital fibre type disproportion

In this congenital myopathy type 1 fibres are smaller than type 2; unlike centronuclear myopathy, the nuclei are in their normal position (Fig. 23.27). The first report was by Brooke in 1973,[53] who suggested from his examination of normal biopsies that a difference greater than 12% in the average size between type 1 and type 2 fibres was abnormal. He then described 12 patients, aged from 11 months to 26 years, whose biopsies showed a greater difference than this, with smaller type 1 fibres. He named the condition congenital fibre type disproportion. Many cases have been reported since then, but those with a small difference, in the region of 12%, have sometimes on follow-up proved to be at the onset of other myopathies.[54] Those in the region of 50% or more have always conformed to the characteristics of a mild, slowly progressive or non-progressive myopathy. The disability does not appear to shorten life, although no case has yet been followed up for a long period. In the oldest patient whom I have seen, a girl of 14, the same discrepancy between the main fibre types persists, but both are larger than they would have been at birth. All patients above the age of two are extremely thin; despite this, muscle strength is only moderately impaired.

Reducing-body myopathy

First described in 1972,[55] this is a very rarely recognised congenital myopathy characterised by inclusion bodies in muscle fibres. The first two patients on record died at 9 months and 2 years 6 months respectively. The inclusions were round or oval, at the edge of a fibre, and filled about a quarter of it. They stained particularly well with menadione-linked α-glycerophosphate as they contained sulphydryl groups able to reduce nitroblue tetrazolium. In ultrastructure the inclusions are composed of particulate matter.[56] A benign form has been described.[57]

Tubular aggregate myopathy

Aggregates of tubules said to be derived from the sarcoplasmic reticulum (Fig. 23.28) are also visible by light microscopy mainly in type 2 fibres. They are seen in sections stained with reduced nicotinamide adenine dinucleotide tetrazolium reductase (NADH-TR) as irregular clumps of reaction product scattered within the muscle fibre

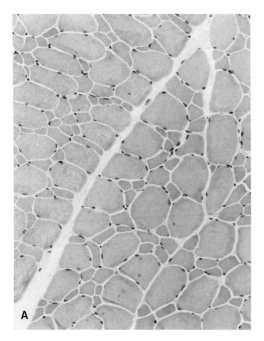

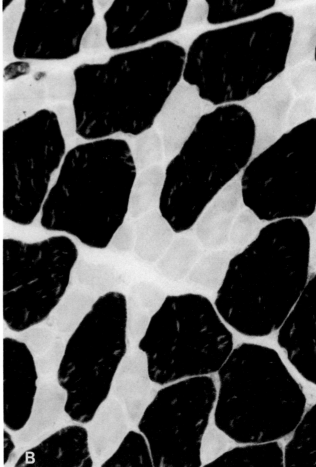

Fig. 23.27a, b Congenital fibre-type disproportion. (**a**) There are two populations of fibres of different size. (**b**) The small fibres are all of type 1 and the large are type 2.
Frozen section (**a**) Haematoxylin-eosin ×160; (**b**) Myosin ATPase 9·4 ×405

and against the sarcolemma. The predilection for type 2 fibres is due to the greater amount of sarcoplasmic reticulum in normal fibres of that type. The first patient reported complained of pain on exercise and weakness of the legs,[58] but the symptomatology in several other cases has been diverse, including a genetically determined slowly progressive myopathy[59] and a myasthenic syndrome. As tubular aggregates have also been found in normal muscle and in patients susceptible to malignant hyperthermia (see p. 649) there is some doubt regarding their specificity and significance.

Other congenital myopathies

The following, mostly very rare, congenital myopathies are listed here, and will be recognisable by the structural characteristics which give them their name:

— 'zebra-body' myopathy
— 'fingerprint-body' myopathy
— sarcotubular myopathy (dilated sarcotubular system)
— familial lysis of type 1 fibres (cores extending across the whole width of a fibre)
— trilaminar muscle fibre disease.

METABOLIC MYOPATHIES

The glycogenoses (glycogen storage diseases)

These are disorders of glycogen metabolism, each characterised by deficiency of one of a number of enzymes; this results in the storage of glycogen in

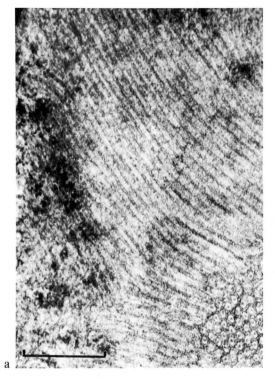

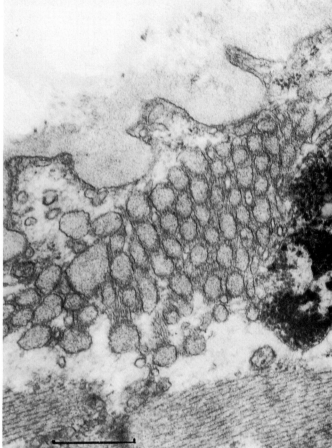

Fig. 23.28a, b (**a**) Tubular aggregates. The tubules run in parallel rows; in cross section (bottom) they are seen to contain a second, central tubule. (**b**) Sometimes more dilated sacs accompany the tubules. Electron micrographs, bar = 0·5 μm

various organs, not always including skeletal muscle. The best known of these enzymes are found in the biochemical sequence in which glycogen is degraded to glucose. The glycogen storage diseases were first reported in the 1920s, and in muscle in the 1930s. But it was not until 1951, when McArdle demonstrated convincingly a block of muscle glycolysis, that interest in muscle glycogen storage disease was awakened.[60] The block was shown a few years later to be due to muscle phosphorylase deficiency. Glycogen in muscle is stored in the cytosol, from which it is soon lost unless the tissue is frozen in liquid nitrogen within minutes of removal; it is stored also in vacuoles derived from lysosomes.

Glycogenosis type 2 (Pompe's disease)

In this type of glycogenosis there is storage of glycogen in many tissues, including skeletal muscle and the myocardium.[61] The missing enzyme is acid maltase, normally present in lysosomes. Typically, the heart is enlarged and there may be pseudohypertrophy of the calf muscles. If there is any suspicion that this form of glycogenosis may be present, the anaesthetist must be alerted to the possibility as cardiac arrest may occur during anaesthesia. The *infantile form* of the disease is fatal by the age of two or three years: invariably there is incapacitating involvement of the muscles of respiration. There is a *childhood form* with later onset, without heart enlargement but still fatal by 15 years of age. In this and in the infantile type all or most fibres are affected. The muscle fibres contain large vacuoles which give a positive reaction for acid phosphatase. The vacuoles vary widely in size. In paraffin sections they contain only a residue of glycogen; much more of the stored glycogen is retained in frozen sections. In addition to glycogen, some vacuoles contain a basophilic substance which stains as acid mucopolysaccharide. The motor innervation is not seriously affected; degeneration of distal sub-terminal motor fibres has been seen on electron microscopy, and glycogen has been noted in Schwann cells in motor nerves. Collateral reinner-vation has not been found.

Adult-onset acid maltase deficiency[62]

This is a much more benign myopathy than the infantile form, as many muscles remain unin-volved and the heart is normal. It may however be incapacitating and painful. Onset is in adult life and the distribution of weakness mainly proximal and truncal. The patient's life span is usually not reduced. The pre-biopsy diagnosis is often limb girdle dystrophy or polymyositis. One-third of patients suffer from ventilatory insufficiency. Ischaemic exercise produces a normal rise in serum lactate, which distinguishes this disease from McArdle's syndrome. Electromyography shows a myopathic response; fibrillation potentials may also occur.

Histology. There is a vacuolar myopathy (Fig. 23.29a) like that in the infantile form; acid mucopolysaccharide deposition is scanty. Fibre type grouping may be seen. Ultrastructurally, glycogen is found both free in the cytoplasm and within lysosomes together with degradation products (Fig. 23.29b).

Glycogenosis type 3 (Cori–Forbes disease; debrancher enzyme deficiency)[63]

The glycogen molecule is large and has many branches to facilitate rapid phosphorylation. En-zymes exist which catalyse both branching and debranching. Absence of the debrancher enzyme is the commonest deficiency but is also the most benign in its effects. The enzyme defect has been detected in several tissues but clinically it causes essentially a mild disorder of the liver in childhood which clears after puberty. The defect is often present in skeletal muscle but only rarely are there any physical signs. Muscle biopsy shows glycogen granules in vacuoles, but electron microscopy

reveals far more glycogen in the cytoplasm than in lysosomes. Ischaemic exercise does not cause a rise in venous lactate, indicating a block in phosphorolytic glycogen breakdown.

Glycogenosis type 4 (Andersen's disease; brancher enzyme deficiency)[64]

This affects many tissues; clinically, it is mani-fested in hepatomegaly and rapidly progressive liver failure in infancy. Skeletal muscle is affected but probably as much by hepatic myopathy as by the glycogenosis.

Glycogenosis type 5 (McArdle's disease; muscle phosphorylase deficiency)[65]

Described by McArdle in 1951, this disease is rare but the impact of its discovery was such that it rapidly became well known.[65] The characteristic clinical presentation is in a young adult who com-plains of severe muscle pain after exercise, relieved by rest. The exercise need only be of brief dura-tion, with a large component of isometric con-traction such as carrying heavy weights, or it may be more sustained, such as climbing stairs or running. However, there are many variations in the mode of presentation; pain on exercise may be absent and the only complaint may be weakness. Myoglobinuria may be induced by exercise due to extensive muscle fibre necrosis. Ischaemic exercise constantly fails to cause a rise in lactate in venous blood.

In McArdle's disease the histochemical test for phosphorylase is negative (Fig. 23.30). This is often wrongly assumed to be due to technical failure. The reaction for this enzyme appears to be all or none, and is not affected in intensity by the slow leaching out of glycogen and phosphorylase that follows excision of the biopsy and continues until the specimen is placed in liquid nitrogen. The biopsy may look normal apart from the PAS and phosphorylase reactions, unless the patient has suffered myoglobinuria, when necrotic and regenerating fibres will be found. With PAS the only positive indication of glycogen increase is in the form of small subsarcolemmal deposits or very narrow subsarcolemmal lines. The presence of material between the muscle fibres that gives a positive reaction with PAS, or a general increase in staining intensity of the whole fibre, is unreliable as a diagnostic observation. The best demonstration of the storage of glycogen in the muscle fibres is by electron microscopy: glycogen particles lie free in masses, sometimes large, under the sarcolemma and in smaller columns between myofibrils. Minor deformities occur in some mitochondria and in the sarcoplasmic reticulum within the deposits.

Glycogenosis type 7 (Tarui's disease; phosphofructokinase deficiency)[66]

Described several years later, the clinical features and histology of Tarui's disease are similar to those of McArdle's disease, but myophosphorylase is present. The deficiency in phosphofructokinase (PFK) can be demonstrated by a histochemical stain. The number of cases reported so far is small (about 30). The condition is of special interest because the partial deficiency of PFK has been found also in red cells, causing haemolysis.

Other glycogenoses

Deficiencies of a number of enzymes producing minimal or overt storage of glycogen have been reported, but all are rare. They include:
— phosphorylase kinase deficiency, which is asymptomatic;
— phosphoglucomutase deficiency, which causes a vacuolar myopathy;
— phosphohexoisomerase deficiency, which has little effect on muscle.

Lactate dehydrogenase deficiency also occurs.

Genetics of glycogenoses. Those cases in which sufficient data are available have an autosomal recessive inheritance pattern.

Lipid storage diseases

That skeletal muscle fibres may contain lipid droplets has been known since the 1850s, when they were called lipid granules and described in the dark (type 1) fibres rather than in the pale (type 2) fibres. An excess of lipid in muscle fibres was described in a familial myopathy a century later.[67] Since then, and particularly since examination of frozen sections of muscle has become a regular

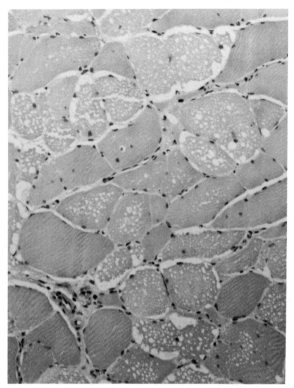

a

Fig. 23.29a, b Acid maltase deficiency. (a) Marked vacuolation of many fibres. (b) A lysosomal vacuole (top left) contains debris and there is abundant free glycogen in the fibre.
(a) Paraffin section, haematoxylin-eosin × 170; (b) Electron micrograph, bar = 1 μm

practice, it has been realised that an excess of triglyceride droplets in type 1 or type 2 fibres occurs as an early response to systemic diseases. It occurs after adrenalectomy for Cushing's syndrome and in drug-induced myopathies, especially those attributable to steroids, and it occurs in acute alcoholic myopathy (Fig. 23.31). In the last two conditions, excess lipid disappears in a matter of months and is replaced by a progressive type 2B fibre atrophy if the intoxications are chronic. Lipid is an important substrate for muscle metabolism both at rest and during prolonged exercise. Triglyceride is as important for the heart as it is for skeletal muscle. The number of droplets present in a normal muscle fibre varies from virtually none to being almost as numerous as the mitochondria, which are of similar size. The lipid is present in the form of bright red droplets when stained by oil red O. The mitochondria also take

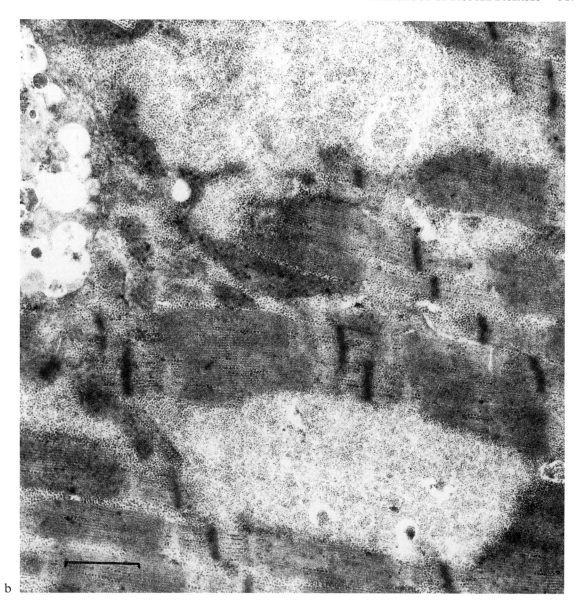

b

this stain by virtue of their phospholipid membranes, but they are only of an inconspicuous dusky colour. In disease, the lipid droplets enlarge. Lipid accumulates in a few fibres of different sizes in various neuromuscular disorders, as though their metabolism were impaired but not to the point of degeneration. Judging from drug-induced myopathies, excessive lipid in the muscle fibre disappears as the muscle recovers.

Lipid storage to a greater degree than in the above conditions is prominent in carnitine deficiency and in a small minority of cases of carnitine palmityl acyl transferase deficiency.

Carnitine deficiency

Carnitine is a protein present in muscle and in other tissues; its function is to transport long chain fatty acids across the inner mitochondrial membrane. When it is deficient, lipids accumulate, mainly in type 1 fibres, in some cases forming abnormally large vacuoles.[68] This type of lipid

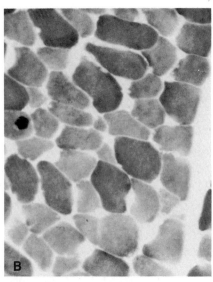

Fig. 23.30a, b McArdle's disease. (**a**) Absent phosphorylase reaction. (**b**) Control phosphorylase showing dark staining of type 2 fibres.
Frozen section × 180

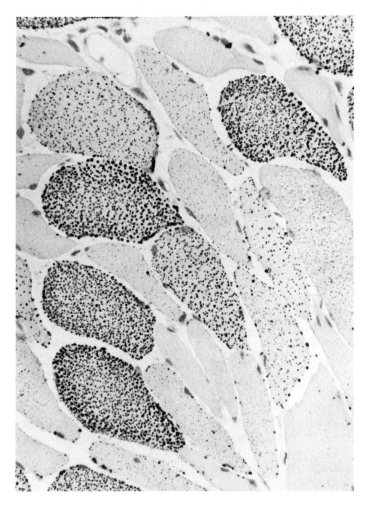

Fig. 23.31 Acute alcoholic myopathy. Type 1 fibres are loaded with triglyceride droplets. There is no sign of atrophy at this stage.
Frozen section, Scharlach R × 180

storage disease may be familial. About 50 cases have been reported. The clinical presentation is often like that in McArdle's syndrome (see p. 645), with exercise intolerance and muscle pain. Treatment by the administration of carnitine has a variable but often good effect. In the last five years there have been rapid advances in knowledge of the biochemistry of the carnitine deficiencies.[69] The lack of numerous enzymes and components of metabolic pathways has been discovered; the deficiencies of these substances interfere with carnitine production and cause secondary carnitine deficiency. Among the best known is acyl coenzyme A dehydrogenase.[70] There are some primary carnitine deficiencies in which the enzyme deficiency is unknown.

Carnitine palmityl acyl transferase deficiency[71]

This enzyme (CPAT) forms part of the chain responsible for the oxidation of long chain fatty acids and is found on both outer and inner aspects of the inner mitochondrial membrane. The disorder may be sporadic or inherited as an autosomal recessive trait. As in carnitine deficiency, the clinical presentation may suggest the diagnosis but the muscle on biopsy may appear entirely normal, for lipid storage occurs but rarely. If there is a combination of pain on exertion and muscle weakness without cramps in the presence of normal histology, the diagnosis may be made on biochemical estimation of the enzyme levels.

MALIGNANT HYPERTHERMIA (MH)[31]

This is a rare and very unusual familial disorder of skeletal muscle, which is asymptomatic until challenged by anaesthesia. The usual triggers are volatile anaesthetics, especially halothane, accompanied by a relaxant, usually suxamethonium. The effect of this form of general anaesthesia is to cause muscle overactivity in the form of continuous rigidity and a rapid rise in core temperature, even up to 46°C. This does not necessarily occur during the first or even second operation on a susceptible patient. If not detected at its very beginning malignant hyperthermia may

be impossible to reverse, and the patient will die. More anaesthetists are now employing core temperature monitoring as a routine and insist on having dantrolene available in the theatre. This is a hydantoin derivative shown first to be of value in porcine MH and now used successfully in the human disorder.

At first, the general view was that MH as a disorder of muscle should have a morphological basis. Open muscle biopsies were made on siblings and parents of victims and an in-vitro test performed measuring contractility of muscle strips exposed in Krebs solution to triggering agents. Reliable means of detecting susceptibility to MH were devised, and investigation showed the results to be compatible with a dominant pattern of inheritance. However, the histology of muscle obtained at the same time was normal in 75% of susceptible patients. Abnormalities were found in the remainder, and characteristically consisted of internal nuclei and 'moth-eaten' and core fibres. The biochemical nature of the disease is unknown. Histology of the muscle biopsy is unhelpful in the diagnosis of MH susceptibility but has revealed some important associations between MH and other inherited muscle disorders. So far most of these have only occurred once or twice, as in the case of Duchenne dystrophy and limb girdle dystrophy, and may be coincidental. In the case of central core disease, however, 8 out of 9 afflicted patients have proved to be MH-susceptible on testing. Families with central core disease should be offered the in-vitro test, if possible, or at least warned to inform their anaesthetist of the association between the disease and MH (see p. 638).

MITOCHONDRIAL MYOPATHIES

These were first described in 1966[72] as another form of non-progressive or slowly progressive congenital myopathy. Two types were recognised originally, both characterised by structural defects of the mitochondria. The mitochondria were either enlarged and deformed, containing crystalline inclusions or forming concentric membranous profiles (Fig. 23.32a), or they were of normal or near normal structure but increased in

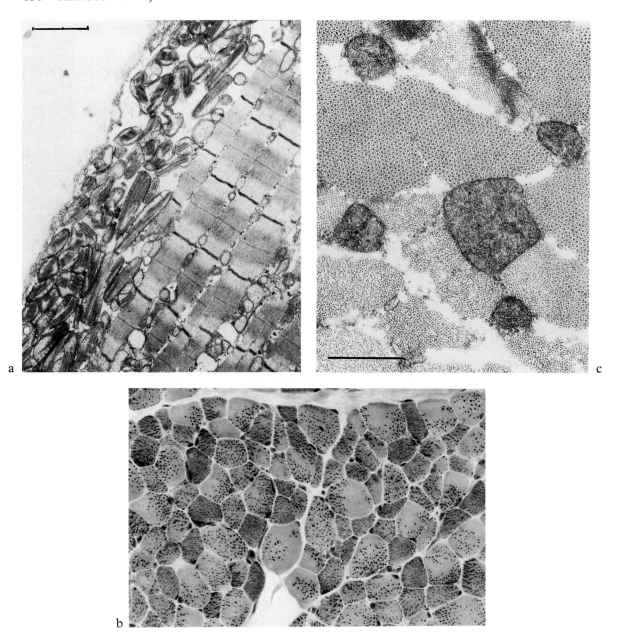

Fig. 23.32a–e Mitochondrial myopathies. (**a**) Ultrastructure of a ragged-red fibre showing abnormal mitochondria with crystalline arrays in a sarcolemmal crescent. (**b**) Pleioconial mitochondria distributed in type 1 and, to a lesser extent, in type 2 fibres. (**c**) The pleioconial mitochondria are of normal structure even when enlarged. (**d**) Ragged-red fibre in longitudinal section. Post-mortem specimen of muscle, received fixed in formalin, thoroughly washed then cut in a cryostat and stained by the modified Gomori method.[43a] (**e**) Two fibres show intense staining and peripheral deposition of mitochondria. These are ragged-red fibres, as seen in the succinate dehydrogenase reaction.
(**a**) Electron micrograph, bar = 2 μm; (**b**) Frozen section, modified Gomori[43a] × 270; (**c**) Electron micrograph, bar = 1 μm; (**d**) Frozen section, modified Gomori × 160; (**e**) succinate dehydrogenase reaction × 580

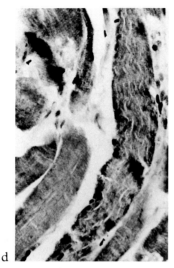

d

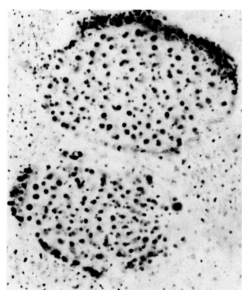

e

realisation that the abnormalities of mitochondrial structure are not primary but are secondary to any one of a large number of possible biochemical deficiencies in the mitochondrion. A full description of the clinical and biochemical aspects of these disorders is beyond the scope of this chapter, but good accounts of both are readily available.[74,75]

Among biochemical factors that continue to be discovered are defects of mitochondrial transport of, for example, fatty acids (see p. 647), various defects of substrate utilisation and defects in the respiratory chain. Although a morphological diagnosis of mitochondrial myopathy can be made, the precise enzyme defect is only identifiable by biochemical techniques.

Mitochondrial myopathy

The mitochondrial abnormalities in this large group of disorders seem to be confined to skeletal muscle in most cases; occasionally cardiac muscle is affected also. The age of onset of symptoms is not constant and may be in infancy, childhood or adult life. There may be exercise intolerance and possibly a myocardial defect. Muscle biopsy rarely reveals megaconial or pleioconial mitochondria (see above). Much more often 'ragged-red' fibres are found:[76] these are best seen in frozen sections stained by the modified Gomori method.[43a] Scattered fibres, perhaps two or three to a medium-power field, stand out because of a broad peripheral red-stained band, which may be continuous, or discontinuously crescentic and irregular (Fig. 23.32d and e). The myofibrils appear to be compressed from without and present an irregular boundary, giving rise to the description of the fibres as ragged-red. With the appropriate stains, mitochondria can be identified in the peripheral deposits and throughout the fibre where they are often accompanied by lipid droplets. Electron microscopy nearly always depicts abnormalities of mitochondrial structure. The presence of 'ragged-red' fibres is characteristic of many mitochondrial myopathies but small numbers of these fibres and of abnormal mitochondria occur in a variety of other disorders, which should not be mistaken for mitochondrial myopathy.

number. The first were named megaconial and the latter pleioconial (Fig. 23.32b and c). At about the same time a mitochondrial myopathy was reported (Luft's disease) in which a newly discovered abnormality of function excited much interest. Measurement of mitochondrial respiration demonstrated gross overactivity resulting in a high metabolic rate in a patient who was euthyroid.[73] Only one other similarly affected patient has been reported since then. Many other mitochondrial myopathies have now been described following the

Mitochondrial encephalomyopathies

Typically, in this group of diseases, a child develops mild muscle weakness and on muscle biopsy a mitochondrial myopathy is diagnosed. Later a slowly progressive disorder of cerebral function develops with apathy and intense depression followed by focal neurological signs and fits. At necropsy the findings are varied: usually a rare encephalopathy such as Canavan's disease, Alpers' cerebral poliodystrophy, Leigh's disease (subacute necrotising encephalomyelopathy) or Zellweger's disease is found (see p. 353).

Abnormal mitochondria, and various metabolic defects,[77] are seen in the brain in these encephalopathies. The best known is pyruvate decarboxylase deficiency in Leigh's disease. In the cases of a brother and sister, aged 9 and 14 years respectively, comparable numbers of 'ragged-red' fibres were found on muscle biopsy, with abnormal mitochondria but no other myopathic features. The boy developed dementia and fits over a long period and died undiagnosed. His sister was mentally normal at the last examination. Such cases are rare but suggest that if obscure encephalopathies are encountered a muscle biopsy may help at least to categorise them.

Progressive external ophthalmoplegia

Progressive external ophthalmoplegia has been known for many years and was the subject of controversy concerning its neurogenic or myopathic nature. In 1951 Kiloh and Nevin[25] showed in a detailed study that the condition was a myopathy and that after ptosis and ophthalmoplegia had been established the myopathy could spread to the shoulders and upper limbs. In 1958 Kearns and Sayre introduced the concept of multi-system disease by reporting ophthalmoplegia associated with retinitis pigmentosa and complete heart block. The definitive paper bringing this syndrome within the scope of the mitochondrial disorders was that by Olson and his colleagues,[76] who introduced the term 'oculocraniosomatic' and demonstrated that limb muscles in progressive external ophthalmoplegia could contain 'ragged-red' fibres.[76,78]

Clinically, progressive external ophthalmoplegia may begin at any age, but the time of onset may be impossible to determine. The progress of the disorder is so insidious that it may not be noticed by either the patient or the family for years. Many cases are familial but there is no constant pattern of inheritance. Many patients refuse biopsy as they have little disability, but may submit when they wish to know the possible genetic consequences. A biopsy of the deltoid seems to be the most suitable for demonstration of the 'ragged-red' fibres.

Biochemical studies of this group of diseases have so far been perplexing. Different defects have been found in clinically identical patients, and some patients with 'ragged-red' fibres have failed to show any enzyme deficiency. The present position seems to be that there are at least two forms of progressive external ophthalmoplegia, namely oculopharyngeal dystrophy and the oculocraniosomatic syndrome, neither of which can be diagnosed until the disorder has progressed beyond the orbit or a limb muscle biopsy shows either rimmed vacuoles (see p. 603) or 'ragged-red' fibres. It is suspected that there is a third familial group in which the deltoid remains normal, and the ophthalmoplegia remains static throughout life, never spreading to other muscles. If genetic advice is to be useful in these purely ocular myopathies, further histological, histochemical and biochemical studies are required.

PERIODIC PARALYSIS

In this disorder, patients suffer from periods of muscle weakness which spontaneously resolve. There are two main types; both are often familial and both are associated with changes in the level of serum potassium.

Hypokalaemic periodic paralysis

This is the more frequent of the two types and the sporadic form is sometimes found in association with thyrotoxicosis. Twice as many males are affected as females, and inheritance is autosomal dominant. Typically, the patient awakens in the early morning unable to move all four limbs; on examination the paralysis appears to be greater in the proximal muscles. The eyes, voice and swallowing are not affected. Serum potassium is low during the attack, falling to 3 mmol/l but it rapidly returns to normal levels (3·8–5 mmol/l) as the paralysis disappears. It is suspected that normal levels of potassium can be reached while weakness is still evident, which would account for the false description of a normokalaemic type. Attacks may last anything from a few hours to three days, but the number of attacks in a lifetime is highly variable. None may occur for several years, but if they are at all frequent fibre necrosis is

induced, weakness becomes permanent and a histological picture develops resembling an indolent dystrophy complicated by large vacuoles (Fig. 23.33a).

Hyperkalaemic periodic paralysis

Also an autosomal dominant disorder, the attacks in this condition are generally milder than in hypokalaemic periodic paralysis. Typically, they are induced by exercise followed by a short period of rest; there may be pain and tingling as well as weakness, usually confined to the legs. The attacks

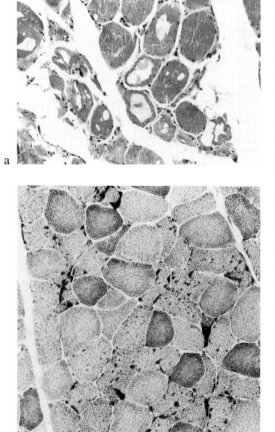

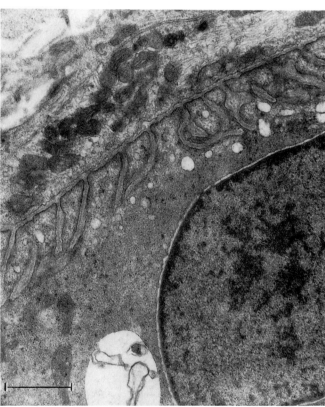

Fig. 23.33a–c (a) Periodic paralysis, late stage. The patient was the father of a young man who had recently developed periodic paralysis. The father's paralysis had become permanent many years previously. The muscle shows gross vacuolar myopathy with fibrosis, fibre size variation and an increase in adipose tissue. (b) A woman of 34 years with hyperkalaemic periodic paralysis. By light microscopy the muscle appeared normal, but on electron microscopy dilated sacs and vesicles are seen near an end-plate and there is a small vacuole near the nucleus (bottom). (c) Thyrotoxic periodic paralysis showing darkly stained tubular aggregates in many type 2 fibres.
(a) Paraffin section, haematoxylin-eosin × 230; (b) Electron micrograph × 9600; (c) Frozen section, NADH-TR × 190

are brief and last for no more than two or three hours, but they are more frequent than in the hypokalaemic variety.

Histology. The essential features are similar in both conditions.[79] Between attacks, in the early stages at least, the muscle is normal. If the effect of the rise or fall of the potassium level on muscle is to be seen, it is advisable to make the biopsy while the serum level is abnormal, although the pathological changes may persist for some time after a serious attack. The presence of vacuoles is characteristic; they are large in hypokalaemic and smaller in hyperkalaemic periodic paralysis. The origin of the vacuoles is suggested by the rare presence of fibres showing dilatation of the sarcoplasmic reticulum (Fig. 23.33b). An occasional finding is the development of tubular aggregates which may be quite abundant in type 2 fibres (Fig. 23.33c). If the motor innervation is stained, enlarged endplates may be seen which persist between attacks. In the later stages of the disease variation in fibre size and internal nuclei may develop. The persistence of a permanent vacuolar myopathy has also been described.

Paramyotonia congenita (of Eulenburg[32])

This rare disorder is considered by some to be a form of periodic paralysis. Myotonia and attacks of weakness are precipitated by cold; some of the patients show features of hyperkalaemic periodic paralysis.

Other causes of periodic paralysis

Periodic paralysis may be induced by a wide range of therapeutic drugs. It may also result from loss of potassium via the gut: a well-known cause of this is the benign villous adenoma of the rectum.

ENDOCRINE MYOPATHIES

The current literature on the endocrine myopathies emphasises two characteristics of these conditions: these are the mildness of the myopathic changes in endocrine diseases generally, when compared with the relative severity of the clinical weakness, and the rapidity of reversal of the symptoms when treatment is started. This must mean that the prime effect of the endocrine deficiency or overactivity is on muscle metabolism and that the effect on structure is secondary and likely to develop late.

Thyroid disease

In *thyrotoxicosis* most patients show excessive weakness but no significant histological changes in the muscles. Reflexes remain brisk. The ophthalmoplegia that may occur in *Graves' disease* is due to enlargement of the extraocular muscles by oedema; this is well demonstrated by orbital CT scans and confirmed histologically by the separation of muscle fibres by oedema fluid (Fig. 23.34b). Some lymphocytes and plasma cells accumulate in the fluid, suggesting a possible immune reaction.

Despite weakness, the early stages of *myxoedema* are not accompanied by myopathy. In severe myxoedema, glycogen is deposited in large subsarcolemmal crescents. In juvenile myxoedema of long duration, similar crescents are found but are composed of glycosaminoglycans (Fig. 23.34a). It is open to speculation whether such deposits are formed within pre-existing glycogen. In 1952 Asboe-Hansen[80] found crescents not only in cases of malignant exophthalmos and myxoedema but in 9 out of 10 patients with thyrotoxicosis. This experience has not been repeated.

In *Hoffmann's syndrome*[80a] (hypothyroid myopathy), which may develop in severe myxoedema, the muscles enlarge, feel firm and contract slowly. The relaxation phase of the deep tendon reflexes is prolonged. Histologically, muscle fibres are large, and may contain contracted myofibrils and large vacuoles (Fig. 23.34c and d).

Thyrotoxic periodic paralysis

This resembles familial hypokalaemic periodic

Fig. 23.34a–d (a) Juvenile myxoedema. The deposits in the muscle fibres are glycosaminoglycans. (b) Graves' disease. Extraocular muscles are separated, presumably by fluid. (c) Hoffmann's syndrome. Enlarged fibres have large oval vacuoles containing debris. (d) Hoffmann's syndrome. Cores contain contracted myofibrils (centre). Paraffin sections: (a, b) Haematoxylin-eosin (a) × 385, (b) × 70; (c, d) PTAH × 450

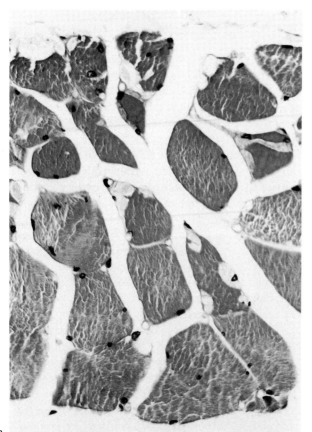

a

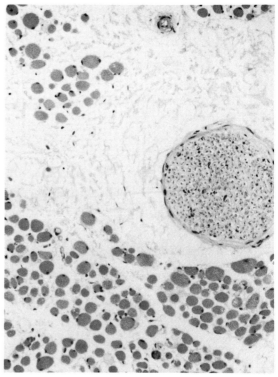

b

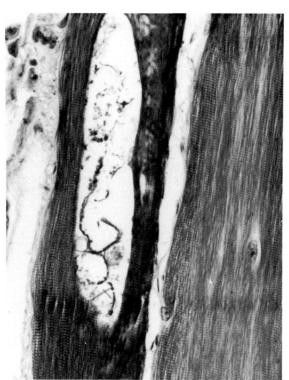

c

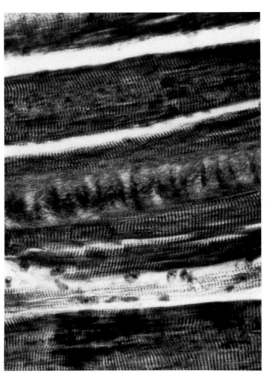

d

paralysis (see above) but with some differences. It is less severe, the vacuoles are less obvious and sometimes are seen only by electron microscopy, and it is usually sporadic. Tubular aggregates may be seen in type 2 fibres. This disorder is not a simple association of two diseases; with resolution of the thyrotoxicosis the attacks of periodic paralysis disappear.

Adrenal disease

In *Addison's disease* there is marked fatigability with rapid reversal on treatment. In the absence of treatment, cachectic atrophy of muscle develops and can be very severe. There is atrophy of all fibre types, but it is most severe in type 2B fibres. The findings in *Cushing's syndrome* are similar to those in, for example, chronic alcoholic myopathy and steroid myopathy (see p. 628): an increase in fibre lipid droplets predominates in one or other fibre type, followed by type 2B fibre atrophy.[81]

Pituitary disease

The findings in *Cushing's disease* due to pituitary adenoma are the same as those in the syndrome due to adrenal disease. In *acromegaly* enlargement of muscles is characteristic, especially of type 1 muscle fibres; internal nuclei may be present. There is no corresponding increase in muscle strength; in fact, the muscles are weaker. The increase in connective tissue in nerves or at common sites of neural compression in the forearm, at the carpal ligament or at the neck of the fibula, may complicate the effect on muscle by causing neurogenic atrophy.

HYPOVITAMINOSES

Vitamin deficiencies have little, if any, effect on muscle structure in man. Experimental vitamin E deficiency in animals produces a histological picture similar to that of muscular dystrophy.

Osteomalacia may be accompanied by a waddling gait and leg weakness that is thought to be a manifestation of osteomalacic myopathy.[82,83] Non-specific atrophy has been reported, and there may be minor changes in the innervation, with sprouting from and elongation of motor end-plates.

MYASTHENIC SYNDROMES

Myasthenia gravis

An early description of the syndrome of extra-ocular and bulbar muscle weakness and fatigability—'bulbar paralysis without anatomical basis'—epitomised the perplexity of physicians at being unable to pinpoint the site of the lesion in such an obviously organic disease, and this remained true even after it was shown to be due to a defect of neuromuscular transmission. At post mortem the thymus was sometimes hyperplastic or even neoplastic, but the muscles at post mortem and at biopsy were normal or contained a few 'lymphorrhages' (small collections of lympho-cytes). Anatomically, it was not until the motor innervation of muscle and especially the motor end-plates were examined systematically in myas-thenia gravis that specific abnormalities could be linked to the disorder.

The clinical features of myasthenia gravis are well known, with a relatively mild form confined to extraocular and bulbar muscles and a generalised form, both exhibiting fatigability. The generalised form may be so severe as to involve the muscles of respiration and require long-term assisted ventilation. Acquired, adult-onset myasthenia gravis can be divided into two main categories; patients with thymoma and those without.[3] The association of the disease with a number of auto-immune disorders led Simpson[84] in 1960 to suggest that myasthenia itself was an autoimmune disorder and could be due to the blocking of acetyl-choline receptors (AChR) at the end-plate by AChR antibodies. This was soon shown to be true in animal experiments, and led to the discovery of antibodies in myasthenic patients. Circulating IgG antibodies to nicotinic AchR are found in 90% of patients with generalised myasthenia gravis but in only 70% of those with longstanding myasthenia restricted to the eye muscles.[3] A variety of therapeutic procedures, including plasmapheresis, are directed towards lowering the antibody levels.[3]

In the late 1950s Coërs and Woolf published their results of in-vivo staining of the innervation in a large number of human muscle disorders,[84a] and described abnormally shaped end-plates in myasthenia gravis. They were simplified, often linear or bifid, sometimes elongated or accompanied by reactive subterminal and ultra-terminal sprouting (Fig. 23.35a). These findings are diagnostic, provided the muscle tissue proper is normal or near normal. The only conditions in which similarly deformed end-plates can occasionally be found are the peripheral neuropathies, but in these the muscle shows partial neurogenic atrophy.

More explicitly, abnormal morphology of the end-plate has been shown in studies in which structural changes were demonstrated at AChR sites.[85,86] These sites lie in the upper parts of the secondary synaptic folds and on the sarcolemmal summits between. When AChR sites are destroyed by antibody action, the folds disintegrate in an irregular way. They shorten, become distorted and disappear (Fig. 23.35b). The effect of this on the shape of the axonic expansions of the end-plate is best seen in light microscopical studies of the motor innervation.

The abnormal end-plates of myasthenia gravis are usually seen in the absence of histological changes in the muscle fibres. On rare occasions they are accompanied by myopathic or neuropathic reactions in the muscle tissue. The best

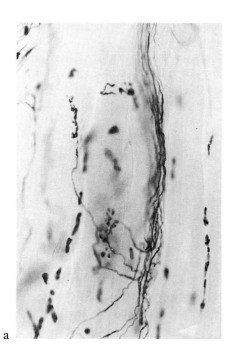

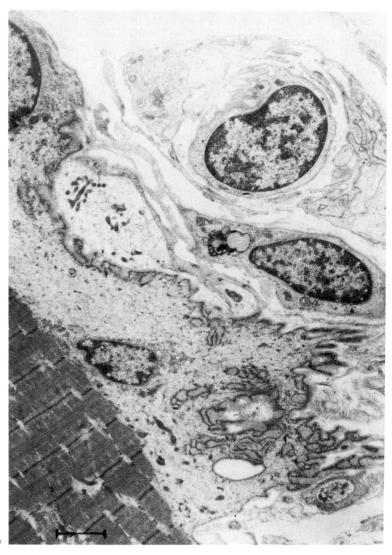

Fig. 23.35a, b (a) Myasthenia gravis. Motor end-plate showing linear elongation and small, deformed expansions.
(b) Myasthenia gravis. Woman, aged 25 years. After birth of her baby she developed weakness of her hand and arms, diplopia at times and ptosis. Deltoid muscle biopsy. The end-plate here shows shortening and distortion of secondary synaptic folds.
(a) Methylene blue × 255; (b) Electron micrograph, bar = 2 μm

known associated disorder is polymyositis, presumably an example of the association between two autoimmune disorders.

For a time, the necrosis, regeneration and inflammation of polymyositis were considered to be part of the spectrum of the histopathology of myasthenia gravis.

Less well known histopathological abnormalities in the muscles in myasthenia gravis are the neuropathic reactions (*neuropathic atrophy*). The simplest is a single fibre atrophy affecting type 1 or type 2 fibres, but not both; this occurs in small areas of muscle. It is likely to be the consequence of end-plate degeneration in the same motor unit which has passed beyond any possibility of regeneration. A more advanced stage of the same process affects small groups of muscle fibres, and finally large group atrophy develops. The unique character of these forms of denervation due to end-plate (more accurately sole-plate) degeneration is that the motor nerves and subterminal axons remain intact,[87] totally unlike the degenerative and regenerative neural reaction due to disease of the lower motor neuron (see p. 590). Affected patients often show permanent muscle wasting irrespective of whether their myasthenia is still active or has 'burnt out'. Such patients are rare in comparison with the number who never show wasting and who recover completely on treatment.

Muscle biopsy is less in demand at present in view of the advance in diagnosis provided by AChR antibody levels. But antibodies are absent in a small proportion of myasthenic patients, and clinical presentations may be atypical. If a biopsy is to be performed it should contain motor end-plates, either in intercostal muscle or deltoid, whether or not these muscles are clinically involved. Preferably, the techniques of staining of the innervation and of studying end-plate ultrastructure should be employed.

Other myasthenic syndromes

Neonatal myasthenia gravis is a distinct entity, due to placental transfer of anti-AChR antibodies.

A rare congenital or *familial myasthenia gravis* is quite different from the adult acquired generalised disease. There are no circulating AChR antibodies but it may be so severe that it causes sudden death in infancy. There are no definite morphological abnormalities at the end-plate, but there is some evidence of failure of resynthesis of acetylcholine.

Myasthenia due to penicillamine. If used in the long-term treatment of rheumatoid arthritis, penicillamine can produce a form of myasthenia in susceptible patients which is identical clinically to adult acquired myasthenia gravis. It improves on withdrawal of the drug. No end-plate abnormalities have been produced experimentally in rats by administration of the drug.

Myasthenic neuromyopathy has been reported recently as if it were a new syndrome. It appears to be similar to the rare neuropathic atrophy described above.

The Eaton–Lambert syndrome.[87a] This differs from myasthenia gravis in a number of ways. It is mainly a disorder of later life and it is commoner in men than in women. The limbs and the trunk muscles are affected; the extraocular and bulbar muscles are affected rarely. Weakness is present during rest but voluntary effort results in an increase in muscle strength followed, after a time, by diminution in strength. A carcinoma, often bronchial, is present in about two-thirds of the patients. AChR antibody levels are normal. The only important structural changes occur in some end-plates, which on carefully controlled measurement show an increase in the area provided by the secondary synaptic folds; both the depth and the number of the folds are increased. Physiologically, the syndrome is explained by the liberation of fewer quanta of acetylcholine by a single nerve stimulus, but the number of quanta released is increased by repetitive stimulation. The primary defect is thus on the axonic side of the end-plate, whereas the myasthenia gravis defect is post-junctional.

MYOADENYLATE DEAMINASE DEFICIENCY[88–90]

This is said to be the commonest enzyme deficiency in muscle and was first described in 1978. It occurs in 1·5% of muscle biopsies, irrespective of the histological diagnosis. 26 cases have been reported in patients who complained of undue fatigue on exertion once they had reached adulthood but who had otherwise normal muscles. Investigation for this deficiency may be advisable in all patients with muscle weakness and cramps. Some adults with the deficiency are totally asymptomatic. Many more investigations are required before its significance can be evaluated. A simple histochemical reaction is available as well as a biochemical assay.

TRAUMA

The mildest form of injury to muscle which concerns the pathologist is that which can be produced by the electromyographer's needle. Experiments have shown that within a few days muscle necrosis of limited extent and an inflammatory reaction can be produced by an electromyography needle, with or without haemorrhage. Such lesions make the diagnosis of muscle disease more difficult (see p. 606).

Compression and haemorrhage

A swelling within the muscle may develop after more severe trauma. A history of injury is usually obtained, but may be forgotten or may not be available in the case of an ill or demented patient. Compression of the calf in a patient deeply unconscious for many hours, for example, a drug addict, an attempted suicide or a chronic alcoholic, may lead to muscle pain of such duration that polymyositis may be suspected and a biopsy performed. Here the effects of direct compression on muscle are complicated by vascular insufficiency and may produce a histological picture resembling polymyositis (see p. 632), in which segmental necrosis of muscle fibres and cellular infiltration may still be active 12 months after the event. These lesions have occasionally been misdiagnosed, clinically and histologically, as sarcomatous.

Compressive blows to muscle do not always lead to haemorrhage, but when they do, a mobile lump may develop in which necrosis, regeneration and fibrosis co-exist. The amount of haemosiderin present varies and may be difficult to find.

Muscle hernia

Other common injuries to muscle are fascial tears, innocuous in themselves but likely to be followed by a herniation of muscle; this presents as a subcutaneous lump unattached to deep structures. The tears tend to occur where the fascia forms a firm wall, as in the anterior tibial compartment, and follows muscle swelling within a confined space. Muscular individuals are more prone to develop hernias. There is evidence that unaccustomed vigorous exercise alone may lead to swelling and pain in the anterior tibial compartment which must be relieved by decompression by means of a long incision in the fascia. This procedure is followed by the formation of a muscle hernia but one that is of controlled proportions. Traumatic herniae are larger and painful, especially when the muscle contracts, when the herniated tissue can be felt to harden. In the course of time muscle swelling disappears and the hernia can be reduced. Histological examination shows merely a sparse peripheral cellular exudate followed by scanty fibrosis.

Muscle rupture

The largest masses that occur in muscle as a result of trauma form when there has been a substantial tear in a muscle belly. It may occur at the lower or upper ends of the calf muscles when the strongly plantar flexed foot comes down so hard on the ground while running or jumping that the foot is suddenly and forcefully dorsiflexed. It may also happen in the biceps brachii when a similar force is exerted in a fight or in gymnastics. The muscle is paralysed for a long time while the separated portions of the muscle belly bunch up to form a round mass. There are many variations depending upon the extent of the tear. Many months are required to provide healing in the form of a fibrous union between the two parts of the muscle. Some masses may be surgically excised at this time. They show interdigitation of muscle fibres and scar tissue; there may be little remaining evidence of haemorrhage but numerous ring fibres form at the severed ends of the muscle fibres (Fig. 22.7, p. 596).

Bone fractures

Muscle damage frequently accompanies bone fractures and causes a pronounced rise in creatine kinase (CK) level. The degree of muscle damage, as in all forms of muscle injury, can be assessed by measuring the CK levels in the serum.

Traumatic and progressive myositis ossificans[91]

Although *traumatic myositis ossificans* is not a true inflammatory disorder, its name remains in the literature, presumably because of its resemblance to the multiple ossifying lesions of *progressive myositis ossificans* in which there may be congenital abnormalities of bone in addition to osteoid and bone formation in muscle, calcification and foci of myositis.[92] The lesions of traumatic myositis ossificans bear some resemblance to this but they are solitary. It appears that severe trauma of muscle, especially with haemorrhage, leads in some individuals to the development of a firm, painful fibroblastic mass within as little as 1–4 weeks. Calcification and ossification eventually

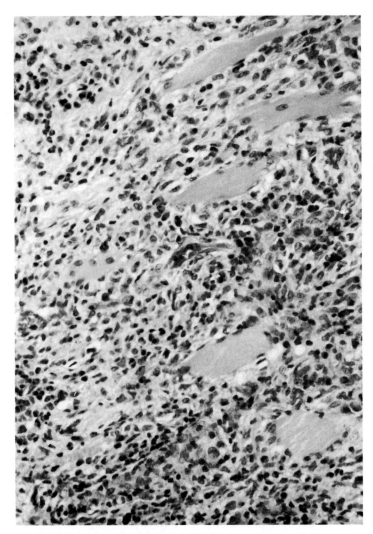

Fig. 23.36 Focal myositis. A few normal and regenerating muscle fibres survive within an intense inflammatory exudate composed of eosinophils, lymphocytes and histiocytes in a fibrous stroma.
Paraffin section, haematoxylin-eosin × 290

develop. The susceptibility of certain individuals to develop this consequence of trauma is not at present understood. The trauma initiating the disorder is either a single acute event or repeated minor injury such as occurs to produce the so-called 'rider's bone' in the origins of the adductor muscles of the thighs. The histopathology of myositis ossificans can bear a strong resemblance to osteogenic sarcoma of soft tissue.[93]

FOCAL INFLAMMATORY LESIONS

Fasciitis

Occasionally an area of skin over muscle becomes very tense and the tissue underneath feels firm; systemic sclerosis may be suspected, or an acute inflammatory myopathy. When a biopsy is performed the disease is seen to involve the fascia, which is greatly thickened from skin to muscle. Histologically, the fascial fibrous tissue is heavily infiltrated by large numbers of lymphocytes, plasma cells and often eosinophils. Eosinophils are also found in polymyositis, but in much smaller numbers. Muscle is said not to be involved by the inflammatory process, but occasionally the latter extends into the superficial muscle fasciculi and this may account to some degree for the muscle weakness. Clinically, joint contractures may follow the induration.

Focal myositis

Rarely, myositis may occur in a single focal area, perhaps 10 cm in diameter, made obvious by swelling and a variable degree of tenderness and pain. The case illustrated in Figure 23.36 involved the lower pectoral region. There were many eosinophils but no fungi or parasites were found.

FIBROMATOSES

This term is used here for proliferative fibroblastic lesions arising in the connective tissue of muscle. They are not true tumours as they are potentially self-limiting yet retain the tumour's ability to invade locally. Their pathogenesis remains unknown.

Proliferative myositis[94]

This condition, which is also known as *nodular fasciitis*, begins as a nodule that grows very rapidly, doubling in size within a matter of days to form a painless lump 2 or 3 cm in diameter, which is freely movable under the skin. Occurring most often in adults, in the shoulder region and trunk, it is very rare in children, if it occurs at all in that age group. The lesion is composed, surprisingly for a freely movable lump, of poorly defined, scar-like tissue within muscle. Histology shows thickening of the perimysium and epimysium, and to a lesser ex-

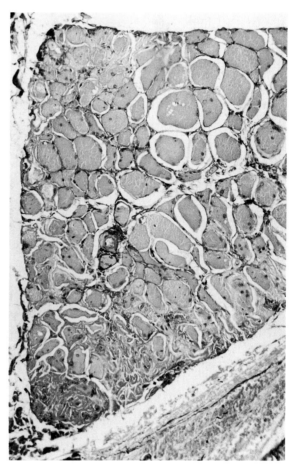

Fig. 23.37 Myosclerosis. Proliferation of endomysial fibrous tissue leads to constriction of individual muscle fibres, regenerative activity and enlargement of nuclei and segmentous vacuolation of other fibres. Formalin fixation has caused shrinkage artefact. Much of the fibrous tissue is recent, but older collagen stains darkly and can be seen occasionally replacing small groups of muscle fibres. Haematoxylin van Gieson × 180

tent of the endomysium, by a proliferation of fibrous tissue in which there are scattered large ovoid cells with prominent nuclei and nucleoli. These cells cannot be ascribed with certainty either to a muscle or a fibrous tissue origin. The effect of the fibrous proliferation is to separate muscle fibres rather than to cause necrosis and regeneration. Only a minority of cases show focal inflammatory cell infiltration: in most it is entirely absent. There is no reason as yet to regard the condition as basically inflammatory, despite the implication of the traditional name. For the present it is best grouped with the fibromatoses whose cause is still unknown.

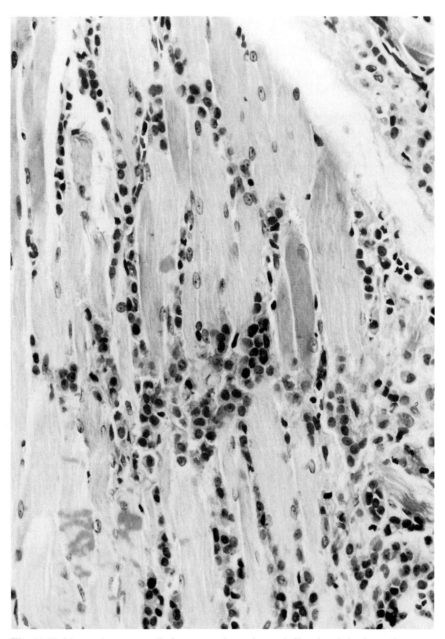

Fig. 23.38 Metastatic tumour cells from a gastric carcinoma infiltrating skeletal muscle. Paraffin section, haematoxylin-eosin × 230

Desmoid tumours

Desmoid means ligament-like, and the pearly white proliferating tissue is thought to originate in aponeuroses. The lesion consists of fibroblasts embedded in collagen. The cells invade and destroy muscle, remnants of which are scattered in the invading tissue. It is this property and the absence of a capsule that distinguishes the mass from a benign fibroma. Mitoses are not common yet growth to 15 cm or more in diameter is possible. Most desmoids originate in the anterior abdominal wall and over 80% occur in women, suggesting the possibility of an endocrine origin. Treatment is by wide excision.

Comparison with keloids has often been made, but the latter remain confined to the skin and subcutaneous tissue. The main differential diagnosis is from neurofibroma (see p. 469). Desmoids must also be distinguished from fibrosarcoma.

Myosclerosis

As the name myosclerosis indicates, a diffuse and dense proliferation of fibrous tissue involves the substance of the affected muscles. The suggestion has been made that it is a form of chronic polymyositis but the pattern of proliferation of the connective tissue suggests that it is primary and has a compressive effect on the included muscle fibres. The condition is much rarer than chronic polymyositis and inflammatory foci are virtually absent from the lesions. The presentation of the disorder may be slow and progressive, or it may be acute, as shown by the contrasting history of two patients. The first, a woman of middle age, had a 20-year history of a gradually developing and ascending hardness of one leg. Biopsy showed fibrous tissue without any characteristics of tumour growth and only a few intact muscle fibres. The second patient was a woman of similar age who complained of recent development of painful swelling of the tongue followed by pain in her forearms. Biopsy showed muscle fibres encircled by swollen endomysial tissue, and some broadening of the perimysium and epimysium (Fig. 23.37).

TUMOURS OF SKELETAL MUSCLE[95]

Haemangiomas, lipomas and angiolipomas are the most frequent benign tumours observed in skeletal muscle. Rhabdomyomas and rhabdomyosarcomas also occur. Granular cell 'myoblastomas' are not truly tumours of muscle but of peripheral nerve (see p. 498).

Involvement of muscle by metastatic carcinoma is uncommon. Mass lesions may form or there may be diffuse infiltration of the muscle by metastatic tumour cells (Fig. 23.38).

A detailed account of tumours of skeletal muscle is in the volume *Bone, Joints and Soft Tissues* of the third edition of *Systemic Pathology*.

REFERENCES

Clinical features

1. Dubowitz V. Muscle disorders in childhood. London: Saunders, 1978.
2. Walton JN. Brain's Diseases of the nervous system. 9th ed. Oxford: Oxford University Press, 1985.
3. Swash M, Schwartz M. Neuromuscular diseases. A practical approach to diagnosis and management 2nd ed. Berlin: Springer, 1988.

Neurogenic muscle disease

4. Kumagai T, Hashizuma Y. Brain Dev 1982; 4: 87.
5. Huang K, Luo Y. J Neurol Sci 1983; 61: 249.
6. Pearn J, Hudgson P. J Neurol Sci 1979; 43: 183.
7. Horton WA, Eldridge R, Brody JA. Neurology 1976; 5: 460.
8. Gajdusek DC, Salazar AM. Neurology 1982; 32: 107.
9. Campbell AMG, Williams ER, Pearce J. Neurology 1969; 19: 1101.

10. Bernat JL, Ochoa JL. J Neurol Neurosurg Psychiatry 1978; 41: 719.

Primary myopathies

11. Rowland LP. N Engl J Med 1988; 318: 1392.
11a. Hoffman EP, Fischbeck KH, Brown RH et al. N Engl J Med 1988; 318: 1368.
11b. Duchenne GB. Arch Gén Méd 1868; Sér 6, 11: 5, 179, 305, 421, 552.
12. Frankel KA, Rosser RJ. Hum Pathol 1976; 7: 375.
13. Mokri B, Engel AG. Neurology 1975; 25: 1111.
14. Kelfer HM, Singer WD, Reynolds RN. Paediatrics 1983; 71: 118.
15. Kloster R. Acta Neurol Scand 1983; 68: 344.
16. Fukuhara N, Suzuki M, Tsubaki T, Kushiro S, Takasawa N. Acta Neuropathol (Berl) 1985; 66: 283.
17. Sandbank U, Sroka H, Kuritzki A, Bornstein B. Isr J Med Sci 1973; 9: 603.

18. Walton JN, Gardner-Medwin D. In: Walton JN, ed. Disorders of voluntary muscle. Edinburgh: Churchill Livingstone, 1981: 500.
19. Bethlem J, van Wijngaarden GK, de Jong J. J Neurol Sci 1973; 18: 351.
20. Emery AEH, Dreifuss FE. J Neurol Neurosurg Psychiatry 1966; 29: 338.
21. Hopkins LC, Jackson JA, Elsas LJ. Ann Neurol 1981; 10: 230.
22. Sumner DW, Crawfurd M dA, Harriman DGF. Brain 1971; 94: 51.
23. Miller JE. Trans Am Acad Ophthalmol Otolaryngol 1971; 75: 1175.
24. Durston JHJ. Br J Ophthalmol 1974; 58: 193.
25. Kiloh LG, Nevin S. Brain 1951; 74: 115.
26. Beckett RS, Netsky MG. Arch Neurol Psychiatry 1953; 69: 64.
27. Little BW, Perl DP. J Neurol Sci 1982; 53: 145.
28. McMenamin JB, Becker LE, Murphy EG. J Pediatr 1982; 100: 692.
29. McMenamin JB, Becker LE, Murphy EG. J Pediatr 1982; 101: 580.
30. Swash M, Fox KP. J Neurol Neurosurg Psychiatry 1975; 38: 91.
31. Harriman DGF. Br J Anaesth 1988; 60: 309.
31a. Thomsen J. Arch Psychiatr Nervenkr 1876; 6: 702.
32. Eulenburg A. Neurol Zentralbl 1886; 5: 265.

Reactive myopathies

33. Mastaglia FL, Br J Hosp Med 1980; (July): 8.
34. Blain PG, Lane RJM. Hosp Update 1986; 12: 217.
35. Blain PG. Adverse Drug React Bull 1984; 104: 384.

Inflammatory myopathies due to known infective agents

36. Whitaker JN. Muscle Nerve 1982; 5: 573.
37. Behan WMH, Behan PO, Draper IT, Williams H. Acta Neuropathol (Berl) 1983; 61: 246.
38. Jolly SS, Pallis C. J Neurol Sci 1971; 12: 155.

Myopathies due to immunological or unknown cause

39. Mastaglia FL, Ojeda VJ. Ann Neurol 1985; 17: 317.
40. Hill DL, Barrows HS. Arch Neurol 1968; 19: 545.
41. Hewlett RH, Brownell B. J Neurol Neurosurg Psychiatry 1975; 38: 1090.
42. Coërs C, Carbone F. Acta Neurol Belg 1966; 66: 353.
43. Lane RJM, Fulthorpe JJ, Hudgson P. J Neurol Neurosurg Psychiatry 1985; 48: 270.
43a. Dubowitz V. Muscle biopsy: a practical approach. 2nd ed. London: Baillière Tindall, 1985.

Congenital myopathies

44. Banker BQ. In: Engel AG, Banker BQ, eds. Myology, basic and clinical. New York: McGraw-Hill, 1986: 2109.
45. Shy GM, Magee KR. Brain 1956; 78: 610.
46. Bethlem J, van Wijngaarden GK, Meijer AEFH, Fleury P. J Neurol Sci 1971; 14: 293.
47. Engel AG, Gomez MR, Groover RJ. Mayo Clin Proc 1971; 46: 666.
48. Currie S, Noronha M, Harriman DGF. In: Abstracts of the Third International Congress on Muscle Diseases. Amsterdam: Excerpta Medica, 1974: 12.
49. Shy GM, Engel WK, Somers JE, Wanko T. Brain 1963; 86: 793.
50. Harriman DGF. Adv Ophthalmol 1970; 23: 55.
51. Spiro AJ, Shy GM, Gonatas NK. Arch Neurol 1966; 14: 1.
52. Harriman DGF, Haleem MA. J Pathol 1972; 108: 237.
53. Brooke MH. In: Kakulas BA, ed. Clinical studies in myology, ICS 295. Amsterdam: Excerpta Medica, 1973: 147.
54. Sulaiman AR, Swick HM, Kinder DS. J Neurol Neurosurg Psychiatry 1983; 46: 175.
55. Brooke MH, Neville HE. Neurology 1972; 22: 829.
56. Huebner G, Pongratz D. Pathologe 1982; 3: 111.
57. Oh SJ, Meyers GJ, Wilson Jr ER, Alexander CB. Muscle Nerve 1983; 6: 278.
58. Morgan-Hughes JA, Mair WGP, Lascelles PT. Brain 1970; 93: 873.
59. Pierobon-Bormioli S, Armani M, Ringel SP et al. Muscle Nerve 1986; 8: 291.

Metabolic myopathies

60. McArdle B. Clin Sci 1951; 10: 13.
61. McAdams AJ, Hug G, Bove KE. Hum Pathol 1974; 5: 463.
62. Engel AG, Gomez MR, Seybold ME, Lambert EH. Neurology 1973; 23: 95.
63. Murase T, Ikeda H, Muro T, Nakao K, Sugita H. J Neurol Sci 1973; 20: 287.
64. Ferguson IT, Mahon M, Cumming WJK. J Neurol Sci 1983; 60: 337.
65. Brownell B, Hughes JT, Goldby FS, Woods HF. J Neurol Sci 1969; 9: 515.
66. Tarui S, Kono N, Kuwajima M, Ikura Y. Monogr Hum Genet 1978; 9: 42.
67. Jordans GHW. Acta Med Scand 1953; 145: 419.
68. Engel AG, Corrado A. Science 1973; 173: 899.
69. Engel AG. In: Engel AG, Banker BQ, eds. Myology. New York: McGraw-Hill, 1986: 1663.
70. Rebouche CJ, Engel AG. Mayo Clin Proc 1983; 58: 533.
71. Argov Z, Di Mauro S. Isr J Med Sci 1983; 19: 552.

Mitochondrial myopathies

72. Shy GM, Gonatas NK, Perez M. Brain 1966; 89: 133.
73. Luft R, Ikkos D. Palamieri G, Ernstek L, Afzelius B. J Clin Invest 1962; 41: 1776.
74. Morgan-Hughes JA. In: Mastaglia FL, Walton JN, eds. Skeletal muscle pathology. Edinburgh: Churchill Livingstone, 1982: 309.
75. Petty RKH, Harding AE, Morgan-Hughes JA. Brain 1986; 109: 915.
76. Olson W, Engel WK, Walsh GO, Einaugler R. Arch Neurol 1972; 26: 193.
77. Shapira Y, Harel S, Russell A. Isr J Med Sci 1977; 13: 161.
78. Karpati G, Carpenter S, Larbrisseau A, Lafontaine R. J Neurol Sci 1973; 19: 133.

Periodic paralysis

79. Faugere MC, Pellisier JF, Toga M. Acta Neuropathol (Berl) 1981; suppl vii: 301.

Endocrine myopathies

80. Asboe-Hansen G, Inersen K, Wichmann R. Acta Endocrinol (Copenh) 1952; 11: 376.
80a. Hoffman J. Dtsch Z Nervenheilkd 1897; 9: 278.
81. Harriman DGF, Reed R. J Pathol 1972; 106: 1.

Hypovitaminoses

82. Smith R, Stern G. Brain 1967; 90: 593.
83. Serratrice G, Pelissier JF, Cros D. Rev Rhum Mal Ostéoartic 1978; 45: 621.

Myasthenic syndromes

84. Simpson JA. Scott Med J 1960; 5: 419.
84a. Coërs C, Woolf AL. The innervation of muscle. Oxford: Blackwell, 1959.
85. Engel AG, Tsujihata M, Lindstrom JM, Lennon VA. Ann NY Acad Sci 1976; 274: 60.
86. Engel AG. Ann Neurol 1984; 6: 519.
87. Brownell B, Oppenheimer DR, Spalding JMK. J Neurol Neurosurg Psychiatry 1972; 35: 311.
87a. Lambert EH, Eaton LM, Rooke ED. Am J Physiol 1956; 187: 612.

Myoadenylate deaminase deficiency

88. Fishbein WN, Armbrustmacher VN, Griffin JL. Science 1978; 299: 545.
89. Goebel HH, Bardosi A, Conrad B, Kuhlendahl HD, Di Mauro S, Rumpf KW. Klin Wochenschr 1986; 64: 342.
90. Fishbein WN, Griffin JL, Armbrustmacher VW. Arch Pathol Lab Med 1980; 104: 462.

Trauma

91. Deluca SA. Am Fam Physician 1985; 32: 127.
92. Smith R, Russell RGG, Woods CG. J Bone Joint Surg [Br] 1976; 58B: 48.
93. Lagier R, Cox JN. Hum Pathol 1975; 6: 653.

Fibromatoses

94. Ushigome S, Takakuwa T, Takagi M, Koizumi H, Morikubo M. Acta Path Jpn 1986; 36: 963.

Tumours

95. Enzinger FM, Weiss SW. Soft tissue tumors. St. Louis, CV Mosby. 1983.

PART 4

Eyes

J. Harry

The eye and associated structures

INTRODUCTION

A knowledge of the embryology, anatomy, histology and physiology of the eye, together with an understanding of some of the problems of clinical ophthalmology, is of great value in appreciating the pathology to be considered in this section. This knowledge is readily accessible in standard textbooks.[1-9] It must be realised, however, that the basic principles of disease apply in ocular tissues as elsewhere, and processes such as inflammation, repair and neoplasia are essentially little different in the eye as compared to other organs in the body. Moreover, many systemic diseases affect the eye[10-11] and some may present with ocular manifestations. This chapter should not be regarded as a comprehensive account of ocular pathology; those with a particular interest are referred to specialist works.[12-18] The main part of the chapter is preceded by a short account of functional anatomy, and a description of the techniques used in the gross examination and processing of excised ocular tissue and enucleated globes. A number of artefacts, which can result in pitfalls and misdiagnosis, are also described.

The chapter concludes with a short *glossary of terms*, some of which are either not mentioned or not defined in the text, yet are used by clinicians and pathologists in the context of ocular disease.

FUNCTIONAL ANATOMY AND METHODOLOGY

FUNCTIONAL ANATOMY

The eye is contained within the fibrofatty tissue of the orbit and moves by means of the extraocular muscles, of which there are six, four recti and two

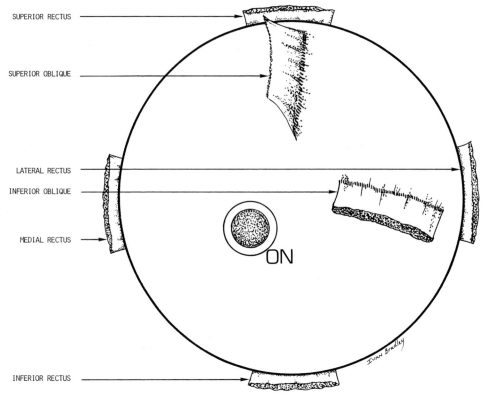

SUPERIOR RECTUS

SUPERIOR OBLIQUE

LATERAL RECTUS
INFERIOR OBLIQUE

MEDIAL RECTUS

ON

INFERIOR RECTUS

Fig. 24.1 Diagram of the extraocular muscles of the right eye as seen from the posterior aspect of the globe. ON: optic nerve.

oblique (Fig. 24.1). From the pathologist's viewpoint, the oblique muscles, superior and inferior, have great practical importance, for their recognition in an enucleated specimen is paramount in confirming the side of the body from which the eye has been removed. The superior oblique has a thin, tendinous insertion and lies transversely across the top of the globe; its cut end is directed towards the medial side. The inferior oblique has a thick, fleshy insertion situated behind the equator and towards the posterior pole.

The transparent media of the eye, namely, the aqueous, the lens, and the vitreous, are contained within three main layers or coats (Fig. 24.2). The outermost is the collagenous corneoscleral envelope comprising the transparent cornea and the opaque, white sclera. The middle coat, the uvea, is vascular and nutritive. It consists of the iris and the ciliary body anteriorly, structures which also contain the involuntary musculature which determines the size of the pupil and,

through the zonular fibres (suspensory ligament), the curvature of the lens. The posterior part of the uvea is the choroid. The innermost layer of the eye is the retina, in which are incorporated the visual receptor cells; the macular region lies at the posterior pole and appears somewhat darker than the surrounding retina due to the underlying pigment epithelium being more heavily pigmented. Nerve fibres leave the eye posteriorly at the optic nerve head. The retina ends anteriorly in front of the equator at the ora serrata and, although not strictly an anatomical boundary, a plane approximately through the ora serrata divides the eye into the anterior and the posterior segments. Aqueous is secreted by the ciliary epithelium, circulates within the anterior ocular compartments (i.e. anterior and posterior chambers), and drains away at the filtration angle into the trabecular meshwork and canal of Schlemm (Fig. 24.3). The vitreous occupies the cavity in the posterior segment behind the lens.

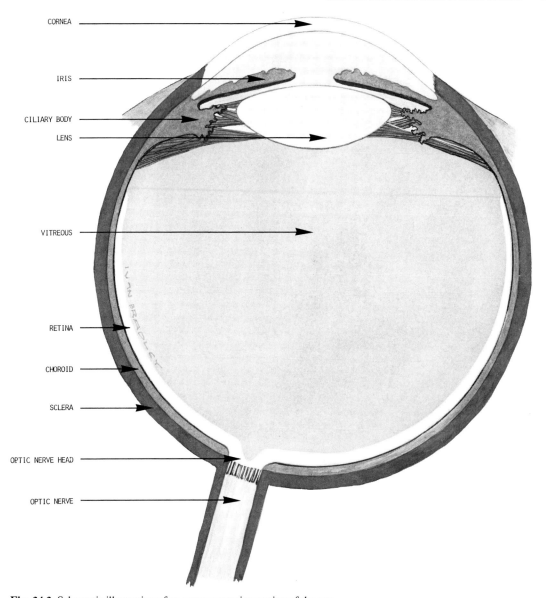

Fig. 24.2 Schematic illustration of an anteroposterior section of the eye.

METHODOLOGY[19]

Tissues and fluids[20-38]

Material removed from the lids, the conjunctiva and the orbit is fixed in formalin and processed in paraffin wax as is material from elsewhere in the body, but it is stressed that lid lesions must be sectioned at right angles to the lid margin whenever this landmark is identified. Trephined corneal discs and excised intraocular tissues, e.g. iridectomy, cyclectomy or trabeculectomy specimens, also are treated no differently from tissue elsewhere. Although justification for them is controversial, uveal and retinal biopsies, and intraocular and orbital fine needle aspirates can be fixed and processed in the usual way, but their interpretation may be difficult. Exenterated orbital contents containing an eye are examined and processed as described under globes (see below). Histological stains are used as with other tissues

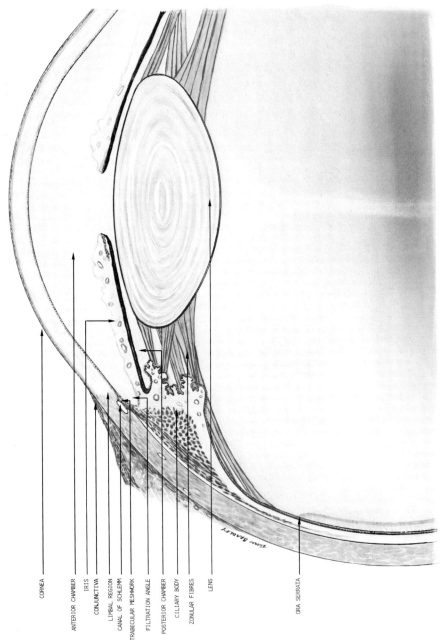

CORNEA

ANTERIOR CHAMBER

IRIS

CONJUNCTIVA

LIMBAL REGION

CANAL OF SCHLEMM

TRABECULAR MESHWORK

FILTRATION ANGLE

POSTERIOR CHAMBER

CILIARY BODY

ZONULAR FIBRES

LENS

ORA SERRATA

Fig. 24.3 Schematic illustration of an anteroposterior section through the anterior segment.

and immunohistochemistry can, on occasion, be extremely useful.[39] Frozen sections may be of value in assessing the surgically excised margins of a lid tumour[40] which has been previously diagnosed by histological study of paraffin embedded material. However, it is not advisable to use frozen sections for the primary diagnosis of ocular, lid, conjunctival and orbital lesions.[41] The microscopic examination of intraocular fluids may be of diagnostic value.[42,43] As a general rule, infected eviscerated specimens should be cultured prior to being fixed for histological study.

Globes (whole eyes)[44]

Fixation. A whole eye removed either at operation or at post-mortem examination is best fixed in neutral buffered formalin for a minimum period of 48 hours. Fixation should be carried out without delay in order to prevent autolysis, which first manifests itself in the retina; folding, detachment and deterioration of the visual receptor cells are the earliest signs of such retinal autolysis. Prior to fixation, the globe must not be opened or punctured. Fixative should never be injected into the vitreous, and at no time must the eye be frozen. After fixation, the eye is washed overnight in tap water; this not only largely removes the formalin, but lessens the risk of artefactual detachment of the retina. In order to restore the natural colour of the specimen prior to gross examination, the eye is then placed in 70% alcohol for at least two hours.

Gross examination. By locating the positions of insertion of both the superior and inferior oblique muscles, the specimen can be identified as either a right or left eye (see p. 670). The global and corneal diameters are measured and any variation from the normal (Table 24.1) recorded. By naked-eye examination or by the use of a dissecting microscope, the external appearances are observed, special note being taken of scars, staphyloma formation and tumours. The position of an intraocular tumour can usually be determined by palpation of the sclera and transillumination of the globe. If there is reason to suspect the presence of a radio-opaque intraocular foreign body the eye must be X-rayed. Using a

Table 24.1 Diameters of the globe and of the cornea in adults.

Globe diameters	
Antero-posterior	24 mm
Horizontal	23·5 mm
Vertical	23 mm
Corneal diameters	
Horizontal	12 mm
Vertical	11 mm

long razor blade (e.g. a Gillette Valet Triple Strip®), the globe is opened anteroposteriorly through the limbus, thus allowing the embedding medium to enter the anterior chamber. Normally, opening of the eye is performed in the horizontal plane unless there is a reason, such as the presence of either a wound or a tumour, why sectioning in another plane would prove advantageous. The portion removed is referred to as the calotte, from its resemblance to a priest's skullcap (Fig. 24.4); it will contain a piece of any such tumour as may be present and if necessary it may be processed rapidly so as to provide a histological diagnosis without delay. If a retinoblastoma is suspected, transverse sections of the surgical cut end of the optic nerve must be taken for histological study to see if there is evidence of tumour infiltration. The opened globe is thoroughly examined and any abnormalities noted (Fig. 24.5). Cataract formation, retinal detachment, tumours, haemorrhages and exudates can all be seen, and the optic nerve head is carefully studied, particular attention being paid as to whether or not it is pathologically cupped. A symmetrical calotte is subsequently removed from the opposite side and the embedded central portion of the globe then forms the main block.

Processing (Table 24.2). If electron microscopical study is required, a portion of tissue can be taken and post-fixed in glutaraldehyde before being transferred to osmium tetroxide. In preparing the specimen for light microscopy decalcification is carried out as necessary and dehydration is achieved by using a series of closely graded alcohols. Embedding may be in either wax or celloidin. The former necessitates the use of a higher temperature, and this can result in shattering of the lens and artefactual changes in the

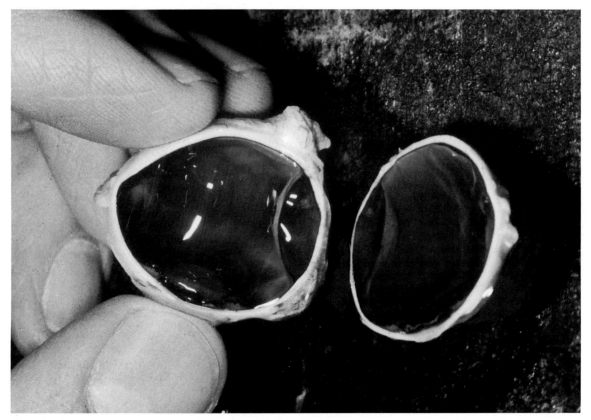

Fig. 24.4 A globe opened anteroposteriorly through the limbus, bisecting an intraocular tumour: a 'calotte' (right) is thus removed, and this can be processed rapidly.
× 2

retina. Celloidin-embedded material is less distorted, but the procedure is lengthy and time consuming; it is not suited to the processing of a tumour where thin sections are required, nor are immunohistochemical studies usually possible. The transparency of a celloidin block, however, allows for continual examination of the specimen at the time of sectioning, and this may be helpful either in the location of a wound or in the search for a small extraocular extension of tumour. Nevertheless, due to its disadvantages celloidin is now rarely used, and with present day laboratory technology, good quality, thin sections can be produced from wax-embedded material without too much difficulty. Staining is performed on eye sections in the same way as on other tissues. A special technique which is sometimes useful in the study of ocular conditions is the preparation of a retinal digest, wherein by digestion with pepsin and trypsin,[45] or trypsin alone, the retinal

vasculature can be left intact, stained, and examined in detail. Such lesions as areas of vaso-obliteration and capillary microaneurysm formation, which are not apparent in other preparations, can be clearly observed by this technique. The need for this type of investigation, however, is infrequent in routine diagnostic pathology.

Microscopy. It is essential that, whatever the nature of any pathological changes, a systematic study of the entire eye section be performed. The corneoscleral envelope, the uvea, the retina, the filtration angle, the lens, the ocular compartments and the optic nerve must all be examined in an orderly and careful manner.

ARTEFACTS

In the examination of any histological preparation of an eye it is important for the histo-

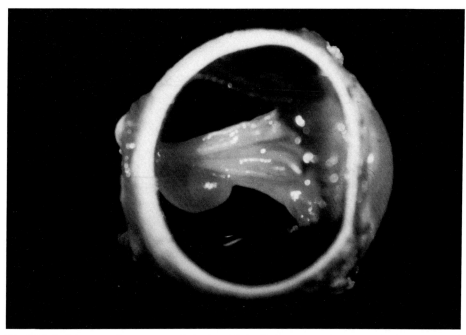

Fig. 24.5 A globe opened anteroposteriorly through the limbus to reveal total detachment of the retina (centre) in which there is cyst formation (the result of degenerative changes). ×3

pathologist to appreciate what is, and what is not, significant.

Artefactual separation or absence of the corneal epithelium is frequently observed. It should be borne in mind that in true corneal ulceration, in addition to the inflammatory changes, there is a gradual shelving from the intact epithelium to the ulcerated area, whereas in an artefact the edge of the remaining epithelium is seen as a sharply demarcated step. Clefts between the corneal lamellae, in the absence of any deposit or extra-cellular fluid, are usually meaningless. Pigment on the anterior capsule of the lens is artefactual unless accompanied by other evidence of iridolenticular adhesion. Large clefts and splits in the lens are usually the result of processing; true cataractous changes take the form of definite vacuoles and globules, or fibrosis and/or calcification.

The neurosensory retina is firmly attached to the pigment epithelium only at the optic nerve head and at the ora serrata. "When is a 'detachment' of the retina an artefact?" is a question that is often posed. If the separation is by either a neoplastic or an exudative process, then the 'detachment' is a true one, but if no such pathology is seen, 'detachment' probably occurred after removal of the globe (Fig. 24.6); in artefactual detachment, very fine granules of pigment from the pigment epithelium are often present on the outer limbs of the visual receptor cells. If the optic nerve has been

Table 24.2 A processing schedule: the globes are processed individually in 4 oz (112 ml) glass jars and the schedule is designed to operate within an 8-hour working day.

Medium	Time
70% Alcohol	4 hours
64 OP Spirit	4 hours
64 OP Spirit	Overnight
74 OP Spirit	1 hour
74 OP Spirit	3 hours
74 OP Spirit	4 hours
74 OP Spirit	Overnight
Chloroform	1 hour
Chloroform	3 hours
Chloroform	4 hours
Chloroform	Overnight
Wax★	1 hour
Wax★	3 hours
Wax★	4 hours
Wax★	Overnight

★ Gurr's pastillated paraffin wax—congealing point 56°C (manufactured by BDH Ltd, Broom Rd, Poole, Dorset, UK).

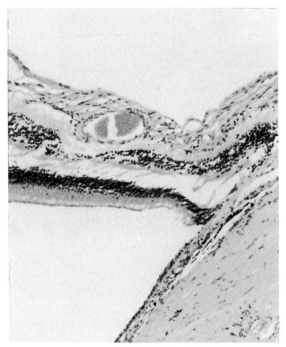

Fig. 24.6 Artefactual detachment of the retina: the neurosensory retina (top) is separated from the pigment epithelium, there is an empty space between the two layers, and pigment is present on the outer limbs of the visual receptor cells.
Haematoxylin-eosin × 110

crushed during enucleation, myelin extrusion is not infrequently seen at the optic nerve head within the eye, and may extend peripherally beneath the retina or even within retinal blood vessels. Microcystic appearances, particularly involving the outer layers of the retina over a wide area, especially posteriorly, are often the sequel to processing in wax.

MINOR OCCASIONAL ALTERATIONS

Following intraocular haemorrhage, blood degradation products are absorbed into the walls of the retinal capillaries, and when stained with haematoxylin and eosin such vessels can easily be misinterpreted as fungal elements.

Calcium oxalate crystals may be deposited within the eye in disorders of oxalate metabolism. They may also be seen in association with degenerative changes, being sometimes present in the lens in advanced cataract, and also in the retina and subretinal fluid in cases of longstanding retinal detachment; in these circumstances they are not considered to have any special significance.

INFLAMMATION

GENERAL CONSIDERATIONS

Ocular inflammatory disease is either infective,[46-59] if produced by bacteria, fungi, viruses, chlamydiae, protozoa and helminths, or immunological,[60-67] when it may involve the eye alone or be part of a systemic immune disorder. This general introduction to these conditions will be followed by more detailed consideration of selected inflammatory diseases.

Bacterial infections. The healthy conjunctival sac may harbour bacteria. Some of these are *saprophytic (e.g. Corynebacterium xerosis)*, but others are potentially *pathogenic (e.g.* staphylococci*)*. The blinking action of the lids, the protection afforded by the lashes, the constant flow of tears which contain immunoglobulins, lysozyme and other antibacterial agents, and also the presence of normal ocular flora, are factors which help to keep the eye free from infection. The mucosal surface of the conjunctiva and cornea, however, may be damaged by minor trauma or by dust and other foreign bodies, and micro-organisms can then gain access to the tissues. Failure of the eyelids to close properly results in *exposure keratitis*, while *neurotrophic keratitis* follows loss of corneal sensation. Any circumstances in which the defence mechanisms are suppressed, and this includes the *acquired immune deficiency syndrome (AIDS)*,[68-75] result in an increased incidence of opportunistic infection.

The Gram-positive bacteria most commonly causing exogenous infection of the eye are *Staphylococcus aureus* and streptococci, including *Streptococcus pneumoniae*. Members of the genera *Haemophilus, Moraxella* and *Proteus, Escherichia coli, Klebsiella pneumoniae* and *Pseudomonas aeruginosa* are among the more important Gram-negative organisms found in ocular disease. In-

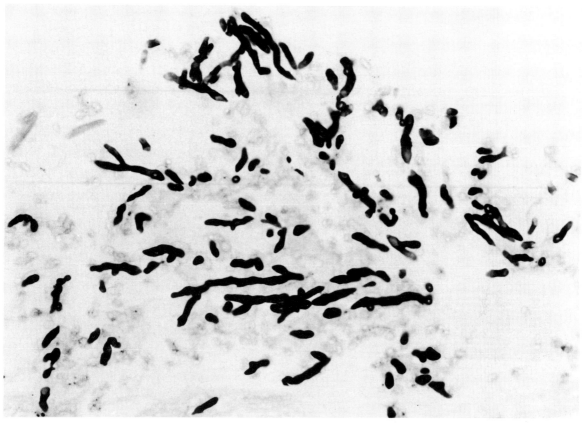

Fig. 24.7 Aspergillus fungal hyphae in a corneal ulcer.
Methenamine (hexamine) silver × 525

fection by *Pseudomonas aeruginosa* provokes a particularly virulent reaction. *Actinomyces israelii* is not uncommonly the cause of local infection in the lacrimal drainage system.

Fungal infections (see p. 682).   Many species of fungi can be isolated from the conjunctival sac of a normal healthy eye, more usually in adults. Foremost among the pathogens which may cause ocular infection are organisms that belong to the *Aspergillus* genus (Fig. 24.7). Ocular mycosis is less common than infection due to either bacteria or viruses, but with the widespread use of antibiotics, chemotherapy and immunosuppression, fungi have come to play an increasingly important rôle in ocular disease. Factors predisposing to localised fungal infection include injury by vegetable matter such as thorns, and the changes in the ocular defence mechanisms which occur in exposure keratitis and dry eye (xerophthalmia).

Viral infections (p. 681–682).   The majority of the viruses that affect the eye produce either follicular conjunctivitis or keratoconjunctivitis. Superimposed infection by bacteria or fungi not infrequently develops, and this complicates the picture. The viruses most commonly seen in ocular infection are members of the *Herpes* and *Adenovirus* groups. *Measles virus* produces keratoconjunctivitis in association with the systemic disease, while many viral infections, if acquired by a mother during pregnancy, may result in congenital abnormalities in the fetus, and the eyes are often affected.

Chlamydial infections (see p. 681). *Chlamydia trachomatis* (TRIC agent) is the most important chlamydial cause of ocular disease. It involves the conjunctiva and cornea primarily. As with virus diseases, secondary infection produced by bacteria and fungi not infrequently develops.

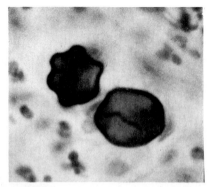

a

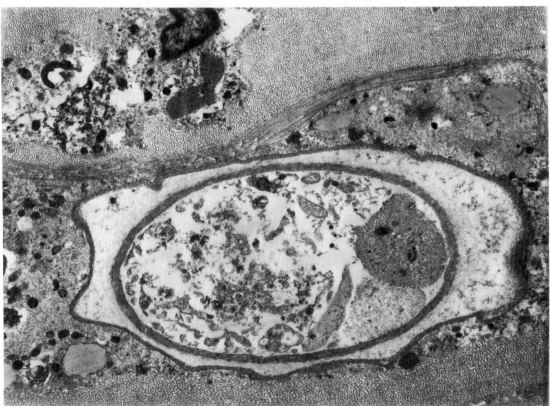

b

Fig. 24.8a, b Cysts of Acanthamoebae.
(**a**) Methenamine (hexamine) silver × 1150; (**b**) Electron micrograph × 10 000

Protozoal infections. *Leishmania* can affect the skin of the lids and also the conjunctiva. Keratitis due to *Acanthamoebae* (Fig. 24.8) has been described,[76] particularly as a complication of the use of contact lenses. In addition to the history of local injury there has usually been exposure to contamination with water from either a pond or a stream in which the free-living amoebae may be present. Corneal infiltration by the sporozoan parasite *Nosema* has been reported.[77] Another protozoon which produces disease of the eye is *Toxoplasma gondii* (see p. 682).

Metazoal infestation (p. 682–683). Among the helminths which affect the ocular structures are *Toxocara canis*, *Onchocerca volvulus* and *Loa loa*.

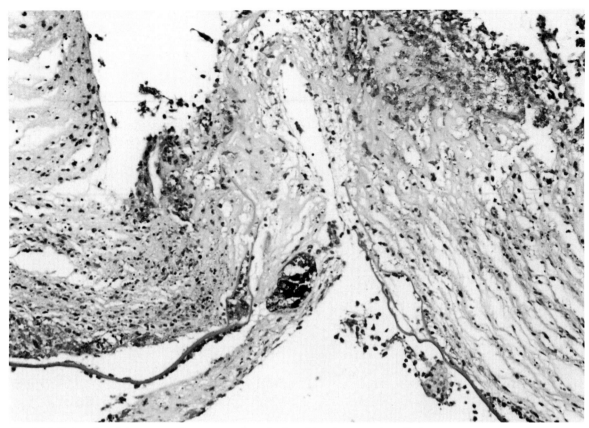

Fig. 24.9 Perforation of the cornea subsequent to ulcerative keratitis: a large number of inflammatory cells is seen and there is incarceration of uveal tissue (centre); disrupted Descemet's membrane is seen on the lower aspect of the cornea. PAS × 200

Hydatid disease is caused by *Echinococcus granulosus*, while other worms, e.g. *Schistosoma*, can produce conjunctival granulomas.

Endophthalmitis. Infection of the interior of the eye can be the result of metastatic spread from an infection elsewhere. However, perforation of the corneoscleral envelope following either corneal infection (Fig. 24.9), an injury or a surgical procedure, is the usual predisposing factor which leads to intraocular suppuration. Most often the infection is bacterial and less frequently fungal. Fungal endophthalmitis, usually due to *Candida albicans*, is seen most frequently in drug addicts.

Inflammation of the orbital tissues. A wide variety of organisms produce orbital cellulitis, which is often secondary to upper respiratory tract infection. The orbit may also be involved in systemic autoimmune diseases. On occasion no obvious cause can be found for orbital inflammation.

Sequelae of inflammation. The sequelae of inflammation, whatever the cause of the latter, vary with the severity of the condition and the site involved. Localised and mild inflammation, particularly of the lids and the conjunctiva, may result in no permanent damage. Severe inflammation, on the other hand, especially if it involves the cornea, the sclera, the uvea, the retina and the intraocular cavities, may cause gross visual disturbance and even blindness. As stated earlier, the principles underlying inflammatory diseases of the eye are essentially little different from those

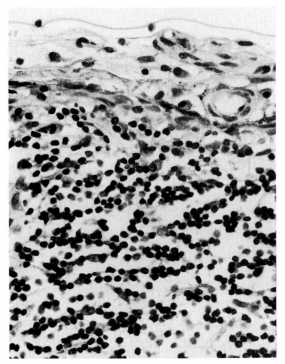

Fig. 24.10 Neovascular tissue on the anterior surface of the iris (rubeosis iridis), which is chronically inflamed. Haematoxylin-eosin × 400

seen elsewhere in the body. Cellular infiltration and exudation are followed by organisation with granulation tissue formation, and later by fibrosis and scarring. If both the palpebral and bulbar conjunctiva are involved to a degree sufficient to produce scarring, adhesions develop (*symblepharon*). Scarring of the cornea results in opacity (*leucoma*). If the inflammatory process has affected the interior of the eye, neovascular tissue may form (Fig. 24.10), and adhesions (*synechiae*) often develop between the iris and the cornea, and/or the lens. Fibrosis, gliosis and calcification can occur, and there is frequently osseous metaplasia with resultant *intraocular bone formation* within which marrow may develop, and on rare occasions there is haemopoiesis. Shrinkage of the globe ultimately follows so that the eye develops a thickened corneoscleral envelope, and the intraocular structures become totally disorganised and largely destroyed (*phthisis bulbi*, Fig. 24.11).

SPECIFIC OCULAR INFLAMMATORY CONDITIONS (INFECTIVE AND IMMUNOLOGICAL)

Granulomas

The commonest granuloma of the lid is *chalazion* (see p. 690), but there are many other causes of granulomatous inflammation, and general principles apply to all of them. Granulomas may occur in the lid and conjunctiva[78] in *sarcoidosis*, the commonest ocular manifestation of which, however, is uveitis; the histological appearances are those of sarcoid as seen elsewhere. There may be lacrimal gland[79] and orbital involvement,[80] and nearly always there is other evidence of the disease. *Tuberculosis* can also involve ocular and adnexal tissue. *Allergic granulomatous inflammation*,[81] characterised histologically by the Splendore–Hoeppli phenomenon, has been observed in the lids and conjunctiva, and in a number of instances fungi or parasites have been implicated as the causative agents. Localised conjunctival granulomas have also been reported in patients with inflammatory disease of the bowel,[82] notably *Crohn's disease*.[83]

Herpes simplex[84]

Herpes simplex virus infections involving the conjunctiva and cornea usually resolve completely, but recurrent attacks often follow. Infection produces intra-epithelial vesicles which break down to give punctate, striate, stellate, dendritic or amoeboid patterns of superficial ulceration. If the virus persists, it penetrates into the corneal stroma and the result is *disciform keratitis*.

Herpes zoster

Varicella–zoster infection, by involving the ophthalmic division of the trigeminal nerve, involves the eyelid, the conjunctiva and the cornea, and there is mucocutaneous ulceration and keratitis. Reactivation of virus, either spontaneous or subsequent to immunosuppression, results in recurrent inflammation.

Cytomegalovirus infection

If acquired during the first trimester of pregnancy,

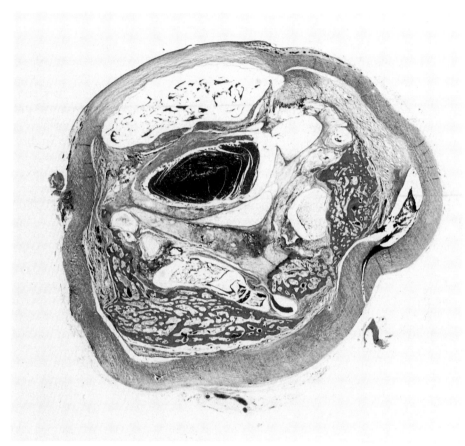

Fig. 24.11 Phthisis bulbi: the corneoscleral envelope is thickened, the intraocular structures are totally disorganised and there is well-developed bone formation (bottom—next to sclera). Cornea at top of field; the dark mass is the lens.
Haematoxylin-eosin ×4

cytomegalovirus causes multiple congenital abnormalities in the fetus; the fetus usually fails to survive. There is involvement particularly of the skeletal system, heart, kidneys, central nervous system and eyes; the eyes show microphthalmos and cataract. Infection also occurs in immuno-logically compromised patients, particularly those who have received renal transplants. Retinitis develops, and this is characterised by the presence of cytomegalic cells, containing a large, intra-nuclear, eosinophilic inclusion body with a surrounding clear halo (the owl's eye appearance) (see Fig. 12.21, p. 338).

Adenovirus infection

Infection of the cornea and conjunctiva may be caused by an adenovirus, usually of type 3, 4, 7, 8 or 10.

Rubella

Rubella (German measles) in a child rarely causes ocular problems, but infection during pregnancy, especially in the first trimester, can result in multiple abnormalities in the fetus. The eyes may be microphthalmic and exhibit iridocyclitis, cataract formation and a pigmentary retinopathy where the pigment epithelium shows alternating areas of hyper- and hypo-pigmentation.

Chlamydia trachomatis (TRIC agent) infection

Ophthalmia neonatorum, inclusion conjunctivitis,

punctate keratoconjunctivitis or trachoma may result from infection by *Chlamydia trachomatis* (TRIC agent: TR = *t*rachoma, IC = *i*nclusion *c*onjunctivitis—the organism causing trachoma is indistinguishable from that producing inclusion conjunctivitis). The most visually destructive of these conditions is trachoma. Follicular keratoconjunctivitis occurs and this is followed by fibrovascular pannus formation and subsequently by extensive and widespread scarring. Useful tests in diagnosing the disease are the demonstration of inclusion bodies in conjunctival scrapings, the isolation of the causative agent in cell cultures and the detection of chlamydial antibody in blood or tears. There is a common association between ocular TRIC infection and chlamydial cervicitis and urethritis.[85]

Ophthalmia neonatorum[86–88]

Ophthalmia neonatorum, by definition, is a purulent discharge from the eye occurring during the first three weeks of life. While gonococci, chlamydia, herpes simplex virus, *Candida albicans* and *Trichomonas vaginalis* have all been implicated, staphylococci and streptococci may equally be responsible for this condition, which can severely damage the cornea.

Histoplasmosis

In association with an initial pulmonary infection, *choroiditis* may develop in the mid-peripheral, macular and peripapillary zones. Healing occurs spontaneously, but for some reason, at present obscure, years later in the macular region, neovascularisation may develop beneath the retinal pigment epithelium and this, together with subsequent haemorrhage, can produce a disciform type of lesion. Histoplasmosis of the eye has also been identified in immunologically compromised hosts.[89]

Toxoplasmosis

Toxoplasma gondii may be found in adults with active or healed, focal retinochoroiditis; many of the lesions represent recurrences of congenital infection. The trophozoites produce a necrotising

retinitis and associated inflammation in the related choroid. A central zone of necrosis is surrounded by lymphocytes, macrophages and occasional giant cells. Older or healed lesions contain encysted forms of the organisms and when these cysts break down, the dormant organisms contained therein escape to infect previously unaffected cells, and the whole process of inflammation and encystment occurs again. It is thought that the destructive aspect of toxoplasma infection is related to an immunologically based reaction, the exact nature of which has not as yet been established.

Nematode endophthalmitis (ocular toxocariasis)[90]

Nematode endophthalmitis is nearly always due to *Toxocara canis* (Fig. 24.12). Generalised systemic infection by this parasite may produce visceral larva migrans, but ocular lesions are not usually associated with symptoms of systemic disease. The eye is infected by larvae passing through either the retinal or the uveal circulation. Bilateral involvement is unknown. The patients are most often children, and there is invariably a history of

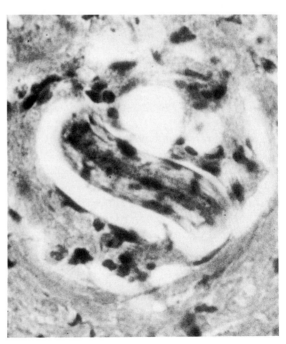

Fig. 24.12 Larva of *Toxocara canis.* Haematoxylin-eosin × 600

contact with puppies. The enzyme-linked immunosorbent assay (ELISA) may be helpful in establishing the diagnosis. Three types of ocular involvement have been described:

1. *Chronic endophthalmitis*, the commonest, where granulomatous inflammation, in which a large number of eosinophils are often seen, surrounds the toxocara larva. The initial lesion is within the retina, but there is spread to involve other intraocular structures and there is associated retinal detachment.
2. *Retinal granuloma*, in which similar inflammatory changes are seen, but the lesion remains localised, usually at the posterior pole, and retinal detachment does not occur.
3. *Peripheral retinitis and pars-planitis*, when the focus of inflammation is situated respectively at the periphery of the retina or within the pars plana of the ciliary body.

Onchocerciasis (African 'river blindness')

Although rarely seen in temperate climates, onchocercal infection of the eye is one of the commonest causes of blindness in the world. The worm (*Onchocerca volvulus*) reaches the anterior segment of the eye from the periorbital skin and conjunctiva, and interstitial keratitis and iridocyclitis develop. In the posterior segment there may be choroidoretinopathy and optic atrophy, but the mechanism by which this involvement comes about is undetermined.

Pemphigus

Catarrhal or purulent conjunctivitis and intra-epithelial bulla formation in the conjunctiva may occur in pemphigus vulgaris.

Pemphigoid (benign mucosal pemphigoid, ocular cicatricial pemphigoid, essential shrinkage of the conjunctiva)[91]

No systemic changes are present in this condition, but there is inflammation and bulla formation in the subepithelial tissue of the conjunctiva, and there is squamous metaplasia of the epithelium with loss of goblet cells. There may also be corneal involvement. Subsequently there is scarring and cicatrisation.

Skin lesions closely resembling those of pemphigoid are seen in *erythema multiforme*, while in the *Stevens–Johnson syndrome* there is associated involvement of the oral and genital mucosa.

Ligneous conjunctivitis (chronic pseudomembranous conjunctivitis)

Ligneous conjunctivitis tends to occur in young children, mainly girls. It is often bilateral and can be complicated by corneal involvement and even perforation of the globe. There may be associated nasopharyngitis and vaginitis. The aetiology is unknown, but either viral infection or auto-

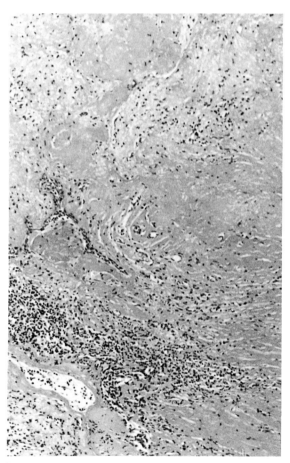

Fig. 24.13 Ligneous conjunctivitis: deposition of fibrin (top) is seen together with granulation tissue. Haematoxylin-eosin × 90

immunity seem to be the most likely causative factors. Histologically, there is a fibrinous deposit associated with an inflammatory cell infiltrate. Subsequently, granulation and connective tissues form, and later a hyalinised mass develops (Fig. 24.13).

Phlyctenular keratoconjunctivitis

Phlyctenular keratoconjunctivitis is caused by a hypersensitivity reaction to bacterial proteins; there is an association with staphylococcal infection. Inflamed nodules occur in the conjunctiva near the limbus, and the cornea may be involved.

Vernal conjunctivitis (spring catarrh)

Reaction to pollen is thought to play an important rôle in the pathogenesis of this self-limiting,

allergic disorder which may be associated with hay fever, asthma and atopic eczema. It is seasonal, occurring primarily in the spring, and usually affects young males. It may involve all the conjunctiva or be localised, particularly to the limbus. Histologically, there is papillary hypertrophy with a subepithelial inflammatory cell infiltrate (Fig. 24.14) in which lymphocytes, plasma cells and a conspicuous number of eosinophils are seen. The surface epithelium may be much thicker than normal, and epithelial processes extend downwards to produce cysts and tubules. In longstanding cases, there is usually an increase in the amount of collagen deep to the surface, and this eventually undergoes hyaline degeneration.

Giant papillary conjunctivitis

Papillae, larger than those seen in vernal conjunctivitis but histologically similar, may occur

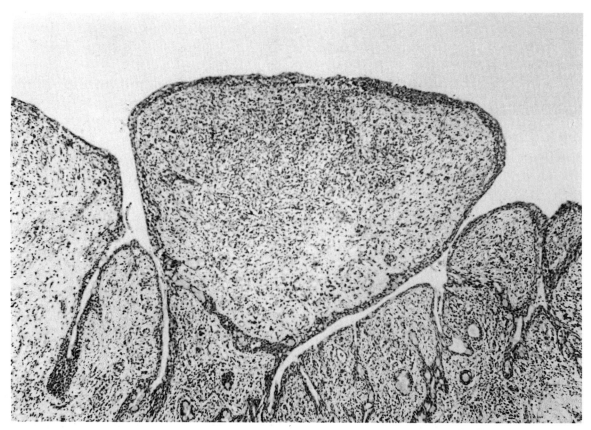

Fig. 24.14 Vernal conjunctivitis: there is papillary hypertrophy and a subepithelial inflammatory cell infiltrate. Haematoxylin-eosin × 85

in the conjunctiva of those who wear contact lenses.

Mooren's ulcer ('corneal melting' syndrome)[92,93]

Ulceration commencing at or near the limbus, possibly involving the entire circumference and slowly spreading across the cornea, is the main feature of this condition. Typically, the ulcer has an overhanging edge, and histological examination reveals chronic inflammation and necrosis. Auto-immunity is the likely cause.

Corneal graft failure

Corneal graft failure in the first few weeks following keratoplasty is due either to defective wound closure, to infection, to local degenerative changes, or to a disturbance in the endothelium consequent upon surgical trauma. Immunological rejection, which is unusual, only manifests itself

later. This is a T-cell mediated response involving cellular rather than humoral mechanisms, and it is characterised by an inflammatory cell infiltrate and vascularisation.

Fuchs' heterochromic cyclitis

Mild, unilateral iridocyclitis, with neovascularisation on the anterior surface of the iris and anterior uveal stromal atrophy, producing heterochromia, are the features of this condition. There may be associated glaucoma and cataract formation.

Sympathetic ophthalmitis (sympathetic ophthalmia)[94-104]

Sympathetic ophthalmitis is a potentially blinding, bilateral, granulomatous, uveal inflammation which can occasionally follow accidental or surgical perforation of one eye (the

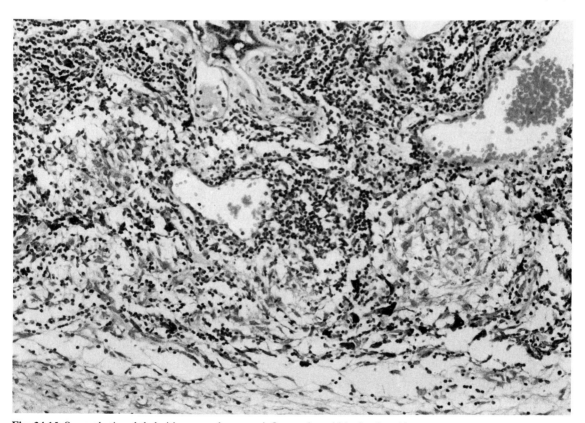

Fig. 24.15 Sympathetic ophthalmitis—granulomatous inflammation within the choroid. Haematoxylin-eosin × 190

exciting eye). Perforation associated with uveal tissue damage is more likely to be followed by development of the condition; ocular infection appears to act as a protection against the disease. Post-traumatic uveitis occurs in the exciting eye and following this (usually after 4–12 weeks, but sometimes earlier or later) inflammation develops in the other eye (*the sympathising eye*). The histological picture of the inflammation is identical in the two eyes. The uveitis is diffuse and granulomatous. There is a dense lymphocytic cellular infiltrate in which there are scattered eosinophils; aggregates of epithelioid cells (Fig. 24.15) and occasional giant cells are present throughout. Necrosis is not seen. Fine granules of uveal pigment can be identified within the phagocytic cells. Granulomas develop between Bruch's membrane and the retinal pigment epithelium (*Dalén–Fuchs' nodules*, Fig. 24.16), but these are not pathognomonic of sympathetic ophthalmitis, as they may be seen in any granulomatous uveitis. The choriocapillaris and the retina are relatively free from inflammation, but typical granulomas are often seen to extend out from the uvea into the neurovascular channels traversing the scleral coat.

The classical theory of its pathogenesis states that sympathetic ophthalmitis is caused by hypersensitivity to uveal pigment liberated during injury. This has been challenged by studies which suggest that an autoimmune reaction to a protein on the membrane of the outer segment of the retinal photoreceptors is responsible. Genetic factors may also play a rôle in the causation of the disorder.

Vogt–Koyanagi–Harada (VKH) syndrome

This comprises two entities: (1) the *Vogt–Koyanagi syndrome* of bilateral panuveitis and meningoencephalitis, together with vitiligo, premature greying of the hair (poliosis) and alopecia, and (2) *Harada's disease*, which exhibits similar ocular and central nervous system changes, but fewer changes in the skin. Histological examination of the eyes shows granulomatous uveitis, as in sympathetic ophthalmitis, but with a heavier plasma cell infiltrate, and involvement of the choriocapillaris; *Dalén–Fuchs' nodules* may be present (see above) and there is extensive, exudative retinal detachment. Viral infection and

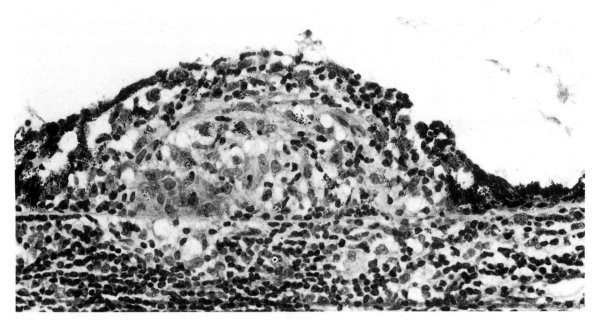

Fig. 24.16 Dalén–Fuchs' nodule: granuloma formation between Bruch's membrane and the retinal pigment epithelium (top); fine granules of uveal pigment are seen within phagocytic epithelioid cells. Haematoxylin-eosin × 430

an immune response to uveal pigment and retinal pigment epithelium have been suggested as causative factors.

Lens-induced endophthalmitis (phacoallergic endophthalmitis)[105]

An inflammatory reaction of an immunological nature initiated by autosensitisation to lens protein may develop when, following either a surgical procedure, such as extracapsular lens extraction, or an injury, lens matter escapes into the ocular cavities. The reaction is usually unilateral, being confined to the operated or injured eye, but on rare occasions it may be bilateral. The inflammation is centred around the lens-iris diaphragm. Polymorphonuclear leucocytes are seen in close relationship to the lens substance, while more peripherally there is an epithelioid and giant cell response (Fig. 24.17); a conspicuous number of eosinophils are also present. The choroid is relatively free from inflammation, but there may be either nodular or diffuse aggregates of inflammatory cells on the inner retinal surface in addition to a retinal perivasculitis.

Rheumatoid arthritis[106,107]

Scleritis is the usual ocular manifestation of rheumatoid arthritis. The anterior sclera is more frequently involved than the posterior, and there may be extension to the cornea. The reaction results in scleral thinning and ectasia, and even perforation (scleromalacia perforans). The basic lesion seen on histological examination is similar to a rheumatoid nodule, with necrosis and granuloma

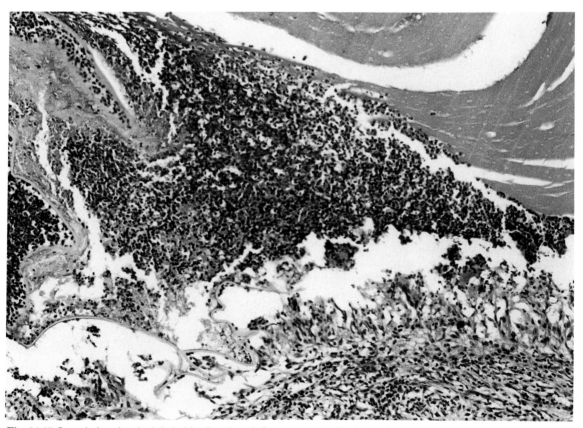

Fig. 24.17 Lens-induced endophthalmitis: there is an inflammatory reaction in relation to the disrupted lens; folded remnants of the lens capsule are seen below and to the left.
Haematoxylin-eosin × 145

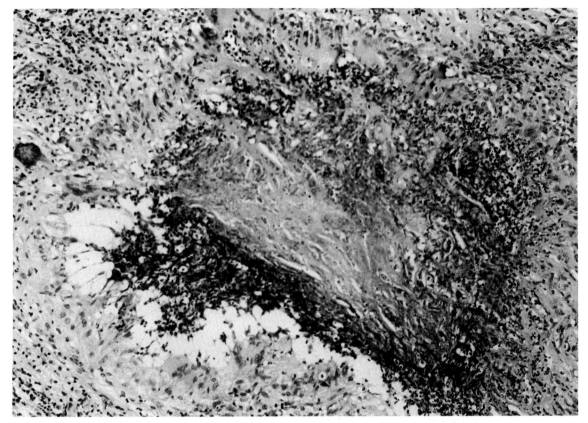

Fig. 24.18 Necrogranulomatous reaction in the sclera. Haematoxylin-eosin × 145

formation—*necrogranulomatous reaction* (Fig. 24.18).

Juvenile rheumatoid arthritis and *ankylosing spondylitis* may be accompanied by uveitis.

Reiter's disease

Non-gonococcal urethritis, with arthritis and conjunctivitis or iridocyclitis, constitutes Reiter's disease. The reaction in the conjunctiva is papillary in nature, there may be an associated keratitis, and the iridocyclitis is non-granulomatous.

Sjögren's syndrome

Dry eye (xerophthalmia), xerostomia and a systemic immune disease, most commonly rheumatoid arthritis, are the characteristics of this syndrome. Secretion by the lacrimal, salivary and conjunctival mucous glands fails, probably due to an autoimmune reaction. There is flattening of the conjunctival epithelium which results in a stratified appearance, and the number of goblet cells is reduced.

Systemic lupus erythematosus[108]

Patients acutely ill with active systemic lupus erythematosus are those most likely to exhibit ocular manifestations. Classically, these take the form of a retinopathy with vasculitis, arteriolar narrowing, venous occlusion, haemorrhages, oedema and 'cotton-wool' spots.

Scleroderma (systemic sclerosis)

Tightness of the lids and dry eye, and retinopathy characterised by haemorrhages, exudates and 'cotton-wool' spots, can be associated with sclero-derma.

Wegener's granulomatosis

Ocular lesions in Wegener's granulomatosis take the form of vasculitis in the eye or orbit. There is often associated involvement of the sinuses.

Polyarteritis nodosa

The characteristic widespread, necrotising arteritis of this disorder can affect almost all the ocular tissues. If the peripheral cornea and sclera are involved, the picture is similar to that in Wegener's granulomatosis and rheumatoid arthritis. There is limbal ulceration and nodular scleritis while haemorrhagic lesions occur in the conjunctiva. Uveitis and retinopathy can develop, and there may also be optic nerve and orbital involvement.

Temporal arteritis (cranial arteritis, giant-cell arteritis) [109,110]

The characteristic feature of temporal arteritis is prominence and tenderness of the superficial temporal artery, biopsy of which shows thickening of the wall by a granulomatous inflammatory reaction (Fig. 24.19). There is narrowing of the vessel lumen, proliferation of the intima, and fragmentation of the internal elastic lamina. Involvement of the vascular supply to the optic nerve head and retina leads to ischaemic necrosis. Not all clinically diagnosed cases show the characteristic histological changes in the temporal

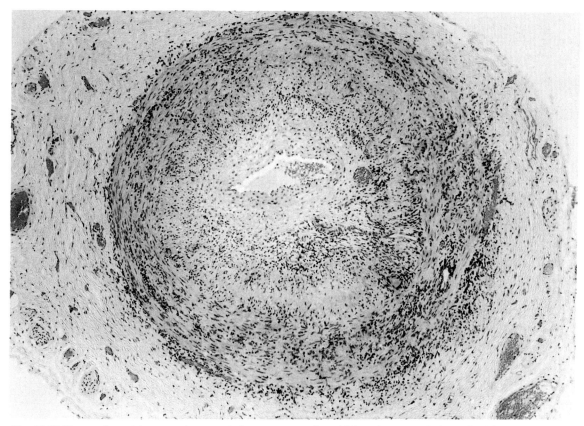

Fig. 24.19 Temporal arteritis: a granulomatous inflammatory reaction with lymphocytes and giant cells, thickening of the vessel wall and narrowing of the lumen. Haematoxylin-eosin ×85

artery, particularly if the biopsy is rather small, as 'skip-areas' of normal artery are not infrequently present between the giant-cell lesions. The erythrocyte sedimentation rate is usually, but not invariably, raised.

Behçet's disease[111]

Acute anterior uveitis with inflammatory exudate in the anterior chamber is the most frequent ocular finding in this disease, the reaction having an immunological basis. There is, however, often associated retinal vasculitis and necrosis, together with papillitis, and subsequently new vessels emanate from the optic nerve head.

Idiopathic inflammation[112]

Very many examples of ocular inflammation, particularly uveitis, are seen in which extensive investigation fails to reveal a cause, there being no evidence of either an infective process or an immune disorder. For so long as their cause remains unknown these cases may be described as idiopathic.

TUMOURS[113-115]

Tumours involving the eyes are divided into two large groups according to whether they arise from outside the eye (extraocular tumours) or from within (intraocular tumours). Lesions resembling tumours, and also cysts, are included here together with true neoplasms.

EXTRAOCULAR TUMOURS[116]

Most extraocular tumours resemble their counterparts elsewhere in the body and for a description of their morphology reference may be made to other sections in Systemic Pathology. Some, however, warrant special consideration.

Eyelid

Basal cell carcinomas are the commonest malignant neoplasms seen in this region and show a pre-

dilection for the lower lid. Squamous cell carcinomas[117,118] also occur as do sebaceous carcinomas[119-122] (Meibomian carcinomas) (Fig. 24.20) which arise most frequently in the upper lid and are, on the whole, more malignant than similar tumours elsewhere. Nodular malignant melanomas[123] carry a worse prognosis if the lid margin is affected than if only the skin of the lid is involved. The majority of lid tumours, however, are benign. A number of lid conditions which are not neoplastic, but which clinically present as tumour-like lesions, are of importance and will be considered here.

Chalazion (Meibomian 'cyst')

A chalazion is not a cyst. It is a granuloma that forms in relation to retained fatty products of secretion of sebaceous glands (Meibomian glands) when these have escaped into the surrounding tissues. The typical histological picture is that of a lipogranuloma (Fig. 24.21). Acute inflammatory cells may be seen in the early stages of development while in older lesions there is fibrosis and scarring.

Molluscum contagiosum

The lesion of molluscum contagiosum is a small nodule that is caused by an unclassified member of the pox group of viruses. The epithelium becomes acanthotic and the affected cells contain inclusions known as molluscum bodies. These intracytoplasmic inclusions are eosinophilic in the deeper cells, which are the first to be involved, but as the cells move upwards, the inclusions become basophilic and replace the cell cytoplasm. Necrotic debris, which eventually forms in the central crater, may be extruded from the surface, and there is often an associated secondary follicular conjunctivitis and superficial punctate keratitis.

Xanthelasma

The presence of lipid-containing histiocytes within the dermis, particularly in relation to skin appendages and blood vessels, constitutes xanthelasma (Fig. 24.22). On occasion there is an associated elevation of serum cholesterol.

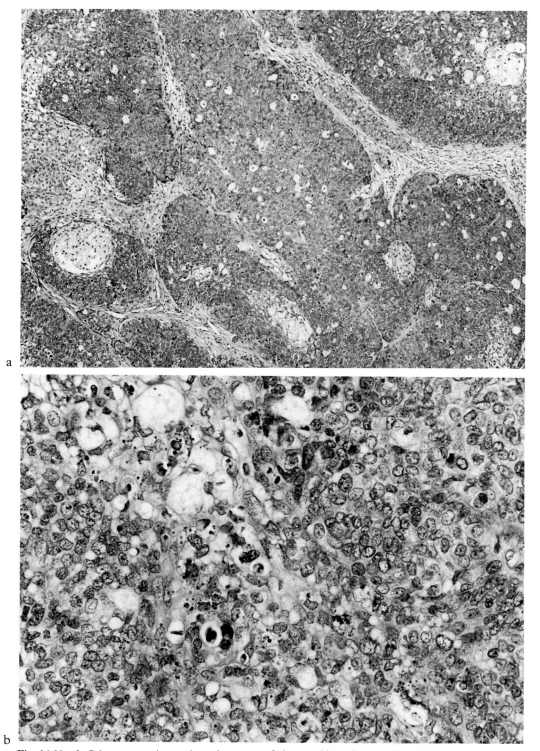

a

b

Fig. 24.20a, b Sebaceous carcinoma: irregular masses of pleomorphic malignant cells exhibiting nuclear hyperchromasia and conspicuous abnormal mitotic activity; numerous 'foamy' lipid-containing cells are present. Haematoxylin-eosin (**a**) ×85; (**b**) ×385

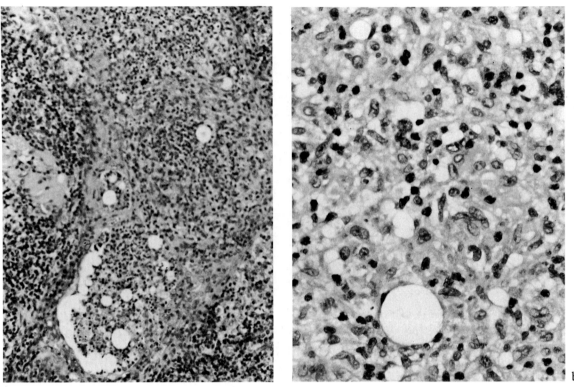

a   b

Fig. 24.21a, b Chalazion; lipogranuloma: fat spaces are seen and there is a granulomatous inflammatory reaction. Haematoxylin-eosin (**a**) × 150; (**b**) × 450

Conjunctiva

Cysts and miscellaneous tumours

Cysts in the conjunctiva usually arise from implantation. Papillomas[124-126] occur most commonly at the corneoscleral junction (limbus), at the eyelid margins, and at the caruncle; multiple and recurrent papillomas are considered to be due to a virus while an unusual variety of conjunctival papilloma is the inverted type, analogous to similar lesions found both in the lacrimal sac and in the upper respiratory passages. A rare condition, known as *hereditary benign intra-epithelial dyskeratosis*, is associated with similar lesions in the oral mucosa. *Dysplastic lesions* of the conjunctival epithelium, which are often associated with either a pinguecula or a pterygium, should be considered as *intra-epithelial neo-plasms*,[127-129] and can be regarded as pre-malignant. Both *in-situ* and *infiltrating squamous cell carcinomas* occur at the limbus, but the

infiltrating lesion carries a more favourable prognosis than similar tumours of the skin. *Muco-epidermoid carcinoma* of the conjunctiva has also been reported.

Lymphomas not infrequently affect the conjunctiva; they resemble the lesions which occur in the orbit and these are discussed more fully later (see p. 696). *Myxomas*[130] of the conjunctiva have been reported. *Kaposi's sarcoma*[131-135] is seen in association with the acquired immune deficiency syndrome (AIDS).

Naevi

The commonest tumours of the conjunctiva are naevi. They are classified in a similar way to cutaneous naevi, which they in many ways resemble. The conjunctival lesion analogous to an intradermal naevus is termed a *subepithelial naevus*. Commonly, proliferating epithelium, which may contain goblet cells, migrates

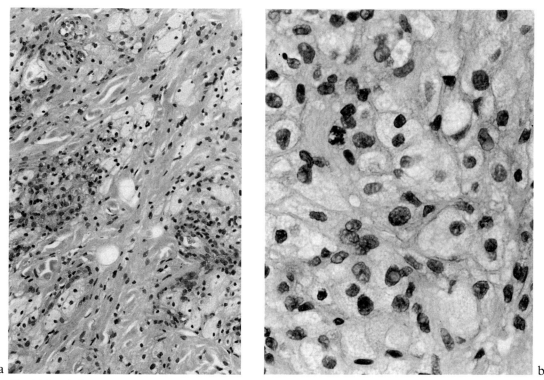

a

b

Fig. 24.22a, b Xanthelasma: foamy lipid-containing histiocytes infiltrate the dermis. Haematoxylin-eosin (**a**) ×130; (**b**) ×550

downwards from the surface with the eventual production of cysts, thus giving rise to '*cystic naevi*' (Fig. 24.23). In addition, conjunctival naevi may become inflamed without this being suggestive of malignant change. *Oculodermal melanocytosis (naevus of Ota)* may also involve the conjunctiva (see p. 699).

Melanosis and intra-epithelial melanocytic neoplasia[136-139]

Secondary melanosis of the conjunctiva may occur in such conditions as Addison's disease or it may follow localised chronic inflammation. Adrenaline (epinephrine), silver, mascara and other foreign material also cause conjunctival pigmentation (*pseudomelanosis*). *Ephelis* (freckle) and *lentigo* occur, as in the skin. Proliferation of melanocytes in the conjunctiva is probably always best regarded as neoplastic, and the term *intra-epithelial melanocytic neoplasia* (Fig. 24.24) may be preferred

to primary acquired melanosis and precancerous melanosis.[140] Such lesions have the potential to develop into in-situ and infiltrating malignant melanomas. If there is involvement only of the basal layer of the epithelium the prognosis is much more favourable than if the entire thickness of the epithelium is affected.

Malignant melanoma[141-143]

Malignant melanomas of the conjunctiva arise either de novo, or from a junctional or compound naevus, or from intra-epithelial melanocytic neoplasia. However, few benign melanotic lesions of the conjunctiva become malignant. Conjunctival melanomas are considered to be less malignant than skin melanomas and, while the depth of invasion is thought to be an important factor, it is not prognostically as important as in cases of melanoma arising in the skin.

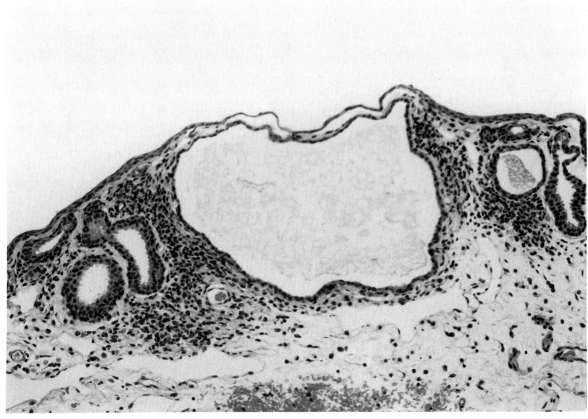

Fig. 24.23 Cystic naevus of conjunctiva: surface epithelium has migrated downwards with the naevus cells to produce cysts. Haematoxylin-eosin × 190

Cornea and sclera

Tumours of the corneoscleral envelope are very unusual. The sclera can, however, be involved in congenital ocular melanocytosis (see p. 699) and the cornea is not infrequently infiltrated by neoplasms arising in adjacent structures. On rare occasions *keloid formation* may follow injury. *Dermoids* and *dermolipomas* are referred to under developmental anomalies (see p. 745).

Orbit

General considerations[144–146]

The different types of tissue found within the orbit are reflected in the wide range of tumours seen. Most expanding lesions are either cystic or inflammatory in origin and are readily diagnosed as such by the histological features observed on microscopy. Neoplasms can originate from fibrous tissue, adipose tissue, blood vessels, nerves, muscle, bone, cartilage, lacrimal gland, lacrimal sac and optic nerve. Lymphomas and metastatic tumours may also be seen. *Dermoid cysts* present in the superotemporal quadrant of the orbit, most often in childhood. *Teratomas* also occur. *Tumours of blood vessels*, particularly cavernous haemangiomas (Fig. 24.25) and haemangiopericytomas[147] (Fig. 24.26), and *nerve sheath tumours* (Fig. 24.27) are among the commonest orbital tumours.

Epithelial tumours of the lacrimal gland[148] are also common and they are histologically similar to those of salivary gland origin. *Pleomorphic adenomas (benign mixed lacrimal tumours)* (Fig.

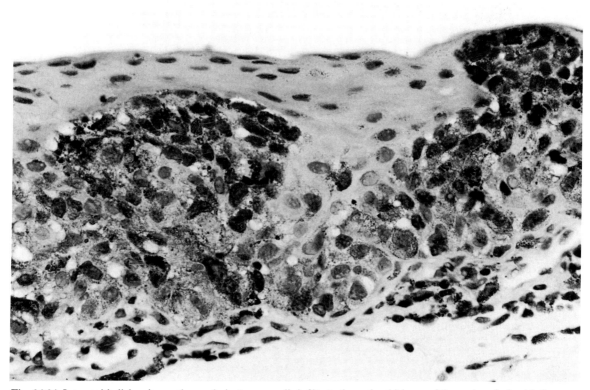

Fig. 24.24 Intra-epithelial melanocytic neoplasia: tumour cells infiltrate the entire thickness of the conjunctival epithelium. Haematoxylin-eosin × 525

24.28) account for just over half of all tumours of this gland. Malignant change can occur in these adenomas to produce *pleomorphic adeno-carcinomas*; such tumours may also arise de novo. The commonest malignant tumour of the lacrimal gland, however, is *adenoid cystic carcinoma* (Fig. 24.29),[149,150] which occurs more often at this site than it does in the salivary glands. *Squamous cell carcinomas, monomorphic adenocarcinomas* and *mucoepidermoid carcinomas* are rare. *Tumours of the lacrimal sac* resemble, and are closely associated with, tumours arising from the nasal mucosa.

Fibrous histiocytomas[151] and *alveolar soft part sarcomas*[152] occur in the orbit. The commonest malignant orbital tumour in children is an *embryonal sarcoma* or *rhabdomyosarcoma* (Fig. 24.30). A *mucocele* usually originates in either the frontal or the ethmoid sinus. *Nodular fasciitis* is basically an inflammatory condition which may affect the episclera and conjunctiva. *Hydatid cysts* can also occur in the orbit.

Optic nerve tumours[153 – 157]

Meningiomas and astrocytomas of the optic nerve can present as orbital lesions and both may be associated with von Recklinghausen's disease (see p. 470). *Meningiomas* (Fig. 24.31) in the orbit are usually the result of extension of intracranial meningiomas, but they can also arise from either the intraorbital or the intracanalicular portion of the optic nerve. Meningiomas can, on very rare occasions, develop elsewhere within the orbit or in the skin, the conjunctiva or the caruncle. Orbital meningiomas occur usually in adults and are more common in females; bilateral involvement has

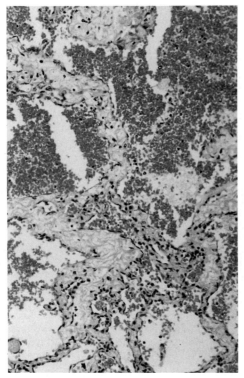

Fig. 24.25 Cavernous haemangioma: the vascular channels are irregular and vary in size. Haematoxylin-eosin × 130

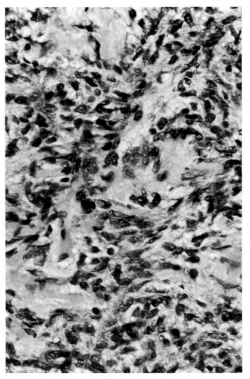

Fig. 24.26 Haemangiopericytoma: solid portion of tumour showing spindle-shaped cells. Haematoxylin-eosin × 385

been reported. Histologically, their appearance is similar to intracranial meningiomas (see p. 462): meningothelial, psammomatous, fibroblastic, angioblastic, and transitional types are seen. The fibroblastic and angioblastic types are, however, unusual in the orbit, and most orbital meningiomas are either meningothelial or transitional. Local recurrence may follow removal, but true malignancy is very rare.

Most *astrocytomas of the optic nerve* (Fig. 24.32)[158] are well-differentiated pilocytic astrocytomas (see p. 435). They usually present in the first decade of life and are slightly more common in females. Proliferation of tumour astrocytes leads to fusiform enlargement of the nerve and visual loss, and there is frequently penetration of the meninges, which become hyperplastic. Meningeal hyperplasia may extend far beyond the limits of the tumour itself and can lead to confusion in diagnosis, particularly if a biopsy is small and un-

representative. Anaplastic astrocytomas (see p. 437) of the optic nerve are extremely rare, occur in adults, and have a very unfavourable prognosis.[159]

Lymphomas and other lymphoproliferative conditions[160–166]

The orbit does not contain any lymphoid tissue and is said to be devoid of lymphatic vessels. Nevertheless, lymphomas and other lymphoproliferative lesions may arise at this site. Orbital lymphomas are classified in the same way as lymphomas in general: most are of B-cell type. Such conditions as *sinus histiocytosis with massive lymphadenopathy, granulocytic sarcomas* with or without associated myeloid leukaemia, and other *leukaemic deposits* have all been reported. *Hodgkin's disease* rarely, if ever, primarily involves orbital tissues.

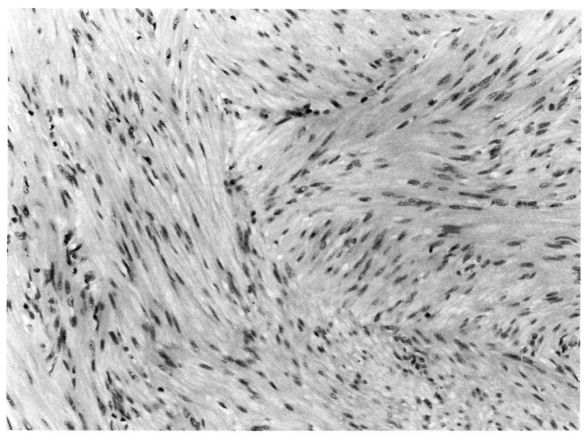

Fig. 24.27 Schwannoma: typical picture of bundles of spindle-shaped cells. Haematoxylin-eosin × 190

Lymphocytic lesions with an *inflammatory basis* occur in the orbit; the presence of germinal follicles helps in their recognition.

Many lymphoproliferative lesions present great diagnostic problems to the pathologist, especially if they are not obviously true lymphomas or do not exhibit germinal follicle formation. Immuno-histochemical studies can help in their diagnosis. It would appear likely that the majority are *low-grade lymphomas*, mostly of lymphoplasmacytoid type; they should be designated as such. While, in certain instances, it would seem appropriate to refer to either a *lymphocytic lesion of indeterminate type* or a *pseudolymphoma*, the terms *pseudotumour* and *benign lymphoma* are confusing and misleading and, in the opinion of some,[167] have no place in modern ocular histopathology. Pseudotumour, however, is a diagnosis not infrequently made by ophthalmologists, and should probably be accepted as a clinical entity.

Secondary tumours

Many orbital tumours are the result of either direct infiltration from neighbouring sites or metastatic spread from a primary tumour elsewhere. *Retinoblastoma* and *uveal melanoma* are the commonest ocular neoplasms which spread to the orbit, but orbital involvement in cancers of local origin may also result from tumours of the lid, the upper respiratory passages and the paranasal sinuses. *Carcinoma* from various sites may metastasise to the orbit, the bronchus being the commonest primary source in males and the breast in females. *Carcinoid tumours*[168] have also been reported.

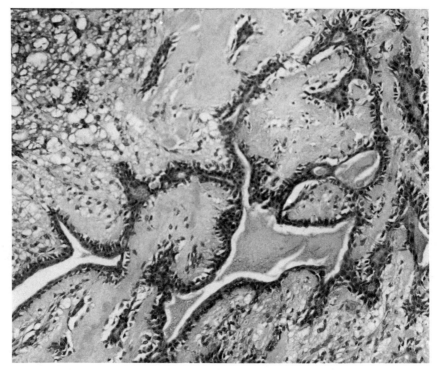

Fig. 24.28 Pleomorphic adenoma of lacrimal gland: irregular epithelium-lined tubular structures are seen, and much of the stroma is hyalinised.
Haematoxylin-eosin × 150

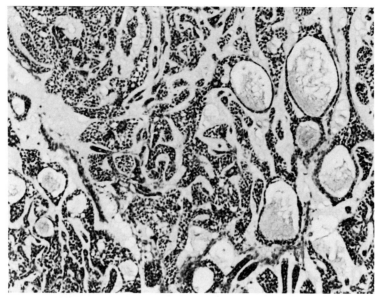

Fig. 24.29 Adenoid cystic carcinoma of lacrimal gland: characteristic cribriform appearance.
Haematoxylin-eosin × 110

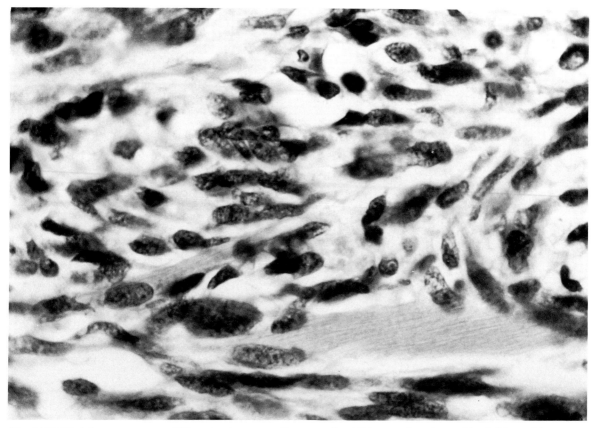

Fig. 24.30 Rhabdomyosarcoma: undifferentiated tumour cells are seen in addition to enlarged strap-like rhabdomyoblasts (bottom).
Haematoxylin-eosin × 1000

INTRAOCULAR TUMOURS[169]

Melanocytomas (naevi)[170,171]

The histogenesis and nomenclature of this group of lesions is a matter for debate. Since naevus cells that originate from melanocytes of surface epithelium (cutaneous or mucosal) are not present within the eye, the term *melanocytoma* is, in some ways, preferable to the more frequently used 'naevus' for benign intraocular neoplasms composed of melanocytic cells. Melanocytomas are variably, but often heavily, pigmented and are found in any part of the uvea. They are composed either of slender spindle-shaped or dendritic cells, or of plump polyhedral or balloon cells with abundant cytoplasm filled with melanin (*magnocellular naevi*). They are not infrequently seen on the anterior surface of the iris (*iris naevi*). They also occur within the ciliary body (Fig. 24.33) or choroid (*ciliary body or choroidal naevi*) where they cause little, if any, stromal thickening and spare the inner capillary vascular network. *Melanocytomas at the optic nerve head*, however, are sizeable swellings. Neither degeneration nor detachment of the overlying retina is associated with benign melanocytic tumours of the choroid.

Congenital ocular melanocytosis (melanosis oculi). In this condition a large number of pigment-containing, dendritic melanocytes are found in the uvea and also in the sclera. When the eyelids and other parts of the skin of the face are involved in addition to the uvea and sclera the condition is known as naevus of Ota. Malignant change may

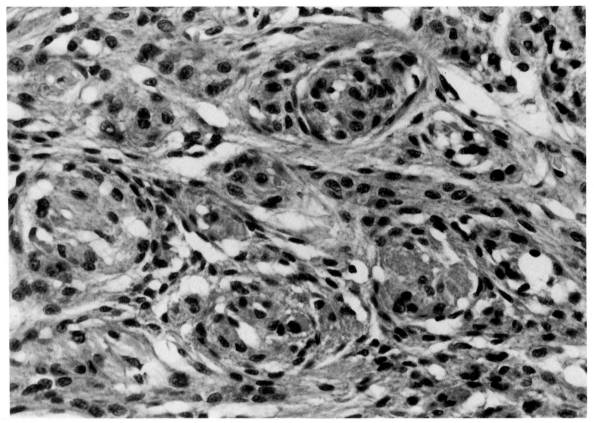

Fig. 24.31 Meningioma: meningothelial type, showing closely packed whorls of meningothelial cells. Haematoxylin-eosin ×525

occur and there is a higher incidence of uveal melanoma in those with such lesions.[172]

Malignant melanoma of the uvea

Malignant melanomas[173-194] affect the choroid, the ciliary body and the iris. Their occurrence in non-Caucasian races is extremely rare.

Malignant melanoma of the choroid (Fig. 24.34). Choroidal melanomas are the commonest primary intraocular malignant neoplasms. Females are slightly more predisposed to such tumours than males. The average age of onset is 50 years. Most choroidal melanomas arise at or near the posterior pole of the eye and while they usually grow as either bilobed, globular or ellipsoid masses (Fig. 24.35), some are more wide-

spread and diffuse, and carry a particularly unfavourable prognosis. There is frequently an associated retinal detachment and degeneration, together with eosinophilic, subretinal exudate. Bruch's membrane is often eroded, and the retina itself may be infiltrated by tumour cells. The pigment and reticulin content of the tumours varies considerably. Necrosis (Fig. 24.36) with associated inflammation may occur, and there may be haemorrhage. Lipid-containing histiocytes are often seen and the tumours not infrequently exhibit a fascicular pattern (Fig. 24.37). On histological grounds, according to Callender's classification,[195a] there are three types of tumour cells:

1. *Spindle A*—cells with small, hyperchromatic, spindle-shaped nuclei, with indistinct nucleoli and indistinct cytoplasm.
2. *Spindle B* (Fig. 24.38)—cells with plump,

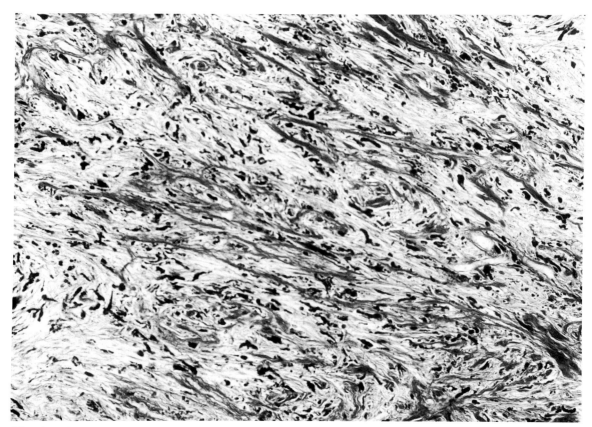

Fig. 24.32 Astrocytoma: the fibrillar processes are clearly seen and there are numerous thick Rosenthal fibres. Phosphotungstic acid haematoxylin × 145

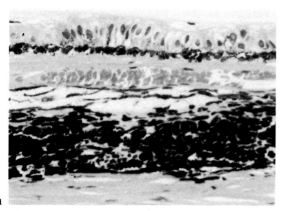

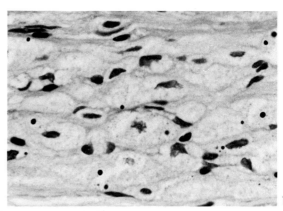

a

b

Fig. 24.33a, b Melanocytoma of the ciliary body: (**a**) The heavily pigmented lesion composed of balloon cells with abundant cytoplasm involves the stroma, but spares the capillary layer. (**b**) Bleached preparation to show the ballooned nature of the tumour cells.
(**a**) Haematoxylin-eosin × 200; (b) Bleached. Haematoxylin-eosin × 520

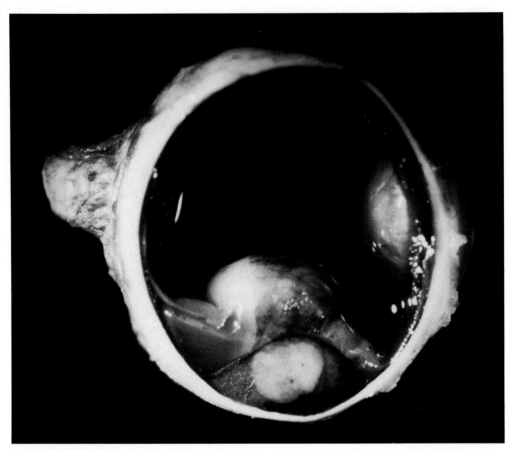

Fig. 24.34 Malignant melanoma of the choroid: the globe has been opened anteroposteriorly through the limbus and a bilobed 'cottage-loaf'-shaped tumour is seen to arise from within the equatorial choroid on one side (bottom of picture).
× 4

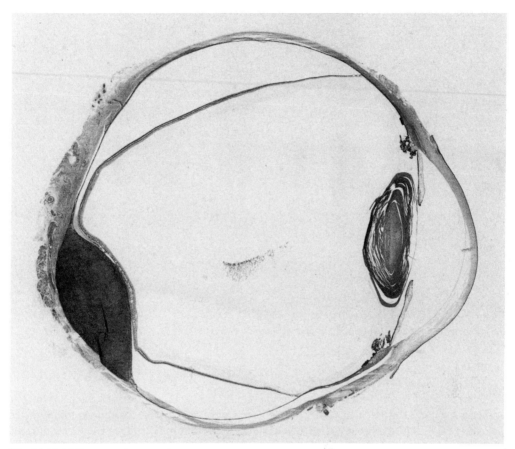

Fig. 24.35 Malignant melanoma of the choroid: section of the eye showing an ellipsoid mass posteriorly (left of picture).
Haematoxylin-eosin ×5

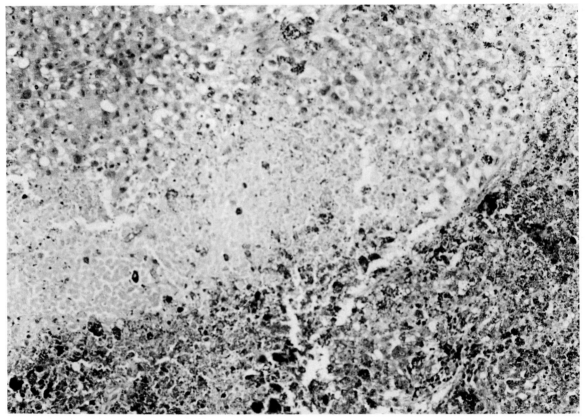

Fig. 24.36 Malignant melanoma of the choroid: an area of necrosis within the tumour. Haematoxylin-eosin × 145

spindle-shaped nuclei, but prominent nucleoli and indistinct cytoplasm.

3. *Epithelioid* (Fig. 24.39)—cells with large, round nuclei, prominent nucleoli and abundant eosinophilic cytoplasm.

A mixture of cell types is usually seen in melanomas, but one type often predominates. From a purely practical viewpoint, however, it may be difficult and even misleading to attempt to distinguish between spindle A and spindle B type cells, and tumours are probably most usefully reported by pathologists as being of spindle cell, epithelioid cell or mixed cell type. The cell type is the most reliable prognostic indicator that can be determined by histological study, being of greater value than either the pigment or the reticulin content, or the degree of mitotic activity. Spindle cell tumours carry a more favourable prognosis than tumours of mixed cell type, necrotic tumours are more malignant than others, and epithelioid tumours carry the worst outlook of all. Three out of four patients with spindle cell melanomas survive 15 years; an unfavourable sign is extrascleral extension or extension into the optic nerve (Fig. 24.40). Size is also important in assessment; small tumours have a better prognosis than large tumours. Metastatic tumour deposits from choroidal malignant melanoma classically occur in the liver.

Malignant melanoma of the ciliary body. Ciliary body melanomas occur usually in the sixth decade of life, and males and females are equally affected. The appearance is of a circumscribed mass and the histological features are similar to choroidal melanomas. Local spread within the eye often involves infiltration of the iris root and the

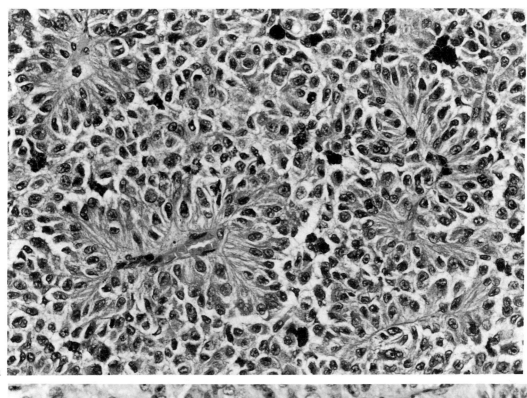

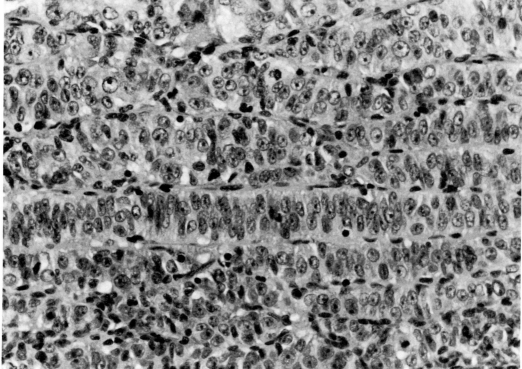

Fig. 24.37a, b Malignant melanoma of the choroid: there is a well-marked fascicular pattern; (**a**) tumour cells radiate around vascular channels; (**b**) tumour cells lie in ribbons.
Haematoxylin-eosin × 385

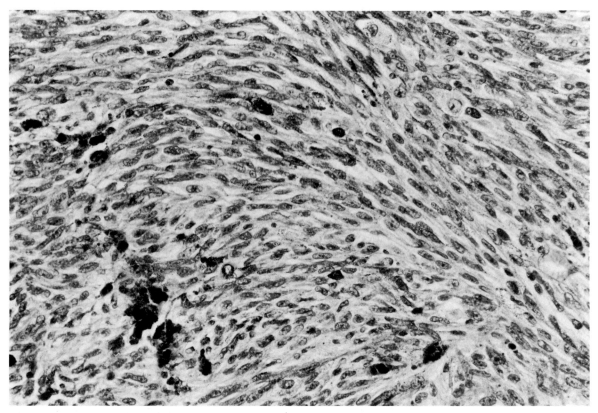

Fig. 24.38 Malignant melanoma of the choroid: typical spindle-shaped cells. Haematoxylin-eosin × 430

choroid. Also, a *'ring' melanoma* may develop; in histological sections of such a tumour there is involvement of the ciliary body on each side of the section. Extrascleral extension can occur and the tumours may metastasise to distant sites, such as the liver and the lungs.

Malignant melanoma of the iris. Iris melanomas often appear to arise from a pre-existing melanocytoma (naevus). They account for about 10% of all uveal melanomas. Most occur in subjects 10–20 years younger than those with melanomas elsewhere in the uvea, and there is equal distribution between the sexes. They usually involve the anterior iris stroma and grow on the anterior surface either as a diffuse plaque or as nodules; there may, however, be involvement of the entire thickness of the iris leaf (Fig. 24.41). Infiltration into the angle of the anterior chamber can

occur, but extrascleral extension and metastasis are rare, and the prognosis is good. Histologically most are of spindle-cell type.

Medulloepithelioma

Medulloepithelioma is a tumour of the ciliary epithelium in children. Formerly it was referred to as diktyoma. Both pigmented and non-pigmented epithelial cells may be present and there is a tubular pattern (Fig. 24.42). If there is associated stromal growth with pluripotential cells becoming neoplastic, heteroplastic elements, particularly cartilage, muscle and brain, may be produced; the result is a *teratoid medulloepithelioma*. Both types of medulloepithelioma may be either benign or malignant; it is often difficult to distinguish one from the other. In the malignant form, while the tubular pattern may be retained, the tumour is

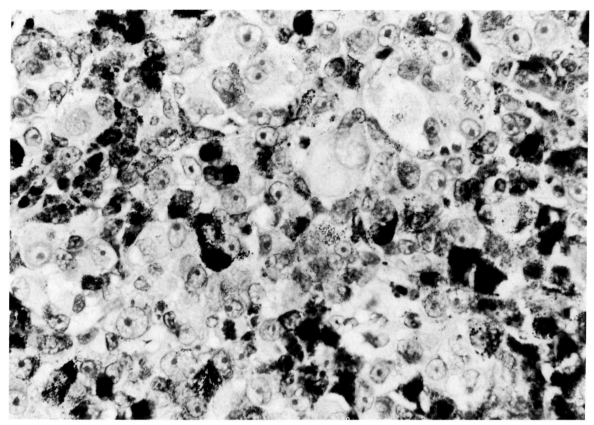

Fig. 24.39 Malignant melanoma of the choroid: epithelioid cells with large round nuclei, prominent nucleoli and abundant cytoplasm.
Haematoxylin-eosin × 665

largely undifferentiated and resembles a retino-blastoma. The presence of numerous mitotic figures and pronounced pleomorphism indicates malignancy, as does local intraocular invasion or extraocular extension. It is advisable, in practical terms, that all medulloepitheliomas be regarded as potentially malignant.

Adenoma and adenocarcinoma

Glandular tumours arise from the ciliary epithelium of adults. There are solid, papillary and pleomorphic types. As with medulloepitheliomas, differentiation of the benign from the malignant can be difficult. Conspicuous mitotic activity, pronounced cellular pleomorphism, local intraocular invasion and extension outside the eye are signs of malignancy.

Fuchs' adenoma

Fuchs' adenoma is a small, discrete, hyperplastic nodule arising from the ciliary epithelium. It is an incidental finding in otherwise normal eyes.

Other epithelial tumours

Tumours may arise from either the pigment epithelium of the iris or the retinal pigment epithelium. They are probably benign, the diagnosis of malignancy rarely, if ever, being justified.

Reactive hyperplasia

Pseudoadenomatous hyperplasia is a reaction seen in eyes previously injured or inflamed. While the ciliary epithelium is most often affected (Fig.

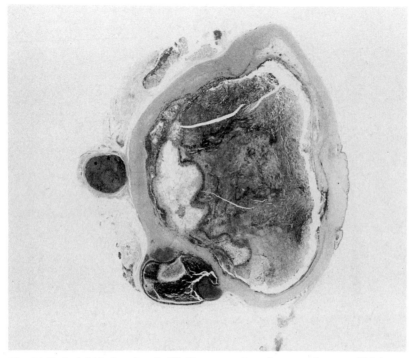

Fig. 24.40 A phthisical eye largely filled by a necrotic malignant melanoma which has infiltrated the optic nerve (left) and has extended outside the globe on one side. Haematoxylin-eosin ×2

24.43), hyperplastic reactions can involve the epithelium of the iris and also the retinal pigment epithelium.

Epithelial cysts[195]

The epithelial layers of both the iris and the ciliary body may split to form a cyst.

Miscellaneous tumours of the uvea

Other tumours which may occur in the uvea include *haemangiomas, leiomyomas, neurogenic tumours (schwannomas and neurofibromas), leiomyosarcomas, rhabdomyosarcomas* and *metastatic tumours* (Fig. 24.44). Metastatic tumours are the commonest group of intraocular neoplasms,[196] and while there is a wide variety of such tumours, the most usual source of choroidal metastases, as of those in the orbit, is the bronchus in males and the breast in females.

Although not neoplastic, it should be borne in mind that *juvenile xanthogranuloma* can affect the uvea, particularly the iris and the ciliary body; the majority of such lesions are in young children.

Retinoblastoma (Figs 24.45 and 24.46)[197–205]

This is the commonest malignant intraocular tumour of children, and it accounts for approximately 1% of deaths from malignant conditions in childhood. It most often develops in the first 3 years of life, is usually multifocal and is frequently bilateral. The survival rate is nowadays 80–90%. It is possible that the neoplastic cells are derived from embryonic nests of neural stem cells or retinoblasts. Undifferentiated areas of tumours are composed of small, round cells with hyperchromatic nuclei and little cytoplasm. Necrosis and calcification are commonly seen, and spontaneous regression may occur. Differentiation occurs, with the formation of *Flexner–Wintersteiner rosettes* (Fig. 24.47), in which the tumour cells are arranged around a central lumen

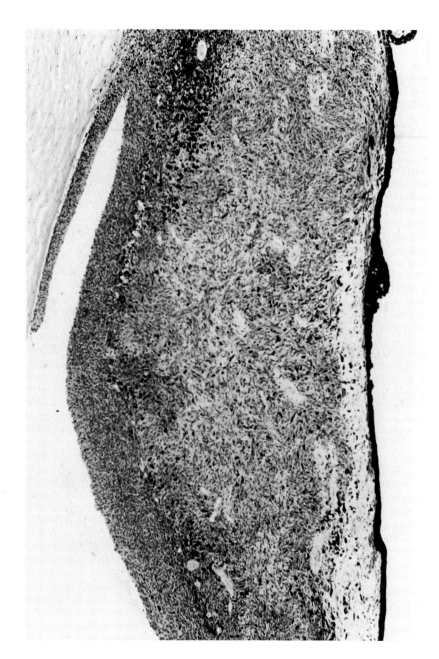

Fig. 24.41 Malignant melanoma of the iris: tumour cells extend from the anterior iris surface to the posterior aspect of the cornea (top right), and there is solid infiltration of the iris leaf. Haematoxylin–eosin × 70

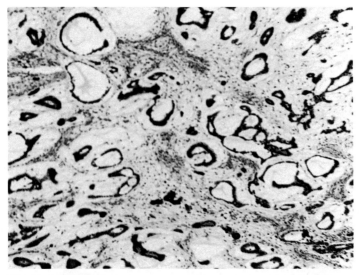

Fig. 24.42 Medulloepithelioma: the neoplastic ciliary epithelium exhibits a tubular pattern.
Haematoxylin-eosin × 70

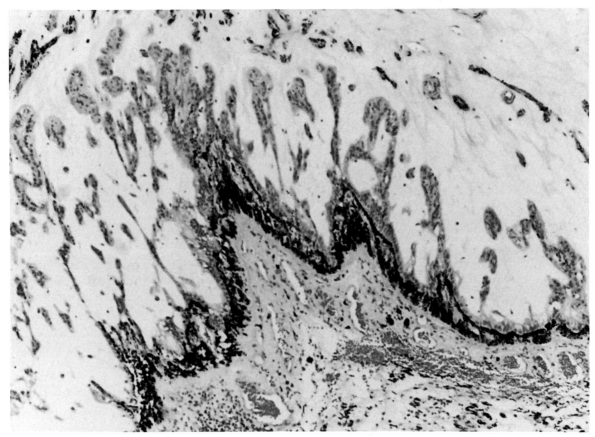

Fig. 24.43 Pseudo-epitheliomatous hyperplasia of the ciliary epithelium.
Haematoxylin-eosin × 95

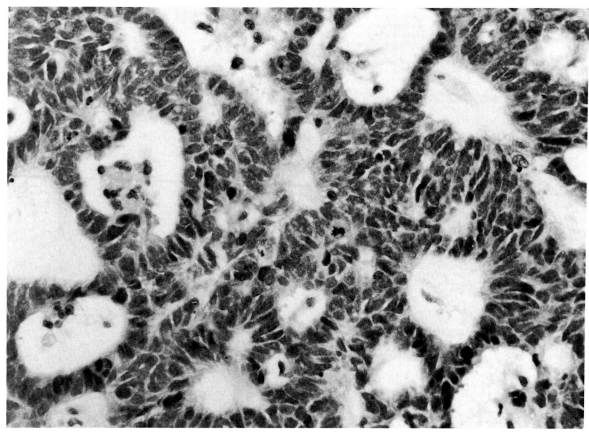

Fig. 24.44 Metastatic adenocarcinoma within the uvea.
Haematoxylin-eosin × 430

which appears to have a limiting membrane similar to the external limiting membrane of the retina. Radial arrangements of cells around a central mass of fibrils are also seen, and these are known as *Homer–Wright rosettes*. 'Fleurettes', which appear to represent abortive photoreceptor structures, can be recognised in some tumours. Pseudorosette formation (Fig. 24.48) is an aggregation of tumour cells around either a blood vessel or an area of necrosis. Growth of retinoblastoma extends into both the subretinal space and the vitreous, the retina usually being detached. Spread can occur along the inner retinal surface and there may be extension into the anterior segment. There may also be infiltration of the choroid and of the optic nerve. Extension of retinoblastoma outside the eye may involve the orbit while distant sites of metastasis include the central nervous system,

bones and lymph nodes. The most important prognostic indicator of a retinoblastoma determinable from routine histological study is the degree of involvement of the optic nerve (Fig. 24.49), the mortality rate being higher if the surgical cut end is infiltrated. Flexner–Wintersteiner rosettes and fleurettes seem to indicate a favourable prognosis; pseudorosette formation has no prognostic significance. Rarely, a retinoblastoma is of the *diffuse infiltrating variety*; usually this occurs in older children and the prognosis is relatively good.

Retinocytoma. A benign variant of retinoblastoma, with well-differentiated cells exhibiting numerous fleurettes, and with no necrosis or mitotic activity, is now recognised and is termed *retinocytoma*.[206]

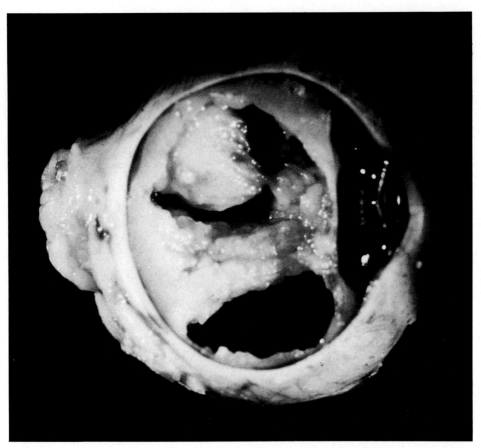

Fig. 24.45 Retinoblastoma: section of a globe opened anteroposteriorly to reveal the tumour occupying much of the posterior segment.
× 4

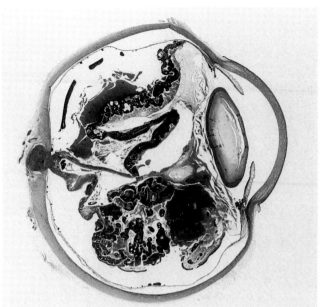

Fig. 24.46 Retinoblastoma: section of an eye showing the tumour involving the posterior segment. Haematoxylin-eosin × 3

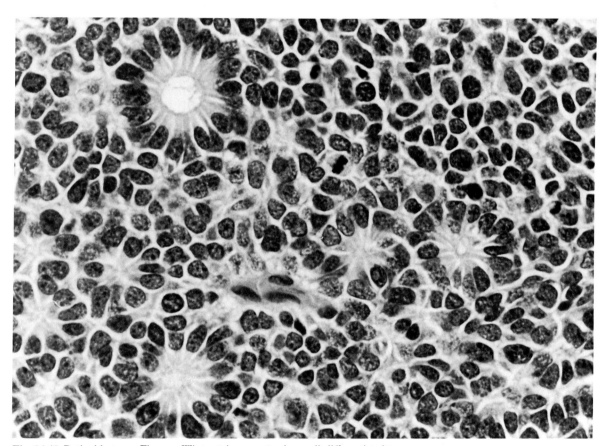

Fig. 24.47 Retinoblastoma: Flexner–Wintersteiner rosettes in a well-differentiated tumour. Haematoxylin-eosin × 850

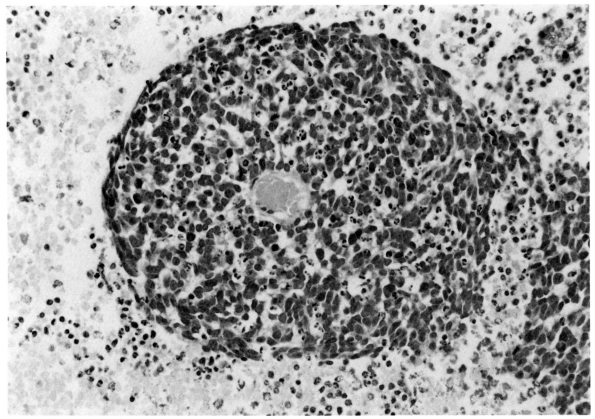

Fig. 24.48 Retinoblastoma: aggregation of tumour cells around a central blood vessel producing a pseudorosette; the adjacent tissue is necrotic.
Haematoxylin-eosin × 430

Phacomatoses

In this group of heredofamilial disorders (see p. 353), the eye is involved together with the skin, the central and peripheral nervous systems, and the viscera. To be considered are *tuberous sclerosis, von Hippel–Lindau angiomatosis, neurofibromatosis, the Sturge–Weber syndrome* and the *Wyburn–Masson syndrome.*

Tuberous sclerosis (Bourneville's disease)[207] (see p. 354). Intraocular lesions occur in about half of the cases of this condition and consist of astrocytic hamartomatous formations involving the optic nerve head and the inner retinal layer.

Von Hippel–Lindau angiomatosis.[208,209] Retinal angiomatosis may be associated with systemic lesions affecting particularly the central nervous system (see p. 355), where angiomatous malformations occur in the cerebellum, medulla, pons and spinal cord. Among other associated conditions there may be renal and pancreatic cysts, adenocarcinoma of the kidney and phaeochromocytoma. The angiomatous malformation in the retina can lead to exudation, haemorrhage and retinal detachment (as occurs in Coats' disease, see p. 721), and eventually to phthisis bulbi.

Neurofibromatosis (von Recklinghausen's disease) (see p. 353). Almost all the ocular tissues can be affected by neurofibromatosis, and meningiomas and astrocytomas of the retina and optic nerve occur more frequently in patients with the disease. Also, any part of the uvea can be involved, and

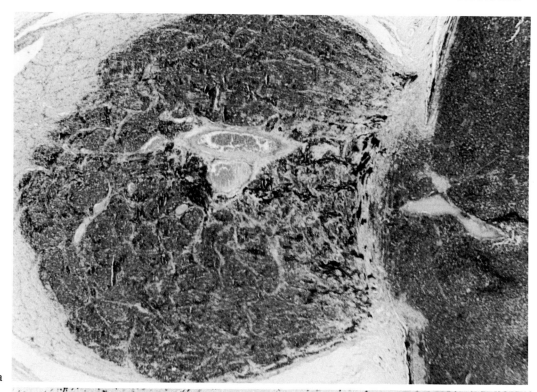

a

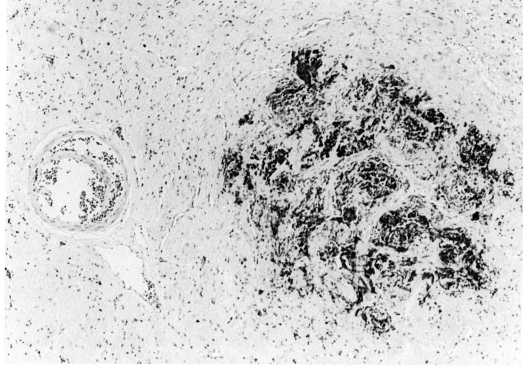

b

Fig. 24.49a, b Retinoblastoma: the optic nerve is infiltrated by tumour.
(**a**) Longitudinal section. (**b**) Transverse section.
Haematoxylin-eosin (**a**) ×30; (**b**) ×110

neurofibromatosis is associated with an increased incidence of congenital glaucoma, melanocytomas and malignant melanomas.

Sturge–Weber syndrome (encephalotrigeminal angiomatosis). In the Sturge–Weber syndrome (see p. 356), facial and intracranial vascular anomalies, and cavernous angioma of the choroid with associated glaucoma, occur, all on the same side.

Wyburn–Masson syndrome. In this syndrome, intracranial racemose angiomatous malformations affecting the midbrain are associated with a similar malformation in the ipsilateral retina. In contrast to other retinal vascular lesions, however, lipid exudation does not occur from the abnormal vessels (see below).

VASCULAR, NEUROLOGICAL AND MUSCULAR DISEASES

Vascular diseases

General considerations[210,211]

The part of the eye mainly affected by vascular diseases is the retina. Before describing the pathology of specific conditions it is beneficial to outline briefly some of the lesions encountered.

Haemorrhages (Fig. 24.50). Trauma, hypertension, inflammation, and haemorrhagic diatheses can all result in extravasation of blood, but haemorrhages also readily occur from abnormal or newly formed vessels. Macroscopically, superficial retinal haemorrhages are flame-shaped or linear because of the arrangement

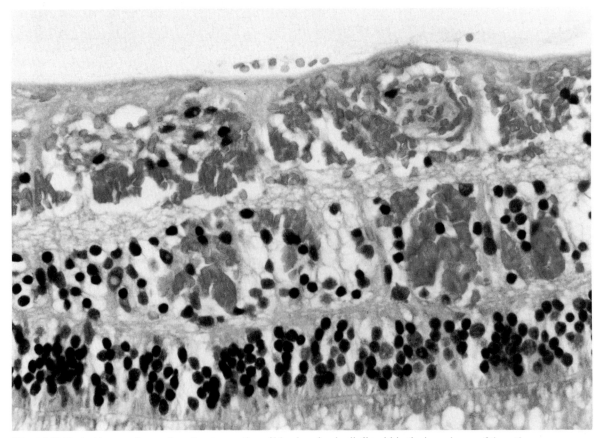

Fig. 24.50 Retinal haemorrhages: there is extravasation of blood, and red cells lie within the inner layers of the retina. Haematoxylin-eosin × 525

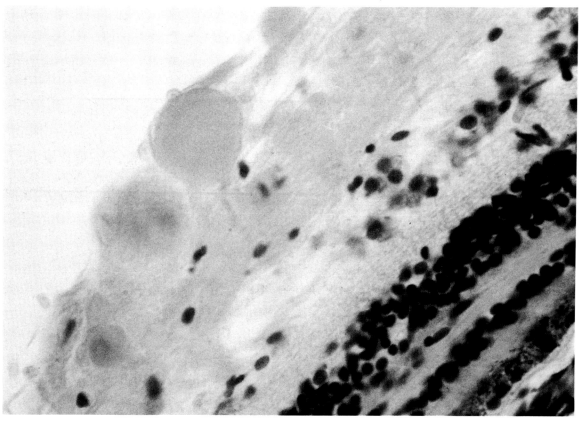

Fig. 24.51 Cytoid bodies: globular structures representing the swollen ends of disrupted axons in the nerve fibre layer (top left).
Haematoxylin-eosin × 950

of the axons in the nerve fibre layer; in contrast, deep haemorrhages are punctate.

Exudates. Exudates either follow structural damage to the endothelial lining of retinal vessels, or develop from abnormal vessels as in diabetes. Leakage of plasma leads to the formation of pools in the outer plexiform layer; the exudates so produced may have a high lipid content, but eventually absorption occurs. Leakage from vessels at the macula can result in *cystoid macular oedema*[212-216] while involvement of the optic nerve head produces *papilloedema*.

'Cotton-wool' spots. Localised lesions known as 'cotton-wool' spots can develop in the nerve fibre layer as the result of focal ischaemia. They consist of aggregates of globular structures known as *cytoid bodies* (Fig. 24.51), representing the swollen ends of disrupted nerve fibres. Following autolysis and phagocytosis, healing occurs with the formation of a glial scar.

Aneurysms. *Leber's miliary aneurysms* represent telangiectasis and varicosity of retinal capillaries. The vessels are excessively permeable and this may lead to the development of Coats' disease (see p. 721). *Microaneurysms* originate either by focal dilatation of a capillary wall or by the fusion of two arms of a capillary loop, and their importance lies in their excessive permeability, which results in serous exudation and haemorrhage. They are seen most often in the retinopathy of diabetes, hypertension, central vein occlusion and macroglobulinaemia.

Neovascularisation. New vessel formation has

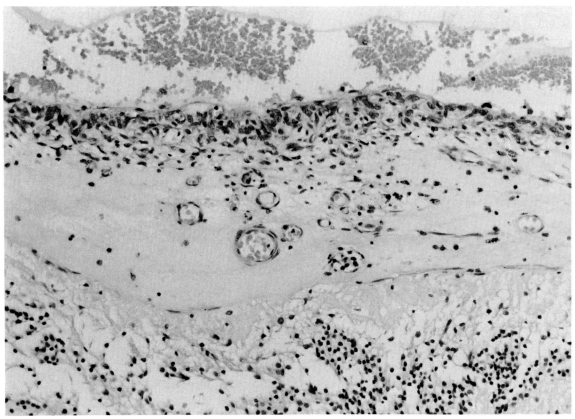

Fig. 24.52 Epiretinal membrane: neovascular tissue (top) on the inner surface of the retina. Haematoxylin-eosin × 190

serious consequences if it occurs at the inner retinal surface and extends into the vitreous where, together with connective tissue proliferation, it results in *epiretinal (preretinal) membrane formation* (Fig. 24.52)[217-222] and *vitreal membrane formation*. The retinopathies of prematurity and of diabetes mellitus, and the occlusion of retinal veins, are important conditions in which this occurs. The same conditions may also give rise to neovascularisation of the iris (Fig. 24.53) and if this extends into the filtration angle, iridocorneal adhesion develops (Fig. 24.54) and this can be followed by glaucoma (*rubeotic or neovascular glaucoma*).

Arteriosclerotic retinopathy

Sclerosed, narrowed vessels (Fig. 24.55) are seen as part of an ageing process, but in the absence of other complicating factors there are no obvious morphological changes in the other retinal elements.

Retinal artery occlusion

The central retinal artery is an end artery, and complete obstruction of the vessel, usually from atherosclerosis, thrombosis, embolism or an inflammatory process, is followed by infarction of the entire retina. Lowering of the blood pressure may also result in ischaemic changes. The retina becomes oedematous and necrotic, and subsequently there is atrophy and gliosis. Occlusion of the main central artery occurs at or behind the lamina cribrosa, but if a main branch vessel is occluded the obstruction is usually at a bifurcation, and infarction of the retina occurs as in central artery occlusion.

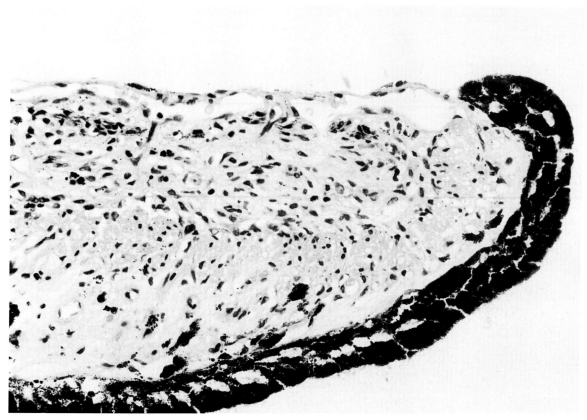

Fig. 24.53 Neovascularisation on the anterior surface of the iris (rubeosis iridis): there is associated slight ectropion uveae, with the pigment layer extending onto the anterior surface of the iris. Haematoxylin-eosin × 430

Retinal vein occlusion

Predisposing factors which can result in occlusion of the central retinal vein include hypertensive vascular disease, abnormal states of the blood such as hyperlipidaemia, polycythaemia and macroglobulinaemia, and vasculitis as is seen in sarcoidosis, Behçet's disease and Eales' disease; not infrequently there is an association with chronic simple glaucoma. Occlusion is thought to occur at the lamina cribrosa, and the effects on the retina are the result of obstructed venous outflow and reduced arterial inflow. If the occlusion is relieved early, there is little, if any, permanent retinal damage; prolonged obstruction can lead to persistent haemorrhages, oedema and cystoid degeneration. About 10–20% of cases of retinal vein occlusion, particularly in the elderly, are followed several months later by glaucoma which develops subsequent to new vessel formation on the anterior iris surface; this condition is known as *thrombotic glaucoma* (rubeotic or neovascular glaucoma). Preretinal vasoproliferation may develop, with resultant vitreal membrane formation. Branch vein occlusion produces similar changes in the area drained by the affected vessel.

Hypertensive retinopathy[223]

Retinopathy in the benign phase of hypertension is unusual, but in the malignant phase there are haemorrhages, 'cotton-wool' spots (see p. 717), serous exudates, and oedema which involves the optic nerve head.

Diabetic retinopathy[224–226]

Diabetes is the commonest cause of proliferative

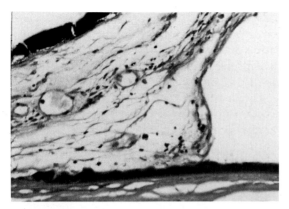

Fig. 24.54 Neovascular tissue in the filtration angle has resulted in iridocorneal adhesion (anterior peripheral synechia).
PAS × 170

retinopathy. The onset of diabetic retinopathy is probably delayed by good control of the metabolic state. In the early stage, the retinopathy can be considered as consisting of background changes which provide the basis for the later development of proliferative lesions. The *background changes* themselves rarely lead to blindness and comprise essentially a microangiopathy involving the arterioles, venules and capillaries. The arterioles exhibit narrowing of their lumen due to hyalinisation of their walls following accumulation of plasma proteins within the vessel wall. The venules become dilated, beaded and sclerosed, and the capillaries exhibit basement membrane thickening, pericyte degeneration and micro-aneurysm formation in addition to focal areas of closure. 'Cotton-wool' spot formation and

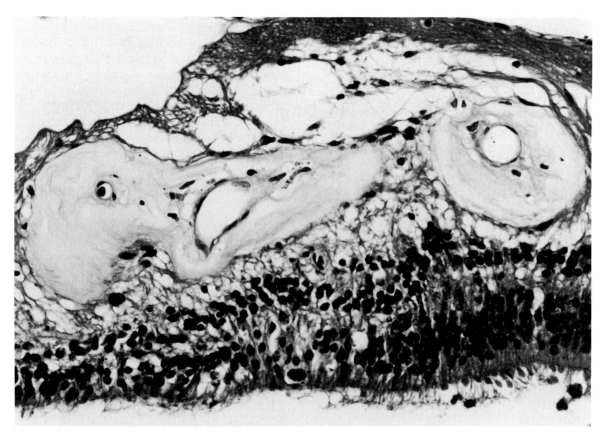

Fig. 24.55 Retinal vascular sclerosis: the vessels have thick walls and narrow lumina.
Gomori's trichrome × 145

neovascularisation follow these background changes. Subsequently, in the *proliferative phase*, in response to retinal hypoxia and the possible release of an angiogenic factor, growth of fibrovascular and glial tissue occurs on the retinal surface and extends into the vitreous. There may be associated haemorrhage, vitreal membrane formation and retinal detachment.

Retinopathy of prematurity[227 – 228]

This disorder, formerly known as *retrolental fibroplasia*, always appears in both eyes, but often to a variable degree. It occurs because the incompletely vascularised retina of an immature, prematurely born infant is susceptible to toxic change induced by high levels of oxygen inhalation. At the onset, there is obliteration of vessels due to oxygen administration which, when discontinued, leads to renewed angioblastic activity and vasoproliferation. This new vessel formation extends into the vitreous, and retinal detachment follows. There may be marked fibrovascular proliferation on the inner surface of the detached retina and the whole mass comes to lie behind the lens, thus producing the fully developed picture of retrolental fibroplasia.

Coats' disease

The term *Coats' type lesion* (or *Coats' syndrome*) is often preferred as the condition may have more than one cause. There may or may not be vascular abnormality as evidenced by telangiectasis or varicosity (*Leber's miliary aneurysms*—see p. 717), sheathing of vessels, and neovascularisation. The changes are nearly always unilateral and usually occur only in males and in the first decade of life. There is intraretinal and subretinal exudate, and the retina becomes detached (Figs 24.56 and 24.57). The basis of the disease appears to be an altered permeability of the retinal capillaries. Pigment and lipid-containing macrophages are seen within the subretinal exudate, and also within the retina, and there is usually conspicuous deposition of cholesterol.

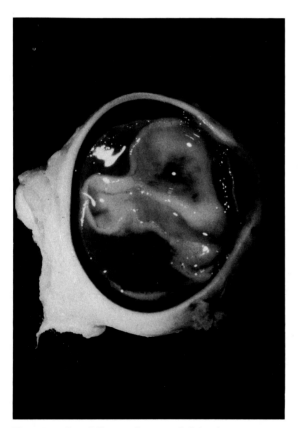

Fig. 24.56 Coats' disease: the opened globe shows detachment of the retina and a subretinal lipid-containing exudate.
× 2

Eales' disease

This generally affects young adult males and is usually unilateral. There is retinal periphlebitis, and neovascularisation and haemorrhage may ensue. The cause of the disease is unknown.

Retinopathy in other conditions

Some of the immune disorders, particularly *systemic lupus erythematosus*, *scleroderma* and *polyarteritis nodosa*, may be associated with a retinopathy, as may *macroglobulinaemia* and *sickle cell disease*.

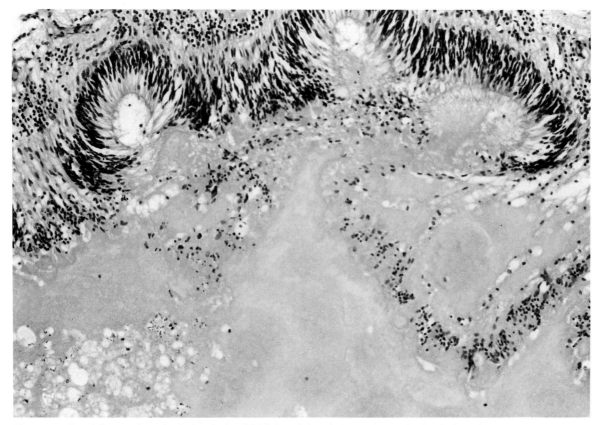

Fig. 24.57 Coats' disease: the retina is detached and folded, and there is intraretinal and subretinal exudate. Haematoxylin-eosin × 145

Neurological diseases

Multiple sclerosis (see p. 255)

Visual impairment, usually unilateral, due to optic nerve involvement often occurs in multiple sclerosis. The pathological changes develop within the axial zone of the retrobulbar portion of the nerve where there is demyelination with degeneration of oligodendrocytes and myelin sheaths, the axons being left relatively intact. There is associated vasocongestion and a mild perivasculitis, while microglial cells phagocytose the myelin debris, and this is followed by an intense astrocytic proliferation with resultant gliosis.

Neuromyelitis optica (Devic's disease)

Neuromyelitis optica is regarded as an acute, virulent form of multiple sclerosis, and it results in bilateral loss of vision. The histological changes in the optic nerves are similar to those seen in multiple sclerosis.

Subacute sclerosing panencephalitis

The focal choroidoretinitis which occurs in this inflammatory condition can cause visual impairment. Visual impairment may also result from cerebral involvement (see p. 212).

Toxic optic neuropathy

In rare instances, *methyl alcohol*, *tobacco* and *drugs* (e.g. tryparsamide) have produced retrobulbar degeneration of the optic nerve.

Muscular diseases

A number of diseases of muscle can involve the

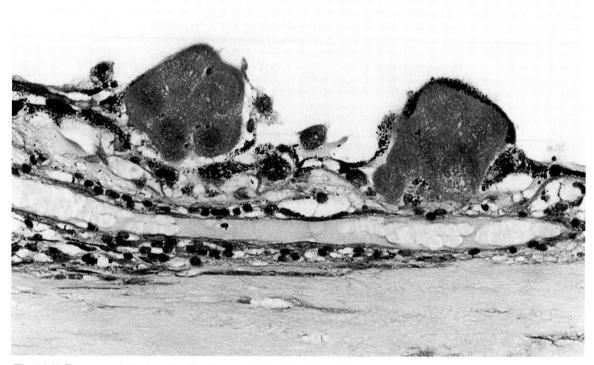

Fig. 24.58 Drusen: nodular deposits of hyaline material on Bruch's membrane. PAS × 525

ocular musculature (see p. 621). *Myasthenia gravis* (see p. 656), produces ptosis and ophthalmoplegia; ptosis is also seen in *myotonic dystrophy* (see p. 624). Some of the other conditions associated with *external ophthalmoplegia* are referred to on page 422.

MISCELLANEOUS DISORDERS OF THE CHOROID AND RETINA

Drusen[229-230]

Deposits of hyaline material on Bruch's membrane are known as drusen (Fig. 24.58), a name derived from the German word *Druse*, meaning a crystallined rock cavity (geode). Drusen may develop as an ageing phenomenon, but are seen in association with retinal detachment, inflammatory and neoplastic lesions, and vascular disorders, and also in phthistical eyes (see p. 680). They should not be confused with *drusen of the optic nerve head*[231] which are thought to be related to axonal degeneration.

Angioid streaks[232]

Angioid streaks are linear brown strands radiating from the optic nerve head. They are bilateral and may be associated with *Paget's disease of bone, pseudoxanthoma elasticum* or the *Ehlers–Danlos syndrome*. They also occur in the absence of any systemic disorder. There is calcification and disruption of Bruch's membrane with proliferation of fibrovascular tissue and atrophy of the pigment epithelium and retinal photoreceptor cells.

Peripheral microcystoid degeneration of the retina

Nearly all adult eyes exhibit this degenerative condition in which cystic lesions are found at the

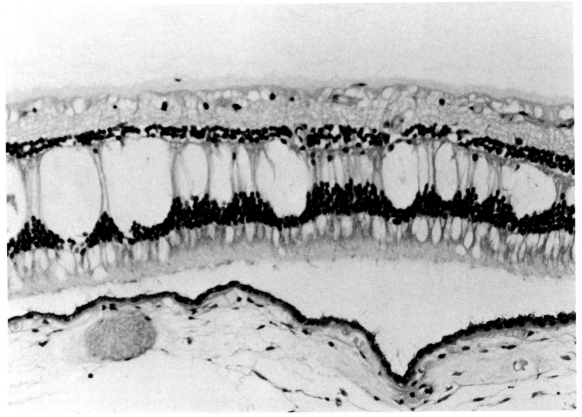

Fig. 24.59 Peripheral microcystic degeneration of the retina: well-circumscribed cystic spaces involve the outer plexiform layer.
Haematoxylin-eosin ×240

retinal periphery (Fig. 24.59), more particularly on the temporal side. Small spaces involve the outer plexiform layer only; large ones affect the inner nuclear and inner plexiform layers also. The walls of the cysts are lined by Müller cells (glial supporting cells characteristic of the nervous portion of the retina). The spaces can enlarge even further, with the consequent development of splits or holes, and retinal detachment may develop.

Senile macular degeneration[233-236]

This occurs, usually bilaterally, in ageing eyes and results from senile vascular disease of the underlying choriocapillaris. Morphologically it may be either *non-disciform* or *disciform*. Disciform degeneration is associated with breaks in Bruch's membrane, which is often calcified, and vascular ingrowth from the choriocapillaris with the sub-

sequent formation of a subretinal fibrovascular plaque. There may be associated haemorrhage, and nests of pigment epithelium cells are seen; degenerative changes occur in the overlying retina, from which vasoproliferation may extend into the subretinal plaque.

Central serous retinopathy

Central serous retinopathy is a self-limiting condition which lasts for a few months. It is of unknown aetiology and may develop in young adults, usually males. It is most often unilateral. The lesion is in the macular region and consists of an accumulation of serous fluid, either between the neurosensory retina and the pigment epithelium, resulting in detachment of the former, or beneath the pigment epithelium itself. The retinal photoreceptors remain normal in appearance.

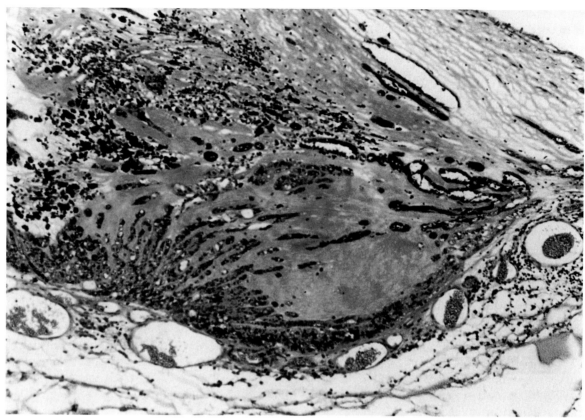

Fig. 24.60 *Ringschwiele*: there is proliferation of retinal pigment epithelium with laminar formation of fibrous tissue. Haematoxylin-eosin × 105

Retinal detachment

The neurosensory retina separates from the pigment epithelium to produce 'detachment' in a variety of pathological conditions. When detachment develops from a rent ('rhegma') or hole in the retina it is known as *rhegmatogenous detachment*. When there is no rent or hole the condition is known as *non-rhegmatogenous detachment*: in these cases the retina becomes 'detached' as the result of an exudative or neoplastic process beneath, or by traction from within the vitreous. The neurosensory retina becomes separated from the blood supply of the choriocapillaris, and the earliest change is degeneration of the rods and cones. The changes then extend to the outer plexiform layer and large cystic spaces are formed. Gliosis and connective tissue proliferation result in tightening and fixed fold formation, and sub-sequently Bruch's membrane thickens and drusen form, while at the periphery and in the pars plana of the ciliary body a *Ringschwiele* (see Glossary, p. 748) may develop (Fig. 24.60).

Retinitis pigmentosa (pigmentary retinopathy)[237–243]

Retinitis pigmentosa is not an inflammatory condition and so the suffix 'itis' is inappropriate, but the alternative term, pigmentary retinopathy, has failed to replace the more traditional and familiar name. The disease displays a multimodal pattern of inheritance, but is usually transmitted as an autosomal recessive trait; it may, however, be either autosomal dominant, X-linked or sporadic. The signs and symptoms appear in early adult life and consist of visual impairment, in which night blindness is a notable feature. Bilateral involvement is usual. Cataract formation is often associated with the disease. Less frequently, other conditions occur with retinitis pigmentosa; they include keratoconus, myopia and Coats' disease. The changes commence in the mid-periphery, but progress to involve the entire retina. Initially, there is degeneration of rods and cones, but eventually all the retinal layers become attenuated and atrophic, and there is gliosis. Melanin pigment, derived from the pigment epithelium, migrates into the neurosensory retina and is deposited in and around the walls of the blood vessels, which are sclerosed. Secondary degenerative changes develop in the optic nerve. Atypical forms of retinitis pigmentosa include central and sectorial types, in which the changes are confined to particular areas of the retina, and *retinitis pigmentosa sine pigmento*, in which there is no pigmentary disturbance. *Leber's congenital amaurosis* is considered to be a congenital form of retinitis pigmentosa.

The pathogenesis of retinitis pigmentosa is obscure. It is a dystrophic condition in which selected mature retinal elements undergo regression and the pigment epithelium is involved along with the neurosensory retina. One theory postulates a primary, genetically induced degeneration of photoreceptors, and another points towards altered function of the retinal pigment epithelium; defective interaction between photoreceptors and pigment epithelium has also been suggested. Pigmentary retinopathy sometimes forms a part of the following syndromes, many of which reflect deficiencies in enzyme synthesis:[244]

1. The mucopolysaccharidoses
   a. Scheie's (MPS type I–S)
   b. Hunter's (MPS type II)[245]
   c. Sanfilippo's (MPS type III)[246,247]
2. Batten–Mayou
3. Laurence–Moon–Bardet–Biedl
4. Bassen–Kornzweig
5. Refsum's
6. Sjögren–Larsson
7. Hallgren's
8. Alström's
9. Usher's
10. Diallinas–Amalric
11. Cockayne's
12. Hallervorden–Spatz
13. Pelizaeus–Merzbacher
14. Alport's
15. Kearns–Sayre
16. Zellweger's[248,249]

Massive gliosis

Gliosis occurs in the retina as a reparative process. Occasionally it can be so massive as to present tumour-like proportions. In this stage it represents formation of hyperplastic scar tissue. The predisposing condition may have occurred years previously.

THE LENS[250]

Cataract (Fig. 24.61)[251–253]

The causes of cataract formation are many and varied. Some may be *congenital* and associated with other developmental anomalies, but the most common are *senile cataracts* and cataracts resulting from *trauma*, with or without perforation of the globe or the retention of an intraocular foreign body. Cataracts may also arise as the result of *drug administration*, such as corticosteroid therapy; they occur in metabolic diseases, particularly diabetes mellitus, and they can also be associated with *diseases of the skin. Inflammatory lesions, neoplasms* and *glaucoma* are among the intraocular conditions which may result in the development of cataract.

In the development of cataract there is *denaturation of lens protein*, which alters the state of hydration; liquefaction develops in the cortex, and *clefts, vacuoles*, and small *hyaline spheres (Morgagnian droplets)* are seen. *Calcification* may occur, and *subepithelial fibrosis* can develop as the result of a metaplastic change in the lens epithelium. The latter can also migrate posteriorly and the cells become swollen subsequent to imbibition of fluid from the liquefied cortex. Certain changes seen in relation to the lens warrant further description.

Morgagnian cataract. This is the name given to the appearance of a shrunken, sclerotic nucleus lying in a fluid cortex.

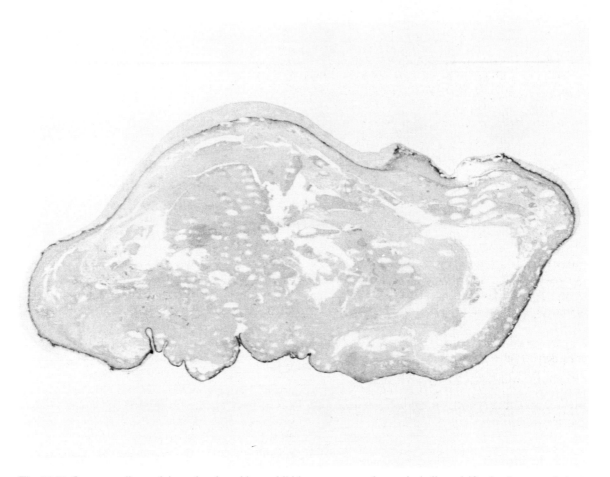

Fig. 24.61 Cataract: a distorted, irregular-shaped lens exhibiting cataractous changes including calcification (seen as a dark linear deposit at the periphery).
Haematoxylin-eosin ×25

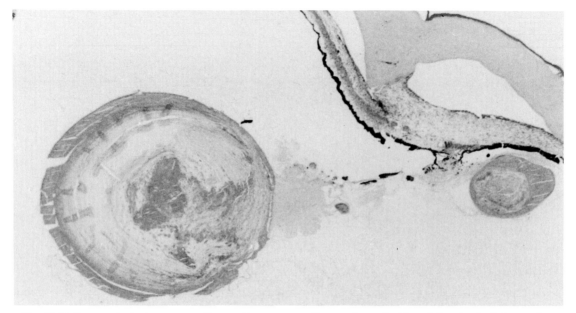

Fig. 24.62 Soemmering's ring cataract: disrupted lens remnants lie posterior to the iris and there is a healed corneal perforation with leucoma adherens (right).
Haematoxylin-eosin × 50

Soemmering's ring cataract. A Soemmering's ring cataract develops after rupture of the lens capsule following either surgery or injury, and is in essence a ring of cataractous material with absence of lens in the central area (Fig. 24.62).

Hirschberg–Elschnig pearls. These are proliferating epithelial cells situated on the lens capsule; they are seen in association with lens remnants.

Pseudoexfoliation of the lens capsule (see capsular glaucoma—p. 731).

Lens dislocation

Dislocation of the lens most commonly follows *trauma*, but it can occur spontaneously where there are defects in the zonular fibres or the ciliary body such as occur in *homocystinuria* (Fig. 24.63) and in the *syndromes of Marfan* and *Weill–Marchesani*.

Intraocular lens implantation[254–261]

Intraocular lens implantation can cause changes in the eye, the nature of which depend upon the type of implant used and its site. Corneal endothelial damage, as evidenced by sparsity of cells, can result in bullous keratopathy and its sequelae, and there may be stromal oedema in addition to thickening, and lamination and/or dehiscence of Descemet's membrane together with cornea guttata and the formation of a thin membrane of fibrous tissue posterior to Descemet's membrane; these changes collectively are known as *pseudophakic keratopathy* (Fig. 24.64) although all may not be seen together in any one specimen. Uveitis, glaucoma and haemorrhage (UGH syndrome), vitreous and retinal detachment, retinal tears and cystoid macular oedema have been described. Infective endophthalmitis due to faulty sterilisation procedures has been reported.

THE VITREOUS

Neovascularisation and vitreal membranes

Inflammatory or haemorrhagic exudate in the vitreous occurs in association with other ocular conditions, while neovascular tissue can proliferate into the vitreous either in the process of organisation of such exudate or alternatively from

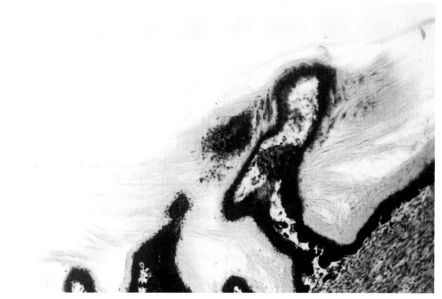

Fig. 24.63 Homocystinuria: thickened zonular fibres are seen in relation to the ciliary epithelium.
Haematoxylin-eosin × 250

a retinopathy (see p. 717). The vitreal membranes so produced have potentially serious deleterious effects on vision, an important mechanism by which this may occur being the development of *traction detachment of the retina.*

Synchysis scintillans

Synchysis scintillans is the presence of golden-

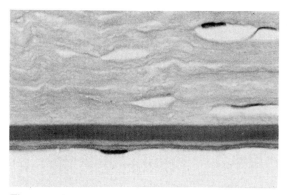

Fig. 24.64 Pseudophakic keratopathy: there is sparsity of corneal endothelium. Descemet's membrane appears slightly thickened and there is a thin membrane of fibrous tissue posteriorly.
PAS × 700

yellow cholesterol crystals in a liquefied vitreous on macroscopical examination of an opened eye. The crystals move freely, but settle in the most dependent position of the globe. The condition is considered to be part of a diffuse deposition of cholesterol within the eye. It is often associated with longstanding detachment of the retina.

Asteroid hyalosis[262–264]

White, round opacities suspended in the vitreous in an otherwise normal eye constitute asteroid hyalosis. As with synchysis scintillans, the condition is observed on macroscopical examination. The opacities are probably either lipids or soaps containing calcium and show no tendency to settle.

GLAUCOMA

Glaucoma is a disease characterised by raised intraocular pressure, pathological cupping of the optic nerve head and damage to retinal and optic nerve fibre bundles. A number of types are recognised, but most cases are due to *impaired outflow of aqueous* consequent upon abnormalities either at the iridocorneal angle or within the tissues of the outflow apparatus.

Congenital glaucoma

Developmental anomalies such as *goniodysgenesis* (malformation of the filtration angle) result in obstruction to the drainage of aqueous, but glaucoma in infants is, on occasion, associated with other disorders, such as the *phacomatoses* (see p. 714).

Open-angle glaucoma—primary (chronic simple glaucoma)

The pathological processes in this type of glaucoma occur within the outflow apparatus. Thickening of the uveal and corneoscleral trabeculae, loss of cellularity in the endothelial meshwork with replacement by hyaline material, and proliferation of endothelial cells are established, recognisable changes, seen by light microscopy. Other, and in some instances more subtle and controversial changes, visualised only by electron microscopy, have been described.[265]

Open-angle glaucoma—secondary

Inflammatory and haemorrhagic debris, macrophages containing material derived from altered lens tissue, tumour cells, pseudoexfoliative capsular material, melanin pigment, or scar tissue may all obstruct the aqueous outflow pathway.

Phacolytic glaucoma. Hypermature, cataractous lens material may escape into the aqueous without there being a demonstrable defect in the lens

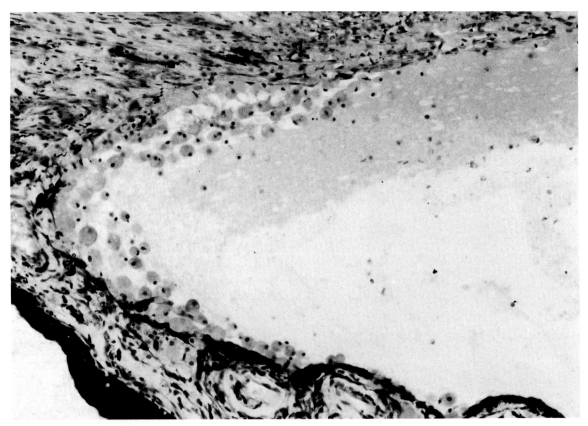

Fig. 24.65 Phacolytic glaucoma: macrophages containing lens material lie within the aqueous at the filtration angle of the anterior chamber.
Haematoxylin-eosin × 190

capsule. There is a macrophage response, phago-cytosis occurs and the accumulation of cells (Fig. 24.65) results in mechanical obstruction to the outflow of aqueous.

Capsular glaucoma.[266,267] Material (pseudo-exfoliative) derived from the capsule or the epithelium of the lens, or from the ciliary epithelium, is deposited on tissue surfaces within the anterior segment, particularly on the lens capsule and zonular fibres, and on the epithelium of the iris and ciliary body. The material is also seen within the aqueous and its outflow system and there is consequent mechanical blockage with sub-sequent glaucoma. The pseudoexfoliative material has a 'Christmas tree' or 'shrub-like' appearance in histological sections (Fig. 24.66).

Pigmentary glaucoma. In myopic patients, usually young adults, the pigment epithelium of the iris may detach and become atrophic. Granules of melanin pigment are extruded and these circulate within the aqueous and become phagocytosed both by macrophages and by trabecular endothelial cells. Inhibition of aqueous drainage results and glaucoma follows.

Contusion angle deformity. Blunt trauma with recession of the filtration angle leads to secondary open-angle glaucoma. In the period immediately following injury this may be due to mechanical ob-struction with inflammatory cells, but in the later stages disorganisation of the trabecular meshwork and the formation of scar tissue impair aqueous drainage.

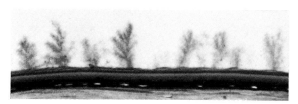

Fig. 24.66 Pseudo-exfoliative material on the lens capsule: the 'Christmas tree' or 'shrub-like' appearance is characteristic.
Methenamine (hexamine) silver × 350

Closed-angle glaucoma—primary

An anatomical abnormality resulting in irido-trabecular contact leads to primary closed-angle glaucoma.

Closed-angle glaucoma—secondary

Secondary closed-angle glaucoma results from inflammatory, vascular and neoplastic diseases which are associated with *neovascularisation* on the anterior surface of the iris. This type of glaucoma is seen also in the *iridocorneal–endothelial (ICE) syndrome*, in which there is iris 'naevus' formation, iris atrophy, formation of peripheral anterior synechiae and corneal endothelial dystrophy with proliferation of endothelial cells and their extension over the anterior surface of the iris.

Effects of raised intraocular pressure

In children, a raised intraocular pressure stretches the corneoscleral envelope diffusely to produce *buphthalmos* (Fig. 24.67), whereas in adults stretching is more localised and *staphylomas* develop, either at the sites of neurovascular channels or in areas weakened by previous inflammation. Sudden elevation of the intraocular pressure produces corneal oedema; the endothelial cells become attenuated and relatively sparse, extracellular fluid accumulates in the stroma, the epithelial cells swell, and bullae form (*bullous keratopathy*) (Fig. 24.68); subsequently there may be infection and keratitis with resultant pannus formation and scarring. If the intraocular pressure is raised over a prolonged period the uvea becomes atrophic. However, the effect of glaucoma on the posterior segment is primarily on the optic nerve head,[268-271] where subsequent to issue destruction, with loss of neurovascular tissue, the lamina cribrosa is either bowed or displaced posteriorly so that a *pathological cup* (Fig. 24.69) develops. In *Schnabel's cavernous optic atrophy*, a cavity in the optic nerve, filled with fluid rich in hyaluronic acid, lies behind the lamina cribrosa. Chronic glaucoma also results in atrophy of the inner layers of the retina, mainly the ganglion cell and nerve fibre layer (Fig. 24.70).

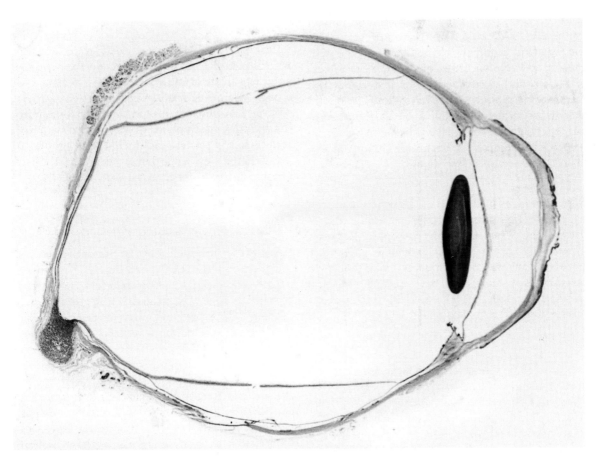

Fig. 24.67 Buphthalmos: section of the enlarged globe, showing its thin corneoscleral envelope.
Haematoxylin-eosin × 6

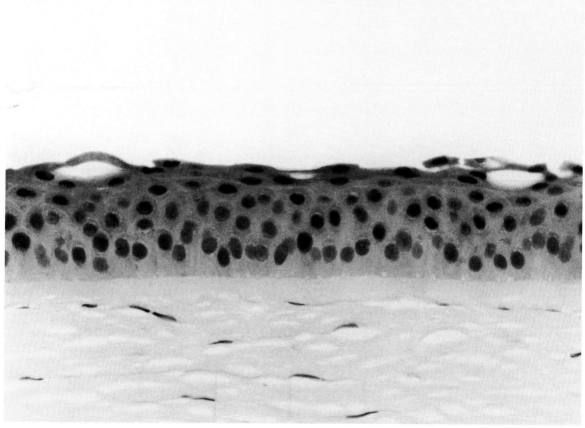

Fig. 24.68 Bullous keratopathy: the epithelium exhibits superficial bulla formation. Haematoxylin-eosin × 525

DEGENERATIVE AND DYSTROPHIC CONDITIONS OF THE CONJUNCTIVA AND CORNEA

Pinguecula and pterygium[272,273]

These conditions can result from repetitive environmental stimuli such as dust and other particulate matter, wind, solar radiation and chemical pollution of the air. A pinguecula is a yellowish elevated focus in the conjunctiva close to the limbus. A pterygium is a wing-shaped mass of thickened conjunctiva that extends across the limbus onto the cornea. Histologically, in both conditions, amorphous, hyaline material is seen in the subepithelial stroma and the fibrocytes are often increased in number, but the essential feature of both lesions is elastotic degeneration of collagen (Fig. 24.71). In addition, a pterygium,

because of its extent, exhibits conspicuous stromal vascularity. In both types of lesion, calcification can occur and the overlying epithelium may become atrophic, hyperplastic, dysplastic or even neoplastic. Gaucher's disease predisposes to the formation of pingueculae.

Hassall–Henle warts

Hassall–Henle warts are localised, well-circumscribed, nodular, flat-topped excrescences on the posterior aspect of the periphery of Descemet's membrane. Their development is regarded as an ageing process.

Arcus senilis

Arcus senilis is the result of ageing, and occurs

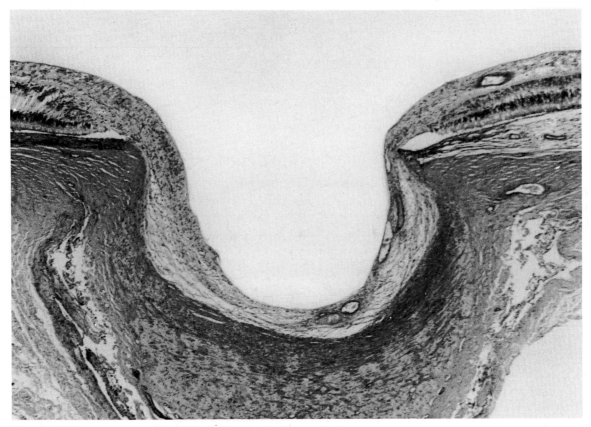

Fig. 24.69 Glaucoma: section of a pathologically cupped optic nerve head.
PAS ×50

locally at the corneal periphery. Separated from the limbus by a clear zone, it is seen in sections as fat droplets in the stromal lamellae. A similar condition may develop in the young (*arcus juvenilis*), usually in association with hyperlipidaemia.

Keratinoid degeneration (spheroidal or Labrador keratopathy, Bietti's nodular keratopathy, climatic droplet keratopathy)

Usually seen in elderly people, this condition is characterised by the presence of hyaline deposits of degenerate collagen in the superficial stroma of the cornea (Fig. 24.72). Similar stimuli to those resulting in pinguecula and pterygium are the predisposing factors (see above).

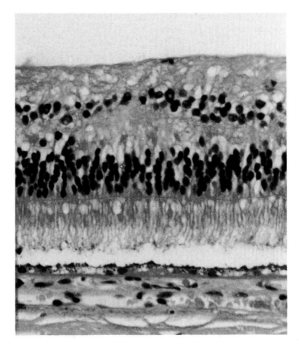

Fig. 24.70 Atrophy of the inner layers of the retina as seen in longstanding glaucoma.
Haematoxylin-eosin ×350

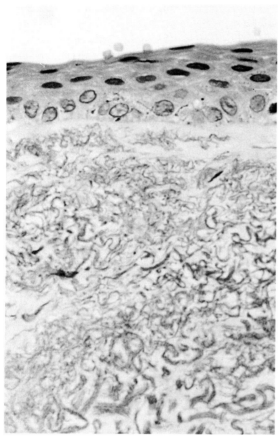

Fig. 24.71 Pinguecula and pterygium: elastotic degeneration of collagen in the subepithelial conjunctival stroma. Haematoxylin-eosin × 700

Band keratopathy

Deposition of calcium in the cornea can occur in any patient with a high level of serum calcium, as with hypervitaminosis D, renal insufficiency, or hyperparathyroidism, but more frequently it develops as a secondary response to a localised inflammatory or degenerative process. The calcium is deposited in the interpalpebral zone as a horizontal band (hence the name), primarily in Bowman's layer, but also on occasion within the superficial stroma (Fig. 24.73), and within the epithelium.

Pannus

Ingrowth of tissue from the limbus into the peripheral part of the cornea, between Bowman's layer and the epithelium, constitutes pannus. It may be of inflammatory origin, following kerato-conjunctivitis, or degenerative, following such conditions as longstanding glaucoma. Histologically, it consists of collagenous or vascularised connective tissue (Fig. 24.74).

Lipid keratopathy

Deposition of lipid in the cornea may occur either in systemic disorders of lipid metabolism or subsequent to corneal vascularisation.

Salzmann's nodular degeneration

Nodular masses of collagen in the superficial corneal stroma, with associated epithelial

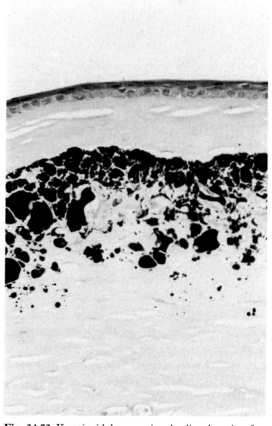

Fig. 24.72 Keratinoid degeneration: hyaline deposits of degenerate collagen are seen in the superficial stroma of the cornea.
Rhodamine B × 200

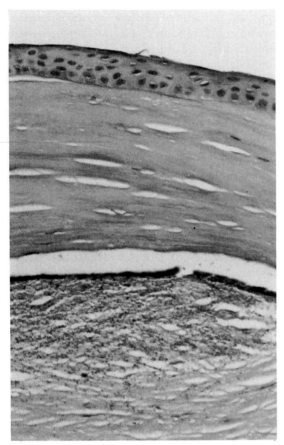

Fig. 24.73 Band keratopathy: calcium is deposited within the disrupted Bowman's layer, and within the superficial stroma of the cornea; there is, in addition, a thick layer of collagenous tissue (pannus) between the epithelium (top) and Bowman's layer.
Haematoxylin-eosin × 250

irregularity and pannus formation, constitute Salzmann's nodular degeneration. The condition follows inflammation or injury.

Amyloid degeneration

In addition to the amyloid seen in lattice dystrophy (see p. 738), the eye may be involved in other forms of local and systemic amyloidosis, amyloid being deposited particularly under the conjunctiva and within the eyelids.

Keratoconus

Keratoconus (Fig. 24.75), which is seen most frequently in girls and young women, is characterised by thinning, scarring and ectasia of the central part of the cornea. The apex of the cone is slightly below and to the nasal side of the cornea. The condition almost always affects both eyes. Its cause is not known. There are ruptures in Bowman's layer, the defects being filled with collagen (Fig. 24.76); the stroma is thinned, and there may be rupture of Descemet's membrane. Corneal oedema may occur as a complication and an intra-epithelial line of iron (*Fleischer's ring*) can form at the base of the cone. In some instances keratoconus is associated with other abnormalities such as Marfan's syndrome, Down's syndrome, and aniridia.

Corneal dystrophies

These are primary, bilateral, heredofamilial

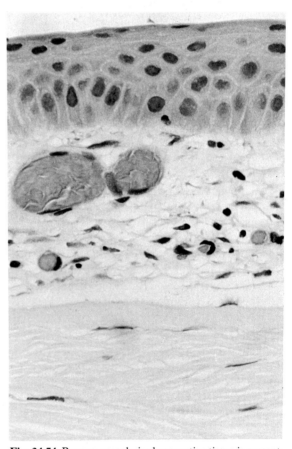

Fig. 24.74 Pannus: vascularised connective tissue is present between the epithelium (above) and Bowman's layer (below).
Haematoxylin-eosin × 550

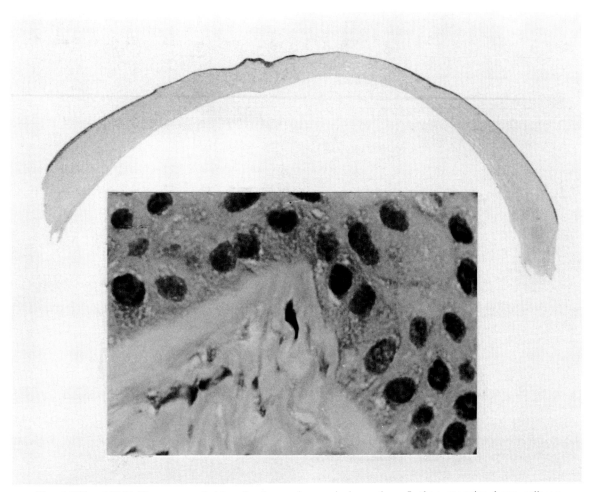

Figs. 24.75 and 24.76 Keratoconus. A thinned and scarred cornea is shown above. In the preparation shown, collagen can be seen to fill the gap between the ends of the disrupted Bowman's layer.
Haematoxylin-eosin × 25 above, × 1350 beneath

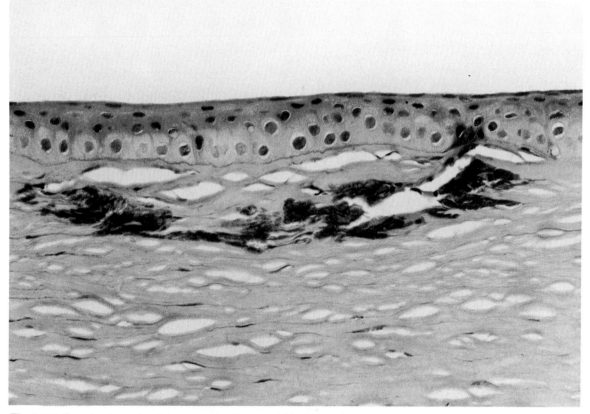

Fig. 24.77 Granular dystrophy of the cornea: hyaline material in the anterior stroma. Masson's trichrome × 430

conditions unaccompanied by systemic disease. They are classified into three main groups, according to whether the initial involvement is in the epithelium, its basement membrane or Bowman's layer (*anterior dystrophies*), in the stroma (*stromal dystrophies*), or in Descemet's membrane or the endothelium (*posterior dystrophies*).

Anterior dystrophies. Characteristically, in the epithelial dystrophies there is intra-epithelial cyst formation, the cysts usually containing degenerate epithelial cells. The epithelial dystrophies include *Meesman's dystrophy* and *Cogan's dystrophy*, and the inherited form of the recurrent erosion syndrome. *Reis–Bücklers dystrophy* involves defects in the epithelial basement membrane with deposition of fibrillary material in Bowman's layer.

Stromal dystrophies. The three classical stromal dystrophies are all progressive, but whereas two of

them, *granular* and *lattice*, are dominantly inherited, the third, *macular*, is transmitted as an autosomal recessive.

(1) *Granular dystrophy*.[274] Discrete opacities appear in the anterior stromal layers of the cornea. Histologically, these are granules of hyaline material (Fig. 24.77) which represents protein secretions from the keratocytes; Masson's trichrome stain colours them a brilliant red. The intervening corneal tissue is normal.

(2) *Lattice dystrophy.* Interlacing or overlapping linear stromal deposits, arranged radially, are seen, and can be shown to be *amyloid* (Fig. 24.78). While lattice dystrophy usually occurs as an isolated condition, on rare occasions it is associated with systemic amyloidosis.

(3) *Macular dystrophy*.[275] In this, the most visually disabling of the stromal dystrophies, the

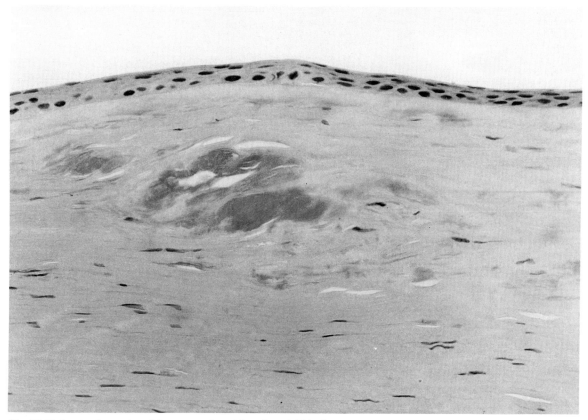

Fig. 24.78 Lattice dystrophy of the cornea: deposition of amyloid in the stroma. Congo red × 430

entire cornea is involved in the accumulation of opaque material which can be demonstrated to be *mucopolysaccharide* (Fig. 24.79). The deposits extend to lie beneath the epithelium and there may also be involvement of the endothelium with the production of excrescences on Descemet's membrane.

Schnyder's dystrophy (central crystalline dystrophy).[276] There are deposits of crystalline material, probably unesterified cholesterol, beneath Bowman's layer in this uncommon dystrophic condition. It is an autosomal dominant disorder, occurring in early life.

Posterior dystrophies. Fuchs' endothelial dystrophy, posterior polymorphous dystrophy and *congenital hereditary endothelial dystrophy* are the important members of this group.

(1) *Fuchs' endothelial dystrophy.* Fuchs' endothelial dystrophy is bilateral, and the characteristic histological changes involve the endothelium and Descemet's membrane. The endothelial cells degenerate and eventually disappear while Descemet's membrane becomes thickened and laminated, and bears irregular, guttate excrescences on its posterior surface (*cornea guttata*—Fig. 24.80). Functional abnormality follows and stromal oedema and bullous keratopathy may develop.

(2) *Posterior polymorphous dystrophy.*[277-278] This dystrophy is also usually bilateral. Descemet's membrane appears thickened, nodular and vesicular, but cornea guttata is not present in the early stages. The endothelial cells take on the appearance of epithelial cells, becoming multilayered and showing microvilli and intercellular

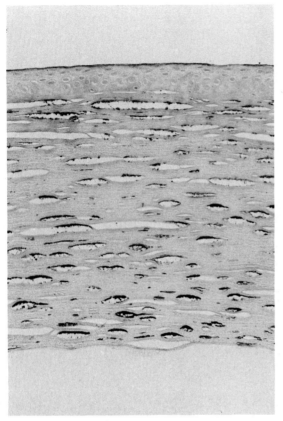

Fig. 24.79 Macular dystrophy of the cornea: mucopolysaccharide is deposited throughout its entire thickness.
Colloidal iron × 200

bridges with tonofibrils; the resulting dysfunction causes stromal and epithelial oedema.

(3) *Congenital hereditary endothelial dystrophy*. In this very rare disorder, fibrous tissue is deposited as a thin layer posterior to Descemet's membrane. The endothelial cells are destroyed and stromal oedema may ensue.

METABOLIC DISORDERS[279]

A number of disorders of metabolism which affect the eye are referred to in other pages of this chapter, but some conditions have not been mentioned. They are, for the most part, considered in detail in other chapters of this volume; the main ocular lesions that they produce are described here.

Mucopolysaccharidoses

Several types of mucopolysaccharidosis (MPS) affect the eyes, resulting in clouding of the cornea, cataract and pigmentary degeneration of the retina (see retinitis pigmentosa, p. 725). The classical form of mucopolysaccharidosis is *Hurler's syndrome* (MPS type I-H, gargoylism), in which a ground-glass appearance of the cornea is due to the deposition of mucopolysaccharides in the

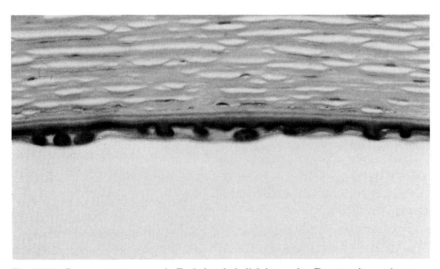

Fig. 24.80 Cornea guttata as seen in Fuchs' endothelial dystrophy: Descemet's membrane (bottom) is thickened and no endothelial cells are visible.
PAS × 250

posterior stroma. The cornea is also cloudy in *Scheie's syndrome* (MPS type I-S). In *Hunter's syndrome* (MPS type II) and *Sanfilippo's syndrome* (MPS type III) the cornea is usually spared.

Sphingolipidoses (see p. 341)

This group of metabolic disorders includes G_{M2} *gangliosidosis type I* (Tay–Sachs disease), G_{M2} *gangliosidosis type II* (Sandhoff's disease),[280] *Niemann–Pick disease*,[281] *metachromatic leucodystrophy, Fabry's disease, Krabbe's disease* and *Gaucher's / disease*. These conditions are characterised by widespread intracellular storage of lipid. The brain cells and retinal ganglion cells are particularly affected, but in Niemann–Pick disease and Fabry's disease the lens and cornea are also involved. Usually, the only ocular manifestation of Gaucher's disease is the development of pingueculae.

Thyrotoxicosis

Dysthyroid exophthalmos is usually, but not invariably, bilateral. There is enlargement of the extraocular muscles, and histologically there is a chronic inflammatory cell infiltrate which involves all the orbital tissues. Ultimately fibrosis develops.

Wilson's disease (hepatolenticular degeneration)

In Wilson's disease (see p. 302),[282] cataract and a *Kayser–Fleischer ring* occur. This ring is due to the presence of copper in and about the periphery of Descemet's membrane.

Hereditary ochronosis[283]

In this disorder, ochronotic pigment (indistinguishable from melanin, but considered to be toxic) is deposited widely throughout the body. Ocular involvement results in deep pigmentation

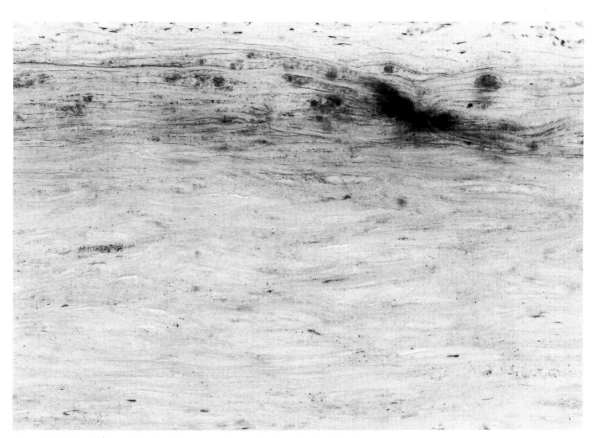

Fig. 24.81 Hereditary ochronosis: ochronotic pigment is deposited within the sclera. Haematoxylin-eosin × 240

of the sclera (Fig. 24.81), mainly at the insertions of the horizontal rectus muscles; lightly pigmented swollen vermiform fibres are seen in the episclera, granular pigmented masses lie beneath, and there are amber structureless globules at the limbus.

TRAUMA

The effect of trauma on the eye varies with the nature and extent of the injury, and may, if the eye has been perforated, also largely depend upon whether or not a foreign body is retained.

Contusion injuries

Contusion injuries result either from direct force applied to the globe or from an indirect force such as that which occurs in other head injuries. Serious sequelae can develop from intraocular haemorrhage and from tears in the uvea (see glaucoma p. 731—contusion angle deformity). Extravasated blood may clear from the anterior chamber, but organisation can occur with the subsequent development of secondary closed-angle glaucoma (*haemorrhagic glaucoma*). Hyphaema (blood in the anterior chamber) from any cause, in the presence of a raised intraocular pressure, produces *blood staining of the cornea* as the breakdown products of disintegrating erythrocytes in the anterior chamber diffuse into the cornea. These products appear under the microscope as small, light-brown to orange, irregular granules. Further breakdown to haemosiderin may occur at a later stage. Retinal damage in the form of oedema and haemorrhages (*commotio retinae*), and of holes and tears, results from blows on the eye. Blows can also cause the lens to become dislocated or cataractous. If they are forceful enough they can rupture the globe, either directly at the point of contact or on the opposite side (contrecoup), or in an area of weakness such as a staphyloma.

Penetrating and perforating injuries[284]

It must be appreciated that a penetrating wound may not necessarily perforate the eye. In the cornea, Bowman's layer, if broken, does not regenerate and damage leaves a permanent scar.

Descemet's membrane has elastic qualities and recoils if disrupted; if the cornea is perforated, a new Descemet's membrane is formed from endothelial cells extending across the deep aspect of the healed wound. A giant cell reaction is often seen in relation to the broken ends of Descemet's membrane. Wounds generally heal well if managed correctly, but serious complications can arise if the wound is neglected, or if there is associated and more widespread damage (Fig. 24.82), such as haemorrhage, disruption and disorganisation of ocular structures, infection, epithelialisation of the anterior segment, or retention of foreign material.

Retrocorneal membrane. Such a membrane formed of fibrous tissue (Fig. 24.83), which may be vascularised, can follow ingrowth of connective tissue subsequent to accidental or surgical per-

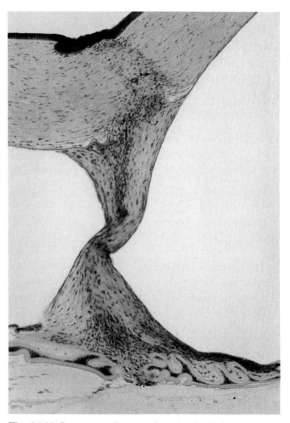

Fig. 24.82 Leucoma adherens: there is a healed corneal perforation, lens remnants are seen below, and a band of scar tissue bridges the anterior chamber. Haematoxylin-eosin × 60

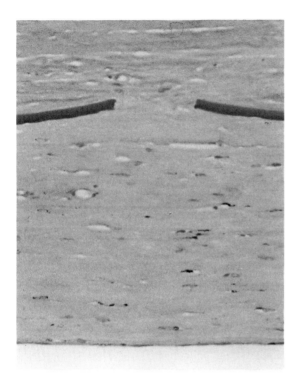

Fig. 24.83 Retrocorneal membrane: there is a break in Descemet's membrane and a thick plaque of fibrous tissue has formed posteriorly (bottom of picture). PAS × 250

foration of the cornea. A similar membrane may also result from organisation of inflammatory or haemorrhagic exudate in the anterior chamber.

Infection. Infection by bacteria or fungi results in postoperative or post-traumatic suppurative endophthalmitis or panophthalmitis.

Epithelialisation of the anterior segment. This occurs when corneal or conjunctival epithelial cells either grow down a wound tract or become implanted into the globe at the time of perforation (Fig. 24.84). Such cells can proliferate to produce an epithelial cyst and subsequently glaucoma may develop due to the prevention of circulation and outflow of aqueous.

Intraocular foreign bodies. Retained intraocular foreign bodies produce complications depending upon the path they take through the eye, the site at which they lodge, and their composition. There

may be extensive damage to ocular tissue with associated haemorrhage. As a general rule, extraneous material in the anterior segment involves less reaction than in the posterior segment, while little reaction occurs if foreign material is lodged in the lens. Many inert substances cause no specific changes if retained within the eye. Two metals which produce serious effects are iron and copper, causing siderosis and chalcosis respectively.

Siderosis bulbi results from the presence of iron-containing foreign bodies (Fig. 24.85). The distribution of iron depends upon the composition, the size and the location of the foreign body, its degree of encapsulation and the time for which it has been retained. The retina and the epithelial structures

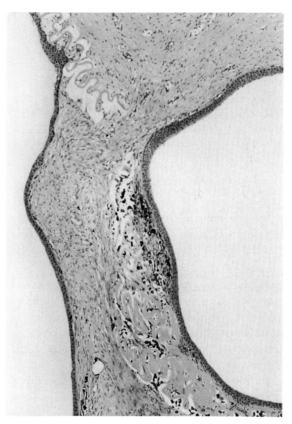

Fig. 24.84 Epithelialisation of the anterior segment: following perforation of the globe, scar tissue has formed within the anterior chamber, and non-keratinised, stratified, squamous epithelium lines the intraocular cavity. Haematoxylin-eosin × 60

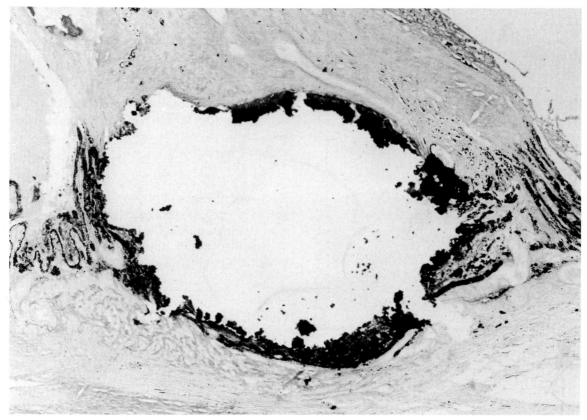

Fig. 24.85 Siderosis bulbi: an iron-containing intraocular foreign body was removed from the ciliary region prior to sectioning; a cavity remains and the surrounding tissue is heavily infiltrated with iron. Perls ×65

of the eye are the sites of election for the early deposition of iron, but eventually all the ocular tissues become impregnated.

Chalcosis is produced by alloys containing less than 85% of copper (pure copper results in intraocular suppuration). A *Kayser–Fleischer ring* develops and birefringent particles are seen to be present on the zonular fibres, in the aqueous, in the vitreous and on the surface of the retina. There is, in addition, a green or red iridescent 'sunflower' cataract.

Sympathetic ophthalmitis and lens-induced end-ophthalmitis. These serious inflammatory conditions can develop as a complication of injuries (see p. 685).

Other types of injury

Localised extraocular or intraocular granulomas may be produced by irritant foreign particles, such as caterpillar hairs (*ophthalmia nodosa*). *Thermal injuries* lead to scarring of all the ocular coats, *chemical injuries* usually damage the conjunctiva and cornea, and *electrical injuries* induce subcapsular opacities in the lens. *Radiation retinopathy*[285] *and optic neuropathy* are characterised by vascular damage with the production of haemorrhages, exudates and 'cotton-wool' spots. *Solar retinopathy* is in reality a burn with coagulation necrosis and pigment disturbance. *Infrared irradiation* can produce cataract and true exfoliation of the lens capsule, in which the capsule splits, the outer aspect curls away, and the cortex becomes opaque. *Lasers*[286,287] are used in industry and in therapeutic procedures; they produce sharply defined changes in the retina with adhesion of the outer layers to the pigment epithelium.

'Battered baby' syndrome (see p. 341). Ocular injuries in this syndrome include dislocation of the lens, cataract, haemorrhages, retinal detachment and glaucoma. This cause of trauma should always be borne in mind if such changes are observed when examining the eyes of infants and young children.

DEVELOPMENTAL ANOMALIES

Lid anomalies

The abnormalities of lid development include ablepharon, colobomas, blepharophimosis, symblepharon and microblepharon. Epicanthic folds are seen in a number of congenital conditions, including *Down's syndrome* and the *Rubinstein–Taybi syndrome* (brachydactylia, facial deformities, cataract, mental retardation and stunted growth).

Dermoids

Dermoids are hamartomatous growths composed of epithelial or connective tissue elements which become entrapped within clefts during embryonic life. They most commonly occur at the corneoscleral junction on the temporal side and may be present in oculoauriculovertebral dysplasia (*Goldenhar's syndrome*). Stratified squamous epithelium is present on the surface and the lesions contain adnexal structures in addition to blood vessels, nerve fibres, muscle and adipose tissue. If adipose tissue is present, the lesion is referred to as a *dermolipoma*.

Osseous choristomas

Choristomatous malformations (malformations composed of tissue not normally present at that site) of bone are occasionally found as solitary lesions in the episclera.

Anophthalmos

If no evagination from the forebrain occurs and no ocular anlage forms, there is congenital absence of the eye, but if an optic vesicle forms, and either does not develop or else regresses, rudiments of an eye may be present.

Synophthalmos

Synophthalmos, an uncommon condition, is characterised by fusion of the orbits and a varying degree of fusion of the two eyes. A single eye (*cyclops*) consequent upon complete fusion of the optic vesicles is extremely rare.

Myopia

Myopia is a developmental abnormality, often transmitted genetically as an autosomal dominant, in which there is an increase in the axial length of the globe. The posterior sclera is thinned and the choroid and retina, particularly at the posterior pole, become atrophic. Microcystoid degeneration, possibly with hole formation, occurs at the retinal periphery and subsequently there may be retinal detachment.

Microphthalmos

Microphthalmos is one of the commonest ocular developmental anomalies, and is related to defective closure of the fetal fissure. It may occur in the absence of other ocular or systemic anomalies (this type includes *nanophthalmos*, when the eye is small but otherwise normal), or there may be other ocular abnormalities such as a persistent hyperplastic primary vitreous or a colobomatous defect, the latter frequently resulting in an *orbital cyst*. There may be an association with maternal rubella, congenital toxoplasmosis, congenital cytomegalovirus infection, craniofacial malformations or chromosomal anomalies.

Microcornea

Microcornea is defined as a cornea of diameter less than 11 mm. It is often seen in conjunction with microphthalmos. It may also be associated with the anterior cleavage syndrome (see below).

Megalocornea

Megalocornea is defined as a cornea of diameter greater than 13 mm. The anomaly may have a genetic basis. It occurs in *Marfan's syndrome*. Other ocular malformations may be associated with it. In the condition of buphthalmos (distension of the eye manifesting congenital glaucoma) the cornea is also enlarged.

Coloboma

The ocular fetal fissure lies in the inferonasal quadrant, and so colobomatous defects occupy this position. Defective closure produces a typical coloboma, and the iris, ciliary body, lens, choroid, retina and optic nerve[288] can all be affected. It is usually an isolated abnormality, but may occur in the *trisomy 13 syndrome* (see below) and in the *thalidomide* and *lysergide* (lysergic acid, LSD) *embryonopathies*.

Aniridia

Aniridia can be considered as a form of atypical iris coloboma. A small rudimentary bud of iris root is present, and so the condition is a hypoplasia rather than an aplasia. Congenital glaucoma occurs in a number of cases and there may be associated cataract formation and macular aplasia. *Nephroblastoma* (Wilms' tumour) develops in a small but significant number of patients with aniridia.

Anterior cleavage syndrome[289]

Under this heading are grouped congenital abnormalities which involve the cornea, the filtration angle and the iris. *Posterior embryotoxon* (a name given to a prominent thickening of Schwalbe's ring because of the bow-like curve of the latter), *Axenfeld's anomaly* (prominent Schwalbe's ring, with strands of iris tissue extending to it), *Reiger's anomaly* (similar to Axenfeld's anomaly, but with hypoplasia of the iris stroma), *iridogoniodysgenesis* (hypoplasia of the anterior iris in addition to Axenfeld's anomaly), *posterior keratoconus* (posterior corneal depression) and *Peter's anomaly* (corneal opacity with adhesion of the iris and/or the lens), are all included in the group.

Developmental anomalies of the lens

Congenital absence of the lens is associated with microphthalmos, and also with cerebral and cranial malformations. *Congenital ectopia lentis* may be part of both *Marfan's syndrome* and *Ehlers–Danlos syndrome*. *Microphakia (spherophakia)* occurs either as an isolated condition or else is present in association with abnormalities of the filtration angle. *Congenital cataracts* arise from a number of causes such as chromosomal abnormalities and maternal viral infections. *Lenticonus*, a conical protrusion of lens substance, is usually posterior and may occur as an isolated abnormality of development.

Persistent hyperplastic primary vitreous

This is almost always unilateral. The affected eye is microphthalmic, the anterior chamber is shallow and there is persistence of the posterior tunica vasculosa lentis. The ciliary processes are elongated and extend inwards, there may be cataract formation and there is a defect in the posterior lens capsule. A mass of retrolental tissue is present, and while this is composed largely of undifferentiated neural and fibrous tissue, there may also be adipose tissue, hyaline material, cartilage and foci of calcification.

Retinal dysplasia

A disorderly formation of the retina may occur either in isolation in one eye, or as a component of such conditions as *Norrie's disease* (see below) and *trisomy 13*. The essential histological feature is the presence of retinal rosettes (Fig. 24.86). The nuclei which outline the rosettes are analogous to the nuclei of the rods and cones, while a membrane that may line the outer margin of the rosettes is analogous to the external limiting membrane.

Norrie's disease

Norrie's disease is a rare condition with an X-linked recessive inheritance pattern. It is characterised by bilateral ocular abnormalities,

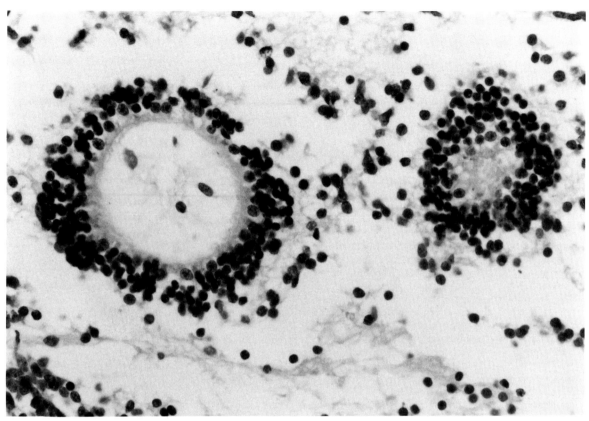

Fig. 24.86 Retinal dysplasia: well-marked rosette formation. Haematoxylin-eosin × 665

deafness and mental retardation. In the posterior segment of the eye, the changes involve the neuro-ectoderm, and, associated with hypoplasia of the sensory retina, there may be retinal dysplasia (see above) together with glial proliferation extending into the vitreous. Secondary changes include retinal detachment and intraocular haemorrhage.

Chromosomal anomalies[290-292]

Trisomy 18 (Edwards' syndrome)[293] and *trisomy 21 (Down's syndrome)* result in ocular abnormalities, but the chromosomal abnormality associated with the most severe ocular changes is *trisomy 13 (Patau's syndrome)*. In trisomy 13 the findings include microphthalmos, corneal abnormalities, filtration angle abnormalities, cataract, colobomatous defects, persistent hyperplastic primary vitreous, retinal dysplasia, and atrophy,

hypoplasia, or a colobomatous defect of the optic nerve.

Albinism[293]

Both the *ocular* and *oculocutaneous forms of albinism* affect the eye, where there is noted to be a lack of pigment in the uvea and retina. The pigment cells themselves are present, but there is diminution of the amount of melanin within them. Most albinism is only partial, total absence of pigment being very rare.

Miscellaneous anomalies

Hamartomatous lesions, particularly in the form of *vascular anomalies* (see phacomatoses, p. 714), occur within the eye. *Retinoschisis* (splitting of the retina) and *retinal detachment* may also be found as developmental defects.

GLOSSARY

Busacca nodules — aggregates of epithelioid cells on the anterior surface of the iris

Cornea guttata — guttate excrescences on the posterior surface of Descemet's membrane

Descemetocele — protrusion of Descemet's membrane through a gap in the corneal stroma

Ectropion uveae — eversion of pigment epithelium of iris onto its anterior surface (often associated with rubeosis iridis)

Endophthalmitis — inflammation involving the intra-ocular structures and the ocular cavities, but excluding the corneo-scleral envelope

Hyphaema — blood in the anterior chamber

Hypopyon — pus in the anterior chamber

Keratic precipitates — aggregates of epithelioid cells on the posterior surface of the cornea

Koeppe nodules — aggregates of epithelioid cells at the pupillary border of the iris

Leucoma — corneal scar

Leucoma adherens — adhesion of intraocular tissue to the deep aspect of a perforating scar of the cornea

Morgagnian droplets — small hyaline spheres in a cataractous lens

Panophthalmitis — inflammation involving all the ocular structures, including the corneo scleral envelope

Phthisis bulbi — shrinkage and disorganisation of the globe, usually the result of severe inflammation or injury

Pseudophakia — the presence within the eye of an artificial lens in place of the natural lens

Rete mirabile — a fine network of new blood vessels emanating from the inner retinal surface

Retinitis proliferans — neovascularisation extending from the retina into the vitreous

Ringschwiele — proliferation of ciliary epithelium and peripheral retinal pigment epithelium, with laminar formation of fibrous tissue, possibly containing some blood vessels

Rubeosis iridis — neovascularisation (fibrovascular tissue) on the anterior surface of the iris

Scleromalacia perforans — a thin, perforated sclera, as may be seen in association with rheumatoid arthritis

Staphyloma — thin, ectatic area of the corneoscleral envelope, lined by atrophic uveal tissue; classified as anterior (corneal), intercalary (limbal), ciliary, equatorial and posterior, according to site

Symblepharon — adhesion of the tarsal to the bulbar conjunctiva

Synechia(e) — intraocular adhesion(s); classified as
anterior (iridicorneal),
and posterior (iridolenticular)

Uveitis — inflammation of the uvea; classified as
anterior (inflammation of the iris and/or the ciliary body, i.e. iritis, cyclitis, iridocyclitis)
and posterior (inflammation of the choroid, i.e. choroiditis).

REFERENCES

Introduction

1. Wolff E. Anatomy of the eye and orbit. 7th ed. London: Lewis, 1976.
2. Fine B, Yanoff M. Ocular histology: a text and atlas. New York: Harper & Row, 1979.
3. Moses RA, ed. Adler's Physiology of the eye. 8th ed. St. Louis: Mosby, 1987.
4. Duke-Elder S, ed. System of ophthalmology, vols 1–15. London: Kimpton, 1958–1976.
5. Duane TD. Clinical ophthalmology. Philadelphia: Harper & Row, 1978–1985.
6. Kanski JJ. Clinical ophthalmology. London: Butterworths, 1984.
7. Miller SJ. Parsons' Diseases of the eye. Edinburgh: Churchill Livingstone, 1984.
8. Spalton DJ, Hitchings RA, Hunter PA. Atlas of clinical ophthalmology. Edinburgh: Churchill Livingstone, 1985.
9. Perkins ES, Hansell P, Marsh RJ. An atlas of diseases of the eye. 3rd ed. Edinburgh: Churchill Livingstone, 1986.
10. Kritzinger EE, Wright BE. Colour atlas of the eye and systemic disease. Chicago: Year Book, 1984.
11. Kanski JJ. The eye in systemic disease. London: Butterworths, 1985.
12. Hogan M, Zimmerman LE. Ophthalmic pathology. Philadelphia: Saunders, 1962.
13. Greer CH. Ocular pathology. 3rd ed. Oxford: Blackwell, 1979.
14. Garner A, Klintworth GK, eds. Pathobiology of ocular disease: a dynamic approach. New York: Dekker, 1982.

15. Yanoff M, Fine BS. Ocular pathology: a text and atlas. 2nd ed. Philadelphia: Harper & Row, 1982.
16. Apple DJ, Rabb MF. Ocular pathology. 3rd ed. St. Louis: Mosby, 1985.
17. Spencer WH, ed. Ophthalmic pathology: an atlas and textbook, vols 1–3. 3rd ed. Philadelphia: Saunders, 1985–1986.
18. Naumann GOH, Apple DJ. Pathology of the eye. Berlin: Springer 1986.

Functional anatomy and methodology

19. Torczynski E. Ophthalmology 1981; 88: 1367.
20. Constable LJ, Chester GH, Horne R, Harriott JF. Br J Ophthalmol 1980; 64: 559.
21. Peyman GA, Juarez CP, Raichand M. Br J Ophthalmol 1981; 65: 723.
22. Ni C, Chang TC, Searl SS, Coughlin-Wilkinson E, Albert DM. Ophthalmology 1981; 88: 1372.
23. Constable IJ, Thompson D, Bockxmeer F van. Trans Ophthalmol Soc UK 1983; 103: 475.
24. Czerniak B, Stanislaw W, Wenancjusz D, Krysztolik Z. Acta Cytol (Baltimore) 1983; 27: 157.
25. Dresner SC, Kennerdell JS, Dekker A. Surv Ophthalmol 1983; 27: 397.
26. Char DH, Miller TR. Am J Ophthalmol 1984; 97: 686.
27. Rootman J, Quenville N, Owen D. Ophthalmology 1984; 91: 708.
28. Kincaid MC, Green WR. Ophthalmology 1984; 91: 719.
29. Foulds WS, Lee WR, Roxburgh STD, Damato BE. Trans Ophthalmol Soc UK 1985; 104: 864.
30. Erie JC, Collyer SK, Campbell RJ. Am J Ophthalmol 1985; 99: 539.
31. Kennerdell JS, Slamovits TL, Dekker A, Johnson BL. Am J Ophthalmol 1985; 99: 547.
32. Folberg R, Augsburger JJ, Gamel JW, Shields JA, Lang WR. Am J Ophthalmol 1985; 100: 654.
33. Norris JL, Stewart WB. Ophthalmology 1985; 92: 34.
34. Augsburger JL, Shields JA, Folberg R, Lang W, O'Hara BJ, Claricci JD. Ophthalmology 1985; 92: 39.
35. Krohel GB, Tobin DR, Chavis RM. Ophthalmology 1985; 92: 666.
36. Karcioglu ZA, Gordon RA, Karcioglu GL. Ophthalmology 1985; 92: 1763.
37. Liu D. Ophthalmology 1985; 92: 1768.
38. Davey CC, Deery ARS. Trans Ophthalmol Soc UK 1986; 105: 78.
39. Messmer EP, Font RL. Ophthalmology 1984; 91: 701.
40. Chalfin J, Putterman AM. Am J Ophthalmol 1979; 87: 802.
41. Harry J. Personal observations, 1986.
42. Green WR. Ophthalmology 1984; 91: 726.
43. Sternberg P, Tiedeman J, Hickingbotham D, McCuen BW, Proia AD. Arch Ophthalmol 1984; 102: 1622.
44. Ashton N. ACP Broadsheet 59, October 1967.
45. Ashton N. Br J Ophthalmol 1963; 47: 521.

Inflammation

46. Smolin G, Tabbara K, Whitcher J. Infectious diseases of the eye. London: Williams & Wilkins, 1984.
47. Fedukowicz HB, Stenson S. External infections of the eye. 3rd ed. Norwalk, Conn.: Appleton-Century-Crofts 1985.
48. Easty DL. Virus disease of the eye. London: Lloyd-Luke, 1985.
49. Darrell RW, ed. Viral diseases of the eye. Philadelphia: Lea & Febiger, 1985.
50. Chandler JW, Gillette TE. Ophthalmology 1983; 90: 585.
51. Smolin G. Trans Ophthalmol Soc UK 1985; 104: 363.
52. Watt PJ, Ward KA. Trans Ophthalmol Soc UK 1985; 104: 367.
53. Seal DV, McGill JI, MacKie IA, Liakos GM, Jacobs P, Goulding NJ. Br J Ophthalmol 1986; 70: 122.
54. Bron AJ, Seal DV. Trans Ophthalmol Soc UK 1986; 105: 18.
55. Watt PJ. Trans Ophthalmol Soc UK 1986; 105: 26.
56. Seal DV. Trans Ophthalmol Soc UK 1986; 105: 32.
57. McGill JI. Trans Ophthalmol Soc UK 1986; 105: 37.
58. Wilson LA. Trans Ophthalmol Soc UK 1986; 105: 43.
59. Easty DL. Trans Ophthalmol Soc UK 1986; 105: 61.
60. Rahi AHS, Garner A. Immunopathology of the eye. Oxford: Blackwell, 1976.
61. Allansmith MR. The eye and immunology. St Louis: Mosby, 1982.
62. Theodore FH, Bloomfield SE, Mondilo BJ. Clinical allergy and immunology of the eye. London: Williams & Wilkins, 1983.
63. Smolin G, O'Connor GR. Ocular immunology. Edinburgh: Churchill Livingstone, 1986.
64. Nussenblatt RB, Salinas-Carmona M, Leake W, Scher I. Am J Ophthalmol 1983; 95: 614.
65. Jakobiec FA, Lefkowitch J, Knowles DM. Ophthalmology 1984; 91: 635.
66. Kaplan HJ, Waldrep JC. Ophthalmology 1984; 91: 655.
67. James DG, Graham E, Hamblin A. Surv Ophthalmol 1985; 30: 155.
68. Holland GN, Gottlieb MS, Yee RD, Schanker HM, Pettit TH. Am J Ophthalmol 1982; 93: 393.
69. Schuman JS, Friedman AH. Trans Ophthalmol Soc UK 1983; 103: 177.
70. Holland GN, Pepose JS, Pettit TH, Gottlieb MS, Yee RD, Foos RY. Ophthalmology 1983; 90: 859.
71. Rosenberg PR, Uliss AE, Friedland GH, Harris CA, Small CB, Klein RS. Ophthalmology 1983; 90: 874.
72. Newman NM, Mandel MR, Gullett J, Fujikawa L. Arch Ophthalmol 1983; 101: 396.
73. Palestine AG, Rodrigues MM, Macher AM et al. Ophthalmology 1984; 91: 1092.
74. Khadem M, Kalish SB, Goldsmith J et al. Arch Ophthalmol 1984; 102: 201.
75. Macher A, Rodrigues MM, Kaplan W et al. Ophthalmology 1985; 92: 1159.
76. Key SN III, Green WR, Willaert E, Stevens AR, Key SN Jr. Arch Ophthalmol 1980; 98: 475.
77. Pinnolis M, Egbert PR, Font RL, Winter FC. Arch Ophthalmol 1981; 99: 1044.
78. Karcioglu ZA, Brear R. Am J Ophthalmol 1985; 99: 68.
79. Weinreb RN. Am J Ophthalmol 1984; 97: 573.
80. Collison JMT, Miller NR, Green WR. Am J Ophthalmol 1986; 102: 302.
81. Ashton N, Cook C. Am J Ophthalmol 1979; 87: 1.
82. Wright P, Trans Ophthalmol Soc UK 1980; 100: 96.
83. Blase WP, Knox DL, Green WR. Br J Ophthalmol 1984; 68: 901.
84. Blodi FC, ed. Herpes simplex infections of the eye—contemporary issues in ophthalmology, vol 1. Edinburgh: Churchill Livingstone, 1984.

85. Oriel JD, Ridgway GL. Current topics in infection series—genital infection by *Chlamydia trachomatis*. London: Arnold, 1982.
86. Pierce JM, Ward ME, Seal DV. Br J Ophthalmol 1982; 66: 728.
87. Ridgway GL. Trans Ophthalmol Soc UK 1986; 105: 41.
88. Rapoza PA, Quinn TC, Kiessling LA, Taylor HR. Ophthalmology 1986; 93: 456.
89. Scholz R, Green WR, Kutys R, Sutherland J, Richards RD. Ophthalmology 1984; 91: 1100.
90. Shields JA. Surv Ophthalmol 1984; 28: 361.
91. Mondino BJ, Brown SI. Ophthalmology 1981; 88: 95.
92. Young RD, Watson PG. Br J Ophthalmol 1982; 66: 341.
93. Murray PI, Rahi AHS. Br J Ophthalmol 1984; 68: 182.
94. Rao NA, Wong VG. Trans Ophthalmol Soc UK 1981; 101: 357.
95. Reynard M, Shulman LA, Azen SP, Minckler DS. Am J Ophthalmol 1983; 95: 216.
96. Font RL, Fine BS, Messmer E, Rowsey JF. Ophthalmology 1983; 90: 66.
97. Jakobiec FA, Marboe CC, Knowles II DM et al. Ophthalmology 1983; 90: 76.
98. Sharp DC, Bell RA, Patterson E, Pinkerton RMH. Arch Ophthalmol 1984; 102: 232.
99. Müller-Hermelink HK, Kraus-Mackiw E, Daus W. Arch Ophthalmol 1984; 102: 1353.
100. Reynard M, Riffenburgh RS, Minckler DS. Br J Ophthalmol 1985; 69: 197.
101. Rao NA, Xu S, Font RL. Ophthalmology 1985; 92: 1660.
102. Chan C-C, Benezra D, Hsu S-M, Palestine AG, Nussenblatt RB. Arch Ophthalmol 1985; 103: 1981.
103. Chan C-C, Nussenblatt RB, Fujikawa LS et al. Ophthalmology 1986; 93: 690.
104. Kaplan HJ, Waldrop CW, Chan WC, Nicholson JKA, Wright JD. Arch Ophthalmol 1986; 104: 240.
105. Rahi AHS. Trans Ophthalmol Soc UK 1982; 102: 395.
106. Young RD, Watson PG. Br J Ophthalmol 1984; 68: 770, 781.
107. Rao NA, Marak GE, Hidayat A. Ophthalmology 1985; 92: 1542.
108. Graham EM, Spalton DJ, Barnard RO, Garner A, Ross Russell RW. Ophthalmology 1985; 92: 444.
109. Albert DM, Searl SS, Craft JL. Ophthalmology 1982; 89: 1111.
110. McDonnell PJ, Moore GW, Miller NR, Hutchins GM, Green WR. Ophthalmology 1986; 93: 518.
111. Michelson JB, Chisari FV. Surv Ophthalmol 1982; 26: 190.
112. Rahi AHS. Trans Ophthalmol Soc UK 1981; 101: 292.

Tumours

113. Reese AB. Tumours of the eye. 3rd ed. New York: Harper & Row, 1976.
114. Jakobiec FA. Ocular and adnexal tumours. Birmingham, Ala.: Aesculapius, 1978.
115. Zimmerman LE, Sobin L, eds. Histological typing of tumours of the eye and adnexa. An international histological classification of tumours, no 24. Geneva: World Health Organization, 1981.
116. Ni C, Albert DM. Int Ophthalmol Clin 1982; 22: (1)entire issue.
117. Caya JG, Hidayat AA, Weiner JM. Am J Ophthalmol 1985; 99: 291.
118. Reifler DM, Hornblass A. Surv Ophthalmol 1986; 30: 349.
119. Wright P, Collin RJO, Garner A. Trans Ophthalmol Soc UK 1981; 101: 214.
120. Rao NA, Hidayat AA, McLean IW, Zimmerman LE. Hum Pathol 1982; 13: 113.
121. Wagoner MD, Beyer CK, Gonder JR, Albert DM. Ann Ophthalmol 1982; 14: 159.
122. Doxanas MT, Green WR. Arch Ophthalmol 1984; 102: 245.
123. Garner A, Koorneef L, Levene A, Collin RJO. Br J Ophthalmol 1985; 69: 180.
124. Lass JH, Jenson AB, Papale JJ, Albert DM. Am J Ophthalmol 1983; 95: 364.
125. Lass JH, Grove AS, Papale JJ, Albert DM, Jenson AB, Lancaster WD. Am J Ophthalmol 1983; 96: 670.
126. McDonnell JM, McDonnell PJ, Mounts P, Wu T-C, Green WR. Arch Ophthalmol 1986; 104: 1801.
127. Waring GO III, Roth AM, Ekins MB. Am J Ophthalmol 1984; 97: 547.
128. Tseng SCG. Ophthalmology 1985; 92: 728.
129. Erie JC, Campbell BJ, Liesegang TJ. Ophthalmology 1986; 93: 176.
130. Pe'er J, Hidayat AA. Am J Ophthalmol 1986; 102: 80.
131. Holland GN, Gottlieb MS, Yee RD, Shanker HM, Pettit TH. Am J Ophthalmol 1982; 93: 393.
132. Holland GN, Pepose JS, Pettit TH, Gottlieb MS, Yee RD, Foos RY. Ophthalmology 1983; 90: 859.
133. Rosenberg PR, Uliss AE, Friedland GH, Harris CA, Small CB, Klein RS. Ophthalmology 1983; 90: 874.
134. Macher AM, Palestine A, Masur H et al. Ophthalmology 1983; 90: 879.
135. Palestine AG, Rodrigues MM, Macher AM et al. Ophthalmology 1984; 91: 1092.
136. Folberg R, McLean IW, Zimmerman LE. Ophthalmology 1984; 91: 673.
137. Folberg R, McLean IW, Zimmerman LE. Hum Pathol 1985; 16: 129.
138. Guillen FJ, Albert DM, Mihm MC Jr. Pathology 1985; 17: 275.
139. Folberg R, McLean IW. Hum Pathol 1986; 17: 652.
140. Cox RW, Harry J. Personal observations, 1986.
141. Crawford LB. Trans Am Ophthalmol Soc 1980; 78: 467.
142. Folberg R, McLean IW, Zimmerman LE. Hum Pathol 1985; 16: 136.
143. Jeffrey IJM, Lucas DR, McEwan C, Lee WR. Histopathology 1986; 10: 363.
144. Henderson JW. Orbital tumours. 2nd ed. New York: Decker, 1980.
145. Shields JA, Bakewell B, Augsburger JJ, Flanagan JC. Arch Ophthalmol 1984; 102: 1606.
146. Shields JA, Bakewell B, Augsburger JJ, Donoso LA, Bernardino V. Ophthalmology 1986; 93: 379.
147. Croxatto JO, Font RL. Hum Pathol 1981; 13: 210.
148. Iwamoto T, Jakobiec FA. Hum Pathol 1982; 13: 236.
149. Gamel JW, Font RL. Hum Pathol 1981; 13: 219.
150. Lee DA, Campbell RJ, Waller R, Ilstrup DM. Ophthalmology 1985; 92: 128.
151. Font RL, Hidayat AA. Hum Pathol 1982; 13: 199.
152. Font RL, Jurco S III, Zimmerman LE. Hum Pathol 1982; 13: 569.
153. Brown GC, Shields JA. Surv Ophthalmol 1985; 29: 239.
154. Wilson WB. Surv Ophthalmol 1981; 26: 109.
155. Marquardt MD, Zimmerman LE. Hum Pathol 1982; 13: 226.

156. Stern B, Jakobiec FA, Houspian EM. Arch Ophthalmol 1980; 98: 505.
157. Marquardt MD, Zimmerman LE. Hum Pathol 1982; 13: 226.
158. West CGH. Br J Neurosurg 1987; 1: 99.
159. Rudd A, Rees JE, Kennedy P et al. J Clin Neuro Ophthalmol 1985; 5: 238.
160. Knowles DM II, Jakobiec FA. Hum Pathol 1983; 13: 148.
161. Jakobiec FA, Iwamoto T, Knowles DM II. Arch Ophthalmol 1982; 100: 84.
162. Garner A, Rahi AHS, Wright JE. Br J Ophthalmol 1983; 67: 561.
163. Knowles DM II, Jakobiec FA. Am J Ophthalmol 1983; 95: 233.
164. Kincaid MC, Green WR. Surv Ophthalmol 1983; 27: 211.
165. van der Gaag R, Koorneef L, van Heerde P et al. Br J Ophthalmol 1984; 68: 892.
166. Ellis JH, Banks PM, Campbell RJ, Liesegang TJ. Ophthalmology 1985; 92: 1311.
167. Harry J, Cox RW. Personal observations, 1986.
168. Ridde PJ, Font RL, Zimmerman LE. Hum Pathol 1982; 13: 459.
169. Lommatzsch PK, Blodi FC, eds. Intraocular tumours; International Symposium under the auspices of the European Ophthalmological Society. New York: Springer, 1983.
170. Juarez CP, Tso MOM. Am J Ophthalmol 1980; 90: 48.
171. Reidy JJ, Apple DJ, Steinmetz RL et al. Surv Ophthalmol 1985; 29: 319.
172. Gonder JR, Shields JA, Albert DM, Augsburger JJ, Lavin PT. Ophthalmology 1982; 89: 953.
173. Packard RBS. Br J Ophthalmol 1980; 64: 565.
174. Zimmerman LE. Trans Ophthalmol Soc UK 1980; 100: 34.
175. Affeldt JC, Minckler DS, Azen SP, Yeh L. Arch Ophthalmol 1980; 98: 1975.
176. McLean IW, Foster WD, Zimmerman LE. Hum Pathol 1982; 13: 123.
177. Gamel JW, McLean IW, Greenberg RA, Zimmerman LE, Lichenstein SJ. Hum Pathol 1982; 13: 893.
178. McLean IW, Foster WD, Zimmerman LE, Gamel JW. Am J Ophthalmol 1983; 96: 502.
179. Gamel JW, McLean IW. Ophthalmology 1984; 91: 679.
180. Zimmerman LE, McLean IW. Ophthalmology 1984; 91: 685.
181. Margo CE, McLean IW. Arch Ophthalmol 1984; 102: 77.
182. Cochran AJ, Foulds WS, Damato BE, Trope GE, Morrison L, Lee WR. Br J Ophthalmol 1985; 69: 171.
183. Seddon JM, Gragoudas ES, Albert DM, Hsieh C-C, Polivogianis L, Friedenberg GR. Am J Ophthalmol 1985; 99: 282.
184. Geisse LJ, Robertson DM. Am J Ophthalmol 1985; 99: 638.
185. Folberg R, Augsburger JJ, Gamel JW, Shields JA, Lang WR. Am J Ophthalmol 1985; 100: 654.
186. Folberg R, Donoso LA, Atkinson B, Ernst CS, Herlyn M, Arbizo VV. Arch Ophthalmol 1985; 103: 275.
187. Donoso LA, Berd D, Augsburger JJ, Mastrangelo MJ, Shields JA. Arch Ophthalmol 1985; 103: 796.
188. Donoso LA, Folberg R, Naids R, Augsburger JJ, Shields JA, Atkinson B. Arch Ophthalmol 1985; 103: 799.
189. Gass JDM. Arch Ophthalmol 1985; 103: 916.
190. Gass JDM. Arch Ophthalmol 1985; 103: 924.
191. Weinhaus RS, Seddon JM, Albert DM, Gragoudas ES, Robinson N. Arch Ophthalmol 1985; 103: 1673.
192. Pach JM, Robertson DM, Taney BS, Martin JA, Campbell RJ, O'Brien PC. Am J Ophthalmol 1986; 101: 325.
193. Donoso LA, Augsburger JJ, Shields JA, Greenberg RA, Gamel J. Arch Ophthalmol 1986; 104: 76.
194. Meecham WJ, Char DH. Arch Ophthalmol 1986; 104: 1626.
195. Shields JA, Kline MW, Augsburger JJ. Br J Ophthalmol 1984; 68: 152.
196. Nelson CC, Hertzberg BS, Klintworth GK. Am J Ophthalmol 1983; 95: 788.
197. Naves AE, Gaisiner PD. Ann Ophthalmol 1981; 13: 1073.
198. Sang DN, Albert DM. Hum Pathol 1982; 13: 133.
199. Lane JC, Klintworth GK. Am J Ophthalmol 1983; 95: 197.
200. Kyritis AP, Tsokos M, Triche TJ, Chader GJ. Nature 1984; 307: 471.
201. Murphee AL, Benedict WF. Science 1984; 223: 1028.
202. Molnar ML, Stefanson K, Morton LS, Tripatti RS, Molnar GK. Am J Ophthalmol 1984; 97: 301.
203. Messmer EP, Font RL, Kirkpatrick JB, Hopping W. Ophthalmology 1985; 92: 167.
204. Donoso LA, Folberg R, Arbizo V. Arch Ophthalmol 1985; 103: 855.
205. Donoso LA, Hamm H, Dietzschuld B, Augsburger JJ, Shields JA, Arbizo V. Arch Ophthalmol 1986; 104: 111.
206. Margo C, Hidayat AA, Kopelman J, Zimmerman LE. Arch Ophthalmol 1983; 101: 1519.
207. Williams R, Taylor D. Surv Ophthalmol 1985; 30: 143.
208. Wing GL, Weiter JJ, Kelly PJ, Albert DM, Gonder JR. Ophthalmology 1981; 88: 1311.
209. Mottow-Lippa L, Tso MOM, Peyman GA, Chejfer G. Ophthalmology 1983; 90: 848.

Vascular, neurological and muscular diseases

210. Ashton N. Trans Ophthalmol Soc UK 1980; 100: 359.
211. Garner A, Kissun RD. Trans Ophthalmol Soc UK 1980; 100: 381.
212. Fine BS, Brucker AJ. Am J Ophthalmol 1981; 92: 466.
213. Tso MOM. Ophthalmology 1982; 89: 902.
214. Eagle RC Jr. Ophthalmology 1984; 91: 613.
215. Yanoff M, Fine BS, Brucker AJ, Eagle RC Jr. Surv Ophthalmol 1984; 28 (suppl): 505.
216. Gass JDM, Anderson DR, Davis EB. Am J Ophthalmol 1985; 100: 82.
217. Kampik A, Kenyon KR, Michels RG, Green WR, de la Cruz Z. Arch Ophthalmol 1981; 99: 1445.
218. Michels RG. Trans Am Ophthalmol Soc 1982; 80: 580.
219. Hiscott PS, Grierson I, Trombetta CJ, Rahi AHS, Marshall J, McLeod D. Br J Ophthalmol 1984; 68: 698.
220. Hiscott PS, Grierson I, McLeod D. Br J Ophthalmol 1984; 68: 708.
221. Hiscott PS, Grierson I, McLeod D. Br J Ophthalmol 1985; 69: 810.
222. Jerdan JA, Michels RG, Glaser BM. Arch Ophthalmol 1986; 104: 286.
223. Tso MOM, Jampol LM. Ophthalmology 1982; 89: 1132.

224. Garner A. J Roy Soc Med 1981; 74: 427.
225. Frank RN. Ophthalmology 1984; 91: 626.
226. Jerdan JA, Michels RG, Glaser BM. Arch Ophthalmol 1986; 104: 286.
227. Ashton N. Br J Ophthalmol 1984; 68: 689.
228. Fryczkowski AW, Peiffer RL, Merritt JC, Kraybill EN, Eifrig DE. Arch Ophthalmol 1985; 103: 224.

Miscellaneous disorders of the choroid and retina

229. Ishibashi T, Patterson R, Ohnishi Y, Inomata H, Ryan SJ. Am J Ophthalmol 1986; 101: 342.
230. Coffey AJH, Brownstein S. Am J Ophthalmol 1986; 102: 164.
231. Tso MOM. Ophthalmology 1981; 88: 1066.
232. Clarkson JG, Altman RD. Surv Ophthalmol 1982; 26: 235.
233. Gartner S, Henkind P. Br J Ophthalmol 1981; 65: 23.
234. Eagle RC Jr. Ophthalmology 1984; 91: 613.
235. Green WR, McDonnell PJ, Yeo JH. Ophthalmology 1985; 92: 615.
236. Tso MOM, Ophthalmology 1985; 92: 628.
237. Bird AC. Trans Ophthalmol Soc UK 1981; 101: 39.
238. Jay M. Br J Ophthalmol 1982; 66: 405.
239. Gartner S, Henkind P. Ophthalmology 1982; 89: 1425.
240. Lahav M, Craft J, Albert DM, Ishii Y. Retina 1982; 2: 65.
241. Szamier RB, Berson EL. Ophthalmology 1985; 92: 271.
242. Rodrigues MM, Wiggert B, Hackett J et al. Ophthalmology 1985; 92: 1165.
243. Albert DM, Pruett RC, Craft JL. Am J Ophthalmol 1986; 101: 655.
244. François J. Surv Ophthalmol 1982; 26: 293.
245. McDonnell JM, Green WR, Maumanee I. Ophthalmology 1985; 92: 1772.
246. Del Monte MA, Maumanee IH, Green WR, Kenyon KR. Arch Ophthalmol 1983; 101: 1255.
247. Lavery MA, Green WR, Jabs EW, Luckenbach MW, Cox JL. Arch Ophthalmol 1983; 101: 1263.
248. Garner A, Fielder AR, Primavesi R, Stevens A. Br J Ophthalmol 1982; 66: 422.
249. Cohen SMZ, Brown III FR, Martyn L et al. Am J Ophthalmol 1983; 96: 488.

The lens

250. Maisel H. The ocular lens: structure, function and pathology. New York: Dekker, 1985.
251. Chylack LT Jr. Ophthalmology 1984; 91: 596.
252. Fagerholm PPP. Trans Ophthalmol Soc UK 1982; L02: 369.
253. Hertzberg R. Trans Ophthalmol Soc UK 1982; 102: 355.
254. McDonnell PJ, Green WR, Maumanee AE, Iliff WJ. Ophthalmology 1983; 90: 386.
255. Apple DJ, Mammalis N, Loftfield K et al. Surv Ophthalmol 1984; 29: 1.
256. McMahon MS, Weiss JS, Riedel KG, Albert DM. Br J Ophthalmol 1985; 69: 452.
257. Drews RC. Trans Ophthalmol Soc UK 1985; 104: 507.
258. Bleckmann H, Lohoff WF. Trans Ophthalmol Soc UK 1985; 104: 512.
259. Wolter JR. Ophthalmology 1985; 92: 135.

260. Champion R, Green WR. Ophthalmology 1985; 92: 1628.
261. Champion R, McDonnell PJ, Green WR. Surv Ophthalmol 1985; 30: 1.

The vitreous

262. Topilow HW, Kenyon KR, Takashi M, Freeman HM, Tolentino FI, Hanninen LA. Arch Ophthalmol 1982; 100: 964.
263. Streeten BW. Arch Ophthalmol 1982; 100: 969.
264. Miller H, Miller B, Rabinowitz H, Zonis S, Nir I. Invest Ophthalmol Vis Sci 1983; 34: 133.

Glaucoma

265. Quigley HA, Addicks EM. Am J Ophthalmol 1980; 90: 854.
266. Bergmanson JPG, Jones WL, Chu LW-F. Br J Ophthalmol 1984; 68: 118.
267. Garner A, Alexander RA. Br J Ophthalmol 1984; 68: 574.
268. Quigley HA, Addicks EM, Green WR, Maumanee AE. Arch Ophthalmol 1981; 99: 635.
269. Minckler DS, Spaeth GL. Surv Ophthalmol 1981; 26: 128.
270. Quigley HA, Hohman RM, Addicks EM, Massof RW, Green WR. Am J Ophthalmol 1983; 95: 673.
271. Maumanee AE. Ophthalmology 1983; 90: 741.

Degenerative and dystrophic conditions of the conjunctiva and cornea

272. Austin P, Jakobiec FA, Iwamoto T. Ophthalmology 1983; 90: 96.
273. Pinkerton OD, Hokama Y, Shigemura LA. Am J Ophthalmol 1984; 98: 225.
274. Rodrigues MM, Streeton BW, Krachmer JH et al. Arch Ophthalmol 1983; 101: 802.
275. Klintworth GK. Trans Ophthalmol Soc UK 1980; 186.
276. Weller RO, Rodger FC. Br J Ophthalmol 1980; 64: 46.
277. Chan C-C, Green WR, Barraquer J, Barraquer-Somers E, de la Cruz Z. Cornea 1982; 1: 155.
278. Polack FM, Bourne WM, Forstos SL, Yamaguchi T. Am J Ophthalmol 1980; 89: 575.

Metabolic disorders

279. Renie WA. In: Goldberg MF, ed. Genetic and metabolic eye disease. 2nd ed. Boston: Little, Brown & Co, 1986.
280. Brownstein S, Carpenter S, Polomeno RC, Little JM. Arch Ophthalmol 1980; 98: 1089.
281. Palmer M, Green WR, Maumanee IH et al. Arch Ophthalmol 1985; 103: 817.
282. Johnson RE, Campbell RJ. Lab Invest 1982; 46: 564.
283. Kampik A, Sani JN, Green WR. Arch Ophthalmol 1980; 98: 1441.

Trauma

284. Winthrop WR, Cleary PE, Minckler DS, Ryan SJ. Br J Ophthalmol 1980; 64: 809.
285. Brown GC, Shields JA, Sanborn G, Augsburger JJ, Savino PJ, Schatz NJ. Ophthalmology 1982; 89: 1494.
286. Thomas EL, Apple DJ, Swartz M, Kavka-Van Norman D. Retina 1984; 4: 22.

287. Rodrigues MM, Spaeth GL, Moster M, Thomas G, Hacket J. Ophthalmology 1985; 92: 1696.

Developmental anomalies

288. Apple DJ, Rabb MF, Walsh PM. Surv Ophthalmol 1983; 27: 3.
289. Shields MB, Buckley E, Klintworth GK, Thresher R. Surv Ophthalmol 1985; 29: 387.

290. Renie WA. In: Goldberg MF, ed. Genetic and metabolic eye disease. 2nd ed. Boston: Little, Brown & Co, 1986.
291. Schmickel RD. Surv Ophthalmol 1980; 25: 37.
292. Calderone JP, Chess J, Borodis G, Albert DM. Br J Ophthalmol 1983; 67: 162.
293. Kinnear PE, Jay B, Witkop CJ. Surv Ophthalmol 1985; 30: 75.